This volume was produced with support from the

Associazione S.P.E.S. Onlus, Bologna

Friends of José Carreras International Leukemia Foundation

Leukemia Clinical Research Foundation

MEDIC Foundation

National Cancer Institute, USA

National Institutes of Health Office of Rare Diseases, USA

University of Chicago Cancer Research Center

The WHO Classification of Tumours of Haematopoietic and Lymphoid Tissues
presented in this book reflects the views of a Working Group
that convened for an Editorial and Consensus Conference at the
International Agency for Research on Cancer (IARC), Lyon
October 25-27, 2007.

Members of the Working Group are indicated
in the List of Contributors on pages 369-374.

Published by the International Agency for Research on Cancer (IARC),
150 cours Albert Thomas, 69372 Lyon Cedex 08, France

Distributed by
WHO Press, World Health Organization, 20 Avenue Appia, 1211 Geneva 27, Switzerland
(Tel: +41 22 791 3264; Fax: +41 22 791 4857; e-mail: bookorders@who.int).

Second print run (20,000 copies)

Format for bibliographic citations:
Swerdlow S.H., Campo E., Harris N.L., Jaffe E.S., Pileri S.A., Stein H., Thiele J., Vardiman J.W. (Eds.):
WHO Classification of Tumours of Haematopoietic and Lymphoid Tissues.
IARC; Lyon 2008

IARC Library Cataloguing in Publication Data

WHO classification of tumours of haematopoietic and lymphoid tissues
Edited by S.H. Swerdlow, E. Campo, N.L. Harris, E.S. Jaffe, S.A. Pileri, H. Stein, J. Thiele, J.W. Vardiman

(World Health Organization classification of tumours)

1. Leukemia – classification 2. Leukemia – genetics 3. Leukemia – pathology
4. Lymphoma – classification 5. Lymphoma – genetics 6. Lymphoma – pathology
I. Swerdlow, Steven H. II. Series

ISBN 978-92-832-2431-0   (NLM Classification: WH 15)

Contents

_____

NOS, not otherwise specified

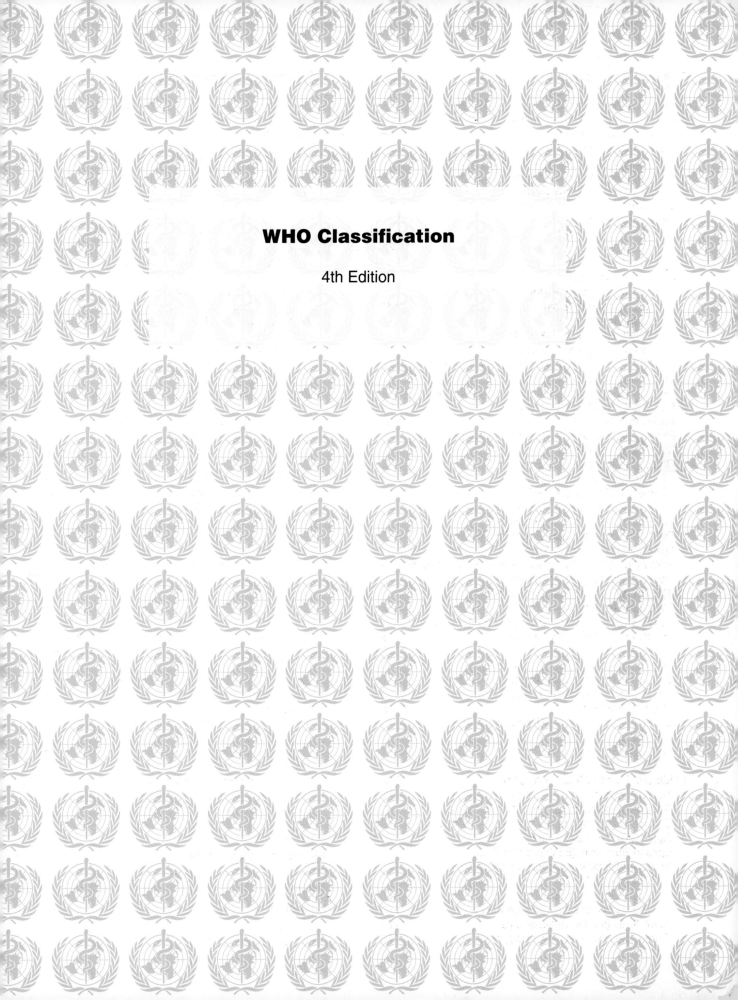

WHO Classification

4th Edition

WHO Classification of tumours of haematopoietic and lymphoid tissues

MYELOPROLIFERATIVE NEOPLASMS

Chronic myelogenous leukaemia, *BCR-ABL1* positive	9875/3
Chronic neutrophilic leukaemia	9963/3
Polycythaemia vera	9950/3
Primary myelofibrosis	9961/3
Essential thrombocythaemia	9962/3
Chronic eosinophilic leukaemia, NOS	9964/3
Mastocytosis	
Cutaneous mastocytosis	9740/1
Systemic mastocytosis	9741/3
Mast cell leukaemia	9742/3
Mast cell sarcoma	9740/3
Extracutaneous mastocytoma	9740/1
Myeloproliferative neoplasm, unclassifiable	9975/3

MYELOID AND LYMPHOID NEOPLASMS WITH EOSINOPHILIA AND ABNORMALITIES OF *PDGFRA*, *PDGFRB* OR *FGFR1*

Myeloid and lymphoid neoplasms with *PDGFRA* rearrangement	*9965/3*
Myeloid neoplasms with *PDGFRB* rearrangement	*9966/3*
Myeloid and lymphoid neoplasms with *FGFR1* abnormalities	*9967/3*

MYELODYSPLASTIC/MYELOPROLIFERATIVE NEOPLASMS

Chronic myelomonocytic leukaemia	9945/3
Atypical chronic myeloid leukaemia, *BCR-ABL1* negative	9876/3
Juvenile myelomonocytic leukaemia	9946/3
Myelodysplastic/myeloproliferative neoplasm, unclassifiable	9975/3
Refractory anaemia with ring sideroblasts associated with marked thrombocytosis	9982/3

MYELODYSPLASTIC SYNDROMES

Refractory cytopenia with unilineage dysplasia	
Refractory anaemia	9980/3
Refractory neutropenia	*9991/3*
Refractory thrombocytopenia	*9992/3*
Refractory anaemia with ring sideroblasts	9982/3
Refractory cytopenia with multilineage dysplasia	9985/3
Refractory anaemia with excess blasts	9983/3
Myelodysplastic syndrome associated with isolated del(5q)	9986/3
Myelodysplastic syndrome, unclassifiable	9989/3
Childhood myelodysplastic syndrome	
Refractory cytopenia of childhood	9985/3

ACUTE MYELOID LEUKAEMIA (AML) AND RELATED PRECURSOR NEOPLASMS

AML with recurrent genetic abnormalities

AML with t(8;21)(q22;q22); *RUNX1-RUNX1T1*	9896/3
AML with inv(16)(p13.1q22) or t(16;16)(p13.1;q22); *CBFB-MYH11*	9871/3
Acute promyelocytic leukaemia with t(15;17)(q22;q12); *PML-RARA*	9866/3
AML with t(9;11)(p22;q23); *MLLT3-MLL*	9897/3
AML with t(6;9)(p23;q34); *DEK-NUP214*	*9865/3*
AML with inv(3)(q21q26.2) or t(3;3)(q21;q26.2); *RPN1-EVI1*	*9869/3*
AML (megakaryoblastic) with t(1;22)(p13;q13); *RBM15-MKL1*	*9911/3*
AML with mutated NPM1	9861/3
AML with mutated CEBPA	9861/3

AML with myelodysplasia-related changes	9895/3
Therapy-related myeloid neoplasms	9920/3

Acute myeloid leukaemia, NOS	9861/3
AML with minimal differentiation	9872/3
AML without maturation	9873/3
AML with maturation	9874/3
Acute myelomonocytic leukaemia	9867/3
Acute monoblastic and monocytic leukaemia	9891/3
Acute erythroid leukaemia	9840/3
Acute megakaryoblastic leukaemia	9910/3
Acute basophilic leukaemia	9870/3
Acute panmyelosis with myelofibrosis	9931/3
Myeloid sarcoma	9930/3

Myeloid proliferations related to Down syndrome

Transient abnormal myelopoiesis	*9898/1*
Myeloid leukaemia associated with Down syndrome	*9898/3*

Blastic plasmacytoid dendritic cell neoplasm	9727/3

ACUTE LEUKAEMIAS OF AMBIGUOUS LINEAGE

Acute undifferentiated leukaemia	9801/3
Mixed phenotype acute leukaemia with t(9;22)(q34;q11.2); *BCR-ABL1*	*9806/3*
Mixed phenotype acute leukaemia with t(v;11q23); *MLL* rearranged	*9807/3*
Mixed phenotype acute leukaemia, B/myeloid, NOS	*9808/3*
Mixed phenotype acute leukaemia, T/myeloid, NOS	*9809/3*
Natural killer (NK) cell lymphoblastic leukaemia/lymphoma	

PRECURSOR LYMPHOID NEOPLASMS

B lymphoblastic leukaemia/lymphoma

B lymphoblastic leukaemia/lymphoma, NOS	*9811/3*

B lymphoblastic leukaemia/lymphoma with recurrent genetic abnormalities	
B lymphoblastic leukaemia/lymphoma with t(9;22)(q34;q11.2); *BCR-ABL1*	*9812/3*
B lymphoblastic leukaemia/lymphoma with t(v;11q23); *MLL* rearranged	*9813/3*
B lymphoblastic leukaemia/lymphoma with t(12;21)(p13;q22); *TEL-AML1 (ETV6-RUNX1)*	*9814/3*
B lymphoblastic leukaemia/lymphoma with hyperdiploidy	*9815/3*
B lymphoblastic leukaemia/lymphoma with hypodiploidy (hypodiploid ALL)	*9816/3*
B lymphoblastic leukaemia/lymphoma with t(5;14)(q31;q32); *IL3-IGH*	*9817/3*
B lymphoblastic leukaemia/lymphoma with t(1;19)(q23;p13.3); *E2A-PBX1 (TCF3-PBX1)*	*9818/3*
T lymphoblastic leukaemia/lymphoma	*9837/3*

MATURE B-CELL NEOPLASMS

Chronic lymphocytic leukaemia/ small lymphocytic lymphoma	9823/3
B-cell prolymphocytic leukaemia	9833/3
Splenic marginal zone lymphoma	9689/3
Hairy cell leukaemia	9940/3
Splenic B-cell lymphoma/leukaemia, unclassifiable	9591/3
Splenic diffuse red pulp small B-cell lymphoma	9591/3
Hairy cell leukaemia-variant	9591/3
Lymphoplasmacytic lymphoma	9671/3
Waldenström macroglobulinemia	9761/3
Heavy chain diseases	9762/3
Alpha heavy chain disease	9762/3
Gamma heavy chain disease	9762/3
Mu heavy chain disease	9762/3
Plasma cell myeloma	9732/3
Solitary plasmacytoma of bone	9731/3
Extraosseous plasmacytoma	9734/3

Extranodal marginal zone lymphoma of mucosa-associated lymphoid tissue (MALT lymphoma)	9699/3
Nodal marginal zone lymphoma	9699/3
Paediatric nodal marginal zone lymphoma	9699/3
Follicular lymphoma	9690/3
Paediatric follicular lymphoma	9690/3
Primary cutaneous follicle centre lymphoma	*9597/3*
Mantle cell lymphoma	9673/3
Diffuse large B-cell lymphoma (DLBCL), NOS	9680/3
T-cell/histiocyte rich large B-cell lymphoma	9688/3
Primary DLBCL of the CNS	9680/3
Primary cutaneous DLBCL, leg type	9680/3
EBV positive DLBCL of the elderly	9680/3
DLBCL associated with chronic inflammation	9680/3
Lymphomatoid granulomatosis	9766/1
Primary mediastinal (thymic) large B-cell lymphoma	9679/3
Intravascular large B-cell lymphoma	9712/3
ALK positive large B-cell lymphoma	9737/3
Plasmablastic lymphoma	9735/3
Large B-cell lymphoma arising in HHV8-associated multicentric Castleman disease	*9738/3*
Primary effusion lymphoma	9678/3
Burkitt lymphoma	9687/3
B-cell lymphoma, unclassifiable, with features intermediate between diffuse large B-cell lymphoma and Burkitt lymphoma	9680/3
B-cell lymphoma, unclassifiable, with features intermediate between diffuse large B-cell lymphoma and classical Hodgkin lymphoma	9596/3

MATURE T-CELL AND NK-CELL NEOPLASMS

T-cell prolymphocytic leukaemia	9834/3
T-cell large granular lymphocytic leukaemia	9831/3
Chronic lymphoproliferative disorder of NK-cells	9831/3
Aggressive NK cell leukaemia	9948/3

Systemic EBV positive T-cell lymphoproliferative disease of childhood	9724/3
Hydroa vacciniforme-like lymphoma	*9725/3*
Adult T-cell leukaemia/lymphoma	9827/3
Extranodal NK/T cell lymphoma, nasal type	9719/3
Enteropathy-associated T-cell lymphoma	9717/3
Hepatosplenic T-cell lymphoma	9716/3
Subcutaneous panniculitis-like T-cell lymphoma	9708/3
Mycosis fungoides	9700/3
Sézary syndrome	9701/3
Primary cutaneous CD30 positive T-cell lymphoproliferative disorders	
Lymphomatoid papulosis	9718/1
Primary cutaneous anaplastic large cell lymphoma	9718/3
Primary cutaneous gamma-delta T-cell lymphoma	*9726/3*
Primary cutaneous CD8 positive aggressive epidermotropic cytotoxic T-cell lymphoma	9709/3
Primary cutaneous CD4 positive small/medium T-cell lymphoma	9709/3
Peripheral T-cell lymphoma, NOS	9702/3
Angioimmunoblastic T-cell lymphoma	9705/3
Anaplastic large cell lymphoma, *ALK* positive	9714/3
Anaplastic large cell lymphoma, ALK negative	9702/3

HODGKIN LYMPHOMA

Nodular lymphocyte predominant Hodgkin lymphoma	9659/3
Classical Hodgkin lymphoma	9650/3
Nodular sclerosis classical Hodgkin lymphoma	9663/3
Lymphocyte-rich classical Hodgkin lymphoma	9651/3
Mixed cellularity classical Hodgkin lymphoma	9652/3
Lymphocyte-depleted classical Hodgkin lymphoma	9653/3

HISTIOCYTIC AND DENDRITIC CELL NEOPLASMS

Histiocytic sarcoma	9755/3
Langerhans cell histiocytosis	9751/3
Langerhans cell sarcoma	9756/3
Interdigitating dendritic cell sarcoma	9757/3
Follicular dendritic cell sarcoma	9758/3
Fibroblastic reticular cell tumour	9759/3
Indeterminate dendritic cell tumour	9757/3
Disseminated juvenile xanthogranuloma	

POST-TRANSPLANT LYMPHOPROLIFERATIVE DISORDERS (PTLD)

Early lesions	
Plasmacytic hyperplasia	9971/1
Infectious mononucleosis-like PTLD	9971/1
Polymorphic PTLD	9971/3
Monomorphic PTLD (B- and T/NK-cell types)*	
Classical Hodgkin lymphoma type PTLD*	

NOS, not otherwise specified.

The italicized numbers are provisional codes for the 4th edition of ICD-O. While they are expected to be incorporated in the next ICD-O edition, they currently remain subject to changes.

The italicized histologic types are provisional entities, for which the WHO Working Group felt there was insufficient evidence to recognize as distinct diseases at this time.

*These lesions are classified according to the leukaemia or lymphoma to which they correspond, and are assigned the respective ICD-O code.

Introduction to the WHO classification of tumours of haematopoietic and lymphoid tissues

N.L. Harris
E. Campo
E.S. Jaffe
S.A. Pileri

H. Stein
S.H. Swerdlow
J. Thiele
J.W. Vardiman

Why classify? Classification is the language of medicine: diseases must be described, defined and named before they can be diagnosed, treated and studied. A consensus on definitions and terminology is essential for both clinical practice and investigation. A classification should contain diseases that are clearly defined, clinically distinctive, non-overlapping (mutually exclusive) and that together comprise all known entities (collectively exhaustive). It should serve as a basis for future investigation, and should be able to incorporate new information as it becomes available. Classification has two aspects: class discovery —the process of identifying categories of diseases, and class prediction —the process of determining which category an individual case belongs to. Pathologists are critical to both processes.

The World Health Organization (WHO) Classification of Tumours of the Haematopoietic and Lymphoid Tissues (4th Edition) was a collaborative project of the European Association for Haematopathology and the Society for Hematopathology. It is a revision and update of the 3rd Edition {1039}, which was the first true worldwide consensus classification of haematologic malignancies. The update, which began in 2006, had an 8-member steering committee composed of members of both societies. The Steering Committee, in a series of meetings and discussions, agreed on a proposed list of diseases and chapters and selected authors, with input from both societies. As with the WHO 3rd edition {897}, the advice of clinical haematologists and oncologists was obtained, in order to ensure that the classification will be clinically useful. Two Clinical Advisory Committees (CAC), one for myeloid neoplasms and other acute leukaemias and one for lymphoid neoplasms, were convened. The meetings were organized around a series of questions, including disease definitions, nomenclature, grading, and clinical relevance. The committees were able to reach consensus on most of the questions posed, and much of the input of the

committees was incorporated into the classification. Over 130 pathologists and haematologists from around the world were involved in writing the chapters. A consensus meeting was held at the headquarters of the IARC in Lyon, France, to make final decisions on the classification and the content of the book.

The WHO classification of tumours of the haematopoietic and lymphoid system is based on the principles initially defined in the "Revised European-American Classification of Lymphoid Neoplasms" (REAL), from the International Lymphoma Study Group (ILSG) {898}. In the WHO classification, these principles have also been applied to the classification of myeloid and histiocytic neoplasms. The guiding principle of the REAL and WHO classifications is the attempt to define "real" diseases that can be recognized by pathologists with available techniques, and that appear be distinct clinical entities. There are 3 important components to this process. First, recognizing that the underlying causes of these neoplasms are often unknown and may vary, this approach to classification uses all available information —morphology, immunophenotype, genetic features, and clinical features— to define diseases. The relative importance of each of these features varies among diseases, depending upon the state of current knowledge, and there is therefore no one "gold standard," by which all diseases are defined. Second, recognizing that the complexity of the field makes it impossible for a single expert or small group to be completely authoritative, and that broad agreement is necessary if a classification is to be accepted, this classification relies on building a consensus among as many experts as possible on the definition and nomenclature of the diseases. We recognize that compromise is essential in order to arrive at a consensus, but believe that the only thing worse than an imperfect classification is multiple competing classifications. Finally, while pathologists must take primary responsibility for developing a

classification, involvement of clinicians is essential to ensure its usefulness and acceptance in daily practice {897}. At the time of publication of the WHO classification (3rd edition), proponents of other classifications of haematologic neoplasms agreed to use the new classification, thus ending decades of controversy over the classification of these tumours {47, 47B, 189, 189A, 190, 673, 775D, 1344A, 1819B}.

As indicated above, there is no one "gold standard," by which all diseases are defined in the WHO classification. Morphology is always important, and many diseases have characteristic or even diagnostic morphologic features. Immunophenotype and genetic features are an important part of the definition of tumours of the haematopoietic and lymphoid tissues, and the availability of this information makes arriving at consensus definitions easier now than it was when only subjective morphologic criteria were available. Immunophenotyping studies are used in routine diagnosis in the vast majority of haematologic malignancies, both to determine lineage in malignant processes and to distinguish benign from malignant processes. Many diseases have a characteristic immunophenotype, such that one would hesitate to make the diagnosis in the absence of the immunophenotype, while in others the immunophenotype is only part of the diagnosis. In some lymphoid and in many myeloid neoplasms a specific genetic abnormality is the key defining criterion, while others lack specific known genetic abnormalities. Some genetic abnormalities, while characteristic of one disease, are not specific (such as *MYC*, *CCND1* or *BCL2* rearrangements or mutations in *JAK2*), and others are prognostic factors in several diseases (such as *TP53* mutations or *FLT3-ITD*). The inclusion of immunophenotypic features and genetic abnormalities to define entities not only provides objective criteria for disease recognition but has identified antigens, genes or pathways that can be targeted for therapy; the success of rituximab, an anti-CD20 molecule, in the treatment of B-cell neoplasms, and of imatinib in the treatment of leukaemias associated with *ABL1* and other rearrangements involving tryosine kinase genes are testament to this approach. Finally, some diseases require knowledge of clinical features – age, nodal versus extranodal presentation, specific anatomic site, and history of cytotoxic and other therapies —to make the diagnosis. Most of the diseases described in the WHO classification are considered to be distinct entities; however, some are not as clearly defined, and these are listed as provisional entities. In addition, borderline categories have been created in this edition for cases that do not clearly fit into one category, so that well-defined categories can be kept homogeneous, and the borderline cases can be studied further.

The WHO classification stratifies neoplasms primarily according to lineage: myeloid, lymphoid, and histiocytic/dendritic cell. A normal counterpart is postulated for each neoplasm. While the goal is to define the lineage of each neoplasm, lineage plasticity may occur in precursor or immature neoplasms, and has recently been identified in some mature haematolymphoid neoplasms. In addition, genetic abnormalities such as *FGFR1*, *PDGFRA* and *PDGFRB* rearrangements may give rise to neoplasms of either myeloid or lymphoid lineage associated with eosinophilia; these disorders are now recognized as a separate group. Precursor neoplasms (acute myeloid leukaemias, lymphoblastic lymphomas/leukaemias, acute leukaemias of ambiguous lineage, and blastic plasmacytoid dendritic cell neoplasm) are considered separately from more mature neoplasms [myeloproliferative neoplasms (MPN), myelodysplastic/myeloproliferative neoplasms, myelodysplastic syndromes, mature (peripheral) B-cell and T/NK-cell neoplasms, Hodgkin lymphoma, and histiocyte/dendritic-cell neoplasms]. The mature myeloid neoplasms are stratified according to their biological features (myeloproliferative, with effective haematopoiesis, versus myelodysplastic, with ineffective haematopoiesis, as well as by genetic features). Within the mature lymphoid neoplasms, the diseases are listed broadly according to clinical presentation (disseminated often leukaemic, extranodal, indolent, aggressive), and to some extent according to stage of differentiation when this can be postulated; however the

order of listing is in part arbitrary, and is not an integral part of the classification.

The 4th edition of the WHO classification incorporates new information that has emerged from basic and clinical investigations in the interval since publication of the 3rd edition. It includes new defining criteria for some diseases, as well as a number of new entities, some defined by genetic criteria —particularly among the myeloid neoplasms— and others by a combination of morphology, immunophenotype, and clinical features. The frequent application of immunophenotyping and genetic studies to peripheral blood, bone marrow, and lymph node samples has also led to the detection of small clonal populations in asymptomatic persons. These include small clones of cells with the *BCR-ABL1* translocation seen in chronic myelogenous leukaemia, small clones of cells with *BCL2-IGH* rearrangement, and small populations of cells that have the immunophenotype of chronic lymphocytic leukaemia (CLL) or follicular lymphoma (monoclonal B lymphocytosis, follicular lymphoma-*in situ*, paediatric follicular hyperplasia with monoclonal B cells). In many cases, it is not clear whether these represent early involvement by a neoplasm, a precursor lesion, or an inconsequential finding. These situations have some analogies to the identification of small monoclonal immunoglobulin components in serum (monoclonal gammopathy of unknown significance). The chapters on these neoplasms include recommendations for dealing with these situations. The recommendations of international consensus groups have been considered, with regard to criteria for the diagnosis of CLL, plasma cell myeloma, Waldenström macroglobulinemia, and new subtypes of cutaneous lymphomas, as well as in the development of new algorithms for the diagnosis of MPN.

A critical feature of any classification of diseases is that it be periodically reviewed and updated to incorporate new information. The Society for Haematopathology and the European Association for Haematopathology now have a more than 10-year record of collaboration and cooperation in this effort. The societies are committed to updating and revising the classification as needed, with input from clinicians and with the collaboration of the WHO. The experience of developing and updating

the WHO classification has produced a new and exciting degree of cooperation and communication among pathologists and oncologists from around the world, which should facilitate continued progress in the understanding and treatment of haematologic malignancies. The multiparameter approach to classification, with an emphasis on defining real disease entites, that has been adopted by the WHO classification, has been shown in international studies to be reproducible; the diseases defined are clinically distinctive, and the uniform definitions and terminology facilitate the interpretation of clinical and translational studies {51, 79}. In addition, accurate and precise classification of disease entities has facilitated the discovery of the genetic basis of myeloid and lymphoid neoplasms in the basic science laboratory.

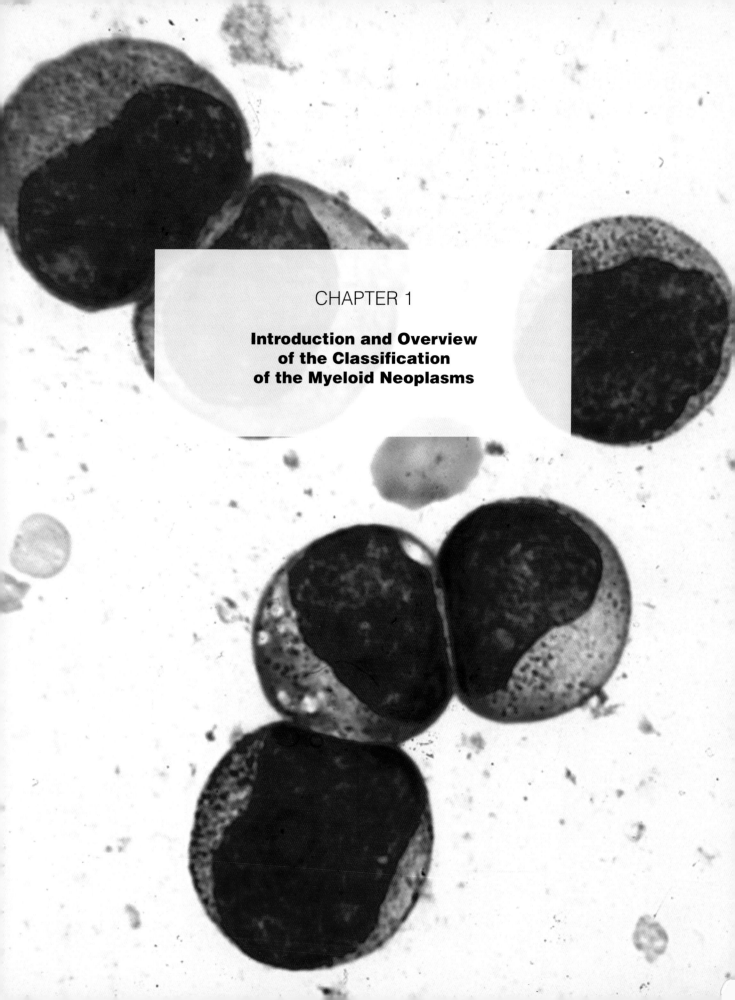

CHAPTER 1

**Introduction and Overview
of the Classification
of the Myeloid Neoplasms**

Introduction and overview of the classification of the myeloid neoplasms

J.W. Vardiman
R.D. Brunning
D.A. Arber
M.M. Le Beau

A. Porwit
A. Tefferi
C.D. Bloomfield
J. Thiele

The WHO Classification of Tumours of the Haematopoietic and Lymphoid Tissues (3rd edition) published in 2001 reflected a paradigm shift in the approach to classification of myeloid neoplasms {1039}. For the first time, genetic information was incorporated into diagnostic algorithms provided for the various entities. The publication was prefaced with a comment predicting future revisions necessitated by rapidly emerging genetic information. The current revision is a commentary on the significant new molecular insights that have become available since the publication of the last classification.

The first entity described in this monograph, chronic myelogenous leukaemia (CML) remains the prototype for the identification and classification of myeloid neoplasms. This leukaemia is recognized by its clinical and morphologic features, and its natural progression is characterized by an increase in blasts of myeloid, lymphoid or mixed myeloid/lymphoid immunophenotype. It is always associated with the *BCR-ABL1* fusion gene that results in the production of an abnormal protein tyrosine kinase (PTK) with enhanced enzymatic activity. This protein is sufficient to cause the leukaemia and also provides a target for protein tyrosine kinase inhibitor (PTKI) therapy that has prolonged the lives of thousands of patients with this often fatal illness {615}. This successful integration of clinical, morphologic and genetic information embodies the goal of the WHO classification scheme.

In this revision, a combination of clinical, morphologic, immunophenotypic and genetic features is used in an attempt to define disease entities, such as CML, that are biologically homogeneous and clinically relevant —the same approach used in the 3rd edition of the classification. Although the previous scheme began to open the door to including genetic abnormalities as criteria to classify myeloid neoplasms, this revision firmly acknowledges that as in CML, recurring genetic abnormalities provide not only objective criteria for recognition of specific entities but also identification of abnormal gene products or pathways that are potential targets for therapy. One example in this revised scheme is the addition of a new subgroup of myeloid neoplasms (Table 1.01) associated with eosinophilia and chromosomal abnormalities that involve the platelet-derived growth factor receptor

Table 1.01 The myeloid neoplasms: major subgroups and characteristic features at diagnosis.

Disease	BM cellularity	% Marrow blasts	Maturation	Morphology	Haematopoiesis	Blood counts	Organomegaly
MPN	Usually increased, often normal in ET	Normal or slightly increased; <10% in chronic phase	Present	Granulocytes, erythroid precursors relatively normal, megakaryocytes abnormal	Effective	Variable; one or more myeloid lineage usually initially increased	Common
Myeloid/lymphoid neoplasms with eosinophilia and abnormalities of *PDGFRA*, *PDGFRB* or *FGFR1*	Increased	Normal or slightly increased; <20% in chronic phase	Present	Relatively normal	Effective	Eosinophilia (≥1.5x10⁹/L)	Common
MDS	Increased, occasionally normocellular or hypocellular	Normal or increased; <20%	Present	Dysplasia in one or more myeloid lineage	Ineffective	Cytopenia(s)	Uncommon
MDS/MPN	Increased	Normal or slightly increased; <20%	Present	Usually one or more lineages dysplastic; JMML often has minimal dysplasia	May vary among lineages	Variable, WBC usually increased	Common
AML	Usually increased	Increased, ≥20%, except in some cases with specific cytogenetic abnormalities or in some cases of erythroleukaemia	Varies, usually minimal	May or may not be associated with dysplasia in one or more lineages	Ineffective or effective	WBC variable, usually anaemia and thrombocytopenia	Uncommon

MPN, myeloproliferative neoplasms; MDS, myelodysplastic syndromes; MDS/MPN, myelodysplastic/myeloproliferative neoplasms; AML, acute myeloid leukaemia; ET, essential thrombocythaemia; JMML, juvenile myelomonocytic leukaemia; WBC, white blood cells.

alpha *(PDGFRA)* or platelet derived growth factor receptor beta *(PDGFRB)* genes —a subgroup defined largely by genetic events that lead to constitutive activation of the receptor tyrosine kinase, PDGFR, and that respond to PTKI therapy {131, 466, 812}. Similar examples are found throughout the classification in each major subgroup, and include not only neoplasms associated with microscopically recognizable chromosomal abnormalities but also with gene mutations without a cytogenetic correlate as well. On the other hand, the importance of careful clinical, morphological and immunophenotypic characterization of each myeloid neoplasm and correlation with the genetic findings cannot be overemphasized. The discovery of activating *JAK2* mutations has revolutionized the approach to the diagnosis of the myeloproliferative neoplasms (MPN) {163, 1044, 1186, 1288}. Yet *JAK2* mutations are not specific for any single clinical or morphologic MPN phenotype, and are also reported in some cases of myelodysplastic syndromes (MDS), myelodysplastic/ myeloproliferative neoplasms (MDS/MPN) and acute myeloid leukaemia (AML). Thus, an integrated, multidisciplinary approach is necessary for the classification of myeloid neoplasms.

With so much yet to learn, there may be some "missteps" as traditional approaches to categorization are fused with more molecularly-oriented classification schemes. Nevertheless, this revision of the WHO classification is an attempt by the authors, editors and the clinicians who served as members of the Clinical Advisory Committee (CAC) to provide an "evidence-based" classification that can be used in daily practice for therapeutic decisions and yet provide a flexible framework for integration of new data.

Prerequisites for classification of myeloid neoplasms by WHO criteria

The WHO classification of myeloid neoplasms relies on the morphologic, cytochemical and immunophenotypic features of the neoplastic cells to establish their lineage and degree of maturation and to decide whether cellular proliferation is cytologically normal or dysplastic or effective or ineffective. The classification is based on criteria applied to initial specimens obtained prior to any definitive therapy, including growth factor therapy, for the myeloid neoplasm. The blast percentage in the peripheral blood, bone marrow and other involved tissues remains of practical importance to categorize myeloid neoplasms and to judge their progression. Cytogenetic and molecular genetic studies are required at the time of diagnosis not only for recognition of specific genetically defined entities, but for establishing a baseline against which future studies can be judged to assess disease progression. Because of the multidisciplinary approach required to diagnose and classify myeloid neoplasms it is recommended that the various diagnostic studies be correlated with the clinical findings and reported in a single, integrated report. If a definitive classification cannot be reached the report should indicate the reasons why and provide guidelines for additional studies that may clarify the diagnosis.

To obtain consistency, the following guidelines are recommended for the evaluation of specimens when a myeloid neoplasm is suspected to be present. It is assumed that this evaluation will be performed with full knowledge of the clinical history and pertinent laboratory data.

Morphology

Peripheral blood: A peripheral blood (PB) smear should be examined and correlated with results of a complete blood count. Freshly made smears should be stained with May-Grünwald-Giemsa or Wright-Giemsa and examined for white blood cell (WBC), red blood cell (RBC) and platelet abnormalities. It is important to ascertain that the smears are well-stained. Evaluation of neutrophil granularity is important when a myeloid disorder is suspected; designation of neutrophils as abnormal based on hypogranular cytoplasm alone should not be considered unless the stain is well-controlled. Manual 200-cell leukocyte differentials of PB smears are recommended in patients with a myeloid neoplasm when the WBC count permits.

Bone marrow aspirate: Bone marrow (BM) aspirate smears should also be stained with May-Grünwald-Giemsa or Wright-Giemsa for optimal visualization of cytoplasmic granules and nuclear chromatin. Because the WHO Classification relies on percentages of blasts and other specific

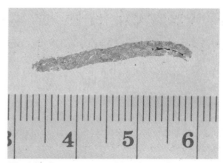
Fig. 1.01 Bone marrow trephine biopsy. Bone marrow trephine biopsies should be at least 1.5 cm in length and obtained at right angles to the cortical bone.

cells to categorize some entities, it is recommended that 500 nucleated BM cells be counted on cellular aspirate smears in an area as close to the particle and as undiluted with blood as possible. Counting from multiple smears may reduce sampling error due to irregular distribution of cells. The cells to be counted include blasts and promonocytes (see definition below), promyelocytes, myelocytes, metamyelocytes, band neutrophils, segmented neutrophils, eosinophils, basophils, monocytes, lymphocytes, plasma cells, erythroid precursors and mast cells. Megakaryocytes, including dysplastic forms, are not included. If a concomitant non-myeloid neoplasm is present, such as plasma cell myeloma, it is reasonable to exclude those neoplastic cells from the count used to evaluate the myeloid neoplasm. If an aspirate cannot be obtained due to fibrosis or cellular packing, touch preparations of the biopsy may yield valuable cytologic information, but differential counts from touch preparations may not be representative. The differential counts obtained from marrow aspirates should be compared to an estimate of the proportions of cells observed in available biopsy sections.

Bone marrow trephine biopsy: The contribution of adequate BM biopsy sections in the diagnosis of myeloid neoplasms cannot be overstated. The trephine biopsy provides information regarding overall cellularity and the topography, proportion and maturation of haematopoietic cells, and allows evaluation of BM stroma. The biopsy also provides material for immunohistochemical studies that may have diagnostic and prognostic importance. A biopsy is essential whenever there is myelofibrosis, and the classification of some entities, particularly MPN, relies heavily on trephine sections. The specimen must be adequate, taken at right angle from the cortical bone and at least 1.5 cm in length to enable the evaluation of at least 10 partially preserved inter-trabecular areas. It should be well-fixed, thinly sectioned at 3–4 micra, and stained with haematoxylin and eosin and/or a stain such as Giemsa that allows for detailed morphologic evaluation. A silver impregnation method for reticulin fibres is recommended and marrow fibrosis graded according to the European consensus scoring system {2214}. A periodic acid-Schiff (PAS) stain may aid in detection of megakaryocytes. Immunohistochemical (IHC) study of the biopsy is often indispensable in the evaluation of myeloid neoplasms and is discussed below.

Blasts: The percentage of myeloid blasts is important for diagnosis and classification of myeloid neoplasms. In the PB the blast percentage should be derived from a 200-cell leukocyte differential and in the BM from a 500-cell count of cellular BM aspirate smears as described above. The blast percentage derived from the BM aspirate should correlate with an estimate of the blast percentage in the trephine biopsy, although large focal clusters or sheets of blasts in the biopsy should be regarded as possible disease progression. Immunohistochemical staining of the BM biopsy for CD34+ blasts often aids in the correlation of aspirate and trephine biopsy findings, although in some myeloid neoplasms the blasts do not express CD34. Flow cytometry determination of blast percentage should not be used as a substitute for visual inspection. The specimen for flow cytometry is often haemodilute, and may be affected by a number of pre-analytic variables, and as noted for the

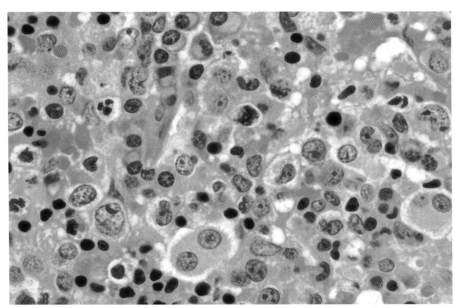

Fig. 1.02 Myelodysplastic syndrome. Bone marrow biopsy section. Bone marrow biopsies should be well-fixed and thin sections (3-4 microns) stained with H&E and/or Giemsa to allow optimal evaluation of histologic details.

biopsy, not all blasts express CD34. Myeloblasts, monoblasts and megakaryoblasts are included in the blast count. Myeloblasts vary from slightly larger than mature lymphocytes to the size of monocytes or larger, with moderate to abundant dark blue to blue-grey cytoplasm. The nuclei are round to oval with finely granular chromatin and usually several nucleoli, but in some nuclear irregularities may be prominent. The cytoplasm may contain a few azurophil granules (Fig 1.03). Monoblasts are large cells with abundant cytoplasm that can be light grey to deeply blue and may show pseudopod formation (Fig 1.04 A,B). Their nuclei are usually round with delicate, lacy chromatin and one or more large prominent nucleoli.

They are usually strongly positive for non-specific esterase (NSE) but have no or only weak myeloperoxidase (MPO) activity. Promonocytes are considered as "monoblast equivalents" when the requisite percentage of blasts is tallied for the diagnosis of acute monoblastic, acute monocytic and acute myelomonocytic leukaemia. Promonocytes have a delicately convoluted, folded or grooved nucleus with finely dispersed chromatin, a small, indistinct or absent nucleolus, and finely granulated cytoplasm (Fig 1.04 C, D). Most promonocytes express NSE and are likely to have MPO activity. The distinction between monoblasts and promonocytes is often difficult, but because the two cell types are summated

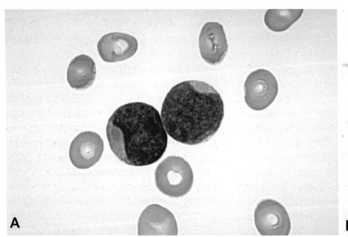

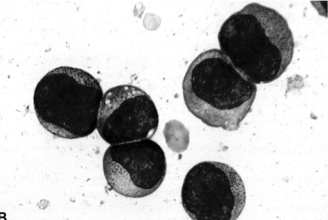

Fig. 1.03 Acute myeloid leukaemia. **A** Agranular myeloblasts. **B** Granulated myeloblasts.

as monoblasts in making the diagnosis of AML, the distinction between a monoblast and promonocyte is not always critical. On the other hand, distinguishing promonocytes from more mature but abnormal leukaemic monocytes can also be difficult, but is critical, because the designation of a case as acute monocytic or acute myelomonocytic leukaemia versus chronic myelomonocytic leukaemia often hinges on this distinction. Abnormal monocytes have more clumped chromatin than a promonocyte, variably indented, folded nuclei and grey cytoplasm with more abundant lilac-colored granules. Nucleoli are usually absent or indistinct (Fig 1.04 E,F). Abnormal monocytes are not considered as monoblast equivalents. Megakaryoblasts are usually of medium to large size with a round, indented or irregular nucleus with finely reticular chromatin and one to three nucleoli. The cytoplasm is basophilic, usually agranular, and may show cytoplasmic blebs (See Chapter 6 on acute myeloid leukaemia, NOS). Small dysplastic megakaryocytes and micromegakaryocytes are not blasts. In acute promyelocytic leukaemia, the blast equivalent is the abnormal promyelocyte. Erythroid precursors (proerythroblasts) are not included in the blast count except in the rare instance of "pure" acute erythroid leukaemia, in which case they are considered as blast equivalents (See Chapter 6 on acute myeloid leukaemia, NOS).

Cytochemistry and other special stains: Cytochemical studies are used to determine the lineage of blasts, although in some laboratories they have been supplanted by immunologic studies using flow cytometry and/or immunohistochemistry. They are usually performed on PB and BM aspirate smears but some can be performed on sections of trephine biopsies or other tissues. Detection of MPO indicates myeloid differentiation but its absence does not exclude a myeloid lineage because early myeloblasts as well as monoblasts may lack MPO. The MPO activity in myeloblasts is usually granular and often concentrated in the Golgi region whereas monoblasts, although usually negative, may show fine, scattered MPO+ granules, a pattern that becomes more pronounced in promonocytes. Erythroid blasts, megakaryoblasts and lymphoblasts are MPO negative. Sudan Black B (SBB) staining parallels MPO but is less specific. Occasional cases of lymphoblastic leukaemia exhibit SBB positivity, in which

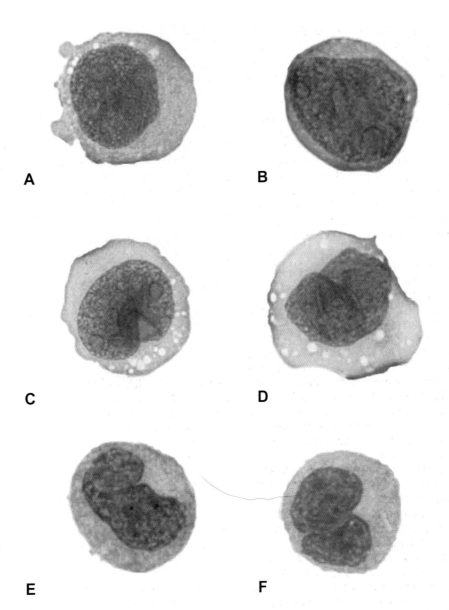

Fig. 1.04 Monoblasts, promonocytes and abnormal monocytes from a case of acute monocytic leukaemia. **A, B** Monoblasts are large with abundant cytoplasm that may contain a few vacuoles or fine granules and have round nuclei with lacy chromatin and one or more variably prominent nucleoli. **C, D** Promonocytes have more irregular and delicately folded nuclei with fine chromatin, small indistinct nucleoli and finely granulated cytoplasm. **E, F** Abnormal monocytes appear immature, yet have more condensed nuclear chromatin, convoluted or folded nuclei, and more cytoplasmic granulation (Courtesy of Dr. J. Goasguen).

case light grey granules are seen rather than the deeply black granules that characterize myeloblasts. The non-specific esterases, α naphthyl butyrate (ANB) and α naphthyl acetate (ANA), show diffuse cytoplasmic activity in monoblasts and monocytes. Lymphoblasts may have focal punctate activity with NSE but neutrophils are usually negative. Megakaryoblasts and erythroid blasts may have some multifocal, punctate ANA positivity, but it is partially resistant to natrium fluoride (NaF) inhibition whereas monocyte NSE is totally

inhibited by NaF. The combination of NSE and the specific esterase, naphthol-ASD-chloroacetate esterase (CAE), which stains primarily cells of the neutrophil lineage and mast cells, permits identification of monocytes and immature and mature neutrophils simultaneously. Some cells, particularly in myelomonocytic leukaemias, may exhibit NSE and CAE simultaneously. While normal eosinophils lack CAE, it may be expressed by neoplastic eosinophils. CAE can be performed on tissue sections as well as PB or marrow aspirate smears.

In acute erythroid leukaemia, a PAS stain may be helpful in that the cytoplasm of the leukaemic proerythroblasts may show large globules of PAS positivity. Well-controlled iron stains should always be performed on the BM aspirate to detect iron stores, normal sideroblasts and ring sideroblasts, the latter of which are defined as erythroid precursors with 5 or more granules of iron encircling one-third or more of the nucleus.

Immunophenotype

Immunophenotypic analysis using either multiparameter flow cytometry or IHC is an essential tool in the characterization of myeloid neoplasms. Differentiation antigens that appear at various stages of haematopoietic development and in corresponding myeloid neoplasms are illustrated in Fig. 1.05, and a thorough description of lineage assignment criteria is provided in the chapters on mixed phenotype acute leukaemia. The techniques employed and the antigens analyzed may vary according to the myeloid neoplasm suspected and the information required to best characterize it as well as by the tissue available. Although often important in the diagnosis of any haematological neoplasm, immunophenotyping in myeloid neoplasms is most commonly required in AML and in determining the phenotype of blasts at the time of transformation of MDS, MDS/MPN and MPN.

Multiparameter flow cytometry is the preferred method of immunophenotypic analysis in AML due to the ability to analyze high numbers of cells in a relatively short period of time with simultaneous recording of information about several antigens for each individual cell. Usually, rather extensive panels of monoclonal antibodies directed against leukocyte differentiation antigens are applied because

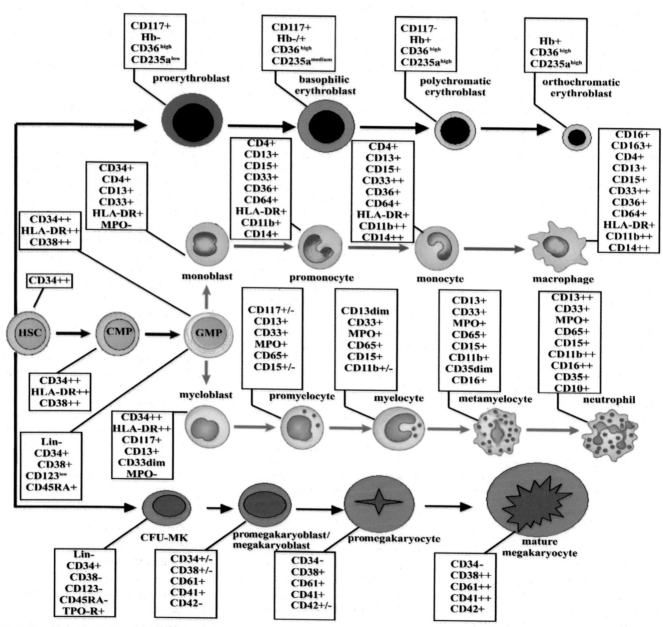

Fig. 1.05 Antigen expression at various stages of normal myeloid differentiation.

the utility of individual markers in identifying commitment of leukaemic cells into the different haematopoietic lineages is limited. Evaluation of expression patterns of several antigens, both membrane and cytoplasmic, is necessary for lineage assignment, to detect mixed phenotype acute leukaemia, and to detect aberrant phenotypes allowing for follow-up of minimal residual disease.

Immunophenotypic analysis has a central role in distinguishing between minimally differentiated acute myeloid leukaemia and acute lymphoblastic leukaemia, and in CML, between myeloid blast phase and lymphoid blast phase. Among AML with recurrent genetic abnormalities, several have characteristic phenotypes. These patterns, described in the respective sections, can help to plan molecular cytogenetic [fluorescence in situ hybridization (FISH)] and molecular investigations in individual patients. Immunophenotypic features of the other AML categories are extremely heterogeneous, probably due to high genetic diversity. Although it has been suggested that expression of certain antigens, such as CD7, CD9, CD11b, CD14, CD56 and CD34 could be associated with an adverse prognosis in AML, their independent prognostic value is still controversial. Aberrant or unusual immunophenotypes have been found in at least 75% of cases of AML. These can be described as cross-lineage antigen expression, maturational asynchronous expression of antigens, antigen overexpression, and the reduction or absence of antigen expression. Similar aberrancies have also been reported in MDS as well, and their presence can be used to support the diagnosis in early or morphologically ambiguous cases of MDS (See Chapter 5). Immunophenotyping by IHC on BM biopsy sections can be applied if marrow cell suspensions are not available for flow cytometry analysis. Antibodies reactive with paraffin-embedded BM biopsy tissue are available for many lineage-associated markers (e.g. MPO, lysozyme, CD3, PAX5, CD33, etc.). As noted previously, CD34 staining of the biopsy can facilitate the detection of blasts and their distribution, provided the blasts express CD34 {1650}. For cases rich in megaloblastoid erythroblasts, immunohistology for glycophorin or haemoglobin may be helpful in distinguishing those cells from myeloblasts (e.g. in cases of RAEB or acute erythroleukaemia), and CD61 or CD42 often aid in the identification of abnormal megakaryocytes.

Genetic studies

The WHO classification includes a number of entities defined in part by specific genetic abnormalities, including gene rearrangements due to chromosomal translocations and to specific gene mutations, so determination of genetic features of the neoplastic cells must be performed if possible. A complete cytogenetic analysis of BM should be performed at the time of initial evaluation to establish the cytogenetic profile, and at regular intervals thereafter to detect evidence of genetic evolution. Additional diagnostic genetic studies should be guided by the diagnosis suspected on clinical, morphologic and immunophenotypic studies. In some cases, reverse transcriptase-polymerase chain reaction (RT-PCR) and/or FISH may detect gene rearrangements that are present in low frequency and not observed in the initial chromosomal analysis, in cases with variants of typical cytogenetic abnormalities, and in cases in which the abnormality is cryptic, such as the FIP1L1-PDGFRA fusion in myeloid neoplasms associated with eosinophilia. Depending on the abnormality, quantitative PCR performed at the time of diagnosis may also provide a baseline against which the response to therapy can be monitored. A number of gene mutations detected by gene sequencing, allele-specific PCR and other techniques have emerged as important diagnostic and prognostic markers in all categories of myeloid neoplasms. Mutations of JAK2, MPL, NRAS, NF1, PTPN11, and KIT in MPN and MDS/MPN, and NPM1, CEBPA, FLT3, RUNX1 and KIT, among others, in AML are important for diagnosis and prognosis, and some, particularly JAK2, FLT3, NPM1 and CEBPA figure importantly in this revised classification. Furthermore, the role of gene over- and under-expression as well as loss of heterozygosity and copy number variants detected by array-based approaches are only now being recognized as important abnormalities that may well influence diagnostic and prognostic models in the near future {1531A}. Nevertheless, microarray profiling studies, although important in the research setting, have not yet been tested in clinical practice.

Revised WHO classification of myeloid neoplasms

Table 1.01 lists the major subgroups of myeloid neoplasms and their characteristic features at diagnosis. The nomenclature for the myeloproliferative entities has been changed from "chronic myeloproliferative diseases" to "myeloproliferative neoplasms" and the subgroup formerly designated as "myelodysplastic/myeloproliferative diseases" has been changed to "myelodysplastic/myeloproliferative neoplasms" to underscore their neoplastic nature. Besides the addition of the new subgroup, "Myeloid and lymphoid neoplasms with eosinophilia and abnormalities of PDGFRA, PDGFRB and FGFR1," new entities have been added and/or diagnostic criteria updated within each subgroup.

Myeloproliferative neoplasms (MPN)

The MPN (Table 1.02) are clonal haematopoietic stem cell disorders characterized by proliferation of one or more of the myeloid lineages (i.e. granulocytic, erythroid, megakaryocytic and mast cell). They are primarily neoplasms of adults that peak in frequency in the 5th to 7th decade, but some subtypes, particularly CML and essential thrombocythaemia (ET), are reported in children as well. The incidence of all subtypes combined is 6–10/100,000 population annually {1053, 1059, 1060}.

Initially, MPN is characterized by hypercellularity of the BM with effective haematopoietic maturation and increased numbers of granulocytes, red blood cells and/or platelets in the PB. Splenomegaly and hepatomegaly are common and caused by sequestration of excess blood cells or proliferation of abnormal haematopoietic cells. Despite an insidious onset each MPN has the potential to undergo a

Table 1.02 Myeloproliferative neoplasms (MPN).

Chronic myelogenous leukaemia, BCR-ABL1 positive (CML)
Chronic neutrophilic leukaemia (CNL)
Polycythaemia vera (PV)
Primary myelofibrosis (PMF)
Essential thrombocythaemia (ET)
Chronic eosinophilic leukaemia, NOS (CEL, NOS)
Mastocytosis
Myeloproliferative neoplasm, unclassifiable (MPN,U)

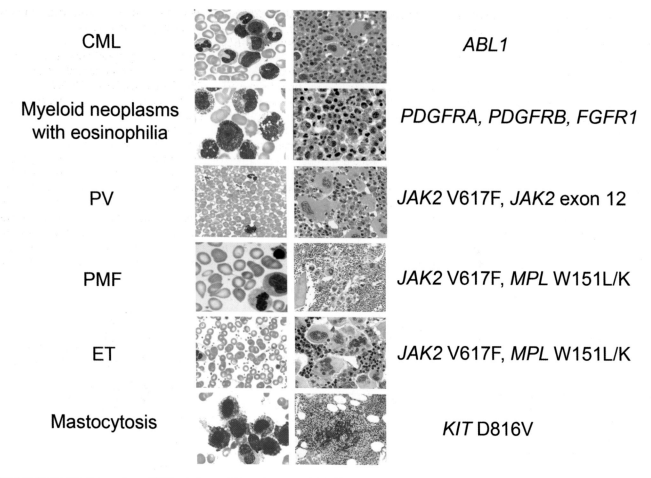

CML			*ABL1*
Myeloid neoplasms with eosinophilia			*PDGFRA, PDGFRB, FGFR1*
PV			*JAK2* V617F, *JAK2* exon 12
PMF			*JAK2* V617F, *MPL* W151L/K
ET			*JAK2* V617F, *MPL* W151L/K
Mastocytosis			*KIT* D816V

Fig. 1.06 Myeloproliferative neoplasms (MPN) and other myeloid neoplasms associated with mutation/rearrangement of tyrosine kinase genes.

stepwise progression that terminates in marrow failure due to myelofibrosis, ineffective haematopoiesis or transformation to an acute blast phase. Evidence of genetic evolution usually heralds disease progression as may increasing organomegaly, increasing or decreasing blood counts, myelofibrosis and onset of myelodysplasia. The finding of 10–19% blasts in the PB or BM generally signifies accelerated disease and 20% or more is sufficient for a diagnosis of blast phase.

Rationale for the diagnosis and classification of MPN

In previous classification schemes the detection of the Philadelphia chromosome and/or *BCR-ABL1* fusion gene was used to confirm the diagnosis of CML whereas the remaining MPN subtypes were diagnosed by their clinical and laboratory features with relatively minor contributions to the diagnosis from morphologic findings. A number of criteria were required not only to distinguish

subtypes of MPN from each other but from reactive granulocytic, erythroid and/ or megakaryocytic hyperplasia.

Revisions in the criteria for classification of MPN in the current scheme have been influenced by two factors —the recent discovery of genetic abnormalities involved in the pathogenesis of *BCR-ABL1* negative MPN and the wider appreciation that histologic features (megakaryocytic morphology and topography, marrow stromal changes, identification of specific cell lineages involved in the proliferation) correlate with clinical features and can be used as criteria to identify MPN subtypes {2177, 2216, 2222}.

Most if not all MPN are associated with clonal abnormalities involving genes that encode cytoplasmic or receptor PTKs. The abnormalities described to date include translocations or point mutations of genes that result in abnormal, constitutively abnormal PTKs that activate signal transduction pathways leading to the abnormal proliferation. In some cases,

these genetic abnormalities, such as the *BCR-ABL1* fusion gene in CML, are associated with consistent clinical, laboratory and morphologic findings that allow them to be utilized as major criteria for classification, whereas others provide proof that the myeloid proliferation is neoplastic rather than reactive.

Acquired somatic mutations of *JAK2*, at chromosome 9p24, have been shown to play a pivotal role in the pathogenesis of many cases of *BCR-ABL1* negative MPN {1044, 1163, 1186, 1287A, 1288}. The most common mutation, *JAK2* V617F, results in a constitutively active cytoplasmic JAK2 that activates signal transducer and activator of transcription (STAT), mitogen activated protein kinase (MAPK) and phosphotidylinositol 3-kinase (PI3K) signaling pathways to promote transformation and proliferation of haematopoietic progenitors (Fig. 1.07). The *JAK2* V617F mutation is found in almost all patients with polycythaemia vera (PV) and in nearly one-half of those with primary myelofibrosis

(PMF) and with essential thrombocythaemia (ET). In the few PV patients who lack the *JAK2* V617F, an activating *JAK2* exon 12 mutation may be found, and in a small proportion of cases of PMF and ET, an activating mutation of *MPL* W515L or W515K is seen. It is important to note that *JAK2* V617F is not specific for any MPN nor does its absence exclude MPN. Furthermore, it has been reported in some cases of MDS/MPN, in rare cases of AML, and in combination with other well-defined genetic abnormalities such as the *BCR-ABL1* {1064}. Thus, diagnostic algorithms for PV, ET and PMF have been altered to take the mutational status of *JAK2* into account as well as to outline the additional laboratory and histologic findings required to reach an accurate classification of cases, regardless of whether the mutation is or is not present.

In addition to the changes in the criteria for PV, ET and PMF, information regarding abnormal PTK function due to rearrangements of the *PDGFRA*, *PDGFRB* or *FGFR1* genes in patients with myeloid neoplasms associated with eosinophilia led to reappraisal and new diagnostic algorithms for those syndromes as well (see below). The appreciation of the role altered PTKs play in the pathogenesis of CML, PV, ET and PMF also argues for the inclusion of similar chronic myeloid proliferations related to PTK abnormalities under the MPN umbrella. Thus, systemic mastocytosis, which has many features in common with other MPN entities and is almost always associated with D816V mutation in the *KIT* gene encoding the receptor PTK, KIT, has been added to this category {2176}. Still, the molecular pathogenesis of nearly half of all cases of ET and PMF, of all cases of chronic neutrophilic leukaemia and a number of myeloid neoplasms associated with eosinophilia remain unknown. For these reliance on clinical, laboratory and morphologic features is essential for diagnosis and classification.

Summary of major changes in the classification of MPN

1. The nomenclature, "myeloproliferative disease" has been changed to "myeloproliferative neoplasm"
2. Mastocytosis has been included in the MPN category
3. Some cases previously meeting the criteria for chronic eosinophilic leukaemia (CEL) may now be categorized as myeloid or lymphoid neoplasms with eosinophilia

and abnormalities of *PDGFRA*, *PDGFRB* or *FGFR1*. If none of these rearrangements are detected, and there is no *BCR-ABL1* fusion gene, they should be categorized as CEL, not otherwise specified.
4. The diagnostic algorithms for PV, ET and PMF have been substantially changed to include information regarding *JAK2* and similar activating mutations as well as pertinent histologic features of the BM biopsy as diagnostic criteria.
5. The threshold of the platelet count for the diagnosis of ET has been lowered to ≥450x10⁹/L.
6. Criteria for CML in accelerated phase have been suggested with the caveat that they have not been fully evaluated in the era of PTKI therapy; studies to determine

their relevance are in progress and revisions may be necessary.

Myeloid and lymphoid neoplasms with eosinophilia and abnormalities of *PDGFRA*, *PDGFRB* or *FGFR1*

Determining the cause of marked, persistent eosinophilia ($\geq 1.5 \times 10^9$/L) in the blood can be challenging and is sometimes clinically urgent because of the potential damage to the heart, lungs, central nervous and other organ systems caused by the eosinophilic infiltration and release of cytokines, enzymes and other proteins. The eosinophils may be derived from the neoplastic clone of a myeloid neoplasm, such as CEL, CML or AML, or they may be reactive due to abnormal

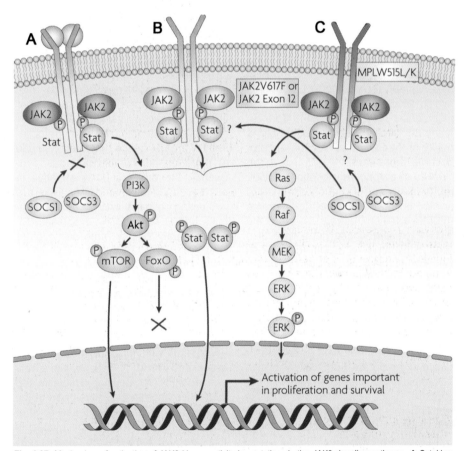

Fig. 1.07 Mechanism of activation of JAK2 kinase activity by mutations in the *JAK2* signaling pathway. **A** Cytokine ligands normally bind cytokine receptors, which results in Janus kinase 2 (JAK2) phosphorylation, recruitment of signal transducer and activator of transcription (Stat) signaling proteins and phosphorylation and activation of downstream signaling pathways including Stat transcription factors, mitogen activated protein kinase (MAPK) signaling proteins, and the phosphotidylinositol 3-kinase (PI3K)–Akt pathway. **B** The *JAK2* V617F and *JAK2* exon 12 mutant kinases bind cytokine receptors, are phosphorylated in the absence of ligand and lead to ligand-independent activation of downstream signaling pathways. **C** By contrast, *MPL* W515L/K mutant thrombopoietin receptors are able to phosphorylate wild-type JAK2 in the absence of thrombopoietin, and result in the activation of signaling pathways downstream of JAK2. Negative regulation of JAK2 signaling is normally mediated by suppressor of cytokine signaling (Socs) proteins, most notably SOCS1 and SOCS3; recent data indicate that the *JAK2* V617F allele might escape negative feedback by SOCS3. Reproduced from {1287A}.

cytokine release from reactive or neoplastic T-cells. In a number of cases, no underlying cause can be found and the clonality of the eosinophils cannot be proven; these cases are appropriately termed "idiopathic hypereosinophilic syndrome" (See Chapters 2 and 3).

Rationale for diagnosis and classification of myeloid and lymphoid disorders with eosinophilia and abnormalities of PDGFRA, PDGFRB or FGFR1

Since the last edition of the WHO classification it has been recognized that many cases of eosinophilia, including a substantial number considered as "idiopathic" are clonal myeloid neoplasms caused by abnormalities in genes that encode the alpha or beta chains of the receptor PTKs, platelet derived growth factor receptor (PDGFR) or fibroblast growth factor receptor 1 (FGFR1). Rearrangements of PDGFRB at chromosome band 5q33 that lead to constitutive activation of the beta moiety of PDGFR were first recognized in cases variably reported as CEL or chronic myelomonocytic leukaemia (CMML) with eosinophilia {131, 812, 2085}. More recently the gene that encodes the alpha moiety of the PDGFR, PDGFRA, at chromosome band 4q12, was found to be involved in cryptic translocations in CEL and in nearly one-half of cases reported as idiopathic hypereosinophilic syndrome {466}. In addition, rearrangements of the FGFR1 tyrosine kinase gene have also been implicated in myeloproliferations with prominent eosinophilia {3, 1354}. However, the clinical and morphologic presentations associated with FGFR1 rearrangement are variable, and include not only presentation as a myeloproliferative neoplasm with eosinophilia, but also as AML and they may even present as, or evolve to, precursor T or B lymphoblastic leukaemia/lymphoma with prominent eosinophils. Cases associated with PDGFRA rearrangements can likewise present as AML or precursor T-cell neoplasms {1469}.

Table 1.03 Myeloid and lymphoid neoplasms with eosinophilia and abnormalities of PDGFRA, PDGFRB, or FGFR1.

| Myeloid and lymphoid neoplasms with PDGFRA rearrangement |
| Myeloid neoplasms with PDGFRB rearrangement |
| Myeloid and lymphoid neoplasms with FGFR1 abnormalities |

Although it might seem most efficient to categorize these cases as CEL within MPN, this would ignore cases with PDGFRB abnormalities that present as CMML as well as cases of FGFR1 and PDGFRA rearrangements that may even have a lymphoid component. To accommodate these translocations, a new subgroup defined largely by the genetic abnormalities of PDGFRA, PDGFRB or FGFR1 has been added (Table 1.03). Detection of one of these abnormalities places the case in this category, regardless of the morphologic classification. Cases of myeloid neoplasms with eosinophilia that lack all of these abnormalities and that meet the criteria for CEL, NOS, in the MPN category should be placed in that group.

Myelodysplastic/myeloproliferative neoplasms (MDS/MPN)

The MDS/MPN (Table 1.04) include clonal myeloid neoplasms that at the time of initial presentation have some clinical, laboratory or morphologic findings that support a diagnosis of MDS, and other findings more consistent with MPN. They are usually characterized by hypercellularity of the BM due to proliferation in one or more of the myeloid lineages. Frequently, the proliferation is effective in some lineages with increased numbers of circulating cells that may be morphologically and/or functionally dysplastic. Simultaneously, one or more of the other lineages may exhibit ineffective proliferation so that cytopenia(s) may be present as well. The blast percentage in the BM and blood is always <20%. Although hepatosplenomegaly is common, the clinical and laboratory findings vary and lie along a continuum between those usually associated with MDS or those usually associated with MPN. Patients with a well-defined MPN who develop dysplasia and ineffective haematopoiesis as part of the natural history of their disease or after chemotherapy should not be placed in this category. Rarely, some patients may present in a transformed stage of an MPN entity in which the chronic phase was not recognized, and may have findings that suggest that they belong to the MDS/MPN group. In such cases, if clinical and laboratory studies fail to reveal the nature of the underlying process, the designation of MDS/MPN, unclassifiable may be appropriate. Patients who have the BCR-ABL1 fusion gene or rearrangements of PDGFRA

Table 1.04 Myelodysplastic/myeloproliferative neoplasms (MDS/MPN).

| Chronic myelomonocytic leukaemia (CMML) |
| Atypical chronic myeloid leukaemia, BCR-ABL1 negative (aCML) |
| Juvenile myelomonocytic leukaemia (JMML) |
| Myelodysplastic/Myeloproliferative neoplasm, unclassifiable (MDS/MPN,U) |
| Provisional entity: Refractory anaemia with ring sideroblasts and thrombocytosis (RARS-T) |

should not be categorized as MDS/MPN, and in contrast to the criteria used in the 3rd edition of the WHO classification, cases of CMML with PDGFRB rearrangements are also excluded.

Rationale for diagnosis and classification of MDS/MPN

This diagnostic category was introduced in the 3rd edition amidst controversy as to whether some entities, particularly CMML, would be better categorized as either MDS or MPN depending on the extent of myeloproliferation as evidenced by the WBC count. Some cases of CMML have low neutrophil counts and only modestly elevated monocyte counts and resemble MDS clinically and morphologically whereas others have markedly elevated WBC counts and organomegaly more in keeping with MPN, yet criteria that clearly distinguish biologically relevant subtypes of CMML remain to be defined.

To date, a few cases of CMML and atypical chronic myeloid leukaemia, BCR-ABL1 negative (aCML) have been reported to demonstrate JAK2 mutations that characterize BCR-ABL1 negative MPN, but the proliferative aspects of most cases of MDS/MPN are related to aberrancies in the RAS/MAPK signaling pathways. In juvenile myelomonocytic leukaemia (JMML) nearly 80% of patients demonstrate mutually exclusive mutations of PTNPN11, NRAS or KRAS, or NF1 {1329, 2096, 2162}, all of which encode signaling proteins in RAS dependent pathways, and approximately 30–40% of cases of CMML and aCML exhibit NRAS mutations {1686, 2311, 2417}. In view of the lack of any specific genetic abnormality to suggest that these entities should be relocated to another myeloid subgroup, they remain in this "mixed" category which acknowledges the overlap that may occur between MDS and MPN. Cases of CMML with eosinophilia associated with PDGFRB rearrangements are excluded, but rare cases of CMML with eosinophilia that do not exhibit such rearrangements should be classified in this category.

The most controversial issue in the subgroup of MDS/MPN is the provisional entity, refractory anaemia with ring sideroblasts and thrombocytosis (RARS-T). The majority (50–60%) of cases of RARS-T studied for *JAK2* V617F carry this mutation {234, 354, 762, 1835, 1839, 1969, 2081, 2139, 2358}. This has prompted the notion that RARS-T should be moved to the MPN group of myeloid neoplasms, whereas others have argued that RARS-T is not an entity at all but merely one of the better recognized MPN entities, such as PMF or ET, in which genetic evolution has led to a dysplastic feature, ring sideroblasts {1966, 2139, 2358}. In a few cases reported, however, the cells of patients with RARS-T, when studied by *in vitro* culture techniques, have growth characteristic more in keeping with MDS than MPN {234, 1835}. An additional question is how to clearly distinguish RARS-T from RARS, in which moderately elevated platelet counts are often reported. This question is more pressing in view of the revised criteria for RARS-T that lowers the platelet threshold from 600x10⁹/L to 450x10⁹/L, in parallel with the revised threshold for ET. It is important to note that the diagnostic criteria for RARS-T include not only the finding of an elevated platelet count in conjunction with anaemia and ring sideroblasts in the BM, but also morphologically abnormal megakaryocytes similar to those of ET or PMF. Only a few patients with RARS and platelet counts in the 450-500x10⁹/L range have been studied for *JAK2* mutations and in most with platelet counts in the lower ranges no mutations have been found. Nevertheless, more studies are needed, and we recommend to test for *JAK2* mutations in patients who have RARS and platelet counts above the normal range. The sum of current information regarding RARS-T argues for its continued placement in the MDS/MPN category, but in view of the debate regarding its precise definition and nature, it is best regarded as a "provisional entity" until more data are available.

Lastly, classification of myeloid neoplasms that carry an isolated isochromosome 17q and that have less than 20% blasts in the PB or BM may prove difficult. Some authors suggest this cytogenetic defect defines a unique disorder characterized by mixed MDS and MPN features associated with prominent pseudo-Pelger-Huët anomaly of the neutrophils, low BM blast count, and a rapidly progressive clinical course. Most cases reported have a prominent monocytic component and meet the criteria for CMML, but in some, the PB monocyte count may not reach the lower threshold for that diagnosis {708, 1437}. In cases that do not fulfill the criteria for CMML or another well defined myeloid category, designation as MDS/MPN, unclassifiable, with isolated isochromosome 17q abnormality, is most appropriate.

Summary of major changes in MDS/MPN

1. Some cases of CMML with eosinophilia are relocated to the category, "Myeloid neoplasms with *PDGFRB* rearrangement"
2. The category, "Atypical CML" has been renamed as "Atypical CML, *BCR-ABL1* negative" to emphasize this disease is not merely a variant of *BCR-ABL1* positive CML.
3. RARS-T remains as a provisional entity, classified as MDS/MPN, unclassifiable, until further data clarifies its appropriate designation. The criteria for its recognition have been modified. The platelet threshold has been lowered to ≥450x10⁹/L, and megakaryocytes with morphology similar to those seen in ET or PMF must be present.

Myelodysplastic syndromes (MDS)

These disorders, usually characterized by the simultaneous proliferation and apoptosis of haematopoietic cells that lead to a normal or hypercellular BM biopsy and PB cytopenia(s), remain among the most challenging of the myeloid neoplasms for proper diagnosis and classification. The general features of MDS, as well as specific guidelines for diagnosis and classification are outlined in Chapter 5.

An important addition to the MDS category (Table 1.05) is the provisional entity, refractory cytopenia of childhood (RCC). This category is reserved for children with MDS who have <2% blasts in their PB and <5% in their BM and persistent cytopenia(s) with dysplasia. In contrast to MDS with refractory cytopenias in adults, the majority of cases of RCC have hypocellular BM biopsy specimens, and the distinction from acquired aplastic anaemia and inherited BM failure syndromes is often challenging {1784}.

An issue appropriate to mention at this point is the criteria used for classification of myeloid neoplasms in which 50% or more of the BM cells are erythroid precursors, and for which acute erythroid leukaemia is considered a possible diagnosis. In such cases, if blasts account for fewer than 20% of WBC in the PB and of all nucleated BM cells, and for less than 20% of the non-erythroid cells in the BM (lymphocytes, plasma cells, etc. are also excluded in this latter calculation), the case is considered as MDS. In this scenario, there is lack of consensus among members of the WHO committee as to whether the MDS should then be classified according to the blast percentage of all nucleated BM cells or according to the blast percentage of all non-erythroid BM cells, but the majority recommends that the MDS be classified using the blast percentage of all marrow nucleated cells. Many cases of refractory anaemia with ring sideroblasts as well as refractory anaemia have marked erythroid proliferation and using the blast percentage of the non-erythroid cells for classification of such cases might cause these to be placed in an unnecessarily high-risk category. On the other hand, if there is severe multilineage dysplasia, very bizarre erythroid morphology, and/or minimal or no maturation to segmented neutrophils, and the blast percentage of total BM cells is not sufficient to place the case into a high-grade MDS category, the case should be flagged for clinical correlation and discussion, with careful follow-up (Table 1.06). More studies are needed however to clarify this controversial issue.

Acute myeloid leukaemia (AML)

AML is a disease resulting from the clonal expansion of myeloid blasts in the PB, BM, or other tissue. It is a heterogeneous disease clinically, morphologically and genetically and may involve only one or

Table 1.05 Myelodysplastic syndromes.

Refractory cytopenia with unilineage dysplasia (RCUD)
    Refractory anaemia (RA)
    Refractory neutropenia (RN)
    Refractory thrombocytopenia (RT)
Refractory anaemia with ring sideroblasts (RARS)
Refractory cytopenia with multilineage dysplasia (RCMD)
Refractory anaemia with excess blasts (RAEB)
Myelodysplastic syndrome with isolated del(5q)
Myelodysplastic syndrome, unclassifiable (MDS,U)
Childhood myelodysplastic syndrome
    Provisional entity: Refractory cytopenia of childhood (RCC)

Table 1.06 Possible diagnoses when erythroid precursors ≥50% of bone marrow nucleated cells.

% Erythroid precursors in bone marrow	Blood/marrow findings	Other findings	Diagnosis
≥50%	≥20% blasts in blood or of all nucleated marrow cells	Case meets criteria for AML with myelodysplasia-related changes	AML with myelodysplasia related changes
≥80% immature erythroid precursors with minimal maturation	Few if any myeloblasts	Minimal if any granulocytic component	Pure erythroid leukaemia
≥50%	<20% blasts in blood; blasts <20% of all nucleated marrow cells	Blasts ≥20% of all non-erythroid* cells in bone marrow	Acute erythroid/myeloid leukaemia
≥50%	<20% blasts in blood, blasts <20% of all nucleated marrow cells	Blasts <20% of all non-erythroid* cells in bone marrow	MDS; classify MDS according to number of blasts in blood and blasts as percentage of all nucleated marrow cells

* Erythroid precursors, lymphoid cells and plasma cells are subtracted from all nucleated marrow cells to calculate the "non-erythroid cells" in the bone marrow.

all myeloid lineages. Worldwide the incidence is approximately 2.5–3 cases per 100,000 population per year, and is reportedly highest in Australia, Western Europe and the United States. The median age at diagnosis is 65 years, with a slight male predominance in most countries. In children less than 15 years of age, AML comprises 15–20% of all cases of acute leukaemia, with a peak incidence in the first 3–4 years of life {559A, 2463A}.

The requisite blast percentage for a diagnosis of AML is 20% or more myeloblasts and/or monoblasts/promonocytes and/or megakaryoblasts in the PB or BM. The diagnosis of myeloid sarcoma is synonymous with AML regardless of the number of blasts in the PB or BM, unless the patient has a prior history of MPN or MDS/MPN, in which case myeloid sarcoma is evidence of acute transformation. The diagnosis of AML can also be made when the blast percentage in the PB and/or BM is less than 20% if there is an associated t(8;21)(q22;q22), inv(16)(p13.1q22), t(16;16)(p13.1;q22) or t(15;17)(q22;q12) chromosomal abnormality, and in some cases of acute erythroid leukaemia when erythroid precursors account for 50% or more of the BM cells and blasts account for 20% or more of the non-erythroid marrow cells (See Chapter on acute myeloid leukaemia, NOS).

Although the diagnosis of AML using the above guidelines is operationally useful to indicate an underlying defect in myeloid maturation, the diagnosis does not necessarily translate into a mandate to treat the patient for AML; clinical factors, including the pace of progression of the disease, must always be taken into consideration when deciding therapy.

Rationale for the WHO diagnosis and classification of AML

The 3rd edition of the WHO classification ushered in the era of formal incorporation of genetic abnormalities in the diagnostic algorithms for the diagnosis of AML. The abnormalities included were mainly chromosomal translocations involving transcription factors and associated with characteristic clinical, morphologic and immunophenotypic features that formed a "clinico-pathologic-genetic" entity. As knowledge regarding leukaemogenesis has increased, so has the acceptance that the genetic abnormalities leading to leukaemia are not only heterogeneous, but complex, and multiple aberrations often cooperate in a multistep process to initiate the complete leukaemia phenotype. Experimental evidence suggests that in many cases, although rearrangement of genes such as RUNX1, CBFB or RARA that encode transcription factors impair myeloid differentiation, a second genetic abnormality is necessary to promote proliferation or survival of the neoplastic clone (Fig. 1.08) {1135A}. Often, the additional abnormalities are mutations of genes such as FLT3 or KIT that encode proteins that activate signal transduction pathways to promote proliferation/survival. A similar multistep process is also evident in AML that evolves from MDS or that has myelodysplasia-related features, often characterized by loss of genetic material and haploinsufficiency of genes. Within the last few years, genetic mutations have also been identified in cytogenetically normal AML {1532}. Some of the mutations, such as those of CEBPA and perhaps NPM1 involve transcription factors, whereas others, including those of FLT3 and NRAS/KRAS, affect signal transduction. Not only have these mutations led to an understanding of leukaemogenesis in cytogenetically normal AML, but they have proved to be powerful prognostic factors {1532}. In summary, genetic abnormalities in AML elucidate the pathogenesis of the neoplasm, provide the most reliable prognostic information, and will likely lead to development of more successful targeted therapy.

One of the challenges in this revision has been how to incorporate important and/or recently acquired genetic information into a classification scheme of AML and yet adhere to the WHO principle of defining homogeneous, biologically relevant entities based not only on genetic studies or their prognostic value, but also on clinical, morphologic and/or immunophenotypic studies. This was particularly problematic for the most frequent and prognostically important mutations in cytogenetically normal AML, mutated FLT3, NPM1 and CEBPA. They have few or variably consistent morphologic, immunophenotypic and clinical features reported to date, and the mutations are not mutually exclusive. For the most part, the framework constructed in the 3rd edition proved flexible enough to incorporate the new entities proposed by members of the WHO committee and the CAC (Table 1.07). The entities initially described in the subgroup "AML with recurring genetic abnormalities" remain with only minor modifications (Table 1.07) and three more entities, characterized by chromosomal translocations associated with fairly uniform morphological and clinical features have been added. Cases with mutated NPM1 and CEBPA are added to the same subgroup as "provisional entities" indicating that more study is needed to fully characterize and establish them as unique entities. Although mutated FLT3 is not included as a separate entity because it is found to be associated with a number of other entities,

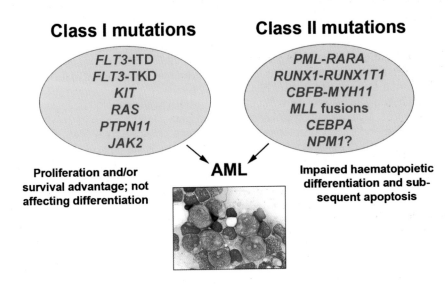

<table>
<tr><td>**Class I mutations**</td><td>**Class II mutations**</td></tr>
</table>

Class I mutations	Class II mutations
FLT3-ITD FLT3-TKD KIT RAS PTPN11 JAK2	PML-RARA RUNX1-RUNX1T1 CBFB-MYH11 MLL fusions CEBPA NPM1?
Proliferation and/or survival advantage; not affecting differentiation	**Impaired haematopoietic differentiation and subsequent apoptosis**

AML

Fig. 1.08 Cooperation between mutations in AML pathogenesis. Modified from {1135A}.

its significance should not be underestimated, and it is essential that it be tested for in all cytogenetically normal patients, including those who demonstrate *NPM1* and *CEBPA* mutations.

Modifications have been made in the subgroup previously termed "AML with multilineage dysplasia." Initially, it was envisioned that this group would encompass biologically unique AML characterized by MDS-like features, including unfavourable cytogenetics, a higher incidence of overexpression of multidrug resistance glycoprotein (ABCB1 or MDR-1) and an unfavourable response to therapy. Dysplasia in ≥50% of cells in two or more haematopoietic lineages was used as a universally-applicable surrogate marker for the myelodysplasia-related features. Although the clinical significance of this group has been verified in some studies, it has been disputed in others in which multivariate analysis showed that multilineage dysplasia had no independent significance in predicting clinical outcome when cytogenetic findings were incorporated in the analysis {69, 869, 2356, 2465}. Accordingly, in this revision, this group has been renamed as "AML with myelodysplasia-related changes." Patients may be assigned to this category if they evolve from previously documented MDS, have specific myelodysplasia-related cytogenetic abnormalities, or lastly, if they exhibit morphologic multilineage dysplasia as defined above. Patients in this latter group with a normal karyotype

should be evaluated for *FLT3*, *NPM1* and *CEBPA* mutations. Currently, however, the clinical significance of a mutation of one or more of these genes in the setting of morphologic multilineage dysplasia is not clear. Future studies may well prove that such cases are better classified according to their genetic abnormalities, but until more data are available, we recommend that such cases be classified as AML with myelodysplasia-related changes (multilineage dysplasia) with the mutational status of the gene appended.

Therapy-related myeloid neoplasms (t-AML/t-MDS and t-AML/t-MDS/MPN) remain in the revised classification as a distinct subgroup. However, most patients who develop therapy-related neoplasms have received therapy with both alkylating agents as well as with topoisomerase II inhibitors, so that a division according to the type of therapy is usually not practical and not recommended in this revision. It has been argued that 90% or more of cases with t-AML/t-MDS or t-AML/t-MDS/MPN have cytogenetic abnormalities similar to those seen in AML with recurrent genetic abnormalities or AML with myelodysplasia-related features and could be assigned to those categories. However, except for patients with t-AML who have inv(16)(p13.1q22), t(16;16)(p13.1;q22) or t(15;17)(q22;q12), in most reported series those with therapy-related myeloid neoplasms have a significantly worse clinical outcome than their *de novo* counterparts with the same genetic abnormalities {36,

Table 1.07 Acute myeloid leukaemia and related myeloid neoplasms.

Acute myeloid leukaemia with recurrent genetic abnormalities
    AML with t(8;21)(q22;q22); *RUNX1-RUNX1T1*
    AML with inv(16)(p13.1q22) or t(16;16)(p13.1;q22); *CBFB-MYH11*
    APL with t(15;17)(q22;q12); *PML-RARA*
    AML with t(9;11)(p22;q23); *MLLT3-MLL*
    AML with t(6;9)(p23;q34); *DEK-NUP214*
    AML with inv(3)(q21q26.2) or t(3;3)(q21;q26.2); *RPN1-EVI1*
    AML (megakaryoblastic) with t(1;22)(p13;q13); *RBM15-MKL1*
    Provisional entity: AML with mutated *NPM1*
    Provisional entity: AML with mutated *CEBPA*
Acute myeloid leukaemia with myelodysplasia-related changes
Therapy-related myeloid neoplasms
Acute myeloid leukaemia, not otherwise specified
    AML with minimal differentiation
    AML without maturation
    AML with maturation
    Acute myelomonocytic leukaemia
    Acute monoblastic/monocytic leukaemia
    Acute erythroid leukaemias
        Pure erythroid leukaemia
        Erythroleukaemia, erythroid/myeloid
    Acute megakaryoblastic leukaemia
    Acute basophilic leukaemia
    Acute panmyelosis with myelofibrosis
Myeloid sarcoma
Myeloid proliferations related to Down syndrome
    Transient abnormal myelopoiesis
    Myeloid leukaemia associated with Down syndrome
Blastic plasmacytoid dendritic cell neoplasms

227, 1886, 2034, 2041}, suggesting some biological differences between the two groups. Furthermore, the study of therapy-related neoplasms may provide valuable insight into the pathogenesis of *de novo* disease by providing clues as to why a few patients develop leukaemia whereas most patients treated with the same therapy do not. Therefore, patients with therapy-related neoplasms should be designated as such, but the specific cytogenetic abnormality should also be listed, for example, "therapy-related AML with t(9;11)(p22;q23)".

Acute myeloid leukaemia, not otherwise specified, encompasses those cases that do not fulfil the specific criteria of any of the other entities. This group accounts for only 25–30% of all AML that are not assigned to one of the more specific categories. As more genetic subgroups are identified, the number of patients that fall into the AML, NOS categories will continue to diminish. Of note is that information used to characterize the subgroups within this category, such as epidemiologic or clinical outcome, is often based on older studies that included patients now assigned to different diagnostic categories, and may not be reliable. Although the proposal to collapse this category into fewer subgroups has been made, the notion that some of these may yet be found to be associated with specific genetic or biologic abnormalities argued to maintain this category.

Myeloid sarcoma, an extramedullary tumour mass consisting of myeloid blasts, is included in the classification as a distinct pathologic entity. However, when myeloid sarcoma occurs *de novo*, the diagnosis is equivalent to a diagnosis of AML, and further evaluation, including genetic analysis, is necessary to determine the appropriate classification of the leukaemia {1742}. When the PB and BM is concurrently involved by AML, these tissues may be used for analysis and further

classification. However, when the myeloid sarcoma precedes evidence of PB or BM involvement, the immunophenotype should be ascertained by flow cytometry and/or immunohistochemistry, and the genotype determined by cytogenetic analysis, or in the absence of fresh tissue, by FISH or molecular analysis for recurrent genetic abnormalities. Myeloid sarcoma may also be the initial indication of relapse in a patient previously diagnosed with AML, or may indicate disease progression to a blast phase in patients with a prior diagnosis of MDS, MDS/MPN or MPN.

Lastly, the unique features of Down syndrome-related myeloid neoplasms has been recognized in a separate listing that includes transient abnormal myelopoiesis and myeloid leukaemias (MDS/AML) associated with Down syndrome.

Summary of major changes in AML

1. AML with recurrent genetic abnormalities.

a) AML with t(8;21)(q22;q22), AML with inv(16)(p13.1q22) or t(16;16)(p13.1;q22), and APL with t(15;17)(q22;q12) are considered as AML regardless of blast count; for all others, blasts ≥20% of PB or of all nucleated BM cells are required.

b) In APL with t(15;17)(q22;q12); *PML-RARA*, variant *RARA* translocations with other partner genes are recognized separately; not all have typical APL features and some have ATRA resistance.

c) The former category, AML with 11q23 (*MLL*) abnormalities has been re-defined as "AML with t(9;11)(p22;q23); *MLLT3-MLL*". Balanced translocations other than that involving *MLLT3* should be specified in the diagnosis. Other abnormalities of *MLL*, such as partial tandem duplication of *MLL* should not be placed in this category.

d) Three new cytogenetically defined entities are added: AML with t(6;9)(p23;q23); *DEK-NUP214*, AML with inv(3)(q21q26.2) or t(3;3)(q21;q26.2); *RPN1-EVI1*; and AML (megakaryoblastic) with t(1;22)(p13;q13); *RBM15-MKL1*.

e) Two provisional entities are added: AML with mutated *NPM1* and AML with mutated *CEBPA*. Although not included as a distinct entity, examination for mutations of *FLT3* is strongly recommended in all cytogenetically normal AML.

2. AML with myelodysplasia-related changes.

a) Name changed from "AML with multilineage dysplasia".

b) Cases of AML are assigned to this category if 1) they have a previous history of MDS and have evolved to AML, 2) they have a myelodysplasia-related cytogenetic abnormality, or 3) if ≥50% of cells in two or more myeloid lineages are dysplastic.

3. Therapy-related myeloid neoplasms. Cases are no longer subcategorized as "alkylating agent related" or "topoisomerase II-inhibitor related" or "other".

4. AML, NOS.

a) Some cases previously assigned to the subcategory of AML, NOS as acute erythroid leukaemia may be re-classified as AML with myelodysplasia-related changes.

b) Cases previously categorized as AML, NOS, acute megakaryoblastic leukaemia should be placed in the appropriate genetic category if they are associated with inv(3)(q21q26.2) or t(3;3)(q21;q26.2); *RPN1-EVI1*, or AML (megakaryoblastic) with t(1;22)(p13;q13); *RBM15-MKL1*. Down syndrome related cases are excluded from this category as well.

5. Myeloid proliferations related to Down syndrome.

New category to incorporate transient abnormal myelopoiesis as well as myeloid leukaemia that is Down syndrome related. MDS related to Down syndrome is considered biologically identical to AML related to Down syndrome.

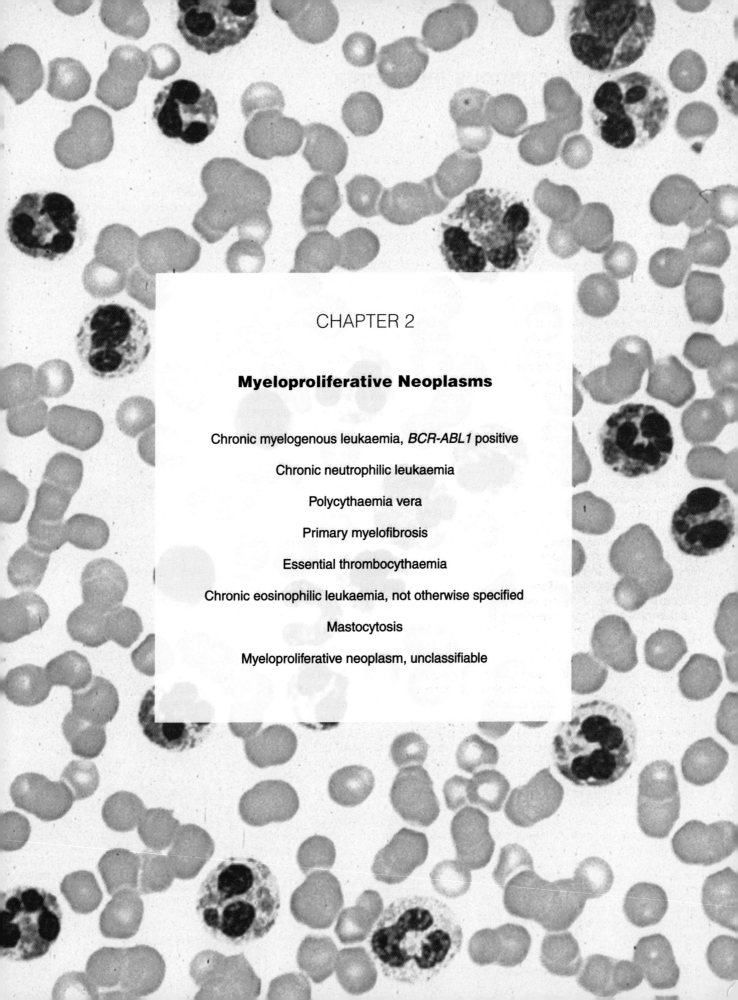

CHAPTER 2

Myeloproliferative Neoplasms

Chronic myelogenous leukaemia, *BCR-ABL1* positive

Chronic neutrophilic leukaemia

Polycythaemia vera

Primary myelofibrosis

Essential thrombocythaemia

Chronic eosinophilic leukaemia, not otherwise specified

Mastocytosis

Myeloproliferative neoplasm, unclassifiable

Chronic myelogenous leukaemia, BCR-ABL1 positive

J.W. Vardiman
J.V. Melo
M. Baccarani
J. Thiele

Definition

Chronic myelogenous leukaemia (CML) is a myeloproliferative neoplasm that originates in an abnormal pluripotent bone marrow (BM) stem cell and is consistently associated with the BCR-ABL1 fusion gene located in the Philadelphia (Ph) chromosome {154, 1455, 1607, 1884}. Although the initial major finding is neutrophilic leukocytosis, the BCR-ABL1 is found in all myeloid lineages as well as in some lymphoid cells and endothelial cells. The natural history of untreated CML is bi- or triphasic: an initial indolent chronic phase (CP) is followed by an accelerated phase (AP), a blast phase (BP) or both.

ICD-O code   9875/3

Synonyms

Chronic granulocytic leukaemia; chronic myeloid leukaemia.

Epidemiology

CML has a worldwide annual incidence of 1–2 cases per 100,000 population. The disease can occur at any age, but the median age at diagnosis is in the 5th and 6th decades of life. There is a slight male predominance {755, 1053, 1826}.

Etiology

Factors predisposing to CML are unknown. Radiation exposure has been implicated in some cases {226, 479}. There does not appear to be an inherited disposition.

Sites of involvement

In CP, the leukaemic cells are minimally invasive and the proliferation is largely confined to haemopoietic tissues, primarily blood, BM and spleen although the liver may be infiltrated as well. In BP, extramedullary tissues, including lymph nodes, skin and soft tissues may show infiltration by blasts {486, 1029, 1534}.

Clinical features

Most patients are diagnosed in CP which usually has an insidious onset. Nearly 20–40% of patients are asymptomatic and are diagnosed when a white blood cell (WBC) count performed at the time of a routine medical examination is found to be abnormal {486, 755, 1942}. Common findings at presentation include fatigue, weight loss, night sweats, splenomegaly and anaemia {486, 1942}. Atypical presentations include marked thrombocytosis unaccompanied by a significantly elevated WBC count as well as initial presentation in BP without a previously detectable CP {34, 486, 1730}. In the absence of curative treatment most patients progress from CP to BP either suddenly or through a transitional AP, although some die in AP without progression. The transformed phases are generally accompanied by worsened performance status and by symptoms related to severe anaemia, thrombocytopenia or marked splenic enlargement {755}.

Morphology

Chronic phase (CP)

In CP the peripheral blood (PB) shows leukocytosis ($12–1000 \times 10^9$/L, median $\sim 100 \times 10^9$/L) due to neutrophils in different stages of maturation with peaks in the percent of myelocytes and segmented neutrophils {486, 755, 1164, 1942, 2067}. There is no significant dysplasia {189, 2458}. Blasts usually account for less than 2% of the WBC {189, 2067}. Absolute basophilia is invariably present and eosinophilia is common {2067}. Absolute monocytosis may be present but the fraction of monocytes is usually <3% {189}, except in rare cases associated with the p190 BCR-ABL1 isoform, in which case monocytosis is nearly always present and confusion with chronic myelomonocytic leukaemia is possible {1458}. The platelet count usually ranges from normal to greater than 1000×10^9/L and thrombocytopenia is uncommon {1942}. The BM cellularity is increased due to granulocytic proliferation with a maturation pattern similar to that in the blood {486, 1534}. In biopsy sections the paratrabecular cuff of immature neutrophils is often 5–10 cells thick in contrast to the normal 2–3 cell layer and the mature neutrophils are situated in the intertrabecular areas. Eosinophils may be prominent. Blasts usually account for less than 5% of the marrow cells in CP and 10% or more indicates disease progression {482}. Erythroid precursors vary but erythroid islands are usually reduced in number and size {2221}. The megakaryocytes of CML are smaller than normal and have hypolobated nuclei ("dwarf megakaryocytes"). Although they may be normal or slightly decreased in number, 40–50% of patients exhibit moderate to extensive megakaryocytic proliferation {296, 775, 2215, 2221}. The initial biopsy

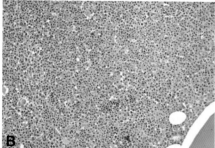

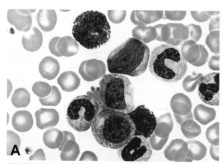

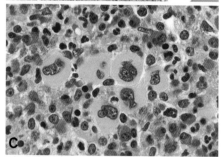

Fig. 2.01 CML, chronic phase. A Peripheral blood smear showing leukocytosis and neutrophilic cells at varying stages of maturation. Basophilia is prominent. No dysplasia is present. B Bone marrow biopsy shows marked hypercellularity due to granulocytic proliferation. C The megakaryocytes in CML are characteristically smaller than normal megakaryocytes.

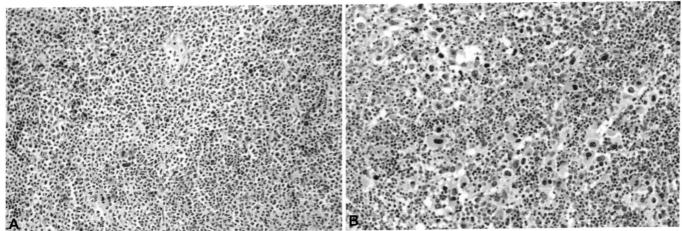

Fig. 2.02 CML chronic phase. There is some variability in the initial bone marrow biopsy of patients with CML. Some authorities {775B} have used the variation in the numbers of megakaryocytes and presence of fibrosis (see Fig. 2.03) as the basis for a histologic classification of CML. **A** Marrow specimen in which granulocytes predominate and megakaryocytes are sparse ("granulocyte rich"). **B** A case with numerous megakaryocytes ("megakaryocyte-rich").

shows moderate to marked reticulin fibrosis in approximately 30% of cases which often correlates with increased numbers of megakaryocytes, larger spleen size and reportedly, a worse prognosis {293, 540, 1217, 2215, 2221}. Pseudo-Gaucher cells and sea-blue histiocytes are commonly observed secondary to increased cell turnover and are derived from the neoplastic clone {35, 2227}. More than 80% of patients have significantly reduced or no iron-laden macrophages {2045}.

In CP the spleen is enlarged due to infiltration of the red pulp cords by granulocytes in different maturation stages. A similar infiltrate may be seen in the hepatic sinusoids and portal areas.

Disease progression/transformed phases in CML

The recognition of disease progression from CP to the transformed stages of AP and BP is important for prognosis and treatment, but the clinical and morphologic boundaries between these stages often overlap and the parameters used to identify them have varied among different investigators {118, 293, 481, 482, 829, 1100, 1941}. Furthermore, there are only scant data relevant to disease progression in the era of protein kinase inhibitor (PTKI) therapy. Bone marrow changes following short and long term PTKI treatment have been extensively studied showing a reduction of granulocytic cellularity, normalization of megakaryopoiesis, regression of fibrosis and increase in apoptosis associated with decrease in proliferative activity {2219}.

Accelerated phase (AP)

In the 3rd edition of the WHO Classification {1039}, it was suggested that the diagnosis of AP could be made if any of the following parameters were present: 1) persistent or increasing WBC ($>10 \times 10^9$/L) and/or persistent or increasing splenomegaly unresponsive to therapy, 2) persistent thrombocytosis ($>1000 \times 10^9$/L) uncontrolled by therapy, 3) persistent thrombocytopenia ($<100 \times 10^9$/L) unrelated to therapy, 4) clonal cytogenetic evolution occurring after the initial diagnostic karyotype, 5) 20% or more basophils in the peripheral blood, and 6) 10–19% myeloblasts in the blood or BM. Criteria 1–4 are more likely to be associated with transition from CP to AP, whereas criteria 5 and 6 more frequently indicate a transition between AP and BP. Although modifications to

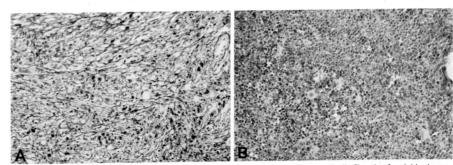

Fig. 2.03 CML, chronic phase. **A** Reticulin stain. Up to 30% of patients may have reticulin fibrosis of variable degree at presentation. **B** The granulocytic proliferation is highlighted by the naphthol-ASD-chloroacetate esterase stain on the biopsy section.

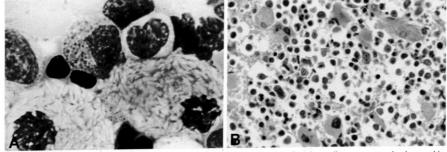

Fig. 2.04 CML, chronic phase. "Pseudo-Gaucher" cells in CML. **A** Pseudo-Gaucher cells are commonly observed in the marrow aspirates of patients with CML. **B** They may also be appreciated as foamy or striated cells in marrow biopsy sections. These histiocytes are secondary to increased cell turnover, are derived from the neoplastic clone and easily distinguishable from the small megakaryocytes (lower margin).

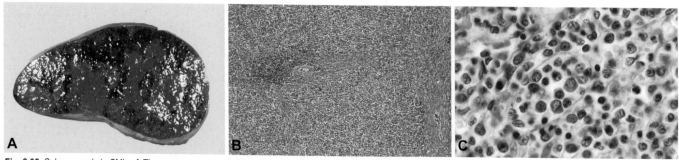

Fig. 2.05 Splenomegaly in CML. **A** The gross appearance of the spleen is solid and uniformly deep red, although areas of infarct may appear as lighter coloured regions. **B** The red pulp distribution of the infiltrate usually compresses and obliterates the white pulp. **C** The leukaemic cells are present in the sinuses as well as in the splenic cords of the red pulp.

these criteria have been suggested and different criteria proposed by others {482}, it is recommended that the parameters listed above still be considered as evidence of disease progression. Whether they or other parameters, such as drug resistance, necessarily indicate shortened survival times or imminent blast transformation is not clear in view of the efficacy of current treatment strategies, and more studies are needed to accurately identify criteria for AP in the face of PTKI therapy. Often in AP the BM is hypercellular and myelodysplasia is seen {1534, 2458}. The increase in myeloid lineage blasts may be readily appreciated with stains for CD34 performed on the biopsy {1650}. Large clusters or sheets of small, abnormal megakaryocytes associated with marked reticulin or collagen fibrosis are commonly

observed and may be considered as presumptive evidence of AP, although these findings are almost always associated with one or more of the other criteria listed above {289, 293, 1534}. The finding of lymphoblasts in the blood or marrow is unusual in AP and should raise concern for lymphoblastic BP {557}.

Blast phase (BP)

The BP may be diagnosed when 1) blasts equal or are greater than 20% of the PB WBC or of the nucleated cells of the BM, or 2) when there is an extramedullary blast proliferation. In approximately 70% of cases, the blast lineage is myeloid and may include neutrophilic, eosinophilic, basophilic, monocytic, megakaryocytic or erythroid blasts or any combination thereof, whereas in approximately 20–30% of

cases the blasts are lymphoblasts {557, 1138, 1558, 1706, 1913, 2454}. In BP the blast lineage may be obvious morphologically but often the blasts are primitive or heterogeneous and cytochemical and immunophenotypic analysis is recommended.

If accumulations of blasts occupy focal but significant areas of the BM, e.g. an entire intertrabecular region, a presumptive diagnosis of BP is warranted, even if the remainder of the BM biopsy shows CP {289}. Immunohistochemical studies for CD34 and/or terminal deoxynucleotidyl transferase (TdT) may help in distinguishing such foci of blasts in BP from the foci of promyelocytes and myelocytes that often are prominent in paratrabecular and perivascular regions during CP. Extramedullary blast proliferations most

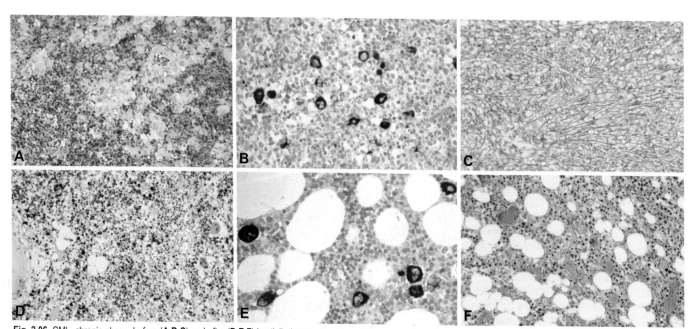

Fig. 2.06 CML, chronic phase, before (**A,B,C**) and after (**D,E,F**) imatinib therapy. Naphthol-ASD-chloroacetate esterase stain of the pre-therapy bone marrow which highlights the granulocytic component (**A**). Dwarf megakaryocytes typical of CML are stained with CD61 (**B**). The silver stain illustrates an increase in the reticulin fibres (**C**). The corresponding stains after 6 months of imatinib therapy (**D, E, F**).

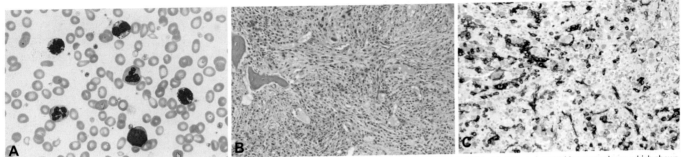

Fig. 2.07 CML, accelerated phase. **A** Peripheral blood smear. Basopils accounted for nearly 30% of the WBC, with occasional blasts. **B** Bone marrow biopsy specimen, which shows area of cellular depletion and prominence of small megakaryocytes. **C** A substantial increase in blasts is well-appreciated with CD34.

commonly present in the skin, lymph node, spleen, bone or central nervous system, but can occur anywhere, and may be of myeloid or lymphoid lineage {1029}.

Immunophenotype

The neutrophils in CP have markedly decreased neutrophil alkaline phosphatase {1640}. In myeloid BP the blasts may have strong, weak or no myeloperoxidase activity but express antigens associated with granulocytic, monocytic, megakaryo-blastic and/or erythroid differentiation. In the majority of cases the myeloid blasts will express one or more lymphoid antigens as well {557, 1138, 1558, 1913}. Most cases of lymphoblastic BP are precursor B in origin but cases of T lymphoblastic origin also occur {1138, 1558, 1913}. In lymphoblastic BP, one or more myeloid antigens are co-expressed on the lymphoblasts in the majority of cases. Approximately 25% of BP cases fulfill criteria for mixed phenotype acute leukaemia (MPAL) {557, 1138, 1558, 1913}, but these are considered as examples of BP and are different from *de novo* MPAL.

Genetics

At diagnosis, 90–95% of cases of CML have the characteristic t(9;22)(q34;q11.2) reciprocal translocation that results in the Ph chromosome [der (22q)] {1607, 1884}. This translocation fuses sequences of the *BCR* gene on chromosome 22 with regions of the *ABL1* gene from chromosome 9 {154}. The remaining cases either have variant translocations that involve a third or even a fourth chromosome in addition to chromosomes 9 and 22, or have a cryptic translocation of 9q34 and 22q11.2 that cannot be identified by routine cytogenetic analysis. In such cases, the *BCR-ABL1* fusion gene is present and can be detected by FISH analysis, RT-PCR or Southern blot techniques {1454}. The

site of the breakpoint in the *BCR* gene may influence the phenotype of the disease {1454}. In CML, the breakpoint in *BCR* is almost always in the major breakpoint cluster region M-BCR, spanning exons 12-16, (previously known as b1-b5) and an abnormal fusion protein, p210, is formed which has increased tyrosine kinase activity {1454}. Rarely, the breakpoint in the *BCR* gene occurs in the µ-BCR region, spanning exons 17-20 (previously known as c1-c4) and a larger fusion protein, p230, is encoded. Patients with this fusion may demonstrate prominent neutrophilic maturation and/or conspicuous thrombocytosis {1454, 1685}. Although breaks in the minor breakpoint region, m-BCR (*BCR* exons 1-2) leads to a shorter fusion protein (p190) and is most frequently associated with Ph positive

ALL, small amounts of the p190 transcript can be detected in >90% of patients with classical p210 CML as well, due to alternative splicing of the *BCR* gene {1907, 2306}. However, this breakpoint may also be seen in rare cases of CML that are distinctive for having increased numbers of monocytes and thus can resemble chronic myelomonocytic leukaemia {1458}.

The enhanced tyrosine kinase activity of BCR-ABL1 is responsible for constitutive activation of several signal transduction pathways {539}. This results in the leukaemic phenotype of CML cells which encompasses deregulated proliferation, reduced adherence to the BM stroma and defective apoptotic response to mutagenic stimuli. The understanding of the abnormal signaling in CML cells led to the design and synthesis of small

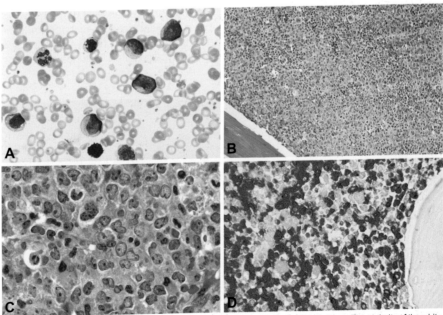

Fig. 2.08 CML, myeloid blast phase. **A** Peripheral blood of a patient with myeloid blast phase. The majority of the white blood cells are blasts. **B,C** Sheets of myeloblasts in the bone marrow biopsy. **D** Myeloperoxidase detected immunohistochemically, proving the myeloid lineage of the blast proliferation.

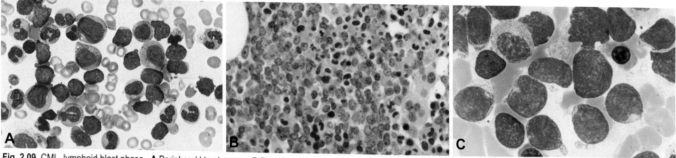

Fig. 2.09 CML, lymphoid blast phase. **A** Peripheral blood smear. **B** Bone marrow biopsy. **C** Marrow aspirate smear.

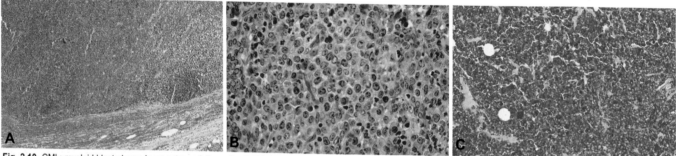

Fig. 2.10 CML, myeloid blast phase, in an extramedullary site. **A,B** Lymph node biopsy obtained from a patient with a history of CML for 3 years. The lymph node architecture is largely effaced by a proliferation of medium to large sized cells. **C** Lysozyme immunohistochemistry confirms the myeloid lineage of the blasts.

molecules that target the tyrosine kinase activity of BCR-ABL1, of which imatinib was the first to be successfully used to treat CML {616, 617}. Imatinib competes with ATP for binding to the BCR-ABL1 kinase domain thus preventing phosphorylation of tyrosine residues on its substrates. Interruption of the oncogenic signal in this way is very effective for control of the disease, particularly when used early in CP. However, the emergence of sub-clones of leukaemic progenitor cells with point mutations that prevent the binding of the inhibitor to the kinase domain of BCR-ABL1 can lead to drug resistance, particularly in AP and BP {1103, 2373}. The second generation compounds nilotinib and dasatinib can circumvent this form of drug failure in the case of most but not all kinase domain mutations associated with imatinib resistance {1103, 2373}.

The molecular basis of disease transformation is still largely unknown. Progression is usually associated with clonal evolution {657, 1487, 1488}, and at the time of transformation to AP or BP, 80% of patients demonstrate cytogenetic changes in addition to the Ph chromosome, such as an extra Ph, +8, +19, or i(17q). Genes shown to be altered in the transformed stages include *TP53*, *RB1*, *MYC*, *p16^{INK4a}* (CDKN2A), *RAS*, *AML1* and *EVI1*, but their role in the transformation, if any, is currently unknown {821, 1455, 1487}. The recent introduction of genome-wide expression profiling by microarray technology has started to reveal other candidate genes associated with the advanced stages, and has also revealed similar gene expression patterns between AP and BP, suggesting that the genetic events leading to transformation in AP and BP occur in late CP or early AP {1608, 1624, 1803}.

Postulated cell of origin

It is currently accepted that CML-CP originates from a pluripotent BM stem cell. However, disease progression may originate in more committed precursors than previously supposed, as myeloid BP has been reported to involve the granulocyte-macrophage progenitor pool rather than the haemopoietic stem cell pool {1474}. Whether the same applies to lymphoid BP is not known.

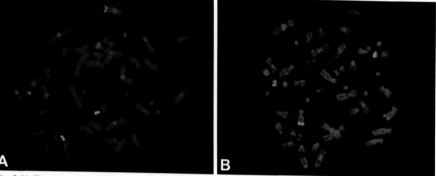

Fig. 2.11 Fluorescence *in situ* hybridization (FISH) with dual color and dual fusion probe on a normal metaphase cell (**A**) and metaphase preparation (**B**) from a patient with t(9;22)(q34;q11.2). A dual color and dual fusion translocation probe is used (VysisR corporation). The *ABL1* and *BCR* probes are labeled with SpectrumOrange and SpectrumGreen respectively. In normal cells (**A**) two orange signals representing the *ABL1* gene at 9q34 and two green signals representing the *BCR* at 22q11.2 are shown. In the patient's CML cells (**B**) one orange (normal 9q34), one green (normal 22q11.2) and two orange/green (yellow) signals, representing derivative 9q34 and 22q11.2, respectively, are detected.

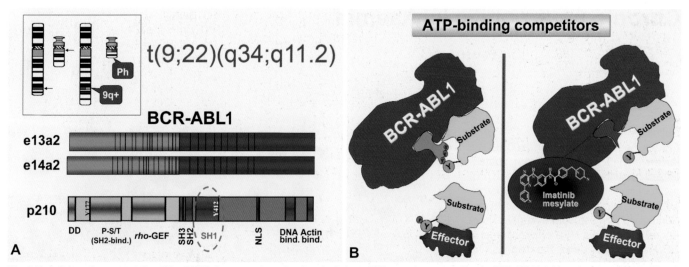

Fig. 2.12 A Schematic representation of the t(9;22) chromosomal translocation, the fusion mRNA transcripts encoded by the *BCR-ABL1* hybrid gene generated in the 22q- or Philadelphia (Ph) chromosome, and the translated BCR-ABL1 fusion protein, whose oncogenic properties rely primarily on its constitutively activated tyrosine kinase encoded by the Src-homology 1 (SH1) domain indicated by the red circle. Some of the other important functional domains contributed by the BCR and ABL1 portions of the oncoprotein are shown. These are the dimerisation domain (DD); Y177 which is the autophosphorylation site crucial for binding to GRB-2; the phospho-Ser and -Thr SH-binding domain; a region homologous to Rho guanidine nucleotide exchange factors (Rho-GEF); the ABL1 regulatory SH3 and SH2 domains; Y412 as the major site of autophosphorylation within the SH1 kinase domain; nuclear localization signals (NLS) and the DNA- and actin-binding domains. **B** Mechanism of action of BCR-ABL1 tyrosine kinase inhibitors. Whereas the physiological binding of ATP to its pocket allows BCR-ABL1 to phosphorylate selected tyrosine residues on its substrates (left diagram), a synthetic ATP mimic such as imatinib fits this pocket (right diagram), but does not provide the essential phosphate group to be transferred to the substrate. The downstream chain of reactions is then halted because, with its tyrosines in the unphosphorylated form, the substrate does not assume the necessary conformation to ensure association with its effector.

Prognosis and predictive factors

Based on historical data prior to any effective therapy, median survival times in CML ranged between 2–3 years {767}. With conventional chemotherapy (busulfan, Hydroxycarbamide) median survival was about 4 years, but progression to AP and BP was only slightly delayed with 10-year overall survival (OS) less than 10% {767, 1948, 2022}. Interferon-α-based regimes delayed progression significantly, with median survival of approximately 6 years and 10-year OS of ~25% {115}. With allogenic stem cell transplant, 10-year OS ranges between 10 and 70%, depending on disease phase, patient age

and donor type {116, 828, 2022}. Three prognostic models based on baseline prognostic variables including age, spleen size, platelet count, the percentage of myeloblasts in PB as well as the percentage of basophils and eosinophils in the PB allowed the calculation of relative risk, hence of the life expectancy, of patients treated with conventional chemotherapy and interferon {905, 1101, 2044} and with imatinib {116, 615}, but not those treated with allogeneic stem cell transplant. Some studies have shown that the predictive values of these models can be further improved by the inclusion of morphologic parameters, particularly the

presence or absence of myelofibrosis {292, 293, 1217, 1218}. Pretransplant myelofibrosis has been reported to be associated with a delayed or failure of haematopoietic reconstitution {293, 2207}. However, in the current era of PTKI therapy, the most important prognostic indicator is the response to treatment at the haematologic, cytogenetic and molecular level {116}. Currently the complete cytogenetic response rate to imatinib is 70–90%, with a 5-year progression free survival and OS between 80–95% {116, 615}.

Chronic neutrophilic leukaemia

B.J. Bain
R.D. Brunning
J.W. Vardiman
J. Thiele

Definition

Chronic neutrophilic leukaemia (CNL) is a rare myeloproliferative neoplasm, characterized by sustained peripheral blood (PB) neutrophilia, bone marrow (BM) hypercellularity due to neutrophilic granulocyte proliferation, and hepatosplenomegaly. There is no Philadelphia (Ph) chromosome or *BCR-ABL1* fusion gene. The diagnosis requires exclusion of reactive neutrophilia and other myeloproliferative neoplasms.

ICD-O code   9963/3

Epidemiology

The true incidence of CNL is unknown, but only about 150 cases have been reported. In one study of 660 cases of chronic leukaemias of myeloid origin, not a single case of CNL was observed {2003}. CNL generally affects older adults, but has also been reported in adolescents {909, 2474, 2504}. The sex distribution is nearly equal {231, 640, 2474, 2504}.

Etiology

The cause of CNL is not known. In up to 20% of reported cases, the neutrophilia was associated with an underlying neoplasm, most usually multiple myeloma {355, 584, 2076}. To date, no cases of CNL associated with myeloma have been reported in which a clonal chromosomal abnormality or evidence of clonality by molecular techniques has been convincingly demonstrated in the neutrophils {2077}. It is thus likely that most cases of CNL associated with myeloma are not autonomous proliferations of the neutrophils, but are secondary to abnormal cytokine release from the neoplastic plasma cells or other cells regulated by the plasma cell population. The same may be true of CNL associated with other neoplasms. However, it should be noted that evolution to acute myeloid leukaemia (AML) occurred in one patient with CNL associated with multiple myeloma {584}.

Sites of involvement

The PB and BM are always involved, and the spleen and liver usually show leukaemic

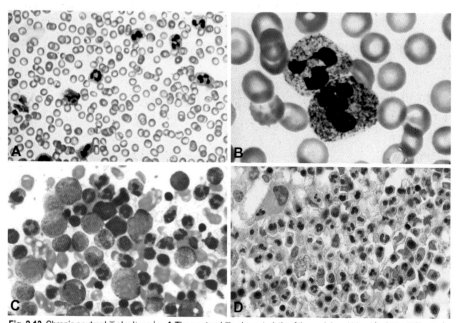

Fig. 2.13 Chronic neutrophilic leukaemia. A The neutrophilia characteristic of the peripheral blood in CNL. B The toxic granulation commonly observed. Reproduced from Anastasi and Vardiman {35A}. C The bone marrow aspirate smear demonstrates neutrophil proliferation from myelocytes to segmented forms with toxic granulation, but no other significant abnormalities. D The bone marrow biopsy specimen is hypercellular, showing a markedly elevated myeloid:erythroid ratio with increased numbers of neutrophils, particularly mature segmented forms.

infiltrates {2257, 2474, 2504}. However, any tissue may be infiltrated by the neutrophils {2257, 2474, 2504}.

Clinical features

The most constant clinical feature reported is splenomegaly, which may be symptomatic. Hepatomegaly is usually present as well {2474, 2504}. A history of bleeding from mucocutaneous surfaces or from the gastrointestinal tract is reported in 25-30% of patients {909, 2504}. Gout and pruritus are other possible symptoms {2504}.

Morphology

The PB smear shows neutrophilia with a white blood cell count ≥25x10⁹/L. The neutrophils are usually segmented, but there may be a substantial increase in band forms as well. In almost all cases, neutrophil precursors (promyelocytes, myelocytes, metamyelocytes) account for fewer than 5% of the white cells, but occasionally, they may account for up to 10% {231, 640, 909, 2474, 2504}. Myeloblasts

are almost never observed in the blood. The neutrophils often appear toxic, with abnormal, coarse granules, but they may also appear normal. Neutrophil dysplasia is not present. Red blood cell and platelet morphology is usually normal. The BM biopsy shows hypercellularity with neutrophilic proliferation. The myeloid:erythroid ratio may reach 20:1 or greater. Myeloblasts and promyelocytes are not increased in percentage at the time of diagnosis, but the percent of myelocytes and mature neutrophils is increased. Erythroid and megakaryocytic proliferation may also occur {231, 2474}. Significant dysplasia is not present in any of the cell lineages and, if found, another diagnosis, such as atypical chronic myeloid leukaemia, should be considered (See Chapter 4). Reticulin fibrosis is uncommon {231, 640, 2474, 2504}. In view of the reported frequency of CNL in association with multiple myeloma, the BM should be examined for evidence of a plasma cell neoplasm {355, 584, 2076, 2077}. If plasma cell abnormalities are present, clonality of the neutrophil lineage should be supported by cytogenetic or molecular techniques before making a diagnosis of CNL. Splenomegaly and hepatomegaly result from tissue infiltration by the neutrophils. In the spleen, the infiltrate is mainly confined to the red pulp; in the liver, the sinusoids, portal areas or both, may be infiltrated {2474, 2504}.

Cytochemistry
The neutrophil alkaline phosphatase score is usually normal or increased, but no other cytochemical abnormality has been reported {909, 2504}.

Genetics
Cytogenetic studies are normal in nearly 90% of patients. In the remaining patients, clonal karyotypic abnormalities may include +8, +9, +21, del(20q), del(11q) and del(12p) {566, 640, 736, 1415, 2466}. Clonal cytogenetic abnormalities may appear during the course of the disease. There is no Ph chromosome or *BCR-ABL1* fusion gene. A variant of chronic myelogenous leukaemia, *BCR-ABL1* positive (CML) has been reported that demonstrates peripheral blood neutrophilia similar to that seen in CNL {1685}. In such cases, a variant BCR-ABL1 fusion protein, p230, is found. Cases with this molecular variant of the *BCR-ABL1* fusion gene should be considered as CML, not CNL. Occasional patients with a *JAK2* mutation have been reported {1083, 1435} and this has sometimes been homozygous {1083}. Complete cytogenetic remission with imatinib was reported in a patient with CNL

Table 2.01 Diagnostic criteria for chronic neutrophilic leukaemia.

1. Peripheral blood leukocytosis, WBC ≥25x10^9/L
    Segmented neutrophils and band forms are >80% of white blood cells
    Immature granulocytes (promyelocytes, myelocytes, metamyelocytes) <10% of white blood cells
    Myeloblasts <1% of white blood cells

2. Hypercellular bone marrow biopsy
    Neutrophilic granulocytes increased in percentage and number
    Myeloblasts <5% of nucleated marrow cells
    Neutrophilic maturation pattern normal
    Megakaryocytes normal or left shifted

3. Hepatosplenomegaly

4. No identifiable cause for physiologic neutrophilia or, if present, demonstration of clonality of myeloid cells
    by cytogenetic or molecular studies
    No infectious or inflammatory process
    No underlying tumour

5. No Philadelphia chromosome or *BCR-ABL1* fusion gene
6. No rearrangement of *PDGFRA*, *PDGFRB* or *FGFR1*
7. No evidence of polycythaemia vera, primary myelofibrosis or essential thrombocythaemia

8. No evidence of a myelodysplastic syndrome or a myelodysplastic/myeloproliferative neoplasm
    No granulocytic dysplasia
    No myelodysplastic changes in other myeloid lineages
    Monocytes <1x10^9/L

and t(15;19)(q13;p13.3), suggesting the possibility of an unidentified fusion gene in some cases {433}.

Postulated cell of origin
Cell of origin is unknown. It is most likely a BM stem cell with limited lineage potential {736, 2466}.

Prognosis and predictive factors
Although generally regarded as a slowly progressive disorder, the survival of patients with CNL is variable, ranging from 6 months to more than 20 years. Usually the neutrophilia is progressive, and anaemia and thrombocytopenia may ensue. The development of myelodysplastic features may signal a transformation of the disease to AML, which has been reported in some patients {909, 2504}. It is not clear whether the transformation was related to previous cytotoxic therapy in the cases reported.

Polycythaemia vera

J. Thiele
H.M. Kvasnicka
A. Orazi
A. Tefferi
G. Birgegard

Definition

Polycythaemia vera (PV) is a chronic myeloproliferative neoplasm (MPN) characterized by increased red blood cell production independent of the mechanisms that normally regulate erythropoiesis. Virtually all patients carry the somatic gain-of-function mutation of the Janus 2 kinase gene, *JAK2* V617F or another functionally similar *JAK2* mutation that results in proliferation not only of the erythroid lineage but of the granulocytes and megakaryocytes as well, i.e. "panmyelosis". Three phases of PV may be recognized: (1) a prodromal, prepolycythaemic phase characterized by borderline to only mild erythrocytosis; (2) an overt polycythaemic phase, associated with a significantly increased red cell mass; and (3) a "spent" or post-polycythaemic myelofibrosis phase (post-PV MF) in which cytopenias, including anaemia, are associated with ineffective haematopoiesis, bone marrow (BM) fibrosis, extramedullary haematopoiesis (EMH), and hypersplenism. The natural progression of PV also includes a low incidence of evolution to a myelodysplastic/preleukaemic phase and/or to acute leukaemia (AML). All causes of secondary erythrocytosis, inheritable polycythaemia and other MPN must be excluded. The diagnosis requires integration of clinical, laboratory and BM histological features as outlined in Table 2.02.

ICD-O code   9950/3

Synonym

Polycythaemia rubra vera.

Epidemiology

The reported annual incidence of PV increases with advanced age and varies from 0.7 to 2.6 per 100 000 inhabitants in Europe and North America, but is much lower in Japan {1059}. Most reports indicate a slight male predominance, with the M:F ratio ranging from 1–2:1 {50, 1389}. The median age at diagnosis is 60 years, and patients younger than 20 years old are only rarely reported {1700}.

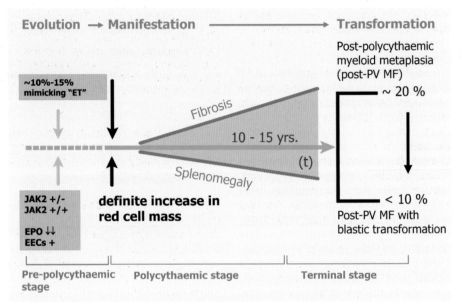

Fig. 2.14 Schematic presentation of the evolution of the disease process in polycythaemia vera.

Etiology

The underlying cause is unknown in most cases. A genetic predisposition has been reported in some families {1778, 2032}. Ionizing radiation and occupational exposure to toxins have been suggested as possible causes in occasional patients {312}.

Sites of involvement

The blood and BM are the major sites of involvement, but the spleen and liver are also affected and are the major sites of EMH in the later stages. However, any organ can be damaged as a result of the vascular consequences of the increased red cell mass.

Table 2.02 Diagnostic criteria for polycythaemia vera (PV). Diagnosis requires the presence of both major criteria and one minor criterion or the presence of the first major criterion together with two minor criteria.

Major criteria

1. Haemoglobin >18.5 g/dL in men, 16.5 g/dL in women or other evidence of increased red cell volume*

2. Presence of *JAK2* V617F or other functionally similar mutation such as *JAK2* exon 12 mutation

Minor criteria

1. Bone marrow biopsy showing hypercellularity for age with trilineage growth (panmyelosis) with prominent erythroid, granulocytic and megakaryocytic proliferation

2. Serum erythropoietin level below the reference range for normal

3. Endogenous erythroid colony formation *in vitro*

---

* Haemoglobin or haematocrit >99th percentile of method-specific reference range for age, sex, altitude of residence or haemoglobin >17 g/dL in men, 15 g/dL in women if associated with a documented and sustained increase of at least 2 g/dL from an individual's baseline value that can not be attributed to correction of iron deficiency, or elevated red cell mass >25% above mean normal predicted value.

Clinical features

The major symptoms of PV are related to hypertension or vascular abnormalities caused by the increased red cell mass. In nearly 20% of patients an episode of venous or arterial thrombosis, such as deep vein thrombosis, myocardial ischaemia or stroke, is documented in the medical history {50} and may be the first manifestation of PV {50, 197, 1389, 2071}. Mesenteric, portal or splenic vein thrombosis and the Budd-Chiari syndrome should always lead to consideration of PV as an underlying cause and may precede the onset of an overt polycythaemic phase {50, 270}. Headache, dizziness, visual disturbances and paraesthesias are major complaints, and pruritus, erythromelalgia and gout are also common. In the full-blown polycythaemic stage physical findings usually include plethora and palpable splenomegaly in 70% and hepatomegaly in 40% of patients {1445, 2071}.

Clinical laboratory studies that aid in confirmation of the diagnosis of PV include subnormal erythropoietin (EPO) levels {223, 1527}, endogenous erythroid colony (EEC) formation {595}, and detection of the *JAK2* V617F or functionally similar mutations, e.g. *JAK2* exon 12 mutations {1981, 2168, 2177}.

Occasionally, patients may present with clinical symptoms suggestive of PV but with a haemoglobin level and/or red cell volume not sufficiently elevated to substantiate the diagnosis. Such patients may be in the pre-polycythaemic phase, which was previously referred to by some authors as "latent PV" or as "pure idiopathic erythrocytosis" {197, 1559, 1715, 1897, 2224}. The detection of a subnormal EPO level, a *JAK2* V617F or functionally similar mutation and/or abnormal EEC formation, in combination with the typical morphologic features described below, will allow the diagnosis of this phase of PV; these features are not found in secondary or spurious polycythaemia. The pre-polycythaemic phase may be expected to become overtly polycythaemic at a later time.

Morphology

The morphological findings in BM biopsy specimens of patients with PV must always be correlated with other clinical and laboratory findings in order to firmly establish the diagnosis {2177}. However, even in the early pre-polycythaemic stage

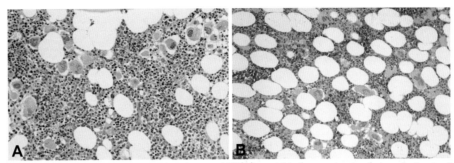

Fig. 2.15 Polycythaemia vera, pre-polycythaemic stage. **A** Mildly hypercellular bone marrow showing a predominance of large megakaryocytes in the bone marrow section. **B** Many large and giant hyperlobulated (ET-like) megakaryocytes in a patient clinically mimicking ET, because of a platelet count in excess of 1000x10⁹/L. Note the only mildly increased granulo- and erythropoiesis (panmyelosis), better demonstrated by naphthol-ASD-chloroacetate esterase reaction.

the morphological findings are of sufficient specificity to allow distinction of PV from secondary polycythaemia as well as other subtypes of MPN {2203}.

Pre-polycythaemic phase and overt polycythaemia

Generally, in the pre-polycythaemic and polycythaemic phases of PV the major features in the peripheral blood (PB) and BM are attributable to effective proliferation in the erythroid, granulocytic and megakaryocytic lineages, i.e. there is panmyelosis. The PB shows a mild to overt excess of normochromic, normocytic red blood cells. If iron deficiency due to bleeding is present, the red cells may be hypochromic and microcytic. Neutrophilia and rarely basophilia may be present. Occasional immature granulocytes may be detectable in the overt polycythaemic phase, but circulating blasts are generally not observed. Because of prominent thrombocytosis, up to 15% of cases of early phase PV may clinically mimic essential thrombocythaemia (ET) {2210} but such cases eventually evolve into an overtly polycythaemic stage {1047, 2007, 2210}.

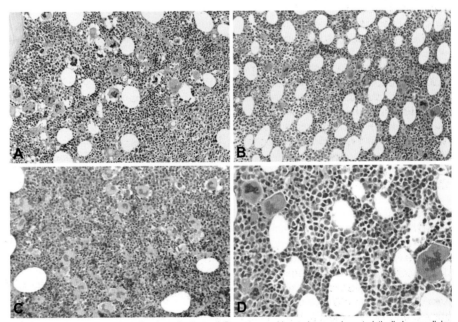

Fig. 2.16 Polycythaemia vera, polycythaemic stage. **A** Bone marrow biopsy shows a characteristically hypercellular marrow during the overt polycythaemic stage. **B** Megakaryocytes revealing different sizes are always a prominent feature. The cells are more easily evaluated by using the PAS reaction. **C** Panmyelosis (trilineage proliferation) as demonstrated by the naphthol-ASD-chloroacetate stain which, by accurately identifying the granulocytic cells (red reaction product), helps in the assessment of the relative proportion of the two major marrow lineages (erythropoietic and granulopoietic). **D** In this disease stage, the megakaryocytes show increased pleomorphism with significant differences in size, but no relevant maturation defects (nuclear-cytoplasmic differentiation). PAS stain.

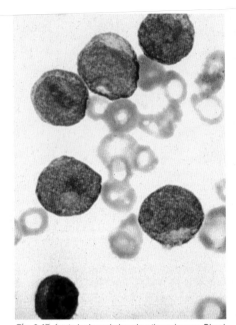

Fig. 2.17 Acute leukaemia in polycythaemia vera. Blood smear from a patient with a long-standing history of PV. The patient had been treated with alkylating agents during the polycythaemic stage. The blasts expressed CD13, CD33, CD117 and CD34, and had a complex karyotype, consistent with therapy-related acute myeloid leukaemia.

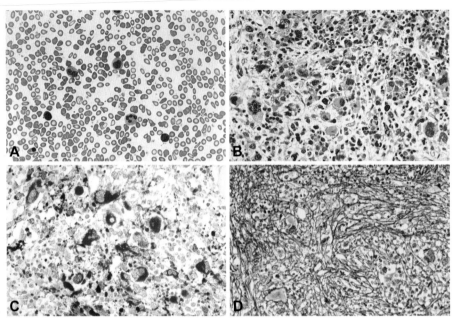

Fig. 2.18 Polycythaemia vera, post-polycythaemic myelofibrosis (post-PV MF) and myeloid metaplasia stage. **A** Peripheral blood smear demonstrates leukoerythroblastosis with numerous teardrop-shaped red blood cells (dacryocytes). **B** Bone marrow shows conspicuously abnormal megakaryocytic proliferation and depletion of the erythroid and granulocytic cells. **C** An immunostain for CD61 illustrates the atypia in the megakaryocytic population, including a population of small immature megakaryocytes. **D** Overt reticulin fibrosis that is invariably present in post-PV MF with myeloid metaplasia.

Bone marrow cellularity has been reported to range from 35–100%, with a median cellularity of about 80% {641}, but characteristically the BM biopsy is hypercellular for the patient's age. A finding that is especially noteworthy is increased cellularity in the subcortical marrow space, an area which is normally hypocellular {775, 2203}. Panmyelosis accounts for the increased cellularity but an increase in the numbers of erythroid precursors and of megakaryocytes is often most prominent {641, 775, 2203}. Erythropoiesis is normoblastic, and granulopoiesis is morphologically normal. The percentage of myeloblasts is not increased. Megakaryocytes are increased in number, particularly in cases with an excess of platelets, and display characteristic morphological abnormalities, such as hyperlobated nuclei, even in the early phase of the disease. The presence of the panmyelosis, which although less prominent in the pre-polycythaemic than in the overt polycythaemic phase, is nevertheless detectable and helps to distinguish early PV from ET, which it may otherwise resemble clinically {2210}. As in the pre-polycythaemic phase, megakaryocytes seen in the polycythaemic stage of PV are clearly distinguishable from those seen in ET.

They typically tend to form loose clusters or to lie close to the bone trabeculae, and often show a significant degree of pleomorphism with a mixture of different sizes. The majority of the megakaryocytes exhibit normally folded or deeply lobulated nuclei, and usually lack significant cytological abnormalities, although a minority show bulbous nuclei and other nuclear abnormalities, particularly when associated with a minor increase in reticulin {2211}. When taking the characteristic histological pattern of PV into account, discrimination of PV from ET and PMF as

well as the distinction from reactive erythrocytosis and thrombocytosis is feasible {2211, 2222}. Reticulin stains will show a normal reticulin fibre network in about 80% of patients, but the remainder display increased reticulin and even borderline to mild collagen fibrosis {297, 641, 775, 1189, 2211} depending on the stage of disease at first diagnosis. Reactive nodular lymphoid aggregates are found in up to 20% of cases {2203}. Stainable iron is lacking in the BM aspirate and biopsy specimens in more than 95% of the cases {641, 2222}.

Table 2.03 Diagnostic criteria for post-polycythaemic myelofibrosis (post-PV MF).

Required criteria

1. Documentation of a previous diagnosis of WHO-defined PV

2. Bone marrow fibrosis grade 2–3 (on 0–3 scale) or grade 3–4 (on 0–4 scale)

Additional criteria (2 are required)

1. Anaemia* or sustained loss of either phlebotomy (in the absence of cytoreductive therapy) or cytoreductive treatment requirement for erythrocytosis

2. Leukoerythroblastic peripheral blood picture

3. Increasing splenomegaly defined as either an increase in palpable splenomegaly of >5 cm from baseline (distance from the left costal margin) or the appearance of newly palpable splenomegaly

4. Development of >1 of 3 constitutional symptoms: >10% weight loss in 6 months, night sweats, unexplained fever (>37.5°C)

---

*Below the reference range for appropriate age, sex, gender and altitude considerations.

"Spent phase" and post-polycythaemic myelofibrosis (post-PV MF)

During the later phases of PV, erythropoiesis progressively decreases. As a consequence, the red blood cell mass normalizes and then decreases, and the spleen further enlarges. Usually these changes are accompanied by corresponding BM alterations {641, 2071}. The most common pattern of disease progression is post-PV MF accompanied by myeloid metaplasia which is characterized by a leukoerythroblastic PB smear, poikilocytosis with teardrop-shaped red blood cells, and splenomegaly due to EMH, as defined in Table 2.03 {143A}. The morphological hallmark of this stage of the disease is overt reticulin and collagen fibrosis of the BM {641, 775, 2203, 2222}. The cellularity varies in this terminal stage, but hypocellular specimens are common. Clusters of megakaryocytes, often with hyperchromatic and very dysmorphic nuclei, are prominent. Erythropoiesis and granulopoiesis are decreased in amount, and are sometimes found, along with megakaryocytes, lying within dilated marrow sinusoids {2203}. Osteosclerosis may also occur {641, 775}. The splenic enlargement is a consequence of EMH, which is characterized by the presence of erythroid, granulocytic and megakaryocytic elements in the splenic sinuses and cords of Billroth. An increase in the number of immature cells may be observed in these stages, but the finding of >10% blasts in the PB or BM or the presence of significant myelodysplasia is unusual, and most likely signals transformation to an accelerated phase and/or a myelodysplastic syndrome (MDS). Cases in which 20% or more blasts are found are considered AML {1701, 2071, 2203, 2222}.

Immunophenotype

No abnormal phenotype has been reported

Genetics

The most frequent genetic abnormality in PV is the somatic gain-of-function mutation JAK2 V617F. Although it occurs in >95% of patients with PV, it is not specific and is found in other MPN as well, but in

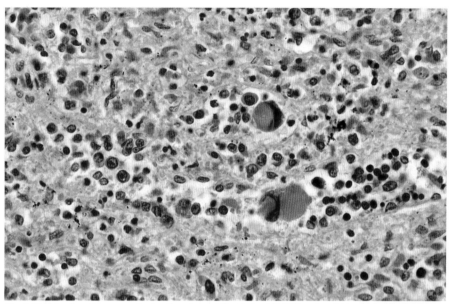

Fig. 2.19 Polycythaemia vera, post-polycythaemic myelofibrosis (post-PV MF) and myeloid metaplasia, splenectomy specimen. The splenic enlargement in the post-polycythaemic phase is due mainly to extramedullary haematopoiesis that occurs in the splenic sinuses, as well as fibrosis and entrapment of platelets and haematopoietic cells in the splenic cords.

lower frequency {163, 1044, 1186, 1288}. The mutation occurs in a haematopoietic stem cell, and is found in all of the myeloid lineages. Hence cells that utilize JAK2 kinase in the intracellular signaling pathway may be hypersensitive to growth factors and other cytokines, including EPO. A functionally similar mutation in exon 12 of JAK2 has also been reported {1981}, so that virtually all patients with PV have a JAK2 aberration. Still, no genetic defect entirely specific to PV has been identified. At diagnosis, cytogenetic abnormalities are detectable in about 20% of patients. The most common recurring abnormalities include +8, +9, del(20q), del(13q) and del(9p); sometimes +8 and +9 are found together {42, 2394}. There is no Philadelphia chromosome or BCR-ABL1 fusion gene. These chromosomal abnormalities are seen with increasing frequency with disease progression and in nearly 80–90% of those with post-PV MF {42}. Almost 100% of those who develop MDS or AML have cytogenetic abnormalities, including those commonly observed in therapy-related MDS and AML (See Chapter 6).

Postulated cell of origin

Haematopoietic stem cell.

Prognosis and predictive factors

With currently available treatment, median survival times >10 years are commonly reported {50, 1215, 1548, 2071}, although controversy persists about the risk factors other than older age {1215, 1389, 1702}. Most patients die from thrombosis or haemorrhage, but up to 20% succumb to myelodysplasia or acute myeloid leukaemia {50, 1389, 2071}.

The factors that predict the risk of thrombosis or haemorrhage are not well defined {1389, 1700, 2071}. The incidence of MDS and acute leukaemic transformation is only 2–3% in patients who have not been treated with cytotoxic agents, but increases to 10% or more following certain types of chemotherapy {704, 1389, 1548, 1701, 1702}.

Primary myelofibrosis

J. Thiele
H.M. Kvasnicka
A. Tefferi
G. Barosi
A. Orazi
J.W. Vardiman

Definition

Primary myelofibrosis (PMF) {1464} is a clonal myeloproliferative neoplasm (MPN) characterized by a proliferation of predominantly megakaryocytes and granulocytes in the bone marrow (BM) that in fully developed disease is associated with reactive deposition of fibrous connective tissue and with extramedullary haematopoiesis (EMH). There is a stepwise evolution from an initial prefibrotic phase {2177} characterized by a hypercellular BM with absent or minimal reticulin fibrosis to a fibrotic phase with marked reticulin or collagen fibrosis in the BM and often osteosclerosis. This fibrotic stage of PMF is characterized by leukoerythroblastosis in the blood with teardrop-shaped red cells, and by hepatomegaly and splenomegaly (Table 2.04).

ICD-O code   9961/3

Synonyms

Chronic idiopathic myelofibrosis (CIMF); Agnogenic myeloid metaplasia (AMM); Myelofibrosis/sclerosis with myeloid metaplasia (MMM); Idiopathic myelofibrosis.

Epidemiology

The overt fibrotic phase is estimated to occur at 0.5–1.5 per 100 000 persons per year {1060, 2167}. It occurs most commonly in the sixth to seventh decade of life, and both sexes are nearly equally affected {2167}. Children are rarely affected {367}.

Etiology

Exposure to benzene or ionizing radiation has been documented in some cases {588}. Rare familial cases of BM fibrosis in young children have been reported. How often this represents an MPN is unknown, but at least some cases appear to represent an autosomal recessive inherited condition {1873}. In other families with a somewhat later age of onset, the features have been consistent with an MPN, suggesting a familial predisposition to PMF {369}.

Sites of involvement

Blood and BM are always involved. In the later stages of the disease, EMH (also known as myeloid metaplasia) becomes prominent, in particular in the spleen {1773}. In the initial stages, randomly distributed CD34+ progenitors are slightly increased in the BM, but not in the peripheral blood (PB). Only in the later stages they appear in large numbers peripherally {1592, 2209}. This increase of CD34+ cells in the PB is a phenomenon largely restricted to overt PMF and is not seen in non-fibrotic polycythaemia vera (PV) or essential thrombocythaemia (ET) {41, 145, 1703}. It has been postulated that EMH is a consequence of the peculiar ability of the spleen to sequestrate the numerous circulating CD34+ cells {2208}. Liver, lymph nodes, kidney adrenal gland, dura mater, gastrointestinal tract, lung and pleura, breast skin and soft tissues are other possible sites of EMH {2167}.

Clinical features

Up to 30% of patients are asymptomatic at the time of diagnosis and are discovered by detection of splenomegaly during a routine physical examination or when a routine blood count discloses anaemia, leukocytosis and/or thrombocytosis. Less commonly, the diagnosis results from discovery of unexplained leukoerythroblastosis or an increased lactate dehydrogenase (LDH) {366, 2167, 2177}. In the initial prefibrotic phase of PMF, the only finding may be marked thrombocytosis mimicking ET {2177, 2201}. Therefore, a sustained thrombocytosis cannot, by itself, discriminate between prefibrotic PMF and ET {2201, 2202, 2204}. Constitutional symptoms may include fatigue, dyspnoea, weight loss, night sweats, low-grade fever

---

Table 2.04 Diagnostic criteria for primary myelofibrosis: diagnosis requires meeting all 3 major and 2 minor criteria.

Major criteria

1. Presence of megakaryocyte proliferation and atypia[a], usually accompanied by either reticulin and/or collagen fibrosis,
   or
   in the absence of significant reticulin fibrosis, the megakaryocyte changes must be accompanied by an increased bone marrow cellularity characterized by granulocytic proliferation and often decreased erythropoiesis (i.e. prefibrotic cellular-phase disease).

2. Not meeting WHO criteria for polycythaemia vera[b], BCR-ABL1+ chronic myelogenous leukaemia[c], myelodysplastic syndrome[d], or other myeloid neoplasms

3. Demonstration of JAK2 V617F or other clonal marker (e.g. MPL W515K/L),
   or
   in the absence of a clonal marker, no evidence that the bone marrow fibrosis or other changes are secondary to infection, autoimmune disorder or other chronic inflammatory condition, hairy cell leukaemia or other lymphoid neoplasm, metastatic malignancy, or toxic (chronic) myelopathies[e]

Minor criteria

1. Leukoerythroblastosis[f]
2. Increase in serum lactate dehydrogenase level[f]
3. Anaemia[f]
4. Splenomegaly[f]

---

[a] Small to large megakaryocytes with an aberrant nuclear/cytoplasmic ratio and hyperchromatic, bulbous, or irregularly folded nuclei and dense clustering.
[b] Requires the failure of iron replacement therapy to increase haemoglobin level to the polycythaemia vera range in the presence of decreased serum ferritin. Exclusion of polycythaemia vera is based on haemoglobin and haematocrit levels, and red cell mass measurement is not required.
[c] Requires the absence of BCR-ABL1.
[d] Requires absence of dyserythropoiesis and dysgranulopoiesis.
[e] Patients with conditions associated with reactive myelofibrosis are not immune to PMF, and the diagnosis should be considered in such cases if other criteria are met.
[f] Degree of abnormality could be borderline or marked.

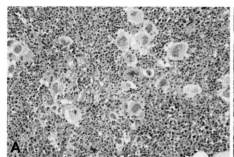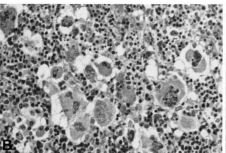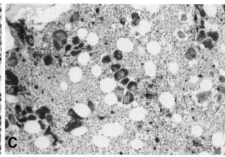

Fig. 2.20 Primary myelofibrosis **A** Prefibrotic-early stage. Megakaryocytic and granulocytic proliferation. Naphthol-ASD-chloroacetate esterase staining visualizes the granulocytic component (red reaction product). Megakaryocytes show extensive clustering and condensed nuclei with conspicuously clumped chromatin and abnormal nuclear-cytoplasmic ratio. **B** Primary myelofibrosis, prefibrotic stage. Megakaryocytic abnormalities are the key finding in diagnosing PMF and in its distinction from other myeloproliferative and reactive disorders. Note the abnormalities of megakaryopoiesis including anisocytosis, abnormal nuclear-cytoplasmic ratios, abnormal chromatin clumping with hyperchromatic nuclei, and plump lobulation of some nuclei (cloud-like nuclei). **C** Following immunohistochemistry for CD61, note abnormal megakaryocytes including the presence of small megakaryocytes.

and bleeding episodes. Gouty arthritis and renal stones due to hyperuricaemia may also occur. Splenomegaly of varying degree is detected in up to 90% of patients and may be massive; nearly 50% have hepatomegaly {143, 366, 367, 1635, 2167}. The *JAK2* V617F mutation may be found in ~50% of patients in the fibrotic phase; its incidence in the prefibrotic stage has not been well studied. Although helpful in distinguishing PMF from reactive conditions that may result in BM fibrosis, the mutation is not specific for PMF but is found in PV and ET as well {2172}.

Morphology

The classical picture of advanced PMF includes a PB smear that shows leuko-erythroblastosis and anisopoikilocytosis (particularly with teardrop-shaped red cells) associated with a hypocellular BM with marked reticulin and/or collagen fibrosis and organomegaly caused by EMH. However, the morphological and clinical findings vary considerably at diagnosis depending on whether the patient is first encountered during the prefibrotic or the fibrotic stage of the disease {2177, 2204}. Because the progressive accumulation of fibrous tissue parallels disease progression, it is important to reproducibly and sequentially grade the amount of BM fibrosis semi-quantitatively by using a scoring system {2214} (Table 2.05).
Prefibrotic and early stage PMF: No registry-based prevalence figures are available for the incidence of the prefibrotic phase of PMF, but series derived from various reference centres reveal that 30–40% of patients are first detected in a prodromal, prefibrotic phase without a significant increase in reticulin and/or collagen fibres

{297, 775, 2202, 2204}. In these cases the BM biopsy is hypercellular with an increase in the number of neutrophils and atypical megakaryocytes. There may be a mild "left shift" in granulopoiesis, but usually metamyelocytes, bands and segmented forms predominate. Myeloblasts are not increased in percentage, and conspicuous clusters of blasts or of CD34+ progenitors are not observed {2202, 2204}. In most cases, erythropoiesis is reduced in quantity, but early erythroid precursors are prominent in some patients {2228}. The megakaryocytes are markedly abnormal, and their histotopography and morphology is the key to the recognition of the prefibrotic stage of PMF. The megakaryocytes often form dense

clusters of variable size that are frequently adjacent to BM vascular sinuses and the bone trabeculae {297, 775, 2204, 2216}. Most megakaryocytes are enlarged, but small megakaryocytes may also be seen, and their detection is greatly facilitated by the use of immunohistochemistry with antibodies reactive with megakaryocytic antigens {2201, 2204}. Deviations from the normal nuclear:cytoplasmic ratio (an expression of defective maturation), abnormal patterns of chromatin clumping with bulbous, "cloud-like" or "balloon-shaped" nuclei, and the frequent occurrence of bare megakaryocytic nuclei are all typical findings. Overall in PMF the megakaryocytes are more atypical than in any other type of MPN. Vascular proliferation is

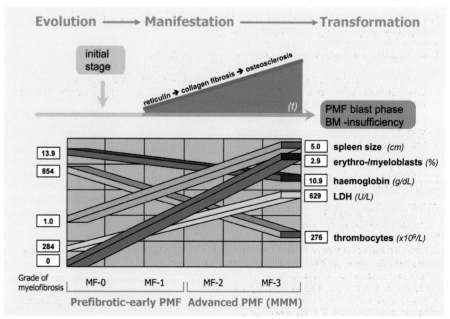

Fig. 2.21 Dynamics of the disease process in primary myelofibrosis (PMF) with associated haematological data (median values) and associated fibre grading.

usual in the BM {1214}, and lymphoid nodules are found in about 20% to 30% {2201, 2204}. Careful BM morphological examination is particularly crucial in distinguishing prefibrotic PMF with accompanying thrombocytosis from ET {712, 796, 2177, 2201, 2216}. Reticulin fibrosis is minimal or even absent (corresponding to grades 0 and 1) during this stage {2214}; if present, it is usually focal and tends to be concentrated around vessels. The majority of cases with prefibrotic and early (reticulin) fibrotic stages of PMF eventually transform into overt fibrotic/sclerotic myelofibrosis associated with EMH {295, 775, 1189, 2204, 2218}.

Fibrotic stage: Most patients with PMF are initially diagnosed in the overt fibrotic stage {143, 366, 1635, 2167}. In this stage the BM biopsy demonstrates clear-cut reticulin or collagen fibrosis (fibrosis grades 2 and 3). The BM may still be focally hypercellular, but more often is normocellular or hypocellular, with patches of active haematopoiesis alternating with hypocellular regions of loose connective tissue and/or fat. Foci of immature cells may be more prominent, although myeloblasts account for <10% of the BM cells {297, 775, 2204}. Atypical megakaryocytes are often the most conspicuous finding; these occur in large clusters or sheets, often within dilated vascular sinuses {295, 2204}. Sometimes the BM is almost devoid of haematopoietic cells, showing mainly dense reticulin or collagen fibrosis, with small islands of haematopoietic precursors situated mostly within the vascular sinuses. Associated with the development of myelofibrosis is a significant proliferation of vessels showing marked tortuosity and luminal distension, often associated with conspicuous intrasinusoidal haematopoiesis {1214, 1347, 1463}. Osteoid seams or appositional new bone formation in bud-like endophytic plaques may be observed {775, 2204}. In this osteosclerotic phase, the bone may form broad, irregular trabeculae that can occupy >50% of the BM space. With exception of allogeneic stem cell transplantation {1592, 2213}, development of myelofibrosis in PMF is not significantly influenced by treatment modalities, and is obviously related to disease progression {295, 2217, 2218}. In patients with a previously established diagnosis of PMF, the finding of 10–19% blasts in the PB and/or BM and the detection by immunohistochemistry of an increased number of CD34+ cells with cluster formation and/or

Table 2.05 Semiquantitative grading of bone marrow fibrosis (MF).

Grading	Description*
MF - 0	Scattered linear reticulin with no intersections (cross-overs), corresponding to normal bone marrow
MF - 1	Loose network of reticulin with many intersections, especially in perivascular areas
MF - 2	Diffuse and dense increase in reticulin with extensive intersections, occasionally with focal bundles of collagen and/or focal osteosclerosis
MF - 3	Diffuse and dense increase in reticulin with extensive intersections and coarse bundles of collagen, often associated with osteosclerosis

*Fibre density should be assessed only in haematopoietic areas.

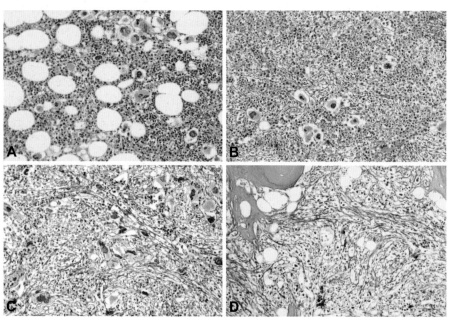

Fig. 2.22 Grading of myelofibrosis (MF) in silver stained bone marrow sections of primary myelofibrosis. **A** MF-0 with no increase in reticulin. **B** MF-1 showing a very loose network of reticulin fibres. **C** MF-2 revealing a more diffuse and dense increase in reticulin fibres and some coarse collagen fibres. **D** MF-3: Coarse bundles of collagen fibres intermingled with dense reticulin accompanied by initial osteosclerosis.

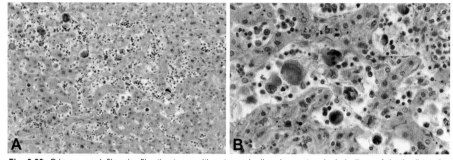

Fig. 2.23 Primary myelofibrosis, fibrotic stage, with extrameduallary haematopoiesis in liver. **A** In the liver, the sinusoids are prominently involved by trilineage proliferation. **B** Megakaryocytes are the hallmark of abnormal intrasinusoidal haematopoiesis.

an a normal endosteal location in the BM {2204, 2209}, indicate an accelerated phase of the disease, whereas ≥20% blasts is considered as acute transformation. Patients with PMF may also present initially in an accelerated phase or an

acute phase. In cases with 20% or more blasts in the PB and/or BM at presentation in which other findings may suggest PMF, the diagnosis of acute leukaemia should be made with only mention of the possible derivation from PMF.

Extramedullary haematopoiesis

The most common site of EMH is the spleen, followed by the liver {1773}. The spleen shows an expansion of the red pulp by erythroid, granulocytic and megakaryocytic cells. Their identification can be aided by immunohistochemistry {1613, 2199}, which also allows an appreciation of an increase in neoangiogenesis {144}. Megakaryocytes are often the most conspicuous component of the EMH. Occasionally large aggregates of megakaryocytes, growing cohesively, can produce macroscopically evident tumoural lesions. In the presence of nodular lesions and, in general, in any advanced stage disease with large amounts of EMH, the possibility of a myeloid sarcoma should be considered and carefully excluded by performing immunohistological studies with CD34 {1773}. The red pulp cords may exhibit fibrosis as well as pooling of platelets. Hepatic sinuses also show prominent EMH, and cirrhosis of the liver may occur {2167}.

Immunophenotype

No abnormal phenotypic features have been reported.

Genetics

No genetic defect specific for PMF has been identified {1832A}. Approximately 50% of patients with PMF exhibit the *JAK2* V617F mutation. Although the presence of the mutation confirms the clonality of the proliferation, it is also found in PV and ET and thus does not distinguish PMF from these MPN {163, 1044, 1064, 1186, 1288}. A functionally similar gain-of-function mutation of *MPL* (*MPL* W515K/L) has been reported in up to 5% of PMF cases, but in occasional cases of ET as well {1689}. Cytogenetic abnormalities occur in up to 30% of patients {630, 1832, 2174}. There is no Philadelphia chromosome or *BCR-ABL1* fusion gene. The presence of either del(13)(q12-22) or der(6)t(1;6) (q21-23;p21.3) is strongly suggestive but not diagnostic of PMF {586}. The most common recurring abnormalities include del (20q), and partial trisomy 1q, although +9 and/or +8 are also reported {630, 1832A, 2174}. Deletions affecting the long arms of chromosomes 7 and 5 occur as well, but may be associated with prior cytotoxic therapy used to treat the myeloproliferative process.

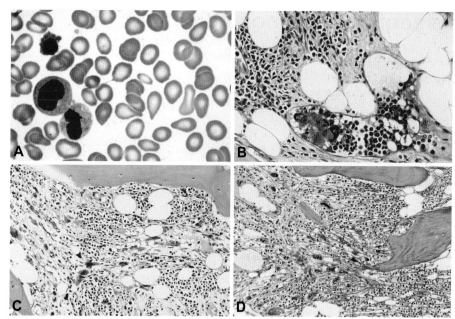

Fig. 2.24 Primary myelofibrosis, fibrotic stage. **A** This peripheral blood smear shows dacryocytes, occasional nucleated red blood cells and immature granulocytes (leukoerythroblastosis). **B** A dilated sinus contains immature haematopoietic elements, most notably megakaryocytes (PAS stain). This intrasinusoidal haematopoiesis together with vascular proliferation is characteristic but not diagnostic of PMF with myeloid metaplasia. **C** Megakaryocytes are often the most conspicuous haematopoietic element in the marrow. Often the cells appear to "stream" through the marrow due to the underlying fibrosis. **D** Marked reticulin and collagen fibrosis associated with a stream-like arrangement of megakaryocytes and initial osteosclerosis is shown (silver stain).

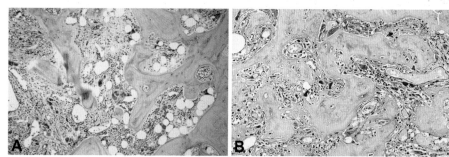

Fig. 2.25 A Primary myelofibrosis, fibrotic stage. Bone marrow biopsy specimen showing hypocellularity, markedly dilated sinuses and severe marrow fibrosis with osteosclerosis, findings typical of advanced stage PMF. **B** PMF with osteomyelosclerosis characterized by broad, irregular bony trabeculae that can occupy up to 50% of the marrow space. Fibrosis, cellular depletion, sinusoidal dilatation and megakaryocytic proliferation are prominent in the intertrabecular areas.

Postulated cell of origin

Haematopoietic stem cell.

Prognosis and predictive factors

The time of survival in patients with PMF ranges from months to decades. The overall prognosis depends on the stage in which PMF is firstly diagnosed {1215, 2204}. The median survival time is approximately 3 to 7 years in patients diagnosed in the fibrotic stage {142, 366, 367, 630, 2167}, which contrasts with a 10- and 15-year relative survival rate of 72% and 59% respectively, in patients diagnosed in the early prefibrotic phase {1215, 1219}. Factors at presentation that adversely affect prognosis include age >70 years, Hb <10 g/dL, platelet count <100x10^6/L, and an abnormal karyotype {142, 143, 366, 630, 1215, 1219, 1832A, 2105, 2174, 2204}. The major causes of morbidity and mortality are BM failure (infection, haemorrhage), thromboembolic events, portal hypertension, cardiac failure and acute leukaemia (AML) {2167}. The reported frequency of AML ranges from 5 to 30% {366, 630, 2167}. Although some cases of AML are related to prior cytotoxic therapy, many have been reported in patients who have never been treated, confirming that AML is part of the natural history of PMF.

Essential thrombocythaemia

J. Thiele
H.M. Kvasnicka
A. Orazi
A. Tefferi
H. Gisslinger

Definition

Essential thrombocythaemia (ET) is a chronic myeloproliferative neoplasm (MPN) that involves primarily the megakaryocytic lineage. It is characterized by sustained thrombocytosis ≥450x10⁹/L in the peripheral blood (PB), increased numbers of large, mature megakaryocytes in the bone marrow (BM), and clinically by episodes of thrombosis and/or haemorrhage. Because there is no known genetic or biological marker specific for ET, other causes for thrombocytosis must be excluded, including other MPN, inflammatory and infectious disorders, haemorrhage and other types of haematopoietic and non-haematopoietic neoplasms. The presence of a *BCR-ABL1* fusion gene excludes the diagnosis of ET.

ICD-O code   9962/3

Synonyms

Primary thrombocytosis; idiopathic thrombocytosis; haemorrhagic thrombocythaemia.

Epidemiology

The true incidence of ET is unknown, but when diagnosed according to the guidelines of the Polycythaemia Vera Study Group (PVSG) {1549}, it is estimated to be 0.6–2.5 per 100 000 persons per year {1055, 1059}. Most cases occur in patients 50–60 years of age, with no major sex predilection. However, a second peak in frequency, particularly in women, occurs at about 30 years of age {705, 902, 1055}. ET can also be seen in children, albeit infrequently {1815}, but must be distinguished from rare cases of hereditary thrombocytosis {585, 2401}.

Sites of involvement

Bone marrow and blood are the principal sites of involvement. The spleen does not show significant extramedullary haematopoiesis (EMH), but is a sequestration site for platelets {705, 902, 2175}.

Etiology

The etiology of ET is unknown.

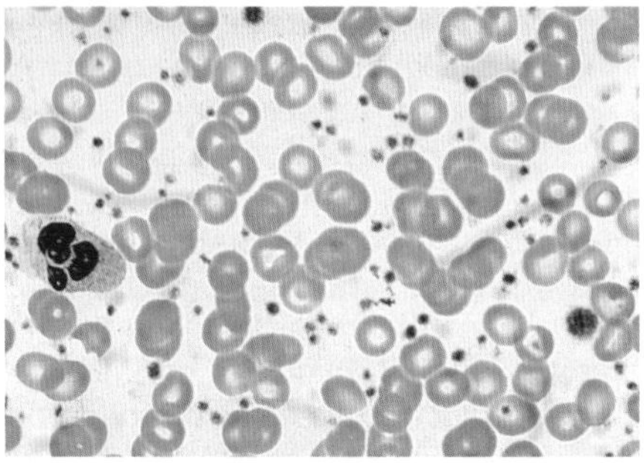

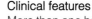

Fig. 2.26 Essential thrombocythaemia, peripheral blood smear. The major abnormality seen is marked thrombocytosis. The platelets show anisocytosis, but are often not remarkably atypical.

Clinical features

More than one half of patients are asymptomatic when a markedly elevated platelet count is discovered fortuitously at the time of a routine PB count {705, 802, 902, 2175}. The remaining patients present with some manifestation of vascular occlusion or haemorrhage {210, 458}. Microvascular occlusion may lead to transient ischaemic attacks, digital ischaemia with paraesthesias, and gangrene {210, 458, 1473, 1829}. Thrombosis of major arteries and veins also occur, and ET may be a cause of splenic or hepatic vein thrombosis as in the Budd-Chiari syndrome. Bleeding occurs most commonly from mucosal surfaces, such as the gastrointestinal tract or upper airway passages {379, 802, 1549, 1955}. If the criteria established by the PVSG for ET are used, mild splenomegaly is present in approximately 50% of patients at diagnosis and hepatomegaly in 15–20% {705, 802, 902, 1549, 2175}. However, when the WHO classification is applied and patients with thrombocytosis associated with the prefibrotic stage of primary myelofibrosis (PMF) are excluded, splenomegaly is seen in only a minority of patients with ET {1215}. Rare patients who meet the criteria for ET have been reported to have nonclonal megakaryocytopoiesis and a lower incidence of thrombotic episodes {901}. Any relationship of such cases to the vast majority of cases of ET that have clonal haematopoiesis is not clear.

Table 2.06 WHO criteria for essential thrombocythaemia (ET): Diagnosis requires meeting all four criteria.

1.   Sustained[a] platelet count ≥450x10⁹/L

2.   Bone marrow biopsy specimen showing proliferation mainly of the megakaryocytic lineage with increased numbers of enlarged, mature megakaryocytes. No significant increase or left-shift of neutrophil granulopoiesis or erythropoiesis

3.   Not meeting WHO criteria for polycythaemia vera,[b] primary myelofibrosis,[c] *BCR-ABL1* positive chronic myelogenous leukaemia[d] or myelodysplastic syndrome[e] or other myeloid neoplasm

4.   Demonstration of *JAK2* V617F or other clonal marker, or in the absence of *JAK2* V617F, no evidence for reactive thrombocytosis[f]

---

[a] Sustained during the work-up process.
[b] Requires the failure of iron replacement therapy to increase haemoglobin level to the polycythaemia vera range in the presence of decreased serum ferritin. Exclusion of polycythaemia vera is based on haemoglobin and haematocrit levels and red cell mass measurement is not required.
[c] Requires the absence of relevant reticulin fibrosis, collagen fibrosis, peripheral blood leukoerythroblastosis, or markedly hypercellular marrow accompanied by megakaryocyte morphology that is typical for primary myelofibrosis including small to large megakaryocytes with an aberrant nuclear/cytoplasmic ratio and hyperchromatic, bulbous or irregularly folded nuclei and dense clustering.
[d] Requires the absence of *BCR-ABL1*.
[e] Requires absence of dyserythropoiesis and dysgranulopoiesis.
[f] Causes of reactive thrombocytosis include iron deficiency, splenectomy, surgery, infection, inflammation, connective tissue disease, metastatic cancer, and lymphoproliferative disorders. However, the presence of a condition associated with reactive thrombocytosis may not exclude the possibility of ET if the first three criteria are met.

In the past, the platelet threshold for the diagnosis of ET was ≥600x10⁹/L {1549}, but some patients have haemorrhagic or thrombotic episodes at lower platelet counts {1272, 1829, 1903}. In order not to compromise the diagnosis in such cases, a number of investigators convincingly argued for a lower platelet threshold for the diagnosis of ET, and the WHO has adopted the recommendation of a platelet count ≥450x10⁹/L, a value that exceeds the 95th percentile for normal platelet counts adjusted for gender and race {1272, 1897, 1903, 2177}. Although this threshold will encompass more patients with ET, it will also include more patients with conditions that mimic ET. It is therefore essential that all criteria listed in Table 2.06 for the diagnosis of ET be met to exclude other neoplastic and non-neoplastic causes of thrombocytosis {2177}. The BM biopsy is particularly helpful in excluding other myeloid neoplasms associated with excessive platelet counts, such as myelodysplastic syndrome (MDS) associated with isolated del (5q), the provisional myelodysplastic/myeloproliferative entity refractory anaemia with ring sideroblasts and thrombocytosis (RARS-T), and the prefibrotic phase of PMF. Although the *JAK2* V617F mutation is found in only 40–50% of cases of ET and is not specific for ET, when present it does exclude reactive thrombocytosis {2177}. Similarly, *in vitro* endogenous erythroid and/or megakaryocytic colony formation, although not specific for ET, also excludes reactive thrombocytosis {594}.

Morphology

The major abnormality seen in the PB is marked thrombocytosis. The platelets often display anisocytosis, ranging from tiny forms to atypical large, giant platelets. Bizarre shapes, pseudopods and agranular platelets may be seen, but are not common. The white blood cell (WBC) count and leukocyte differential are usually normal, although a borderline elevation in the WBC count may occur {705, 802, 902, 2175}. Basophilia is usually absent or minimal {1549}. The red blood cells are usually normocytic and normochromic unless recurrent haemorrhage has caused iron deficiency, in which case they may be hypochromic and microcytic. Leukoerythroblastosis and teardrop-shaped red blood cells are not seen in ET {2175}.

In most cases, the BM core biopsy shows a normocellular or moderately hypercellular BM {775, 2216}. The most striking abnormality is a marked proliferation of megakaryocytes with a predominance of large to giant forms displaying abundant, mature cytoplasm, and deeply lobulated and hyperlobulated (stag-horn like) nuclei. The megakaryocytes are usually dispersed throughout the BM but may occur in loose clusters. Bizarre, highly atypical megakaryocytes, such as those observed in PMF, are not found in ET and if present, the diagnosis of ET should be questioned {712, 796, 2200, 2205}. Proliferation of erythroid precursors may be found in a few cases, particularly if the patient has experienced haemorrhages, but granulocytic proliferation is highly unusual; if present, the increase in granulopoiesis is usually only of mild degree. There is no increase in myeloblasts nor is myelodysplasia observed. The network of reticulin fibres is normal or only minimally increased in ET, and the finding of significant reticulin fibrosis or any collagen fibrosis excludes the diagnosis of ET {712, 775, 796, 2177, 2205, 2216}. Bone marrow aspirate smears also reveal the markedly increased numbers of megakaryocytes of large size with hyperlobulated nuclei and, in the background, large sheets of platelets. Emperipolesis of BM elements is frequently observed in ET, but is not a specific finding. Stainable iron is present in the aspirated BM specimens of 40–70% of patients at diagnosis {1549}.

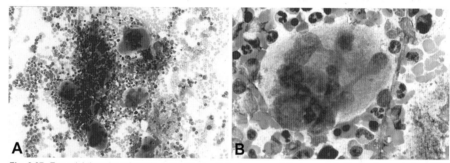

Fig. 2.27 Essential thrombocythaemia, bone marrow aspirate smear. **A** An increase in the number and size of the megakaryocytes. **B** Note the deeply lobulated megakaryocytic nuclei, as well as large pools of platelets. Note that the aspirate smears fail to reveal the overall marrow architecture and distribution of the megakaryocytes that can be only seen in the biopsy.

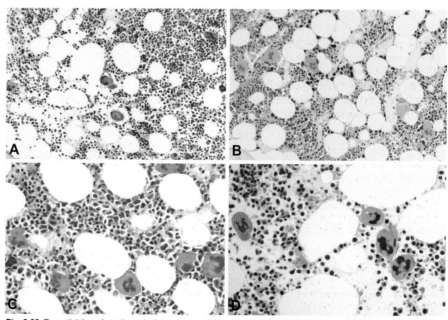

Fig. 2.28 Essential thrombocythaemia, bone marrow biopsy. **A** Normocellular bone marrow with an increased number of large to giant megakaryocytes. **B** No significant increase in erythropoiesis or granulopoiesis (naphthol-ASD-chloroacetate esterase stain: granulocytic cells are stained in red by the reaction product). **C** The enlarged megakaryocytes (PAS staining). They reveal abundant amounts of mature cytoplasm and deeply lobulated and hyperlobulated (stag-horn-like) nuclei. **D** The large to giant megakaryocytes may show arrangement into small, loose clusters.

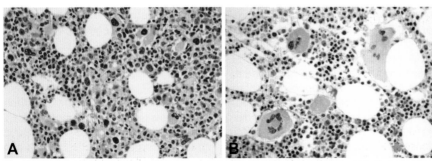

Fig. 2.29 Chronic myelogenous leukaemia (**A**) compared to (**B**) essential thrombocythaemia. CML often presents with an elevated platelet count and, in cases in which the white blood cell count is not markedly elevated, may be confused with ET. The PAS reaction highlights the small size of the megakaryocytes together with their condensed hypolobulated nuclei in CML (**A**). These features allow for an easy separation from ET, in which the megakaryocytes are large to giant and conspicuously hyperlobulated (**B**).

The morphological findings in the BM biopsy are essential to distinguish ET from other MPN, myeloid disorders and reactive conditions that present with sustained thrombocytosis. The finding of even a mild degree of combined granulocytic and erythroid proliferation should raise consideration of prodromal stage polycythaemia vera (PV) {2210}, and the finding of granulocytic proliferation associated with bizarre, highly atypical megakaryocytes should prompt concern for the prefibrotic stage of PMF {2201, 2223}. Significant dyserythropoiesis or dysgranulopoiesis suggest a diagnosis of MDS rather than ET. The large megakaryocytes with hyperlobulated nuclei of ET contrast with the medium-sized monolobated megakaryocytes associated with del (5q) as an isolated chromosomal abnormality in MDS and with the small, dysplastic megakaryocytes associated with the inv(3)(q21q26.2) or t(3;3)(q21;q26.2) chromosomal abnormality. Lastly, some patients with chronic myelogenous leukaemia (CML) may initially present with thrombocytosis without leukocytosis and can mimic ET clinically. Although the large megakaryocytes of ET can be easily distinguished from the small "dwarf" megakaryocytes of CML, cytogenetic and/ or molecular genetic analysis to exclude a *BCR-ABL1* fusion gene is recommended for all patients in whom a diagnosis of ET is considered {1841}.

Immunophenotype
No aberrant phenotype has been described.

Genetics
No molecular genetic or cytogenetic abnormality specific for ET is known. Approximately 40–50% of cases carry the *JAK2* V617F or a functionally similar mutation {163, 1044, 1064, 1186, 1288}. These mutations are not specific for ET and are found in PV and PMF as well. A gain-of-function mutation of *MPL*, *MPL* W515K/L, has been reported in 1% of cases of ET {1689}. None of these mutations are found in cases of reactive thrombocytosis. An abnormal karyotype is found in only 5–10% of patients with ET when diagnosed according to the previous PVSG criteria {1549}. There is no consistent abnormality, but those reported include +8, abnormalities of 9q, and del(20q) {939, 1682}. Although isolated del(5q) has also been reported in ET, careful morphologic examination is required to distinguish such cases from MDS associated with this abnormality {1682}.

Postulated cell of origin
Haematopoietic stem cell.

Prognosis and predictive factors
ET is an indolent disorder characterized by long symptom-free intervals, interrupted by occasional life-threatening thromboembolic or haemorrhagic episodes {705, 802, 902, 1215, 1549, 2175}. Although after many years a few patients with ET may develop BM fibrosis associated with myeloid metaplasia (EMH), such progression is uncommon {297, 775, 1189, 2220}. Precise diagnostic guidelines for diagnosing post-ET MF are given in Table 2.07. Strict adherence to those and other WHO criteria {143A, 2177} is necessary to prevent diagnostic confusion associated with early PMF accompanied by thrombocytosis {365}. Transformation of ET to acute myeloid leukaemia or MDS occurs in <5% of patients, and when it does occur is likely related to previous cytotoxic therapy {705, 802, 902, 1800}. Median survivals of 10–15 years are commonly reported. Because ET usually occurs late in middle age, the life expectancy is near normal for many patients {1215, 1702, 2200, 2430}. Finally, it is noteworthy that the majority of clinical studies are based on previous diagnostic guidelines {1549} that fail to differentiate clearly between the early prefibrotic stages of PMF with accompanying thrombocytosis and ET according to the WHO classification {1215, 2200, 2205}. A substantial difference in overall prognosis has been reported when these two different classification systems are applied to the same patient population {1215}.

Table 2.07 WHO diagnostic criteria for post-essential thrombocythaemia myelofibrosis (post-ET MF).

Required criteria
1. Documentation of a previous diagnosis of WHO-defined essential thrombocythaemia
2. Bone marrow fibrosis grade 2–3 (on 0–3 scale) or grade 3–4 (on 0–4 scale)

Additional criteria (2 are required)
1. Anaemia* or ≥2 g/dL decrease from baseline haemoglobin level
2. A leukoerythroblastic peripheral blood picture
3. Increasing splenomegaly defined as either an increase in palpable splenomegaly of >5 cm from baseline (distance from the left costal margin) or the appearance of newly palpable splenomegaly
4. Increased LDH (above reference level)
5. Development of >1 of 3 constitutional symptoms: >10% weight loss in 6 months, night sweats, unexplained fever (>37.5 °C)

*Below the reference range for appropriate age, gender, and altitude considerations.

Chronic eosinophilic leukaemia, not otherwise specified

B.J. Bain
D.G. Gilliland
J.W. Vardiman
H.-P. Horny

Definition

Chronic eosinophilic leukaemia (CEL) is a myeloproliferative neoplasm (MPN) in which an autonomous, clonal proliferation of eosinophil precursors results in persistently increased numbers of eosinophils in the peripheral blood (PB), bone marrow (BM) and peripheral tissues, with eosinophilia being the dominant haematological abnormality. Organ damage occurs as a result of leukaemic infiltration or the release of cytokines, enzymes or other proteins by the eosinophils. Chronic eosinophilic leukaemia, not otherwise specified, (CEL, NOS) excludes patients with a Philadelphia (Ph) chromosome, *BCR-ABL1* fusion gene or rearrangement of *PDGFRA*, *PDGFRB* or *FGFR1*.

In CEL, NOS the eosinophil count is ≥1.5x10^9/L in the blood. There are fewer than 20% blasts in the PB or BM. To make a diagnosis of CEL, there should be evidence for clonality of the eosinophils or an increase in myeloblasts in the PB or BM. In many cases however, it is impossible to prove clonality of the eosinophils, in which case, if there is no increase in blast cells, the diagnosis of "idiopathic hypereosinophilic syndrome" is made. The idiopathic hypereosinophilic syndrome (idiopathic HES) is defined as eosinophilia (≥1.5x10^9/L) persisting for at least 6 months, for which no underlying cause can be found, and which is associated with signs of organ involvement and dysfunction {443, 2382}; there is no evidence for eosinophil clonality. It is a diagnosis of exclusion, and may include some cases of true eosinophilic leukaemia that cannot currently be recognized, as well as cases of cytokine-driven eosinophilia that are due to the abnormal release of eosinophil growth factors, e.g. interleukin (IL) 2, 3 and 5, for unknown reasons {128, 443, 1971, 2072, 2382}.

ICD-O code   9964/3

Synonym

Hypereosinophilic syndrome (not recommended).

Epidemiology

Due to the previous difficulty in distinguishing CEL from idiopathic HES, the true incidence of these diseases is unknown, although they are rare. Many patients who would until recently have been classified as having idiopathic HES can now be shown to have CEL associated with a *FIP1L1-PDGFRA* fusion gene {466}. Since this condition occurs mainly in adult men, the male dominance and the peak incidence in the fourth decade previously described in "HES" {443, 1971, 2072, 2382} are now explained, at least in part. The epidemiological features of cases of HES that remain idiopathic have not yet been clearly defined.

Sites of involvement

CEL is a multisystem disorder. The PB and BM are always involved. Tissue infiltration by the eosinophils, and release of cytokines and humoral factors from the eosinophil granules lead to tissue damage in a number of organs, but the heart, lungs, central nervous system, skin and gastrointestinal tract are commonly involved. Evidence of splenic and hepatic involvement is present in 30–50% of patients {443, 1971, 2072, 2382}.

Clinical features

Sometimes eosinophilia is detected incidentally in patients who are otherwise asymptomatic. In other patients, constitutional symptoms, such as fever, fatigue, cough, angioedema, muscle pains, pruritus and diarrhoea are found. The most serious clinical findings relate to endomyocardial fibrosis, with ensuing restrictive cardiomegaly. Scarring of the mitral/tricuspid valves leads to valvular regurgitation and formation of intracardiac thrombi, which may embolize to the brain or elsewhere. Peripheral neuropathy, central nervous system dysfunction, pulmonary symptoms due to lung infiltration, and

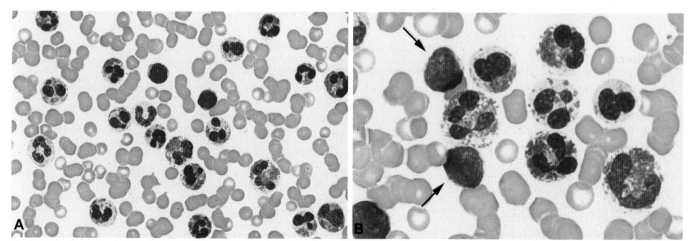

Fig. 2.30 Reactive eosinophilia in a patient with ALL. **A** Peripheral blood of a patient with ALL. The elevation of the white blood cell count is due primarily to eosinophils, with only an occasional lymphoblast. **B** The lymphoblasts (arrows) are clearly appreciated in the blood smear.

rheumatological findings are other frequent manifestations {443, 1971, 2072, 2382}.

Morphology

In CEL, NOS the most striking feature in the PB is eosinophilia, there being mainly mature eosinophils with only small numbers of eosinophilic myelocytes or promyelocytes {443, 710, 1200, 1971, 2072, 2382}. There may be a range of eosinophil abnormalities, including sparse granulation with clear areas of cytoplasm, cytoplasmic vacuolation, nuclear hypersegmentation or hyposegmentation, and enlarged size. These changes may be seen in cases of reactive as well as of neoplastic eosinophilia, however, and are thus not very helpful in deciding whether a case is likely to be CEL {128}. Neutrophilia often accompanies the eosinophilia, and some cases have monocytosis. Mild basophilia has been reported {710}. Blast cells may be present but are less than 20%.

The BM is hypercellular due in part to eosinophilic proliferation {289, 443, 710, 1200, 2382}. In most cases, eosinophil maturation is orderly, without a disproportionate increase in myeloblasts. Charcot-Leyden crystals are often present. Erythropoiesis and megakaryocytopoiesis are usually normal. The finding of increased numbers of myeloblasts (5–19%) supports a diagnosis of CEL, as does the observation of dysplastic features in other cell lineages. Marrow fibrosis is seen in some cases {289, 710}. Any tissue may show eosinophilic infiltration and Charcot-Leyden crystals are often present. Fibrosis is a common finding, and is caused by the degranulation of the eosinophils with the release of eosinophil basic protein and eosinophil cationic proteins {443, 1931, 2382}.

Differential diagnosis

Diagnosis requires positive evidence of the leukaemic nature of the condition and exclusion of cases of MPN with rearrangement of *PDGFRA*, *PDGFRB* or *FGFR1*. The diagnostic process often starts with exclusion of reactive eosinophilia. A detailed history, physical examination, blood count and blood film are essential. Conditions to be excluded include parasitic infection, allergies, pulmonary diseases such as Loeffler's syndrome, cyclical eosinophilia, skin diseases such as angiolymphoid hyperplasia, collagen vascular disorders and Kimura's

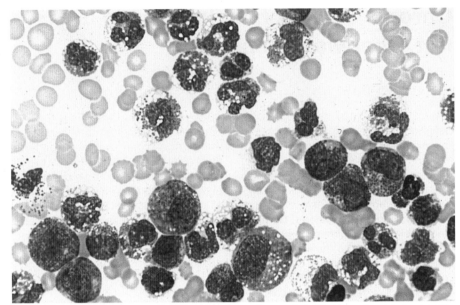

Fig. 2.31 Chronic eosinophilic leukaemia. Peripheral blood smear from a patient with a history of persistent eosinophilia. Immature as well as mature eosinophils are present. Cytogenetic analysis showed trisomy of chromosome 10.

disease {128, 1931}. In addition, a number of neoplastic disorders such as T-cell lymphoma, Hodgkin lymphoma, systemic mastocytosis, acute lymphoblastic leukaemia and other MPN may be associated with abnormal release of IL2, IL3, IL5 or GM-CSF and a secondary eosinophilia that mimics CEL {128, 1168, 1172, 1450, 1616, 1924, 1931, 2461}; in systemic mastocytosis there can also be eosinophils belonging to the neoplastic clone. The BM should be carefully inspected for any process which might explain the eosinophilia as a secondary reaction, such as vasculitis, lymphoma, acute lymphoblastic leukaemia, systemic mastocytosis or granulomatous disorders. Some cases of persistent eosinophilia are due to the abnormal release of cytokines by T-cells that

are immunophenotypically aberrant and that may or may not be clonal {286, 1156, 2024}. When such an aberrant T-cell population is present, the case is not CEL nor is it idiopathic HES. If the monocyte count is >1x10⁹/L a diagnosis of chronic myelomonocytic leukaemia with eosinophilia may be more appropriate, but if there are dysplastic features and >10% neutrophil precursors in the PB and no monocytosis, a diagnosis of atypical chronic myeloid leukaemia with eosinophilia should similarly be considered.

The distinction between CEL, NOS, and idiopathic HES is important. Idiopathic HES can be diagnosed only in fully investigated patients and only when (i) there is an eosinophil count of ≥1.5x10⁹/L persisting for at least 6 months; (ii) reactive

Table 2.08 Diagnostic criteria of chronic eosinophilic leukaemia (myeloproliferative neoplasm with prominent eosinophilia).

1. There is eosinophilia (eosinophil count ≥1.5x10⁹/L)
2. There is no Ph chromosome or *BCR-ABL1* fusion gene or other myeloproliferative neoplasm (PV, ET, PMF) or MDS/MPN (CMML or aCML)
3. There is no t(5;12)(q31-35;p13) or other rearrangement of *PDGFRB*
4. There is no *FIP1L1-PDGFRA* fusion gene or other rearrangement of *PDGFRA*
5. There is no rearrangement of *FGFR1*
6. The blast cell count in the peripheral blood and bone marrow is less than 20% and there is no inv(16)(p13.1q22) or t(16;16)(p13.1;q22) or other feature diagnostic of AML
7. There is a clonal cytogenetic or molecular genetic abnormality, or blast cells are more than 2% in the peripheral blood or more than 5% in the bone marrow

*If a patient has eosinophilia but these criteria are not met the diagnosis may be reactive eosinophilia, idiopathic hypereosinophilia or idiopathic hypereosinophilic syndrome.

eosinophilia is excluded by appropriate thorough investigation; (iii) AML, MPN, MDS, MPN/MDS and systemic mastocytosis are excluded; (iv) a cytokine-producing, immunophenotypically-aberrant, T-cell population is excluded; (v) and there is tissue damage as a result of hypereosinophilia. If criteria i-iv are met but there is no tissue damage, the appropriate diagnosis is idiopathic hypereosinophilia.

Patients in whom a diagnosis of idiopathic hypereosinophilia or idiopathic HES is made should be kept under regular review since evidence may subsequently emerge that the condition is leukaemic in nature. Treatment may also be necessary.

Cytochemistry
Cytochemical stains can be used to identify eosinophils but they are not essential for diagnosis. Partial degranulation can lead to eosinophils having reduced peroxidase content.

Immunophenotype
No specific immunophenotypic abnormality has been reported in CEL.

Genetics
No single or specific cytogenetic or molecular genetic abnormality has been identified in CEL, NOS. Cases with rearrangement of *PDGFRA*, *PDGFRB* or *FGFR1* are specifically excluded. The detection of a Ph chromosome or *BCR-ABL1* fusion gene indicates one of the rare cases of chronic myelogenous leukaemia with dominant eosinophilia, rather than CEL. Even when eosinophilia occurs in conjunction with a chromosomal abnormality that is usually myeloid neoplasm-associated, it may be difficult to decide

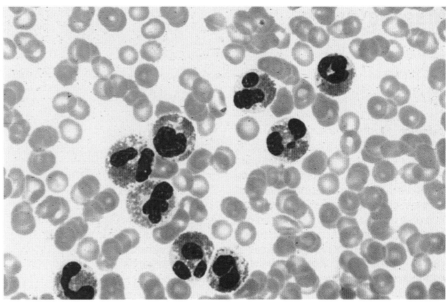

Fig. 2.32 Idiopathic HES. A blood smear of a patient with cardiac failure, leukocytosis and hypereosinophilia.

whether the eosinophils are part of the clonal process, since reactive eosinophilia can occur in patients with myeloid neoplasms {711}. However, the finding of a recurring karyotypic abnormality that is usually observed in myeloid disorders, such as +8 or i(17q), does support the diagnosis of CEL {128, 1692}. Occasional patients have a *JAK2* mutation {1064}. X-linked polymorphism analysis of the *PGK* or *HUMARA* genes can occasionally be used in female patients to demonstrate clonality {392, 1350}.

Postulated cell of origin
The cell of origin is a haemopoietic stem cell, but the lineage potential of the affected cell may be variable.

Prognosis and predictive factors
Survival is quite variable. In some series in which patients with idiopathic HES as well as those with probable eosinophilic leukaemia were included, 5-year survival rates approached 80% {443, 1971, 2072, 2382}. Marked splenomegaly, as well as the finding of blasts in the blood or increased blasts in the BM, cytogenetic abnormalities and dysplastic features in other myeloid lineages have been reported to be unfavourable prognostic findings {443, 1971, 2072, 2382}.

Mastocytosis

H.-P. Horny*
D.D. Metcalfe
J.M. Bennett
B.J. Bain

C. Akin
L. Escribano
P. Valent

Definition

Mastocytosis is due to a clonal, neoplastic proliferation of mast cells that accumulate in one or more organ systems. It is characterized by the presence of multifocal compact clusters or cohesive aggregates/infiltrates of abnormal mast cells. The disorder is heterogeneous, ranging from skin lesions that may spontaneously regress to highly aggressive neoplasms associated with multiorgan failure and short survival (Table 2.09). Subtypes of mastocytosis are recognized mainly by the distribution of the disease and clinical manifestations. In cutaneous mastocytosis (CM), the mast cell infiltration remains confined to the skin, whereas systemic mastocytosis (SM) is characterized by involvement of at least one extracutaneous organ with or without evidence of skin lesions. Mastocytosis should be strictly separated from mast cell hyperplasia or mast cell activation states without morphological and/or molecular abnormalities that characterize the neoplastic proliferation.

ICD-O codes

Cutaneous mastocytosis (urticaria pigmentosa)	9740/1
Diffuse cutaneous mastocytosis	9740/1
Solitary mastocytoma of skin	9740/1
Indolent systemic mastocytosis	9741/1
Systemic mastocytosis with AHNMD**	9741/3
Aggressive systemic mastocytosis	9741/3
Mast cell leukaemia	9742/3
Mast cell sarcoma	9740/3
Extracutaneous mastocytoma	9740/1

**AHNMD, associated haematological clonal non-mast cell disorder

Synonym
Mast cell disease.

Epidemiology
Mastocytosis may occur at any age. Cutaneous mastocytosis is most common in children and may be present at birth. About 50% of afflicted children develop typical skin lesions before 6 months of age. In adults, CM is less frequently diagnosed than in children {2055, 2436}. A slight male predominance has been reported in CM. SM is generally diagnosed after the second decade of life; the male to female ratio has been reported to vary from 1:1 to 1:3 {181, 1465, 1694}.

Sites of involvement
Approximately 80% of patients with mastocytosis have evidence of skin involvement {1687}. In SM the bone marrow (BM) is almost always involved, so morphological and molecular analysis of a BM biopsy specimen is strongly recommended to confirm or exclude the diagnosis {287, 290, 971, 1275}. Rarely, the peripheral blood (PB) shows leukaemia due to significant numbers of circulating mast cells {972, 1484}. Other organs that may be involved in SM include the spleen, lymph nodes, liver and gastrointestinal tract mucosa, but any tissue may be affected {287, 966, 968, 973, 1275, 1334, 1466, 1694}. Skin lesions occur in more than 50% of SM patients, and are more often observed in those with an indolent course.

Table 2.09 Classification of mastocytosis.

1. Cutaneous mastocytosis (CM)
2. Indolent systemic mastocytosis (ISM)
3. Systemic mastocytosis with associated clonal haematological non-mast-cell lineage disease (SM-AHNMD)
4. Aggressive systemic mastocytosis (ASM)
5. Mast cell leukaemia (MCL)
6. Mast cell sarcoma (MCS)
7. Extracutaneous mastocytoma

For the participants of the Year 2000 Working Group Conference on Mastocytosis who were involved in the definition of criteria and WHO classification of mastocytosis: C Akin, KF Austen, JM Bennett, RD Brunning, L Escribano, H-P Horny, K Lennert, CY Li, JB Longley, G Marone, DD Metcalfe, R Nunez, MR Parwaresch, LB Schwartz, K Sotlar, WR Sperr, P Valent, JW Vardiman, K Wolff.

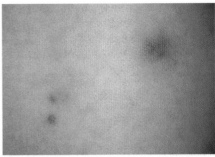
Fig. 2.33 Cutaneous mastocytosis. Darier's sign. The skin lesions of all forms of cutaneous mastocytosis may urticate when stroked. A palpable wheal appears a few moments after the physical stimulation, due to the release of histamine from the mast cells.

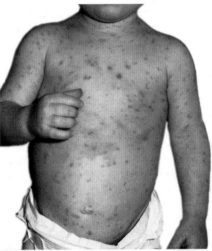
Fig. 2.34 Cutaneous mastocytosis. Numerous typical macular and maculopapular pigmented lesions of urticaria pigmentosa in a young child.

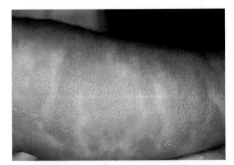
Fig. 2.35 Diffuse cutaneous mastocytosis. Thickened, reddish "peau chagrine" lesions characteristic of diffuse cutaneous mastocytosis. This variant occurs almost exclusively in children.

In contrast, aggressive variants of SM often present without skin lesions {971}. However, some SM patients without skin lesions may on occasion present with an indolent form of SM, most often isolated BM mastocytosis.

Clinical features

Cutaneous mastocytosis includes several distinct clinico-histopathological entities. Lesions of all forms of CM may urticate when stroked ("Darier's sign") and most show intraepidermal accumulation of melanin pigment. The term "urticaria pigmentosa" macroscopically describes these two clinical features. Blistering ("bullous mastocytosis") does not represent a separate subtype but rather an exaggeration of urticaria. Blistering is usually seen in patients less than 3 years of age, and may be associated with all forms of paediatric CM {1687, 2055, 2436}.

Symptoms in SM at presentation have been grouped into 4 categories: 1) constitutional symptoms (fatigue, weight loss, fever, diaphoresis), 2) skin manifestations (pruritus, urticaria, dermatographism), 3) mediator-related systemic events (abdominal pain, gastrointestinal distress, flushing, syncope, headache, hypotension, tachycardia, respiratory symptoms) and 4) musculoskeletal complaints (bone pain, osteopenia/osteoporosis, fractures, arthralgias, myalgias) {181, 2290}. These symptoms range from mild in many patients to severe, life-threatening mediator-related events in others. Symptoms may also be related to organ impairment (due to mast cell infiltrates), particularly in patients with high-grade aggressive or leukaemic disease variants.

Physical findings in SM at diagnosis may include splenomegaly (often minimal), while lymphadenopathy and hepatomegaly are found at significantly lower frequencies {966, 968, 973, 1275, 1466}. Organomegaly is often absent in the most common variant, indolent systemic mastocytosis (ISM), but is usually present, along with impaired organ function, in aggressive systemic mastocytosis (ASM) and in leukaemic variants. Severe systemic symptoms may occur in patients with ISM following extensive release and generation of biochemical mediators including histamine, eicosanoids, proteases and heparin. For example, gastrointestinal symptoms such as peptic ulcer disease or diarrhoea are more commonly attributed to release of biologically active mediators than to

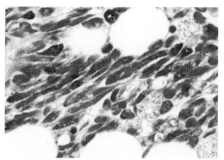

Fig. 2.36 Indolent systemic mastocytosis. Dense infiltrate consisting mainly of spindle-shaped slightly hypogranular mast cells.

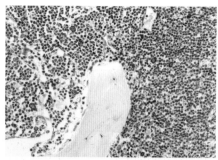

Fig. 2.37 Mast cell hyperplasia (round, loosely scattered, mature-appearing cells) in a case of lymphoplasmacytic lymphoma with packed bone marrow infiltration.

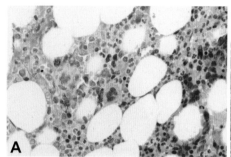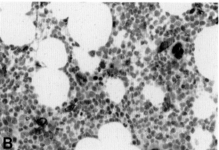

Fig. 2.38 Indolent systemic mastocytosis. **A** Loosely scattered spindle-shaped hypogranular mast cells without tendency to aggregate. Diagnosis is facilitated when additional immunostaining and molecular analysis are performed. **B** Immunostaining with CD25 shows an atypical immunophenotype of mast cells with membrane associated reactivity.

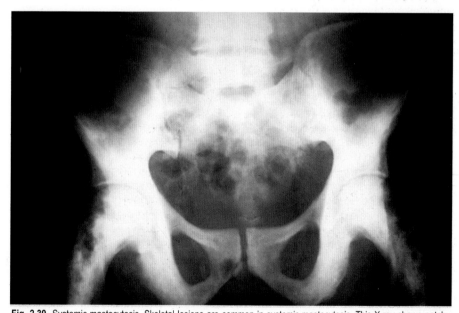

Fig. 2.39 Systemic mastocytosis. Skeletal lesions are common in systemic mastocytosis. This X-ray shows patchy osteosclerosis, osteoporosis and multiple lytic lesions in the femur.

infiltration of the gastrointestinal tract by excessive numbers of abnormal mast cells {181, 1334, 2288}.

Haematological abnormalities in SM include anaemia, leukocytosis, blood eosinophilia (a frequent finding), neutropenia, and thrombocytopenia {130, 287, 713, 971, 1162, 1687}. Bone marrow failure is encountered only in patients with aggressive or leukaemic disease variants. Significant numbers of circulating mast cells are rarely observed and are suggestive of mast cell leukaemia {2290}. In up to 30% of cases with SM, an associated, clonal haematological, non-mast cell lineage disease (AHNMD) is diagnosed before,

Table 2.10 Criteria for cutaneous and systemic mastocytosis.

Cutaneous mastocytosis (CM)*

Skin lesions demonstrating the typical clinical findings of UP/MPCM, diffuse cutaneous mastocytosis or solitary mastocytoma, and typical histological infiltrates of mast cells in a multifocal or diffuse pattern in an adequate skin biopsy. In addition, a diagnostic prerequisite for the diagnosis of CM is the absence of features/criteria sufficient to establish the diagnosis of SM.

*Updated and slightly modified criteria for skin involvement in mastocytosis have recently been suggested {47A}.

Systemic mastocytosis (SM)

The diagnosis of SM can be made when the major criterion and one minor criterion or at least three minor criteria are present.

Major criterion:

Multifocal, dense infiltrates of mast cells (≥15 mast cells in aggregates) detected in sections of bone marrow and/or other extracutaneous organ(s).

Minor criteria:

1. In biopsy sections of bone marrow or other extracutaneous organs, >25% of the mast cells in the infiltrate are spindle-shaped or have atypical morphology or, of all mast cells in bone marrow aspirate smears, >25% are immature or atypical.

2. Detection of an activating point mutation at codon 816 of *KIT* in bone marrow, blood or another extracutaneous organ.

3. Mast cells in bone marrow, blood or other extracutaneous organs express CD2 and/or CD25 in addition to normal mast cell markers.

4. Serum total tryptase persistently exceeds 20 ng/mL (unless there is an associated clonal myeloid disorder, in which case this parameter is not valid).

---

simultaneously with, or after the diagnosis of SM. In principle, any defined myeloid or lymphatic malignancy may occur as the AHNMD, but myeloid neoplasms predominate, and chronic myelomonocytic leukaemia (CMML) is most common {971, 975, 2056, 2066, 2095, 2290}. In patients with SM-AHNMD, clinical symptoms and disease course relate both to the associated haematological disorder and to SM {1977, 2290}.

Serum tryptase levels are used in the evaluation and monitoring of patients with mastocytosis. The finding of a persistently elevated serum total tryptase >20 ng/mL is suggestive of SM and is used as a "minor" criterion for diagnosis, unless there is an associated clonal myeloid non-mast cell disorder, in which case this parameter is not valid. Serum tryptase levels are normal to slightly elevated in most patients with CM and have also been found to be independent of the patient's tryptase haplotype {1977, 2290}.

Morphology

The diagnosis of mastocytosis requires demonstration of multifocal clusters or cohesive aggregates/infiltrates of mast cells in an adequate BM biopsy specimen (Table 2.10). The histological pattern of the mast cell infiltrate may vary according to the tissue sampled {130, 290, 713, 966, 968, 973, 1162, 1466}. A diffuse interstitial infiltration pattern is defined as loosely scattered mast cells in the absence of compact aggregates. It must be noted, however, that this pattern is also observed in reactive mast cell hyperplasia and in cases of myelomastocytic leukaemia, a term used for cases with advanced myeloid neoplasms in whom elevated numbers of immature atypical mast cells are found, but criteria for SM are not met {2065}. In patients with the diffuse infiltration pattern it is therefore impossible to establish the diagnosis of mastocytosis without additional studies including the demonstration of an aberrant immunophenotype and/or detection of an activating point mutation in *KIT* {977, 978, 1198, 2056, 2057}. In contrast, the presence of multifocal compact mast cell infiltrates or a diffuse-compact mast cell infiltration pattern is highly compatible with the diagnosis of mastocytosis during first inspection. However, additional immunohistochemical and molecular studies are strongly recommended even in these cases.

In tissue sections stained with H&E, normal/reactive mast cells usually are loosely scattered throughout the sample, and display round to oval nuclei with clumped chromatin, a low nuclear/cytoplasmic ratio, and nucleoli that are absent or indistinct. The mast cell cytoplasm is abundant and usually filled with small, faintly visible granules. Dense aggregates of mast cells are only very exceptionally detected in reactive states or in patients treated with stem cell factor (SCF) {1275, 1694, 2290}. In smear preparations, mast cells are readily visible in Romanowsky stains as medium-sized round or oval cells with plentiful cytoplasm, containing densely packed metachromatic granules and round or oval nuclei. In normal/reactive states, mast cells are easily distinguished from the smaller metachromatic

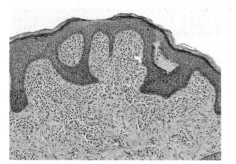

Fig. 2.40 Typical skin lesion of a child with urticaria pigmentosa. Aggregates of mast cells fill the papillary dermis and extend as sheets into the reticular dermis.

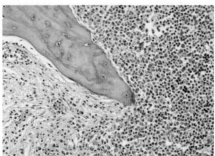

Fig. 2.41 Systemic mastocytosis. One region of the bone marrow is occupied by mast cells with fibrosis, whereas the adjacent area is hypercellular, with panmyelosis.

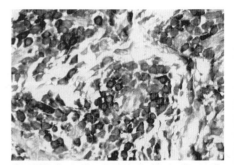

Fig. 2.42 Systemic mastocytosis. Mast cells usually demonstrate metachromatic granules when stained with Giemsa or, as in this case, with toluidine blue.

Table 2.11 Subclassification of cutaneous mastocytosis.

1. Urticaria pigmentosa (UP)/maculopapular cutaneous mastocytosis (MPCM)
2. Diffuse cutaneous mastocytosis
3. Solitary mastocytoma of skin

basophils which have segmented nuclei, and larger and fewer granules. With enzyme cytochemistry, mast cells react strongly with naphthol-ASD-chloroacetate esterase (CAE) but do not express myeloperoxidase. In mastocytosis, the cytology of mast cells varies, but abnormal cytologic features are almost always detected, including marked spindling and hypogranularity {2290}.

Cytomorphological atypia is pronounced in high-grade lesions of mastocytosis, with the occurrence of metachromatic blast cells being a usual feature of mast cell leukaemia {2290}. The finding of frequent mast cells with bi- or multilobated nuclei ("promastocytes") usually indicates an aggressive mast cell proliferation, although these cells may be seen at low frequency in other subtypes of the disease {2290}. Mitotic figures in mast cells do occur, but are infrequent even in the aggressive or leukaemic variants of SM.

To assess mast cell numbers with conventional staining procedures, Giemsa or toluidine blue are employed to detect the metachromatic mast cell granules and CAE is also helpful {2290}. However, the most specific methods for identification of immature or atypical mast cells in tissue sections utilize immunohistochemical staining for tryptase/chymase and CD117 and, for neoplastic mast cells, CD2 and CD25. The morphologic features of the common subtypes of mastocytosis are described below.

Cutaneous mastocytosis (CM)

The diagnosis of CM requires the demonstration of typical clinical findings and histological proof of abnormal mast cell infiltration of the dermis (Table 2.10). In cases of isolated CM, there is no evidence of systemic involvement using such parameters as elevated levels of total serum tryptase or organomegaly. Recently, consensus criteria for the diagnosis of CM have been further refined, and three major variants of CM are now recognized (Table 2.11) {2286}.

Table 2.12 Criteria for variants of systemic mastocytosis.

1. Indolent systemic mastocytosis (ISM)
Meets criteria for SM. No "C" findings (see below). No evidence of an associated non-mast cell lineage clonal haematological malignancy/disorder (AHNMD). In this variant, the mast cell burden is low and skin lesions are almost invariably present.

1.1 Bone marrow mastocytosis
As above (ISM) with bone marrow involvement, but no skin lesions.

1.2 Smouldering systemic mastocytosis
As above (ISM), but with 2 or more "B" findings but no "C" findings.

2. Systemic mastocytosis with associated clonal haematological non-mast cell lineage disease (SM-AHNMD)
Meets criteria for SM and criteria for an associated, clonal haematological non-mast cell lineage disorder, AHNMD (MDS, MPN, AML, lymphoma, or other haematological neoplasm that meets the criteria for a distinct entity in the WHO classification).

3. Aggressive systemic mastocytosis (ASM)
Meets criteria for SM. One or more "C" findings. No evidence of mast cell leukaemia. Usually without skin lesions.

3.1 Lymphadenopathic mastocytosis with eosinophilia
Progressive lymphadenopathy with peripheral blood eosinophilia, often with extensive bone involvement, and hepatosplenomegaly, but usually without skin lesions. Cases with rearrangement of *PDGFRA* are excluded.

4. Mast cell leukaemia (MCL)
Meets criteria for SM. Bone marrow biopsy shows a diffuse infiltration, usually compact, by atypical, immature mast cells. Bone marrow aspirate smears show 20% or more mast cells. In typical MCL, mast cells account for 10% or more of peripheral blood white cells. Rare variant: aleukaemic mast cell leukaemia – as above, but <10% of white blood cells are mast cells. Usually without skin lesions.

5. Mast cell sarcoma (MCS)
Unifocal mast cell tumour. No evidence of SM. Destructive growth pattern. High-grade cytology.

6. Extracutaneous mastocytoma
Unifocal mast cell tumour. No evidence of SM. No skin lesions. Non-destructive growth pattern. Low-grade cytology.

"B" findings
1. Bone marrow biopsy showing >30% infiltration by mast cells (focal, dense aggregates) and/or serum total tryptase level >200 ng/mL.
2. Signs of dysplasia or myeloproliferation, in non-mast cell lineage(s), but insufficient criteria for definitive diagnosis of a haematopoietic neoplasm (AHNMD), with normal or only slightly abnormal blood counts.
3. Hepatomegaly without impairment of liver function, and/or palpable splenomegaly without hypersplenism, and/or lymphadenopathy on palpation or imaging.

"C" findings
1. Bone marrow dysfunction manifested by one or more cytopenia (ANC <1.0x10^9/L, Hb <10 g/dL, or platelets <100x10^9/L), but no obvious non-mast cell haematopoietic malignancy.
2. Palpable hepatomegaly with impairment of liver function, ascites and/or portal hypertension.
3. Skeletal involvement with large osteolytic lesions and/or pathological fractures.
4. Palpable splenomegaly with hypersplenism.
5. Malabsorption with weight loss due to GI mast cell infiltrates.

Urticaria pigmentosa (UP)/maculopapular cutaneous mastocytosis (MPCM)

This is the most frequent form of CM. In children, the lesions of UP tend to be larger and papular. Histopathology typically reveals aggregates of spindle-shaped mast cells filling the papillary dermis and extending as sheets and aggregates into the reticular dermis, often in perivascular and periadnexal positions {2436}. A sub-variant, usually occurring in young children, presents as non-pigmented, plaque-forming lesions. In adults, the lesions are disseminated, and tend to be red or brown-red and macular or maculopapular. Histopathology of adult UP tends to reveal

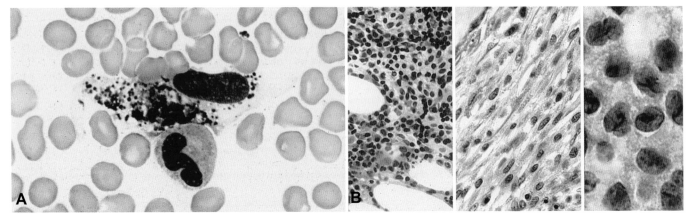

Fig. 2.43 A Bone marrow smear of a patient with indolent systemic mastocytosis. The cell is atypical, with an indented nucleus in an eccentric location, and cytoplasm that shows an elongated extrusion with irregular distribution of granules. **B** Systemic mastocytosis. The cells may have bland nuclei with moderate amounts of pale cytoplasm, spindled shapes that resemble fibroblasts, or lobulated nuclei with abundant clear cytoplasm. The latter cells may resemble monocytes or histiocytes, and are more commonly seen in aggressive mast cell lesions.

fewer mast cells than observed in children. The number of lesional mast cells may sometimes overlap with the upper range of mast cell numbers found in normal or inflamed skin. In some cases, examination of multiple biopsies and immunohistochemical analysis may be necessary to establish the diagnosis of CM {2286, 2436}.

Diffuse cutaneous mastocytosis

This clinically remarkable subvariant of CM is much less frequent than UP and presents almost exclusively in childhood. Here the skin is diffusely thickened and may have a *peau chagrine* or *peau d'orange* (orange peel) appearance. There are no individual lesions. In patients with clinically less obvious infiltration of the skin, the biopsy usually shows a band-like infiltrate of mast cells in the papillary and upper reticular dermis. In massively infiltrated skin, the histological picture may be the same as that seen in solitary mastocytoma {2055, 2436}.

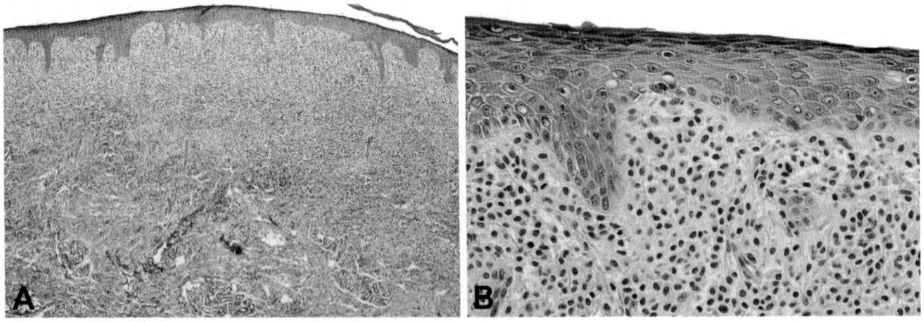

Mastocytoma of skin

This occurs as a single lesion, almost exclusively in infants, without predilection of site. The histologic picture is one of sheets of mature-appearing highly metachromatic mast cells with abundant cytoplasm that densely infiltrate the papillary and reticular dermis. These mast cell infiltrates may extend into the subcutaneous tissues {1154}. Cytological atypia is not detected. This allows separation of mastocytoma from an extremely rare mast cell sarcoma of the skin {1958}.

Systemic mastocytosis (SM)

The prerequisites for the diagnosis of SM are outlined in Table 2.10. In most cases, aggregates of atypical mast cells are readily found in tissue sections. The criteria for variants of SM are given in Table 2.12.

Bone marrow

In most cases of SM, multifocal, sharply demarcated compact infiltrates of mast cells are the most common and easily detectable feature in the BM biopsy. The infiltrates are found predominantly in paratrabecular and/or perivascular locations {290, 965, 971, 977, 978, 1198}. The focal lesions are comprised of varying numbers of mast cells, intermingled with varying numbers of lymphocytes, eosinophils, histiocytes, and fibroblasts. These diagnostic "mixed" infiltrates are often

Fig. 2.44 Mastocytoma of skin. An isolated lesion from the wrist of an infant. **A** The papillary and reticular dermis are filled with mast cells. **B** At higher magnification, the bland appearance of the mast cell infiltrate can be appreciated.

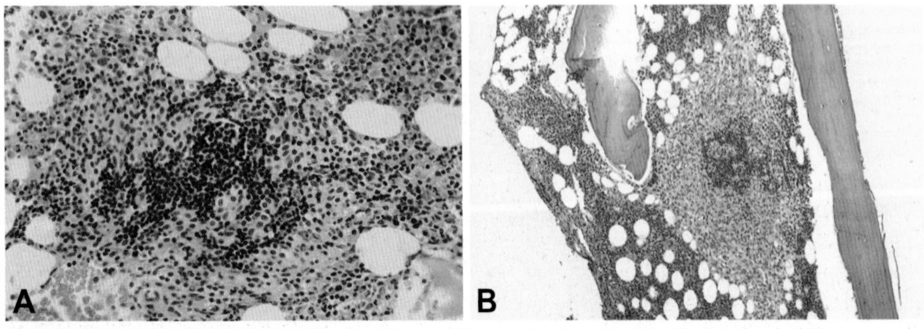

Fig. 2.45 Systemic mastocytosis, bone marrow biopsy. **A** The focal lesions of mast cells often consist of a central core of lymphocytes, surrounded by polygonal mast cells with pale, faintly granular cytoplasm, with reactive eosinophils at the outer margin of the lesion. **B** The lesions are often well-circumscribed, and may occur in paratrabecular or perivascular locations, but may be randomly distributed in the intertrabecular regions as well.

seen in ISM and generally show either a central core of lymphocytes surrounded by mast cells, or a central compact mast cell aggregate with a broad rim of lymphocytes {965}. In other cases, the lesions are more monomorphic and are mainly composed of spindle-shaped mast cells that abut or stream along the bony trabeculae {977, 978}. Significant reticulin fibrosis and thickening of the adjacent bone are frequently observed. Sometimes, the BM space is diffusely replaced by compact mast cell infiltrates, which may resemble sheets of fibroblasts {971}. Marked reticulin or even collagen fibrosis is frequently observed in such cases {971, 977, 978}. Usually, there is a mixture of both spindle-shaped and round mast cells. Rarely, compact infiltrates may exclusively consist of round hypergranular mast cells, which meets the criteria for so-called tryptase-positive round cell infiltration of BM (TROCI-BM) {976}. In contrast to spindle-shaped tryptase-expressing cells that are always mast cells, the round tryptase-positive cells in TROCI are either mast cells (coexpression of CD117 and chymase), neoplastic basophils (primary or secondary basophilic leukaemia) or myeloblasts in the setting of a tryptase-positive acute myeloid leukaemia.

Careful inspection of the BM not affected by mastocytosis is of crucial importance. Often, the unaffected BM is unremarkable with a normal distribution of fat cells and haematopoietic precursors. Such cases usually either belong to ISM with involvement of skin and BM, or represent isolated mastocytosis of the BM. However, in other cases the BM not directly infiltrated by mast cells may be extremely hypercellular due to the proliferation of cells of non-mast cell lineages, including neutrophils, monocytes, or less frequently, eosinophils or blast cells. Depending on the type of proliferating cells, these findings may be reactive (myeloid hyperplasia), or may indicate the presence of a coexisting haematopoietic neoplasm such as acute myeloid leukaemia, a myeloproliferative neoplasm, a myelodysplastic syndrome or myelodysplastic/myeloproliferative neoplasm, or chronic eosinophilic leukaemia. Lymphoproliferative diseases, such as plasma cell myeloma or malignant lymphoma, are less frequently seen {110, 969, 971, 975, 1147, 1484, 2056, 2066, 2095}. In all such cases, the associated haematologic disease should be classified according to established WHO criteria. It is important to note whether there is increased cellularity of the marrow or disturbed maturation of haematopoietic cells, because, even if criteria for a coexisting myeloid neoplasm are not completely fulfilled, hypercellularity or abnormal myeloid maturation patterns could be associated with an unfavourable outcome (progression to ASM or SM-AHNMD) or with a smouldering variant of SM in which the outcome is uncertain {2290}. Interpretation of findings must include consideration that reactive, nonclonal mast cell hyperplasia may accompany a variety of haematological disorders, including myeloid and especially lymphoid neoplasms, such as lymphoplasmacytic lymphoma or hairy cell leukaemia {2290}. In such reactive states, the predominantly round mast cells lack major cytological atypia, and are almost always loosely scattered throughout the tissues, a finding that clearly contrasts with the compact aggregates of neoplastic spindle-shaped mast cells found in mastocytosis {2290}.

The documentation of BM involvement accompanying SM is usually established by examination of a BM trephine biopsy specimen. However, the analysis of marrow aspirate smears does provide useful

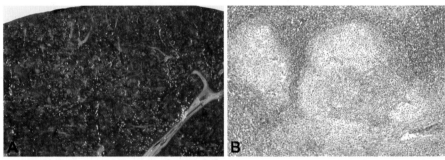

Fig. 2.46 Systemic mastocytosis, spleen. **A** Spleen from a patient with systemic mastocytosis. **B** Aggregates of mast cells may be seen in the red or white pulp, or both. In this case, mast cells are seen in a perifollicular location.

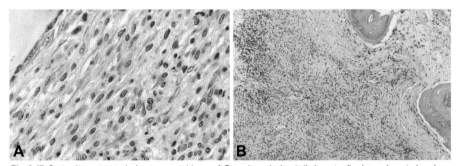

Fig. 2.47 Systemic mastocytosis, bone marrow biopsy. **A** Densely packed, spindled mast cells along a bony trabeculum. **B** Often, the monomorphic, spindled mast cells are accompanied by fibrosis, and may replace large areas of the bone marrow biopsy specimen. Osteosclerosis often accompanies such lesions.

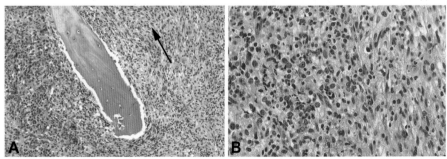

Fig. 2.48 SM-AHNMD (acute myeloid leukaemia). **A** The streaming, spindled cells of a large mast cell aggregate can be seen on one side of the bony trabeculum (arrow), whereas a monotonous population of blast cells is seen on the opposite side. **B** The spindled cells of mast cell disease abut on a large aggregate of blasts.

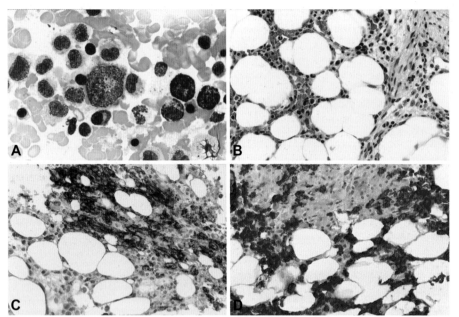

Fig. 2.49 Systemic mastocytosis with associated hairy cell leukaemia. **A** Bone marrow aspirate smear with hairy cells and atypical mast cells. **B** The spindled mast cells are present adjacent to the hairy cell infiltrate in the interstitial regions of the marrow. Although hairy cell leukaemia may occasionally assume a spindled morphology, in this case the mast cell tryptase illustrated in (**C**) clearly demonstrates the mast cell origin of the spindled cells, and an immunostain for CD20 identifies the hairy cells in (**D**).

additional information and is crucial for the diagnosis of mast cell leukaemia and of some subvariants of SM-AHNMD {2290}. In ISM, most mast cells are found within the thicker regions of the aspirated crushed fragments. Mast cells in ISM, which should always be assessed in the thin regions and at a fair distance from BM particles, usually comprise <1% of all nucleated marrow cells. This is in contrast to mast cell leukaemia, where mast cell numbers by definition equal or exceed 20% of all nucleated cells in aspirate smears {290, 977, 978, 2290}.

Lymph node

Lymph nodes appear to be rarely involved in SM in that significant lymphadenopathy is unusual. The mast cell infiltrates within lymph nodes may involve any of the anatomical compartments but particularly involve the paracortical areas. Mast cell infiltrates can be either focal or diffuse, but rarely totally efface preexisting architecture. Hyperplasia of germinal centres, evidence of angioneogenesis, tissue eosinophilia, plasmacytosis and reticulin/collagen fibrosis usually accompany the mast cell infiltrates {968, 1466}. In a few patients, lymphadenopathy is marked, with a progressive clinical course mimicking malignant lymphoma. If significant blood eosinophilia is present, such cases

have been reported to belong to a defined subset of ASM, namely "lymphadenopathic SM with eosinophilia" {1484, 2290}. In such cases, studies for rearrangement of *PDGFRA* are recommended, and if present, the case should be reassigned to the category of myeloid neoplasm with eosinophilia and rearrangement of *PDGFRA*.

Spleen

The white and red pulp of the spleen may be involved in SM, with rare cases showing preferential infiltration of the lymphoid follicles of the white pulp {973}. Here, mast cell infiltrates often present as focal

granulomatoid lesions in the paratrabecular and parafollicular areas, or within the lymphatic follicles, or as diffuse infiltrates within the red pulp. As in other tissue sites, eosinophilia and fibrosis are frequently observed in areas of mast cell infiltration. In some cases, an associated haematological disorder may be present, but this is often difficult to diagnose using splenic tissues alone {973, 1466}.

Liver

Liver involvement in SM usually presents with disseminated small granulomatoid foci of mast cells within the periportal tracts and as loosely scattered mast cells within the sinusoids. Severe liver involvement is only rarely seen in SM. Widening and fibrosis of periportal areas is commonly found, but fully developed cirrhosis is rare {966, 1466}.

Gastrointestinal (GI) tract mucosa

Involvement of the GI tract mucosa by mastocytosis is frequently suspected clinically but may only rarely be assessed morphologically. As in other tissues, at least one compact mast cell infiltrate is required to support the diagnosis of SM. In typical cases, these mast cells show an abnormal immunophenotype with expression of CD25, and an activating point mutation of *KIT* is present. Due to the frequency of CD25-positive lymphocytes, careful examination of the tissue is necessary to avoid false positive results. To evaluate a GI biopsy for mastocytosis, both anti-tryptase and anti-CD117 antibodies should be applied in order to avoid false positive results due to strong background staining when only anti-tryptase antibodies are used. A few

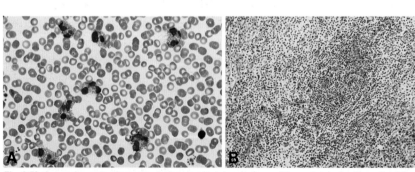

Fig. 2.50 Aggressive systemic mastocytosis subvariant, lymphadenopathic mastocytosis with eosinophilia. **A** The peripheral blood smear of a patient with systemic mastocytosis. The peripheral blood smear shows eosinophilia. **B** Lymph node biopsy. The lymph node is infiltrated by mast cells with a significant infiltrate by eosinophils. The patient expired of heart failure, secondary to eosinophilic infiltration and myocardial fibrosis. Such cases should always be evaluated for rearrangement of *PDGFRA*, and if present, should be as a myeloid neoplasm with eosinophilia associated with rearrangement of *PDGFRA*.

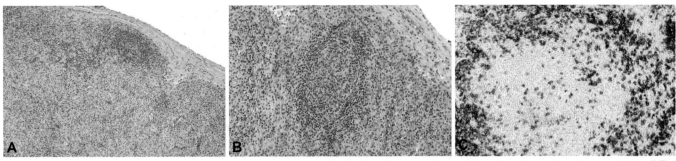

Fig. 2.51 Systemic mastocytosis, lymph node biopsy. **A** Lymph node biopsy that is diffusely infiltrated by neoplastic mast cells, leaving only a remnant of a normal follicle. **B** The infiltrate often is parafollicular in distribution. **C** An immunohistochemical stain for mast cell tryptase illustrates the parafollicular distribution of the mast cell infiltrate in the same biopsy.

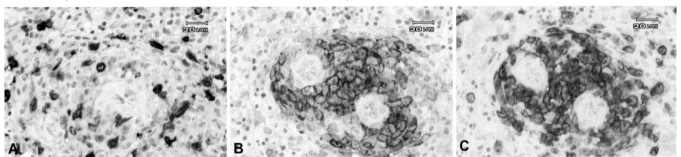

Fig. 2.52 Perivascular accumulation of mast cells stained for mast cell tryptase (**A**), CD117 (**B**) and CD25 (**C**) in the bone marrow of a patient with systemic mastocytosis.

exceptional cases exhibit a diffuse compact infiltration of the lamina propria mucosae by atypical mast cells, and this may resemble inflammatory bowel disease or malignant lymphoma at first glance. Altogether, four patterns of involvement of the GI tract mucosa by mastocytosis can be discriminated {171}: 1) Loosely scattered mast cells without dense aggregates but with an atypical immunophenotype and an activating point mutation of *KIT*, usually in the setting of SM of some duration and involving the BM, 2) Slight increase in loosely-scattered mast cells with occasional dense aggregates and an atypical immunophenotype with expression of CD25, usually associated with an activating point mutation of *KIT*, 3) Diffuse compact infiltration of the mucosa by atypical mast cells, resembling the aggressive variant of SM in other tissues {171} and 4) Localized mast cell sarcoma (based on one published case with involvement of the ascending colon) {1176}.

Skeletal lesions

The frequency of bone changes varies with the subtype of disease. While pure diffuse osteosclerosis is unusual in ISM (about 6%), it is observed in about one third of patients with ASM. The most common radiological finding associated with ISM consists of concurrent osteosclerotic and osteolytic lesions (45%). Osteopenia

or osteoporosis is another frequent finding in patients with mastocytosis, and may occur in any variant.

Mast cell leukaemia (MCL)

In mast cell leukaemia, mast cells equal or exceed 20% of all nucleated cells in aspirate smears {290, 977, 978, 2290}. In this rare and highly aggressive form of SM, the BM reveals a diffuse, compact infiltrate with marked reduction of fat cells and normal haematopoietic precursors. The mast cells often show signs of marked atypia with hypogranular cytoplasm, irregularly shaped monocytoid or bilobated nuclei (promastocytes), and may even present as metachromatic blasts {2290}. In some cases, the nucleoli may be prominent. In typical cases, mast cells account for 10% or more of the circulating nucleated cells. If mast cells comprise less than 10% the circulating cells, the diagnosis of an "aleukaemic" variant of MCL is appropriate {2289}.

Mast cell sarcoma (MCS)

Mast cell sarcoma is extremely rare and characterized by a localized and destructive growth of highly atypical mast cells, which can be identified only after

application of appropriate immunohistochemical markers, particularly anti-tryptase and anti-CD117. Although initially localized, distant spread followed by a terminal phase resembling MCL is seen after a short interval. Mast cell sarcomas have been reported to occur in the larynx, large bowel, meninges, bone and skin {265, 970, 1176}.

Extracutaneous mastocytoma

This localized tumour consists of an accumulation of mature-appearing granulated strongly metachromatic mast cells, in contrast to the highly atypical mast cells observed in a mast cell sarcoma. Extracutaneous mastocytoma is exceptionally rare, and the reported cases involved the lung {398}.

Immunophenotype

Mast cells co-express CD9, CD33, CD45, CD68 and CD117 but lack several myelomonocytic antigens, including CD14, CD15 and CD16, as well as most T- and B-cell related antigens {974, 977, 978, 1073, 1292, 1687, 2290}. Virtually all mast cells, irrespective of stage of maturation or neoplastic state, react with antibodies against tryptase; a cell not expressing tryptase cannot be identified as a mast cell immunohistochemically. Chymase is expressed in a subpopulation of mast cells. Chymase is highly specific but much less sensitive for the identification of atypical and immature mast cells than CD117, whereas CD117 expression is a highly sensitive but rather nonspecific marker of mast cells. Neoplastic mast cells show a similar antigen profile to that of normal mast cells, but in contrast to normal mast cells, they also coexpress CD2 or CD2 and CD25. These latter observations are of considerable value in the diagnosis and in the differential diagnosis of mastocytosis and related tumours, and can be applied in immunohistochemical as well as in flow cytometry studies {650, 1655, 2057}. The application of anti-CD25 antibodies has been found particularly useful in the histopathological evaluation for suspected SM. However, CD2-positive T-cells are usually present in tissues and must be taken into account before an atypical CD2-positive mast cell population can be properly identified. Altogether, it can be assumed in the routine diagnostic evaluation of mastocytosis that cells expressing tryptase/chymase and CD117 are mast cells, and cells coexpressing tryptase/chymase, CD117 and CD2/CD25 are neoplastic mast cells {2057}. CD25 expression may be inconstant or even undetectable on mast cells in some rare subvariants of the disease, such as well-differentiated SM or in a subgroup of patients with mast cell leukaemia {14}.

Genetics

Mastocytosis is frequently associated with somatic activating point mutations within *KIT* {2176}. In most cases, codon 816 mutations in the tyrosine kinase domain are detectable. Rare familial cases with germline mutations of *KIT* have been reported {14, 15, 1331, 1332, 1333, 1557, 2176}. In patients with SM-AHNMD additional genetic defects are detected, depending on the type of AHNMD.
Somatic point mutations of the *KIT* proto-oncogene that encodes the tyrosine kinase receptor for SCF are detected as recurring abnormalities in mastocytosis {14, 15, 1331, 1332, 1333, 1557, 1656, 2176}. The most commonly observed mutation shows substitution of Val for Asp at codon 816 (D816V). This mutation results in ligand-independent activation of KIT tyrosine kinase and provides relative resistance to the prototypical tyrosine kinase inhibitor imatinib {995, 1557}.

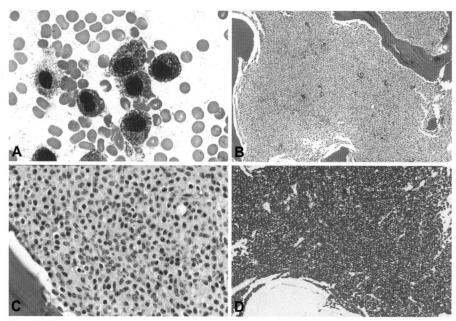

Fig. 2.53 Mast cell leukaemia. **A** Peripheral blood smear. Note the bilobed nuclei and relatively poorly-granulated cytoplasm often seen in this aggressive form of mastocytosis. **B** The bone marrow biopsy is diffusely infiltrated by the neoplastic mast cells. **C** demonstrates the "clear cell" appearance that is due to the poor granulation of the cytoplasm that is typical of immature mast cells of mast cell leukaemia. **D** An immunohistochemical stain for mast cell tryptase in mast cell leukaemia.

The D816V mutation is identified in the mast cells of 95% or more of adults with SM when sensitive methods are used, including nested PNA-PCR or PCR on pooled micro-dissected single mast cells. Other activating point mutations of exon 17, such as D816Y, D816H and D816F are rarely seen {756, 1332, 1333, 2056}. The D816V mutation is seen in only about one third of CM in paediatric patients {14, 1331, 1332} and the frequency of point mutations other than D816V is significantly higher in CM than in SM. In patients with SM-AHNMD, additional genetic defects may be detected, depending on the type of AHNMD. For example, in SM associated with AML, the *RUNX1-RUNX1T* fusion gene may be found, whereas in cases of

SM associated with myeloproliferative neoplasms, *JAK2* V617F may be found. The detection of the *FIP1L1-PDGFRA* fusion gene has been reported in patients with mast cell proliferation and eosinophilia {2286}. Although patients presenting with elevated serum tryptase levels, clonal BM eosinophilia with a *FIP1L1-PDGFRA* fusion gene and a few scattered atypical mast cells have been described as having an unusual variant of SM {130, 713, 1162}, most of these patients do not fulfill SM criteria, particularly as compact mast cell infiltrates are missing, and they are best classified as a myeloid neoplasm with eosinophilia and rearrangement of *PDGFRA* (See Chapter 3) {2287}.

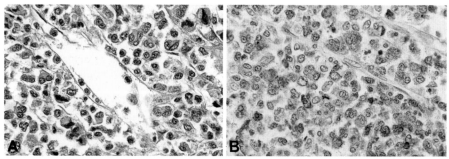

Fig. 2.54 Mast cell sarcoma. **A** This tumour is comprised of poorly differentiated neoplastic cells that show no cytological evidence of mast cell differentiation. **B** The immunohistochemical detection of mast cell tryptase confirms the mast cell origin of the tumour.

Postulated cell of origin

Haematopoietic stem cells.

Prognosis and predictive factors

In children, CM usually has a favourable outcome and may regress spontaneously before or during puberty. In adults, cutaneous lesions generally do not regress and are, in contrast to a previous belief, often associated with SM, usually the indolent variant. One study identified predictors of a poorer prognosis as late onset of symptoms, absence of CM, thrombocytopenia, elevated lactate dehydrogenase (LDH), anaemia, BM hypercellularity, qualitative PB smear abnormalities, elevated alkaline phosphatase and hepatosplenomegaly. The percentage and morphology of mast cells in BM smears have been identified as additional important and independent predictors of survival in mastocytosis {2290}.

Currently, there is no cure for SM, and the prognosis depends on the disease category {2287, 2288}. Patients with high-grade (aggressive) disease including mast cell leukaemia may survive only a few months, whereas those with indolent SM usually have a normal life expectancy {2287, 2288}. SM patients with cutaneous involvement usually also follow an indolent course, whereas patients with aggressive disease often have no skin lesions {2290}. However, isolated BM mastocytosis as a subvariant of ISM with excellent prognosis also presents without cutaneous lesions. If there is an associated haematological malignancy, the clinical course and prognosis are usually dominated by this related haematological malignancy {975}. Patients with aggressive SM generally show a rapid clinical course with a survival of only a few years. MCS shows a progressive course with death within months. Patients with ASM, MCL and MCS are thus candidates for cytoreductive therapies.

Myeloproliferative neoplasm, unclassifiable

H.M. Kvasnicka
B.J. Bain
J. Thiele
A. Orazi
H.-P. Horny
J.W. Vardiman

Definition

The designation, myeloproliferative neoplasm, unclassifiable (MPN, U) should be applied only to cases that have definite clinical, laboratory and morphological features of an MPN but that fail to meet the criteria for any of the specific MPN entities, or that present with features that overlap two or more of the MPN categories. Most cases of MPN, U, will fall into one of three groups: 1) Early stages of polycythaemia vera (PV), primary myelofibrosis (PMF) or essential thrombocythaemia (ET) in which the characteristic features are not yet fully developed; 2) Advanced stage MPN, in which pronounced myelofibrosis, osteosclerosis, or transformation to a more aggressive stage (i.e. increased blasts and/or dysplasia) obscures the underlying disorder {775, 1216, 2206, 2216, 2222}; or, 3) Patients with convincing evidence of an MPN in whom a coexisting neoplastic or inflammatory disorder obscures some of the diagnostic clinical and/or morphological features. The presence of a Philadelphia (Ph) chromosome, BCR-ABL1 fusion gene or rearrangement of PDGFRA, PDGFRB or FGFR1 genes excludes the diagnosis of MPN,U.

The diagnosis MPN,U should not be used when clinical data necessary for proper classification are insufficient or not available, when the bone marrow (BM) specimen is of inadequate quality or size for accurate evaluation {1216, 2216, 2222}, or when there has been recent cytotoxic or growth factor therapy —problems that account for the majority of the unclassifiable cases encountered in routine practice. In such cases it is often preferable to describe the morphological findings, and to suggest additional clinical and laboratory procedures that are needed to further classify the process, including adequate peripheral blood (PB) and BM biopsy and aspirate specimens. When a diagnosis of MPN, U is made, the report should summarize the reason for the difficulty in reaching a more specific diagnosis, and, if possible, specify which of the MPN can be excluded from consideration.

If a case does not have the features of one of the well-defined entities, the possibility that it is not an MPN must be strongly considered. A reactive BM response to infection and inflammation, toxins, chemotherapy, and administration of growth factors, cytokines and immunosuppressive agents may closely mimic MPN and must be excluded. Furthermore, a number of other haematopoietic and non-haematopoietic neoplasms, such as lymphoma or metastatic carcinoma, may infiltrate the marrow and cause reactive changes, including dense fibrosis and osteosclerosis that can be misconstrued as an MPN {2206}. Detection of a clonal cytogenetic abnormality, a JAK2 V617F or other functionally similar JAK2 mutation, or an MPL (MPL W515K/L) mutation will distinguish an MPN from such reactive conditions, although not all cases of MPN, U express a currently recognized genetic marker {2171, 2177}. In addition, the defining characteristics of each MPN must be considered with the realization that, as with any other biological process, variations do occur, and they may progress through different stages so that the clinical and morphological manifestations of the disease will change with time {2177, 2216}.

ICD-O code   9975/3

Epidemiology

The exact incidence of MPN, U is unknown, but some reports indicate that the percentage of unclassifiable cases account for as many as 10–15% of all cases of MPN {775, 2222}. The frequency varies

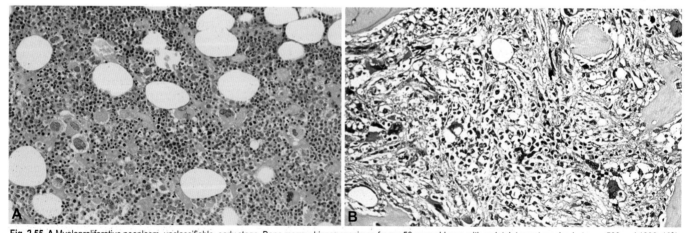

Fig. 2.55 A Myeloproliferative neoplasm, unclassifiable, early stage. Bone marrow biopsy specimen from a 50-year-old man with a platelet count ranging between 500 and 1000x10⁹/L for many months and with a haemoglobin concentration of 17 g/dL. A bone marrow biopsy demonstrates a hypercellular marrow with an increased number of enlarged, mature appearing megakaryocytes and a slight increase in the number of erythroid precursors. **B** Myeloproliferative neoplasm, unclassifiable, late fibrotic stage. A bone marrow biopsy specimen from a 65-year-old female with leukocytosis, pancytopenia and marked splenomegaly. The specimen shows hypocellularity and fibrosis with osteosclerosis and the presence of markedly atypical megakaryocytes.

significantly according to the experience of the diagnostician and the specific classification system and criteria utilized to classify MPN {1216, 2216}.

Etiology
The cause is unknown.

Sites of involvement
Similar to the other MPN.

Clinical features
The clinical features of MPN, U are similar to those seen in the other MPN. In patients with early, unclassifiable disease, organomegaly may be minimal or absent, but splenomegaly and hepatomegaly may be massive in those with advanced disease in whom BM specimens are characterized by marked myelofibrosis and/or increased numbers of blasts {2216}. The haematological values are also variable, and range from mild leukocytosis and moderate to marked thrombocytosis, with or without accompanying anaemia, to severe cytopenias due to BM failure. Some patients with MPN, U present with otherwise unexplained portal or splanchnic vein thrombosis.

Morphology
Many cases that are diagnosed as MPN, U belong to very early stage disease in which the differentiation between ET, the prefibrotic stage of PMF, and the prepolycythaemic stages of PV is difficult {1216, 2223, 2224}. Often, the PB smear in such cases shows thrombocytosis and variable neutrophilia. The haemoglobin concentration may be normal, mildly decreased or borderline increased. The BM biopsy specimen frequently shows hypercellularity and often prominent megakaryocytic proliferation, with variable amounts of granulocytic and erythroid proliferation {2216, 2223, 2224}. If the guidelines suggested in the previous sections for each specific MPN are carefully applied with close attention paid to the megakaryocytic morphology and histotopography, most cases can be accurately assigned to a specific subtype; but if not, the designation of MPN, U is preferable until careful follow-up data or additional laboratory studies provide evidence leading to a precise diagnosis.
In late-stage disease, the BM specimens may reveal dense fibrosis and/or osteomyelosclerosis, indicating a terminal or burnt-out stage, and distinction between the post-polycythaemic stage of PV

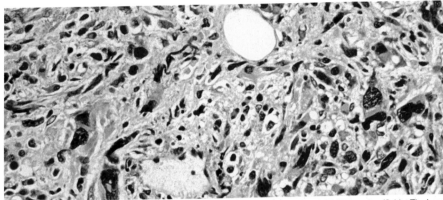

Fig. 2.56 Myeloproliferative neoplasm, unclassifiable, with features simulating an MDS/MPN, unclassifiable. The bone marrow biopsy shows the presence of severe dysmegakaryopoiesis: the dysplastic appearance of this case was therapy-related, a consequence of hydroxycarbamide given to a PV patient in late stage.

(post-PV MF) or rarely ET (post-ET MF) {143A} and the overt fibrotic-osteosclerotic stage of PMF may be impossible if there is no previous history or histology for review {2203, 2206, 2216, 2222}. Although chronic myelogenous leukaemia (CML) may also be accompanied by marked myelofibrosis, the small size of the megakaryocytes will alert the morphologist to the correct diagnosis, and cytogenetic and molecular genetic demonstration of the Ph chromosome or the BCR-ABL1 fusion gene will confirm the diagnosis of CML {775, 2216, 2222}.
More than 10% blasts in the PB or BM and/or the finding of significant myelodysplasia generally indicates a transition of the disease to a more aggressive, often terminal blast phase. If the initial diagnostic specimen has features of a myeloproliferative process that cannot be specifically categorized, but shows 10–19% blasts in the PB or BM, the diagnosis of an accelerated stage of an MPN, U, is appropriate. Immunohistochemical staining of the BM biopsy sections for CD34 may be of diagnostic value in these cases by demonstrating increased numbers and/or clusters of blasts {2216, 2222}. If blasts account for 20% or more of the peripheral white blood cells or nucleated BM cells in the initial specimen, then the diagnosis is acute leukaemia, and the suggestion that the case may be a blast transformation of a previous but unclassifiable MPN is appropriate. Myelodysplastic features may appear during the natural progression of an MPN even without prior cytoreductive therapy. However, if the initial pretreatment specimen demonstrates myelodysplasia, the diagnosis of a myelodysplastic syndrome or of

a myelodysplastic/myeloproliferative neoplasm, including the provisional entity, refractory anaemia with ring sideroblasts and thrombocytosis, should be considered {127, 129, 865, 1245, 1406, 2082, 2169}.

Immunophenotype
No abnormal phenotype has been reported for this group of patients.

Genetics
There is no cytogenetic or molecular genetic finding specific for this group. There is no Philadelphia chromosome, BCR-ABL1 fusion gene, or rearrangement of PDGFRA, PDGFRB or FGFR1. Some cases with a mutation of JAK2 as a sole genetic abnormality do not meet the criteria for a specific MPN or any other specific disease category, and are thus best categorized as MPN, U.

Postulated cell of origin
Haematopoietic stem cell.

Prognosis and predictive factors
In patients with the initial stages of an MPN that is unclassifiable, follow-up studies performed at intervals of 4–6 months will often provide sufficient information for a more precise classification {2216, 2222}. Such patients in the early stages of disease will have a prognosis similar to those of the group into which their disease eventually evolves. Patients with advanced disease in whom the initial process is no longer recognizable due to BM fibrosis or blastic infiltration would be expected to have a poor prognosis.

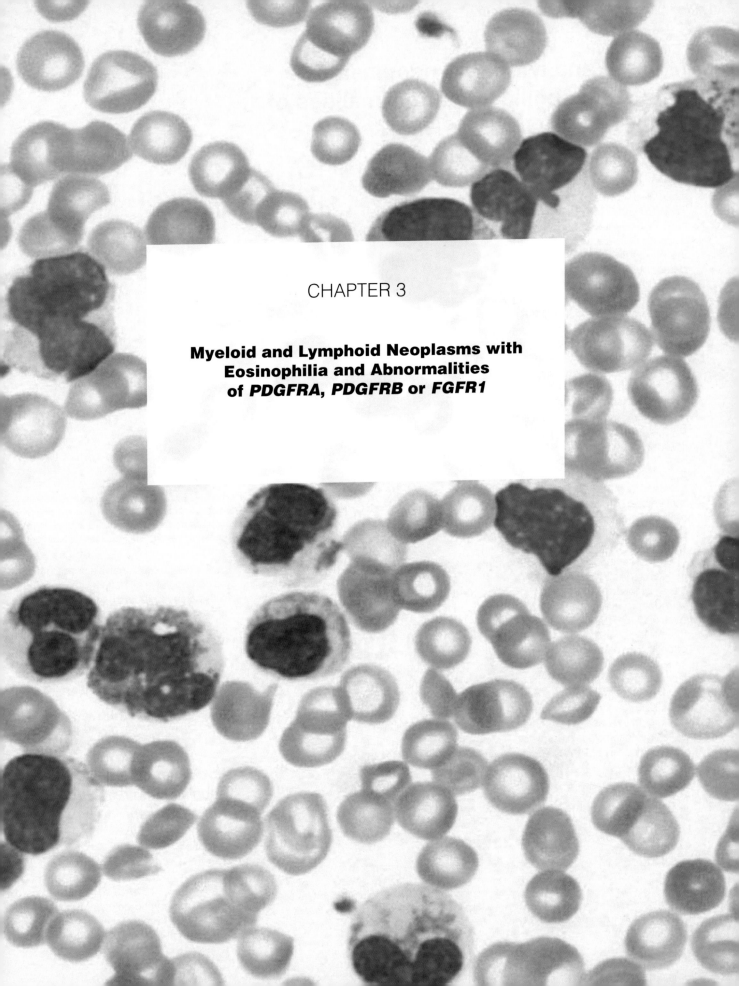

CHAPTER 3

**Myeloid and Lymphoid Neoplasms with
Eosinophilia and Abnormalities
of *PDGFRA*, *PDGFRB* or *FGFR1***

Myeloid and lymphoid neoplasms with eosinophilia and abnormalities of *PDGFRA, PDGFRB* or *FGFR1*

B.J. Bain
D.G. Gilliland
H.-P. Horny
J.W. Vardiman

Myeloproliferative and lymphoid neoplasms associated with rearrangement of *PDGFRA, PDGFRB* and *FGFR1* constitute three rare specific disease groups, which have some shared features and some that differ. All result from formation of a fusion gene encoding an aberrant tyrosine kinase. Eosinophilia is characteristic but not invariable. It has been established that, in the case of *PDGFRA* and *FGFR1*-related neoplasms, the cell of origin is a mutated pluripotent (lymphoid-myeloid) stem cell. It is possible that this is also true for *PDGFRB*-related neoplasms, but this has yet to be established.

All three disorders can present as a chronic myeloproliferative neoplasm (MPN), but the frequency of manifestation as a lymphoid neoplasm varies. The clinical and haematological features are also influenced by the partner gene involved. In the case of *PDGFRA*-related disorders, presentation is usually as chronic eosinophilic leukaemia (CEL) with prominent involvement of the mast cell lineage and sometimes of the neutrophil lineage. Less often, presentation is as acute myeloid leukaemia (AML) or precursor-T lymphoblastic lymphoma (T-LBL), in both instances with accompanying eosinophilia. In the case of *PDGFRB*-related disease, the features of the MPN are more variable but are often those of chronic myelomonocytic leukaemia (CMML) with eosinophilia. Proliferation of aberrant mast cells can again be a feature. Acute transformations that have been described to date have been myeloid. In the case of *FGFR1*-related disease, a lymphomatous presentation is common, particularly T-LBL with accompanying

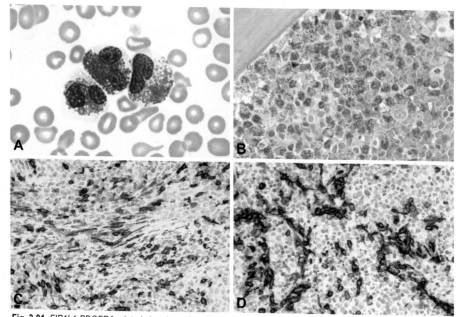

Fig. 3.01 *FIP1L1-PDGFRA*-related chronic eosinophilic leukaemia. **A** Peripheral blood film showing three moderately degranulated eosinophils, Romanowsky stain. **B** Trephine biopsy section. Abundant eosinophils and eosinophil precursors, Giemsa stain. **C** Trephine biopsy section. Abundant mast cells, many of which are spindle-shaped, forming small loose clusters, Mast cell tryptase staining. **D** Trephine biopsy section. CD25 expression in the mast cells.

eosinophilia. Other patients have had CEL, precursor-B lymphoblastic leukaemia/lymphoma or AML.

The importance of recognizing these disorders is that the aberrant tyrosine kinase activity can make the disease responsive to tyrosine kinase inhibitors. This hope has already been realized for MPN with rearrangement of *PDGFRA* or *PDGFRB*, which are responsive to imatinib and some related tyrosine kinase inhibitors. Similar specific therapy has not yet been developed for *FGFR1*-related disease. Relevant cytogenetic analysis,

molecular genetic analysis or both should be carried out in all patients in whom MPN with eosinophilia is suspected and also in patients presenting with an acute leukaemia or lymphoblastic lymphoma with eosinophilia. Recognition of *PDGFRA*-related disease usually requires molecular genetic analysis, since the majority of cases result from a cryptic deletion, whereas cytogenetic analysis will reveal the causative abnormality in the case of *PDGFRB*- and *FGFR1*-related disease.

Myeloid and lymphoid neoplasms with PDGFRA rearrangement

Definition
The most common MPN associated with *PDGFRA* rearrangement is that associated with *FIP1L1-PDGFRA* formed as a result of a cryptic deletion at 4q12 {466} (Table 3.01). Presentation is generally as CEL but can be as AML, T-LBL or both

Table 3.01 Diagnostic criteria of an MPN* with eosinophilia associated with *FIP1L1-PDGFRA*.

A myeloproliferative neoplasm with prominent eosinophilia
    AND
Presence of a *FIP1L1-PDGFRA* fusion gene[†]

---

* Patients presenting with acute myeloid leukaemia or lymphoblastic leukaemia/lymphoma with eosinophilia and a *FIP1L1-PDGFRA* fusion gene are also assigned to this category.

[†] If appropriate molecular analysis is not available, this diagnosis should be suspected if there is a Ph-negative MPN with the haematological features of chronic eosinophilic leukaemia associated with splenomegaly, a marked elevation of serum vitamin B12, elevation of serum tryptase and increased bone marrow mast cells.

simultaneously {1469}. Acute transformation can follow presentation as CEL. Organ damage occurs as a result of leukaemic infiltration or the release of cytokines, enzymes or other proteins by the eosinophils and possibly also by mast cells. The peripheral blood (PB) eosinophil count is markedly elevated (in cases reported to date it has almost always been ≥1.5x10⁹/L) although it should be noted that, in some series of patients, investigation was confined to patients with eosinophilia. There is no Ph chromosome or *BCR-ABL1* fusion gene. Except when there is transformation to acute leukaemia, there are <20% blasts in the PB and bone marrow (BM).

ICD-O code

The provisional code proposed for the fourth edition of ICD-O is *9965/3*.

Synonyms

Chronic eosinophilic leukaemia; chronic eosinophilic leukaemia with *FIP1L1-PDGFRA*; myeloproliferative variant of the hypereosinophilic syndrome.

Epidemiology

The *FIP1L1-PDGFRA* syndrome is rare. It is considerably more common in men than women; the M:F ratio is ~17:1. Its peak incidence is between 25 and 55 years (median age of onset in late 40s) with reported cases ranging in age from 7 to 77 years {131}.

Etiology

The cause is unknown, although several cases have been reported following cytotoxic chemotherapy {1625, 2157} and a case of chronic myeloid leukaemia with a *BCR-PDGFRA* fusion gene also followed combination chemotherapy {1906}.

Sites of involvement

CEL associated with *FIP1L1-PDGFRA* is a multisystem disorder. The PB and BM are always involved. Tissue infiltration by eosinophils, and release of cytokines and humoral factors from the eosinophil granules lead to tissue damage in a number of organs, but the heart, lungs, central and peripheral nervous system, skin and gastrointestinal tract are commonly involved. The spleen is enlarged in the majority of patients.

Clinical features

Patients usually present with fatigue or pruritus, or with respiratory, cardiac or

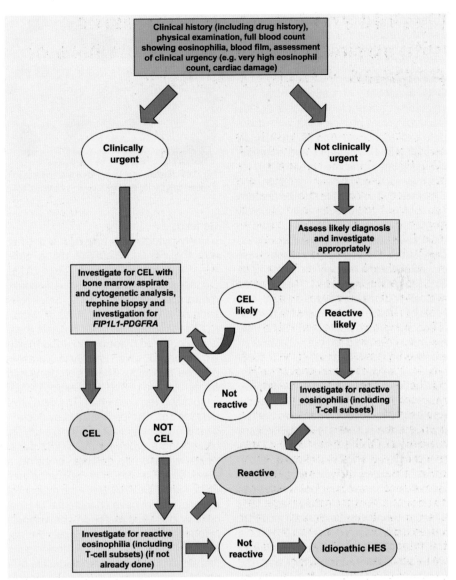

Fig. 3.02 Flow diagram showing the diagnostic process in hypereosinophilia. CEL, chronic eosinophilic leukaemia. The definitive diagnosis is shown within blue circles/ovals.

gastrointestinal symptoms {466, 1391, 2309}. The majority of patients have splenomegaly, and a minority have hepatomegaly. The most serious clinical findings relate to endomyocardial fibrosis, with ensuing restrictive cardiomyopathy. Scarring of the mitral/tricuspid valves leads to valvular regurgitation and formation of intracardiac thrombi, which may embolize. Venous thromboembolism and arterial thromboses are also observed. Pulmonary disease is restrictive and related to fibrosis; symptoms include dyspnoea and cough; there may also be an obstructive element. Serum tryptase is increased (>12 ng/ml), usually to a lesser extent than in mast cell disease but with some overlap. Levels of serum vitamin B12 are

markedly elevated {2309}. *FIP1L1-PDGFRA*-associated CEL is very responsive to imatinib, the gene product being 100-fold more sensitive than BCR-ABL1 {466}.

Morphology

The most striking feature in the PB is eosinophilia, the eosinophils being mainly mature with only small numbers of eosinophil myelocytes or promyelocytes. There may be a range of eosinophil abnormalities, including sparse granulation with clear areas of cytoplasm, cytoplasmic vacuolation, smaller than normal granules, immature granules that are purplish on a Romanowsky stain, nuclear hypersegmentation or hyposegmentation and increased eosinophil size {466, 2309}.

These changes may, however, be seen in cases of reactive as well as of neoplastic eosinophilia {128} and, in some cases, of FIP1L1-PDGFRA-associated CEL, the eosinophil morphology is close to normal. Only a minority of patients have any increase in peripheral blast cells {2309}. Neutrophils may be increased, while basophil and monocyte counts are usually normal {1854}. Anaemia and thrombocytopenia are sometimes present. Any tissue may show eosinophilic infiltration, and Charcot-Leyden crystals may be present. The BM is hypercellular with markedly increased eosinophils and precursors. In most cases, eosinophil maturation is orderly, without a disproportionate increase in blasts, but in a minority the percentage of blast cells is increased. There may be necrosis and Charcot-Leyden crystals, particularly in those cases where the disease is becoming more acute {466}. Bone marrow mast cells are often but not always increased on trephine biopsy {1163, 1688} and mast cell proliferation should be recognized as a feature of FIP1L1-PDGFRA-associated MPN. The mast cells may be scattered or in loose non-cohesive clusters or in cohesive clusters {1163, 1688}. Many cases have a marked increase in CD25+ spindle-shaped atypical mast cells, and in occasional cases morphological features are indistinguishable from those of systemic mastocytosis. Reticulin is increased {1163}. Patients presenting with AML or T-LBL have had coexisting eosinophilia (PB counts 1.4–17.2x10⁹/L) and in the majority of cases pre-existing eosinophilia was also documented {1469}.

Cytochemistry

Cytochemical stains are not essential for diagnosis. The reduced granule content of eosinophils can lead to reduced peroxidase content and inaccurate automated eosinophil counts.

Immunophenotype

Eosinophils may show immunophenotypic evidence of activation such as expression of CD23, CD25 and CD69 {1163}. The mast cells in this syndrome are usually CD2-negative CD25-positive {1162} but sometimes are CD2-negative CD25-negative {1469} and occasionally CD2-positive CD25-positive {1469}. In comparison, the mast cells of systemic mastocytosis are almost always CD25-positive and are CD2-positive in about two thirds of cases.

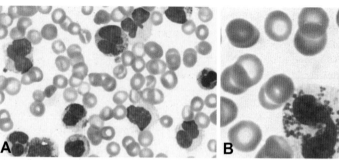

Fig. 3.03 Myeloid neoplasm with eosinophilia associated with *PDGFRB* rearrangement. Peripheral blood film of a patient with t(5;12) showing numerous abnormal eosinophils; eosinophils were 40% of leukocytes.

Genetics

Usually cytogenetic analysis is normal, with the FIP1L1-PDGFRA fusion gene resulting from a cryptic del(4)(q12). Occasionally there is a chromosomal rearrangement with a 4q12 breakpoint such as t(1;4)(q44;q12) {466} or t(4;10)(q12;p11) {2163}. In other patients there is an unrelated cytogenetic abnormality, e.g. trisomy 8, which is likely to represent disease evolution. The fusion gene can be detected by RT-PCR, nested RT-PCR often being required {466}. The causative deletion can also be detected by fluorescence in situ hybridization (FISH) analysis, often using a probe for the CHIC2 gene, which is uniformly deleted, or using a break-apart probe that encompasses FIP1L1 and PDGFRA. Since the majority of patients do not have an increase of blast cells or any abnormality on conventional cytogenetic analysis, it is usually the detection of the FIP1L1-PDGFRA fusion gene that permits the definitive diagnosis of a myeloid neoplasm. Cytogenetic abnormalities appear to be more common when evolution to AML has occurred {1469}.

Postulated cell of origin

The cell of origin appears to be a pluripotent haemopoietic stem cell able to give rise to eosinophils and in some patients neutrophils, monocytes, mast cells, T cells and B cells {1854}. The detection of the fusion gene in a lineage does not necessarily correlate with morphological evidence of involvement of that lineage. Lymphocytosis, for example, is not usual, even in those with apparent involvement of the B or the T lineage {1854}. In chronic phase disease, involvement is predominantly of eosinophils and to a lesser extent mast cells and neutrophils. Acute phase disease may be myeloid or T lymphoblastic {1469}.

Prognosis and predictive factors

Since FIP1L1-PDGFRA-associated CEL and its imatinib responsiveness were recognized for the first time only in 2003 {466}, the long-term prognosis is not yet known. However, prognosis appears favourable if cardiac damage has not already occurred and imatinib treatment is available. Imatinib resistance can develop, e.g. as a result of a T674I mutation (which is equivalent to the T315I mutation that can occur in the BCR-ABL1 gene) {466, 844}. Alternative tyrosine kinase inhibitors such as PKC412 and sorafenib may be effective in these patients {468, 1297, 2103}. Patients presenting as AML or T lymphoblastic lymphoma can achieve sustained complete molecular remission with imatinib {1469}.

Variants

A number of possible molecular variants of FIP1L1-PDGFRA-associated CEL have been recognized in which there are other fusion genes incorporating part of PDGFRA. A male patient with imatinib-responsive CEL was found to have a KIF5B-PDGFRA fusion gene associated with a complex chromosomal abnormality involving chromosomes 3, 4 and 10 {1979}, and a female patient had a CDK5RAP2-PDGFRA fusion gene associated with ins(9;4)(q33;q12q25) {2354}. A male patient with t(2;4)(p24;q12) and a STRN-PDGFRA fusion gene {497} and another with t(4;12)(q2?3;p1?2) and an ETV6-PDGFRA fusion gene, both with the haematological features of CEL, responded to low-dose imatinib {497}.

Patients with t(4;22)(q12;q11) and a BCR-PDGFRA fusion gene, four cases of which have been described, have disease characteristics intermediate between those of FIP1L1-PDGFRA-associated eosinophilic leukaemia and those of BCR-ABL1-positive chronic myelogeneous leukaemia; eosinophilia may or may not be prominent {162, 765, 1906, 2266}. Accelerated phase {162} and T {162} and B lymphoblastic transformation {2266} have been reported. The condition is imatinib-sensitive {1906, 2266}.

Myeloid neoplasms with PDGFRB rearrangement

Definition
A distinctive type of myeloid neoplasm occurs in association with rearrangement of PDGFRB at 5q31~33 (Table 3.02). Usually there is t(5;12)(q31~33;p12) with formation of an ETV6-PDGFRB fusion gene {812, 1134}. In uncommon variants, other translocations with a 5q31~33 breakpoint lead to the formation of other fusion genes, also incorporating part of PDGFRB (Table 3.03). In cases with t(5;12), and in the variant translocations, there is synthesis of an aberrant, constitutively activated tyrosine kinase. The haematological features are most often those of CMML (usually with eosinophilia) but some patients have been characterized as atypical chronic myeloid leukaemias (aCML) (usually with eosinophilia), CEL and MPN with eosinophilia {131, 2085}; single cases have been reported of AML, probably superimposed on chronic idiopathic myelofibrosis {2245}, and of juvenile myelomonocytic leukaemia {1513}, the latter associated with a variant fusion gene. Eosinophilia is usual but not invariable {2085}. Acute transformation can occur, often in a relatively short period of time. MPN with PDGFRB rearrangement is sensitive to tyrosine kinase inhibitors such as imatinib {64}.

ICD-O code
The provisional code proposed for the fourth edition of ICD-O is 9966/3.

Synonym
Chronic myelomonocytic leukaemia with eosinophilia associated with t(5;12).

Epidemiology
This neoplasm is considerably more common in men (M:F=2:1) and has a wide age range (8–72 years) with the peak incidence being in middle-aged adults; median age of onset is in the late 40s {2085}.

Table 3.02 Diagnostic criteria of MPN associated with ETV6-PDGFRB fusion gene or other rearrangement of PDGFRB.

A myeloproliferative neoplasm, often with prominent eosinophilia and sometimes with neutrophilia or monocytosis *AND*
Presence of t(5;12)(q31~q33;p12) or a variant translocation* or, demonstration of an ETV6-PDGFRB fusion gene or of rearrangement of PDGFRB
* Because t(5;12)(q31~q33;p12) does not always lead to an ETV6-PDGFRB fusion gene, molecular confirmation is highly desirable. If molecular analysis is not available, this diagnosis should be suspected if there is a Ph-negative MPN associated with eosinophilia and with a translocation with a 5q31-33 breakpoint.

Table 3.03 Molecular variants of MPN associated with ETV6-PDGFRB. Modified from {131}.

Translocation	Fusion gene	Haematological diagnosis
t(1;3;5)(p36;p21;q33)	WDR48-PDGFRB	CEL
der(1)t(1;5)(p34;q33), der(5)t(1;5)(p34;q15), der(11)ins(11;5)(p12;q15q33)	GPIAP1-PDGRFB	CEL
t(1;5)(q21;q33)	TPM3-PDGFRB	CEL
t(1;5)(q23;q33)	PDE4DIP-PDGFRB	MPD/MDS with eosinophilia
t(4;5;5)(q23;q31;q33)	PRKG2-PDGFRB	Chronic basophilic leukaemia
t(3;5)(p21-25;q31-35)	GOLGA4-PDGFRB	
t(5;7)(q33;q11.2)	HIP1-PDGFRB	CMML with eosinophilia
t(5;10)(q33;q21)	CCDC6-PDGFRB	aCML with eosinophilia, MPD with eosinophilia
t(5;12)(q31-33;q24)	GIT2-PDGFRB	CEL
t(5;14)(q33;q24)	NIN-PDGFRB	Ph-negative CML (13% eosinophils)
t(5;14)(q33;q32)	KIAA1509-PDGFRB	CMML with eosinophilia
t(5;15)(q33;q22)	TP53BP1-PDGFRB	Ph-negative CML with prominent eosinophilia
t(5;16)(q33;p13)	NDE1-PDGFRB	CMML
t(5;17)(q33;p13)	RABEP1-PDGFRB	CMML
t(5;17)(q33;p11.2)	SPECC1-PDGFRB	JMML

aCML, atypical chronic myeloid leukaemia; CEL, chronic eosinophilic leukaemia; CML, chronic myeloid leukaemia; CMML, chronic myelomonocytic leukaemia; JMML, juvenile myelomonocytic leukaemia; MPD/MDS, myeloproliferative/myelodysplastic syndrome; MPN, myeloproliferative neoplasm.

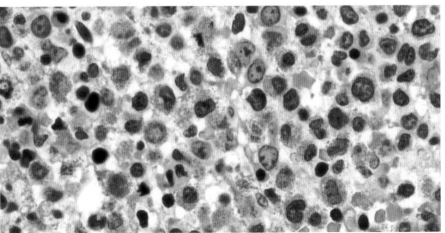

Fig. 3.04 Myeloid neoplasm with eosinophilia associated with PDGFRB rearrangement. Trephine biopsy section from a patient with t(5;12) showing a marked increase in eosinophils.

Sites of involvement

MPN associated with t(5;12)(q31~33;p12) is a multisystem disorder. The PB and BM are always involved. The spleen is enlarged in the majority of patients. Tissue infiltration by eosinophils and release of cytokines, humoral factors or granule contents by eosinophils can contribute to tissue damage in a number of organs.

Clinical features

Patients often have splenomegaly, with hepatomegaly being present in a minority. Some patients have skin infiltration and some have cardiac damage leading to cardiac failure. Serum tryptase may be mildly or moderately elevated. The great majority of patients who have been treated with imatinib have been found to be responsive.

Morphology

The white cell count is increased. There may be anaemia and thrombocytopenia. There is a variable increase of neutrophils, eosinophils, monocytes and eosinophil and neutrophil precursors. Rarely, there is a marked increase in basophils {2355}. The BM is hypercellular as a result of active granulopoiesis (neutrophilic and eosinophilic). Bone marrow trephine biopsy may show, in addition, an increase of mast cells and these may be spindle-shaped {503, 2355}. Bone marrow reticulin may be increased {2355}. In chronic phase disease, the blast cell count is less than 20% in the PB and BM.

Cytochemistry

The eosinophils, neutrophils and monocytes show the expected cytochemical reactions for cells of these lineages.

Immunophenotype

Immunophenotypic analysis of the mast cells has shown expression of CD2 and CD25, as is also observed in the majority of cases of mast cell disease {2355}.

Genetics

Cytogenetic analysis usually shows t(5;12) (q31~33;p12) with the translocation resulting in formation of an ETV6-PDGFRB fusion gene {812} (previously known as TEL-PDGFRB). In one patient ETV6-PDGFRB resulted from a four-way translocation, t(1;12;5;12)(p36;p13;q33;q24) {489}, and in another occurred in association with ins(2;12)(p21;q?13q?22) {512}. The 5q breakpoint is sometimes assigned to 5q31 and sometimes to 5q33, although the gene map locus of PDGFRB gene is 5q31-32.

Not all translocations characterized as t(5;12)(q31;p13) lead to ETV6-PDGFRB fusion. Cases without a fusion gene are not assigned to this category of MPN and, importantly, are not likely to respond to imatinib; in such cases an alternative leukaemogenic mechanism is upregulation of interleukin 3 (IL3) {467}. RT-PCR, using primers suitable for all known breakpoints, is therefore recommended to confirm ETV6-PDGFRB {498} but if molecular analysis is not available a trial of imatinib is justified in patients with an MPN associated with t(5;12).

Postulated cell of origin

The cell of origin appears to be a multipotent haemopoietic stem cell, which is able to give rise to neutrophils, monocytes, eosinophils and probably mast cells.

Prognosis and predictive factors

Pre-imatinib, the median survival was less than 2 years. There are not yet reliable data on survival of imatinib-treated patients, but in a small series (10 patients) the median survival was 65 months {512}. Median survival is likely to improve as patients are recognized and started on appropriate treatment at diagnosis rather than when cardiac damage or transformation has already occurred.

Variants

A number of molecular variants of MPN with ETV6-PDGFRB fusion have been reported {131, 2085}. In addition, a patient who acquired eosinophilia at relapse of AML was found to have acquired t(5;14) (q33;q22) with a TRIP11-PDGFRB fusion gene. A number of other patients have rearrangement of PDGFRB but with the second gene involved being unknown. Complex rearrangements appear to be common (e.g. a small inversion as well as translocation) {2085}. Because of the therapeutic implications, FISH (break-apart FISH with a PDGFRB probe) is indicated in all patients with a presumptive diagnosis of MPN who have a 5q31~33 breakpoint, particularly, but not only, if there is eosinophilia. However, FISH analysis does not always demonstrate rearrangement of PDGFRB, even when it is detectable on Southern Blot analysis {2085}. Molecular analysis is not indicated if there is no 5q31~33 breakpoint on classical cytogenetic analysis since all cases reported to date have had a cytogenetically detectable abnormality.

Myeloid and lymphoid neoplasms with FGFR1 abnormalities

Definition

Haematological neoplasms with FGFR1 rearrangement are heterogeneous. They are derived from a pluripotent haematopoietic stem cell, although in different patients or at different stages of the disease the neoplastic cells may be precursor cells or mature cells. Presentation can be as an MPN or, in transformation, as AML, T or B lineage lymphoblastic lymphoma/leukaemia or mixed phenotype acute leukaemia (MPAL) (Table 3.04).

ICD-O code

The provisional code proposed for the fourth edition of ICD-O is 9967/3.

Synonyms

8p11 myeloproliferative syndrome, 8p11 stem cell syndrome, 8p11 stem cell leukaemia/lymphoma syndrome.

Epidemiology

This neoplasm occurs across a wide age range (3–84 years) but most patients are young, with a median age of onset of

---

Table 3.04 Diagnostic criteria of MPN or acute leukaemia associated with FGFR1 rearrangement.

A myeloproliferative neoplasm with prominent eosinophilia and sometimes with neutrophilia or monocytosis
OR
Acute myeloid leukaemia or precursor T-cell or precursor B-cell lymphoblastic leukaemia/lymphoma (usually associated with peripheral blood or bone marrow eosinophilia)
AND
Presence of t(8;13)(p11;q12) or a variant translocation leading to FGFR1 rearrangement demonstrated in myeloid cells, lymphoblasts or both

around 32 years {1354}. In contrast to MPN with rearrangement of *PDGFRA* and *PDGFRB*, there is only a moderate male predominance (1.5:1).

Sites of involvement
Tissues primarily involved are BM, PB, lymph nodes, liver and spleen. Lymphadenopathy is the result of infiltration by either lymphoblasts or myeloid cells.

Clinical features
Some patients present as lymphoma with mainly lymph node involvement, while others present with myeloproliferative features, such as splenomegaly and hypermetabolism, and yet others with features of AML or myeloid sarcoma {3, 1006, 1354}. Systemic symptoms such as fever, weight loss and night sweats are often present {131}.

Morphology
Presentation may be as CEL, AML, T-LBL or, least often, precursor B lymphoblastic leukaemia/lymphoma. Cases of acute leukaemia/lymphoblastic lymphoma may be of mixed phenotype. In patients who present with CEL, there may be subsequent transformation to AML (including myeloid sarcoma), T or B lineage lymphoblastic leukaemia/lymphoma or MPAL. Lymphoblastic lymphoma appears to be more common in patients with t(8;13) than in those with variant translocations {1354}. Patients who present in chronic phase usually have eosinophilia and neutrophilia and, occasionally, monocytosis. Those who present in transformation are often also found to have eosinophilia. Overall, about 90% of patients have PB or BM eosinophilia {1354}. The eosinophils belong to the neoplastic clone, as do the lymphoblasts and myeloblasts in cases in transformation. Basophilia is not usual but patients with *BCR-FGFR1* fusion may have basophilia {1879}. An association with polycythaemia vera has been observed in three patients with t(6;8)/*FGFR1OP1-FGFR1* fusion {1770, 2340}.

T precursor lymphoblastic lymphoma characteristically shows eosinophilic infiltration within the lymphoma.

Cases should be classified as leukaemia/lymphoma associated with *FGFR1* rearrangement, followed by further details of the specific presentation, e.g. "leukaemia/lymphoma associated with *FGFR1* rearrangement/chronic eosinophilic leukaemia, T precursor lymphoblastic lymphoma" or "leukaemia/lymphoma associated with *FGFR1* rearrangement/myeloid sarcoma".

Cytochemistry
Neutrophil alkaline phosphatase score is often low, but cytochemistry is not important in the diagnosis.

Immunophenotype
Immunophenotypic analysis is not useful in chronic phase disease, but is important to demonstrate the T or B lineage of precursor B-cell or precursor T-cell leukaemia/lymphoma.

Genetics
A variety of translocations with an 8p11 breakpoint can underlie this syndrome. Secondary cytogenetic abnormalities occur, among which trisomy 21 is most often observed. Depending on the partner chromosome, a variety of fusion genes incorporating part of *FGFR1* are formed. All fusion genes encode an aberrant tyrosine kinase (Table 3.05).

Table 3.05 Chromosomal rearrangements and fusion genes reported in MPN associated with *FGFR1* rearrangement*. Modified from {131}.

Cytogenetics	Molecular genetics	N[†]
t(8;13)(p11;q12)	ZNF198-FGFR1	21
t(8;9)(p11;q33)	CEP110-FGFR1	8
t(6;8)(q27;p11-12)	FGFR1OP1-FGFR1	6
t(8;22)(p11;q11)	BCR-FGFR1	5
t(7;8)(q34;p11)	TRIM24-FGFR1	1
t(8;17)(p11;q23)	MYO18A-FGFR1	1
t(8;19)(p12;q13.3)	HERVK-FGFR1	1
ins(12;8)(p11;p11p22)	FGFR1OP2-FGFR1	1

* In addition, *FGFR1* rearrangement has been found in association with t(8;12)(p11;q15) and t(8;17)(p11;q25) but the suspected involvement of *FGFR1* in t(8;11)(p11;p15) was not confirmed.
[†] Numbers updated from MacDonald and Cross {1354}.

Postulated cell of origin
The cell of origin is a pluripotent lymphoid-myeloid haematopoietic stem cell.

Prognosis and predictive factors
The prognosis is currently poor. There is no established tyrosine kinase inhibitor therapy for MPN with *FGFR1* rearrangement, although PKC142 was effective in one case {400}. Interferon has induced a cytogenetic response in several patients {1354, 1402}. Until specific therapy is developed, haematopoietic stem cell transplantation should be considered, even in those who present in chronic phase.

CHAPTER 4

Myelodysplastic/Myeloproliferative Neoplasms

Chronic myelomonocytic leukaemia

Atypical chronic myeloid leukaemia, *BCR-ABL1* negative

Juvenile myelomonocytic leukaemia

Myelodysplastic/myeloproliferative neoplasm, unclassifiable

Chronic myelomonocytic leukaemia

A. Orazi
J.M. Bennett
U. Germing
R.D. Brunning
B.J. Bain
J. Thiele

Definition

Chronic myelomonocytic leukaemia (CMML) is a clonal haematopoietic malignancy that is characterized by features of both a myeloproliferative neoplasm and a myelo-dysplastic syndrome. It is characterized by: 1) persistent monocytosis >1x10^9/L in the peripheral blood (PB); 2) absence of a Philadelphia (Ph) chromosome and *BCR-ABL1* fusion gene; 3) no rearrange-ment of *PDGFRA* or *PDGFRB* (should be specifically excluded in cases with eosinophilia); 4) fewer than 20% blasts (promonocytes are considered as blast equivalents) in the PB and bone marrow (BM); and 5) dysplasia involving one or more myeloid lineages. However, if con-vincing myelodysplasia is not present, the diagnosis of CMML can still be made if the other requirements are met, and an acquired, clonal cytogenetic or molecular genetic abnormality is present in the BM cells, or if the monocytosis has persisted for at least 3 months and all other causes of monocytosis, such as the presence of malignancy, infection or inflammation, have been excluded. CMML is further subdivided into two subsets, CMML-1 and CMML-2, depending on the number of blasts plus promonocytes in the PB and BM. The clinical, haematological and mor-phological features of CMML are hetero-geneous, and vary along a spectrum from predominantly myelodysplastic to mainly myeloproliferative in nature. In contrast with the *BCR-ABL1* negative myeloproliferative

Table 4.01 Diagnostic criteria for chronic myelomonocytic leukaemia.

1.	Persistent peripheral blood monocytosis >1x10^9/L
2.	No Philadelphia chromosome or *BCR-ABL1* fusion gene
3.	No rearrangement of *PDGFRA* or *PDGFRB* (should be specifically excluded in cases with eosinophilia)
4.	Fewer than 20% blasts* in the blood and in the bone marrow
5.	Dysplasia in one or more myeloid lineages. If myelodysplasia is absent or minimal, the diagnosis of CMML may still be made if the other requirements are met, and: - an acquired, clonal cytogenetic or molecular genetic abnormality is present in the haemopoietic cells, *or* - the monocytosis has persisted for at least 3 months *and* - all other causes of monocytosis have been excluded.

* Blasts include myeloblasts, monoblasts and promonocytes. Promonocytes are monocytic precursors with abundant light grey or slightly basophilic cytoplasm with a few scattered, fine lilac-coloured granules, finely-distributed, stippled nuclear chromatin, variably prominent nucleoli, and delicate nuclear folding or creasing, and in this classification are equivalent to blasts. Abnormal monocytes which can be present both in the peripheral blood and bone marrow are excluded from the blast count.

neoplasms, *JAK2* V617F mutation is un-common in CMML {1058, 2082}.

ICD-O code   9945/3

Epidemiology

There are no reliable incidence data for CMML, because in some epidemiological surveys CMML is grouped with chronic myeloid leukaemias and in others is regarded as a myelodysplastic syndrome (MDS) {108}. In one study in which CMML accounted for 31% of the cases of MDS, the incidence of MDS was estimated to be approximately 12.8 cases per 100 000 persons per year {2414}. The median age

at diagnosis is 65–75 years, with a male predominance of 1.5–3:1 {48, 683, 777, 2047, 2102}.

Etiology

The etiology of CMML is unknown. Occu-pational and environmental carcinogens and ionizing irradiation are possible causes in some cases {108, 2026}.

Sites of involvement

The PB and BM are always involved. The spleen, liver, skin and lymph nodes are the most common sites of extramedullary leukaemic infiltration {48, 683, 777}.

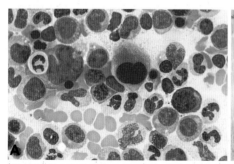 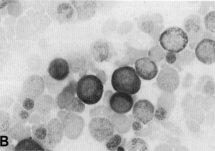 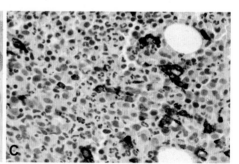

Fig. 4.01 Chronic myelomonocytic leukaemia-1. **A** In the Wright-Giemsa stained preparation, the dysplastic granulocytic component is obvious. **B** The monocytic component is appreciated with the special stains, naphthol-ASD-chloroacetate esterase reaction combined with alpha naphthyl butyrate esterase (monocytes brown, neutrophils blue, dual staining cells have mixture of blue and brown). **C** Bone marrow biopsy section stained by CD163. Note the positivity in scattered monocytic cells as well as the strong staining of the bone marrow macrophages. Immunohistochemistry can be used to identify monocytes in tissue sections, but is less sensitive than cytochemistry applied to bone marrow aspirate smears.

Clinical features

In the majority of patients, the white blood cell (WBC) count is increased at the time of diagnosis, and the disease appears as an atypical myeloproliferative neoplasm. In other patients, however, the WBC is normal or slightly decreased with variable neutropenia and the disease resembles MDS. The incidence of the most common presenting complaints of fatigue, weight loss, fever and night sweats is similar in the two groups of patients, as is the rate of infection and of bleeding due to thrombocytopenia {48, 683, 777, 2047, 2102}. Although splenomegaly and hepatomegaly may be present in either group, they are more frequent (up to 50%) in patients with leukocytosis {777}.

Morphology and cytochemistry

Peripheral blood monocytosis is the hallmark of CMML. By definition, monocytes are always >1x10⁹/L and usually range from 2 to 5x10⁹/L, but may exceed 80x10⁹/L {48, 683, 1396, 1471}. Monocytes are almost always >10% of leukocytes {189, 2003}. The monocytes generally are mature, with unremarkable morphology, but can exhibit abnormal granulation, or unusual nuclear lobation or chromatin pattern {1185}. The latter cells are best termed abnormal monocytes —a designation used to describe monocytes that are immature, but, in comparison to promonocytes (and monoblasts), have denser chromatin, nuclear convolutions and folds, and a more greyish cytoplasm. Blasts and promonocytes may also be seen, but if the sum of blasts plus the promonocytes is 20% or more, the diagnosis is AML rather than CMML. Other changes in the PB are variable. The WBC may be normal or slightly decreased, with neutropenia, but in nearly one half of patients it is increased due not only to monocytosis but also to neutrophilia {777, 1396, 1645}. Neutrophil precursors (promyelocytes, myelocytes) usually account for <10% of the leukocytes {189, 2003}. Dysgranulopoiesis, including neutrophils with hypolobated or abnormally lobated nuclei or abnormal cytoplasmic granulation, is present in most cases, but may be less prominent in patients with leukocytosis than those with a normal or low WBC {1185, 1396}. It may be difficult in some cases to distinguish between hypogranular neutrophils and dysplastic monocytes. Mild basophilia is sometimes present. Eosinophils are usually normal or slightly increased in number, but in some cases eosinophilia may be striking. CMML with eosinophilia may be diagnosed when the criteria for CMML are present, but in addition the eosinophil count in the PB is ≥1.5x10⁹/L. Patients in this category may have complications related to the degranulation of the eosinophils. These "hypereosinophilic" cases of CMML may

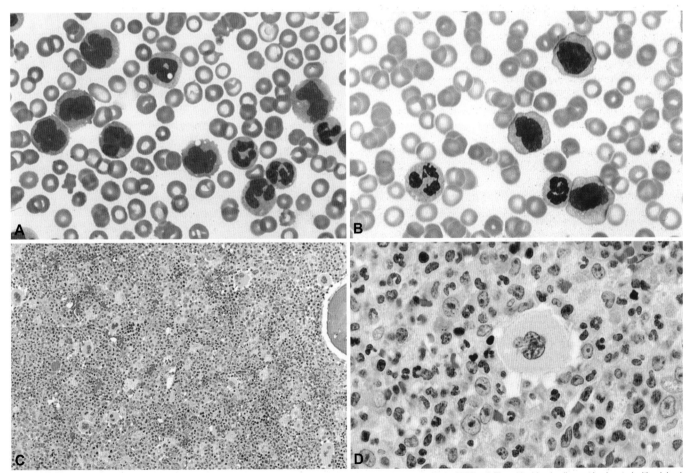

Fig. 4.02 Chronic myelomonocytic leukaemia-1. The degree of leukocytosis, neutrophilia and dysplasia is variable in CMML. **A** The white blood cell count is elevated with minimal dysplasia in the neutrophil series. **B** A normal white blood cell count with absolute monocytosis, neutropenia and dysgranulopoiesis. **C** A bone marrow biopsy specimen from a patient with CMML-1. Often, the granulocytic component is most obvious in the biopsy specimen, and monocytes may not be readily appreciated. **D** The folded nuclei and delicate nuclear chromatin characteristic of monocytes can be appreciated among the granulocytes.

closely resemble cases of myeloid neoplasms with eosinophilia associated with specific cytogenetic/molecular genetic abnormalities involving *PDGFRA* or *PDGFRB* genes, for which such cases should always be examined. These disorders are considered separately from CMML. Mild anaemia, often normocytic but sometimes macrocytic, is common. Platelet counts vary, but moderate thrombocytopenia is often present. Atypical, large platelets may be observed {48, 1396}.

The BM is hypercellular in over 75% of cases, but normocellular and even hypocellular specimens also occur {1471, 2102}. Granulocytic proliferation is often the most striking finding in the BM biopsy but an increase in erythroid precursors may be seen as well {189, 1471}. Monocytic proliferation is invariably present, but can be difficult to appreciate in the biopsy or on BM aspirate smears. Cytochemical and immunohistochemical studies that aid in the identification of monocytes and their less mature forms are strongly recommended when the diagnosis of CMML is suspected {2170}. Dysgranulopoiesis, similar to that found in the blood, is present in the BM of most patients with CMML, and dyserythropoiesis (e.g. megaloblastic changes, abnormal nuclear contours, ring sideroblasts) is observed in over one half of patients {777, 1396, 1471}. Micromegakaryocytes and/or megakaryocytes with abnormally lobated nuclei are found in up to 80% of patients {1396, 1471}.

A mild to moderate increase in the amount of reticulin fibres is seen in the BM of nearly 30% of patients with CMML {1406}. Nodules composed of mature plasmacytoid dendritic cells (plasmacytoid monocytes) in the BM biopsy have been reported in 20% of cases {1649}. These cells have round nuclei, finely dispersed chromatin, inconspicuous nucleoli and a rim of eosinophilic cytoplasm. The cytoplasmic membrane is usually distinct, with well-defined cytoplasmic borders. This imparts a cohesive appearance to the infiltrating cells. Apoptotic bodies, often within starry sky histiocytes, are frequently present. The relationship of the plasmacytoid dendritic cell proliferation to the leukaemic cells has been considered uncertain {120, 655, 895, 967}. A recent study, however, has shown that they are clonal, neoplastic in nature, and closely related to the associated myeloid neoplasm {2335}.

The splenic enlargement in CMML is usually due to infiltration of the red pulp by leukaemic cells. Lymphadenopathy is uncommon, but when it occurs, it may signal transformation to a more acute phase, and the lymph node may show diffuse infiltration by myeloid blasts. Sometimes, there is lymph node and (less commonly) splenic involvement by a diffuse infiltration of plasmacytoid dendritic cells. In some patients generalized lymphadenopathy due to tumoural proliferations of plasmacytoid dendritic cells may be

the presenting manifestation of CMML. Blast cells plus promonocytes usually account for fewer than 5% of the peripheral blood leukocytes and fewer than 10% of the nucleated BM cells at the time of diagnosis. A higher number of blasts (plus promonocytes) than this may identify patients who have a poor prognosis or a greater risk of rapid transformation to acute leukaemia {48, 682, 683, 833, 2102, 2170, 2443}. Thus, it is recommended that CMML be further divided into two subcategories, depending on the number of blasts (plus promonocytes) found in the PB and BM, as follows:

CMML-1
Blasts (including promonocytes) <5% in the PB, <10% in the BM;

CMML-2
Blasts (including promonocytes) 5–19% in the PB or 10–19% in the BM, or when Auer rods are present irrespective of the blast plus promonocyte count.

The value of this approach has been recently confirmed {780}.
Cytochemical or immunophenotypic studies are strongly recommended whenever the diagnosis of CMML is considered. When performed on PB and BM aspirate smears, alpha naphthyl acetate esterase or alpha naphthyl butyrate esterase, used alone or in combination with naphthol-ASD-chloroacetate esterase (chloroacetate

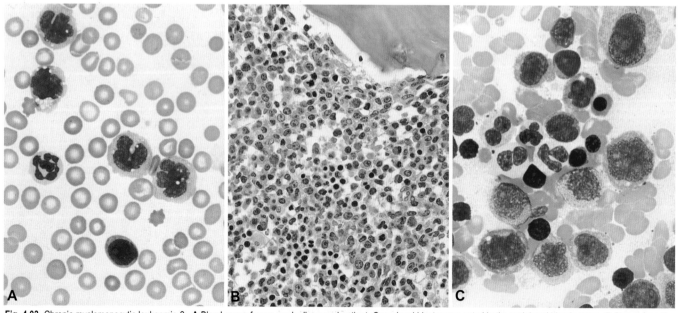

Fig. 4.03 Chronic myelomonocytic leukaemia-2. **A** Blood smear from a newly diagnosed patient. Occasional blasts were noted in the peripheral blood smear. **B** Biopsy from the same patient. The immaturity of the bone marrow elements can be readily appreciated. **C** Blasts and promonocytes account for 12% of the marrow cells (aspirate smear).

esterase, CAE) is extremely useful to assess the monocytic component.

Immunophenotype

The PB and BM cells usually express the expected myelomonocytic antigens, such as CD33 and CD13, with variable expression of CD14, CD68 and CD64 {243, 1377, 2442}. The PB and BM monocytes often express aberrant phenotypes with two or more aberrant features by flow cytometric analysis. Some, such as decreased expression of CD14, may reflect relative monocyte immaturity. Other aberrant characteristics include overexpression of CD56, aberrant expression of CD2 or decreased expression of HLA-DR, CD13, CD15, CD64 or CD36. There may be aberrant phenotypic features on maturing granulocytic cells and neutrophils may also show aberrant scatter properties. An increased percentage of CD34+ cells or an emerging blast population with aberrant immunophenotype has been associated with early transformation to acute leukaemia (AML) {626, 2442, 2459}.
Immunohistochemistry on tissue sections for the identification of monocytic cells is relatively insensitive as compared with cytochemistry or flow cytometry. The most reliable markers are CD68R and CD163 {1649}. Lysozyme used in conjunction with cytochemistry for CAE can also facilitate the identification of monocytic cells, which are lysozyme-positive but negative for CAE, in contrast with the granulocytic precursor cells, which are positive for both. An increased percentage of CD34+ cells detected by immunohistochemistry has also been associated with transformation {1649}.
The plasmacytoid dendritic cells associated with CMML have a characteristic immunophenotype. They are positive for CD123, CD14, CD43, CD68, CD68R, CD45RA, CD33 (weakly) and CD4. Granzyme B is also regularly expressed, but TIA1 and perforin are not. Variable CD56 expression is seen in a minority of the cases, while T-cell-associated antigens such as CD2 and CD5 can also be present.

Genetics

Clonal cytogenetic abnormalities are found in 20–40% of patients with CMML, but none is specific {48, 683, 684, 777, 867, 2102, 2170, 2260}. The most frequent recurring abnormalities include +8, -7/del(7q) and structural abnormalities of 12p. As many as 40% of patients exhibit point

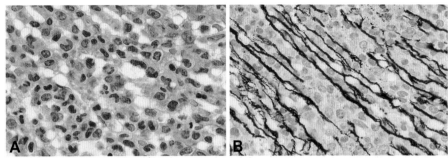

Fig. 4.04 Chronic myelomonocytic leukaemia. Some degree of fibrosis may be seen in up to 30% of cases. **A,B** These photomicrographs illustrate reticulin fibrosis in a marrow biopsy specimen of a patient with CMML.

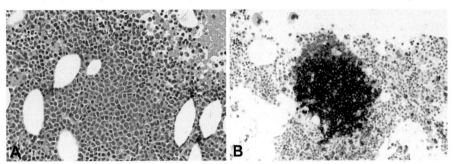

Fig. 4.05 Chronic myelomonocytic leukaemia. **A** Nodules composed of plasmacytoid dendritic cells in the bone marrow of a patient with CMML. **B** CD123 is positive in plasmacytoid dendritic cells.

mutations of *RAS* genes at diagnosis or during the disease course {1686, 2118, 2417}. The appropriate categorization of haematological neoplasms associated with isolated isochromosome 17q is uncertain at this time. Although a proportion of cases meet the criteria for CMML, others may be more appropriately categorized as MDS/MPN, unclassifiable {708, 1437}. Abnormalities of 11q23 are uncommon in CMML, and instead suggest the diagnosis of AML.
Cases of MDS/MPN with eosinophilia associated with t(5;12)(q31~33;p12) and an *ETV6-PDGFRB* fusion gene, which were formerly included in the CMML category, are now considered a distinct entity. Cases resembling CMML may express the p190 BCR-ABL1 isoform and should be classified as chronic myelogenous leukaemia (CML). Thus, if a t(9;22)(q34;q11.2) is not detected by cytogenetic analysis it is insufficient to use only PCR analysis for the presence of p210 to exclude CML.

Postulated cell of origin

Haemopoietic stem cell.

Prognosis and predictive factors

Survival of patients with CMML is reported to vary from one to more than 100 months, but the median survival time in most series

is 20–40 months {48, 682, 683, 777, 779, 833, 2047, 2102, 2170, 2443}. Progression to AML occurs in approximately 15–30% of cases. A number of clinical and haematological parameters, including splenomegaly, severity of anaemia and degree of leukocytosis, have been reported to be important factors in predicting the course of the disease. However, in virtually all studies, the percentage of PB and BM blasts is the most important factor in determining survival {48, 480, 682, 683, 777, 780, 833, 2047, 2102, 2170, 2443}.

Atypical chronic myeloid leukaemia, *BCR-ABL1* negative

J.W. Vardiman
J.M. Bennett
B.J. Bain
R.D. Brunning
J. Thiele

Definition

Atypical chronic myeloid leukaemia, *BCR-ABL1* negative (aCML) is a leukaemic disorder with myelodysplastic as well as myeloproliferative features at the time of initial diagnosis. It is characterized by principal involvement of the neutrophil lineage with leukocytosis resulting from an increase of morphologically dysplastic neutrophils and their precursors. However, multilineage dysplasia is common and reflects the stem cell origin of aCML. The neoplastic cells do not have a *BCR-ABL1* fusion gene.

ICD-O code   9876/3

Synonym

Atypical chronic myeloid leukaemia.

Epidemiology

The exact incidence of aCML is not known, but is reported to be only 1–2 cases for every 100 cases of *BCR-ABL1* positive CML {2003}. Patients with aCML tend to be elderly. In the few series reported to date, the median age at diagnosis is the seventh or eighth decade of life but the disease has been reported in teenagers as well {266, 928, 1208, 1396, 2003}. The reported male:female ratio varies, but based on the larger series reported, is approximately 1:1 {266, 928, 1208, 1396}.

Sites of involvement

The peripheral blood (PB) and bone marrow (BM) are always involved; splenic and hepatic involvement are also common.

Clinical features

There are only a few reports of the clinical features of patients with aCML. Most patients have symptoms related to anaemia or sometimes to thrombocytopenia, whereas in others the chief complaint is related to splenomegaly {266, 928, 1208, 1396, 2003}.

Morphology and cytochemistry

The white blood cell (WBC) count is always ≥13x10⁹/L {189} but median values ranging from 24–96x10⁹/L have been reported and some patients have WBC

Table 4.02 Diagnostic criteria for atypical chronic myeloid leukaemia, *BCR-ABL1* negative (aCML).

- Peripheral blood leukocytosis (WBC ≥ 13x10⁹/L) due to increased numbers of neutrophils and their precursors with prominent dysgranulopoiesis
- No Ph chromosome or *BCR-ABL1* fusion gene
- No rearrangement of *PDGFRA* or *PDGFRB*
- Neutrophil precursors (promyelocytes, myelocytes, metamyelocytes) ≥10% of leukocytes
- Minimal absolute basophilia; basophils usually <2% of leukocytes
- No or minimal absolute monocytosis; monocytes <10% of leukocytes
- Hypercellular bone marrow with granulocytic proliferation and granulocytic dysplasia, with or without dysplasia in the erythroid and megakaryocytic lineages
- Less than 20% blasts in the blood and in the bone marrow

counts in excess of 300x10⁹/L {266, 928, 1208, 1396, 2003}. Blasts are usually less than 5% and always less than 20% of leukocytes. Neutrophil precursors (promyelocytes, myelocytes and metamyelocytes) usually comprise 10–20% or more of the leukocyte differential. Although the absolute monocyte count may be increased, the percentage of monocytes rarely exceeds 10. Basophilia may be observed but is not prominent {189, 266, 928, 1396, 2003}. The major feature that characterizes aCML is dysgranulopoiesis, which is often pronounced. Acquired Pelger-Huët or other nuclear abnormalities, such as abnormally clumped nuclear chromatin or bizarrely segmented nuclei, and abnormal cytoplasmic granularity may be observed in the neutrophils. Moderate anaemia is frequent and the red blood cells may show changes indicative of dyserythropoiesis, including macroovalocytosis. The platelet count is variable, but thrombocytopenia is

common {189, 928, 1396, 2003}.
The BM biopsy is hypercellular due to an increase of neutrophils and their precursors. Blasts may be modestly increased in number, but are always less than 20%; large sheets or clusters of blasts are not present. Dysgranulopoiesis is a constant finding and the changes in the neutrophil lineage observed in the BM are similar to those described for the blood. Megakaryocytes may be decreased, normal or increased in number, but in most cases some dysmegakaryopoiesis is present, including small megakaryocytes and micromegakaryocytes and/or megakaryocytes with hypolobulated or non-lobulated nuclei {266, 928}. Usually the M:E ratio is greater than 10:1, but in some cases erythroid precursors account for over 30% of the BM cells. Dyserythropoiesis is present in at least 50% of cases {189, 266, 928}. Increased reticulin fibres are seen in some cases at the time of diagnosis, or may

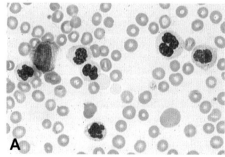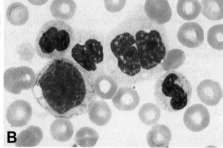

Fig. 4.06 Atypical chronic myeloid leukaemia. **A** An elevated WBC count in the peripheral blood. **B** Marked dysplasia and immature granulocytes. Cytogenetic studies revealed a +8, but no Ph-chromosome, and no *BCR-ABL1* fusion gene was detected by FISH.

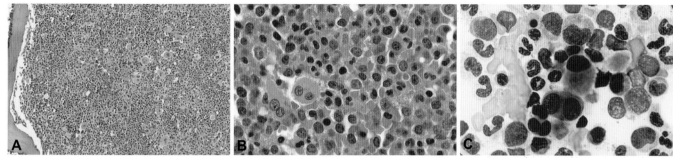

Fig. 4.07 Atypical chronic myeloid leukaemia. **A** Bone marrow biopsy shows hypercellularity, due to granulocytic proliferation. **B** Note an increase in the number of megakaryocytes, with small, abnormal forms. From the biopsy alone, the morphology would be difficult to differentiate from *BCR-ABL* positive chronic myelogenous leukaemia. **C** Bone marrow aspirate smear. Dysplasia in the granulocytic and the megakaryocytic lineages is evident.

appear later in the course of the disease. Most cases reported as the "syndrome of abnormal chromatin clumping" can be considered as a variant of aCML {276, 680, 1007}. These are characterized in the PB and BM by a high percentage of neutrophils and precursors that exhibit exaggerated clumping of the nuclear chromatin.

No specific cytochemical abnormality has been reported to date, although stains to detect a significant monocytic component can be useful to exclude chronic myelomonocytic leukaemia (CMML). A nonspecific esterase reaction performed on a BM aspirate may identify significantly more monocytes than are appreciated by routine stains. Leukocyte alkaline phosphatase scores may be low, normal or elevated, and thus are not useful for diagnosis {1208, 1396}.

Immunophenotype
No specific immunophenotypic characteristics have been reported to date. As with cytochemistry, immunohistochemical studies for CD14 or CD68R on biopsy sections may help to identify monocytes; finding a significant BM monocytosis should call the diagnosis of aCML into question.

Genetics
Karyotypic abnormalities are reported in up to 80% of patients with aCML. The most common abnormalities are +8 and del(20q), but abnormalities of chromosomes 13, 14, 17, 19 and 12 are commonly reported as well {266, 928, 1396}. Rarely, patients whose neoplastic cells have an isolated isochromosome 17q may have features of aCML although most will fulfill the criteria for CMML {1437}.

There is no *BCR-ABL1* fusion gene. Cases with rearrangement of *PDGFRA* or *PDGFRB* genes are also specifically excluded. The activating *JAK2* V617F mutation has been reported in some cases of aCML {1064,1287}. Approximately 30% of cases are associated with acquired mutations of *NRAS* or *KRAS* {2311}.

Some cases of t(8;9)(p22;p24) with the *PCM1-JAK2* fusion gene have been reported as "aCML" {259, 1833} but data currently available suggest they have eosinophilia and lack myelodysplasia and may be better regarded as chronic eosinophilic leukaemia. Meticulous description of the morphology of atypical myeloid proliferations associated with various genetic defects will be necessary to assign them to appropriate categories.

Postulated cell of origin
Bone marrow haematopoietic stem cell.

Prognosis and predictive factors
Patients with aCML fare poorly. The series reported to the present time include only small numbers of patients, but median survival times range from 14–29 months {266, 928, 1208, 2003}. Age >65 years, female sex, WBC >50x10^9/L thrombocytopenia, and Hb <10g/dL have been reported to be adverse prognostic findings {266, 928}. However, patients who receive BM transplantation may have an improved outcome {1178}. In approximately 15–40% of patients, aCML evolves to acute myeloid leukaemia, whereas the remainder die of marrow failure {266, 1208}.

Juvenile myelomonocytic leukaemia

I. Baumann
J.M. Bennett
C.M. Niemeyer
J. Thiele
K. Shannon

Definition

Juvenile myelomonocytic leukaemia (JMML) is a clonal haematopoietic disorder of childhood characterized by proliferation principally of the granulocytic and monocytic lineages. Blasts plus promonocytes account for <20% of cells in peripheral blood (PB) and bone marrow (BM). Erythroid and megakaryocytic abnormalities are frequently present {32, 303, 1477}. BCR-ABL1 is absent, whereas mutations involving genes of the RAS/MAPK pathway are characteristic.

ICD-O code   9946/3

Synonym

Juvenile chronic myelomonocytic leukaemia.

Epidemiology

The incidence of JMML is estimated to be approximately 1.3 per million children 0–14 years of age per year. It accounts for less than 2–3 % of all leukaemias in children, but for 20-30% of all cases of myelodysplastic and myeloproliferative disease in patients <14 years of age {907, 1704}. The age at diagnosis ranges from one month to early adolescence, but 75% of cases occur in children <3 years of age {345, 1346, 1595}. Boys are affected nearly twice as frequently as girls. Approximately 10% of cases occur in children with the clinical diagnosis of neurofibromatosis type 1 (NF1) {345, 1595, 2101}.

Etiology

The cause of JMML is not known. Rare cases have been reported in identical twins {1705}. The association between NF1 and JMML has long been established {345, 1595, 2101}. In contrast to adults who have NF1, children with NF1 are reported to have a 200- to 500-fold increased risk of developing myeloid malignancy, mainly JMML {1595}. Occasionally young infants with Noonan syndrome develop a JMML-like disorder, which resolves without treatment in some cases and behaves more aggressively in others {121}. These children carry germline mutations in PTPN11, the gene encoding the protein tyrosine phosphatase SHP2 {2162} or in KRAS {1974}.

Sites of involvement

The PB and BM always show evidence of myelomonocytic proliferation. Leukaemic infiltration of the liver and spleen is found in virtually all cases. Although any tissue may be infiltrated, lymph node, skin and the respiratory tract are other common sites of involvement {345, 1346, 1595}.

Clinical features

Most patients present with constitutional symptoms or evidence of infection {345, 1346, 1595}. There is generally marked hepatosplenomegaly. Occasionally spleen size is normal at diagnosis but rapidly increases thereafter. About half the patients

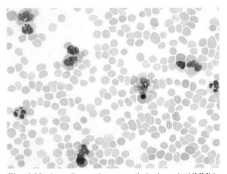

Fig. 4.08 Juvenile myelomonocytic leukaemia (JMML). Peripheral blood smear showing abnormal monocytes with cytoplasmic vacuoles and two normoblasts.

have lymphadenopathy. In addition, leukaemic infiltrates may give rise to markedly enlarged tonsils. Signs of bleeding are frequent and about a quarter of the patients have skin rashes. Café au lait spots are noted in patients with NF1.

A remarkable feature of many JMML cases is a markedly increased synthesis of haemoglobin F, specifically in cases with a normal karyotype {345, 1595}. Additional features include polyclonal hypergammaglobulinaemia and the presence of autoantibodies {345, 1595}. The clinical and laboratory features of JMML sometimes closely mimic infectious diseases, including those due to Epstein-Barr virus, cytomegalovirus, human herpesvirus 6 and others {1376, 1596, 1751}. Appropriate laboratory testing including molecular studies and in vitro cultures may be required to exclude infections as a cause for the clinical and haematologic findings.

In vitro, there is marked hypersensitivity of myeloid progenitor cells to GM-CSF {644}; this has become the hallmark of the disease, and represents an important diagnostic tool.

Morphology and cytochemistry

The PB is the most important specimen in proving the diagnosis. It generally shows leukocytosis, thrombocytopenia and often anaemia {345, 1346, 1595}. The median reported white blood count (WBC) varies from 25–30x10^9/L, but rarely is >100x10^9/L. The leukocytosis is comprised mainly of neutrophils, with some immature cells, such as promyelocytes and myelocytes,

Table 4.03 Diagnostic criteria of juvenile myelomonocytic leukaemia*.

1. Peripheral blood monocytosis >1x10^9/L

2. Blasts (including promonocytes)** are <20% of the leukocytes in the blood and of the nucleated bone marrow cells

3. No Ph chromosome or BCR-ABL1 fusion gene

4. Plus two or more of the following:
   - Haemoglobin F increased for age
   - Immature granulocytes in the peripheral blood
   - WBC count >10x10^9/L
   - Clonal chromosomal abnormality (may be monosomy 7)
   - GM-CSF hypersensitivity of myeloid progenitors in vitro

*Modified from {1596}.
**In this classification, promonocytes are equivalent to blasts.

as well as of monocytes. Blasts (including promonocytes) usually account for fewer than 5% of the white cells, and always less than 20%. Eosinophilia and basophilia are observed in a minority of cases. Nucleated red blood cells are often seen. Red blood cell changes include macrocytosis, particularly in patients with monosomy 7, but normocytic red cells are more common, and microcytosis due to iron deficiency or acquired thalassaemia phenotype {961} may be seen as well. Although platelet counts are variable, thrombocytopenia is usual and may be severe {345, 1346, 1595, 1705}.

Bone marrow findings are not by themselves diagnostic. The BM aspirate and biopsy are hypercellular with granulocytic proliferation, although in some patients erythroid precursors may predominate {1595, 1705}. Monocytes in the BM are often less impressive than in the PB, generally accounting for 5–10% of the BM cells. Blasts (including promonocytes) account for <20% of the BM cells, and Auer rods are never seen. Most often dysplasia is minimal. However, dysgranulopoiesis, including pseudo Pelger-Huët neutrophils or hypogranularity may be noted in some cases and erythroid precursors may be enlarged. Megakaryocytes are often reduced in number, but marked megakaryocytic dysplasia is unusual {345, 1595, 1705}. Reticulin fibrosis has been noted in some patients {345}.

Leukaemic infiltrates are common in the skin where myelomonocytic cells infiltrate the superficial and deep dermis. In the lung, leukaemic cells spread from the capillaries of the alveolar septa into alveolae, and in the spleen they infiltrate the red pulp, and have a predilection for trabecular and central arteries. In the liver, the sinusoids and the portal tracts are infiltrated.

No specific cytochemical abnormalities have been reported in JMML. In BM aspirate smears, cytochemical stains for alpha naphthyl acetate esterase or butyrate esterase, alone or in combination with naphthol-ASD-chloroacetate esterase, may be helpful in detection of the monocytic component. Although leukocyte alkaline phosphatase scores are reported to be elevated in about 50% of patients, this test is not helpful in establishing the diagnosis {1346}.

Immunophenotype

No specific immunophenotypic abnormalities have been reported in JMML. In extramedullary tissues, the monocytic component

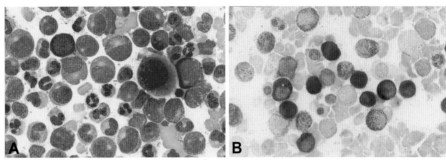

Fig. 4.09 Juvenile myelomonocytic leukaemia. A The bone marrow aspirate smear usually reflects the changes noted in the blood, but the monocyte component is difficult to appreciate. B A combined alpha napthyl acetate esterase and naphthol-ASD-chloroacetate esterase reaction identifies the granulocytic (blue reaction product) and the monocytic component (brown reaction product). A few cells contain both products.

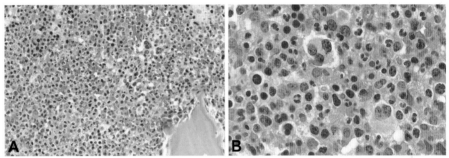

Fig. 4.10 Juvenile myelomonocytic leukaemia. A The bone marrow is hypercellular with granulocytic proliferation. B The megakaryocytes are reduced in number, but appear morphologically normal in the biopsy. Blasts are not substantially increased in number.

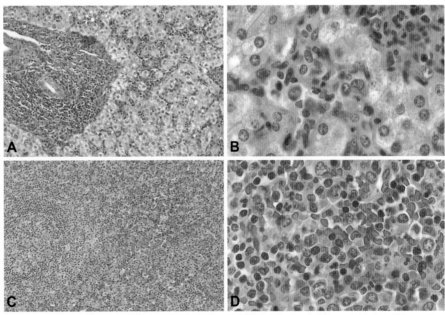

Fig. 4.11 Juvenile myelomonocytic leukaemia. The leukaemic infiltrate in the liver is in the portal regions (A) as well as in the hepatic sinusoids (B). C The leukaemic infiltrate in the red pulp of the spleen encroaches upon the germinal centre. D The infiltrate is comprised mainly of immature and mature neutrophils and monocytes.

is best detected by immunohistochemical techniques that detect lysozyme and CD68R. However, individual cases may show almost exclusively infiltration by myeloperoxidase-positive granulopoietic precursor cells.

Genetics

Karyotyping studies show monosomy 7 in about 25% of patients, other abnormalities in 10%, and a normal karyotype in 65% {1595}. Philadephia chromosome and the *BCR-ABL1* fusion gene are absent.

There is evidence that JMML is, at least in part, due to aberrant signal transduction resulting from mutations of components of the RAS/MAPK signaling pathway. Somatic mutations in *PTPN11* occur in 35% of patients {1329, 2162}, and oncogenic mutation of the *RAS* genes, *NRAS* and *KRAS2,* and of *NF1* are each seen in approximately 20% {2162}. Mutations in *PTPN11*, the *RAS* genes and *NF1* are largely mutually exclusive, suggesting that pathological activation of RAS dependent pathways plays a central role in the pathophysiology of the disease.

In JMML cells of children with NF1, uniparenteral disomy results in duplication of the mutant *NF1* allele {714, 2096}. Since the *NF1* gene product, neurofibromin, is a negative modulator of RAS function, the loss of the normal *NF1* allele is associated with RAS hyperactivity {1997}.

Postulated cell of origin
Haematopoietic stem cell.

Prognosis and predictive factors
Although JMML rarely transforms into acute leukaemia, it is a rapidly fatal disorder for most children if left untreated. The median survival time without allogeneic stem cell transplantation (HSCT) is about one year. Low platelet count, age above 2 years at diagnosis and high haemoglobin F at diagnosis are the main predictors of short survival {345, 1595, 1705}. In the absence of effective treatment, most children

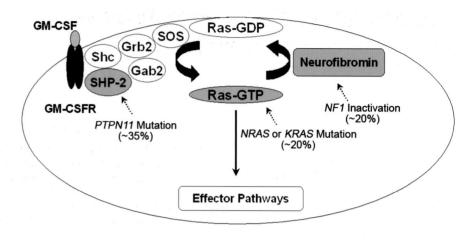

Fig. 4.12 Molecular lesions In Ras signaling proteins in JMML. GM-CSF normally binds to its receptor, induces heterodimerization, and assembles a complex of signaling molecules and adapters that includes Shc and Grb. These proteins, in turn, recruit Gab2, SHP-2 and SOS, which catalyzes guanine nucleotide exchange on Ras and increases intracellular levels of Ras-GTP. Once activated, Ras-GTP interacts with a number of downstream effectors. The GTPase activating proteins p120GAP and neurofibromin bind to Ras-GTP and accelerate conversion of Ras-GTP to Ras-GDP. Hypersensitivity to GM-CSF is a cellular hallmark of JMML that results from a number of distinct genetic mechanisms. Mutations in *PTPN11* increase SHP-2 phosphatase activity and enhance Ras signaling. Similarly, cancer-associated amino acid substitutions in *NRAS* or *KRAS2* result in mutant Ras proteins that accumulate in the active, GTP-bound conformation. Finally, inactivation of the *NF1* tumour suppressor gene deregulates Ras signaling through loss of neurofibromin.

die from organ failure, such as respiratory failure, due to leukaemic infiltration.

Haematopoietic stem cell transplant (HSCT) from a related or unrelated HLA compatible donor can cure about half the patients {1326}. Relapse is the major cause of treatment failure. There is clear evidence that graft versus leukaemia effect plays an important role, since a substantial proportion of children can be cured after a failed HSCT by donor lymphocyte infusion and immunomodulatory therapy {1787}. The role of anti-leukaemic therapy prior to HSCT is currently uncertain.

Myelodysplastic/myeloproliferative neoplasm, unclassifiable

J.W. Vardiman
J.M. Bennett
B.J. Bain
I. Baumann
J. Thiele
A. Orazi

Definition

Myelodysplastic/myeloproliferative neoplasm, unclassifiable, (MDS/MPN, U) meets the criteria for the MDS/MPN category in that, at the time of initial presentation, there are clinical, laboratory and morphological features that overlap both MDS and MPN. Cases classified as MDS/MPN, U do not meet the criteria for chronic myelomonocytic leukaemia, juvenile myelomonocytic leukaemia or atypical chronic myeloid leukaemia. The finding of a BCR-ABL1 fusion gene or of rearrangement of PDGFRA, PDGFRB or FGFR1 excludes the diagnosis of MDS/MPN, U.

It is important that the designation MDS/MPN, U not be used for patients with a previous, well-defined MPN who develop dysplastic features in association with transformation to a more aggressive phase. However, MDS/MPN, U may include some patients in whom the chronic phase of an MPN was not previously detected, and who initially present in transformation with myelodysplastic features. If the underlying MPN cannot be identified, the designation of MDS/MPN, U is appropriate. If there has been any recent cytotoxic or growth factor therapy, follow-up clinical and laboratory observations are essential to demonstrate that the peripheral blood (PB) and bone marrow (BM) changes are not due to the treatment.

ICD-O code   9975/3

Synonyms

Mixed myeloproliferative/myelodysplastic syndrome, unclassifiable; "overlap" syndrome, unclassifiable.

Sites of involvement

The BM and PB are always involved; spleen, liver and other extramedullary tissues may be involved.

Clinical features

The clinical features of MDS/MPN, U overlap those found in diseases of the MDS and MPN categories {129, 1588, 2311}.

Table 4.04 Diagnostic criteria for myelodysplastic/myeloproliferative neoplasm, unclassifiable (MDS/MPN, U).

- The case has clinical, laboratory and morphological features of one of the categories of MDS (refractory cytopenia with unilineage dysplasia, refractory anaemia with ring sideroblasts, refractory cytopenia with multilineage dysplasia, refractory anaemia with excess of blasts) and <20% blasts in the blood and bone marrow
  and
- Has prominent myeloproliferative features, e.g. platelet count $\geq 450\times10^9$/L associated with megakaryocytic proliferation, or WBC count $\geq 13\times10^9$/L, with or without prominent splenomegaly
  and
  Has no preceding history of an underlying MPN or of MDS, no history of recent cytotoxic or growth factor therapy that could explain the myelodysplastic or myeloproliferative features, and no Philadelphia chromosome or BCR-ABL1 fusion gene, no rearrangement of PDGFRA, PDGFRB or FGFR1, and no isolated del(5q), t(3;3)(q21;q26) or inv(3)(q21q26)
  or
- The patient has de novo disease with mixed myeloproliferative and myelodysplastic features and cannot be assigned to any other category of MDS, MPN or of MDS/MPN.

Morphology and cytochemistry

These disorders are characterized by proliferation of one or more myeloid lineages that is ineffective, dysplastic or both and simultaneously, by effective proliferation, with or without dysplasia, in one or more of the other myeloid lineages. Laboratory features usually include anaemia of variable severity, with or without macrocytosis and often dimorphic red blood cells on the peripheral smear. In addition, there is evidence of effective proliferation in one or more lineages, either as thrombocytosis (platelet count $\geq 450\times10^9$/L) or leukocytosis (white blood cell count $\geq 13\times10^9$/L). Neutrophils may show dysplastic features and there may be giant or hypogranular platelets. Blasts account for <20% of the leukocytes in the PB and of the nucleated cells of the BM, and a finding of ≥ 10% blasts in the PB or BM likely indicates transformation to a more aggressive stage. The BM biopsy specimen is hypercellular and may show proliferation in any or all of the myeloid lineages. However, dysplastic features are simultaneously present in at least one cell line.

Cytochemical findings may be similar to those seen in MDS or in MPN.

Immunophenotype

May be similar to findings in MDS and/or MPN.

Genetics

There is no cytogenetic or molecular genetic finding specific for this group. A Philadelphia chromosome and BCR-ABL1 fusion gene should always be excluded prior to making the diagnosis of MDS/MPN, U. Cases with rearrangements of PDGFRA, PDGFRB or FGFR1 or with isolated del(5q) or t(3;3) (q21;q26) or inv(3)(q21q26) are excluded from this category as well. In difficult cases, the presence of a JAK2 V617F mutation may help to confirm a haematopoietic neoplasm, though the significance of such mutations in this entity is uncertain. Occasional cases with isolated del(5q) and JAK2 V617F mutation have been reported to have features that overlap MDS and MPN {1005}.

Postulated cell of origin

Haematopoietic stem cell.

Refractory anaemia with ring sideroblasts (RARS) associated with marked thrombocytosis

Definition

In the third edition of the WHO Classification, RARS-T, previously also referred to as essential thrombocythaemia (ET) with ring sideroblasts, was proposed as a provisional entity to encompass patients who have the clinical and morphological features of the myelodysplastic syndrome,

RARS, but who also have marked thrombocytosis associated with abnormal megakaryocytes similar to those observed in the *BCR-ABL1* negative MPN, such as ET or early-stage primary myelofibrosis (PMF) {865, 1077, 2109}. However, some investigators have suggested that RARS-T is not a unique entity but instead represents cases of other subtypes of MDS or well-defined MPN that have acquired ring sideroblasts as a secondary form of dysplasia {1966}. It is not clear whether RARS-T is a distinct entity, one end of the spectrum of RARS, a progression of RARS due to an additional acquired genetic abnormality, or less likely, the occurrence of two rare diseases in the same patient. Therefore, until these questions are more clearly answered, RARS-T remains a provisional entity.

In support of a myeloproliferative component to this neoplasm, the majority of cases reported as RARS-T have shown the *JAK2* V617F mutation, or much less commonly, the *MPL* W515K/L mutation {234, 354, 762, 1835, 1839, 1969, 2081, 2139, 2358}. On the other hand, the few reported cases with this mutation that have been studied for endogenous colony formation *in vitro* have demonstrated a pattern more akin to that of MDS {234, 1835}. Thus it may be that the provisional designation of an MDS/MPN accurately reflects the underlying biology in a substantial proportion of the patients {762}; more study is needed to further clarify this disorder.

Cases with isolated del(5q),t(3;3)(q21;q26) or inv(3)q21q26) are excluded from this category, as are cases with a *BCR-ABL1* fusion gene. In addition, if there has been a prior diagnosis of an MPN without ring sideroblasts, or there is evidence that the ring sideroblasts might be a consequence of therapy or represent disease progression in a patient with features that meet the criteria of another well-defined MPN, this designation should not be used.

ICD-O code

9982/3

Morphology

These cases have features of RARS (anaemia with no blasts in the PB and dysplastic, ineffective erythroid proliferation often with megaloblastoid features, ring sideroblasts ≥15% of the erythroid precursors, and <5% blasts in the BM) and thrombocytosis with a platelet count ≥450x10⁹/L associated with proliferation

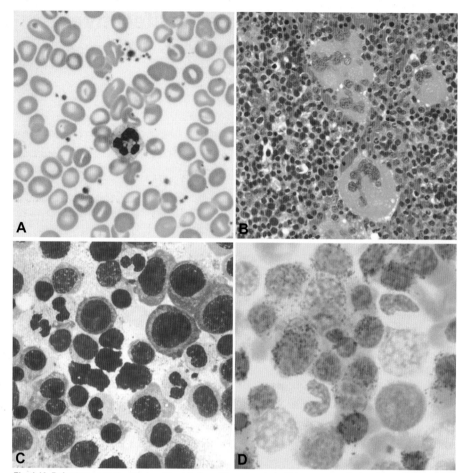

Fig. 4.13 Refractory anaemia with ring sideroblasts and thrombocytosis. This sequence of microphotographs illustrate blood and bone marrow of a 62-year-old man who presented with severe anaemia and a platelet count of 850x10⁹/L. **A** Abnormal red cells and thrombocytosis. **B** Erythroid proliferation and abnormal megakaryocytes resembling megakaryocytes seen in ET. **C** Mild dyserythropoiesis. **D** The majority of erythroid precursors were ring sideroblasts.

of large atypical megakaryocytes similar to those observed in *BCR-ABL1* negative MPN (See Chapter 2).

The minimum platelet count required for inclusion has been lowered to 450x10⁹/L from 600x10⁹/L for consistency with the defining criterion for ET, and because several studies have demonstrated that patients with platelet counts lower than 600x10⁹/L may have biological features, including *JAK2* V617F mutations, similar to those with counts ≥600x10⁹/L {354}. It is important to note that the criteria for RARS-T includes morphologically abnormal megakaryocytes similar to those observed in ET and in PMF. This criterion should aid in distinguishing RARS-T from those cases of RARS commonly reported to have a modest increase in their platelet count. Nevertheless, we recommend testing for *JAK2* V617F when the platelet count is elevated in patients with RARS until the borderline between RARS and RARS-T is more clearly defined.

Genetics

The recent discovery that up to 60% of patients with RARS-T harbour the *JAK2* V617F mutation (an incidence similar to that found in ET and PMF) or less commonly, the *MPL* W515K/L mutation, not only elucidates the reason for the proliferative aspect of RARS-T but also would seem to move it closer to the MPN category {234, 354, 762, 1835, 1839, 1969, 2081, 2139, 2358}. Thus, studies for *JAK2* V617F, and, if indicated, for the *MPL* W515K/L mutation should always be performed in such cases.

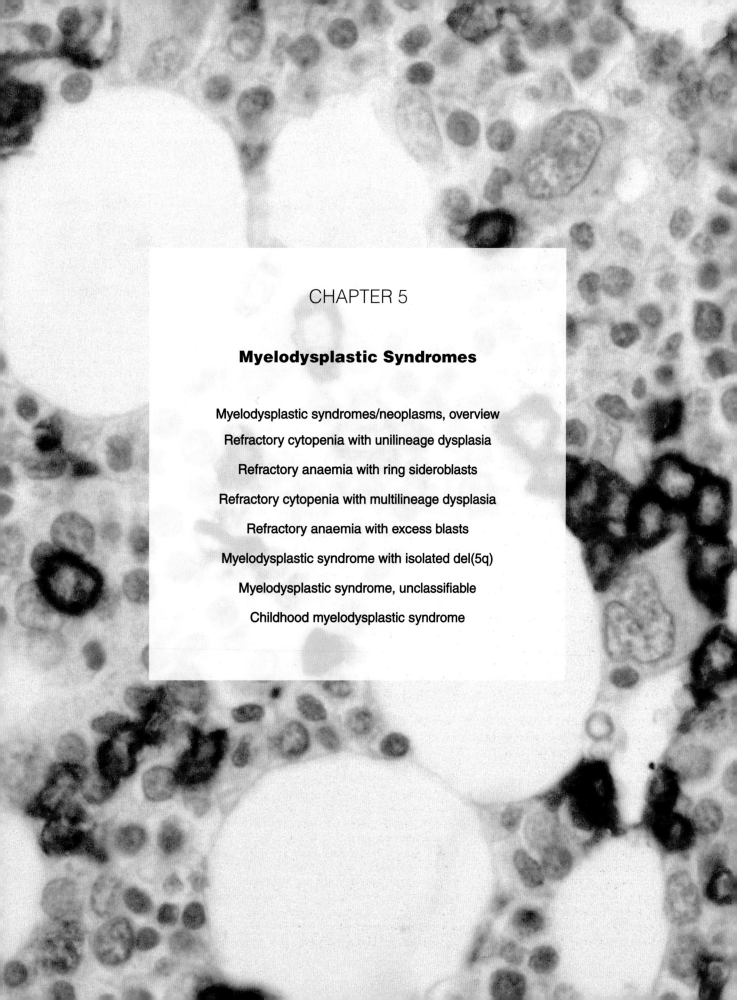

CHAPTER 5

Myelodysplastic Syndromes

Myelodysplastic syndromes/neoplasms, overview

R.D. Brunning
A. Orazi
U. Germing
M.M. Le Beau

A. Porwit
I. Baumann
J.W. Vardiman
E. Hellstrom-Lindberg

Definition

The myelodysplastic syndromes (MDS) are a group of clonal haematopoietic stem cell diseases characterized by cytopenia(s), dysplasia in one or more of the major myeloid cell lines, ineffective haematopoiesis, and increased risk of development of acute myeloid leukaemia (AML) {190, 353, 2310}. There is an enhanced degree of apoptosis which contributes to the cytopenias {260}. The thresholds for cytopenias as recommended in the International Prognostic Scoring System (IPSS) for risk stratification in the MDS are haemoglobin <10g/dL, absolute neutrophil count (ANC) <1.8x10^9/L and platelets <100x10^{9}L {833, 833A}. Values above these thresholds are, however, not exclusionary for a diagnosis of MDS if definitive morphologic and/or cytogenetic findings are present {2327}. The dysplasia may be accompanied by an increase in myeloblasts in the peripheral blood (PB) and bone marrow (BM) but the number is <20%, which is the requisite threshold recommended for the diagnosis of AML. It is important to recognize that the threshold of 20% blasts in the PB or BM for the distinction of AML from MDS does not represent a therapeutic mandate for treating patients with 20% blasts as acute leukaemia. A treatment decision to manage the patient as AML or MDS must be based on several factors including age, prior history of a myelodysplastic syndrome, overall clinical assessment and tempo of the process, which are the same determinant factors for patients with 30% blasts. Although progression to AML is the natural course in many cases of MDS, the percentage of patients who progress varies substantially in the various subtypes; a higher percentage of MDS with increased myeloblasts transforms to AML {781, 1371}. Although the majority of MDS are characterized by progressive BM failure, the biologic course in some patients, e.g. refractory anaemia with unilineage dysplasia (RA) and refractory anaemia with ring sideroblasts (RARS), is prolonged and indolent with a very low incidence of evolution to AML {781, 1370, 2327}.

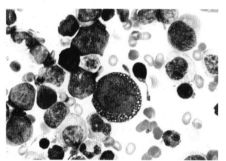

Fig. 5.01 Bone marrow smear from a patient with parvovirus B19 infection showing marked erythroid hypoplasia with occasional giant erythroblasts with dispersed chromatin and fine cytoplasmic vacuoles.

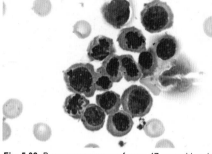

Fig. 5.02 Bone marrow smear from a 47-year-old male with pancytopenia being chronically poisoned with arsenic. There is marked dyserythropoiesis.

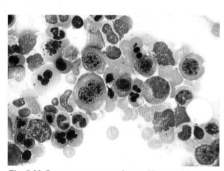

Fig. 5.03 Bone marrow smear from a 57-year-old woman who received several chemotherapeutic agents for breast carcinoma including folic acid antagonists.

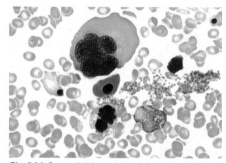

Fig. 5.04 Congenital dyserythropoietic anaemia. Marked dyserythropoiesis in a marrow smear from a patient with congenital dyserythropoiesis, type III.

Epidemiology

Myelodysplastic syndromes occur principally in older adults with a median age of 70 years, with a non-age corrected annual incidence of 3–5/100 000 persons but rising to >20/100 000 among those over the age of 70 years {109, 783}. Approximately 10 300 incident cases of MDS were diagnosed in 2003 in the USA {1351}. There is a male predominance. Therapy-related myelodysplastic syndromes are discussed in Chapter 6.

Clinical features

The majority of patients present with symptoms related to cytopenia(s); most of the patients are anaemic and transfusion-dependent. Less frequent are neutropenia and/or thrombocytopenia. Organomegaly is infrequently observed.

Etiology

Primary or *de novo* MDS occurs without a known history of chemotherapy or radiation exposure. Possible etiologies for primary MDS include benzene exposure at levels well above the minima allowed by most government agencies, cigarette smoking, exposure to agricultural chemicals or solvents and family history of haematopoietic neoplasms {2113}. Some inherited haematological disorders, such as Fanconi anaemia, dyskeratosis congenita, Shwachmann-Diamond syndrome and Diamond-Blackfan syndrome are also associated with an increased risk of MDS.

Morphology

The morphological classification of MDS is principally based on the percent of blasts in the BM and PB, the type and degree of dysplasia and the presence of ring sideroblasts {190}. The cytopenias generally correspond to the dysplastic lineage, but discordance may be present (Table 5.01) {2327}. To determine the blast percentage in the BM, a 500-cell differential of all nucleated cells in a smear or trephine imprint is recommended and in the PB, a 200-leukocyte differential. In severely cytopenic patients, buffy coat smears of PB may facilitate performing the differential.

The characteristics of the dysplasia are relevant when distinguishing between the various types of MDS and may be important in predicting biology. In addition, some cytogenetic abnormalities are associated with characteristic dysplastic features, e.g. isolated del(5q) and hypolobated and non-lobated megakaryocyte nuclei and del(17p) with hypolobated neutrophil nuclei {1237}.

Assessment of the degree of dysplasia may be problematic depending on the quality of the smear preparations and the stain. Poor quality smears may result in misinterpretation of the presence or absence of dysplasia particularly in assessing neutrophil granulation. Because of the critical importance of recognition of dysplasia to the diagnosis of an MDS, the necessity of high quality slide preparations cannot be overemphasized. Slides for the assessment of dysplasia should be made from freshly obtained specimens; specimens exposed to anticoagulants for more than two hours are unsatisfactory.

As a general precaution, no patient should be diagnosed as having MDS without knowledge of the clinical and drug history and no case of MDS should be reclassified while the patient is on growth factor therapy, including erythropoietin. In addition, cytopenia(s) in the absence of dysplasia should not be interpreted as an MDS. A presumptive diagnosis of MDS may be made in the absence of dysplasia if certain cytogenetic abnormalities are present (See Genetics). Persistent cytopenia without dysplasia and without one of the specific cytogenetic abnormalities considered as presumptive evidence of MDS should be viewed as the recently described "idiopathic cytopenia of undetermined significance" (ICUS), and the patient's haematologic and cytogenetic status should be carefully monitored {2422}.

In an attempt to more accurately predict clinical behaviour, cases of MDS without

Table 5.01 Peripheral blood and bone marrow findings in myelodysplastic syndromes (MDS).

Disease	Blood findings	Bone marrow findings
Refractory cytopenias with unilineage dysplasia (RCUD) Refractory anaemia (RA); Refractory neutropenia (RN); Refractory thrombocytopenia (RT)	Unicytopenia or bicytopenia[1] No or rare blasts (<1%)[2]	Unilineage dysplasia: ≥10% of the cells in one myeloid lineage <5% blasts <15% of erythroid precursors are ring sideroblasts
Refractory anaemia with ring sideroblasts (RARS)	Anaemia No blasts	≥15% of erythroid precursors are ring sideroblasts Erythroid dysplasia only <5% blasts
Refractory cytopenia with multilineage dysplasia (RCMD)	Cytopenia(s) No or rare blasts (<1%)[2] No Auer rods <1x10⁹/L monocytes	Dysplasia in ≥10% of the cells in ≥ two myeloid lineages (neutrophil and/or erythroid precursors and/or megakaryocytes) <5% blasts in marrow No Auer rods ±15% ring sideroblasts
Refractory anaemia with excess blasts-1 (RAEB-1)	Cytopenia(s) <5% blasts[2] No Auer rods <1x10⁹/L monocytes	Unilineage or multilineage dysplasia 5-9% blasts[2] No Auer rods
Refractory anaemia with excess blasts-2 (RAEB-2)	Cytopenia(s) 5–19% blasts Auer rods ±[3] <1x10⁹/L monocytes	Unilineage or multilineage dysplasia 10–19% blasts Auer rods ±[3]
Myelodysplastic syndrome – unclassified (MDS-U)	Cytopenias ≤1% blasts [2]	Unequivocal dysplasia in less than 10% of cells in one or more myeloid cell lines when accompanied by a cytogenetic abnormality considered as presumptive evidence for a diagnosis of MDS (See Table 5.04) <5% blasts
MDS associated with isolated del(5q)	Anaemia Usually normal or increased platelet count No or rare blasts (<1%)	Normal to increased megakaryocytes with hypolobated nuclei <5% blasts Isolated del(5q) cytogenetic abnormality No Auer rods

[1] Bicytopenia may occasionally be observed. Cases with pancytopenia should be classified as MDS-U.

[2] If the marrow myeloblast percentage is <5% but there are 2-4% myeloblasts in the blood, the diagnostic classification is RAEB 1. Cases of RCUD and RCMD with 1% myeloblasts in the blood should be classified as MDS, U.

[3] Cases with Auer rods and <5% myeloblasts in the blood and <10% in the marrow should be classified as RAEB 2.

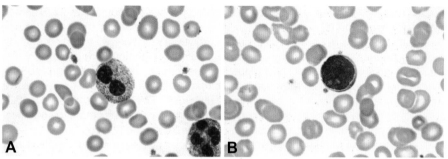

Fig. 5.05 A Blood smear from a patient on granulocyte colony stimulating factor. A neutrophil with a bilobed nucleus and increased azurophilic granulation. **B** The same specimen as (**A**) showing a myeloblast.

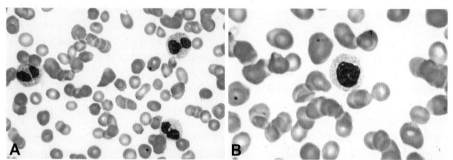

Fig. 5.06 A Dysgranulopoiesis. Blood smear from a patient with refractory cytopenia with multilineage dysplasia (RCMD) and a complex karyotype including del(17p) showing three neutrophils with bilobed nuclei. **B** Higher magnification of the same smear showing a neutrophil with a non-lobulated nucleus.

an increase in blasts are recognized as manifesting either unilineage or multilineage dysplasia. In RA and RARS, the dysplasia is generally confined to the erythroid lineage. Unilineage dysplasia may also occur in the neutrophils, refractory neutropenia (RN), and megakaryocytes, refractory thrombocytopenia (RT), but these processes are much less frequent than unilineage dysplasia involving the

erythroid cells. In refractory cytopenia with multilineage dysplasia (RCMD) with or without ring sideroblasts, significant dysplastic features are recognized in two or more of the major myeloid cell lineages. The recommended requisite percentage of cells manifesting dysplasia to qualify as significant is ≥10% {1864} in the erythroid precursors and granulocytes. Significant megakaryocyte dysplasia is defined as

≥10% dysplastic megakaryocytes based on evaluation of at least 30 megakaryocytes in smears or sections. Future studies may result in modification of this recommendation {1420}. Micromegakaryocytes and multinucleate megakaryocytes are the most reliable dysplastic findings in the megakaryocyte series {1420, 2327}.

Although the majority of patients with MDS and unilineage dysplasia present with a single cytopenia, this revised classification allows for bicytopenia in refractory cytopenia with unilineage dysplasia (RCUD) and RARS (Table 5.02). The majority of patients with RCMD have 2 cytopenias {1864}.

Characteristics of dysplasia
Dyserythropoiesis is manifest principally by alterations in the nucleus including budding, internuclear bridging, karyorrhexis, multinuclearity and megaloblastoid changes; cytoplasmic features include ring sideroblasts, vacuolisation and periodic acid-Schiff positivity, either diffuse or granular (Table 5.03). Dysgranulopoiesis is characterized primarily by nuclear hypolobation (pseudo Pelger-Huët) and hypersegmentation, cytoplasmic hypogranularity, pseudo Chediak-Higashi granules and small size. Megakaryocyte dysplasia is characterized by micromegakaryocytes with hypolobated nuclei, non-lobated nuclei in megakaryocytes of all sizes, and multiple, widely-separated nuclei. Megakaryocytic dysplasia may be more readily appreciated in BM sections than smears and both types of specimens should be evaluated.

The characteristics of the dysplasia may be relevant in predicting biology of a myelodysplastic disorder and the relationship to specific cytogenetic abnormalities, e.g. 5q- syndrome {2327}. Unilineage dysplasia is observed in RCUD and RARS. Multilineage dysplasia involving two or three of the myeloid cell lines is more frequently observed in the high-grade MDS and is used to distinguish RCMD from RCUD {1864}. Similarly, the presence of multilineage dysplasia is used to separate RARS from RCMD with ring sideroblasts, the latter of which has a similar clinical course to RCMD. An increased number of ring sideroblasts, occasionally >15% of the erythroid precursors, may be observed in refractory anaemia with excess blasts (RAEB). The defining criteria of RAEB-1 or RAEB-2 dictate the classification in such cases.

Table 5.02 Summary of cytopenias and dysplasia characteristics in MDS without an increase of marrow blasts.

Cytopenia(s)	Dysplasia	Categories
Unicytopenia Bicytopenia	Unilineage	Refractory cytopenia with unilineage dysplasia (RCUD) Refractory anaemia (RA) Refractory neutropenia (RN) Refractory thrombocytopenia (RT)
Unicytopenia Bicytopenia	Unilineage and ≥15% ring sideroblasts	Refractory anaemia with ring sideroblasts (RARS)
Pancytopenia	Unilineage	Myelodysplastic syndrome, unclassified (MDS-U)
Unicytopenia Bicytopenia Pancytopenia	Multilineage (≥2 myeloid cells lines)	Refractory cytopenia with multilineage dysplasia (RCMD)
Unicytopenia Bicytopenia Pancytopenia	Multilineage and ≥15% ring sideroblasts	Refractory cytopenia with multilineage dysplasia (RCMD)

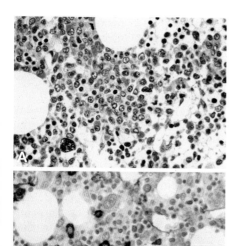

Fig. 5.07 A Abnormal localization of immature precursors. Bone marrow section from a case of RAEB-1 contains a focus of immature myeloid precursors. **B** A focus of immature cells in a bone marrow biopsy from a case of RAEB-2 reacted with antibody to CD34. A majority of the immature cells are positive.

The relationship between cytopenias, type of dysplasia, and classification is summarized in Table 5.02.

The significance of the Auer rod in myeloid disorders has historically been somewhat uncertain. For several decades its detection was viewed as virtually diagnostic of AML. There was no specificity applied to it with the introduction of the concept of MDS by the FAB group. In the revised FAB classification of 1982 it was viewed as evidence of a high-grade MDS, refractory anaemia with excess of blasts in transformation, (RAEB T), irrespective of the blast percentage in the PB or BM {190}. In the prior WHO Classification of the MDS it was considered as evidence

of RAEB-2 or CMML-2 in the context of MDS or MDS/MPN regardless of the blast percentage. This concept is retained in the present classification. Cases of MDS with <5% blasts in the BM and <1% in the PB may rarely have Auer rods. These cases have been reported to be associated with an adverse prognosis {2415}.

Differential diagnostic considerations

A major problem in the diagnosis of MDS is the determination whether the presence of myelodysplasia is due to a clonal disorder or is the result of some other factor. The presence of dysplasia is not in itself definitive evidence of a clonal disorder. There are several nutritional, toxic and other factors which may cause myelodysplastic changes, including but not limited to vitamin B12 and folic acid deficiency, essential element deficiencies and exposure to heavy metals, particularly arsenic and several commonly used drugs and biologic agents {260}. The antibiotic cotrimoxazole may cause marked neutrophil nuclear hypolobation indistinguishable from the changes observed in MDS. In some patients on multiple drugs it may be difficult to identify the causative agent of the neutrophil changes {1136, 2141}. Congenital haematological disorders such as congenital dyserythropoietic anaemia must also be considered as a cause of dysplasia when it is confined to the erythroid cells. Parvovirus B19 infection may be associated with erythroblastopenia with giant megaloblastoid erythroblasts; the immunosuppression agent mycophenolate mofetil may also be associated with erythroblastopenia. Chemotherapeutic agents may result in marked dysplasia of all myeloid cell lineages. Granulocyte colony-stimulating factor result in morphologic alterations in the neutrophils, including marked hypergranularity and

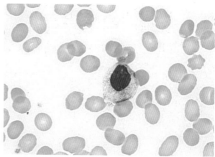

Fig. 5.10 Neutrophil with a non-lobated nucleus (pseudo Pelger-Huët) in a blood smear from a patient on co-trimoxazole. Approximately 50 percent of the neutrophils had a similar appearance.

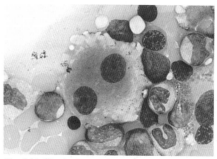

Fig. 5.11 Binucleate megakaryocyte in a bone marrow smear from a patient with a two-year history of refractory thrombocytopenia. There is a central granulomere and a peripheral hyalomere.

striking nuclear hypolobation {1968}; blasts may be observed in the PB and may reach levels of 9–10% and rarely higher in patients with no evidence of AML or MDS. The BM blast percentage is generally normal, but may be increased as well. Paroxysmal nocturnal haemoglobinuria may also present with features similar to MDS. As a result of all these possibilities, it is extremely important to be aware of the clinical history including exposure to drugs or chemicals and consider non-clonal disorders as possible etiologies when evaluating cases with myelodysplasia, particularly those cases with no increase in blasts. Repeated BM biopsies, including cytogenetic studies, over a period of several months may be necessary in difficult cases.

Histopathology

The value of the BM biopsy in MDS is well established {1647}. It may aid in confirming a suspected diagnosis by excluding reactive conditions in which dyshaematopoietic changes may also be observed; it can also increase the diagnostic accuracy and helps in refining the IPSS score {2328}. Assessment of BM cellularity and stromal reactions, e.g. fibrosis, are additional

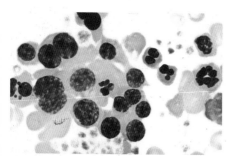

Fig. 5.08 Myelodysplastic dyserythropoiesis. Bone marrow smear from an adult male with refractory cytopenia with multilineage dysplasia (RCMD) and complex cytogenetic abnormalities including del(17p) and del(5q).

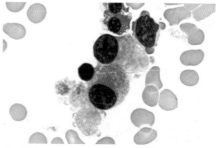

Fig. 5.09 Dysplastic megakaryocytes. Bone marrow aspirate smear from a 37-year-old male with pancytopenia showing megakaryocytes with dysplastic features.

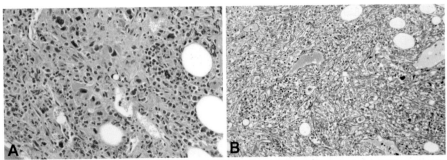

Fig. 5.12 A Bone marrow biopsy from a case of MDS (RAEB) with myelofibrosis. Several micromegakaryocytes are present. **B** Reticulin stain on a marrow biopsy from a case of MDS with myelofibrosis. There is a marked increase in reticulin fibres.

important diagnostic features of the biopsy. The BM in MDS is usually hypercellular or normocellular; the cytopenias result from the ineffective haematopoiesis. Histologically, aggressive MDS may be characterized by the presence of aggregates (3–5 cells) or clusters (>5 cells) of blasts in BM biopsies usually localized in the central portion of the BM away from the vascular structures and endosteal surfaces of the bone trabeculae. These are frequently present in RAEB. The blasts can also be identified by immunohisto-chemistry with antibody to CD34, an antigen expressed in progenitor cells and

early precursor BM cells in the majority of cases. Anti-CD34 can be used to demonstrate pathologic accumulations of blasts both singly and in clusters in aggressive subtypes of myeloid neoplasms {2050}. With some fixatives, CD34 will also immunoreact with megakaryocytes in MDS. Immunohistologic analysis with anti-CD34 may be especially useful in cases of MDS with fibrosis or hypocellular marrows as well as therapy-related cases to assess blast percentage. In these instances the presence of fibrosis or fatty changes in the BM may make accurate characterization of the process very difficult.

Hypoplastic MDS
In a minority of the cases of MDS, approximately 10%, the BM is hypocellular. These cases have been referred to as hypoplastic MDS. This group, which has no independent prognostic significance *per se*, may lead to difficulties in the differential diagnosis with aplastic anaemia {834, 1648}. In addition, anti-thymocyte globulin and other therapies used for aplastic anaemia have been used with some degree of success in this subgroup {260, 1302, 2477, 2478}. It is also important when considering the diagnosis of hypoplastic MDS to exclude toxic myelopathy and autoimmune disorders.

MDS with myelofibrosis
Significant degrees of myelofibrosis are observed in approximately 10% of the cases of MDS. These cases have been referred to as MDS with fibrosis {1246}. Most of the cases with fibrosis have excess of blasts and an aggressive clinical course. Such cases may erroneously be considered low-grade MDS if only the blast count determined from the BM aspirate, which is usually diluted with PB, is evaluated. In the fibrotic group, as in other

cases of MDS with inadequate aspirates, the blast determination requires a BM biopsy and immunohistochemical studies for CD34 may prove invaluable.

Immunophenotyping
Published studies on immunophenotyping by flow cytometry in MDS have focused on several strategies, including determining the size and immunophenotype of the blast population and assessing the maturation pattern of the myeloid cell population. More specifically, these studies included immunophenotyping of CD34+ cells, application of scoring systems, and pattern recognition strategies using multicolor analysis and comparison with normal/reactive PB and BM.

There is generally good correlation between the percentage of blasts as determined by morphologic examination of routine smear or imprint or immunohistologic preparations and percentage of CD34+ cells determined by flow cytometry (FC). However, in some cases there may be significant discordance due to significant myelofibrosis and haemodilute samples. As a result, FC percentages of CD34+ cells cannot replace differential counts on smears. However, FC may be informative if abnormal phenotypes of CD34+ cells are detected; this could be additional evidence of dysplasia. In addition, an emerging pathological population of CD34 or CD117 cells in low-grade MDS could suggest evolution of the disease {1622}.

Maturation patterns of erythropoietic, granulocytic, and monocytic differentiation in the normal/reactive BM, as well as the immunophenotype of the mature cells in PB have been thoroughly described using four-color FC. Erythroid abnormalities as determined by the pattern of expression of H-ferritin, CD71 and CD105 in glycophorin A (GPA) positive nucleated cells reportedly can predict morphological erythroid dysplasia with 98% sensitivity {550}. Aberrant maturation patterns in granulopoiesis could predict morphological dysplasia and abnormal cytogenetics in approximately 90% of cases {1212}. Thus, flow cytometry results correlate well with morphology and cytogenetics in MDS. However, in cases with borderline dysplasia by morphology and no cytogenetic abnormalities, FC results are highly suggestive for MDS only if there are three or more aberrant features in erythropoietic, granulocytic or monocytic maturation; single aberrant features by FC are not

Table 5.03 Morphologic manifestations of dysplasia.

Dyserythropoiesis
  Nuclear
    Nuclear budding
    Internuclear bridging
    Karyorrhexis
    Multinuclearity
    Nuclear hyperlobation
    Megaloblastic changes
  Cytoplasmic
    Ring sideroblasts
    Vacuolization
    Periodic acid-Schiff positivity

Dysgranulopoiesis
  Small or unusually large size
  Nuclear hypolobation
   (pseudo Pelger-Huët; pelgeroid)
  Irregular hypersegmentation
  Decreased granules; agranularity
  Pseudo Chediak-Higashi granules
  Auer rods

Dysmegakaryocytopoiesis
  Micromegakaryocytes
  Nuclear hypolobation
  Multinucleation (normal megakaryocytes are
    uninucleate with lobulated nuclei)

significant. Cases with inconclusive morphologic and cytogenetic findings and three or more aberrant features by flow cytometry should be reevaluated over several months for definitive morphologic or cytogenetic evidence of MDS.

Genetics

Cytogenetic and molecular studies have a major role in the evaluation of patients with MDS in regard to prognosis, determination of clonality {833, 1641}, and the recognition of cytogenetic, morphologic, and clinical correlates. Clonal cytogenetic abnormalities are observed in ~50% of MDS cases. Myelodysplastic syndromes associated with an isolated del(5q) occur primarily in women, are characterized by megakaryocytes with non-lobated or hypolobated nuclei, refractory macrocytic anaemia, normal or increased platelet count, and a favourable clinical course, and are recognized as a specific type of MDS in this classification. The occurrence of 17p loss is associated with MDS or AML with pseudo Pelger-Huët anomaly, small vacuolated neutrophils, *TP53* mutation and unfavourable clinical course; it is most common in therapy-related MDS {1237}. Complex karyotypes (≥3 abnormalities) typically include chromosomes 5 and/or 7 [-5/del(5q), -7/del(7q)], and are generally associated with an unfavourable clinical course. Several other cytogenetic findings appear to be associated with characteristic morphologic abnormalities such as isolated del(20q) with involvement of erythroid cells and megakaryocytes, and abnormalities of chromosome 3 [inv(3)(q21q26.2) or t(3;3)(q21;q26.2)], which are associated with MDS and AML with increased abnormal megakaryocytes {289, 866, 1207}.

Some clonal cytogenetic abnormalities occuring in MDS are not definitive evidence for this disorder in the absence of morphological criteria, e.g. -Y, +8 or del(20q) as the sole abnormality. The other abnormalities listed in Table 5.04 in the presence of a refractory cytopenia, but no morphologic evidence of dysplasia, are considered presumptive evidence for MDS. It is recommended that these patients be followed carefully for emerging morphological evidence of MDS. FISH provides increased sensitivity in monitoring such patients, once a recurring abnormality has been identified.

Postulated cell of origin

Haematopoietic stem cell.

Prognosis and predictive factors

The morphological subtypes of MDS can be generally categorized into three risk groups based on duration of survival and incidence of evolution to AML. The low-risk groups are RCUD and RARS. The intermediate-risk groups are RCMD with or without ring sideroblasts and RAEB-1. Patients with RAEB-2 constitute the high-risk group. It should be noted that patients with bicytopenia in RCUD and RARS have been reported to have a shorter survival than patients with one cytopenia {2327}. Patients with one cytopenia in the context of RCMD had a longer survival than patients with two cytopenias {2327}.

The importance of cytogenetic studies as a prognostic indicator in MDS has been recognized and codified by the International Myelodysplastic Syndrome Working Group {833}. Three major risk categories of cytogenetic findings have been defined: i) good risk —normal karyotype, isolated del(5q), isolated del (20q) and -Y; ii) poor risk —complex abnormalities, i.e., ≥3 abnormalities, or abnormalities of chromosome 7; and iii) intermediate risk —all other abnormalities.

A scoring system for predicting survival and evolution to AML based on percent BM blasts, type of cytogenetic abnormalities, and degree and number of cytopenias has been proposed by this group (Table 5.05) {833, 833A}. Four risk groups based on this scoring system are recognized: low, 0; INT (intermediate)-1, 0.5–1.0; INT-2, 1.5–2.0; and high, ≥2.5. In general, the higher-risk groups are related to higher BM blast percentage, more unfavourable cytogenetic findings and more

severe degree of cytopenia.

Consideration of age improves predictability of survival; patients younger than 60 years of age have improved survival in the individual risk categories compared with patients older than 60 years.

The cytogenetic subgrouping of the IPSS system also has an independent value in predicting the outcome of allogeneic stem cell transplantation in patients with MDS {532}.

Table 5.04 Recurring chromosomal abnormalities and their frequency in the myelodysplastic syndromes at diagnosis.

Abnormality	MDS	t-MDS
Unbalanced		
+8*	10%	
-7 or del(7q)	10%	50%
-5 or del(5q)	10%	40%
del(20q)*	5-8%	
-Y*	5%	
i(17q) or t(17p)	3-5%	
-13 or del(13q)	3%	
del(11q)	3%	
del(12p) or t(12p)	3%	
del(9q)	1-2%	
idic(X)(q13)	1-2%	
Balanced		
t(11;16)(q23;p13.3)		3%
t(3;21)(q26.2;q22.1)		2%
t(1;3)(p36.3;q21.2)	1%	
t(2;11)(p21;q23)	1%	
inv(3)(q21q26.2)	1%	
t(6;9)(p23;q34)	1%	

* The presence of these abnormalities as the sole cytogenetic abnormality in the absence of morphologic criteria is not considered definitive evidence for MDS. In the setting of persistent cytopenias of undetermined origin, the other abnormalities shown are considered presumptive evidence of MDS in the absence of definitive morphologic features.

Table 5.05 International Prognostic Scoring System (IPSS) for MDS {833,833A}. See Prognosis and predictive factors for interpretation.

Score	0	0.5	1	1.5	2
Prognostic variables					
% bone marrow blasts	<5%	5–10%		11–19%	20–30%*
Karyotype**	Good	Intermediate	Poor		
Cytopenias***	0–1	2–3			

*This group is recognized as AML in the WHO classification.
**Karyotype: Good = normal, -Y, del(5q), del(20q);
Poor = complex (≥3 abnormalities) or chromosome 7 anomalies;
Intermediate = other abnormalities
***Cytopenias: Hgb <10g/dL
Neutrophils <1.8x10⁹/L
Platelets <100x10⁹/L

Refractory cytopenia with unilineage dysplasia

R.D. Brunning
R.P. Hasserjian
A. Porwit
J.M. Bennett

A. Orazi
J. Thiele
E. Hellstrom-Lindberg

Definition

Refractory cytopenia with unilineage dysplasia (RCUD) is intended to encompass those myelodysplastic syndromes (MDS) which present with a refractory cytopenia with unilineage dysplasia and includes refractory anaemia (RA), refractory neutropenia (RN) and refractory thrombocytopenia (RT). Although refractory anaemia with ring sideroblasts is also characterized by unilineage dysplasia, it is considered as a distinct entity of its own. Refractory bicytopenia may be included in the RCUD category if accompanied by unilineage dysplasia. It is recommended that refractory pancytopenia with unilineage dysplasia be placed in the category of myelodysplastic syndrome, unclassifiable (MDS-U). The recommended level for dysplasia is ≥10% in the cell lineage affected. The recommended levels for defining cytopenias are haemoglobin <10g/dL, absolute neutrophil count (ANC) <1.8x10⁹/L and platelet count <100x10⁹/L {833, 833A}. However, values above these levels do not exclude MDS if definitive morphologic and/or cytogenetic evidence of MDS is present. The type of cytopenia in the majority of cases will correspond to the type of unilineage dysplasia, e.g. anaemia and erythroid dysplasia, although discordance between type of cytopenia and cell lineage dysplasia may be observed {2327}. Some of the cases previously classified as MDS-U may be included in this category, e.g. RN, RT. All non-clonal causes for the dysplasia must be explored and excluded before the diagnosis of MDS is established. These include, but are not limited to, drug and toxin exposure, growth factor therapy, viral infections, immunologic disorders, congenital disorders, vitamin deficiencies and possible essential element deficiencies, such as copper deficiency {837}. Excessive zinc supplementation has also been reported to be associated with severe cytopenia and dysplastic changes {1010}. If a clonal cytogenetic abnormality is not present, there should be a period of observation of six months from initial examination before a diagnosis of MDS is established unless more definitive morphologic or genetic evidence emerges during the observation period.

The presence of peripheral blood (PB) blasts essentially excludes a diagnosis of RCUD although in an occasional case a rare blast may be identified: patients with the findings of RCUD and 1% blasts in the PB and <5% in the bone marrow (BM) on two successive evaluations should be placed in the category of MDS-U because of the uncertain biology of this constellation of findings. Patients with 2–4% blasts in the PB and <5% blasts in the BM should be classified as refractory anaemia with excess blasts-1 (RAEB-1) if other criteria for MDS are present. The number of cases with these findings is very low and these patients should be carefully observed for increasing BM blast percentage {1165}. Refractory cytopenia with unilineage dysplasia should not be equated with "Idiopathic cytopenia of undetermined significance" (ICUS) which lacks the minimal morphologic or genetic criteria requisite for a diagnosis of MDS and should not be considered as such {2422}.

Synonym

Refractory anaemia.

Epidemiology

Refractory cytopenia with unilineage dysplasia comprises 10–20% of all cases of MDS {782, 1371}. It is primarily a disease of older adults; the median age is around 65–70 years. There is no significant sex predilection. The vast majority of RCUD cases are RA. Refractory neutropenia and refractory thrombocytopenia are rare and extreme caution should be used in making either of these diagnoses.

Sites of involvement

The PB and BM are the principal sites of involvement.

Clinical features

In RCUD, the presenting symptoms are related to the type of cytopenia. The cytopenias are refractory to haematinic therapy, but may be responsive to growth factors {983}.

Morphology

Refractory anaemia
(ICD-O code 9980/3)

In the PB in RA, the red blood cells are usually normochromic, normocytic or normochromic, macrocytic. Unusually, there is anisochromasia or dimorphism with a

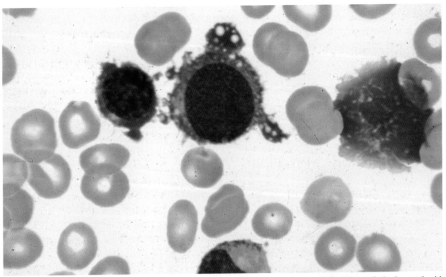

Fig. 5.13 Refractory anaemia. This bone marrow smear specimen shows dysplastic features only in the erythroid precursors; occasional erythroblasts show vacuolated cytoplasm and slightly megaloblastoid nuclei.

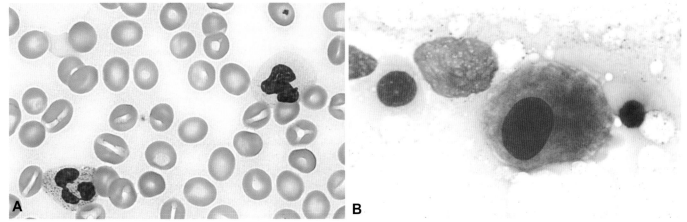

Fig. 5.14 A Refractory neutropenia. Blood smear from a 56-year-old male; the neutrophil in the lower left is normal appearing with well-granulated cytoplasm and a normally segmented nucleus. The neutrophil in the upper right is dysplastic with moderately hypogranular cytoplasm and occasional Döhle bodies. The nucleus shows retarded segmentation. Approximately half of the neutrophils were dysplastic. Cytogenetic studies showed an extra copy of chromosome 8 and pericentric inversion of chromosome 12. **B** A dysplastic megakaryocyte in a marrow smear from a 27-year-old male with a two year history of refractory thrombocytopenia. There is asynchronous nuclear cytoplasmic development with a well-granulated cytoplasm and a non-lobated immature nucleus. Cytogenetic studies at this time showed a missing Y chromosome. There was subsequent evolution at which time cytogenetic studies showed a missing Y, additional 9 and deletion 13.

population of hypochromic red blood cells. Anisocytosis and poikilocytosis vary from none to marked. Blasts are rarely seen and, if present, account for <1% of the white blood cells. The neutrophils and platelets are usually normal in number and morphology. However, some degree of either neutropenia or thrombocytopenia may be present.

The erythroid precursors in the BM in RA vary from decreased to markedly increased; dyserythropoiesis varies from slight to moderate; unequivocal evidence of dysplasia must be present in 10% or more erythroid precursors. Dyserythropoiesis is manifest principally by alterations in the nucleus including budding, internuclear bridging, karyorrhexis, multinuclearity and megaloblastoid changes; cytoplasmic features include vacuolization and periodic acid-Schiff positivity, either diffuse or granular. Ring sideroblasts may be present but are <15% of erythroid precursors. Myeloblasts account for <5% of the nucleated BM cells. The neutrophils and megakaryocytes are normal or may show minimal dysplasia, but always <10% in either cell line. The BM biopsy is generally hypercellular due to increased erythroid precursors, but may be normocellular or even hypocellular.

Refractory neutropenia
(ICD-O code 9991/3)
Refractory neutropenia is characterized by ≥10% dysplastic neutrophils in the PB or BM; the dysplasia is principally manifest as nuclear hypolobation and hypogranulation.

Neutropenia secondary to drug therapy, toxic exposure, infectious processes, immune mechanisms, or other causative factors must be excluded. The other myeloid cell lines do not show significant dysplasia (<10%).

Refractory thrombocytopenia
(ICD-O code 9992/3)
Refractory thrombocytopenia is characterized by ≥10% dysplastic megakaryocytes of at least 30 megakaryocytes evaluated: hypolobate megakaryocytes, binucleate and multinucleate megakaryocytes and micromegakaryocytes are the most reliable and reproducible features of megakaryocyte dysplasia. Dysplastic megakaryocytes may be more evident in sections than smears and usually well exceed the 10% threshold. The megakaryocytes may be increased or decreased. The other myeloid cell lines do not show significant dysplasia (<10%). Distinction from chronic autoimmune thrombocytopenia is critical and may be extremely difficult clinically and morphologically. Cytogenetic studies may be of considerable aid in this distinction {866}.

Immunophenotype
In refractory anaemia aberrant immunophenotypic features of erythropoietic precursors can be found by flow cytometry analysis {550}. There are no data on RN and RT.

Genetics
Cytogenetic abnormalities may be observed in up to 50% of cases of refractory anaemia {782}. Several different acquired clonal chromosomal abnormalities may be observed, and although useful for establishing a diagnosis of RA, they are not specific. The abnormalities generally associated with RA include del(20q), +8 and abnormalities of 5 and/or 7. The number of reported cases of RN and RT is too low to allow for generalizations, although del(20q) has been reported in RT {866, 1938}.

Postulated cell of origin
Haematopoietic stem cell.

Prognosis and predictive factors
The clinical course is protracted; the median survival of patients with RA in one series was approximately 66 months and the rate of progression to AML at 5 years was approximately 2% {782}. In another study, the median survival for patients over 70 years of age with RA, RARS and MDS with del(5q) was not significantly different from the non-affected population {1371}. Approximately 90–95% of patients with RA have low or intermediate International Prognostic Scoring System (IPSS) scores {833, 833A}. Approximately 80–85% have good to intermediate cytogenetic profiles {782, 1371}. Most patients with RT have low IPSS scores and 90% of the patients live more than two years {1938}.

Refractory anaemia with ring sideroblasts

R.P. Hasserjian
N. Gattermann
J.M. Bennett
R.D. Brunning
J. Thiele

Definition

Refractory anaemia with ring sideroblasts (RARS) is a myelodysplastic syndrome (MDS) characterized by anaemia, morphologic dysplasia in the erythroid lineage and ring sideroblasts comprising ≥15% of the bone marrow (BM) erythroid precursors. There is no significant dysplasia in non-erythroid lineages. Myeloblasts comprise <5% of the nucleated BM cells and are not present in the peripheral blood (PB). Secondary causes of ring sideroblasts must be excluded.

ICD-O code   9982/3

Epidemiology

RARS accounts for 3–11% of MDS cases. It occurs primarily in older individuals with a median age of 60–73 years and has a similar frequency in males and females {267, 782, 1371}.

Etiology

Ring sideroblasts represent erythroid precursors with abnormal accumulation of iron within mitochondria, including some deposited as mitochondrial ferritin {352, 827}. Primary defects of haem synthesis (such as the δ-aminolevulinic acid synthetase defect in hereditary X-linked sideroblastic anaemia) can largely be excluded because protoporphyrin IX, the end product of porphyrin synthesis, is not decreased in RARS {1209}. Furthermore, acquired mutations in genes of the haem synthetic pathway have not been demonstrated in RARS {2084}. Therefore, a primary defect

of mitochondrial iron metabolism is suspected. This defect may be caused by somatic mutations or deletions in nuclear or mitochondrial DNA. Potentially analogous congenital disorders include the Pearson marrow-pancreas syndrome, which features sideroblastic anaemia and is caused by congenital large deletions of mitochondrial DNA {478}. Somatic point mutations of mitochondrial DNA have been identified in the BM of some patients with RARS {763} but it remains to be established whether they cause the sideroblastic phenotype {1422}. Clonality of CD34-positive progenitor cells and erythroid and granulocytic elements has been demonstrated in RARS patients by X-chromosome inactivation analysis {549, 2126}. Stem cells from RARS patients display poor erythroid colony formation *in vitro* and manifest abnormal iron deposition at a very early stage of erythroid development {444, 2178}. This evidence suggests that RARS represents a clonal stem cell defect that manifests as abnormal iron metabolism in the erythroid lineage and results in ineffective erythropoiesis.

Sites of involvement

The PB and BM are the principal sites of involvement. The liver and spleen may show evidence of iron overload.

Clinical features

The presenting symptoms are related to anaemia, which is usually of moderate degree; some patients may additionally be thrombocytopenic or neutropenic. There

may be symptoms related to progressive iron overload.

Morphology

Patients typically present with normochromic macrocytic or normochromic normocytic anaemia. The red blood cells in the PB smear may manifest a dimorphic pattern with a major population of normochromic red blood cells and a minor population of hypochromic cells. Blasts are not present in the PB. The BM aspirate smear shows an increase in erythroid precursors with erythroid lineage dysplasia, including nuclear lobation and megaloblastoid features. Granulocytes and megakaryocytes show no significant dysplasia (<10% dysplastic forms). Haemosiderin-laden macrophages are often abundant. Myeloblasts are less than 5% of the nucleated BM cells. On an iron-stained aspirate smear, 15% or more of the red cell precursors are ring sideroblasts, as defined by 5 or more iron granules encircling one third or more of the nucleus. The BM biopsy is normocellular to markedly hypercellular, usually with a marked erythroid proliferation. Megakaryocytes are normal in number and morphology.

Ring sideroblasts are frequently observed in other types of MDS {776, 1078}. For example, cases with ring sideroblasts that have excess blasts in the PB or BM are classified as refractory anaemia with excess of blasts (RAEB). When ring sideroblasts are 15% or more of the erythroid precursors but there are 10% or more dysplastic cells in any non-erythroid lineage,

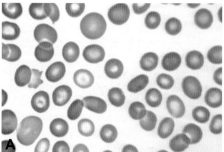
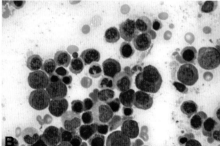
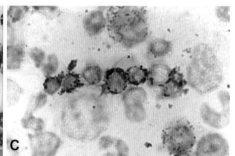

Fig. 5.15 Refractory anaemia with ring sideroblasts. **A** Blood smear with dimorphic red blood cells and macrocytes (Wright-Giemsa). **B** Bone marrow aspirate smear showing a marked erythroid proliferation with a dysplastic binucleate form (Wright-Giemsa). **C** Iron stain of bone marrow aspirate showing numerous ring sideroblasts.

and blasts are <1% in the PB and <5% in the BM with no Auer rods or monocytosis, the case is classified as refractory cytopenia with multilineage dysplasia (RCMD). Such patients have inferior survival to patients with RARS.

Non-neoplastic causes of ring sideroblasts, including alcohol, toxins (lead and benzene), drugs (isoniazid), zinc administration, copper deficiency and congenital sideroblastic anaemia, must be excluded {20}.

Immunophenotype
In refractory anaemia with ring sideroblasts, aberrant immunophenotypic features of erythropoietic precursors can be found by flow cytometry analysis {550}.

Genetics
Clonal chromosomal abnormalities are seen in 5–20% of cases of RARS and, when present, typically involve a single chromosome {267, 776, 778}.

Postulated cell of origin
Haematopoietic stem cell.

Prognosis and predictive factors
Approximately 1–2% of cases of RARS evolve to acute myeloid leukaemia. The reported overall median survival is 69–108 months {549, 778}.

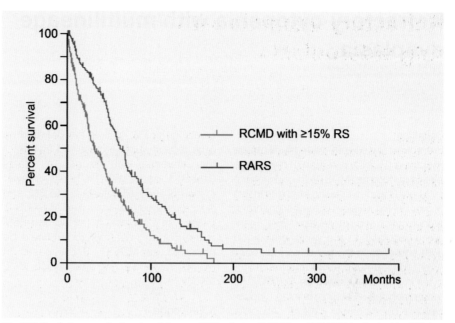

Fig. 5.16 Survival curves after long-term follow-up of 167 patients with RARS and 318 RCMD patients with ≥15% ring sideroblasts (RS), showing inferior survival for the patients with ring sideroblasts and multilineage dysplasia (p=0.00005)(Data from the Dusseldorf MDS registry).

Refractory cytopenia with multilineage dysplasia

R.D. Brunning
J.M. Bennett
E. Matutes
A. Orazi
J.W. Vardiman
J. Thiele

Definition

Refractory cytopenia with multilineage dysplasia (RCMD) is a type of myelodysplastic syndrome (MDS) with one or more cytopenias and dysplastic changes in two or more of the myeloid lineages: erythroid, granulocytic, megakaryocytic {1864}. There are <1% blasts in the peripheral blood (PB) and <5% in the bone marrow (BM); Auer rods are not present and the monocytes in the PB are less than 1×10^9/L. The recommended levels for defining cytopenias are haemoglobin <10g/dL, absolute neutrophil count <1.8×10^9/L and platelet count <100×10^9/L {833, 833A}. However, values in excess of these thresholds are not exclusionary of a diagnosis of MDS if definitive morphologic and/or cytogenetic findings are consistent with a diagnosis, e.g. complex cytogenetic abnormalities. The thresholds for dysplasia are ≥10% in each of the affected cell lines. In assessing dysplasia it is recommended that 200 neutrophils and precursors and 200 erythroid precursors be evaluated in smear and/or trephine imprint preparations. The neutrophil dysplasia may be evaluated in PB or BM smears. At least 30 megakaryocytes should be evaluated for dysplasia in BM smears or sections. In some cases, dysplastic megakaryocytes may be more readily identified in sections than smears. In particular the presence of micro-megakaryocytes should be noted. Cases with multilineage dysplasia and 2–4%

blasts in the PB, <5% in the BM, and no Auer rods should be classified as refractory anaemia with excess of blasts (RAEB)-1; cases with 1% blasts or fewer in the PB and <5% blasts in the BM, and Auer rods should be classified as RAEB-2; cases with 1% blasts in the PB and <5% in the BM and no Auer rods should be classified as MDS-U. Some cases of RCMD have ≥15% ring sideroblasts {782, 1371}.

ICD-O code   9985/3

Epidemiology

Refractory cytopenia with multilineage dysplasia occurs in older individuals; the median age is approximately 70 years. There is a slight predominance of males. The peak incidence for males is 70–74 years, for females 75–79 years {782}. It accounts for ~30% of cases of MDS {782, 1371}.

Sites of involvement

Blood and bone marrow.

Clinical features

Most patients present with evidence of BM failure with cytopenia of two or more myeloid cell lines.

Morphology

The BM is usually hypercellular. Neutrophil dysplasia is characterized by

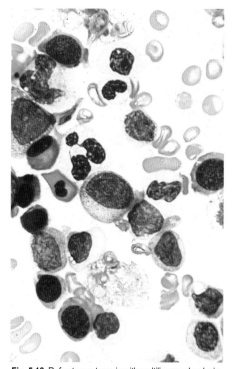

Fig. 5.18 Refractory cytopenia with multilineage dysplasia. Bone marrow smear shows evidence of dysplasia in both the erythroid precursors and the neutrophils. The mature neutrophils are small and have hypolobulated nuclei.

hypogranulation and/or nuclear hyposegmentation with marked clumping of the nuclear chromatin (pseudo Pelger-Huët nuclei). The nuclear hyposegmentation may occur as two clumped nuclear lobes connected by a thin chromatin strand (pince-nez type) or markedly clumped non-lobated nuclei. Myeloblasts account for <5% of the BM cells. In some cases there is a marked increase in erythroid precursors. Erythroid precursors may show cytoplasmic vacuoles and marked nuclear irregularity, including internuclear chromatin bridging, multilobation, nuclear budding, multinucleation and megaloblastoid nuclei. The vacuoles are usually poorly defined and dissimilar to the sharply demarcated vacuoles observed in toxic alterations such as alcoholism. The vacuoles may be periodic acid-Schiff (PAS) positive; there may also be diffuse cytoplasmic PAS positivity. In RCMD,

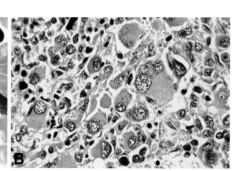

Fig. 5.17 Refractory cytopenia with multilineage dysplasia and complex cytogenetic abnormalities. **A** Bone marrow smear from a 37-year-old male with pancytopenia shows erythroid precursors with megaloblastoid nuclei and a red cell precursor with the nucleus encircled by Pappenheimer bodies (iron granules); ring sideroblasts were present in an iron stained smear. **B** Bone marrow section from the specimen in (**A**). Megakaryocytes are markedly increased and many have dysplastic features.

variable numbers of ring sideroblasts may be identified. Megakaryocyte abnormalities which may be observed include non-lobated nuclei, hypolobated nuclei, binucleate or multinucleate megakaryocytes and micromegakaryocytes; the micromegakaryocyte is defined as a megakaryocyte approximately the size of a promyelocyte or smaller with a non-lobated or bilobed nucleus and is the most reliable and reproducible dysplastic feature in the megakaryocyte series {1420}.

Immunophenotype
See Chapter on myelodysplastic syndromes/neoplasms, overview.

Genetics
Clonal cytogenetic abnormalities including trisomy 8, monosomy 7, del(7q), monosomy 5, del(5q), and del(20q), as well as complex karyotypes, may be found in up to 50% of patients with RCMD {782, 833}.

Postulated cell of origin
Haematopoietic stem cell.

Prognosis and predictive factors
The clinical course varies. The majority of patients with RCMD has International Prognostic Scoring System (IPSS) scores in the intermediate category {833, 833A}. Prognostic factors relate to the degree of cytopenia and dysplasia. The frequency of acute leukaemia evolution at two years is ~10% in RMCD {782}. The overall median survival is approximately 30 months. Patients with complex karyotypes have survivals similar to patients with refractory anaemia with excess of blasts (RAEB) {782}.

Refractory anaemia with excess blasts

A. Orazi
R.D. Brunning
R.P. Hasserjian
U. Germing
J. Thiele

Definition
Refractory anaemia with excess blasts (RAEB) is a myelodysplastic syndrome (MDS) with 5–19% myeloblasts in the bone marrow (BM) or 2–19% blasts in the peripheral blood (PB). Because of differences in survival and incidence of evolution to acute myeloid leukaemia (AML), two categories of RAEB are recognized: RAEB-1, defined by 5–9% blasts in the BM or 2–4% blasts in the PB, and RAEB-2, defined by 10–19% blasts in the BM or 5–19% blasts in the PB {833}. The presence of Auer rods in blasts qualifies a case as RAEB-2 irrespective of the blast percentage {781}.

ICD-O code   9983/3

Epidemiology
This disease affects primarily individuals over 50 years of age. It accounts for approximately 40% of all patients with MDS.

Etiology
The etiology is unknown. Exposure to environmental toxins, including pesticides, petroleum derivatives and some heavy metals increases risk, as does cigarette smoking {2113A}.

Sites of involvement
Blood and bone marrow.

Clinical features
Most patients initially present with symptoms related to BM failure, including anaemia, thrombocytopenia and neutropenia.

Morphology
The PB smear frequently shows abnormalities in all three myeloid cell lines, including red cell anisopoikilocytosis, large, giant or hypogranular platelets and abnormal cytoplasmic granularity and nuclear segmentation of the neutrophils. Blasts are commonly present. The BM is usually hypercellular. The degree of dysplasia may vary. Erythropoiesis may be increased with macrocytic/megaloblastoid changes. The erythroid precursors may

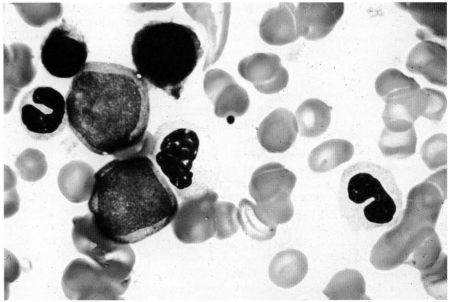

Fig. 5.19 Refractory anaemia with excess blasts-1 (RAEB-1). Bone marrow smear. The mature neutrophils in this case show nuclear hypolobulation (pseudo Pelger-Huët nuclei) and cytoplasmic hypogranularity.

show dyserythropoiesis including the presence of abnormally lobulated nuclei and internuclear bridging. Granulopoiesis is frequently increased and shows variable degrees of dysplasia. This is characterized primarily by small size neutrophils with nuclear hypolobation (pseudo Pelger-Huët nuclei) or nuclear hypersegmentation, cytoplasmic hypogranularity and/or pseudo Chediak-Higashi granules. Megakaryopoiesis is variable in quantity but is frequently normal to increased. The megakaryocytes often show a tendency to cluster. Dysmegakaryopoiesis is almost invariably present and is usually characterized by the presence of abnormal forms predominantly of small size, including micromegakaryocytes {2226}. However, megakaryocytes of all sizes as well as forms with multiple widely-separated nuclei can also occur. The BM biopsy shows alteration of the normal histotopography. Both erythropoiesis and megakaryopoiesis appear frequently dislocated towards the paratrabecular areas that are normally predominantly occupied by granulopoietic cells.
In a minority of cases the BM appears normocellular or hypocellular. RAEB cases with hypocellular BM represent only a small proportion of cases of hypoplastic MDS, since most of these cases do not show an increased number of blasts and belong to the group of refractory cytopenia with unilineage dysplasia (RCUD) or less commonly to refractory cytopenia with multilineage dysplasia (RCMD). The BM biopsy can be very useful in documenting the presence of an excess of blasts particularly in cases with suboptimal aspirate smears such as those associated with a hypocellular and/or fibrotic BM. Blasts in RAEB often tend to form cell clusters or aggregates that are usually located away from bone trabeculae and vascular structures, a histologic finding formerly referred to as abnormal localization of immature precursors (ALIP). Immunohistochemical staining for CD34 may be particularly helpful in their identification.

RAEB with fibrosis (RAEB-F):
In about 15% of patients with MDS, the BM shows a significant degree of reticulin fibrosis. Such cases have been termed MDS with fibrosis (MDS-F) {1246, 1406}.

Since myelofibrosis can be seen also in cases of therapy-related MDS, myeloproliferative neoplasms, and, rarely, in reactive dyshaematopoietic conditions (e.g. HIV-related myelopathy) these conditions need to be excluded. Because of the lack of consensus on the degree of fibrosis necessary to characterize a case as MDS-F, it is still unclear whether fibrosis represents an independent prognostic parameter {2083}. The current working definition of MDS-F requires diffuse coarse reticulin fibrosis with or without concomitant collagenization, associated with dysplasia in at least two cell lineages {2083, 2312}. Most of the cases defined as MDS-F belong to the RAEB category (RAEB-F). The presence of an excess of blasts in these cases can usually be demonstrated using immunohistochemistry, particularly for CD34. The BM smears are usually inadequate. A characteristic finding in RAEB-F is an increased number of megakaryocytes with a spectrum of cell size (including micromegakaryocytes) and a high degree of dysplasia {1246}. Cases of RAEB-F may morphologically overlap acute panmyelosis with myelofibrosis (APMF) previously referred to as acute (malignant) myelofibrosis. APMF is distinct from RAEB-F by its abrupt onset with fever and bone pain {1651, 2225}.

Immunophenotype

Flow cytometry in RAEB often shows increased numbers of cells positive for precursor cell associated antigens CD34 and/or CD117. These cells are usually positive for CD38, HLA-DR and myeloid-associated antigens CD13 and/or CD33. Asynchronous expression of granulocytic maturation antigens CD15, CD11b and/or CD65 can be seen in the blast population. Aberrant expression of CD7 on blast cells is seen in 20% of cases and CD56 is present in 10% of cases, while expression of other lymphoid markers is rare {1210, 1623}.

In tissue sections, CD34 immunohistochemistry may be used to confirm the presence of an increased number of blasts; it allows the appreciation of their arrangement into clusters or aggregates, a characteristic finding seen in most of the cases of RAEB {2050}. Antibodies such as CD61 or CD42b can aid in the identification of micromegakaryocytes and other small dysplastic forms, which are particularly numerous in cases of RAEB-F {1246, 2226}.

Genetics

A variable percentage of cases of RAEB (30–50%) have clonal cytogenetic abnormalities, including +8, -5, del(5q), -7, del(7q) and del(20q). Complex karyotypes may also be observed {782}.

Postulated cell of origin

Haematopoietic stem cell.

Prognosis and predictive factors

Refractory anaemia with excess blasts is usually characterized by progressive BM failure with increasing cytopenias. Approximately 25% of cases of RAEB-1 and 33% of patients with RAEB-2 progress to AML; the remainder succumb to the sequelae of BM failure. The median survival is approximately 16 months for RAEB-1 and 9 months for RAEB-2 {781}. CD7 expression has been associated with poor prognosis {1623}.

RAEB-2 patients with 5–19% blasts in the PB have a median survival of 3 months similar to that of myelodysplasia-related AML {2114}. In contrast, cases defined as RAEB-2 based only on the presence of Auer rods, have a prognosis which is similar to that seen in cases of RAEB-2 with 2–4% peripheral blasts (median survival, 12 months) {2114}.

Myelodysplastic syndrome with isolated del(5q)

R.P. Hasserjian
M.M. Le Beau
A.F. List
J.M. Bennett
J. Thiele

Definition
Myelodysplastic syndrome with isolated del(5q) is a myelodysplastic syndrome (MDS) characterized by anaemia with or without other cytopenias and/or thrombocytosis and in which the sole cytogenetic abnormality is del(5q). Myeloblasts comprise <5% of nucleated bone marrow (BM) cells and <1% of peripheral blood (PB) leukocytes and Auer rods are absent.

ICD-O code   9986/3

Synonym
Myelodysplastic syndrome with 5q deletion (5q- syndrome).

Epidemiology
MDS with isolated del(5q) occurs more often in women, with a median age of 67 years.

Etiology
Presumed loss of a tumour suppressor gene in the deleted region. Possible candidates include the early growth response 1 (*EGR1*) and α-catenin (*CTNNA1*) genes and as-yet-unidentified gene(s) in 5q32 {256, 1075, 1324}. The *RPS14* gene that encodes a ribosomal protein has been proposed as a candidate in the 5q- syndrome, raising the possibility that a defect in ribosomal protein function causes that disorder {256, 635, 1075, 1324}.

Sites of involvement
Blood and bone marrow.

Clinical features
The most common symptoms are usually related to anaemia, which is often severe and usually macrocytic. Thrombocytosis is present in one third to one half of patients, while thrombobocytopenia is uncommon {794, 1417}.

Morphology
The BM is usually hypercellular or normocellular and frequently exhibits erythroid hypoplasia {2362}. Megakaryocytes are increased in number and are normal to slightly decreased in size with conspicuously

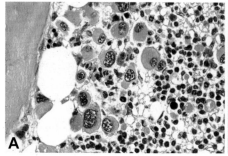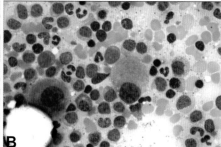

Fig. 5.20 Myelodysplastic syndrome with isolated del(5q). **A** Bone marrow section. Numerous megakaryocytes of various sizes are present. Several have hypolobated nuclei. **B** Bone marrow aspirate smear. Two megakaryocytes with hypolobated, rounded nuclei are present.

non-lobated and hypolobated nuclei. In contrast, dysplasia in the erythroid and myeloid lineages is uncommon {257, 794}. The term "5q- syndrome" has been used to designate a subset of cases with macrocytic anaemia, normal or elevated platelet count and BM erythroid hypoplasia {257, 2362}. The number of blasts in the BM is <5% and in the PB is <1%.

Genetics
The sole cytogenetic abnormality involves an interstitial deletion of chromosome 5; the size of the deletion and the breakpoints are variable, but bands q31-q33 are invariably deleted. If any additional cytogenetic abnormality is present (with the exception of a loss of the Y chromosome), the case should not be placed in this category. It has been recently reported that a small subset of patients with isolated del(5q) may show a concomitant *JAK2* V617F mutation. Until more data are collected for such cases and their clinical behaviour and response to therapy such as lenalidomide are clarified, it is prudent to classify them as MDS with isolated del(5q) (rather than in the MDS/MPN category) and to note the presence of the *JAK2* V617F in the diagnosis {1005}.

Postulated cell of origin
Haematopoietic stem cell. FISH analysis has confirmed presence of the del(5q) abnormality in differentiating erythroid, myeloid, and megakaryocytic cells, but generally not in mature lymphoid cells {39, 219}.

Prognosis and predictive factors
This disease is associated with a median survival of 145 months, with transformation to acute myeloid leukaemia occurring in <10% of patients {794}. Patients with del(5q) associated with other chromosomal abnormalities or with excess blasts have an inferior survival and are excluded from this diagnosis {794}. Recently, the thalidomide analogue lenalidomide has been shown to benefit MDS patients with isolated del(5q) as well as del(5q) with additional cytogenetic abnormalities. Transfusion independence was achieved in two thirds of patients and was closely linked to suppression of the abnormal clone {795, 1320}.

Myelodysplastic syndrome, unclassifiable

A. Orazi
R.D. Brunning
I. Baumann
R.P. Hasserjian

Definition

Myelodysplastic syndrome, unclassifiable (MDS-U) is a subtype of MDS which initially lacks findings appropriate for classification into any other MDS category. Three possible situations which qualify patients for inclusion in this category are listed under "morphology".

ICD-O code   9989/3

Synonym

Myelodysplastic syndrome, NOS.

Epidemiology

The incidence of myelodysplastic syndrome, unclassifiable, is unknown.

Sites of involvement

The peripheral blood (PB) and bone marrow (BM) are the principal sites of involvement.

Clinical features

Patients present with symptoms similar to those seen in the other myelodysplastic syndromes.

Morphology

There are no specific morphological findings. The diagnosis of myelodysplastic syndrome, unclassifiable, can be made in the following instances:

1. Patients with the findings of refractory cytopenia with unilineage dysplasia (RCUD) or refractory cytopenia with multilineage dysplasia (RCMD) but with 1% blasts in the PB qualify for MDS-U {1165}.

2. Cases of MDS with unilineage dysplasia which are associated with pancytopenia. In contrast, the RCUD category only allows for a single cytopenia or bi-cytopenia.

3. Patients with persistent cytopenia(s) with 1% or fewer blasts in the blood and fewer than 5% in the BM, unequivocal dysplasia (Table 5.03) in less than 10% of the cells in one or more myeloid lineages, and who have cytogenetic abnormalities considered as presumptive evidence of MDS (Table 5.04) are placed in this category. MDS-U patients should be carefully followed for evidence of evolution to a more specific MDS type.

Genetics

See Table 5.04.

Postulated cell of origin

Haematopoietic stem cell.

Prognosis and predictive factors

If characteristics of a specific subtype of MDS develop later in the course of the disease, the case should be reclassified accordingly. In cases diagnosed as MDS, U, it is unknown both the percentage of patients which transform to acute myeloid leukaemia as well as the disease survival. Cases with features otherwise consistent with a diagnosis of RCUD or RCMD, but in which 1% blasts are detected in the peripheral blood, have been shown to have a prognosis which is intermediate between RCUD (or RCMD) and that of refractory anaemia with excess blasts (RAEB) {1165}.

Childhood myelodysplastic syndrome

I. Baumann
C.M. Niemeyer
J.M. Bennett
K. Shannon

Myelodysplastic syndrome (MDS) is very uncommon in children, accounting for less than 5% of all haematopoietic neoplasms in patients less than 14 years of age (Table 5.06) {908, 910, 1595A, 2079A}. The *de novo* or primary form of MDS in children should be distinguished from cases of "secondary MDS" that follow congenital or acquired bone marrow (BM) failure syndromes and from therapy-related MDS that follows cytotoxic therapy for a previous neoplastic or non-neoplastic condition. Furthermore, although MDS associated with Down syndrome has been reported to account for 20–25% of cases of childhood MDS in the past {2079A}, this disorder is now considered as a unique biologic entity synonymous with Down syndrome-related myeloid leukaemia and distinct from other cases of childhood MDS (See Chapter 6).

Many of the morphologic, immunophenotypic and genetic features observed in MDS in adults are also seen in childhood forms of the disease but there are some significant differences reported, particularly in patients who do not have increased blasts in their peripheral blood (PB) or

BM. For example, the subtypes of refractory anaemia with ring sideroblasts and MDS associated with isolated del (5q) chromosomal abnormality are exceedingly rare in children {1595A}. Isolated anaemia, which is the major presenting manifestation of refractory anaemia (RA) in adults, is uncommon in children, who are more likely to present with neutropenia and thrombocytopenia {908, 1109}. In addition, hypocellularity of the BM is more commonly observed in childhood MDS than in older patients. Therefore, some children have findings that do not readily fit into the "low grade" MDS categories. To address these differences, a provisional entity, refractory cytopenia of childhood (RCC) is introduced and defined below.

For children with MDS in whom there are 2–19% blasts in the PB or 5–19% blasts in the BM, the same criteria utilized for adults with refractory anaemia with excess blasts (RAEB) should be applied. Currently, in contrast to adult MDS, there are no available studies that have investigated the prognostic significance of distinguishing RAEB-1 and RAEB-2 in children, but it is recommended that this distinction be made for future investigation. Children with RAEB generally have relatively stable PB counts for weeks or months. Some cases diagnosed in children as acute myeloid leukaemia (AML) with 20–29% blasts in the PB and/or BM that have myelodysplasia-related changes, including cases with myelodysplasia-related cytogenetic abnormalities (See Chapter 6) may also have slowly progressive disease. These cases, considered as refractory anaemia with excess blasts in transformation in the French-American-British cooperative classification, may lack the clinical features of acute leukaemia and behave more like MDS than AML {908}, thus follow-up PB and BM studies are often necessary to measure the pace of the disease in such cases. Children who present with a PB and/or BM disorder associated with t(8;21)(q22;q22), inv(16)(p13.1q22) or t(16;16)(p13.1;q22) or t(15;17)(q22;q12) should be considered to have AML regardless of the blast count.

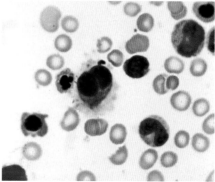

Fig. 5.21 Refractory cytopenia of childhood (RCC). Bone marrow smear showing abnormal nuclear lobulation of an erythropoietic precursor cell and a small megakaryocyte with a bi-lobed nucleus.

Refractory cytopenia of childhood (RCC)

Definition

Refractory cytopenia of childhood (RCC) is a myelodysplastic syndrome (MDS) characterized by persistent cytopenia with <5% blasts in the BM and <2% blasts in the PB {908}. Although the presence of dysplasia is required for the diagnosis, the cytological evaluation of dysplasia by itself constitutes only one aspect of the morphological diagnosis of RCC. The evaluation of an adequate BM trephine biopsy specimen is indispensable for the diagnosis of RCC in children. About 75% of children with RCC show considerable hypocellularity of the BM {1784}. Consequently, it may be very challenging to differentiate hypocellular RCC from other BM failure disorders, especially from acquired aplastic anaemia and inherited BM failure disorders. Down syndrome-related myeloid neoplasms are excluded from this diagnosis. The WHO Working Group assigned RCC to a group of provisional entities.

ICD-O code   9985/3

Synonym

Refractory anaemia of childhood.

Epidemiology

RCC is the most common subtype of MDS in childhood accounting for about 50% of

---

Table 5.06 Incidence of haematological malignancies in children 0 - 14 years. Combined data from Denmark 1980–1991 and British Columbia 1982–1996 {907, 908}.

	N	%	Incidence[2]
ALL	815	79	38.5
AML[1]	115	11	5.4
MDS[1]	38	4	1.8
Myeloid leukaemia of DS	19	2	0.9
JMML	25	2	1.2
CML	13	1	0.6
PV/ET	3	0	0.1
Unclassified	3	0	0.1
Total	1031	100	48.7

ALL, acute lymphoblastic leukaemia; AML, acute myeloid leukaemia; MDS, myelodysplastic syndrome; JMML, juvenile myelomonocytic leukaemia; CML, chronic myelogenous leukaemia; PV, polycythaemia vera; ET, essential thrombocythaemia
[1] Excluding Down syndrome (DS)
[2] per million population per year

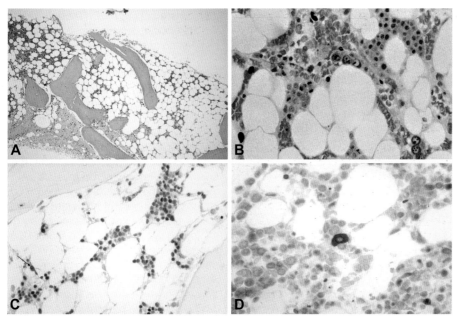

Fig. 5.22 Refractory cytopenia of childhood (RCC). Bone marrow biopsies. **A** This specimen shows the patchy distribution of haematopoiesis in RCC. **B** Cluster of proerythroblasts without maturation. **C** Left shifted erythropoietic island with naphthol-ASD-chloracetate esterase positive mast cells and very few positive granulopoietic cells. **D** CD61 immunohistochemical stain showing a positive megakaryocyte within an erythropoietic island. CD61 may be very helpful in detecting dysplastic megakaryocytes to aid in confirming the diagnosis of RCC.

the cases {1704, 1784}. It is diagnosed in all age groups and affects boys and girls with equal frequency {1109}.

Sites of involvement
Blood and BM are always affected. Generally, spleen, liver and lymph nodes are not sites of initial manifestation.

Clinical features
The most common symptoms are malaise, bleeding, fever and infection {1109}. Lymphadenopathy secondary to local or systemic infection may be present, but hepatosplenomegaly is generally not a feature of RCC. In up to 20% of patients, no clinical signs or symptoms are reported {1109}. Congenital abnormalities of different organ systems may be present.
Three quarters of patients have a platelet count below 150x10^9/L, while anaemia with a haemoglobin concentration of less than 10 g/dL is noted in about half of the affected children {1109}. Macrocytosis of red cells evaluated according to the patient's age is seen in most. The white blood count is generally decreased with severe neutropenia noted in about 25% {1109}.

Etiology
The etiology is unknown in most cases.

Morphology
The classical picture of RCC is a PB smear that shows red blood cell anisopoikilocytosis and macrocytosis. Anisochromia may be present. Platelets often display anisocytosis and occasionally giant platelets can be detected. Neutropenia with pseudo-Pelger-Huët nuclei and/or hypogranularity of neutrophil

cytoplasm may be noted. Blasts are absent or account for less than 2% of the white blood cells.
On BM aspirate smears dysplastic changes should be present in two different myeloid cell lineages, or exceed 10% in one single cell line (Table 5.07). Erythroid abnormalities include nuclear budding, multinuclearity, karyorrhexis, internuclear bridging, cytoplasmic granules and macrocytic changes. Cells of granulocytic lineage may exhibit hyposegmentation with pseudo-Pelger-Huët nuclei, hypo-/agranularity of the cytoplasm, macrocytic (giant) bands and cytoplasmic-nuclear maturation asynchrony. Myeloblasts account for fewer than 5% of the BM cells. Megakaryocytes are usually absent or very low in number. The detection of micromegakaryocytes is a strong indicator of RCC. Ring sideroblasts are not found.
In RCC with normo- or hypercellular BM specimens there is slight to moderate increase of erythropoiesis with accumulation of immature precursor cells, mainly proerythroblasts. Increased numbers of mitoses indicate ineffective erythropoiesis. Granulopoiesis appears slightly to moderately decreased and cells of granulocytic lineage are loosely scattered. Blasts account for less than 5% of the BM cells, and CD34 staining on the biopsy is useful for verification of the blast percentage. Megakaryocytes may be normal, decreased or increased in number and display dysplasia with non-lobulated nuclei, abnormally separated nuclear

Table 5.07 Minimal diagnostic criteria for refractory cytopenia of childhood.

	Erythropoiesis	Granulopoiesis	Megakaryopoiesis
Bone marrow aspirate	Dysplastic changes* and/or megaloblastoid changes in at least 10% of erythroid precursors	Dysplastic changes# in at least 10% of granulocytic precursors and neutrophils; <5% blasts	Unequivocal micromegakaryocytes, other dysplastic changes§ in variable numbers
Bone marrow biopsy	A few clusters of at least 20 erythroid precursors. Stop in maturation with increased numbers of proerythroblasts. Increased numbers of mitoses.	No minimal diagnostic criteria	Unequivocal micromegakaryocytes; immunohistochemistry is obligatory (CD61, CD41), other dysplastic changes§ in variable numbers
Peripheral blood		Dysplastic changes# in at least 10% of neutrophils; <2% blasts	

---
* Abnormal nuclear lobulation, multinuclear cells, nuclear bridges,
# Pseudo-Pelger-Huët cells, hypo-or agranularity, giant bands (In cases of severe neutropenia this criteria may not be fulfilled).
§ Megakaryocytes of variable size with separated nuclei or round nuclei. The absence of megakaryocytes will not exclude refractory cytopenia of childhood.

Table 5.08
Comparison of morphological criteria of hypoplastic refractory cytopenia of childhood and aplastic anaemia in childhood.

Refractory cytopenia of childhood

	Bone marrow biopsy	Bone marrow aspirate cytology
Erythropoiesis	Patchy distribution Left shift Increased mitoses	Nuclear lobulation Multinuclearity Megaloblastoid changes
Granulopoiesis	Marked decrease Left shift	Pseudo-Pelger-Huët anomaly Agranulation of cytoplasm Hypogranulation of cytoplasm Nuclear-cytoplasmic maturation defects
Megakaryopoiesis	Marked decrease Dysplastic changes Micromegakaryocytes	Micromegakaryocytes Multiple separated nuclei Small round nuclei
Lymphocytes	May be increased focally or dispersed	May be increased
CD34+ cells	No increase	

Aplastic anaemia in childhood

	Bone marrow biopsy	Bone marrow aspirate cytology
Erythropoiesis	Lacking or single small focus with less than 10 cells with maturation	Lacking or very few cells, without dysplasia or megaloblastoid change
Granulopoiesis	Lacking or marked decrease, very few small foci with maturation	Few maturing cells with no dysplasia
Megakaryopoiesis	Lacking or very few, no dysplastic megakaryocytes	Lacking or few non-dysplastic megakaryocytes
Lymphocytes	May be increased focally or dispersed	May be increased
CD34+ cells	No increase	

lobes and characteristic micromegakaryocytes. There is no increase in reticulin fibres.

The majority of patients with RCC show a marked decrease of BM cellularity, down to 5–10% of the normal age matched value. The morphologic findings are similar to those observed in the normally cellular or hypercellular cases. Immature erythroid precursors form one or several islands consisting of at least 10 cells. This patchy pattern of erythropoiesis is usually accompanied by sparsely distributed granulopoiesis. Megakaryocytes are significantly decreased or absent. Although micromegakaryocytes may be rare or not always found, they should be searched for carefully as they are important in establishing the diagnosis. Multiple sections prepared from the biopsy may be helpful in identification of abnormal megakaryocytes and immunohistochemistry to identify micromegakaryocytes is obligatory. Fatty tissue between the areas of haematopoiesis can mimic aplastic anaemia (Table 5.08). Therefore at least two biopsies at least two weeks apart are recommended to facilitate the detection of representative BM spaces containing foci of erythropoiesis.

Differential diagnosis
In children, a variety of non-haematological disorders such as viral infections, nutritional deficiencies and metabolic diseases can give rise to secondary myelodysplasia, thereby mimicking RCC (Table 5.09). In the absence of a cytogenetic marker the clinical course of cases suspected of RCC has to be carefully evaluated before a clear-cut diagnosis can be made. The haematological differential diagnosis includes acquired aplastic anaemia, inherited BM failure diseases and paroxysmal nocturnal haemoglobinuria (PNH). In contrast to RCC, acquired aplastic anaemia presents with adipocytosis of the BM spaces with few scattered myeloid cells; there are no erythroid islands with increased numbers of immature erythroblasts, no granulocytic dysplasia and no micromegakaryocytes (Table 5.08). Contrary to what is sometimes reported in adults with aplastic anaemia, at presentation, acquired aplastic anaemia of childhood does not have megaloblastic features; following immunosuppressive therapy, the histological pattern of acquired aplastic anaemia can no longer be separated from that observed in RCC. The inherited BM failure disorders such as Fanconi anaemia, dyskeratosis congenita, Shwachman-Diamond syndrome, amegakaryocytic thrombocytopenia or pancytopenia with radioulnar synostosis show overlapping morphological features with RCC. They have to be excluded by medical history, physical examination and the appropriate laboratory and molecular studies before a definite diagnosis of RCC can be made. The clinical picture of PNH is rare in childhood, although PNH clones in the absence of haemolysis or thrombosis may be observed in children with RCC {2292}. The relation between RCC with two or more dysplastic lineages and refractory cytopenia with multilineage dysplasia (RCMD) has not yet been evaluated. Currently it is recommended that children who otherwise fit the criteria for RCMD be considered as RCC until such studies clarify whether the number of lineages involved is an important prognostic discriminator in childhood MDS.

Immunophenotype
Micromegakaryocytes can be missed easily in H&E stained BM trephine biopsy sections but can be more readily appreciated by the expression of platelet glycoproteins like CD61 (glycoprotein IIIa), CD41 (glycoprotein IIb/IIIa) or von Willebrand factor. Myeloblasts do not account for more than 5% of the BM cells, and detection of 5% or more CD34, myeloperoxidase, lysozyme and CD117 positive blast

cells may indicate progression to high grade MDS. Clusters of myeloblasts are not seen in RCC.

Genetics

The genetic changes predisposing to MDS in childhood remain largely obscure. The presumed underlying mechanism may also give rise to subtle phenotypic abnormalities noted in many children with MDS. Monosomy 7 is the most common cytogenetic abnormality {1109, 1704, 1784}. Other cytogenetic abnormalities including complex karyotypes may also be observed. Most cases of RCC show a normal karyotype irrespective of BM cellularity. There is no difference in morphology between cases with or without monosomy 7.

Postulated cell of origin

Haematopoietic stem cell with multilineage potential.

Prognosis and predictive factors

Karyotype is the most important factor for progression to advanced MDS. Patients with monosomy 7 have a significantly higher probability of progression than patients with other chromosomal abnormalities or normal karyotype {1109}.

Table 5.09
Disorders which may present with morphological features indistinguishable from refractory cytopenia of childhood.

- Infections (e.g. cytomegalovirus, herpes viruses, parvovirus B19, visceral leishmaniasis)
- Vitamin deficiency (e.g. deficiency of vitamin B12, folate, vitamin E)
- Metabolic disorders (e.g. mevalonate kinase deficiency)
- Rheumatic disease
- Autoimmune lymphoproliferative disorders (e.g. FAS deficiency)
- Mitochondrial deletions (Pearson syndrome)
- Inherited bone marrow failure disorders (e.g. Fanconi anaemia, dyskeratosis congenita, Shwachmann-Diamond syndrome, amegakaryocytic thrombocytopenia, thrombocytopenia with absent radii, radioulnar synostosis, Seckel syndrome)
- Paroxysmal nocturnal haemoglobinuria (PNH)
- Acquired aplastic anaemia during haematological recovery

Spontaneous disappearance of monosomy 7 and cytopenia has been reported in infants, but remains a rare event {1380}. In contrast to monosomy 7, patients with trisomy 8 or normal karyotype may experience a long stable course of their disease. Currently, haematopoietic stem cell transplantation (HSCT) is the only curative therapy and is the treatment of choice for patients with monosomy 7 or complex karyotypes early in the course of their disease. In view of a low transplant-related mortality HSCT can also be recommended for patients with other karyotypes if a suitable donor is available {1784, 2104}.

An expectant approach with careful observation may be reasonable for patients in the absence of transfusion requirements, severe cytopenia or infections. Because early BM failure can at least in part be mediated by T-cell immunosuppression of haematopoiesis, immunosuppressive therapy can be a successful therapy strategy for improving outlook in some children with RCC {2033, 2471}.

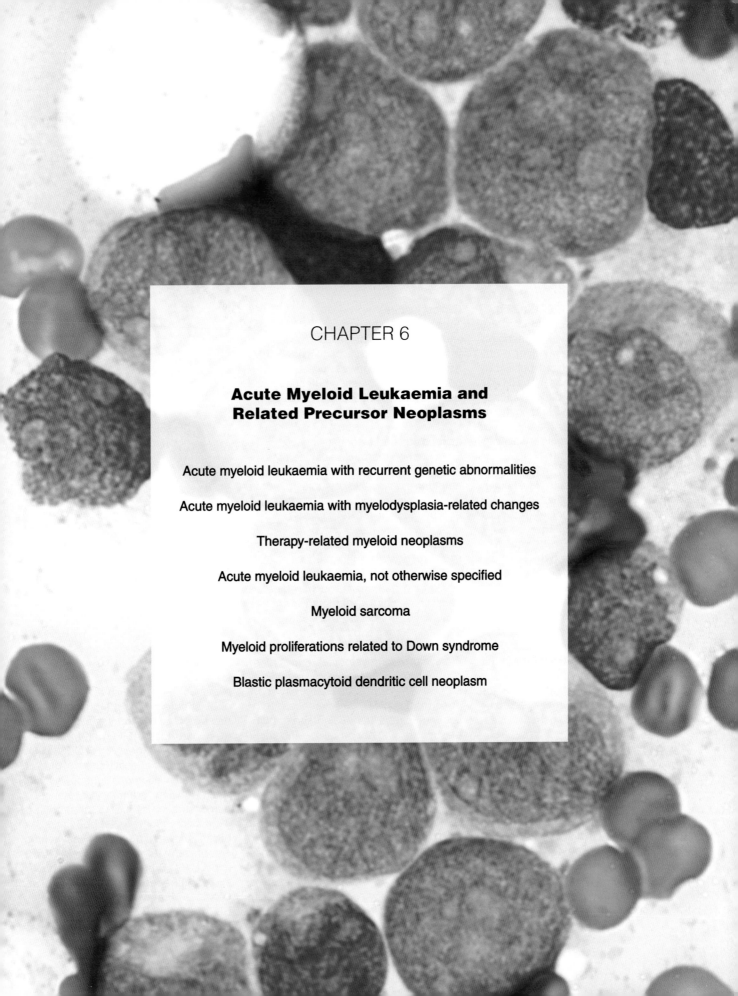

CHAPTER 6

Acute Myeloid Leukaemia and Related Precursor Neoplasms

Acute myeloid leukaemia with recurrent genetic abnormalities

Acute myeloid leukaemia with myelodysplasia-related changes

Therapy-related myeloid neoplasms

Acute myeloid leukaemia, not otherwise specified

Myeloid sarcoma

Myeloid proliferations related to Down syndrome

Blastic plasmacytoid dendritic cell neoplasm

D.A. Arber   J.W. Vardiman
R.D. Brunning   A. Porwit
M.M. Le Beau   J. Thiele
B. Falini   C.D. Bloomfield

Acute myeloid leukaemia with recurrent genetic abnormalities

AML with balanced translocations/inversions

This group is characterized by recurrent genetic abnormalities of prognostic significance. The most commonly identified are balanced abnormalities: t(8;21)(q22;q22), inv(16)(p13.1q22) or t(16;16)(p13.1;q22), t(15;17)(q22;q12) and t(9;11)(p22;q23) {306, 721, 848, 2036}. Each of these structural chromosome rearrangements creates a fusion gene encoding a chimaeric protein that is required, but usually not sufficient, for leukaemogenesis {2063}. Many of these disease groups have characteristic morphological and immunophenotypic features {65}. The categories of acute myeloid leukaemia (AML) with t(8;21)(q22;q22), inv(16)(p13.1q22) or t(16;16)(p13.1;q22) or t(15;17)(q22;q12) are considered as acute leukaemias without regard to blast cell count. It is not yet clear if all cases with t(9;11)(p22;q23), t(6;9)(p23;q34), inv(3)(q21q26.2), t(3;3) (q21;q26.2) or t(1;22)(p13;q13) should be categorized as AML when the blast cell count is <20%. Many of the translocations are detected by RT-PCR which has a higher sensitivity (1×10^{-5}) than cytogenetic analysis (1×10^{-2}). Cases of therapy-related AML/myelodysplastic syndrome (MDS) may also have the balanced translocations and inversions that are described in this section, but these should be diagnosed as therapy-related AML/MDS with the associated genetic abnormality noted.

Acute myeloid leukaemia with t(8;21)(q22;q22); RUNX1-RUNX1T1

Definition

Acute myeloid leukaemia, with t(8;21) (q22;q22); *RUNX1-RUNX1T1* is an AML generally showing maturation in the neutrophil lineage.

ICD-O code   9896/3

Epidemiology

The t(8;21)(q22;q22) is found in ~5% of cases of AML and in 10% of the prior acute myeloblastic leukaemia with maturation (M2) category of the French-American-British classification. It occurs predominantly in younger patients.

Clinical features

Tumour manifestations, such as myeloid sarcomas, may be present at presentation. In such cases the initial bone marrow (BM) aspiration may show a misleading low number of blast cells, but should be diagnosed as AML despite a blast percentage in the BM of <20.

Morphology and cytochemistry

The common morphological features include the presence of large blasts with abundant basophilic cytoplasm, often containing numerous azurophilic granules and perinuclear clearing or hofs. A few blasts in many cases show very large granules (pseudo-Chédiak-Higashi granules), suggesting abnormal fusion. Auer rods are frequently found and appear as a single long and sharp rod with tapered ends; they may be detected in mature neutrophils. In addition to the large blast cells, some smaller blasts, predominantly in the peripheral blood (PB), may be found. Promyelocytes, myelocytes and mature neutrophils with variable dysplasia are present in the BM. These cells may show abnormal nuclear segmentation (e.g. pseudo-Pelger-Huët nuclei) and/or cytoplasmic staining abnormalities, including homogeneous pink coloured cytoplasm in neutrophils. Dysplasia of other cell lines, however, is uncommon. Eosinophil precursors are frequently increased, but they do not exhibit the cytological or cytochemical abnormalities characteristic of AML associated with abnormalities of chromosome 16; basophils and/or mast cells are sometimes present in excess. A monocytic component is usually minimal or absent. Erythroblasts and megakaryocytes are morphologically normal. Rare cases with a BM blast percentage <20 occur. These should be classified as AML and not as MDS.

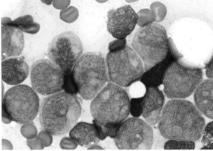

Fig. 6.01 Acute myeloid leukaemia with t(8;21)(q22;q22). Bone marrow blasts showing abundant granular cytoplasm with perinuclear clearing and large orange-pink granules.

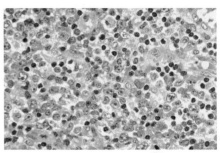

Fig. 6.02 Myeloid sarcoma. Biopsy of an orbital mass from a child with AML with a t(8;21)(q22;q22). There are eosinophil precursors scattered in the predominant blast population.

Immunophenotype

Most cases of AML with the (8;21)(q22;q22) translocation display a characteristic immunophenotype with a subpopulation of blast cells showing high intensity expression of CD34, together with HLA-DR, myeloperoxidase (MPO) and CD13, but relatively weak expression of CD33 {1140, 1775}. There are usually signs of granulocytic differentiation with subpopulations of cells showing granulocytic maturation demonstrated by CD15 and/or CD65 expression. Sometimes populations of blasts showing maturation asynchrony are present (e.g. co-expressing CD34 and CD15). These leukaemias frequently express the lymphoid markers CD19 and PAX5, and may express cytoplasmic CD79a {996, 1155, 2236}. Some cases are terminal deoxynucleotidyl transferase (TdT) positive; however, TdT expression is generally weak. CD56 is expressed in a fraction of cases and may have adverse prognostic significance {123}.

Genetics

The genes for both heterodimeric components of core binding factor (CBF), *RUNX1* (also known as *AML1* or *CBFA*) and *CBFB* are involved in rearrangements associated with acute leukaemias {2063}. The t(8;21) (q22;q22) involves the *RUNX1* gene, which encodes core-binding factor subunit alpha and the *RUNX1T1* (*ETO*) gene {608, 1294, 1733}. The *RUNX1-RUNX1T1* fusion transcript is consistently detected in patients with t(8;21)(q22;q22) AML. The CBF transcription factor is essential for haematopoiesis, and transformation by *RUNX1-RUNX1T1* likely results from transcriptional repression of normal *RUNX1* target genes via aberrant recruitment of nuclear transcriptional co-repressor complexes. Over 70% of patients show additional chromosome abnormalities: e.g. loss of a sex chromosome or del(9q) with loss of 9q22. Secondary cooperating mutations of *KRAS* or *NRAS* are common (30%) in paediatric CBF-associated leukaemias {808}. Mutations of *KIT* occur in 20–25% of cases {1696}.

Postulated normal couterpart

Myeloid stem cell with predominant neutrophil differentiation.

Prognosis and predictive factors

Acute myeloid leukaemia with t(8;21) (q22;q22) is usually associated with a good response to chemotherapy and a high complete remission rate with long-term disease-free survival when treated with high dose cytarabine in the consolidation phase {228, 848}. Some factors appear to adversely affect prognosis including CD56 expression and the presence of *KIT* mutations {123, 1696}.

Acute myeloid leukaemia with inv(16)(p13.1q22) or t(16;16)(p13.1;q22); CBFB-MYH11

Definition

Acute myeloid leukaemia with inv(16) (p13.1q22) or t(16;16)(p13.1;q22); *CBFB-MYH11* is an AML that usually shows monocytic and granulocytic differentiation and characteristically abnormal eosinophil component in the BM {1258, 1393, 2063}.

ICD-O code   9871/3

Synonym

Acute myeloid leukaemia with abnormal marrow eosinophils.

Epidemiology

Either inv(16)(p13.1q22) or t(16;16) (p13.1;q22) is found in 5–8% of all cases of AML. They can occur in all age groups but are found predominantly in younger patients.

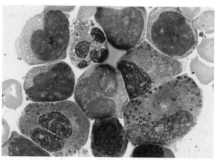

Fig. 6.04 Acute myeloid leukaemia with associated inv(16)(p13.1q22). Abnormal eosinophils, one with large basophilic coloured granules, are present.

Clinical features

Myeloid sarcomas may be present at initial diagnosis or at relapse and may constitute the only evidence of relapse in some patients.

Morphology and cytochemistry

In these cases, in addition to the usual morphological features of acute myelo-monocytic leukaemia, the BM shows a variable number of eosinophils (usually increased, but sometimes <5%) at all stages of maturation without significant maturation arrest. The most striking abnormalities involve the immature eosinophilic granules, mainly evident at the promyelocyte and myelocyte stages. The abnormalities are usually not present at later stages of eosinophil maturation. The eosinophilic granules are often larger than those normally present in immature eosinophils, purple-violet in colour, and in some cells are so dense that they obscure the cell

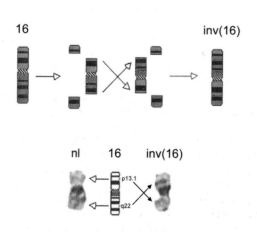

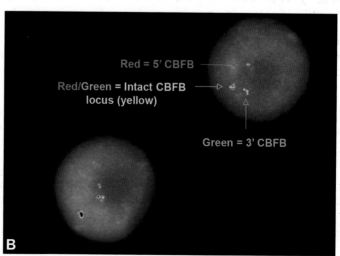

Fig. 6.03 Acute myeloid leukaemia with inv(16)(p13.1q22). **A** The inversion 16 results from breakage and rejoining of bands 16p13.1 and 16q22. G-banded normal (nl) chromosome 16 and inv(16) are shown. **B** Dual color fluorescence *in situ* hybridization: the 5' region of *CBFB* is labeled in red; the 3' region in green. A normal chromosome 16 has the 5' and 3' regions contiguous to each other resulting in a single yellow or overlapping red/green signals. The inversion 16 splits the *CBFB* locus resulting in separate red and green signals. Both interphase cells have one normal 16 chromosome and one inv(16).

morphology. The mature eosinophils may occasionally show nuclear hyposegmentation. The naphthol-ASD-chloroacetate esterase reaction, which is normally negative in eosinophils, is characteristically faintly positive in these abnormal eosinophils. Such a reaction is not seen in eosinophils of AML with the t(8;21)(q22;q22). Auer rods may be observed in myeloblasts. At least 3% of the blasts show myeloperoxidase (MPO) reactivity. The monoblasts and promonocytes usually show non-specific esterase reactivity, although it may be weaker than expected or even absent in some cases. In addition to the predominant monocytic and eosinophil components, the neutrophils in the BM are usually sparse, with a decreased number of mature neutrophils. The PB is not different from other cases of acute myelomonocytic leukaemia; eosinophils are not usually increased, but an occasional case has been reported with abnormal and increased eosinophils in the PB. While the majority of cases of inv(16)(p13.1q22) have been identified as having abnormal eosinophils, in some cases they are rare and difficult to find. Occasional cases with this genetic abnormality lack the eosinophilia or show only myeloid maturation without a monocytic component or only monocytic differentiation. Not infrequently, the blast percentage is only at the threshold level of 20% or occasionally lower. Cases with inv(16)(p13.1q22) or t(16;16);(p13.1;q22) and less than 20% BM blasts should be diagnosed as AML. The BM trephine biopsy is usually hypercellular, but may occasionally be normocellular.

Immunophenotype

Most of these leukaemias are characterized by a complex immunophenotype with the presence of multiple blast populations: immature blasts with high CD34 and CD117 expression and populations differentiating towards granulocytic (CD13, CD33, CD15, CD65, MPO positive) and monocytic (CD14, CD4, CD11b, CD11c, CD64, CD36 and lysozyme positive) lineages. Maturation asynchrony is often seen. Co-expression of CD2 with myeloid markers has been frequently documented but it is not specific for this diagnosis.

Genetics

The inv(16)(p13.1q22) found in the vast majority of this subtype and the less common t(16;16)(p13.1;q22) both result in the fusion of the CBFB gene at 16q22 to the MYH11 gene at 16p13.1 {2006}. MYH11 codes for a smooth muscle myosin heavy chain {506}. The CBFB gene codes for the core binding factor (CBF) beta subunit, a heterodimeric transcription factor known to bind the enhancers of T-cell receptor (TCR), cytokine genes, and other genes. The CBFB subunit heterodimerises with CBFA, the gene product of RUNX1, one of the genes involved in AML with t(8;21)(q22;q22). Occasionally cytological features of AML with abnormal eosinophils may be present without karyotypic evidence of a chromosome 16 abnormality, the CBFB-MYH11 being nevertheless demonstrated by molecular genetic studies {1533, 1882}. By conventional cytogenetic analysis, the inv(16)(p13.1q22)/t(16;16) (p13.1;q22) is a subtle rearrangement that may be overlooked when metaphase preparations are suboptimal. Thus, at diagnosis, the use of FISH and RT-PCR methods may be necessary to document the genetic alteration. Secondary cytogenetic abnormalities occur in approximately 40% of cases, with +22, +8 (10–15% each), and del(7q) or +21(~5%) most commonly observed {1390}. Trisomy 22 is fairly specific for inv(16)(p13.1q22) patients, being very rarely detected with other primary aberrations in AML, whereas +8 is commonly seen in patients with other primary aberrations. Rare cases of AML and chronic myelogenous leukaemia with both inv(16)(p13.1q22) and t(9;22)(q34;q11.2) have been reported, and this finding in chronic myelogenous leukaemia is usually associated with accelerated or blast phase of the disease {2454}. Mutations of KIT occur in approximately 30% of cases {1696}.

Postulated normal counterpart

Haematopoietic stem cell with potential to differentiate into granulocytic and monocytic lineages.

Prognosis and predictive factors

Clinical studies have shown that patients with AML with inv(16)(p13.1q22) or t(16;16) (p13.1;q22) achieve longer complete remissions when treated with high dose cytarabine in the consolidation phase {848, 1530}. However, older patients have decreased survival and those with KIT mutations have a higher risk of relapse and worse survival {546, 1696}. Patients with +22 as a secondary abnormality have been reported to have improved outcome {1390, 1962}.

Acute promyelocytic leukaemia with t(15;17)(q22;q12); PML-RARA

Definition

Acute promyelocytic leukaemia [APL or AML with t(15;17)(q22;q12)] is an AML in which abnormal promyelocytes predominate. Both hypergranular or "typical" APL and microgranular (hypogranular) types exist.

ICD-O code   9866/3

Synonym

AML with t(15;17)(q22;q12).

Epidemiology

Acute promyelocytic leukaemia comprises 5–8% of AML {2078}. The disease can occur at any age but patients are predominantly adults in mid-life.

Clinical features

Typical and microgranular APL are frequently associated with disseminated intravascular coagulation (DIC). In microgranular APL, unlike typical APL, the leukocyte count is very high, with a rapid doubling time.

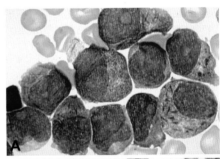

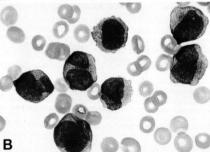

Fig. 6.05 Acute promyelocytic leukaemia. A Hypergranular type in bone marrow smear. There are several abnormal promyelocytes with intense azurophilic granulation. Several of the promyelocytes contain numerous Auer rods (faggot cells). B Microgranular variant, in peripheral blood smear. There are several abnormal promyelocytes with lobulated, almost cerebriform nuclei. The cytoplasm contains numerous small azurophilic granules; other cells appear sparsely granular.

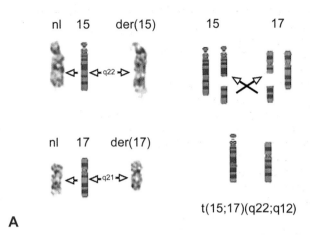

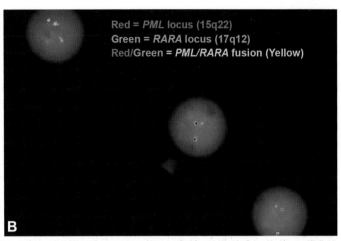

Red = *PML* locus (15q22)
Green = *RARA* locus (17q12)
Red/Green = *PML/RARA* fusion (Yellow)

t(15;17)(q22;q12)

A

B

Fig. 6.06 Acute promyelocytic leukaemia with t(15;17)(q22;q12). **A** The translocation 15;17 results from breakage and reunion of bands 15q22 and 17q12. G-banded normal (nl) 15 and 17 chromosomes (left) and the derivative (der) 15 and 17 resulting from the translocation are shown on the right. **B** Dual color fluorescence *in situ* hybridization with probes *PML* (15q22) and *RARA* (17q12) demonstrate the presence of a *PML/RARA* fusion resulting from the 15;17 translocation. Each of the three interphase cells has one separate red (*PML*) signal, one separate green (*RARA*) signal, and one yellow or overlapping red/green signal consistent with the presence of a *PML/RARA* gene fusion.

Morphology and cytochemistry

The nuclear size and shape in the abnormal promyelocytes of hypergranular APL are irregular and greatly variable; they are often kidney-shaped or bilobed. The cytoplasm is marked by densely-packed or even coalescent large granules, staining bright pink, red or purple in Romanowsky stains. The cytoplasmic granules may be so large and/or numerous that they totally obscure the nuclear cytoplasmic margin. In some cells, the cytoplasm is filled with fine dust-like granules. Characteristic cells containing bundles of Auer rods ("faggot cells") randomly distributed in the cytoplasm are present in most cases. Myeloblasts with single Auer rods may also be observed. Auer rods in hypergranular APL are usually larger than in other types of AML and they may have a characteristic morphology at the ultrastructural level with a hexagonal arrangement of tubular structures with a specific periodicity of approximately 250 mm in contrast to the 6–20 laminar periodicity of Auer rods in other types of AML. The MPO reaction is always strongly positive in all the leukaemic promyelocytes, with the reaction product covering the entire cytoplasm and often the nucleus. The non-specific esterase reaction is weakly positive in approximately 25% of cases. Only occasional obvious leukaemic promyelocytes may be observed in the PB.

Cases of microgranular (hypogranular) APL are characterized by distinct morphological features such as apparent paucity or absence of granules, and predominantly bilobed nuclear shape {811}.

The apparent hypogranular cytoplasm relates to the submicroscopic size of the azurophilic granules. This may cause confusion with acute monocytic leukaemia on Romanowsky stained smears; however, a small number of the abnormal promyelocytes showing clearly visible granules and/or bundles of Auer rods (faggot cells) can be identified in many cases. The leukocyte count is frequently markedly elevated in the microgranular variant of APL with numerous abnormal microgranular promyelocytes in contrast to typical APL. The MPO reaction is strongly positive contrasting with the weak or negative reaction in monocytes. Abnormal promyelocytes with deeply basophilic cytoplasm have been described mainly in the relapse phase in patients who have been previously treated with all-*trans* retinoic acid (ATRA). The BM biopsy is usually hypercellular. The abnormal promyelocytes have relatively abundant cytoplasm with numerous granules; occasionally Auer rods may be identified in well-prepared specimens. The nuclei are frequently convoluted.

Immunophenotype

Acute promyelocytic leukaemia with the t(15;17)(q22;q12) (hypergranular or "typical" variant) is characterized by low expression or absence of HLA-DR, CD34, leukocyte integrins CD11a, CD11b and CD18, a homogeneous, bright expression of CD33, and heterogeneous expression of CD13. Many cases show expression of CD117, although sometimes weak. The granulocytic differentiation markers CD15 and CD65 are negative or only

weakly expressed {1654, 1678} and CD64 expression is common. In cases with microgranular morphology or bcr3 transcript of the *PML-RARA* fusion gene there is frequent expression of CD34 and CD2, at least on a fraction of cells {653}. Approximately 20% of APL cases express CD56, which has been associated with a worse outcome {690}. Using immunocytochemistry, antibodies against the *PML* gene product show a characteristic nuclear multigranular pattern with nucleolar exclusion, in contrast to the speckled relatively large nuclear bodies seen in normal promyelocytes or blasts from other types of AML {662}.

Genetics

In addition to its therapeutic impact, the sensitivity of APL cells to ATRA has led to the discovery that the retinoic acid receptor alpha *(RARA)* gene on 17q12 fuses with a nuclear regulatory factor gene on 15q22

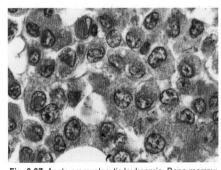

Fig. 6.07 Acute promyelocytic leukaemia. Bone marrow biopsy. Abnormal promyelocytes with abundant hypergranulated cytoplasm. The nuclei are generally round to oval. Several of the nuclei are irregular and invaginated.

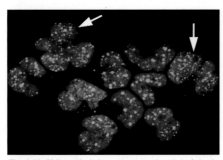

Fig. 6.08 PML antibody in acute promyelocytic leukaemia showing a characteristic nuclear multigranular pattern with nucleolar exclusion.

(promyelocytic leukaemia or *PML* gene) giving rise to a *PML-RARA* fusion gene product {506, 529, 1452}. Rare cases of APL lacking the classic t(15;17)(q22;q12) on routine cytogenetic studies have been described with complex variant translocations involving both chromosomes 15 and 17 with an additional chromosome or with submicroscopic insertion of *RARA* into *PML* leading to the expression of the *PML-RARA* transcript; these latter cases are considered as cryptic or masked t(15;17) (q22;q12) {847}. Morphological analysis shows no major differences between the t(15;17)(q22;q12) positive group and the *PML-RARA* positive patients without t(15;17)(q22;q12). Secondary cytogenetic abnormalities are noted in ~40% of cases, with +8 being the most frequent (10–15%). Mutations involving *FLT3*, including internal tandem duplication (ITD) and tyrosine kinase domain mutations (TKD) occur in 34–45% of APL. *FLT3*-ITD mutations are most common and are associated with a higher white blood cell count, microgranular blast cell morphology and involvement of the bcr3 breakpoint of *PML* {318, 747, 1199}.

Postulated normal counterpart
Myeloid stem cell with potential to differentiate to granulocytic lineage.

Prognosis and predictive factors
Acute promyelocytic leukaemia has a particular sensitivity to treatment with ATRA, which acts as a differentiating agent {342, 2152}. The prognosis in APL, treated optimally with ATRA and an anthracycline is more favourable than for any other AML cytogenetic subtype, and cases of relapsed or refractory APL show a generally good response with arsenic trioxide therapy {607, 685}. Expression of CD56 is associated with a less favourable prognosis while

the prognostic significance of *FLT3*-ITD mutations in this disease remains unclear {690, 1199}.

Variant *RARA* translocations in acute leukaemia
A subset of cases, often with morphological features resembling acute promyelocytic leukaemia, show variant translocations involving *RARA*. These variant fusion partners include *ZBTB16* (previously known as promyelocytic leukaemia zinc finger gene or *PLZF*) at 11q23; the nuclear matrix associated gene *(NUMA1)* at 11q13; the nucleophosmin gene *(NPM1)* at 5q35 and *STAT5B* at 17q11.2 {2488}.
Some cases with variant translocations were initially reported as having APL morphology {1914}. However, the t(11;17) (q23;q12); *ZBTB16-RARA* subgroup shows some morphological differences with a predominance of cells with regular nuclei, many granules, usual absence of Auer rods, an increased number of Pelgeroid neutrophils and strong MPO activity {1914}. The initial cases of APL associated with t(5;17)(q35;q12) had a predominant population of hypergranular promyelocytes and a minor population of hypogranular promyelocytes; Auer rods were not identified by light microscopy {476}. Some acute promyelocytic leukaemia variants, including t(11;17)(q23;q12) with *ZBTB16-RARA* and cases with *STAT5B-RARA* fusions are resistant to ATRA {1452}. APL with the t(5;17)(q35;q12) appears to respond to ATRA {1452}.
Cases with these variant translocations should be diagnosed as AML with a variant *RARA* translocation.

Acute myeloid leukaemia with t(9;11)(p22;q23); MLLT3-MLL

Definition
Acute myeloid leukaemia with t(9;11) (p22;q23); *MLLT3-MLL* is usually associated with monocytic features.

ICD-O code   9897/3

Synonym
Acute myeloid leukaemia, 11q23 abnormalities.

Epidemiology
The t(9;11)(p22;q23) may occur at any age, but is more common in children, being

present in 9–12% of paediatric and 2% of adult AML {306, 721}.

Clinical features
Patients may present with disseminated intravascular coagulation. They may have extramedullary myeloid (monocytic) sarcomas and/or tissue infiltration (gingiva, skin).

Morphology and cytochemistry
There is a strong association between acute monocytic and myelomonocytic leukaemias and t(9;11)(p22;q23), although occasionally the t(9;11) is detected in AML with or without maturation. Monoblasts and promonocytes typically predominate. Monoblasts are large cells, with abundant cytoplasm which can be moderately to intensely basophilic and may show pseudopod formation. Scattered fine azurophilic granules and vacuoles may be present. The monoblasts usually have round nuclei with delicate lacy chromatin, and one or more large prominent nucleoli. Promonocytes have a more irregular and delicately convoluted nuclear configuration; the cytoplasm is usually less basophilic and sometimes more obviously granulated, with occasional large azurophilic granules and vacuoles. Monoblasts and promonocytes usually show strong positive nonspecific esterase reactions. The monoblasts often lack MPO reactivity.

Immunophenotype
Cases of AML with the t(9;11)(p22;q23) in children are associated with strong expression of CD33, CD65, CD4 and HLA-DR, while expression of CD13, CD34 and CD14 is usually low {491}.
Most AML cases with 11q23 abnormalities express the NG2 homologue (encoded by *CSPG4*), a chondroitin sulfate molecule reacting with the Mab 7.1 {2456}. Most adult AML cases with 11q23 abnormalities express some markers of monocytic differentiation including CD14, CD4, CD11b, CD11c, CD64, CD36 and lysozyme, while variable expression of immature markers such as CD34 and CD117 and of CD56 has been reported {1541}.

Genetics
Molecular studies have identified a human homologue of the Drosophila trithorax gene designated *MLL (HRX)*, that results in a fusion gene in translocations involving 11q23 {114}. The MLL protein is a histone methyltransferase that assembles in protein complexes that regulate gene tran-

scription via chromatin remodeling. The t(9;11)(p22;q23) involving *MLLT3 (AF9)* is the most common *MLL* translocation in AML and appears to represent a distinct entity. Secondary cytogenetic abnormalities are common with t(9;11) (p22;q23), with +8 most commonly observed, but do not appear to influence survival {306, 1531}.

Postulated normal counterpart
Haematopoietic stem cell with multilineage potential.

Prognosis and predictive factors
Acute myeloid leukaemia with the t(9;11)(p22;q23) has an intermediate survival and one that is superior to AML with other 11q23 translocations {1531, 1891}. Cases with the t(9;11) and <20% blasts must be monitored closely for development of more definite evidence of AML.

Variant *MLL* translocations in acute leukaemia
Over 80 different translocations involving *MLL* are now described in adult and paediatric acute leukaemia, with over 50 translocation partner genes now characterized {1470, 2008}. Translocations involving *MLLT2 (AF4)*, resulting predominantly in acute lymphoblastic leukaemia (ALL), and *MLLT3 (AF9)*, resulting predominantly in AML, are the most common. Other *MLL* translocations that commonly result in AML include the *MLLT1 (ENL)*, *MLLT10 (AF10)*, *MLLT4 (AF6)* and *ELL* as partner genes. Other than the *MLL-ELL* fusion resulting from the t(11;19)(q23;p13.1), which is most often associated with only AML, these fusions occur predominantly in AML, but may be seen in ALL as well. Up to one third of *MLL* translocations in AML are not detectable on conventional karyotype analysis, and FISH or other molecular studies may be necessary to identify these variant translocations {2008}. AML with these fusions usually have myelomonocytic or monoblastic morphologic and immunophenotypic features. While in the past all of these translocations were encompassed by the category of AML with 11q23 abnormalities, the diagnosis should now specify the specific abnormality and should be limited to cases with 11q23 balanced translocations involving *MLL*. For example, a case of AML with an *MLL-ENL* fusion would be diagnosed as acute myeloid leukaemia with t(11;19)(q23;p13.3); *MLL-ENL*. Acute myeloid leukaemia with cytogenetic

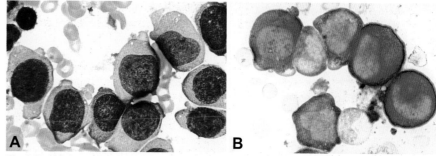

Fig. 6.09 AML (monoblastic) with t(9;11)(p22;q23). Bone marrow smears. **A** Several monoblasts, some with very abundant cytoplasm and fine myeloperoxidase negative azurophilic granules are present. **B** Non-specific esterase reaction showing intensely positive monoblasts.

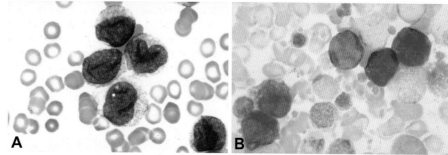

Fig. 6.10 AML (monocytic) with t(9;11)(p22;q23). Bone marrow smears. **A** There are several monoblasts and promonocytes with very pale cytoplasm containing numerous fine azurophilic granules. The promonocytes have delicate nuclear folds. **B** Non-specific esterase stain. The promonocytes are intensely reactive.

abnormalities associated with prior therapy or myelodysplasia, such as t(2;11) (p21;q23) or t(11;16)(q23;p13.3), should be diagnosed as therapy-related AML or AML with myelodysplasia-related changes (See Chapter on therapy-related myeloid neoplasms).

Acute myeloid leukaemia with t(6;9)(p23;q34); DEK-NUP214

Definition
Acute myeloid leukaemia with the t(6;9) (p23;q34); *DEK-NUP214* is an AML with or without monocytic features that is often associated with basophilia and multilineage dysplasia {1714, 2035}.

ICD-O code
The provisional code proposed for the fourth edition of ICD-O is *9865/3*.

Epidemiology
The t(6;9)(p23;q34) is detected in 0.7–1.8% of AML, and occurs in both children and adults with a median age of 13 years in childhood and 35 years in adults {306, 2035, 2036}.

Clinical features
Acute myeloid leukaemia with t(6;9) (p23;q34) usually presents with anaemia and thrombocytopenia, and often with pancytopenia. In adults, the presenting white blood cell count is generally lower than other AML types with a median white blood cell count of 12x10⁹/L {2035}.

Morphology and cytochemistry
The BM blasts of AML with t(6;9)(p23;q34) may have morphologic and cytochemical features of any FAB subtype of AML other than acute promyelocytic leukaemia and acute megakaryoblastic leukaemia, with AML with maturation and acute myelomonocytic leukaemia the most common {28, 1676, 2035}. Auer rods are present in approximately one third of cases. Blasts are myeloperoxidase positive and may be positive or negative for non-specific esterase. Therefore, there are no features specific to the blast cell population in this entity. Marrow and PB basophilia, defined as >2%, is generally uncommon in AML, but is seen in 44-62% of cases of AML with t(6;9)(p23;q34). In addition, most cases show evidence of granulocytic and erythroid dysplasia, with megakaryocytic dysplasia possibly less common. Ring sideroblasts

are present in a subset of cases. The percentage of BM blasts is variable, and some cases may present with less than 20% blasts.

Immunophenotype
The blasts have a non-specific myeloid immunophenotype with consistent expression of myeloperoxidase, CD13, CD33, CD38 and HLA-DR {28, 1676, 2035}. Most cases also express CD117, CD34 and CD15 while a subset of cases express the monocyte-associated marker CD64 and approximately half are terminal deoxynucleotidyl transferase (TdT) positive. Other lymphoid antigen expression is uncommon.

Genetics
The t(6;9)(p23;q34) results in a fusion of *DEK* on chromosome 6 with *NUP214 (CAN)* on chromosome 9. The resulting nucleoporin fusion protein acts as an aberrant transcription factor as well as altering nuclear transport by binding to soluble transport factors {1949}. The t(6;9) is the sole clonal karyotypic abnormality in the vast majority of cases, but some patients will have the t(6;9)(p23;q34) in association with a complex karyotype {2035}. *FLT3*-ITD mutations are very common in AML with t(6;9)(p23;q34) occurring in 69% of paediatric cases and 78% of adult cases {1676, 2035}. *FLT3*-TKD mutations appear to be uncommon in this entity.

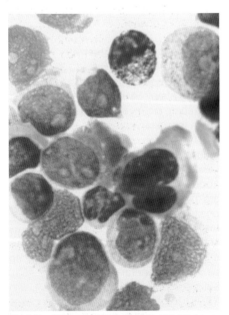

Fig.6.11 AML with t(6;9)(p23;q34). The blasts are admixed with dysplastic erythroid precursors and scattered basophils (centre, right).

Postulated normal counterpart
Haematopoietic stem cell with multilineage potential.

Prognosis and predictive factors
Acute myeloid leukaemia with t(6;9) (p23;q34) in both adults and children has a generally poor prognosis, similar to other AML with unfavourable cytogenetic abnormalities. Elevated white blood cell counts are most predictive of shorter overall survival and increased BM blasts are associated with shorter disease-free survival. Based on limited data, allogeneic stem cell transplantation may be associated with better overall survival compared to patients with no stem cell transplantation {2035}.Cases with t(6;9)(p23;q34) and <20% blasts must be monitored closely for development of more definite evidence of AML.

Acute myeloid leukaemia with inv(3)(q21q26.2) or t(3;3)(q21;q26.2); RPN1-EVI1

Definition
Acute myeloid leukaemia with inv(3) (q21q26.2) or t(3;3)(q21;q26.2); *(RPN1-EVI1)* is an AML that may present *de novo* or arise from a prior MDS. It is often associated with normal or elevated PB platelet counts and has increased atypical BM megakaryocytes with mono- or bi-lobated nuclei and associated multilineage dysplasia {225, 1983, 2131}.

ICD-O code
The provisional code proposed for the fourth edition of ICD-O is *9869/3*.

Epidemiology
Acute myeloid leukaemia with inv(3) (q21q26.2) or t(3;3)(q21;q26.2) represents 1–2% of all AML {306, 2036}. It occurs most commonly in adults with no sex predilection.

Clinical features
Patients most commonly present with anaemia and a normal platelet count, although marked thrombocythaemia occurs in 7–22% of patients {845, 1983}. Patients may present *de novo* or have a prior MDS. A subset of patients present with hepatosplenomegaly, but lymphadenopathy is uncommon {1983, 2004, 2189}.

Morphology and cytochemistry
Peripheral blood changes may include hypogranular neutrophils with a pseudo-Pelger-Huët anomaly, with or without associated peripheral blasts. Red cell abnormalities are usually mild without teardrop cells. Giant and hypogranular platelets are common and bare megakaryocyte nuclei may be present {225}. The BM blasts of AML with inv(3)(q21q26.2) or t(3;3) (q21;q26.2) may have morphologic and cytochemical features of any FAB subtype of AML other than acute promyelocytic leukaemia with acute myeloid leukaemia without maturation, acute myelomonocytic leukaemia and acute megakaryoblastic leukaemia morphologies most common {715, 1983}. A subset of cases has less than 20% blast cells at the time of diagnosis, including cases with features of chronic myelomonocytic leukaemia. Multilineage dysplasia of non-blast cell BM elements is a frequent finding with atypical megakaryocytes most common {715, 1054, 1983}. Megakaryocytes may be normal or increased in number with many small (<30 μm) monolobed or bilobed forms, but other dysplastic megakaryocytic forms may also occur. Dysplasia of maturing erythroid cells and neutrophils is also common. Marrow eosinophils, basophils and/or mast cells may be increased. The BM biopsy shows increased small, hypolobated megakaryocytes. Bone marrow cellularity is variable with some cases presenting as hypocellular AML. Marrow fibrosis is variable.

Immunophenotype
Immunophenotypic studies of AML with inv(3)(q21q26.2) or t(3;3)(q21;q26.2) are limited. The blast cells generally express CD13, CD33, HLA-DR, CD34 and CD38. Blast cells of some cases also aberrantly express CD7 and a subset may express megakaryocytic markers such as CD41 and CD61. Aberrant expression of lymphoid markers other than CD7 appears uncommon {2004}.

Genetics
A variety of abnormalities of the long arm of chromosome 3 occur in myeloid malignancies, with inv(3)(q21q26.2) and t(3;3) (q21;q26.2) being the most common. The abnormalities involve the oncogene *EVI1* at 3q26.2, or its longer form *MDS1-EVI1*, and *RPN1* at 3q21. RPN1 may act as an enhancer of *EVI1* expression resulting in increased cell proliferation, and impaired

cell differentiation; it induces haematopoietic cell transformation {1236, 1609, 2125}. Other cytogenetic aberrations involving 3q26.2, such as t(3;21)(q26.2;q22) resulting in an *EVI1-RUNX1* fusion and usually seen in therapy-related disease, are not included in this disease category. Secondary karyotypic abnormalities are common with inv(3)(q21q26.2) and t(3;3) (q21;q26.2) with monosomy 7 most common, occurring in approximately half of cases, followed by 5q deletions and complex karyotypes {1983}. These abnormalities may precede the development of the 3q26.2 abnormality {1609}.

Patients with AML with inv(3)(q21q26.2) or t(3;3)(q21;q26.2) show overexpression of *EVI1* and *GATA2*, but these findings do not appear to be specific for the genetic abnormality {1236, 1609}.

Patients with chronic myelogenous leukaemia may acquire inv(3)(q21q26.2) or t(3;3)(q21;q26.2), and such a finding usually portends accelerated or blast phase of their disease. Cases with both t(9;22) (q34;q11.2) and inv(3)(q21q26.2) or t(3;3) (q21;q26.2) are best considered as aggressive phases of chronic myelogenous leukaemia, rather than AML with inv(3) (q21q26.2) or t(3;3)(q21;q26.2).

Postulated normal counterpart
Haematopoietic stem cell with multilineage potential.

Prognosis and predictive factors
AML with inv(3)(q21q26.2) or t(3;3) (q21;q26.2) is an aggressive disease with short survival {715, 1834, 1983}. Two patients with AML with inv(3)(q21q26.2) were reported to show a response to arsenic trioxide with thalidomide, with one achieving complete remission {1824}. Cases with inv(3)(q21q26.2) or t(3;3)(q21;q26.2) and <20% blasts must be monitored closely for development of more definite evidence of AML.

Acute myeloid leukaemia (megakaryoblastic) with t(1;22)(p13;q13); RBM15-MKL1

Definition
Acute myeloid leukaemia with t(1;22) (p13;q13); *RBM15-MKL1* is an AML generally showing maturation in the megakaryocyte lineage.

ICD-O code
The provisional code proposed for the fourth edition of ICD-O is *9911/3*.

Epidemiology
The t(1;22)(p13;q13) is an uncommon abnormality in AML, representing <1% of all cases. It most commonly occurs in infants without Down syndrome, with a female predominance.

Clinical features
Acute myeloid leukaemia with t(1;22) (p13;q13) is a *de novo* AML restricted to infants and young children (3 years or less) with most cases occurring in the first 6 months of life (median, 4 months). The vast majority of cases present with marked organomegaly, especially hepatosplenomegaly. Patients also have anaemia, and usually have thrombocytopenia and a moderately elevated white blood cell count.

Morphology and cytochemistry
The PB and BM blasts of AML with t(1;22) (p13;q13) are similar to those of acute megakaryoblastic leukaemia of AML, NOS. Small and large megakaryoblasts may be present and they may be admixed with more morphologically undifferentiated blast cells with a high nuclear-cytoplasmic ratio resembling lymphoblasts. The megakaryoblasts are usually of medium to large size (12-18 μm) with a round, slightly irregular or indented nucleus with fine reticular chromatin and one to three nucleoli. The cytoplasm is basophilic, often agranular, and may show distinct blebs or pseudopod formation. Micromegakaryocytes are common, but dysplastic features of granulocytic and erythroid cells are not usually present. The BM biopsy is usually normocellular to hypercellular with reticulin and collagenous fibrosis usually present. Cases may show a stromal pattern of BM infiltration mimicking a metastatic tumour {205, 341}. Cytochemical stains for Sudan black B (SBB) and MPO are consistently negative in the megakaryoblasts. A subset of cases will have less then 20% BM blasts, but a low blast cell count due to difficulties aspirating BM secondary to fibrosis should be excluded.

Immunophenotype
The megakaryoblasts express one or more of the platelet glycoproteins: CD41 (glycoprotein IIb/IIIa), and/or CD61 (glycoprotein IIIa). The more mature platelet-associated

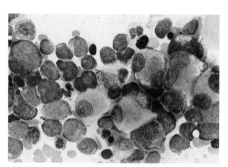

Fig. 6.12 AML with inv(3)(q21q26.2). Bone marrow aspirate with increased blasts and atypical, monolobated megakaryocytes.

marker CD42 (glycoprotein Ib) is less frequently present. The myeloid-associated markers CD13 and CD33 may be positive. CD34, the pan-leukocyte marker CD45, and HLA-DR are often negative; CD36 is characteristically positive. Blasts are negative with MPO antibodies. Lymphoid markers and terminal deoxynucleotidyl transferase (TdT) are not expressed. Cytoplasmic expression of CD41 or CD61 is more specific and sensitive than surface staining; the higher specificity is due to possible adherence of platelets to blast cells in other types of AML, which may be misinterpreted as positive staining by flow cytometry.

Genetics
Patients should have karyotypic evidence of t(1;22)(p13;q13) or molecular genetic evidence of a *RBM15-MKL1* fusion. In most cases, t(1;22)(p13;q13) occurs as the sole karyotypic abnormality. This translocation results in a fusion of RNA-binding motif protein-15 (*RBM15*) (also known as *OTT*) and megakaryocyte leukaemia-1 (*MKL1*) (also known as *MAL*) {1352}. *RBM15* encodes RNA recognition motifs and a spen paralog and ortholog C-terminal (SPOC) domain, while *MKL1* encodes a DNA-binding motif involved in chromatin organization. The fusion gene may modulate chromatin organization, HOX-induced differentiation and extracellular signaling pathways {1461}.

Postulated normal counterpart
Myeloid stem cell with predominant megakaryocytic differentiation.

Prognosis and predictive factors
Although early reports suggested a poor prognosis for AML with t(1;22)(p13;q13) {205, 341}, more recent studies have found the patients to respond well to intensive

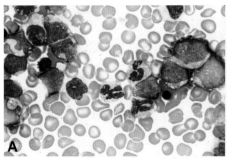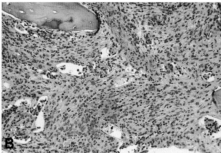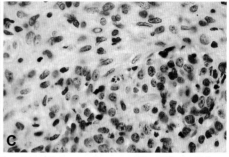

Fig. 6.13 Acute myeloid leukaemia with associated t(1;22)(p13;q13). **A** Bone marrow smear from a 3.5-month-old child contains a heteromorphous population of blasts. **B** Bone marrow section shows extensive replacement of marrow by intertwining bundles of blast cells. **C** High magnification of the specimen shows blasts without differentiating features.

AML chemotherapy with long disease-free survival {620}. Cases with the t(1;22) (p13;q13) and <20% blasts on aspirate smears should be correlated with the biopsy to exclude BM fibrosis as a cause of a falsely low blast cell count. If this is excluded, these patients must be monitored closely for development of more definite evidence of AML, such as the presence of extramedullary disease or myeloid sarcoma.

AML with gene mutations

In addition to translocations and inversions, specific gene mutations also occur in AML. They include frequent mutations of fms-related tyrosine kinase 3 *(FLT3)*, nucleophosmin *(NPM1)* and, less commonly, mutations of the *CEBPA* gene (encoding the CCAAT/enhancer binding protein-α), *KIT, MLL, WT1, NRAS* and *KRAS*. Alone or in combination, mutations of *FLT3, NPM1* and *CEBPA* have been reported in patients with AML with a normal karyotype where they have prognostic significance in the context of most current therapies, although they may be seen in patients with abnormal karyotypes as well {1532}.

FLT3, located at 13q12, encodes a tyrosine kinase receptor that is involved in haematopoietic stem cell differentiation and proliferation. *FLT3* is expressed on these progenitor cells as well as on the blast cells in most cases of AML. *FLT3* mutations may occur with any AML type (20–40% of all cases) and in MDS, but are most common in AML with t(6;9) (p23;q34), acute promyelocytic leukaemia and AML with a normal karyotype {1184, 2035}. The two primary types of *FLT3* mutations are internal tandem duplications *(FLT3-ITD)* within the juxtamembrane domain (75–80%) and mutations affecting codons 835 or 836 of the second tyrosine

kinase domain (TKD) (20–35%). While *FLT3* mutations may occur in association with recurrent cytogenetic abnormalities, such as t(6;9)(p23;q34) and t(15;17)(q22;q12), they may also occur with other so-called cooperating mutations. *FLT3*-ITD mutations are associated with an adverse outcome, but the significance of the less common *FLT3*-TKD mutations remains controversial {117, 1447, 2396}. Detection of *FLT3*-ITD is important because the prognosis of most cytogenetically normal AML subtypes correlates with the presence or absence of this mutation. *KIT*, located at 4q11-12, is a member of the type III tyrosine kinase family and encodes a 145-kD transmembrane glycoprotein. Gain-of-function mutations of *KIT* occur in a variety of diseases, including gastrointestinal stromal tumours, germ cell tumours, mastocytosis and AML. Mutations of *KIT* have been shown to have prognostic significance among AML with t(8;21)(q22;q22) and inv(16)(p13.1q22)/ t(16;16)(p13.1;q22), in which they are associated with a poor prognosis {1696}. These *KIT* mutations most commonly occur within exon 8 and 17. To date, *WT1* mutations have been shown to confer a poor prognosis in AML patients with a normal karyotype {1696A}, but there is less compelling evidence of prognostic significance for the less frequent mutations of *MLL, NRAS* and *KRAS*. Molecular studies have shown that the *MLL* gene is rearranged more frequently than is revealed by conventional cytogenetic studies. A partial tandem duplication of *MLL* has been reported in 5–10% of adults with a normal karyotype {313, 603} and in patients with isolated trisomy 11 {314}. Its adverse prognostic significance in patients with a normal karyotype is reported to be eliminated in patients receiving an autologous stem cell transplant in first remission {2395}.

NPM1 mutations occur in about one third of adult AML and *CEBPA* mutations in

6–15% of all AML. *NPM1* mutations are typically heterozygous and the leukaemia cells retain a wild-type allele {667}. They usually occur at exon 12 of the *NPM1* gene {666} but rarely involve exon 9 or 11 {17}. About 40 mutation variants have been described {667}, the most common being mutation A, a TCTG tetranucleotide duplication at positions 956 to 959, which accounts for 70–80% of adult AML with *NPM1* mutation. Independent of type, *NPM1* mutations generate common alterations at the C-terminus of NPM in leukaemic mutants, i.e. replacement of tryptophan(s) at position 288 and 290 and creation of a nuclear export signal (NES) motif, which mediates aberrant localization of NPM to the cytoplasm {667}.

CEBPA (CCAAT/enhancer-binding protein-α) mutations occur only in AML and are usually biallelic mutations. The normal gene encodes a transcription factor involved in control of proliferation and differentiation of myeloid progenitors. While mutations may occur throughout the whole gene sequence, two general categories of mutation occur: out-of-frame insertions and deletions in the N-terminal region and in-frame insertions and deletions in the C-terminal region. Mutations of *NPM1* and *CEBPA* are frequently observed in AML with a normal karyotype and, in the absence of *FLT3*-ITD, are associated with a favourable prognosis {216, 602, 1970, 2198, 2331}. In view of the frequency of these mutations, their prognostic significance, and their association with certain morphologic and clinical features, it has been suggested that they may identify unique subsets of AML. Therefore, two new provisional entities, AML with mutated *NPM1* and AML with mutated *CEBPA* are proposed. These have been given provisional status because they have been only recently described and more study is required to confirm these categories as

Table 6.01 Molecular genetic alterations affecting clinical outcome of AML patients in specific cytogenetic groups.

Genetics	Cytogenetics	Prognostic significance
KIT mutations	t(8;21)(q22;q22)	DFS and RFS significantly shorter for patients with KIT mutations (especially those in exon 17) compared with wild-type KIT patients {233A, 2009A} CIR and RI significantly higher for patients with KIT mutations compared with patients with wild-type KIT {310A, 1696} EFS significantly shorter for patients with KIT mutations (especially those in exon 17) compared with patients with wild-type KIT {233A, 1969A} OS significantly shorter for patients with KIT mutations (especially those in exon 17) compared with patients with wild-type KIT {233A, 310A, 1969A, 2009A} No significant difference in OS between patients with and without KIT mutations {1696}
KIT mutations	inv(16)(p13.1q22)/ t(16;16)(p13.1;q22)	RR worse for patients with KIT mutations in exon 8 compared with patients with wild-type KIT {338A} CIR higher and OS worse for patients with KIT mutations in exon 17 compared with patients with wild-type KIT {1696} No significant difference in EFS, RI, RFS and OS between patients with and without KIT mutations {233A, 310A}
FLT3-ITD	Normal*	CRD and DFS significantly shorter for patients with FLT3-ITD compared with patients without FLT3-ITD {193A, 216, 736A, 2394A} EFS significantly shorter for patients with FLT3-ITD compared with patients without FLT3-ITD {233B} OS significantly shorter for patients with FLT3-ITD compared with patients without FLT3-ITD {193A, 216, 736A} No significant difference in OS between patients with and without FLT3-ITD {233B, 2394A}
FLT3-ITD with no expression of wild-type FLT3 allele	Normal	DFS and OS significantly shorter for patients with FLT3-ITD and no expression of wild-type FLT3 allele compared with patients without FLT3-ITD {2394A}
FLT3-TKD	Normal	DFS significantly shorter for patients with FLT3-TKD compared with patients with wild-type FLT3 alleles {2396}
MLL-PTD	Normal	CRD (but not OS) significantly shorter for patients with MLL-PTD compared with patients without MLL-PTD {313, 603} No difference in DFS and OS between patients with and without MLL-PTD receiving intensive treatment including autologous SCT {2395}
CEBPA mutations	Normal	CRD and OS significantly longer for patients with CEBPA mutations compared with patients with wild-type CEBPA genes {216, 737} No significant difference in OS between patients with and without CEBPA mutations {233B} EFS significantly shorter for patients with CEBPA mutations compared with patients with wild-type CEBPA genes {233B}
Cytoplasmic localization of NPM	Normal	CR rate of patients with cytoplasmic localization of NPM not significantly different from CR rate of patients with nuclear localization of NPM in univariable analysis. Cytoplasmic localization of NPM was an independent favourable prognostic factor for CR achievement in multivariate logistic-regression model including WBC, age, NPM localization and FLT3 mutations {666}
NPM1 mutations	Normal	CR rate significantly better for patients with NPM1 mutations than for patients with wild-type NPM1 genes {1970} No significant difference in CR rates between patients with and without NPM1 mutations {139A, 233B} DFS and RFS significantly longer for patients with NPM1 mutations compared with patients with wild-type NPM1 genes {602, 2198} No significant difference in RFS between patients with and without NPM1 mutations {139A, 233B, 1970} EFS significantly longer for patients with NPM1 mutations compared with patients with wild-type NPM1 genes {1970} No significant difference in EFS between patients with and without NPM1 mutations {139A, 233B} No significant difference in OS between patients with and without NPM1 mutations {139A, 233B, 602, 1970, 2198}
NPM1 & FLT3-ITD mutations	Normal	CR rates, EFS, RFS, DFS and OS significantly better for patients with NPM1 mutations who lack FLT3-ITD compared with patients with NPM1 mutations and FLT3-ITD or those with wild-type NPM1 genes with or without FLT3-ITD. NPM1 mutations do not seem to significantly affect poor prognosis of patients with FLT3-ITD {602, 1970, 2198} No significant differences in EFS and OS between patients with NPM1 mutations and no FLT3-ITD compared with patients with NPM1 mutations and FLT3-ITD and those with wild-type NPM1 genes with or without FLT3-ITD {139A}
WT1 mutations	Normal	Failure to achieve a CR with standard induction chemotherapy for patients with WT1 mutations and FLT3-ITD {2120A}. DFS and OS significantly shorter for patients with WT1 mutations compared with patients with wild-type WT1 alleles {1696A}
BAALC expression	Normal	CR rate and rate of primary resistant disease significantly worse for patients with high expression of the BAALC gene in blood compared with patients with low expression of the BAALC gene {135B} No significant difference in CR rates between patients with high and patients with low expression of the BAALC gene {135A, 216} DFS, EFS, RR and OS significantly worse and CIR significantly higher for patients with high expression of the BAALC gene in blood compared with patients with low expression of the BAALC gene {135A, 135B, 216}
ERG expression	Normal	CR rates, EFS, CIR, and OS significantly worse for patients with high expression of the ERG gene in blood compared with patients with low expression of the ERG gene {1390A, 1390B}
MN1 expression	Normal	OS and RFS significantly shorter and RR higher for patients with high expression of the MN1 gene compared with patients with low expression of the MN1 gene {937A}

Modified by Dr Mrózek from Mrózek and Bloomfield {1531A} and Mrózek et al. {1532} with permission.
EFS, event-free survival; RFS, relapse-free survival; OS, overall survival; CIR, cumulative incidence of relapse; RI, relapse incidence; DFS, disease-free survival; RR, risk of relapse; FLT3-ITD, internal tandem duplication of the FLT3 gene; FLT3-TKD, mutations in the tyrosine kinase domain of the FLT3 gene; CRD, complete remission duration; MLL-PTD, partial tandem duplication of the MLL gene; SCT, stem cell transplantation; CR, complete remission; *, Normal karyotype.

disease entities rather than prognostic factors. A small number of AML will show both *NPM1* and *CEBPA* mutations, which would not fit well into the proposed classification structure. In addition, the prognostic significance of the chromosome aberrations reported to occur in 5–15% of AML with *NPM1* or *CEBPA* mutations is not yet clear. Therefore, the presence of any of the recurrent translocations or inversions should be identified in any AML diagnosis. In addition, because of the adverse prognostic impact of *FLT3* mutations in AML with *NPM1* mutations, mutation analysis of *FLT3* should always be performed with *NPM1* and *CEBPA*.

These mutations are not detectable by cytogenetic analysis and are usually detected by PCR. Detection of cytoplasmic NPM by immunohistochemistry correlates well with the molecular method {664}, but similar immunohistochemical surrogate tests are not currently available for all known mutations.

Acute myeloid leukaemia with mutated *NPM1*

Definition
Acute myeloid leukaemia with mutated *NPM1* carries mutations that usually involve exon 12 of the *NPM1* gene. Aberrant cytoplasmic expression of nucleophosmin (NPM) is a surrogate marker of this gene mutation {666}. This AML type frequently has myelomonocytic or monocytic features and typically presents *de novo* in older adults with a normal karyotype.
The WHO Working Group assigned this lesion to a group of provisional entities.

ICD-O code   9861/3

Synonym
Acute myeloid leukaemia with cytoplasmic nucleophosmin (NPMc+ AML).

Epidemiology
NPM1 mutation is one of the most common recurring genetic lesions in AML {283, 602, 666, 667, 2198, 2331}. Prevalence increases with age, occurring in 2–8% of childhood AML and 27%–35% of adult AML. *NPM1* mutations occur in 45–64% of adult AML with a normal karyotype {283, 351, 439, 666, 2198, 2331}. This disease appears to show a female predominance.

Clinical features
Acute myeloid leukaemia with *NPM1* mutation usually presents without a history of a MDS or MPN {666}. Patients often exhibit anaemia and thrombocytopenia, but often have higher white blood cell and platelet counts than other AML types {602}. Patients may show extramedullary involvement, the most frequently affected sites being gingiva, lymph nodes and skin.

Morphology and cytochemistry
There is a strong association between acute myelomonocytic and acute monocytic leukaemia and *NPM1* mutation {666, 667}; notably, 80–90% of acute monocytic leukaemias show *NPM1* mutation.

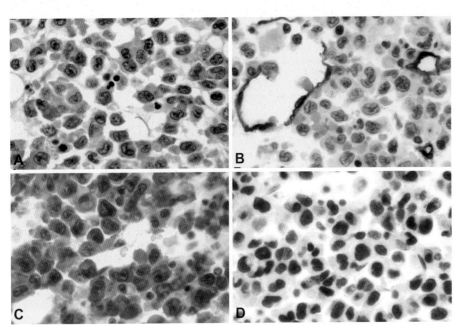

Fig. 6.14 Acute myeloid leukaemia with *NPM1* mutations and myelomonocytic features. **A** Bone marrow biopsy showing complete replacement by large blasts with abundant cytoplasm and folded nuclei. **B** Leukaemic cells are CD34-negative. **C** Leukaemic cells show aberrant cytoplasmic expression of nucleophosmin (NPM). **D** Expression of C23/nucleolin is restricted to the nucleus.

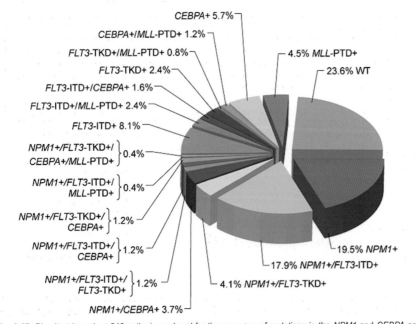

Fig. 6.15 Pie chart based on 246 patients analyzed for the presence of mutations in the *NPM1* and *CEBPA* genes, *FLT3*-ITD, *FLT3*-TKD and *MLL*-PTD. Each sector indicates the percentage of patients harbouring one or more of the aforementioned mutations. WT indicates patients with only wild-type alleles of genes tested. From Mrozek *et al.* {1532} and adapted from Dohner *et al.* {602}.

However, *NPM1* mutations are also detected in AML with and without maturation and in acute erythroid leukaemia. A subset of cases shows multilineage dysplasia. These cases usually have a normal karyotype and the blast cells are CD34 negative. The BM biopsy is usually markedly hypercellular. Bone marrow blast percentages are generally higher in AML with mutated *NPM1* than in other acute myeloid leukaemias with a normal karyotype {602}.

The diagnosis relies on the identification of the genetic lesion by molecular techniques and/or immunohistochemical detection in paraffin sections of aberrant cytoplasmic expression of NPM {667}. Immunostaining with anti-NPM antibodies reveals involvement of two or more BM lineages (myeloid, monocytic, erythroid, megakaryocytic) in the vast majority of AML with *NPM1* mutation {1698}. The variability of BM cell types showing *NPM1* mutations accounts for the wide morphological spectrum of this leukaemia.

Immunophenotype

In addition to myeloid antigens (CD13, CD33, MPO), the blasts in AML with *NPM1* mutation frequently express markers of monocytic differentiation, including CD14, CD11b and the macrophage-restricted CD68. The most striking immunophenotypic feature of AML with *NPM1* mutation, which is independent of the degree of maturation of leukaemic cells, is the lack of expression of CD34 {666}. By immunohistochemistry on paraffin sections, antibodies against NPM show the characteristic aberrant expression of the protein in the cytoplasm of leukaemic cells {666}. In contrast, positivity for C23/nucleolin (another major nucleolar protein) is restricted to the nucleus of leukaemic cells. Immunohistochemical detection of cytoplasmic NPM is predictive of *NPM1* mutations {664}, since the mutations cause critical changes in the structure of NPM native protein (characteristically located in the nucleolus), leading to its increased export from the nucleus and aberrant accumulation in the cytoplasm.

Genetics

Acute myeloid leukaemia with *NPM1* mutation is usually associated with a normal karyotype, however, 5–15% of AML with *NPM1* mutation show chromosomal aberrations {666, 667}, including +8 and del(9q) {2198}. *NPM1* mutations are usually

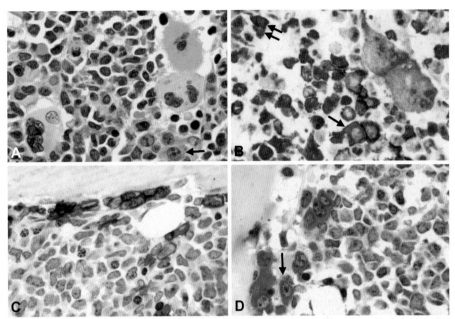

Fig. 6.16 Multilineage involvement in AML with *NPM1* mutations. **A** Bone marrow biopsy. Massive replacement by myeloid blasts with maturation; there are also megakaryocytes and occasional immature erythroid cells (arrow). **B** The same case as (**A**). Myeloid blasts (double arrows), megakaryocytes and immature erythroid cells (arrow) show aberrant cytoplasmic positivity for NPM (blue). Immature erythroid cells (arrow) are double-stained for glycophorin (brown) and NPM (blue). **C** Bone marrow biopsy. Minimally differentiated acute myeloid leukaemia with *NPM1* mutations; occasional immature glycophorin-positive erythroid cells are present. **D** The same case as (**C**). Myeloid blasts and immature erythroid cells (arrow) show cytoplasmic expression of NPM.

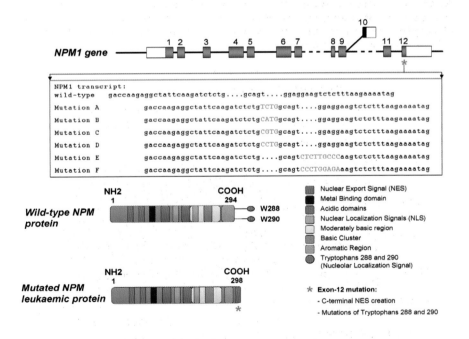

Fig. 6.17 Acute myeloid leukaemia with *NPM1* mutations. Mutations usually occur at exon 12 of the *NPM1* gene. The first identified *NPM1* mutations (A to F) are shown {666}. Mutation A is the most frequent, accounting for 70–80% of cases. All mutations result in common changes at the C-terminus (COOH) of the wild-type NPM protein. These changes (asterisk in the NPM mutated protein) consist of replacement of tryptophan(s) at position 288 and 290 and creation of a new export signal (NES) motif, which are both responsible for the increased nuclear export and aberrant cytoplasmic accumulation of the NPM mutants.

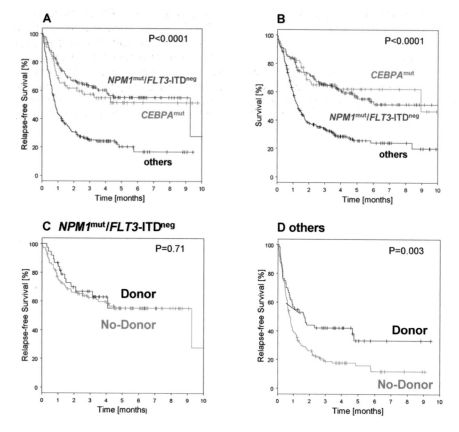

Fig. 6.18 Prognosis of AML patients. **A,B** The genotypes *NPM1^mut/FLT3*-ITD^neg and *CEBPA^mut* are favourable prognostic markers. **C,D** Univariate donor *versus* no-donor analysis on relapse-free survival of AML with normal karyotype in first complete remission, according to genotype. The donor group was defined by the availability of a HLA-matched family donor comprising a match in the loci HLA-A, HLA-B and HLA-DR. **C** Results in AML with favourable genotype *NPM1^mut/FLT3*-ITD^neg; (**D**) the results in AML with adverse genotypes *FLT3*-ITD^pos and *NPM1^wt/CEBPA^wt/FLT3*-ITD^neg; Only AML with adverse genotypes (**D**) benefit from allogeneic stem cell transplantation. From Schlenk RF *et al.* {1962A}

favourable prognosis to AML with a chromosomal aberration or with multilineage dysplasia.

Acute myeloid leukaemia with mutated *CEBPA*

Definition
Acute myeloid leukaemia with mutated *CEBPA* usually meets criteria for AML with maturation or AML without maturation, but some cases may show myelomonocytic or monoblastic features. This leukaemia usually presents *de novo*.
The WHO Working Group assigned this lesion to a group of provisional entities.

ICD-O code   9861/3

Epidemiology
CEBPA mutations occur in 6–15% of *de novo* AML and in 15–18% of AML with normal karyotypes {216, 737, 1280}. There are no apparent age or sex differences between *CEBPA* mutated and non-mutated AML {2040}.

Clinical features
Acute myeloid leukaemia with mutated *CEBPA* tends to have higher haemoglobin levels, lower platelet counts, lower lactate dehydrogenase levels and higher PB blast cell counts when compared to *CEBPA* non-mutated AML. This leukaemia type also has a lower frequency of lymphadenopathy and myeloid sarcoma {216, 737}.

Morphology and cytochemistry
There are no distinctive morphologic features of AML with normal karyotype and *CEBPA* mutations, but the vast majority of cases have features of either AML without or with maturation. Less commonly, cases have monocytic or myelomonocytic features. Three percent or more of the blasts are myeloperoxidase or Sudan black B positive, and most cases are non-specific esterase negative.

Immunophenotype
Leukaemic blasts usually express one or more of the myeloid-associated antigens, CD13, CD33, CD65, CD11b, and CD15. There is usually expression of HLA-DR and CD34 on the majority of blasts. Monocytic markers such as CD14 and CD64 are usually absent. CD7 is present in 50–73% of cases, while expression of

mutually exclusive of the recurrent genetic abnormalities that define the AML entities described in the preceding section {665} and with partial tandem duplications of *MLL* and *CEBPA* mutations, although concurrence of these abnormalities with mutated *NPM1* have been reported {602, 2198}. About 40% of AML with *NPM1* mutations also carry *FLT3*-ITD {666}. *NPM1* mutations appear to precede *FLT3*-ITD and these leukaemias are more genetically stable during disease evolution {439, 2198}. AML with cytoplasmic mutated *NPM1* shows a distinct gene expression profile characterized by up-regulation of *HOX* genes {19, 2331} that differs from that of other AML types, including AML with *MLL* rearrangement {1539}.

Postulated normal counterpart
Haematopoietic stem cell {1394}.

Prognosis and predictive factors
Acute myeloid leukaemia with mutated *NPM1* typically shows a good response to induction therapy {666}. Acute myeloid leukaemia with mutated *NPM1* and a normal karyotype, in the absence of a *FLT3*-ITD mutation, has a characteristically favourable prognosis {283, 602, 1970, 2198, 2331}. The coexistence of *FLT3*-ITD mutations is associated with a poorer prognosis, but these patients still appear to have an improved prognosis compared to AML that is *NPM1* negative and *FLT3*-ITD positive {746}. Younger individuals with AML and a normal karyotype exhibiting the genotype *NPM1* mutated/*FLT3*-ITD negative show a prognosis that is comparable to that of AML with t(8;21)(q22;q22) or inv(16) (p13.1q22) and may possibly be exempted from allogeneic stem cell transplantation in first complete remission {602}. It is not known whether a *NPM1* mutated/*FLT3*-ITD negative genotype also confers a

CD56 or other lymphoid antigens is uncommon {216, 1308}.

Genetics
Seventy percent of AML with *CEBPA* mutation have a normal karyotype. *FLT3*-ITD mutations occur in 22–33% of cases.

Postulated normal counterpart
Haematopoietic stem cell.

Prognosis
Acute myeloid leukaemia with a normal karyotype and *CEBPA* mutation is associated with a favourable prognosis, similar to that of AML with inv(16)(p13.1q22) or t(8;21)(q22;q22). The significance of *FLT3*-ITD on the prognosis of this group is currently unclear, with small studies suggesting either no impact or a negative impact on prognosis {737, 1780}. Although uncommon, the prognostic significance of AML with *CEBPA* mutations and other chromosomal aberrations remains unclear.

Acute myeloid leukaemia with myelodysplasia-related changes

D.A. Arber
R.D. Brunning
A. Orazi
B.J. Bain

A. Porwit
J.W. Vardiman
M.M. Le Beau
P.L. Greenberg

Definition

Acute myeloid leukaemia (AML) with myelodysplasia-related changes is an acute leukaemia with 20% or more peripheral blood (PB) or bone marrow (BM) blasts with morphological features of myelodysplasia or a prior history of a myelodysplastic syndrome (MDS) or myelodysplastic/myeloproliferative neoplasm (MDS/MPN), or MDS-related cytogenetic abnormalities, and absence of the specific genetic abnormalities of AML with recurrent genetic abnormalities. Patients should not have a history of prior cytotoxic or radiation therapy for an unrelated disease. Therefore, there are three possible reasons for assigning cases to this subtype: AML arising from previous MDS or MDS/MPN; AML with an MDS-related cytogenetic abnormality; and AML with multilineage dysplasia. A given case may be assigned to this subtype for one, two or all three reasons (Table 6.02).

ICD-O code   9895/3

Synonym

Acute myeloid leukaemia with multilineage dysplasia.

Epidemiology

This category of AML with myelodysplasia-related changes occurs mainly in elderly patients and is rare in children {913, 1269}. Although the definition of multilineage dysplasia is variable in the literature, this category appears to represent 24–35% of all cases of AML {69, 869, 1493, 2465}.

Clinical features

Patients with AML with myelodysplasia-related changes often present with severe pancytopenia. Some cases with 20–29% blasts, especially those arising from MDS or in childhood, may be slowly progressive. These cases, with relatively stable PB counts for weeks or months, considered refractory anaemia with excess blasts in transformation in the French-American-British Cooperative Group classification, may behave clinically in a manner more similar to MDS than to AML.

Morphology and cytochemistry

Most, but not all cases in this category of AML have morphological evidence of multilineage dysplasia which must be assessed on well-stained smears of PB and BM. To classify an AML as having myelodysplasia-related changes based on

morphology, dysplasia must be present in at least 50% of the cells in at least two BM cell lines. Dysgranulopoiesis is characterized by neutrophils with hypogranular cytoplasm, hyposegmented nuclei (pseudo-Pelger-Huët anomaly) or bizarrely segmented nuclei. In some cases, these features may be more readily identified on PB than BM smears. Dyserythropoiesis is characterized by megaloblastosis, karyorrhexis and nuclear irregularity, fragmentation or multinucleation. Ring sideroblasts, cytoplasmic vacuoles and periodic acid-Schiff (PAS) positivity are additional features of dyserythropoiesis. Dysmegakaryopoiesis is characterized by micromegakaryocytes and normal sized or large megakaryocytes with non-lobulated or multiple nuclei. Dysplastic megakaryocytes may be more readily appreciated in sections than smears {69, 742}.

Some cases will not have sufficient non-blast cell BM elements to adequately assess for multilineage dysplasia or have sufficient non-blast cells but do not meet the criteria described above for a morphologic diagnosis of AML with multilineage dysplasia. These cases are diagnosed as AML with myelodysplasia-related changes by the detection of MDS-related cytogenetic abnormalities and/or by a prior history of MDS.

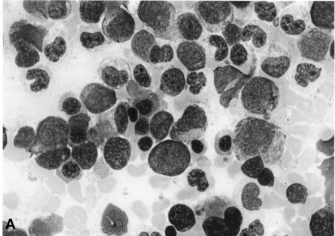
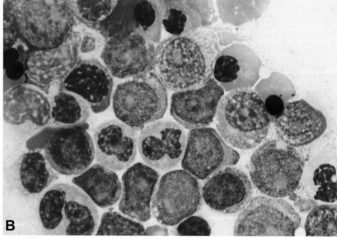

Fig. 6.19 Acute myeloid leukaemia with myelodysplasia-related changes (multilineage dysplasia). The marrow aspirate shows numerous agranular blasts as well as admixed hypogranular neutrophils with clumped nuclear chromatin and erythroid precursors with irregular nuclear contours. **A** A small, hypolobated megakaryocyte is present at the bottom. **B** A higher magnification of another case showing more irregular nuclear features of erythroid precursors and neutrophils with clumped nuclear chromatin.

Immunophenotype

Immunophenotyping results are variable due to the heterogeneity of the underlying genetic changes. In cases with aberrations of chromosomes 5 and 7, a high incidence of CD34, terminal deoxynucleotidyl transferase (TdT), and CD7 expression has been reported {2324}. In cases with antecedent MDS, CD34+ cells frequently constitute only a subpopulation of blasts and may have a stem-cell related immunophenotype with low expression of CD38 and/or HLA-DR. Blasts often express pan-myeloid markers (CD13, CD33). There is frequently aberrant expression of CD56 and CD7 {1623}. The maturing myeloid cells may show patterns of antigen expression differing from those seen in normal myeloid development, and there may be alterations in the light scatter properties of maturing cells, particularly neutrophils. There is an increased incidence of multi-drug resistance glycoprotein (MDR-1) expression in the blast cells {1206, 1268, 1269}.

Genetics

Chromosome abnormalities are similar to those found in MDS and often involve gain or loss of major segments of certain chromosomes with complex karyotypes and -7/del(7q) and -5/del(5q) being most common {1269, 1530, 1641}. Additional abnormalities that are considered sufficient for inclusion in this category are given in Table 6.03. While trisomy 8 and del(20q) are also common in MDS, these findings are not considered to be disease-specific and are not, by themselves, sufficient to consider a case as AML with myelodysplasia-related changes. Similarly, loss of the Y chromosome is a non-specific finding in older men and should not be considered sufficient for cytogenetic evidence of this disease category. Balanced translocations are less common in this disorder, but when they occur are often translocations involving 5q32-33. The t(3;5)(q25;q34) is associated with multilineage dysplasia and a younger age at presentation than most other cases in this disease group {66}. In addition, AML with inv(3)(q21q26.2), t(3;3)(q21;q26.2) or with t(6;9)(p23;q34) may show evidence of multilineage dysplasia, but these are now recognized as distinct entities in the AML with recurrent genetic abnormalities group and should be classified as such. However, cases with the specific 11q23 rearrangements, t(11;16)(q23;p13.3) and t(2;11)(p21;q23), if not associated with prior cytotoxic therapy, should be classified in this group rather than as a variant translocation of 11q23.

Cases of AML with multilineage dysplasia may carry NPM1 and/or FLT3 mutations {2356}. Most NPM1 mutated cases would be expected to have a normal karyotype, CD34-negative blasts and no history of prior MDS {2015}. However, the presence of an MDS-associated karyotypic abnormality should take diagnostic precedence over the detection of an NPM1 or CEBPA mutation for classification purposes until the significance of such rare genetic combinations is clarified. In patients with AML with multilineage dysplasia and a normal karyotype, information regarding the mutational status of NPM1, CEBPA and FLT3 may provide important prognostic information, and the presence of these mutations should be noted along with the diagnosis of AML with myelodysplasia-related changes (multilineage dysplasia) {2356}.

Differential diagnosis

The principal differential diagnoses are refractory anaemia with excess blasts, acute erythroid leukaemia, acute megakaryoblastic leukaemia and the other categories of AML, not otherwise specified (NOS). Careful blast cell counts, adherence to the diagnostic criteria for morphological dysplasia and evaluation for MDS-related cytogenetic abnormalities should resolve most cases, with this category having priority over the purely morphologic categories of AML, NOS. For example, a case with ≥20% BM myeloblasts, multilineage dysplasia, ≥50% BM erythroid precursors and monosomy 7 should be considered as AML with myelodysplasia-related changes rather than acute erythroid leukaemia. Similarly, a case with 20% or more BM megakaryoblasts and multilineage dysplasia would be considered AML with myelodysplasia-related changes (megakaryoblastic type).

Postulated normal counterpart

Multipotent haematopoietic stem cell.

Prognosis and predictive factors

Acute myeloid leukaemia with myelodysplastic features generally has a poor prognosis with a lower rate of achieving complete remission than other AML types {69, 742, 1269, 1493, 2465}. While there are no overall prognostic differences

Table 6.02 Criteria for the diagnosis of AML with myelodysplasia-related features.

≥20% blood or marrow blasts
AND
Any of the following
Previous history of myelodysplastic syndrome
Myelodysplastic syndrome-related cytogenetic abnormality (see Table 6.03)
Multilineage dysplasia
AND
Absence of both
Prior cytotoxic therapy for an unrelated disease
Recurring cytogenetic abnormality as described in AML with recurrent genetic abnormalities.

Table 6.03 Cytogenetic abnormalities sufficient to diagnose AML with myelodysplasia-related features when ≥20% PB or BM blasts are present.

Complex karyotype*
Unbalanced abnormalities
-7/del(7q)
-5/del(5q)
i(17q)/t(17p)
-13/del(13q)
del(11q)
del(12p)/t(12p)
del(9q)
idic(X)(q13)
Balanced abnormalities
t(11;16)(q23;p13.3)**
t(3;21)(q26.2;q22.1)**
t(1;3)(p36.3;q21.1)
t(2;11)(p21;q23)**
t(5;12)(q33;p12)
t(5;7)(q33;q11.2)
t(5;17)(q33;p13)
t(5;10)(q33;q21)
t(3;5)(q25;q34)

* ≥3 unrelated abnormalities, none of which are included in the AML with recurrent genetic abnormalities subgroup; such cases should be classified in the appropriate cytogenetic group.
** These abnormalities most commonly occur in therapy-related disease and therapy-related AML should be excluded before using these abnormalities as evidence for a diagnosis of AML with myelodysplasia-related features.

between cases with and without prior MDS {69}, recognition of cases with prior MDS and relatively low blast counts may identify cases with less clinically aggressive disease. Some cases with prior MDS and 20–29% BM blasts, considered refractory anaemia with excess blasts in transformation in the French-American-British Cooperative Group classification, may behave in a manner more similar to MDS than other AML. These cases, as well as cases with myelodysplasia and just under 20% blasts, require regular monitoring of PB counts and BM morphology for changes suggesting disease progression to overt AML.

Although AML with multilineage dysplasia is generally associated with a poor prognosis, several studies have not found morphology to be a significant parameter when using multi-variant analysis that also incorporates the results of cytogenetic analysis, high risk cytogenetic abnormalities being more significantly associated with prognosis {869, 2356, 2465}. Therefore, multilineage dysplasia should be considered as a possible indicator of high risk cytogenetic abnormalities, but in the absence of such abnormalities, may not be important. In such cases, fluorescence *in situ* hybridization (FISH) studies for MDS-related abnormalities may be useful. It is currently unclear whether a *NPM1* positive/*FLT3*-negative genotype in AML with multilineage dysplasia confers the same good prognosis as in other AML with *NPM1* mutations. Cases of AML with multilineage dysplasia and *NPM1* mutations usually do not have adverse cytogenetic findings or a history of prior MDS {2015}. However, the clinical impact of mutation status versus the presence of multilineage dysplasia requires more investigation. Therefore, it is not yet clear how cases of AML with multilineage dysplasia without prior MDS or MDS-related cytogenetic abnormalities and with an *NPM1* mutation or a *CEBPA* mutation should be classified. However, as noted

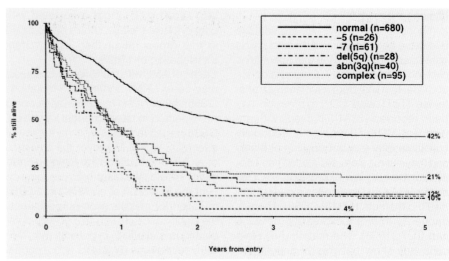

Fig. 6.20 Survival curve for cases of acute myeloid leukaemia with adverse cytogenetic findings in the MRC-AML 10 trial. Reproduced from Grimwade D *et al.* {848}.

above, at this time cases of AML with MDS-related cytogenetic findings and one of these mutations should be diagnosed as AML with myelodysplasia-related changes as well as noting the mutation detected.

Diagnostic terminology

Because there are different pathways to a diagnosis of AML with myelodysplasia-related changes, which upon further study may have clinical differences, it is recommended that the reason(s) for diagnosing a case as such be included in the diagnosis. For example, a case diagnosed solely on morphology would be considered "AML with myelodysplasia-related changes (multilineage dysplasia)"; a case arising from previously diagnosed

MDS without associated dysplasia identified at the time of AML diagnosis would be considered "AML with myelodysplasia-related changes (following previous MDS)"; and a case with prior MDS, dysplastic features and monosomy 7 would be considered "AML with myelodysplasia-related changes (following previous MDS, MDS-associated cytogenetic abnormality and multilineage dysplasia). Cases with *NPM1*, *CEPBA* and/or *FLT3* mutations should also indicate the mutation finding (i.e. "AML with myelodysplasia-related changes (multilineage dysplasia) and *NPM1* mutation"). Finally, because of the possible clinical heterogeneity of cases with low blast cell counts (20–29%), the blast count should be clearly stated in the report.

Therapy-related myeloid neoplasms

J.W. Vardiman   E. Matutes
D.A. Arber   I. Baumann
R.D. Brunning   J. Thiele
R.A. Larson

Definition
This category includes therapy-related acute myeloid leukaemia (t-AML), myelodysplastic syndrome (t-MDS) and myelodysplastic/myeloproliferative neoplasms (t-MDS/MPN) occurring as late complications of cytotoxic chemotherapy and/or radiation therapy administered for a prior neoplastic or non-neoplastic disorder. Although some patients may be diagnosed morphologically as t-MDS, t-MDS/MPN or t-AML according to the number of blasts present, all of these therapy-related neoplasms are best considered together as a unique clinical syndrome. Excluded from this category is transformation of MPN since it is often not possible to determine if this is disease evolution or therapy-related.

ICD-O code   9920/3

Synonym
Therapy-related acute myeloid leukaemia, NOS.

Epidemiology
Therapy-related t-AML/t-MDS and t-AML/t-MDS/MPN account for 10–20% of all cases of AML, MDS and MDS/MPN {1278, 1433, 1536}. The incidence among patients treated with cytotoxic agents varies according to the underlying disease and the treatment strategy. Any age group may be affected but the risk associated with alkylating agent or radiation therapy generally increases with age whereas the risk for those treated with topoisomerase II inhibitors is similar across all ages {651, 1278}.

Etiology
Therapy-related neoplasms are thought to be the consequence of mutational events induced by cytotoxic therapy. Some individuals may have a heritable predisposition due to polymorphisms in genes that affect drug metabolism or DNA-repair mechanisms, but for most cases the underlying pathogenesis remains uncertain {1899}. Cytotoxic agents commonly implicated are listed in the Table 6.04. Although other

therapies such as hydroxycarbamide (hydroxyurea), radioisotopes, L-asparaginase and haematopoietic growth factors have been suggested to be leukaemogenic, their primary role in therapy-related haematologic neoplasms, if any, is not clear. Characteristic clinical, morphologic and genetic features often relate to the previous therapy received.

Sites of involvement
Peripheral blood (PB) and bone marrow (BM) are the principle sites of involvement.

Clinical features
Nearly an equal number of patients give a history of treatment for a previous haematological malignancy as for a non-haematological solid tumour. However, 5–20% of patients are reported to have received cytotoxic therapy for a non-neoplastic disease. A similar number develop a therapy-related myeloid neoplasm after high dose chemotherapy and autologous haematopoietic stem cell transplant for a previously treated malignancy {1433, 2041}. Two subsets of t-AML/t-MDS and t-AML/t-MDS/MPN are generally recognized. The most common occurs 5–10 years after exposure to alkylating agents and/or ionizing radiation. Patients often present with t-MDS and evidence of BM failure with one or multiple cytopenias, although a minority will present with t-MDS/MPN or with overt t-AML. This category is commonly associated with unbalanced loss of genetic material, often involving chromosomes 5 and/or 7. The second category of t-AML/t-MDS and t-AML/t-MDS/MPN encompasses 20–30% of patients, has a latency period of about 1–5 years, and follows treatment with agents that interact with DNA topoisomerase II (topoisomerase II inhibitors). Most patients in this subset do not have a myelodysplastic phase but present initially with overt acute leukaemia that is often associated with a balanced chromosomal translocation {651, 1716, 2041}. Although it may be useful to consider t-AML/t-MDS and t-AML/t-MDS/MPN as being alkylating agent and/or radiation-related or as topoisomerase II inhibitor-related,

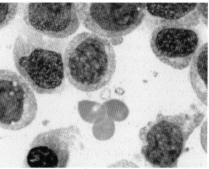

Fig. 6.21 Therapy-related AML with t(9;11)(p22;q23). This patient developed t-AML less than one year following institution of therapy for osteosarcoma. The therapy included both alkylating agents and topoisomerase II inhibitors.

in practice many patients have received polychemotherapy that includes both classes of drugs and the boundary between the two categories is not always sharp {2041}.

Morphology
The majority of patients present with t-AML/t-MDS associated with multilineage dysplasia. Commonly, but not invariably in such cases, a history of prior therapy with alkylating agents and/or radiation therapy is elicited and cytogenetic studies reveal abnormalities of chromosomes 5 and/or 7, or a complex karyotype. Nevertheless, dysplasia may be seen in some cases with balanced translocations as well. The PB shows one or more cytopenias. Anaemia is almost always present and red cell morphology is characterized in most cases by macrocytosis and poikilocytosis. Dysplastic changes in the neutrophils include abnormal nuclear lobation, particularly hypolobation, and cytoplasmic hypogranulation. Basophilia is frequently present {1472}. The BM may be hypercellular, normocellular or hypocellular, and slight to marked BM fibrosis occurs in approximately 15% of cases. Dysgranulopoiesis and dyserythropoiesis are present in most patients. Ring sideroblasts are reported in up to 60% of cases and in some cases exceed 15% of the erythroid precursors. Megakaryocytes vary in num-

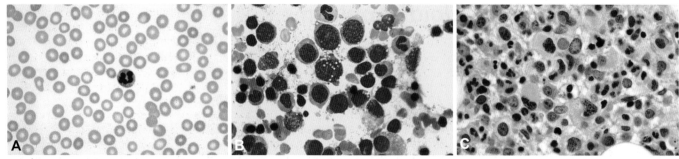

Fig. 6.22 Therapy-related MDS/AML. This 42-year-old man was treated with ABVD therapy for classical Hodgkin lymphoma but relapsed 16 months later and was given salvage chemotherapy and radiotherapy. Two years later he presented with pancytopenia in the PB (**A**), a BM aspirate (**B**) and BM biopsy (**C**) showed increased blasts and multilineage dysplasia. A complex karyotype included loss of chromosomes 5 and 7.

ber but dysplastic forms of variable size with mono- or hypolobated or widely separated nuclei are seen in the majority of cases {1472, 1647}. The percentage of blasts also varies but in patients presenting with a myelodysplastic phase almost 50% will have less than 5% BM blasts {1472, 2026}. About 5% of patients have features of MDS/MPN, such as chronic myelomonocytic leukaemia {2026}. Although patients presenting with myelodysplasia and cytopenias may be designated as t-MDS or t-AML depending on their morphology and blast counts, such subclassification may lack clinical significance {2026}.

In 20–30% of cases, the first manifestation of therapy-related myeloid neoplasm is overt acute leukaemia without a preceding myelodysplastic phase. Often, but not invariably, these cases follow topoisomerase II inhibitor therapy. The majority of the cases are associated with balanced recurrent chromosomal translocations that frequently involve 11q23 (*MLL*) or 21q22 (*RUNX1*), and have morphology that resembles *de novo* acute leukaemia

associated with these chromosomal abnormalities {36, 1886, 2034} although a few cases may present as MDS or have dysplastic features as well. Many cases fall in the categories of acute monoblastic leukaemia or myelomonocytic leukaemia, but cases with granulocytic differentiation also occur. Cases morphologically (and cytogenetically) identical to those observed in all of the subtypes of AML with recurring cytogenetic abnormalities have been described, including acute promyelocytic leukaemia. Such cases should be designated as t-AML with the appropriate cytogenetic abnormality indicated, e.g. t-AML with t(9;11)(p21;q23). Cases of lymphoblastic leukaemia (ALL) also occur in this group, usually associated with a t(4;11)(q21;q23) chromosomal abnormality {1022, 1984}.

Immunophenotype

There are no specific immunophenotypic findings in t-AML/MDS or in t-AML/t-MDS/ MPN. Immunophenotyping studies reflect the heterogeneity of the underlying morphology and often show changes similar

to their *de novo* counterparts {68}. Blasts are generally CD34+ and express pan-myeloid markers (CD13, CD33). There is frequent aberrant expression of CD56 and/or the lymphoid-associated marker CD7. The maturing myeloid cells may show patterns of antigen expression that differ from that seen in normal myeloid development, and there may be alterations in the light scatter properties of maturing cells, particularly neutrophils.

Genetics

The leukaemic cells of over 90% of patients with t-AML/t-MDS show an abnormal karyotype. The cytogenetic abnormalities often correlate with the latent period between the initial therapy and the onset of the leukaemic disorder and with the previous cytotoxic therapy {1254, 1433, 1716, 1886, 2041}. Approximately 70% of patients harbour unbalanced chromosomal aberrations, mainly whole or partial loss of chromosomes 5 and/or 7, that are often associated with one or more additional chromosomal abnormalities [e.g. del(13q), del(20q), del(11q), del(3p), -17, -18, -21, +8] in a complex karyotype. These changes are usually associated with a long latent period, a preceding myelodysplastic phase or t-AML with dysplastic features, and alkylating agent and/or radiation therapy. The remaining 20–30% of patients have balanced chromosomal translocations that involve rearrangements of 11q23 [including t(9;11)(p22;q23) and t(11;19) (q23;p13)], 21q22 [including t(8;21) (q22;q22) and t(3;21)(q26.2;q22.1)] and other abnormalities such as t(15;17) (q22;q12) and inv(16)(p13.1q22). The balanced translocations are generally associated with a short latency period, most often present as overt AML without a preceding myelodysplastic phase, and

Table 6.04 Cytotoxic agents implicated in therapy-related haematologic neoplasms*.

Alkylating agents
Melphalan, cyclophosphamide, nitrogen mustard, chlorambucil, busulfan, carboplatin, cisplatin, dacarbazine, procarbazine, carmustine, mitomycin C, thiotepa, lomustine, etc.

Ionizing radiation therapy
Large fields including active bone marrow

Topoisomerase II inhibitors
Etoposide, teniposide, doxorubicin, daunorubicin, mitoxantrone, amsacrine, actinomycin
*Topoisomerase II inhibitors may also be associated with therapy-related lymphoblastic leukaemia

Others
Antimetabolites: thiopurines, mycophenolate, fludarabine
Antitubulin agents (usually in combination with other agents): vincristine, vinblastine, vindesine, paclitaxel, docetaxel

are associated with prior topoisomerase II inhibitor therapy.

Postulated normal counterpart
Haematopoietic stem cell.

Prognosis and predictive factors
The prognosis of t-AML/t-MDS and t-AML/t-MDS/MPN is generally poor, although it is strongly influenced by the associated karyotypic abnormality as well as the comorbidity of the underlying malignancy or disease for which cytotoxic therapy was initially required. Overall, 5-year survival of less than 10% is commonly reported. Cases associated with abnormalities of chromosome 5 and/or 7 and a complex karyotype have a particularly poor outcome, with a median survival time of less than one year regardless of whether they present as overt acute leukaemia or as t-MDS {1472, 2026}. In contrast to *de novo* MDS, some reports have suggested that neither the blast percentage nor subclassification have a significant impact on clinical outcome, and the designation of t-AML/t-MDS or t-AML/t-MDS/MPN may be more appropriate {1472, 2026}. Patients with balanced translocations generally have a better prognosis, but, except for those with t(15;17)(q22;q12) and inv(16)(p13.1q22) or t(16;16)(p13.1;q22), median survival times are shorter than for their *de novo* counterparts {36, 227, 1886, 2034, 2041}.

It should be noted that occasional patients assigned to the category of therapy-related myeloid neoplasms represent coincidental disease and would be expected to behave like other *de novo* disease.

D.A. Arber
R.D. Brunning
A. Orazi
A. Porwit

L. Peterson
J. Thiele
M.M. Le Beau

Acute myeloid leukaemia, not otherwise specified

The category of acute myeloid leukaemia, not otherwise specified (AML, NOS) encompasses those cases that do not fulfil criteria for inclusion in one of the previously described groups with recurrent genetic abnormalities, myelodysplasia-related changes or that are therapy-related. These tumours are felt to be derived from haematopoietic stem cells. The clinical relevance of some subgroups of AML, NOS is of questionable significance {69, 2153} but they are retained in the classification because they define criteria for the diagnosis of AML across a diverse morphologic spectrum and include the unique diagnostic criteria for erythroleukaemia. Mutation analysis and cytogenetic studies are recommended for cases in this category and may offer more prognostic significance than the morphologic subtypes. The primary basis for subclassification within this category is the morphological and cytochemical/immunophenotypic features of the leukaemic cells that indicate the major lineages involved and the degree of maturation. The defining criterion for AML is 20% or more myeloblasts in the peripheral blood (PB) or bone marrow (BM); the promonocytes in AML with monocytic differentiation are considered blast equivalents. The classification of acute erythroid leukaemia is unique and is based on the percentage of abnormal erythroblasts for pure erythroid leukaemia and the percentage of myeloblasts among non-erythroid cells for the erythroid/myeloid type. It is recommended that the blast percentage in the BM be determined from a 500 cell differential count using an acceptable Romanowsky stain. In the PB, the differential should include 200 leukocytes; if there is a marked leukopenia, buffy coat smears can be used. Should an aspirate smear not be obtainable due to BM fibrosis and if the blasts express CD34, immunohistochemical detection of CD34 on biopsy sections may provide valuable information and may allow the diagnosis of AML if the 20% blast threshold is met. The major criteria required for this category are based on examination of BM aspirates, PB smears, and BM trephine biopsies. The recommendations for classification are applicable only to specimens obtained prior to chemotherapy. It should be noted that most of the epidemiologic data cited for each AML, NOS entity has been largely gathered from studies using the prior FAB classification scheme, and may not directly apply to series of patients classified by the WHO system, in which most patients will be classified into other, more specific entities, and for which sufficient epidemiologic data is not yet available.

Acute myeloid leukaemia with minimal differentiation

Definition

Acute myeloid leukaemia with minimal differentiation is an AML with no evidence of myeloid differentiation by morphology and light microscopy cytochemistry. The myeloid nature of the blasts is demonstrated by immunological markers and/or ultrastructural studies including ultrastructural cytochemistry. Immunophenotyping studies are essential in all cases to distinguish this disease from acute lymphoblastic leukaemia (ALL).

ICD-O code   9872/3

Epidemiology

These cases comprise <5% of cases of AML. The disease may occur at any age, but most patients are either infants or older adults.

Clinical features

Patients with AML, minimally differentiated usually present with evidence of BM failure with anaemia, thrombocytopenia and neutropenia. There may be leukocytosis with a markedly increased number of blasts.

Morphology and cytochemistry

The blasts are usually of medium size with dispersed nuclear chromatin, round or slightly indented nuclei with one or two nucleoli. The cytoplasm is agranular with

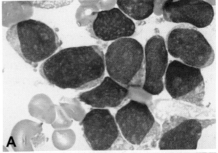
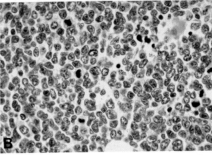

Fig. 6.23 Acute myeloblastic leukaemia, minimal differentiated. **A** Bone marrow smear. The blasts vary in size, amount of cytoplasm and prominence of nucleoli. There are no differentiating features. **B** Bone marrow section. This bone marrow is completely replaced by blasts without differentiating features.

a varying degree of basophilia. Less frequently, the blasts are small with more condensed chromatin, inconspicuous nucleoli and scanty cytoplasm resembling lymphoblasts. The cytochemical reactions for myeloperoxidase (MPO), Sudan Black B (SBB) and naphthol-ASD-chloroacetate esterase (CAE) are negative (<3% positive blasts); α naphthyl acetate and butyrate esterases are negative or may show a non-specific weak or focal reaction distinct from that of monocytic cells {186, 1084, 1880}. In some unusual cases of AML with minimal differentiation there may be a residual normal population of maturing neutrophils. These cases may resemble AML with maturation, but are distinguished by the absence of MPO or SBB positivity in the blasts and the absence of Auer rods. The BM sections are usually markedly hypercellular with poorly differentiated blasts. With sensitive ultrastructural studies, MPO, CAE activity may be demonstrated in small granules, endoplasmic reticulum, Golgi area and/or nuclear membranes.

Immunophenotype
Most cases express early, haematopoietic-associated antigens (such as CD34, CD38 and HLA-DR) and lack antigens associated with myeloid and monocytic maturation, such as CD11b, CD15, CD14, CD64 and CD65. Blast cells usually express CD13 and/or CD117 while expression of CD33 is found in approximately 60% of cases. Blasts are negative for B- and T-associated cytoplasmic lymphoid markers cCD3, cCD79a and cCD22. MPO is negative by cytochemistry, but may be positive in a fraction of blasts by flow cytometry or immunohistochemistry. Nuclear terminal deoxynucleotidyl transferase (TdT) is positive in approximately 50% of cases. Expression of CD7 has been reported in approximately 40% of cases, while expression of other membrane, lymphoid-associated markers is rare.

Genetics
No unique chromosomal abnormality has been identified in AML with minimal differentiation. The most common abnormalities previously reported are complex karyotypes and unbalanced abnormalities, such as -5/del(5q), -7/del(7q), +8 and del(11q), but the presence of some of these abnormalities would now place the case in the category of AML with myelodysplasia-related changes. Mutations of *RUNX1 (AML1)* occur in 27% of cases and 16–22% of cases have *FLT3* mutations.

Differential diagnosis
The differential diagnosis includes ALL, acute megakaryoblastic leukaemia, mixed phenotype acute leukaemia and more rarely, the leukaemic phase of large cell lymphoma. Immunophenotyping studies are essential to distinguish these conditions.

Acute myeloid leukaemia without maturation

Definition
Acute myeloid leukaemia without maturation is characterized by a high percentage of BM blasts without significant evidence of maturation to more mature neutrophils. Blasts constitute ≥90% of the non-erythroid cells. The myeloid nature of

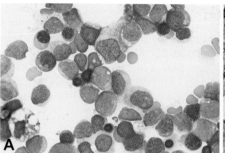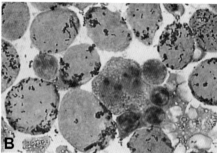

Fig. 6.24 Acute myeloid leukaemia without maturation. Bone marrow smear. **A** The cells are predominantly myeloblasts; occasional myeloblasts contain azurophilic granules or Auer rods. There is no evidence of maturation beyond the myeloblast stage. **B** Myeloperoxidase reaction showing numerous myeloblasts with strong peroxidase reactivity. There are several peroxidase negative erythroid precursors in the centre.

the blasts is demonstrated by MPO or SBB (3% or more of blasts) positivity and/or Auer rods.

ICD-O code 9873/3

Epidemiology
Acute myeloid leukaemia without maturation comprises 5–10% of cases of AML. It may occur at any age but the majority of patients are adults; the median age is approximately 46 years.

Clinical features
The patients usually present with evidence of BM failure with anaemia, thrombocytopenia and neutropenia. There may be a leukocytosis with markedly increased blasts.

Morphology and cytochemistry
Some cases of AML without maturation are characterized by obvious myeloblasts, some of which have azurophilic granulation and/or unequivocal Auer rods. In other cases, the blasts resemble lymphoblasts and lack azurophilic granules: MPO and SBB positivity are present in a variable number of blasts, but always in at least 3%. The BM biopsy sections are usually markedly hypercellular although normocellular or hypocellular cases may occur.

Immunophenotype
Acute myeloid leukaemia without maturation usually presents with a population of blasts expressing MPO and one or more of myeloid-associated antigens such as CD13, CD33 and CD117. CD34 and HLA-DR are positive in approximately 70% of cases. There is generally no expression of markers associated with granulocytic maturation such as CD15 and CD65 or monocytic markers such as CD14 and

CD64. CD11b is expressed in a fraction of cases. Blasts are negative for B- and T-associated cytoplasmic lymphoid markers: cCD3, cCD79a and cCD22. CD7 is found in ~30% of cases, while expression of other membrane, lymphoid-associated markers such as CD2, CD4, CD19 and CD56 has been described in 10–20% of cases.

Genetics
There is no demonstrated association between AML without maturation and specific recurrent chromosomal abnormalities. The immunoglobulin heavy chain gene and T-cell receptor chain genes, in most cases, are in a germline configuration.

Differential diagnosis
The differential diagnosis includes ALL in cases with blast cells lacking granules or having a low percentage of MPO-positive blasts, and AML with maturation in cases with a higher percentage of MPO-positive blasts.

Acute myeloid leukaemia with maturation

Definition
Acute myeloid leukaemia with maturation is characterized by the presence of ≥20% blasts in the BM or PB and evidence of maturation (≥10% maturing cells of neutrophil lineage); cells of monocyte lineage comprise <20% of BM cells.

ICD-O code 9874/3

Epidemiology
Acute myeloid leukaemia with maturation comprises approximately 10% of cases of AML {69}. It occurs in all age groups;

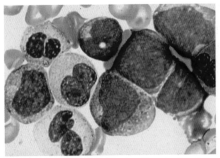

Fig. 6.25 Acute myeloid leukaemia with maturation. Bone marrow smear. In addition to the myeloblasts, there are several more mature neutrophils; one neutrophil has a pseudo Pelger-Huët nucleus.

20% of patients are <25 years of age and 40% are ≥60 years of age {2078}.

Clinical features

Patients often present with symptoms r elated to anaemia, thrombocytopenia and neutropenia. The white blood cell count is variable as is the number of blasts.

Morphology and cytochemistry

Blasts with and without azurophilic granulation are present. Auer rods are frequently present. Promyelocytes, myelocytes and mature neutrophils comprise at least 10% of the BM cells; variable degrees of dysplasia are frequently present. Eosinophil precursors are frequently increased but do not exhibit the cytological or cytochemical abnormalities characteristic of the eosinophils in acute myelomonocytic leukaemia associated with inv(16)(p13.1q22). Basophils and/or mast cells are sometimes increased. The BM biopsy is usually hypercellular.

Immunophenotype

Leukaemic blasts in AML with maturation usually express one or more of the myeloid-associated antigens, CD13, CD33, CD65, CD11b and CD15. There is often expression of HLA-DR, CD34 and/or CD117, which may be present only in a fraction of blasts. Monocytic markers such as CD14 and CD64 are usually absent. CD7 is present in 20–30% of cases, while expression of CD56, CD2, CD19 and CD4 is uncommon (~10% of cases).

Genetics

There is no demonstrated association between AML with maturation and specific recurrent chromosomal abnormalities.

Differential diagnosis

The differential diagnosis includes refractory anaemia with excess blasts in cases with a low blast percentage, AML without maturation when the percentage of blasts is high, and acute myelomonocytic leukaemia in cases with increased monocytes.

Acute myelomonocytic leukaemia

Definition

Acute myelomonocytic leukaemia is an acute leukaemia characterized by the proliferation of both neutrophil and monocyte precursors. The PB or BM has ≥20% blasts (including promonocytes); neutrophils and their precursors and monocytes and their precursors each comprise at least 20% of BM cells. This arbitrary minimal limit of 20% monocytes and their precursors distinguishes acute myelomonocytic leukaemia from cases of AML with or without maturation in which some monocytes may be present. A high number (usually ≥5x10⁹/L) of monocytic cells may be present in the PB.

ICD-O code   9867/3

Epidemiology

Acute myelomonocytic leukaemia comprises 5–10% of cases of AML. It occurs in all age groups but is more common in older individuals; the median age is 50 years. There is a male:female ratio of 1.4:1 {2078}.

Clinical features

Patients typically present with anaemia and thrombocytopenia, fever and fatigue. The white blood cell count may be high with numerous blasts and promonocytes.

Morphology and cytochemistry

The monoblasts are large cells, with abundant cytoplasm which can be moderately to intensely basophilic and may show pseudopod formation. Scattered fine azurophilic granules and vacuoles may be present. The monoblasts usually have round nuclei with delicate lacy chromatin and one or more large prominent nucleoli. Promonocytes have a more irregular and delicately convoluted nuclear configuration; the cytoplasm is usually less basophilic and sometimes more obviously granulated, with occasional large azurophilic granules and vacuoles. Monocytes and promonocytes may not always be readily distinguishable in routinely stained BM smears. The PB typically shows an increase in monocytes, which are often more mature than those in the BM. The monocytic component may be more evident in the PB than in the BM. At least 3% of the blasts should show MPO positivity. The monoblasts, promonocytes, and monocytes are typically non-specific esterase (NSE) positive, although in some cases reactivity may be weak or absent. If the cells meet morphologic criteria for monocytes, absence of NSE does not exclude the diagnosis. Double staining for NSE and CAE or MPO may show dual positive cells.

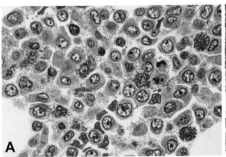
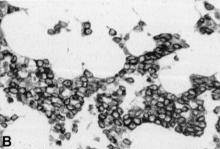
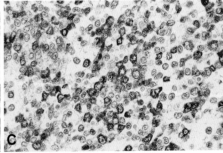

Fig. 6.26 Acute myeloid leukaemia with maturation. **A** Bone marrow biopsy illustrates myeloblasts with abundant cytoplasm and azurophilic granules. Occasional blasts contain an Auer rod. Scattered eosinophils are present. **B,C** Bone marrow biopsies, showing numerous blasts with intense myeloperoxidase activity (**B**) and lysozyme positivity (**C**).

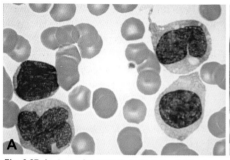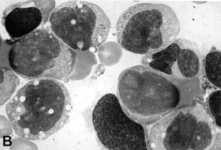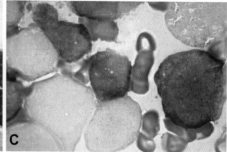

Fig. 6.27 Acute myelomonocytic leukaemia. **A** Blood smear, myeloblast, monoblast and promonocytes. **B** Bone marrow smear. Myeloblasts and several more mature monocytes including promonocytes. **C** Non-specific esterase reaction on a bone marrow smear. Several NSE positive cells are present. The non-reacting cells are predominantly myeloblasts and neutrophil precursors.

Immunophenotype

These leukaemias generally show several populations of blasts variably expressing myeloid antigens CD13, CD33, CD65 and CD15. One of the blast populations is usually also positive for some markers characteristic of monocytic differentiation such as CD14, CD4, CD11b, CD11c, CD64, CD36, macrophage-restricted CD68 (PGM1), CD163 and lysozyme. In particular, co-expression of CD15 and strong CD64 is characteristic of monocytic differentiation. There is often also a population of immature blasts that express CD34 and/or CD117. Most cases are positive for HLA-DR, approximately 30% for CD7, while expression of other lymphoid-associated markers is rare.

Genetics

Myeloid-associated, non-specific cytogenetic abnormalities, e.g. +8, are present in the majority of the cases.

Differential diagnosis

The major differential diagnoses include AML with maturation, acute monocytic leukaemia and chronic myelomonocytic leukaemia. The distinction from the other AML types is based on the cytochemical

findings and percent of monocytic cells. The differential diagnosis with chronic myelomonocytic leukaemia is critical and relies on the proper identification of promonocytes.

Acute monoblastic and monocytic leukaemia

Definition

Acute monoblastic leukaemia and acute monocytic leukaemia are myeloid leukaemias in which 80% or more of the leukaemic cells are of monocytic lineage including monoblasts, promonocytes and monocytes; a minor neutrophil component, <20%, may be present. Acute monoblastic leukaemia and acute monocytic leukaemia are distinguished by the relative proportions of monoblasts and promonocytes. In acute monoblastic leukaemia, the majority of the monocytic cells are monoblasts (typically ≥80%). In acute monocytic leukaemia, the majority of the monocytic cells are promonocytes.

ICD-O code   9891/3

Epidemiology

Acute monoblastic leukaemia comprises <5% of cases of AML. It may occur at any age but is most common in young individuals. Extramedullary lesions may occur. Acute monocytic leukaemia comprises <5% of cases of AML; the male:female ratio is 1.8:1. It is more common in adults (median, 49 years) {2078}.

Clinical features

Bleeding disorders are common presenting features. Extramedullary masses, cutaneous and gingival infiltration, and central nervous system (CNS) involvement are common.

Morphology and cytochemistry

Monoblasts are large cells, with abundant cytoplasm which can be moderately to intensely basophilic and may show pseudopod formation. Scattered fine azurophilic granules and vacuoles may be present. The monoblasts usually have round nuclei with delicate lacy chromatin, and one or more large prominent nucleoli. Promonocytes have a more irregular and delicately convoluted nuclear configuration; the cytoplasm is usually less basophilic and sometimes more obviously granulated, with occasional large azurophilic granules and vacuoles. Auer rods are rare in acute monoblastic leukaemia and, when present, are usually in cells identifiable as myeloblasts. Haemophagocytosis (erythrophagocytosis) may be observed and suggests an associated t(8;16)(p11.2;p13.3) chromosomal abnormality {2079}. Haemophagocytosis with an associated t(8;16)(p11.2;p13.3) may also be observed in AML with maturation. The monoblasts and promonocytes usually show intense non-specific esterase activity in most cases. In up to 10–20% of cases of acute monoblastic leukaemia, the

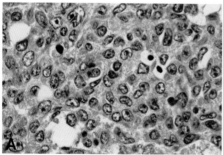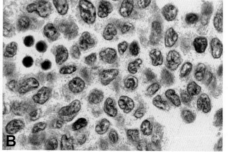

Fig. 6.28 A Acute monoblastic leukaemia. Bone marrow biopsy showing complete replacement by a population of large blasts with abundant cytoplasm. The nuclei are generally round to oval; occasional nuclei are distorted. **B** Acute monocytic leukaemia. Bone marrow section. The nuclear folds in the promonocytes are prominent.

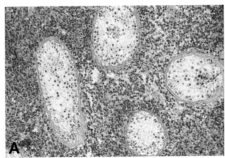
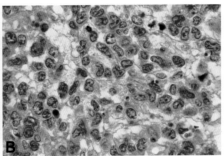

Fig. 6.29 Acute monocytic leukaemia, testicular infiltration. **A** Low magnification of a biopsy of a testis from a patient with acute monocytic leukaemia. There is extensive expansion and infiltration of the space between the seminiferous tubules. **B** The monocytic cells have relatively abundant cytoplasm and very dispersed chromatin.

non-specific esterase reaction is negative or very weakly positive. In some of these, immunophenotyping may be necessary to establish monocytic differentiation. Monoblasts are typically MPO negative; promonocytes may show some scattered MPO positivity. The BM biopsy in acute monoblastic leukaemia is usually hypercellular with a predominant population of large, poorly differentiated blasts with abundant cytoplasm. Nucleoli may be prominent. The promonocytes in acute monocytic leukaemia show nuclear lobulation. The extramedullary lesion may be predominantly of monoblasts or promonocytes or an admixture of two cell types.

Immunophenotype
By flow cytometry, these leukaemias variably express myeloid antigens CD13, CD33 (often very bright), CD15 and CD65. There is generally expression of at least two markers characteristic of monocytic differentiation such as CD14, CD4, CD11b, CD11c, CD64, CD68, CD36 and lysozyme. CD34 is positive only in 30% of cases, while CD117 is more often expressed. Almost all cases are positive for HLA-DR. MPO may be expressed in acute monocytic leukaemia and less often in monoblastic leukaemia. Aberrant expression of CD7 and/or CD56 is found in 25–40% of cases. By immunohistochemistry in paraffin-embedded BM biopsy specimens and in extramedullary myeloid (monoblastic) sarcomas, MPO, CAE are typically negative but may be weakly positive. Lysozyme is often positive, but is relatively non-specific. Macrophage-specific CD68 and CD163 are often positive and appear to be more specific for monocytic differentiation.

Genetics
Myeloid-associated, non-specific cytogenetic abnormalities are present in the majority of the cases. The t(8;16)(p11.2;p13.3) may be associated with acute monocytic leukaemia or acute myelomonocytic leukaemia and, in the majority of cases, is associated with haemophagocytosis by leukaemic cells, particularly erythrophagocytosis and coagulopathy {2079}.

Differential diagnosis
The major differential diagnosis of acute monoblastic leukaemia includes AML without maturation, AML minimally differentiated and acute megakaryoblastic leukaemia. Extramedullary myeloid (monoblastic) sarcomas may be confused with malignant lymphoma or soft tissue sarcomas. Occasional cases resemble prolymphocytic leukaemia; they are readily distinguished by immunophenotypic analysis and cytochemistry. The major differential diagnosis of acute monocytic leukaemia includes chronic myelomonocytic leukaemia, acute myelomonocytic leukaemia and microgranular acute promyelocytic leukaemia (APL). These

can be distinguished with well-stained smears. The differential diagnosis with chronic myelomonocytic leukaemia is critical and relies on the proper identification of promonocytes and their inclusion as blast equivalents. The abnormal promyelocytes in APL are intensely MPO and CAE positive whereas the monocytes are weakly reactive or negative.

Acute erythroid leukaemia

Definition
Acute erythroid leukaemias are acute leukaemias that are characterized by a predominant erythroid population. Two subtypes are recognized based on the presence or absence of a significant myeloid (granulocytic) component:
Erythroleukaemia (erythroid/myeloid) is defined by the presence in the BM of ≥50% erythroid precursors in the entire nucleated cell population and ≥20% myeloblasts in the non-erythroid cell population, i.e. the myeloblasts are calculated as a percent of the non-erythroid cells.
Pure erythroid leukaemia represents a neoplastic proliferation of immature cells (undifferentiated or proerythroblastic in appearance) committed exclusively to the erythroid lineage (≥80% of BM cells) with no evidence of a significant myeloblastic component {753}.

ICD-O code   9840/3

Epidemiology
Erythroleukaemia (erythroid/myeloid) is predominantly a disease of adults {2078}. It comprises <5% of cases of AML. Pure erythroid leukaemia is extremely rare and can occur at any age, including childhood.

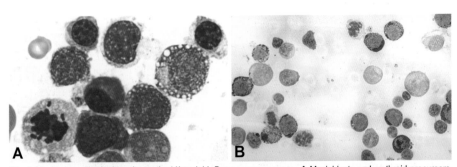

Fig. 6.30 Acute erythroleukaemia, erythroid/myeloid. Bone marrow smear. **A** Myeloblasts and erythroid precursors with dyserythropoietic changes are present. **B** Bone marrow smear. Periodic acid-Schiff reaction. There are several erythroid precursors at varying stages of maturation with PAS-positive cytoplasm. The more immature precursors have a coarsely granular-globular reaction; the later stage precursors have a diffuse cytoplasmic positivity.

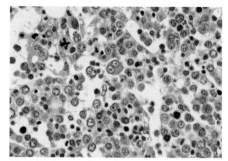

Fig. 6.31 Acute erythroid leukaemia, erythroid/myeloid. Bone marrow biopsy. There is a population of erythroid precursors and myeloblasts reflecting the dual lineage proliferation. A binucleate megakaryocyte is present.

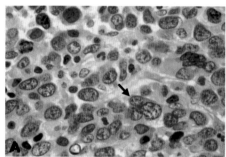

Fig. 6.32 Pure erythroid leukaemia. Bone marrow smear with numerous very immature erythroid precursors; these cells have cytoplasmic vacuoles which occasionally coalesce.

Clinical features

The clinical features of the erythroid leukaemias are not unique but profound anaemia and circulating erythroblasts are common. Erythroleukaemia (erythroid/myeloid) may present *de novo* or evolve from MDS or, less commonly, from chronic myeloproliferative neoplasms (MPN).

Morphology and cytochemistry

Erythroleukaemia (erythroid/myeloid)

All maturation stages of the erythroid precursors may be present, frequently with a shift to immaturity. The erythroid precursors are dysplastic with megaloblastoid nuclei and/or bi- or multinucleated forms; the cytoplasm in the more immature cells frequently contains poorly demarcated vacuoles, which may coalesce. Large multinucleated erythroid cells may be present. The myeloblasts are of medium size, often containing a few cytoplasmic granules and occasionally Auer rods and are similar to the myeloblasts in AML with and without maturation. Dysplastic changes of maturing neutrophils and megakaryocytes are common. The iron stain may show ring sideroblasts and the periodic acid–Schiff (PAS) stain may be positive in the erythroid precursors either in a globular or diffuse pattern. The MPO, CAE and SBB stains may be positive in the myeloblasts. The BM biopsy in erythroid/myeloid leukaemia is usually hypercellular. There may be prominent megakaryocytic dysplasia.

Pure erythroid leukaemia

The undifferentiated form of pure erythroid leukaemia is usually characterized by the presence of medium to large size erythroblasts usually with round nuclei, fine chromatin and one or more nucleoli

(proerythroblast); the cytoplasm is deeply basophilic, often agranular and frequently contains poorly demarcated vacuoles which are often PAS-positive. Occasionally the blasts are smaller and resemble the lymphoblasts of ALL. The cells are negative for MPO and SBB; they show reactivity with α-naphthyl acetate esterase, acid phosphatase and PAS, the latter usually in a block-like staining pattern. In the BM biopsies of pure acute erythroid leukaemia the cells appear undifferentiated.

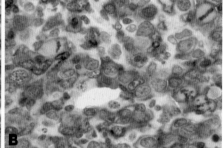

Fig. 6.33 Pure erythroid leukaemia. Bone marrow section. **A** A predominant population of very immature erythroid precursors, some of which are multilobated (arrow). **B** The immature erythroid precursors and mitotic figures show positivity for glycophorin A.

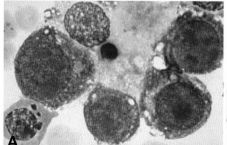

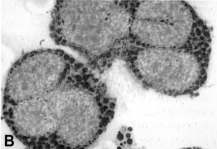

Fig. 6.34 Pure erythroid leukaemia. **A** Bone marrow smear shows four abnormal proerythroblasts. The erythroblasts are large with finely dispersed chromatin, prominent nucleoli and cytoplasmic vacuoles, some of which are coalescent. **B** The cytoplasm of the proerythroblasts shows intense globular PAS staining.

Immunophenotype

Erythroleukaemia (erythroid/myeloid)

The erythroblasts in erythroleukaemia generally lack myeloid-associated markers and are negative with anti-MPO; they react with antibodies to haemoglobin A and glycophorin, but the more immature cells may be negative. An aberrantly low expression of CD71 may be present. The immunophenotype of the myeloid population usually corresponds to that of AML without differentiation or AML with minimal differentiation.

Pure erythroid leukaemia

The more differentiated forms can be detected by the expression of glycophorin and haemoglobin A and absence of MPO and other myeloid markers; the blasts are often negative for HLA-DR and CD34, but may be positive for CD117. The more immature forms are usually negative for glycophorin or this is only weakly expressed in a minority of blasts. Other markers such as carbonic anhydrase 1, Gero antibody against the Gerbich blood group or CD36 are usually positive as they detect erythroid progenitors at earlier stages of differentiation. However, CD36 is not specific for erythroblasts and may be expressed by monocytes and megakaryocytes. Antigens associated with megakaryocytes (CD41 and CD61) are typically negative, but may be partially expressed in some cases. Immunohistochemistry to haemoglobin A or glycophorin may be helpful in establishing cell origin in biopsy specimens.

Genetics
There is no specific chromosome abnormality described in this type of AML. Complex karyotypes with multiple structural abnormalities are common, with -5/del(5q), -7/del(7q) and +8 the most common {1282}. However, cases with -5/del(5q), -7/del(7q) and/or complex chromosomal abnormalities should be classified as AML with myelodysplasia-related changes if the other requirements for that category are satisfied.

Differential diagnosis
Erythroleukaemia (erythroid/myeloid) should be distinguished from refractory anaemia with excess blasts (RAEB), AML with myelodysplasia-related changes, AML with maturation with increased erythroid precursors and reactive erythroid hyperplasia following therapy or administration of erythropoietin. A BM differential count of all nucleated cells should be performed. If the overall percentage of blast cells is ≥20% and multilineage dysplasia is present in ≥50% of the cells of two or more lineages, a diagnosis of AML with myelodysplasia-related changes should be made. When there are <20% total blasts and the erythroid precursors are ≥50% of all cells, the differential count of non-erythroid cells should be calculated. If blasts are ≥20% of non-erythroid cells, the diagnosis is erythroleukaemia (erythroid/myeloid); if <20%, the diagnosis is usually MDS. The differential diagnosis of pure erythroid leukaemia includes megaloblastic anaemia due to vitamin B12 or folate deficiency. In equivocal cases, a trial of B12 or folate therapy should be considered.

Pure erythroid leukaemia without morphologic evidence of erythroid maturation may be difficult to distinguish from other types of AML, particularly megakaryoblastic leukaemia, and also from ALL or lymphoma. Lack of expression of lymphoid antigens will exclude the latter diagnoses. Distinction from megakaryoblastic leukaemia is the most difficult; if the immunophenotype is characteristic of

erythroid precursors, a diagnosis can be established, however some cases are ambiguous and there may be cases with concurrent erythroid-megakaryocytic involvement.

Prognosis and predictive factors
Erythroid/myeloid leukaemia is generally associated with an aggressive clinical course. The morphologic findings may evolve to a more predominant myeloblast picture. Pure erythroid leukaemia is usually associated with a rapid clinical course.

Acute megakaryoblastic leukaemia

Definition
Acute megakaryoblastic leukaemia is an acute leukaemia with 20% or more blasts of which at least 50% are of megakaryocyte lineage; however, this category excludes cases of AML with myelodysplasia-related changes, AML with t(1;22)(p13;q13), inv(3)(q21q26.2), t(3;3)(q21;q26.2) and Down syndrome-related cases.

ICD-O code   9910/3

Epidemiology
Acute megakaryoblastic leukaemia occurs in both adults and children. This is an uncommon disease comprising <5% of cases of AML.

Clinical features
Patients present with cytopenias, often thrombocytopenia, although some may have thrombocytosis. Dysplastic features in the neutrophils, erythroid precursors, platelets and megakaryocytes may be present. Hepatosplenomegaly is infre-

quent. An association between acute megakaryoblastic leukaemia and mediastinal germ cell tumours has been observed in young adult males {1594}.

Morphology and cytochemistry
The megakaryoblasts are usually of medium to large size (12–18 µm) with a round, slightly irregular or indented nucleus with fine reticular chromatin and one to three nucleoli. The cytoplasm is basophilic, often agranular, and may show distinct blebs or pseudopod formation. In some cases the blasts are predominantly small with a high nuclear-cytoplasmic ratio resembling lymphoblasts; large and small blasts may be present in the same patient. Occasionally, the blasts occur in small clusters. Circulating micromegakaryocytes, megakaryoblastic fragments, dysplastic large platelets and hypogranular neutrophils may be present. Micromegakaryocytes are small cells with 1 or 2 round nuclei with condensed chromatin and mature cytoplasm; these should not be counted as blasts. In some patients, because of extensive BM fibrosis resulting in a "dry tap", the percent of BM blasts is estimated from the BM biopsy. Imprints of the biopsy may also be useful. Although acute megakaryoblastic leukaemia may be associated with extensive fibrosis, this is not an invariant finding. The histopathology of the biopsy varies from cases with a uniform population of poorly differentiated blasts to a mixture of poorly differentiated blasts and maturing dysplastic megakaryocytes; varying degrees of reticulin fibrosis may be present. Cytochemical stains for SBB, CAE and MPO are consistently negative in the megakaryoblasts; the blasts may show reactivity with PAS and for acid phosphatase and punctate or focal nonspecific esterase reactivity.

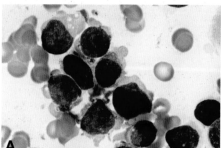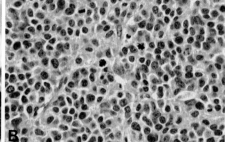

Fig. 6.35 Acute megakaryoblastic leukaemia. A Bone marrow smear from a 22-month-old child with complete replacement by poorly differentiated blasts. B Bone marrow section.

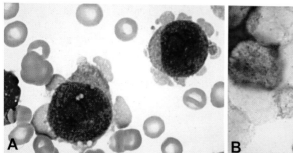

Fig. 6.36 Acute megakaryoblastic leukaemia. A Bone marrow smear. The two megakaryoblasts are large cells with cytoplasmic pseudopod formation; portions of the cytoplasm are "zoned" with granular basophilic areas and clear cytoplasm. Nucleoli are unusually prominent. B Bone marrow smear reacted with antibody to CD61 (platelet glycoprotein IIIa). The cytoplasm of the megakaryoblasts is intensely reactive.

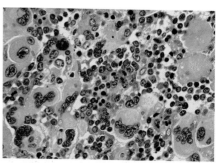

Fig. 6.37 Acute megakaryoblastic leukaemia. Bone marrow biopsy shows virtually complete replacement by a population of blasts and well-differentiated megakaryocytes. There is a minor population of erythroid precursors.

Immunophenotype

The megakaryoblasts express one or more of the platelet glycoproteins: CD41 (glycoprotein IIb/IIIa), and/or CD61 (glycoprotein IIIa). The more mature platelet-associated marker CD42 (glycoprotein Ib) is less frequently present. The myeloid-associated markers, CD13 and CD33, may be positive. CD34, the pan-leukocyte marker CD45, and HLA-DR are often negative, especially in children; CD36 is characteristically positive. Blasts are negative with the anti-MPO antibody and with other markers of granulocytic differentiation. Lymphoid markers and TdT are not expressed, but there may be aberrant expression of CD7. Cytoplasmic expression of CD41 or CD61 is more specific and sensitive than surface staining, due to possible adherence of platelets to blast cells, which may be misinterpreted as positive staining by flow cytometry. In cases with fibrosis, immunophenotyping on BM trephine biopsies is particularly important for diagnosis. Megakaryocytes and in some cases megakaryoblasts can be recognized by a positive reaction with antibodies to von Willebrand's factor, the platelet glycoproteins (CD61, CD42b) and LAT (linker of activation of T-cells); the detection of platelet glycoproteins is the most lineage specific but detection is highly dependent on procedures used for fixation and decalcification.

Genetics

There is no unique chromosomal abnormality associated with acute megakaryoblastic leukaemia in adults. Complex karyotypes typical of MDS, inv(3) (q21q26.2) and t(3;3)(q21q26.2) can all be associated with megakaryoblastic/megakaryocytic differentiation {507, 1637}

but these cases are all assigned to other categories of AML (See AML with recurrent genetic abnormalities).

In young males with mediastinal germ cell tumours and acute megakaryoblastic leukaemia, several cytogenetic abnormalities have been observed of which i(12p) is characteristic.

Differential diagnosis

The differential diagnosis includes minimally differentiated AML, AML with myelodysplasia-related changes, acute panmyelosis with myelofibrosis, ALL, pure erythroid leukaemia and blastic transformation of chronic myelogenous leukaemia or megakaryoblastic crisis of any MPN. In the latter two conditions, there is usually a history of a chronic phase and splenomegaly is an almost constant finding. Some metastatic tumours in the BM, particularly in children, e.g. alveolar rhabdomyosarcoma, may resemble acute megakaryoblastic leukaemia. In general, acute megakaryoblastic leukaemia represents a proliferation predominantly of megakaryoblasts, whereas acute panmyelosis is characterized by a trilineage proliferation, i.e. granulocytes, megakaryocytes and erythroid precursors. The distinction between acute megakaryoblastic leukaemia, acute panmyelosis with fibrosis and AML with myelodysplasia-related changes is not always clear.

Prognosis and predictive factors

The prognosis of this category of acute megakaryoblastic leukaemia is usually poor when compared to other AML types as well as in comparison to AML with t(1;22)(p13;q13) {620, 1637} and acute megakaryoblastic leukaemia in Down syndrome.

Acute basophilic leukaemia

Definition

Acute basophilic leukaemia is an AML in which the primary differentiation is to basophils.

ICD-O code   9870/3

Epidemiology

This is a very rare disease with a relatively small number of reported cases, comprising <1% of all cases of AML.

Clinical features

As in other acute leukaemias, patients present with features related to BM failure and may or may not have circulating blasts. In addition, cutaneous involvement, organomegaly, lytic lesions and symptoms related to hyperhistaminemia may be present.

Morphology and cytochemistry

The circulating PB and BM blasts are of medium size with a high nuclear-cytoplasmic ratio, an oval, round or bilobed nucleus characterized by dispersed chromatin and one to three prominent nucleoli. The cytoplasm is moderately basophilic and contains a variable number of coarse basophilic granules which are positive in metachromatic stains; vacuolation of the cytoplasm may be present. Mature basophils are usually sparse. Dysplastic features in the erythroid precursors may be present. Electron microscopy shows that the granules contain structures characteristic of basophil precursors; they contain an electron-dense particulate substance, are internally-bisected; e.g. have a theta character, or contain crystalline material arranged in a pattern of scrolls or lamellae, the latter finding is more typical of mast cells. Coexistence of basophil and mast cell granules may be identified in the same immature cells {1732}. The most characteristic cytochemical reaction is metachromatic positivity with toluidine blue. In addition, the blasts usually show a diffuse pattern of staining with acid phosphatase and, in some cases, PAS-positivity in blocks or lakes; the blasts are often negative by light microscopy for SBB, MPO, CAE and non-specific esterase. The BM trephine biopsy shows diffuse replacement by blast cells.

Immunophenotype

Leukaemic blasts express myeloid markers such as CD13 and/or CD33, and are usually positive for CD123, CD203c and CD11b, but negative for other monocytic markers. Blasts may express CD34 and in contrast to normal basophils may be positive for HLA-DR but are negative for CD117. Immunophenotypic detection of abnormal mast cells expressing CD117, mast cell tryptase and CD25 will distinguish mast cell leukaemia from acute basophilic leukaemia. Usually blasts show expression of CD9. Some cases may be positive for membrane CD22 and/or TdT. Other membrane and cytoplasmic, lymphoid-associated markers are usually negative {1295,2074}.

Genetics

There is no consistent chromosomal abnormality identified in these cases. AML with t(6;9)(p23;q34) is specifically excluded as are cases associated with a *BCR-ABL1* fusion gene.

Differential diagnosis

The differential diagnosis includes blast phase of MPN, other AML subtypes with basophilia such as AML with t(6;9) (p23;q34), mast cell leukaemia and, more rarely, a subtype of ALL with prominent coarse granules. The clinical features and cytogenetic pattern will distinguish cases presenting *de novo* from those resulting from transformation of chronic myelogenous leukaemia and from other AML subtypes with basophilia. Immunological markers will distinguish between granulated ALL and acute basophilic leukaemia and light microscopic cytochemistry for myeloperoxidase and electron microscopy will distinguish acute basophilic leukaemia from other leukaemias.

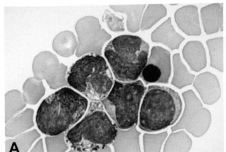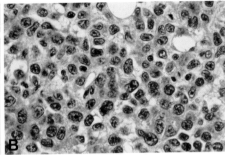

Fig. 6.38 Acute basophilic leukaemia. Bone marrow smear. **A** Blasts and immature basophils. The basophil granules vary from large coarse granules to smaller granules. **B** Bone marrow trephine biopsy. The blasts are poorly differentiated.

Prognosis and predictive factors

Since this is a rare type of acute leukaemia, there is little information on survival. The cases observed have generally been associated with a poor prognosis.

Acute panmyelosis with myelofibrosis

Definition

Acute panmyelosis with myelofibrosis (APMF) is an acute panmyeloid proliferation with increased blasts and accompanying fibrosis of the BM {168, 2120} that does not meet criteria for AML with myelodysplasia-related changes.

ICD-O code   9931/3

Synonyms

Acute (malignant) myelofibrosis, acute (malignant) myelosclerosis.

Epidemiology

Acute panmyelosis with myelofibrosis is a very rare form of AML. APMF occurs *de novo*. It is primarily a disease of adults but has also been reported in children.

Clinical features

Patients present acutely with severe constitutional symptoms including weakness and fatigue; fever and bone pain are also frequently observed. Pancytopenia is always present. There is no or minimal splenomegaly. The clinical evolution is usually rapidly progressive {2225}.

Morphology and cytochemistry

The PB shows pancytopenia which is usually marked. The red blood cells show no or minimal anisopoikilocytosis and variable macrocytosis; rare erythroblasts can be seen but teardrop-shaped cells (dacryocytes) are not observed.

Occasional neutrophil precursors including blasts may be identified. Dysplastic changes in myeloid cells are frequent. Abnormal platelets may be noted. Bone marrow aspiration is frequently unsuccessful; either no BM is obtained or the specimen is suboptimal. Bone marrow biopsy supplemented with immunohistology is required for diagnosis {2124, 2225}. The BM biopsy is hypercellular and shows, within a diffusely fibrotic stroma, an increased proliferation of erythroid precursors, granulocyte precursors and megakaryocytes (panmyelosis), which is variable in terms of the relative proportion of each given component. Characteristic findings include foci of immature haematopoietic cells including blasts associated with conspicuously dysplastic megakaryocytes predominately of small size with eosinophilic cytoplasm showing variable degrees of cytological atypia including the presence of hypolobulated or non-lobulated nuclei with dispersed chromatin. Micromegakaryocytes may be present but should not be counted as blasts. The visibility of the small megakaryocytes may be accentuated with the PAS stain and immunohistochemistry {2225}. The overall frequency of blasts in APMF marrows is uncertain. Based on BM biopsy, a median value of 22.5% was found in a recent study {1651}. Most cases have a range of 20–25%. The degree of myelofibrosis is variable. In most patients there is a marked increase in reticulin fibres with coarse fibres; frank collagenous fibrosis is, however, uncommon.

Immunophenotype

If sufficient BM specimen is obtained for immunologic markers or circulating blasts are present in the PB, the cells show phenotypic heterogeneity, with varying degrees of expression of myeloid-associated antigens. The blasts usually express the progenitor/early precursor-associated marker CD34 and one or more myeloid-associated antigens: CD13, CD33 and CD117 {1651, 2124, 2225}. Myeloperoxidase is usually negative in the blasts. In some cases a proportion of immature cells express erythroid antigens. Immunohistochemistry can facilitate the identification of the relative proportions of the various myeloid components on the biopsy specimen and is generally used to confirm the multilineage nature of the proliferation. This is usually done by employing a panel of antibodies which includes myeloperoxidase, lysozyme, anti-megakaryocytic markers (CD61, CD42b, CD41 or anti-von Willebrand's factor) and erythroid markers such as glycophorin and haemoglobin A. These confirm the presence of panmyelosis and allow exclusion of specific "unilineage"-predominant proliferations, such as acute megakaryoblastic leukaemia.

Genetics

If sufficient specimen for cytogenetic analysis is obtained, the results are usually abnormal. The detection of a complex karyotype, frequently involving chromosomes 5 and/or 7 [-5/del(5q), -7/del(7q)] {2225}, means that the case is assigned to AML with myelodysplasia-related changes, not to acute panmyelosis.

Differential diagnosis

The major differential diagnosis of APMF includes other types of AML with associated BM fibrosis including acute megakaryoblastic leukaemia {1651}. Usually less problematic is the distinction from primary myelofibrosis (PMF), post-polycythaemia vera myelofibrosis, post-essential thrombocythaemia myelofibrosis, and from other neoplasms that can be encountered in a myelofibrotic BM such as metastatic malignancies with a desmoplastic stromal reaction. The distinction between AML, particularly cases of AML with myelodysplasia-related changes with multilineage dysplasia and myelofibrosis and acute megakaryoblastic leukaemia with myelofibrosis, and APMF may be difficult,

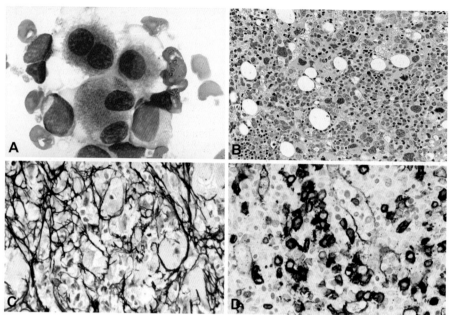

Fig. 6.39 Acute panmyelosis with myelofibrosis. **A** A marrow trephine imprint. There are several megakaryocytes with hypolobulated nuclei and blast forms. **B** The marrow is markedly hypercellular with increased fibrosis with a heterogeneous mixture of cells that include atypical megakaryocytes. **C** An increase in reticulin fibrosis. **D** Immunohistochemistry for CD34 shows an increase in blast cells.

particularly if no specimen suitable for cytogenetic analysis can be obtained.

If the proliferative process is predominantly one cell type, i.e. myeloblasts, and there is associated myelofibrosis, the case should be classified as AML with a specific subtype, e.g. AML-myelodysplasia-related, and then designated with the qualifying phrase "with myelofibrosis". Acute megakaryoblastic leukaemia is associated with the presence of ≥20% blasts, of which at least 50% are megakaryoblasts. In contrast, the blasts of APMF are more heterogenous, poorly differentiated and express CD34. The majority of blasts do not display megakaryocytic reactivity, and the proliferative process involves all of the major BM cell lines.

Particularly difficult is the distinction between APMF and cases of MDS associated with both an excess of blasts and myelofibrosis (RAEB-F), since the latter cases can share most of the morphological findings seen in APMF. Clinically, APMF can be separated from MDS by its more abrupt onset with fever and bone pain. In APMF,

histology of the BM shows more numerous megakaryocytes and, on average, a higher number of blasts than what are found in RAEB. Cases of RAEB-2-F, except for their usually less acute clinical presentation, may be indistinguishable from APMF {1651}. APMF is distinguished from PMF by the more numerous blast cells in the former and the distinct cytological characteristics of the megakaryocytes in the latter (See Chapter 2). The presence of a metastatic malignancy or, rarely a lymphoid disorder can be excluded by studies with appropriate antibodies.

Postulated normal counterpart

Haematopoietic stem cell. The fibroblastic proliferation is secondary.

Prognosis and predictive factors

The disease is usually associated with poor response to chemotherapy and usually only a few months survival {1651, 2124}.

Myeloid sarcoma

S.A. Pileri
A. Orazi
B. Falini

Definition

A myeloid sarcoma is a tumour mass consisting of myeloid blasts with or without maturation occurring at an anatomical site other than the bone marrow (BM). Infiltrates of any site of the body by myeloid blasts in leukaemic patients are not classified as myeloid sarcoma unless they present with tumour masses in which the tissue architecture is effaced.

ICD-O code   9930/3

Synonyms

Extramedullary myeloid tumour; granulocytic sarcoma; chloroma

Epidemiology

There is a predilection for males and last decades of life. The male:female ratio is 1.2:1. The median age is 56 years (range, 1 month–89 years) {663, 1742}.

Etiology

The same as for acute myeloid leukaemia (AML) and myeloproliferative neoplasms (MPN).

Sites of involvement

Almost every site of the body can be involved, the skin, lymph node, gastrointestinal tract, bone, soft tissue and testis being more frequently affected {663, 1742}. In less than 10% of cases, myeloid sarcoma presents at multiple anatomical sites {663, 1742}.

Clinical features

Myeloid sarcoma may occur *de novo*: its detection should be considered as the equivalent of a diagnosis of AML. It may precede or coincide with AML or represent acute blastic transformation of myelodysplastic syndromes (MDS), MPN or MDS/MPN {663, 1742}.

Finally, myeloid sarcoma may also be the initial manifestation of relapse in a patient with previously diagnosed AML, regardless of blood or BM findings {1742}.

Morphology

A myeloid sarcoma most commonly consists of myeloblasts with or without features of promyelocytic or neutrophilic maturation that partially or totally efface the tissue architecture. In a significant

proportion of cases, it displays myelomonocytic or pure monoblastic morphology {663, 1742}. Tumours with trilineage haematopoiesis or predominantly erythroid precursors or megakaryoblasts are rare and may occur in conjunction with transformation of MPN {1742}.

Cytochemistry

On imprints, cytochemical stains for myeloperoxidase (MPO), naphthol-ASD-chloroacetate esterase (CAE) and non-specific esterase (NSE) may assist in differentiating granulocytic lineage (MPO+, CAE+) from monoblastic forms (NSE+). In addition, CAE reaction can be applied to routine sections, although the results may depend on fixation and decalcifying agents.

Immunophenotype

On immunohistochemistry in paraffin sections, CD68/KP1 is the most commonly expressed marker, followed in decreasing frequency by MPO, CD117, CD99, CD68/PG-M1, lysozyme, CD34, terminal deoxynucleotidyl transferase (TdT), CD56, CD61/LAT/von Willebrand antigen, CD30,

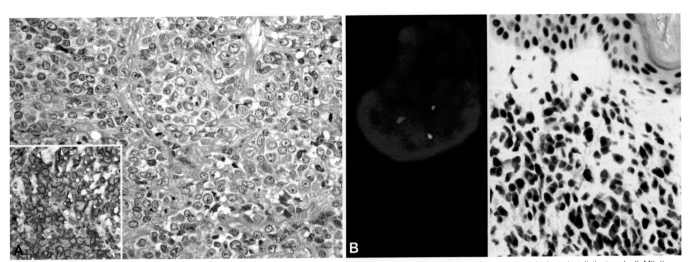

Fig. 6.40 Myeloid sarcoma. **A** The tumour consists of blasts with scant cytoplasm and round-oval nuclei with finely-dispersed chromatin and minute but distinct nucleoli. Mitotic figures are numerous. Neoplastic cells strongly express MPO (inset). **B** (left) Interphase FISH with the CBFB (core binding factor beta) dual color: break apart rearrangement probe in a sample showing splitting of the gene (one red and one green signal lay apart in the nucleus, while the normal CBFB allele appear as a red/green fusion spot). **B** (right) (skin) Staining for nucleophosmin (NPMc). Leukaemic cells infiltrating the derma show, in addition to the expected nuclear positivity, an aberrant cytoplasmic expression of NPM which reveals the presence of *NPM1* gene mutation. Cells of the overlying epidermis show a nuclear-restricted positivity for NPM.

glycophorin, and CD4 {1742}. Foci of plasmacytoid dendritic cell differentiation (CD123+) are occasionally observed in cases carrying inv(16) {1742}. The combination of the above mentioned markers allows the recognition of tumours with a more immature myeloid phenotype, as well as of cases with myelomonocytic, monoblastic, erythroid or megakaryocytic differentiation. Exceptionally, aberrant antigenic expressions are observed (cytokeratins, B- or T-cell markers). Cases that meet criteria for mixed phenotype AML are not classified as myeloid sarcoma (See Chapter 7). Flow cytometric analysis on cell suspensions reveals positivities for CD13, CD33, CD117 and MPO in tumours with myeloid differentiation, and for CD14, CD163 and CD11c in the monoblastic ones.

Genetics

By FISH and/or cytogenetics, chromosomal aberrations are detected in about 55% of cases. They include monosomy 7, trisomy 8, *MLL*-rearrangement, inv(16), trisomy 4, monosomy 16, 16q-, 5q-, 20q- and trisomy 11 {1742}. About 16% of cases carry evidence of *NPM1* mutations as shown by aberrant cytoplasmic NPM expression {663, 666}. The t(8;21)(q22;q22) observed in paediatric series seems to be less frequent in adulthood {1742, 1978}.

Differential diagnosis

The major differential diagnosis is with malignant lymphoma. The diagnosis of myeloid sarcoma is validated by the results of cytochemical and/or immunophenotypic analyses. These allow the distinction of myeloid sarcoma from: lymphoblastic lymphoma, Burkitt lymphoma, diffuse large B-cell lymphoma, small round cell tumours, particularly in children, and blastic plasmacytoid dendritic cell neoplasm {1742}. These tumours must be distinguished from non-effacing tissue infiltrates by AML or MPN.

Postulated normal counterpart

Haematopoietic stem cell.

Prognosis and predictive factors

The clinical behaviour and response to therapy seem not to be influenced by any of the following factors: age, sex, anatomical site(s) involved, *de novo* presentation, clinical history related to AML, MDS or MPN, histological features, immunophenotype and cytogenetic findings {1742}. Patients who undergo allogeneic or autologous BM transplantation seem to have a higher probability of prolonged survival or cure {268, 1742}.

Myeloid proliferations related to Down syndrome

I. Baumann
C.M. Niemeyer
R.D. Brunning
D.A. Arber
A. Porwit

Individuals with Down syndrome (DS) have an increased risk of leukaemia compared to non-DS individuals {716, 2365}. The increased risk is variously estimated at 10 to 100 fold. The increased risk extends into the adult years. In addition to the increased incidence, the ratio of acute lymphoblastic leukaemia (ALL) to acute myeloid leukaemia (AML) in DS children less than 4 years of age is approximately equal, 1.0:1.2, compared to non-DS children in the same age group in which the ratio is 4:1. There is an approximately 150 fold increase in AML in DS children less than 5 years of age; 70% of the cases of AML in DS children less than 4 years of age are acute megakaryoblastic leukaemia in contrast to the 3–6% incidence of this form of leukaemia in non-DS children. The acute megakaryoblastic leukaemia which occurs in DS children has somewhat unique morphologic, immunophenotypic, molecular and clinical characteristics which distinguish it from other forms of acute megakaryoblastic leukaemia, including *GATA1* mutations {835, 1362}. These various features serve as the rationale for the recognition of this form of leukaemia as a distinct type in the WHO classification. In addition to the unique characteristics of the predominant form of AML in DS children less than 4 years of age, approximately 10% of DS neonates manifest a haematologic disorder referred to as transient abnormal myelopoiesis or transient myeloproliferative disorder which may be morphologically indistinguishable from the predominant form of AML in DS children {271, 1409}. This disorder resolves spontaneously over a period of several weeks to 3 months. In 20–30% of the affected cases, non-remitting acute megakaryoblastic leukaemia subsequently develops in 1 to 3 years. It is important to recognize that although the aforementioned disorders have received the most attention in DS patients, they occur in a specific age group and other forms of acute leukaemia, both ALL and AML, affect DS individuals. The overall increased risk for DS individuals includes all types. The same approach for characterizing the specific type of leukaemia in DS patients must include the same careful morphologic, immunophenotypic, cytogenetic and molecular evaluation as in non-DS individuals to ensure that appropriate therapy is administered {2489}.

Transient abnormal myelopoiesis

Definition
Transient abnormal myelopoiesis (TAM) is a unique disorder of Down syndrome (DS) newborns that presents with clinical and morphologic findings indistinguishable from AML. The blasts have morphologic and immunologic features of megakaryocytic lineage.

ICD-O code
The provisional code proposed for the fourth edition of ICD-O is *9898/1*.

Synonym
Transient myeloproliferative disorder.

Epidemiology
Transient abnormal myelopoiesis occurs in approximately 10% of DS newborns: it uncommonly occurs in phenotypically normal neonates with trisomy 21 mosaicism.

Clinical features
At presentation, thrombocytopenia is most common; other cytopenias are less frequently encountered. There may be a marked leukocytosis and the percentage of blasts in the peripheral blood (PB) may exceed the blast percentage in the bone marrow (BM). Hepatosplenomegaly may be present. Rarely, clinical complications include cardiopulmonary failure, hyperviscosity, splenic necrosis and progressive hepatic fibrosis {592}. The process in the majority of patients undergoes spontaneous remission within the first three months of life; a few children experience life threatening or even fatal clinical complications.

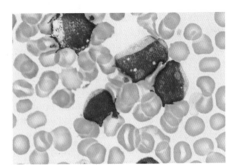

Fig. 6.41 Blood smear from a one day-old infant with Down syndrome and transient abnormal myelopoiesis. The PB contained 55% blasts. Cytogenetic study showed trisomy 21 as the sole abnormality. The process resolved spontaneously over a period of four weeks.

Morphology and immunophenotype
The morphologic and immunophenotypic features of TAM are similar to those of the blasts in most cases of DS AML. Peripheral blood and BM blasts often have basophilic cytoplasm with coarse basophilic granules and cytoplasmic blebbing suggestive of megakaryoblasts. Some patients have PB basophilia; erythroid and megakaryocytic dysplasia is often present in the BM {271}. Blasts in TAM display a characteristic immunophenotype {1251}. In most cases the blasts are positive for CD34, CD56, CD117, CD13, CD33, CD7, CD4 dim, CD41, CD42, TPO-R, IL-3R, CD36, CD61, CD71, and are negative for myeloperoxidase, CD15, CD14 and glycophorin A. The blasts in approximately 30% of cases are positive for HLA-DR.
Antibodies to CD41 and CD61 may be particularly useful in identifying cells of megakaryocytic lineage in immunohistologic preparations.

Genetics
In addition to trisomy 21, acquired *GATA1* mutations are present in blast cells of TAM {835, 942, 2347}. While gene array studies have suggested differences in expression between AML of DS and TAM, these findings have not yet been confirmed {258, 1298, 1439}.

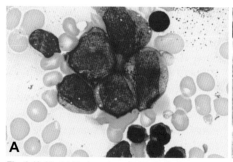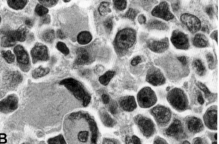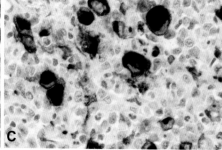

Fig. 6.42 Myeloid leukaemia associated with Down syndrome in a two year-old child. **A** Bone marrow smear. The PB and BM smears contained multiple blasts as illustrated. Many of the blasts contained numerous coarse basophilic coloured granules, which were myeloperoxidase negative. Cytogenetic study at this time showed trisomy 8 in addition to trisomy 21. **B** Bone marrow trephine biopsy from the same patient. There are numerous blasts and occasional megakaryocytes including one with a non-lobated nucleus. **C** An immuno-histologic reaction with CD-61 antibody. There are numerous reacting cells including obvious megakaryocytes and several smaller cells.

Prognostic and predictive factors

Although the disorder is characterized by a high rate of spontaneous remission, non-transient AML develops 1 to 3 years later in 20–30% of these children {2503}. Indications for chemotherapy in TAM are not firmly established.

Myeloid leukaemia associated with Down syndrome

Definition

Individuals with DS have a 50 fold increase in incidence of acute leukaemia during the first 5 years of life compared to non-DS individuals. Acute myeloid leukaemia in DS is usually an acute megakaryoblastic leukaemia, accounting for 50% of cases of acute leukaemia in DS

individuals beyond the neonatal period. There are no biological differences in DS individuals between myelodysplastic syndrome (MDS) and overt AML; therefore, a comparable diagnostic differentiation algorithm is not relevant and would have no prognostic or therapeutic consequences. Since this type of disease is unique to children with DS the term myeloid leukaemia of DS encompasses both MDS and AML.

ICD-O code

The provisional code proposed for the fourth edition of ICD-O is *9898/3*.

Epidemiology

The great majority of children with DS with myeloid leukaemia are under 5 years of life. About 1–2% of children with DS will develop AML during the first 5 years of

life. Children with DS account for ~20% of all paediatric patients with AML/MDS {271, 592, 908}. Myeloid leukaemia of DS occurs in 20–30% of children with a prior history of TAM and the leukaemia usually occurs 1–3 years after TAM.

Sites of involvement

Blood and BM are the principle sites of involvement. Extramedullary involvement, mainly of spleen and liver, is almost always present.

Clinical features

The disorder manifests predominantly in the first 3 years of life. The clinical course in children with less than 20% blast cells in the BM appears to be relatively indolent and presents initially with a period of thrombocytopenia. A preleukaemic phase comparable to refractory cytopenia of childhood (RCC) generally preceeds MDS with excess blasts or overt leukaemia.

Morphology

In the pre-leukaemic phase, which can last for several months, the disease has the features of RCC (See Chapter 5) lacking a significant increase of blasts. Erythroid cells are macrocytic. Dysplastic features may be more pronounced than in primary refractory cytopenia.

In cases of AML, blasts and occasionally erythroid precursors are usually present in the PB. Erythrocytes often show considerable anisopoikilocytosis, sometimes dacryocytes. The platelet count is usually decreased and giant platelets may be observed.

In the BM aspirate, the morphology of the leukaemic blasts shows particular features with round to slightly irregular nuclei and a moderate amount of basophilic

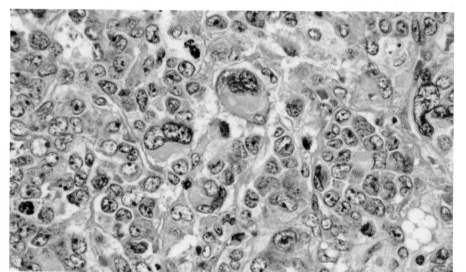

Fig. 6.43 Section of an abdominal lymph node from a child with Down syndrome and acute megakaryoblastic leukaemia. The node is completely replaced by blasts with occasional megakaryocytes, some of which are dysplastic.

cytoplasm; cytoplasmic blebs may be present. The cytoplasm of a variable number of blasts contains coarse granules resembling basophilic granules. The granules are generally myeloperoxidase negative. Erythroid precursors often show megaloblastic changes as well as dysplastic forms, including bi- or trinucleated cells and nuclear fragments. Dysgranulopoiesis may be present.

The BM core may show a dense network of reticulin fibres, making adequate BM aspiration difficult or impossible. Erythropoiesis may be increased in cases with a low blast percentage and decreases with disease progression. Maturing cells of neutrophil lineage are usually decreased. In cases with a dense blast cell infiltration rare dysplastic megakaryocytes may be seen. In other cases of acute megakaryoblastic leukaemia, megakaryocytes may be markedly increased with clusters of dysplastic small forms, micromegakaryocytes and occasionally an increase in promegakaryocytes.

Immunophenotype

Leukaemic blasts in acute megakaryocytic leukaemia of DS display a similar immunophenotype to blasts in TAM {1251}. In most cases, the blasts are positive for CD117, CD13, CD33, CD7, CD4, CD42, TPO-R, IL-3R, CD36, CD41, CD61, CD71, and are negative for myeloperoxidase, CD15, CD14 and glycophorin A. However, in contrast to TAM, CD34 is negative in 50% of cases and approximately 30% of cases are negative for CD56 and CD41. Leukaemic blasts in other types of AML in DS display phenotypes corresponding to the particular AML category.

Antibodies to CD41 and CD61 may be particularly useful in identifying cells of megakaryocytic lineage in immunohistologic preparations.

Genetics

In addition to trisomy 21, somatic mutations of the gene encoding the transcription factor *GATA1* are considered pathognomonic of transient abnormal myelopoieisis

of Down syndrome (TAM) or MDS/AML of DS {835, 942, 1362}. Children above the age of 5 with myeloid leukaemia may not have *GATA1* mutations and such cases should be considered as "conventional" MDS or AML. Trisomy 8 is a common cytogenetic abnormality in myeloid leukaemia of DS occurring in 13–44% of patients {908, 918}. Monosomy 7 is very rare in DS-associated myeloid leukaemia.

Postulated normal counterpart

Haematopoietic stem cell.

Prognostic and predictive factors

Clinical outcome for young children with DS and myeloid leukaemia with *GATA1* mutations is unique and is associated with a better response to chemotherapy and very favourable prognosis compared to non-DS children with AML {1250}. The children should be treated on DS-specific protocols. Myeloid leukaemia in older DS children with *GATA1* mutation has a poorer prognosis comparable to AML in patients without DS {751}.

Blastic plasmacytoid dendritic cell neoplasm

F. Facchetti
D.M. Jones
T. Petrella

Definition

Blastic plasmacytoid dendritic cell (BPDC) neoplasm is a clinically aggressive tumour derived from the precursors of plasmacytoid dendritic cells (also known as professional type 1 interferon producing cells or plasmacytoid monocytes), with a high frequency of cutaneous and bone marrow (BM) involvement and leukaemic dissemination.

ICD-O code   9727/3

Synonyms

Blastic NK-cell lymphoma {1039}, agranular CD4+ natural killer cell leukaemia {277}, blastic natural killer leukaemia/lymphoma {576}, agranular CD4+CD56+ haematodermic neoplasm {1736}/tumour {920}.

Epidemiology

This is a rare form of haematologic neoplasm, without any known racial or ethnic predilection. It has a male/female ratio of 3.3:1; most patients are elderly, with a mean/median age at diagnosis of 61–67 years, but it can occur at any age, including childhood {702, 920, 1031}.

Etiology

There are currently no clues to the etiology of BPDC, but its association with myelodysplasia in some cases may suggest a related pathogenesis. There is no association with Epstein-Barr virus (EBV).

Sites of involvement

The disease tends to involve multiple sites, with a predilection for skin (almost 100% of cases), followed by BM and peripheral blood (PB)(60–90%), and lymph nodes (40–50%) {920, 1735}.

Clinical features

The patients usually present with asymptomatic solitary or multiple skin lesions that can be nodules, plaques, or bruise-like areas. Regional lymphadenopathy at presentation is common (20%); PB and BM involvement can be minimal at presentation, but invariably develops with progression of disease. Cytopenias (especially thrombocytopenia) can occur at diagnosis, and in a minority of cases can be severe, indicating BM failure {702, 920}.

Following initial response to chemotherapy, relapses invariably occur, involving skin alone, or skin associated with other sites, including soft tissues and the central nervous system. In most cases a fulminant leukaemic phase ultimately develops {702}.

About 10–20% of cases of BPDC are associated with or develop into a myelomonocytic leukaemia or acute myeloid leukaemia {702, 920, 924, 1142, 1735, 1830}. These second leukaemias can evolve from underlying myelodysplasia, or appear suddenly upon progression or relapse {702, 924, 1142}.

BPDC must be distinguished from the occasional association of a myeloid neoplasia (especially chronic myelomonocytic leukaemia) with massive nodal or extra-nodal localization of plasmacytoid dendritic cells, in which the plasmacytoid dendritic cells are morphologically mature and CD56 negative {2335}.

Morphology

BPDC is usually characterized by a diffuse, monomorphous infiltrate of medium-sized blast cells with irregular nuclei, fine chromatin and one to several small nucleoli. The cytoplasm is usually scant and appears grey-blue and agranular on Giemsa stain. Mitoses are variable in number, but rarely prominent; angioinvasion and coagulative necrosis are absent. In cutaneous infiltrates, tumour cells predominantly occupy the dermis, sparing the epidermis, but eventually extending to subcutaneous fat. Lymph nodes are diffusely involved in the interfollicular areas and medulla, with a leukaemic pattern of infiltration.

Bone marrow biopsy may show either a mild interstitial infiltrate only detectable by immunophenotyping, or massive infiltration; residual haematopoietic tissue may exhibit dysplastic features, especially in megakaryocytes {1735}. On PB and BM smears tumour cells may show cytoplasmic microvacuoles localized along the cell membrane and pseudopodia.

Cytochemistry

The neoplastic cells in BPDC are negative with non-specific esterase, and myeloperoxidase cytochemical stains.

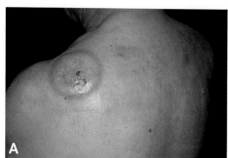
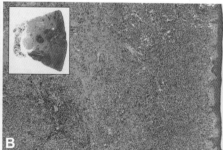
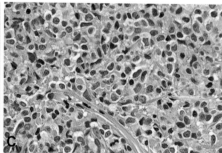

Fig. 6.44 Blastic plasmacytoid dendritic cell neoplasm. **A** Skin tumour and plaques. **B** The infiltrate diffusely involves the dermis and extends to subcutaneous fat, but spares the epidermis. **C** The neoplastic cells are medium-sized, with fine chromatin and scanty cytoplasm, reminiscent of undifferentiated blasts.

Immunophenotype

Tumour cells express CD4, CD43, CD45RA and CD56, as well as the plasmacytoid dendritic cell-associated antigens CD123 (interleukin-3 α-chain receptor), BDCA-2/CD303, TCL1, CLA (cutaneous lymphocyte-associated antigen) and the interferon-α dependent molecule MxA {92, 920, 924, 1735-1737, 1739, 1747, 1830, 2279}. Rarely, the CD56 antigen can be negative, which does not rule out the diagnosis if CD4, CD123 and TCL1 are present. Tumours that share some but not all immunophenotypic features of BPDC may be better classified as "acute leukaemia of ambiguous lineage".

CD68 (an antigen typically found on normal plasmacytoid dendritic cells) is expressed in 50% of cases, in the form of small cytoplasmic dots {1735, 1739}. Among lymphoid and myeloid-associated antigens, CD7 and CD33 are relatively common; and some cases have shown expression of CD2, CD36 and CD38, while CD3, CD5, CD13, CD16, CD19, CD20, CD79a, LAT (linker for activation of T cells), lysozyme and myeloperoxidase are regularly negative. Granzyme B, which is regularly found in normal plasmacytoid dendritic cells, has been demonstrated on flow immunophenotyping and mRNA analysis in BPDC {395, 820}, but it is mostly negative on tissue sections, similarly to other cytotoxic molecules such as perforin and TIA1.

Terminal deoxynucleotidyl transferase (TdT) is expressed in about one third of cases, with positivity ranging between 10% and 80% of cells; CD34 and CD117 are negative. EBV antigens or EBV-encoded small nuclear RNA (EBER) are not found.

Except for CD56 and TdT, the immunophenotype of BPDC largely overlaps with that of plasmacytoid dendritic cells occurring in reactive lymph nodes and tonsils {654}. Because other haematologic neoplasms (such as acute myeloid leukaemia, extranodal NK/T-cell lymphoma, nasal type and mature T-cell lymphomas), with or without skin involvement, may express CD56 with or without CD4, an extensive immunohistochemical and/or genetic analysis is mandatory before a definitive diagnosis of BPDC is made {92, 173, 386, 920, 1386}.

Genetics

T-cell and B-cell receptor genes are usually germline {92, 1735, 1830}, except for a few cases that showed T-cell receptor

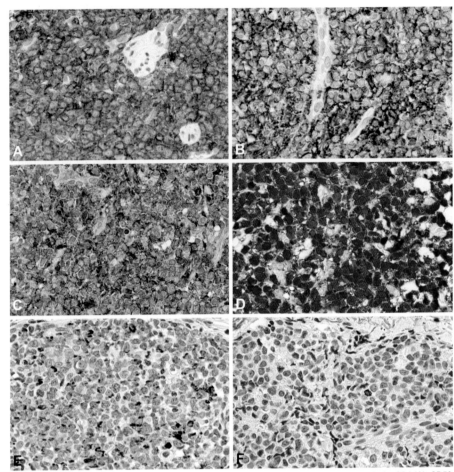

Fig. 6.45 Blastic plasmacytoid dendritic cell neoplasm. The neoplastic cells show immunoreactivity for CD4 (**A**), CD56 (**B**), CD123 (**C**), TCL1 (**D**) and CD68 (**E**), but are negative for the cytotoxic marker TIA1 (**F**).

gamma rearrangement {920, 1735}. Two thirds of patients with BPDC have an abnormal karyotype; specific chromosomal aberrations are lacking, but complex karyotypes are common; six major recurrent chromosomal abnormalities have been recognized, including 5q21 or 5q34 (72%), 12p13 (64%), 13q13-21 (64%), 6q23-qter (50%), 15q (43%) and loss of chromosome 9 (28%) {1279, 1737, 1830}. Gene expression profiling and array-based comparative genomic hybridization have shown recurrent deletions of regions on chromosome 4 (4q34), 9 (9p13-p11 and 9q12-q34) and 13 (13q12-q31) that contain several tumour suppressor genes with diminished expression (RB1, LATS2), while elevated expression of the products of the oncogenes HES6, RUNX2 and FLT3 is not associated with genomic amplification {578}.

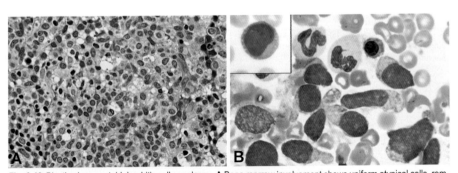

Fig. 6.46 Blastic plasmacytoid dendritic cell neoplasm. **A** Bone marrow involvement shows uniform atypical cells, reminiscent of lymphoblasts. Leukaemic cells in bone marrow aspirate (**B**) and PB (inset). The blasts show finely-dispersed chromatin and abundant cytoplasm that contain microvacuoles (inset).

Postulated normal counterpart

The normal counterpart is the precursor of the plasmacytoid dendritic cells.

Data on antigen {395, 396, 820, 920, 924, 1031, 1051, 1736, 1739, 2279} and chemokine receptor expression {185}, *in vitro* functional assays {185, 396}, gene expression profiling {578}, as well as on the tumour-derived cell line CAL-1 {1361} all point toward a derivation from the precursors of a special subset of dendritic cells, the plasmacytoid dendritic cells {356, 857, 2059}. These cells are distinguished by their production of high amounts of α-interferon in humans {357}; in the past, they have been defined with many different terms, such as lymphoblast, T-associated plasma cell, plasmacytoid T-cell and plasmacytoid monocyte {654}. The immunophenotypic heterogeneity with regards to TdT and the association with myeloid disorders suggests a multilineage potential for some cases of BPDC.

Prognosis and predictive factors

The clinical course is aggressive, with a median survival of 12–14 months, irrespective of the initial pattern of disease. Most cases (80–90%) show an initial response to multiagent chemotherapy, but relapses with subsequent resistance to drugs are regularly observed. Long-lasting remissions have been documented in sporadic cases, usually occurring in young patients who have been treated with acute leukaemia-type induction therapy, followed by allogeneic stem cell transplantation in first complete remission {92, 920, 1735}.

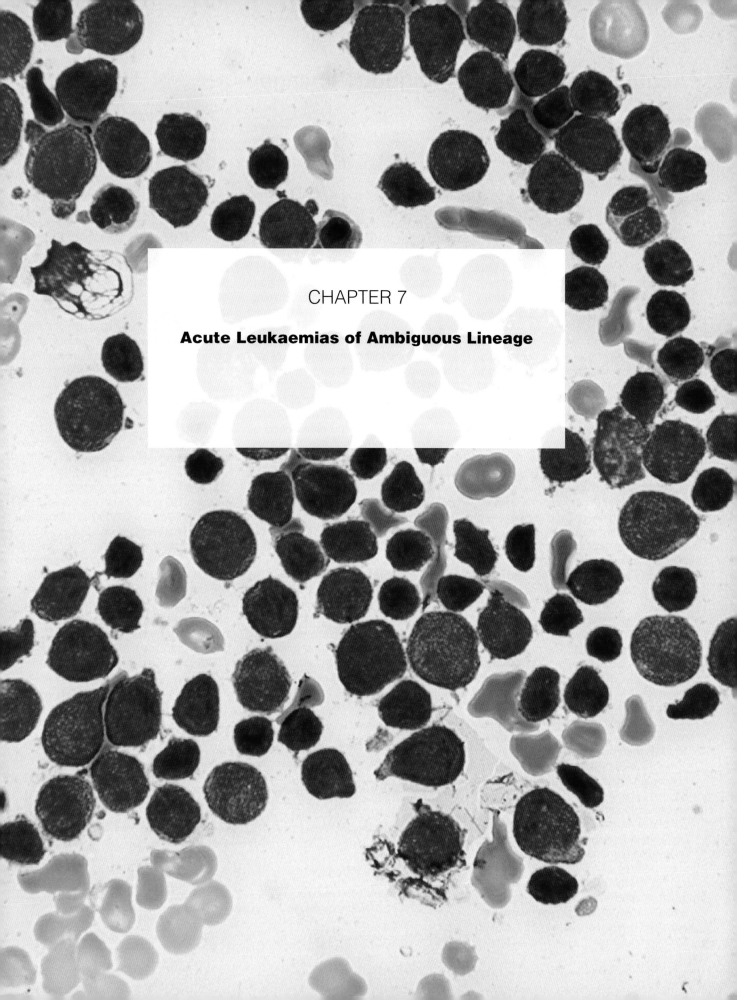

CHAPTER 7

Acute Leukaemias of Ambiguous Lineage

Acute leukaemias of ambiguous lineage

M.J. Borowitz
M.-C. Béné
N.L. Harris
A. Porwit
E. Matutes

Acute leukaemias of ambiguous lineage encompass those leukaemias that show no clear evidence of differentiation along a single lineage. They include leukaemias with no lineage-specific antigens (acute undifferentiated leukaemia, AUL) and those with blasts that express antigens of more than one lineage to such a degree that it is not possible to assign the leukaemia to any one lineage with certainty (mixed phenotype acute leukaemias, MPAL). The latter can either contain distinct blast populations, each of a different lineage, or one population with multiple antigens of different lineages on the same cells, or a combination.

Historically, there has been confusion both in the terminology and definition of MPAL. The term acute bilineal (or bilineage) leukaemia has been applied to leukaemias containing separate populations of blasts of more than one lineage, and the term biphenotypic leukaemia to those containing a single population of blasts coexpressing antigens of more than one lineage {885, 1267, 1427, 2119}, although sometimes the latter term also encompassed bilineal leukaemia. Here the term mixed phenotype acute leukaemia applies to this group of lesions in general, and, as defined below, the more specific terms B/myeloid (B/MY) and T/myeloid (T/MY) leukaemia to refer to leukaemias containing the two lineages specified, irrespective of whether one or more than one population of blasts is seen.

Some well-defined myeloid leukaemic entities may have immunophenotypic features that might suggest that they be classified as B/myeloid (B/MY) or T/myeloid (T/MY) leukaemias. However, MPAL, as defined here, excludes cases that can be classified in another category, either by genetic or clinical features. These specifically include cases with the recurrent acute myeloid leukaemia (AML)-associated translocations t(8;21), t(15;17) or inv(16); the first of these especially frequently expresses multiple B-cell markers {2236}. In addition, cases of leukaemia with *FGFR1* mutations are not considered T/MY leukaemias. Cases of chronic myelogenous leukaemia (CML) in blast crisis, MDS-related AML and therapy-related AML should be classified primarily as such, even if they have a mixed phenotype, with a secondary notation that they have a mixed phenotype.

The diagnosis of ambiguous lineage leukaemias rests on immunophenotyping. Flow cytometry is the preferred method for establishing the diagnosis, especially when a diagnosis of MPAL is dependent upon demonstrating coexpression of lymphoid and myeloid differentiation antigens on the same cell. Cases in which the diagnosis rests on demonstration of two distinct leukaemic populations with a different phenotype may also be established by immunohistochemistry in tissue sections, or with cytochemical stains for myeloperoxidase on smears coupled with flow cytometry to detect a leukaemic B or T lymphoid population.

The myeloid component of an MPAL can be recognized in one of three ways:

1) When there are two or more distinct populations of leukaemic cells, one of which would meet immunophenotypic criteria for acute myeloid leukaemia (with the exception that this population need not comprise 20% of all nucleated cells)

2) When there is a single population of blasts that by itself would meet criteria for B acute lymphoblastic leukaemia (B-ALL) or T acute lymphoblastic leukaemia (T-ALL) and the blasts also express myeloperoxidase, most frequently shown by flow cytometric positivity, on blast cells coexpressing lymphoid markers. The myeloid lineage antigens CD13, CD33 and CD117 are not specific enough to allow identification of a mixed phenotype leukaemia.

3) When there is a single population of cells that by itself would meet criteria for B or T-ALL in which the blasts also show unequivocal evidence of monoblastic differentiation: either diffuse positivity for non-specific esterase or expression of more than one monocytic marker such as CD11c, CD14, CD36, CD64 or lysozyme. The first of these three instances would previously have been considered "bilineage leukaemia" while alternatives 2 and 3 represent what would have been termed "biphenotypic leukaemia".

The T-cell component of an MPAL is recognized by strong expression of cytoplasmic CD3, either on the entire blast population, or on a separate subpopulation of leukaemic cells. Surface CD3, though rare, also indicates T-cell lineage. Expression of cCD3 is best determined by flow cytometry using relatively bright fluorophores such as phycoerythrin or allophycocyanin, and should be as bright or nearly as bright as that of normal residual T cells present in the sample. T-cell lineage can also be demonstrated by CD3 expression on blasts by immunohistochemistry on bone marrow biopsies, though it should be noted that polyvalent

Table 7.01 Requirements for assigning more than one lineage to a single blast population.

Myeloid lineage
Myeloperoxidase (flow cytometry, immunohistochemistry or cytochemistry)
or
Monocytic differentiation (at least 2 of the following: NSE, CD11c, CD14, CD64, lysozyme)

T lineage
Cytoplasmic CD3 (flow cytometry with antibodies to CD3 epsilon chain; immunohistochemistry using polyclonal anti-CD3 antibody may detect CD3 zeta chain, which is not T-cell specific)
or
Surface CD3 (rare in mixed phenotype acute leukaemias)

B lineage (multiple antigens required)
Strong CD19 with at least 1 of the following strongly expressed: CD79a, cytoplasmic CD22, CD10
or
Weak CD19 with at least 2 of the following strongly expressed: CD79a, cytoplasmic CD22, CD10

T-cell antibodies used in immunohistochemistry also react with the zeta (ζ) chain of the T-cell receptor present in the cytoplasm of NK-cells, and are thus not absolutely T-cell specific.

In contrast to what is described above with myeloid and T-cell lineages, no single marker is sufficiently specific to indicate B-cell differentiation with certainty, so that a constellation of findings is needed. B-cell differentiation can be recognized when there is a distinct subpopulation of cells that by itself meets criteria for B-ALL. When only one population of cells is present, then B-lineage assignment requires either 1) strong CD19 expression coupled with strong expression of at least one of the following antigens: CD10, CD79a or cCD22; or 2) weak CD19 expression coupled with strong expression of at least two of the following: CD10, CD79a and cCD22. Rarely, a case may be assigned as B lineage even if CD19 is negative, though care must be taken when doing this because of the relative lack of specificity of CD10 and CD79a.

Cases of MPAL based on one criterion at diagnosis (e.g. "biphenotypic leukaemia") may change over time or at relapse to the other ("bilineage leukaemia"), or vice versa. Also, following therapy, persistent disease or relapse may occur as either pure ALL or AML. Some cases of what has been termed "lineage switch" {1684, 1825} may reflect this phenomenon.

Ambiguous lineage leukaemias are rare and account for less than 4% of all cases of acute leukaemia. Many cases of what have been reported as undifferentiated leukaemia can be demonstrated to be leukaemias of unusual lineages, and many cases of what have been reported as biphenotypic acute leukaemias may in fact represent acute lymphoid or myeloid leukaemias with cross-lineage antigen expression, so that the actual frequency may even be lower. These leukaemias occur both in children and adults but more frequently in the latter, although some subtypes of MPAL may be more common in children {1145, 1671}.

A variety of genetic lesions have been reported in ambiguous lineage leukaemias, especially MPAL. Two of these, the t(9;22) (q34;q11) BCR-ABL1 translocation, and translocations associated with the MLL gene occur frequently enough and are associated with distinctive features that they are considered as separate entities.

Acute undifferentiated leukaemia

Definition
Acute undifferentiated leukaemia expresses no markers considered specific for either lymphoid or myeloid lineage. Before categorizing a leukaemia as undifferentiated, it is necessary to perform immunophenotyping with a comprehensive panel of monoclonal antibodies in order to exclude leukaemias of unusual lineages, such as those derived from myeloid or plasmacytoid dendritic cell precursors, NK-cell precursors, basophils or even non-haematopoietic tumours.

ICD-O code   9801/3

Synonyms
Acute leukaemia, NOS; stem cell acute leukaemia.

Epidemiology
These leukaemias are very rare, and nothing substantial is known about their frequency.

Sites of involvement
Bone marrow and blood. There are too few cases to know whether there is a predilection for other sites.

Clinical features
There are no features that distinguish this from other acute leukaemias.

Morphology
The blasts have no morphologic features of myeloid differentiation.

Cytochemistry
The blasts are negative for myeloperoxidase and esterase.

Immunophenotype
These leukaemias typically express no more than one membrane marker of any given lineage. By definition, they lack the T or myeloid lineage specific markers cCD3 and MPO and do not express B-cell specific markers such as cCD22, cCD79a or strong CD19. They also lack specific features of other lineages such as megakaryocytes or plasmacytoid dendritic cells. Blasts often express HLA-DR, CD34, and/or CD38 and may be positive for terminal deoxynucleotidyl transferase.

Genetics
There are too few cases described to know whether any consistent genetic lesions occur.

Postulated normal counterpart
Haematopoietic stem cell.

Prognosis and predictive factors
While anecdotal experience generally considers these leukaemias to be of poor prognosis, information is too scanty to make any definitive statements.

Mixed phenotype acute leukaemia with t(9;22) (q34;q11.2); BCR-ABL1

Definition
This is a leukaemia meeting the criteria for MPAL in which the blasts also have the t(9;22) translocation or BCR-ABL1 rearrangement. Some patients with chronic myeloid leukaemia may develop or even present with a mixed blast phase that would meet criteria for MPAL, however this diagnosis should not be made in patients known to have had CML.

ICD-O code
The provisional code proposed for the fourth edition of ICD-O is 9806/3.

Epidemiology
Although this is the most common recurrent genetic abnormality seen in mixed phenotype acute leukaemia, it is a rare leukaemia, probably accounting for less than 1% of acute leukaemias. It occurs in both children and adults, but is more common in adults {338, 1145}.

Clinical features
Patients present with features similar to those of other patients with acute leukaemia. Though there are not enough data to be certain, it is likely that they present with high white blood cell counts, similar to patients with Ph+ ALL.

Morphology
Many cases show a dimorphic blast population, one resembling lymphoblasts and the other myeloblasts, although some cases have no distinguishing features. Cases generally do not show significant myeloid maturation; care should be taken about making this diagnosis in a case of

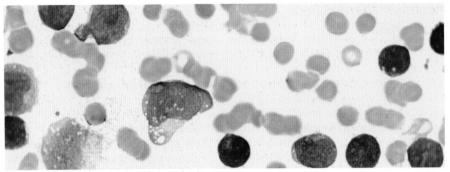

Fig. 7.01 B/myeloid leukaemia with t(9;22)(q34;q11.2). The blasts vary from small lymphoid appearing blasts to large blasts with dispersed chromatin, prominent nucleoli and a moderate amount of pale cytoplasm.

myeloid leukaemia with maturation that also expresses lymphoid markers, because such a pattern may be seen in patients with blast phase of CML.

Immunophenotype
The great majority of cases have blasts meeting criteria for B and myeloid lineage, as described above, though some cases have T and myeloid blasts. Triphenotypic leukaemia has also rarely been reported.

Genetics
All cases have either the t(9;22) detected by classical karyotyping, or the *BCR-ABL1* translocation detected by FISH or PCR. Many cases have additional cytogenetic abnormalities, and often have complex karyotypes.

Postulated normal counterpart
Multipotent haematopoietic stem cell. There is no evidence that this leukaemia derives from a different cell from other cases of Ph+ acute leukaemia.

Prognosis and predictive factors
This type of leukaemia has a poor prognosis; it appears to be worse than that of other patients with MPAL {1145}. It is not clear whether the prognosis is worse than that of patients with Ph+ ALL, or if different therapy can improve outcome. There are no known factors among patients with this leukaemia that can predict who will do better or worse. It would be expected that imatinib and related tyrosine kinase inhibitors might be useful in the treatment of this type of leukaemia; however, there are no data available to state this with certainty.

Mixed phenotype acute leukaemia with t(v;11q23); MLL rearranged

Definition
This is a leukaemia meeting requirements for mixed phenotype acute leukaemia in which the blasts also have a translocation involving the *MLL* gene. Many cases of ALL with *MLL* translocations express myeloid-associated antigens, but these should not be considered MPAL unless they meet the specific criteria noted above.

ICD-O code
The provisional code proposed for the fourth edition of ICD-O is *9807/3*.

Epidemiology
This is a rare leukaemia that is more common in children than in adults. As with ALL or AML with *MLL* rearrangements, this leukaemia is relatively more common in infancy {1145, 1671}.

Clinical features
Patients present similarly to other patients with acute leukaemia. As with other acute leukaemias with *MLL* translocations, high white blood cell counts are common.

Morphology
Most commonly these leukaemias display a dimorphic blast population, with one population clearly resembling monoblasts and the other resembling lymphoblasts. However, in other cases they may have no distinguishing features and appear only as undifferentiated blast cells. Cases in which the entire blast population is monoblastic are more likely to be AML with an *MLL* translocation.

Immunophenotype
In the majority of cases it is possible to recognize a lymphoblast population with a CD19-positive, CD10-negative B precursor (pro-B) immunophenotype, frequently positive for CD15. Expression of other B markers such as CD22 and CD79a is often weak. In addition to this, cases also fulfil criteria for myeloid lineage as defined above, most commonly via demonstration of a separate population of myeloid, and usually monoblastic leukaemic cells {1671, 2371}. Coexpression of myeloperoxidase on lymphoid blasts is rare. *MLL* translocations can also produce T-ALL, so that it is theoretically possible that T/myeloid leukaemias could occur, although these have not been reported.

Genetics
All cases have rearrangements of the *MLL* gene, with the most common partner gene being *AF4* on chromosome 4 band q21 {338, 1671}. Translocations t(9;11) and t(11;19) have also been reported. The rearrangement may be detected either by standard karyotyping or by FISH with an *MLL* breakapart probe or, less commonly, by PCR. Cases with deletions of chromosome 11q23 detected by karyotyping should not be considered in this category. The *MLL* translocation may be the only lesion present or there may be other secondary cytogenetic or molecular abnormalities although no additional genetic lesions common to multiple cases have been described.

Prognosis and predictive factors
This is a poor prognosis leukaemia {1145, 2371}. Patients with B/myeloid leukaemia with *MLL* translocations are often treated differently from patients diagnosed with ALL with *MLL* translocations, but there is no evidence that this is necessary or helpful.

Mixed phenotype acute leukaemia, B/myeloid, NOS

Definition
This leukaemia meets criteria for assignment to both B and myeloid lineage as described above, but in which the blasts lack the above-mentioned genetic abnormalities.

ICD-O code

The provisional code proposed for the fourth edition of ICD-O is *9808/3*.

Epidemiology

This is a rare leukaemia, probably accounting for about 1% of leukaemias overall. It can be seen both in children and adults but it is more common in adults.

Clinical features

There are no unique clinical features.

Morphology

Most cases have blasts with no distinguishing features, morphologically resembling ALL, or have dimorphic populations with one resembling lymphoblasts and the other resembling myeloblasts.

Immunophenotype

Blasts meet the criteria for both B-lymphoid and myeloid lineage assignment listed above. Myeloperoxidase-positive myeloblasts or monoblasts commonly also express other myeloid-associated markers including CD13, CD33 or CD117. Expression of more mature markers of B-cell lineage such as CD20 is rare but may occur, particularly when a separate population of B-cell lineage is identified {2371}.

Genetics

Most cases of B/myeloid leukaemia have clonal cytogenetic abnormalities. Many different lesions have been demonstrated, though none is of such frequency to suggest specificity for this group of leukaemias. Lesions that have been seen in more than a single case include del(6p),

12p11.2 abnormalities, del (5q), structural abnormalities of 7, and numerical abnormalities including near tetraploidy {338, 1671}. Complex karyotypes may be seen. There are insufficient data in the literature to suggest that B/myeloid and T/myeloid leukaemias have different frequencies of different genetic lesions, once the t(9;22) and *MLL* rearrangements have been accounted for.

Postulated normal counterpart

Multipotential haematopoietic stem cell. There is growing evidence of a possible relationship between B-cell and myeloid development suggesting either involvement of a common precursor, or of a precursor of one lineage that has reactivated a differentiation program of the other {1127, 1240}.

Prognosis and predictive factors

B/myeloid leukaemia is generally considered a poor prognosis leukaemia. Many patients meeting criteria for B/myeloid leukaemia have the unfavourable genetic lesions and it has been suggested that this accounts for their poor prognosis {1145}. Whether adverse cytogenetic features entirely explains the poor outcome is not definitively established {1267, 2371}.

Mixed phenotype acute leukaemia, T/myeloid, NOS

Definition

This leukaemia meets criteria for assignment to both T and myeloid lineage as described above, but in which the blasts lack the above mentioned genetic abnormalities.

ICD-O code

The provisional code proposed for the fourth edition of ICD-O is *9809/3*.

Epidemiology

This is a rare leukaemia, probably accounting for less than 1% of leukaemias overall. It can be seen both in children and adults. It may be relatively more frequent in children than is B/myeloid acute leukaemia.

Clinical features

There are no unique clinical features.

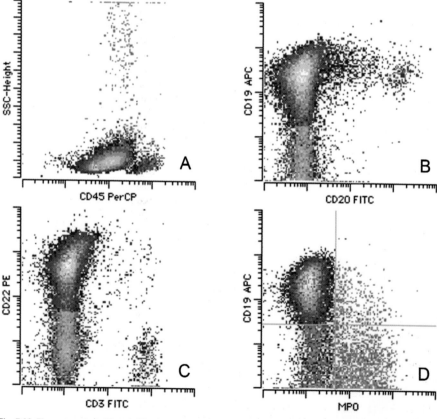

Fig. 7.02 Flow cytometry in B/myeloid leukaemia. **A** CD45 vs Side scatter display showing a major population of dim CD45+ blasts. B lymphoblasts are blue, residual normal B cells red and myeloperoxidase positive cells (including both blasts and residual normal cells) green. **B,C** The B-cell markers CD19 and CD22 are strongly expressed on the B lymphoid blasts, at levels comparable to that seen with residual normal B-cells (in red). **D** Most of the B-cell blasts lack MPO and many though not all of the B-negative blasts are MPO positive. There is a small population of blasts coexpressing CD19 and MPO.

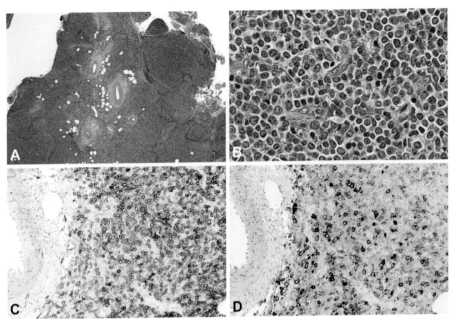

Fig. 7.03 T/myeloid leukaemia infiltrating a lymph node. **A, B** Diffuse replacement of node by a population of cells with high nucleus/cytoplasm ratios and fine chromatin histologically indistinguishable from lymphoblastic lymphoma/leukaemia. **C** Immunoperoxidase stain for CD3, showing staining of the majority of the blast cells. **D** Immunoperoxidase stain for myeloperoxidase. Distinct staining of a subpopulation of cells with round nuclei, indicating that they are part of the neoplasm, and not infiltrating granulocytes.

Morphology

Most cases have blasts with no distinguishing features, morphologically resembling ALL, or have dimorphic populations, with one resembling lymphoblasts and the other resembling myeloblasts.

Immunophenotype

Blasts meet the criteria for both T-lymphoid and myeloid lineage assignment listed above. Myeloperoxidase-positive myeloblasts or monoblasts commonly also express other myeloid-associated markers including CD13, CD33 or CD117. In addition to cCD3, the T-cell component frequently expresses other T-cell markers including CD7,CD5, and CD2. Expression of surface CD3 may occur when a separate population of T-cell lineage is identified {2371}.

Genetics

Most cases have clonal chromosomal abnormalities, although none is of such frequency to suggest specificity for this group of leukaemias. There are insufficient data in the literature to suggest that B/MY and T/MY leukaemias have different frequencies of different genetic lesions, once the t(9;22) and *MLL* rearrangements have been accounted for.

Postulated normal counterpart

Multipotential haematopoietic stem cell. There is growing evidence of a possible relationship between T-cell and myeloid development suggesting either involvement of a common precursor, or of a lymphoid precursor that has reactivated a myeloid differentiation program {1127, 1240}.

Prognosis and predictive factors

T/myeloid leukaemia is generally considered a poor prognosis leukaemia, although data are limited on the outcome of these patients distinct from other MPAL patients. Patients with T/myeloid leukaemia have not been treated uniformly, although combinations of myeloid-directed and lymphoid-directed therapy have been tried, and some patients may respond to one or the other.

Mixed phenotype acute leukaemia, NOS - rare types

Some cases of leukaemia have been seen in which leukaemic blasts show clear-cut evidence of both T and B lineage commitment as defined above. This is a very rare phenomenon, with a frequency that is likely lower than what has been reported in the literature. As strictly applied, the most recent EGIL criteria for biphenotypic leukaemia (scores higher than 2 in more than one lineage), which assigned 2 points to CD79a expression {53, 187} would likely overestimate the incidence of B/T leukaemia because CD79a can be detected in T-ALL {1750}. In assigning B lineage to a case of T-cell leukaemia, CD79a and CD10 should not be considered as evidence of B-cell differentiation. There have also been a few cases with evidence of trilineage (B, T and myeloid lineage) assignment. Overall there are too few cases of either of these to make any specific statements about clinical features, genetic lesions or prognosis.

To date, there have been no reports of B or T/megakaryocytic or B or T/erythroleukaemias. Because it has been suggested that erythroid and megakaryocytic lineages are the earliest to branch off from the pluripotent haematopoietic stem cell, leaving progenitor cells with T, B and myeloid potential {11}, neoplasms of these combinations of lineages may not occur. If they

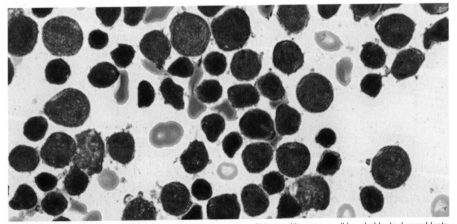

Fig. 7.04 T/myeloid leukaemia. There is a dimorphic population of blasts with many small lymphoblasts; larger blasts also have high nucleus/cytoplasm ratio, fine chromatin and inconspicuous nucleoli.

do occur, it is possible that the definitions used here might not detect all cases, as these leukaemias would not be expected to express MPO.

Other ambiguous lineage leukaemias

Under some circumstances leukaemias may express combinations of markers that do not allow classification as either AUL or MPAL as defined above, yet definitive classification along a single lineage may be difficult. Examples of such cases might include cases that express T-cell-associated but not T-cell-specific markers such as CD7 and CD5 without cytoplasmic CD3, along with myeloid-associated antigens such as CD33 and CD13 without myeloperoxidase. Such cases are best considered acute unclassifiable leukaemias. With more extended panels containing newer, less commonly used markers, such leukaemias might be able to be classified.

Natural killer cell lymphoblastic leukaemia/ lymphoma
This neoplasm has been very difficult to define, and there is considerable confusion in the literature. Contributing to the confusion is that many cases reported as NK leukaemia because of the expression of N-CAM (CD56) are now recognized to represent cases of plasmacytoid dendritic cell leukaemia {1735, 1736}. Similarly, the entity of myeloid/NK-cell acute leukaemia {1980, 2129}, which has been suggested to be of precursor NK origin {1660} has a primitive immunophenotype that cannot be distinguished from acute myeloid leukaemia with minimal differentiation, and until further evidence emerges these should be considered as cases of AML. Early in development, NK-cell progenitors express no specific markers {733} or express markers that overlap with those seen in T-cell ALL, including CD7, CD2 and even CD5 and cytoplasmic CD3 {2070}, so that distinguishing between T-ALL and NK-cell tumours may be difficult. More mature but more specific markers such as CD16 are rarely expressed in any acute leukaemia, while some markers that might be considered relatively more specific, but still expressed on NK progenitors, such as CD94 or CD161 {733} are not commonly tested. Some well characterized cases of NK precursor tumours with lymphomatous

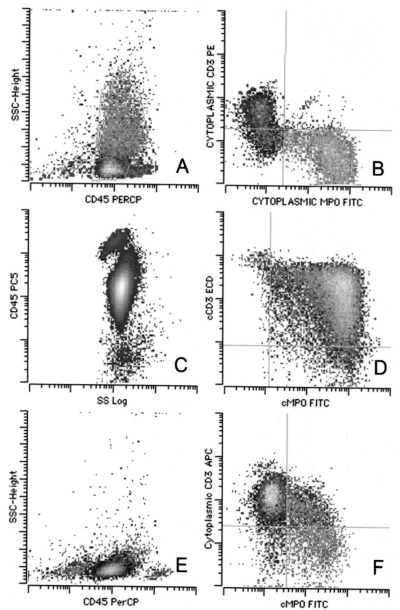

Fig. 7.05 Flow cytometry in several cases of T/myeloid leukaemia (**A,C,E** Gating on all cells. **B,D,F** Gating on blasts, with normal T cells superimposed in violet). **A,B** T/MY leukaemia with two separate populations of T (blue) and myeloid (green) blasts ("Bilineage leukaemia"). The CD45/SSC displayed in (**A**) shows that the myeloid and T-cell populations have distinct light scatter profiles. Residual normal T-cells are shown in violet, and show that cCD3 in the T-ALL is comparable in intensity to the normal cells. **C,D** T/MY leukaemia with a single population of blasts (red) coexpressing both cCD3 and MPO ("biphenotypic leukaemia"). Normal T-cells are again in violet. There is a wide range of cCD3 expression, but the brightest blasts are about as bright as normal T-cells. **E,F** T/MY leukaemia in which both coexpression (red) and separate populations of T (blue) and myeloid (green) blasts can be seen. Neither the term biphenotypic nor bilineage would readily fit this leukaemia.

presentations that expressed NK-specific CD94 1A transcripts have been described {1306}. It is hoped that wider availability of more specific NK markers including panels of antibodies against killer immunoglobulin-like receptors (KIRs) will help clarify this disease, but until then this is best considered a provisional entity. The diagnosis of precursor NK lymphoblastic leukaemia/

lymphoma may be considered in a case that expresses CD56 along with immature T-associated markers such as CD7 and CD2 and even including cCD3, provided that it lacks B-cell and myeloid markers, T-cell and *IG* receptor genes are in the germline configuration {1128, 1174, 1660} and blastic plasmacytoid dendritic cell leukaemia has been excluded.

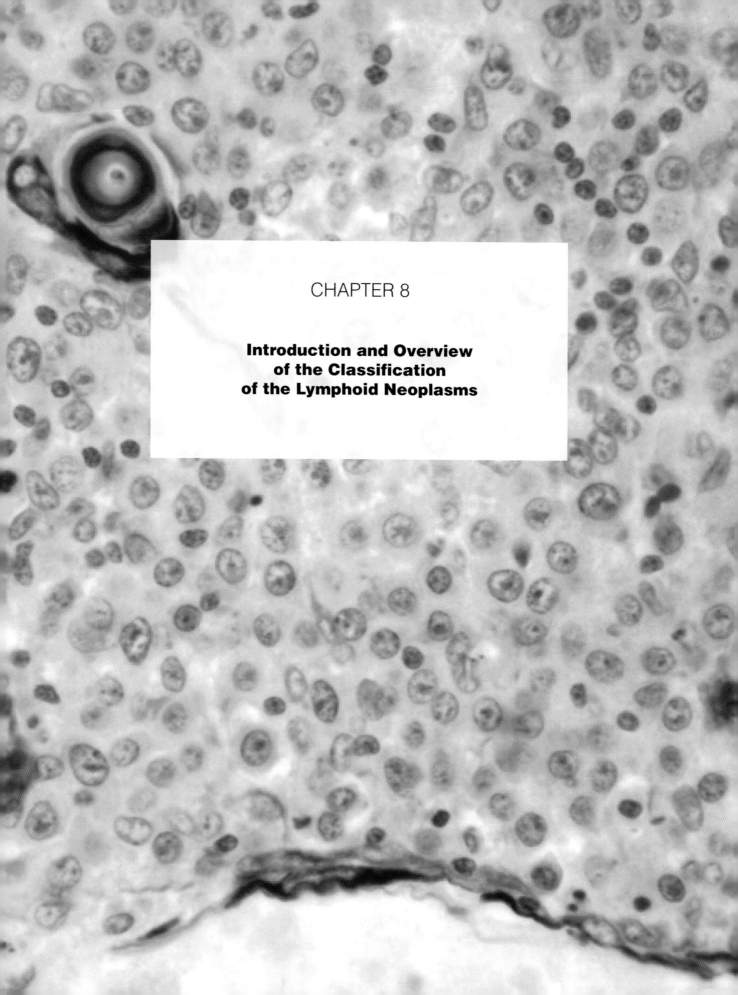

CHAPTER 8

**Introduction and Overview
of the Classification
of the Lymphoid Neoplasms**

Introduction and overview of the classification of the lymphoid neoplasms

E.S. Jaffe
N.L. Harris
H. Stein
E. Campo
S.A. Pileri
S.H. Swerdlow

Definition

B cell and T/NK cell neoplasms are clonal tumours of mature and immature B cells, T cells or natural killer (NK) cells at various stages of differentiation. Because NK cells are closely related, and share some immunophenotypic and functional properties with T cells, these two classes of neoplasms are considered together.

B-cell and T-cell neoplasms in many respects appear to recapitulate stages of normal B-cell or T-cell differentiation, so that they can be to some extent classified according to the corresponding normal stage. However, some common B-cell neoplasms, e.g. hairy cell leukaemia, do not clearly correspond to a normal B-cell differentiation stage. Some neoplasms may exhibit lineage heterogeneity, or even more rarely, lineage plasticity {1037, 1357}. Thus, the normal counterpart of the neoplastic cell cannot at this time be the sole basis for the classification.

Pathobiology of lymphoid neoplasms and the normal immune system

There are two major arms of the immune system that differ, both in the nature of the target and the type of the immune response, known as the innate and adaptive immune responses. Cells of the innate immune system represent a first line of defense, a primitive response. Cells of the innate immune system include NK cells, CD3+ CD56+ T-cells or NK-like T-cells, and γδ T cells. These cells play a role in barrier defenses involving mucosal and cutaneous immunity. They do not need to encounter antigen in the context of the major histocompatibility complex (MHC), and thus do not require antigen presenting cells to initiate an immune response. The adaptive immune system is a more sophisticated type of immune response. It is specific for a particular pathogen; two key features of the adaptive immune response are specificity and memory. This contrasts with innate immune responses which are non-specific for the target, and do not require or lead to immunological memory.

B-cell lymphomas: lymphocyte differentiation and function

B-cell neoplasms tend to mimic stages of normal B-cell differentiation, and the resemblance to normal cell stages is a major basis for their classification and nomenclature.

Normal B-cell differentiation begins with precursor B cells known as progenitor B cells/B lymphoblasts (blast cells that are the precursors of the entire B-cell line), which undergo immunoglobulin *VDJ* gene rearrangement and differentiate into mature surface immunoglobulin (sIg) positive (IgM+ IgD+) naïve B cells via pre-B cells with cytoplasmic μ heavy chains and immature IgM+ B cells. Naïve B cells, that are often CD5+, are small resting lymphocytes that circulate in the peripheral blood (PB) and also occupy primary lymphoid follicles and follicle mantle zones (so-called recirculating B cells) {1004A, 1152A}. Most cases of mantle cell lymphoma are thought to correspond to CD5 positive naïve B cells {994A}.

On encountering antigen that fits their surface Ig receptors, naïve B cells undergo transformation, proliferate, and ultimately mature into antibody-secreting plasma cells and memory B cells. Transformed cells formed from naïve B cells that have encountered antigen may mature directly into plasma cells that produce the early IgM antibody response to antigen. T-cell independent maturation can take place outside of the germinal centre {424}. It is debated whether somatic hypermutation of the *IGH@* genes occurs during this

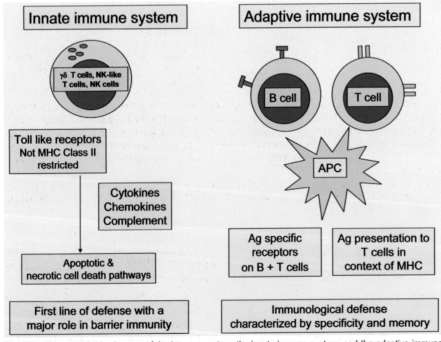

Fig. 8.01 There are two main arms of the immune system, the innate immune system, and the adaptive immune system. Diagram shows respective roles of lymphocyte subpopulations in the innate and adaptive immune responses. NK cells, NK-like T cells, and γδ T cells function with other cell types including granulocytes and macrophages as a first line of defense. These cells have cytotoxic granules (shown in red) containing perforin and granzymes. The innate immune system lacks specificity and memory. In the adaptive immune system, B cells and T cells recognize antigens (Ag) through specific receptors, immunoglobulin (Ig) and the T-cell receptor complex (TCR) respectively. Antigen presentation to T cells must take place via antigen-presenting cells (APC) in the context of the appropriate major histocompatibility complex (MHC) Class II antigens. Figure modified from {1035}.

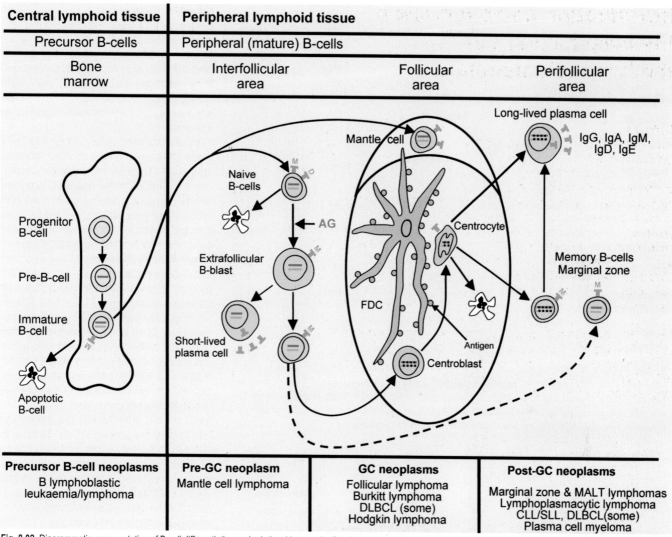

Central lymphoid tissue	Peripheral lymphoid tissue		
Precursor B-cells	Peripheral (mature) B-cells		
Bone marrow	Interfollicular area	Follicular area	Perifollicular area

Precursor B-cell neoplasms	Pre-GC neoplasm	GC neoplasms	Post-GC neoplasms
B lymphoblastic leukaemia/lymphoma	Mantle cell lymphoma	Follicular lymphoma Burkitt lymphoma DLBCL (some) Hodgkin lymphoma	Marginal zone & MALT lymphomas Lymphoplasmacytic lymphoma CLL/SLL, DLBCL(some) Plasma cell myeloma

Fig. 8.02 Diagrammatic representation of B-cell differentiation and relationship to major B-cell neoplasms. B-cell neoplasms correspond to stages of B-cell maturation, even though the precise cell counterparts are not known in all instances. Precursor B-cells that mature in the bone marrow may undergo apoptosis or develop into mature naïve B-cells that, following exposure to antigen and blast transformation, may develop into short-lived plasma cells or enter the germinal centre (GC) where somatic hypermutation and heavy chain class switching occur. Centroblasts, the transformed cells of the GC, either undergo apoptosis or develop into centrocytes. Post-GC cells include both long-lived plasma cells and memory/marginal zone B-cells. Most B-cells are activated within the GC, but T-cell independent activation can take place outside of the germinal centre and also probably leads to memory type B-cells. Monocytoid B-cells, many of which lack somatic hypermutation, are not illustrated.
DLBCL, diffuse large B-cell lymphoma; CLL/SLL, chronic lymphocytic leukaemia/small lymphocytic lymphoma; MALT, mucosa-associated lymphoid tissue; AG, antigen; FDC, follicular dendritic cell. Red bar, immunoglobulin heavy chain gene *(IGH@)* rearrangement; blue bar, immunoglobulin light chain gene *(IGL)* rearrangement; black insertions in the red and blue bars indicate somatic hypermutation.

extrafollicular maturation. Other antigen-exposed B cells migrate into the centre of a primary follicle, proliferate, and fill the follicular dendritic cell (FDC) meshwork, forming a germinal centre {1325A, 1355A}. Germinal centre centroblasts express low levels of sIg, and also switch off expression of BCL2 protein; thus, they and their progeny are susceptible to death through apoptosis {1828A}. Centroblasts express CD10 and BCL6 protein, a nuclear transcription factor that is expressed by both centroblasts and centrocytes. BCL6 is not expressed in naïve B cells and is switched

off in memory B cells and plasma cells {1346, 1760}.
In the germinal centre, somatic hypermutation occurs in the immunoglobulin heavy and light chain variable *(IGV)* region genes; these mutations may result in a non-functional gene, or a gene that produces antibody with lower or higher affinity for antigen than the native *IG* gene. Also in the germinal centre some cells switch from IgM to IgG or IgA production. Through these mechanisms, the germinal centre reaction gives rise to the higher affinity IgG or IgA antibodies of the

late primary or secondary immune response {1356A}. The *BCL6* gene also undergoes somatic mutation in the germinal centre, however, at a lower frequency than is seen in the *IG* genes {1698A}. Ongoing *IGV* region gene mutation with intraclonal diversity is a hallmark of germinal centre cells, and both *IGV* region gene mutation and *BCL6* mutation serve as markers of cells that have been through the germinal centre. Most diffuse large B-cell neoplasms (DLBCL) are composed of cells that at least in part resemble centroblasts and that have mutated *IGV*

Table 8.01 Immunophenotypic features of common mature B-cell neoplasms.

Neoplasm	sIg; cIg	CD5	CD10	CD23	CD43	CD103	BCL6	IRF4/ MUM1	Cyclin D1	ANXA1
CLL/SLL	+;-/+	+	-	+	+	-	-	(+PC)	-	-
LPL	+/-;+	-	-	-	-/+	-	-	+*	-	-
Splenic MZL	+;-/+	-	-	-	-	-	-	-	-	-
HCL	+;-	-	-	-	-	+	-	-	+/-	+
Plasma cell myeloma	-;+	-	-/+	-	-/+	-	-	+	-/+	-
MALT lymphoma	+;+/-	-	-	-/+	-/+	-	-	+*	-	-
Follicular lymphoma	+;-	-	+/-	-/+	-	-	+	-/+#	-	-
MCL	+;-	+	-	-	+	-	-	-	+	-
Diffuse large B-cell lymphoma	+/-;-/+	-***	-/+##	NA	-/+	NA	+/-##	+/-**	-	-
Burkitt lymphoma	+;-	-	+	-	+/-	NA	+	-/+	-	-

+, >90% of cases +; +/-, >50% of cases +; -/+, <50% of cases +; -, <10% of cases +. IRF4/MUM1, interferon regulating factor 4; ANXA1, Annexin A1; PC, proliferation centres; *, plasma cell component positive; #, some grades 3a and 3b; ##, DLBCL of germinal centre B-cell type (GCB) express CD10 and BCL6; **, DLBCL of activated B-cell type (ABC) are typically positive for IRF4/MUM1; ***, some DLBCL are CD5+; NA, not applicable; LPL, lymphoplasmacytic lymphoma; MZL, marginal zone lymphoma; MCL, mantle cell lymphoma.

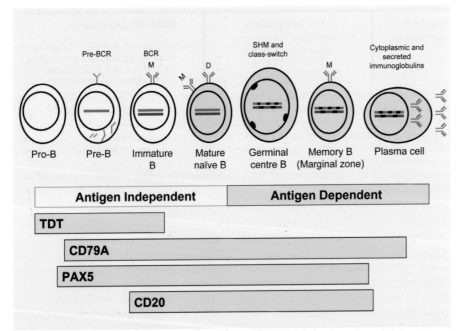

Fig.8.03 Schematic diagram showing phenotype of B lymphocytes at varying stages of maturation. TDT is a feature of early lymphoid precursors, including both B and T lymphoblasts, as well as the blasts in some cases of acute myeloid leukaemia. CD79A and PAX5 appear at the time of heavy chain gene rearrangement. CD20 is not expressed until the stage of immunoglobulin light chain gene *(IGL)* rearrangement. TDT, terminal deoxynucleotidyl transferase; SHM, somatic hypermutation; Red bar, *IGH@* rearrangement; blue bar, *IGL* rearrangement; Pre-BCR, pre-B-cell receptor consisting of a IG heavy chain and the surrogate light chain (which is composed of two linked small peptides VpreB and λ5, represented in green); BCR, B cell receptor of mature B cells; Red bar and blue bar with black insertions, rearranged *IGH@* and *IGL* genes with somatic hypermutation.

genes, consistent with a derivation from cells that have been exposed to the germinal centre. Burkitt lymphoma cells are BCL6+ and have mutated *IGH* genes, and are thus also thought to correspond to a germinal centre blast cell. Both Burkitt and DLBCL correspond to proliferating cells, and are clinically aggressive tumours.

Centroblasts mature to centrocytes, and these cells are seen predominantly in the light zone of the germinal centre. Centrocytes express sIg that has an altered antibody combining site as compared with that of their progenitors, based both on somatic mutations and heavy chain class switching. Centrocytes with mutations that result in increased affinity are rescued from apoptosis and they re-express BCL2 protein {1355A}. Through interaction with surface molecules on FDC's and T-cells, such as CD23 and CD40 ligand, centrocytes switch off BCL6 protein expression {346, 1760}, and differentiate into either memory B-cells or plasma cells {1355A}. BCL6 and IRF4/MUM1 are reciprocally expressed, with IRF4/MUM1 being positive in late centrocytes and plasma cells {661, 1914A}. IRF4/MUM1 plays a critical role in down-regulating BCL6 expression {1914A}. Follicular lymphomas are tumours of germinal centre B-cells (centrocytes and centroblasts) in which the germinal centre cells fail to undergo apoptosis, in most cases due to a chromosomal rearrangement, t(14;18), that prevents the normal switching off of BCL2 protein expression. Centrocytes usually predominate over centroblasts, and these neoplasms tend to be indolent.

Post-germinal centre memory B-cells circulate in the PB and comprise at least some of the cells in the follicular marginal zones of lymph nodes, spleen and mucosa-associated lymphoid tissue (MALT). Marginal zone B-cells of this compartment typically express pan-B antigens, surface IgM with only low level IgD and lack both CD5 and CD10 {2064A, 2293B}. Plasma cells produced in the germinal centre enter the PB and home to the bone marrow (BM). They contain predominantly IgG or IgA; they lack sIg and CD20, but express IRF4/MUM1, CD79a, CD38 and CD138. Both memory B-cells and long-lived plasma cells have mutated *IGV* region genes, but do not continue to undergo mutation. Post-germinal centre B-cells retain the ability to home to tissues in which they have undergone antigen

Table 8.02 Immunophenotypic features of common mature T-cell and NK-cell neoplasms.

Neoplasms	CD3	CD4	CD8	CD7	CD5	CD2	TIA1	GrB Per	CD30	CD25	CD56	CD16	CD57	BCL6	CD10	EBV	EMA
T-PLL	+	+	+/-	+	+	+	-	-	-	-	-	-	-	-	-	-	-
T-LGL	+	-	+	-/+	-/+	+	+	+	-	-	-	+	+	-	-	-	-
ATLL	+	+	-	-	+	+	-	-	-/+	++	-	-	-	-	-	-	-
Agg NK	+ c	-	-/+	-	-	+	+	+	-	-	+	-	-	-	-	+	-
ENK/T, Nasal type	+ c	-	-/+	-	-	+	+	+	-	-	+	-	-	-	-	+	-
EATL	+	-	-/+	+	-	+	+	+	-/+	-/+	-/+#	-	-	-	-	-	-/+
HSTL	+*%	-	+/-	+	-	+	+	-	-	-	+	-	-	-	-	-	-
SPTCL	+	-	+	+	-/+	+	+	+	-	-	-	-	-	-	-	-	-
MF/SS	+	+	-/+	-/+	+/-	+	-	-	-	-	-	-	-	-	-	-	-
Primary cutaneous γδ T-cell lymphoma	+*	-	-/+	-/+	-	+	+	+	-	-	+	-	-	-	-	-	-
Primary cutaneous CD30+ LPD	+	+	-	-	+/-	+	+	-+	+	-	-	-	-	-	-	-	+/-
AITL	+	+	-	+	+	+	-	-	-	-	-	-	-	+/-	+/-	-**	-
PTCL, NOS##	+	+/-	-/+	-/+	-/+	+	-	-	-/+	-	-	-	-^	-^	-^	-	-
ALCL, ALK+	-/+	+/-	-/+	-/+	+/-	+/-	+	+	++	++	+/-	-	-	-	+	-	++
ALCL, ALK-	+/-	+/-	-/+	-/+	+/-	+/-	+/-	+/-	++	++	+/-	-	-	-	-	-	+

c, cytoplasmic CD3 only, restricted to CD3 ε; *, T-cell receptor γδ; %, a minority of cases expresses the αβ T-cell receptor. #, CD56 is expressed in the monomorphic type of EATL or Type II; **, EBV is absent in neoplastic cells, but is nearly always present in a subpopulation of background B-cells; ##, PTCL, NOS is not a single disease, but a heterogeneous group, and therefore, a variety of immunophenotypic profiles can be seen. ^, a subset of PTCL, NOS are derived from follicular helper T-cells (T_FH), and often express CD57, CD10 and BCL6; T-PLL, T-cell prolymphocytic leukaemia; T-LGL, T-cell large granular lymphocytic leukaemia; ATLL, adult T-cell leukaemia/ lymphoma; Agg NK, aggressive NK-cell leukaemia; ENK/T-nasal type, extranodal NK/T-cell lymphoma, nasal-type; EATL, enteropathy-associated T-cell lymphoma; HSTL, hepatosplenic T-cell lymphoma; SPTCL, subcutaneous panniculitis-like T-cell lymphoma; MF/SS, mycosis fungoides and Sézary syndrome; primary cutaneous CD30+ LPD, primary cutaneous CD30+ T-cell lymphoproliferative disease, including primary cutaneous anaplastic T-cell lymphoma; AILT, angioimmunoblastic T-cell lymphoma; PTLC, NOS, peripheral T-cell lymphomas, not otherwise specified; ALCL, anaplastic large cell lymphoma. GrB, granzyme B; Per, perforin.

play an important role in preventing autoimmunity. Tregs express high density CD25, and the transcription factor FOXP3, in combination with CD4. Adult T-cell leukaemia/lymphoma (ATLL), has been linked to Treg cells based on expression of both CD25 and FoxP3, and this finding helps to explain the marked immunosuppression associated with ATLL {1862A}.

Recent studies have tried to relate the pathological or clinical manifestations of T-cell lymphomas to cytokine or chemokine expression by the neoplastic cells, or accompanying accessory cells within the lymph node. For example, the hypercalcemia associated with ATLL has been linked to secretion of factors with osteoclast-activating activity {664, 1358}. The haemophagocytic syndrome seen in some T-cell and NK-cell malignancies has been associated with secretion of both cytokines and chemokines, in the setting defective cytolytic function {737, 1276}.

Genetics

Several mature B-cell neoplasms have characteristic genetic abnormalities that are important in determining their biologic features and can be useful in differential diagnosis. These include the t(11;14) in mantle cell lymphoma, t(14;18) in follicular lymphoma, t(8;14) and variants in Burkitt lymphoma, and t(11;18) in MALT lymphoma {515, 1104, 1285}. The t(11;14) is seen in both mantle cell lymphoma and a fraction of cases of plasma cell myeloma, but minor differences in the translocation exist, involving different portions of the immunoglobulin heavy chain gene (IGH@) {199}. The most common paradigm for translocations involving the IGH@ on 14q, is that a cellular proto-oncogene comes under the influence of the IGH@ promoter. For example, in follicular lymphoma, the overexpression of BCL2 blocks apoptosis in germinal centre B-cells. The t(11;18), common in MALT lymphoma, results in a fusion gene, API2/MALT1 {574, 1837, 2109A}. The expression of API2 inhibits the activity of several caspases. The partner gene, MALT1, activates the NFκB pathway, as do other translocations found in MALT lymphoma, such as t(1;14) and t(14;18).

Only a few T-cell neoplasms have thus far been associated with specific genetic abnormalities. Anaplastic large cell lymphoma, ALK+, is defined by translocations involving the ALK (anaplastic lymphoma kinase) gene on chromosome 5, (t(2;5) and variants {582, 1229}). Hepatosplenic T-cell lymphoma is associated with

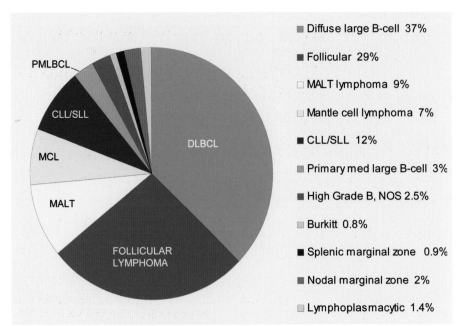

- ■ Diffuse large B-cell 37%
- ■ Follicular 29%
- □ MALT lymphoma 9%
- ▨ Mantle cell lymphoma 7%
- ■ CLL/SLL 12%
- ▨ Primary med large B-cell 3%
- ■ High Grade B, NOS 2.5%
- ▨ Burkitt 0.8%
- ■ Splenic marginal zone 0.9%
- ■ Nodal marginal zone 2%
- □ Lymphoplasmacytic 1.4%

Fig. 8.06 Relative frequencies of B-cell lymphoma subtypes in adults. Significant differences exist in different geographic regions. However, diffuse large B-cell lymphoma (DLBCL) and follicular lymphoma are the most common subtypes irrespective of geographic or ethnic group. Note that these figures underestimate the incidence of CLL/SLL, as only patients presenting clinically with lymphoma were included. MCL, mantle cell lymphoma; CLL/SLL, chronic lymphocytic leukaemia/small lymphocytic lymphoma; PMLBCL, primary mediastinal large B-cell lymphoma; SMZL, splenic marginal zone lymphoma; NMZL, nodal marginal zone lymphoma. Data based on {51}.

isochromosome 7q. However, the molecular pathogenesis of most other T-cell and NK-cell neoplasms remains to be defined. Multiple other genetic tools have been brought to bear on the study of mature lymphoid neoplasms. These include comparative genomic hybridisation (CGH), and the newer and more sensitive technique of array CGH, both of which can identify areas of deletion or amplification within the genome {165-167}. Gene expression microarrays can interrogate the expression of thousands of genes at the RNA level, helping to elucidate pathways of activation and transformation {509, 510, 513, 701, 1507, 1867, 1944}. Most recently, studies have begun to explore changes at the epigenetic level that control the expression of multiple genes {1314}.

Principles of classification

The classification of lymphoid neoplasms is based on utilisation of all available information to define disease entities {898}. Morphology and immunophenotype are sufficient for the diagnosis of most lymphoid neoplasms. However, no one antigenic marker is specific for any neoplasm, and a combination of morphologic features and a panel of antigenic markers are necessary for correct diagnosis. Most B-cell lymphomas have characteristic

immunophenotypic profiles that are very helpful in diagnosis. However, immune profiling is somewhat less helpful in the subclassification of T-cell lymphomas.

In addition, while certain antigens are commonly associated with specific disease entities, these associations are not entirely disease-specific. For example, CD30 is a universal feature of ALCL, but can be expressed in other T-cell and B-cell lymphomas and classical Hodgkin lymphoma (CHL). Similarly, while CD56 is a characteristic feature of nasal NK/T-cell lymphoma, it can be seen in other T-cell lymphomas, and in plasma cell neoplasms {208, 701, 1325}. Within a given disease entity, variation in immunophenotypic features can be seen. For example, most hepatosplenic T-cell lymphomas are of $\gamma\delta$ T-cell phenotype, but some cases are of $\alpha\beta$ derivation. Likewise, some follicular lymphomas are CD10-negative. Additionally, the presence of an aberrant immunophenotype may suggest or help to confirm a diagnosis of malignancy {1034}.

While lineage is a defining feature of most lymphoid malignancies, in recent years there has been a greater appreciation of lineage plasticity within the haematopoietic system. Lineage switch, or demonstration of multiple lineages is most often encountered in immature haematolymphoid neoplasms,

but also can be seen rarely in mature lymphomas {451A, 675A, 880A}.

Genetic features are playing an increasingly important role in the classification of lymphoid malignancies, and for many of the small B-cell lymphomas and leukaemias, recurrent genetic alterations have been identified. However, the molecular pathogenesis of most T-cell and NK-cell lymphomas remains unknown. Genetic studies, in particular PCR studies of IGH@ and T-cell receptor (TCR) gene rearrangements and fluorescence in situ hybridization (FISH), are valuable diagnostic tools, both for determination of clonality in B-cell and T-cell proliferations (aiding in the differential diagnosis with reactive hyperplasia), and in identifying translocations associated with some disease entities.

The WHO classification emphasizes the importance of knowledge of clinical features, both for accurate diagnosis, as well as for the definition of some diseases, such as marginal zone lymphoma of MALT type versus nodal or splenic marginal zone lymphoma, mediastinal large B-cell lymphoma versus DLBCL, and most mature T-cell and NK-cell neoplasms. Diagnosis of lymphoid neoplasms should not take place in a vacuum, but in the context of a complete clinical history.

Lymphoid malignancies range in their clinical behaviour from low grade to high grade. However, within any one entity a range in clinical behaviour can be seen. Moreover, histological or clinical progression is often encountered during a patient's clinical course. For these reasons, the WHO classification does not attempt to stratify lymphoid malignancies in terms of grade. Both morphology and immunophenotype often change over time, as the lymphoid neoplasm undergoes clonal evolution with the acquisiton of additional genetic changes. In addition, evolution over time does not necessarily lead to the development of a more aggressive lymphoma. For example, patients with DLBCL can relapse with a more indolent clonally related follicular lymphoma. Some of these clonal evolutions can be unexpected and not obviously connected, such as the development of a plasmacytoma in a patient with CHL {1042B}.

Traditionally, classical Hodgkin lymphomas (CHL) have been considered separately from so-called "non-Hodgkin lymphomas." However, with the recognition that CHL is of B-cell lineage, greater overlap has been appreciated between CHL and many forms of B-cell malignancy. The 4th edition of the WHO classification recognizes these grey zones, and provides for the recognition of cases that bridge the gap between these various forms of lymphoma {2265}.

Epidemiology

Precursor lymphoid neoplasms including B lymphoblastic leukaemia/lymphoma (B-ALL/LBL) and T lymphoblastic leukaemia/lymphoma (T-ALL/LBL) are primarily diseases of children. 75% of cases occur in children under six years of age. Approximately 85% of cases presenting as ALL are of precursor B-cell type, whereas lymphoblastic malignancies of precursor T-cell type more often present as lymphoma, with mediastinal masses. A male predominance is seen in lymphoblastic malignancies of both B-cell and T-cell lineages.

Mature B-cell neoplasms comprise over 90% of lymphoid neoplasms worldwide {51, 79}. They represent approximately 4% of new cancers each year. They are more common in developed countries, particularly the United States, Australia, New Zealand and Western Europe. The most recent survey from the Surveillance, Epidemiology and End Results (SEER) program in the United States indicated an incidence rate per 100 000 persons per year of 33.65 for all lymphoid neoplasms, 26.13 for B-cell neoplasms, 1.79 for all T-cell neoplasms, and 2.67 for Hodgkin lymphoma {1525A}. The most common types are follicular lymphoma and DLBCL, which together make up more than 60% of all lymphomas exclusive of Hodgkin lymphoma and plasma cell myeloma {37, 51}. The incidence of lymphomas, in particular B-cell lymphomas, is increasing worldwide, with more than 280 000 cases occurring annually each year {2112A}. The individual B-cell neoplasms vary in their relative frequency in different parts of the world. Follicular lymphoma is more common in the United States (35% of non-Hodgkin lymphomas) and Western Europe, and is uncommon in South America, Eastern Europe, Africa and Asia. Burkitt lymphoma is endemic in equatorial Africa, where it is the most common childhood malignancy, but it comprises only 1–2% of lymphomas in the United States and Western Europe. The median age for all types of mature B-cell neoplasms is in the 6th and 7th decades, but mediastinal large B-cell

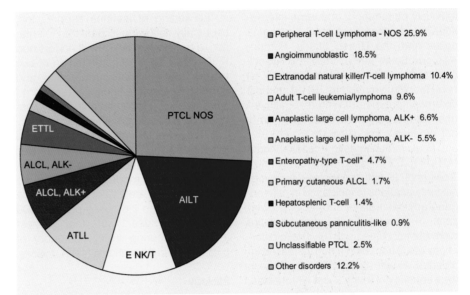

Fig. 8.07 Relative frequencies of mature T-cell lymphoma subtypes in an adult patient population. Significant differences exist in different geographic regions. However, peripheral T-cell lymphoma, not otherwise specified (NOS) and AITL are two of the most common subtypes internationally. * Note that the category of enteropathy-type T-cell lymphoma (ETTL)* used in this study was not equivalent to enteropathy-associated T-cell lymphoma (EATL) as defined in this monograph. ETTL was utilized largely as a generic category for most T-cell lymphomas involving the intestine, inclusive of EATL and γδ T-cell lymphomas. Data courtesy of J. Vose and The International Peripheral T-Cell Lymphoma Project {57A}.

lymphoma has a median age of ~35 years. Of the mature B-cell lymphomas, only Burkitt lymphoma and DLBCL occur with any significant frequency in children. Most types have a male predominance (52–55%), but mantle cell lymphoma has a striking male predominance (74%), while females predominate in follicular lymphoma (58%) and most particularly in primary mediastinal large B-cell lymphoma (66%). Primary mediastinal large B-cell lymphoma and classical Hodgkin lymphoma of the nodular sclerosis subtype have similar clinical profiles at presentation, most commonly affecting adolescent and young adult females. These common clinical features first prompted consideration that these lymphomas might be related {1870, 1944, 2265}

One major known risk factor for mature B-cell neoplasia appears to be an abnormality of the immune system, either immunodeficiency or autoimmune disease. Although evidence of immune system abnormalities are lacking in most patients with mature B-cell neoplasms, immunodeficient patients have a markedly increased incidence of B-cell neoplasia, particularly DLBCL and Burkitt lymphoma {193, 331, 1569}. Major forms of immunodeficiency currently include infection with the human immunodeficiency virus (HIV), iatrogenic immunosuppression to prevent

allograft rejection or graft versus host disease (GVHD) and primary immune deficiencies. Some autoimmune diseases are also associated with an increased risk of lymphoma, particularly B-cell lymphomas in patients with lymphoepithelial sialadenitis or Hashimoto thyroiditis {1114, 1116}. Mutations in genes controlling lymphocyte apoptosis have been linked to a risk for both autoimmune disease and lymphoma (mainly B-cell types). Patients with the autoimmune lymphoproliferative syndrome, which usually is caused by germline mutations in *FAS*, have an increased risk for B-cell lymphomas and Hodgkin lymphomas {2108}. Somatically acquired *FAS* gene mutations also have been reported in some sporadic B-cell lymphomas, most commonly marginal zone lymphomas {855}. Recent studies employing molecular epidemiology have identified polymorphisms in a number of immunoregulatory genes that appear to impact both risk of lymphoma and prognosis within a patient cohort {359A, 1248A, 2358C}. Molecular epidemiology is a relatively recent area of investigation and more data will be accumulated in the coming years. For example, a recent study found increased risk associated with polymorphisms in certain drug metabolizing enzymes {16A}.

Mature T-cell and NK-cell neoplasms are

relatively uncommon. In a large international study that evaluated lymphoma cases from the United States, Europe, Asia and South Africa, T-cell and NK-cell neoplasms accounted for only 12% of all non-Hodgkin lymphomas {51}. The most common subtypes of mature T-cell lymphomas are peripheral T-cell lymphoma, not otherwise specified (NOS) (25.9%) and angioimmunoblastic T-cell lymphoma (AITL) (18.5%), respectively {57A}.

T-cell and NK-cell lymphomas show significant variations in incidence in different geographical regions and racial populations. In general, T-cell lymphomas are more common in Asia {616}. These differences result from both a true increased incidence, as well as a relative decrease in the frequency of many B-cell lymphomas, such as follicular lymphoma. One of the main risk factors for T-cell lymphoma in Japan is the virus, human T-cell leukaemia virus type I (HTLV-I). In endemic regions of southwestern Japan, the seroprevalence of HTLV-I is 8–10%. The cumulative life-time risk for the development of adult T-cell leukaemia/lymphoma (ATLL) is 6.9% for a seropositive male and 2.9% for a seropositive female {683}. Other regions with a relatively high seroprevalence for HTLV-I include the Caribbean basin, where Blacks are primarily affected over other racial groups {760}. Differences in viral strain also may affect the incidence of the disease {523, 1345}.

Another major factor influencing the incidence of T-cell and NK-cell lymphomas is racial predisposition. EBV-associated NK and T-cell neoplasms, including extranodal NK/T-cell lymphoma, nasal type, aggressive NK leukaemia, and paediatric EBV+ T-cell and NK-cell lymphomas are much more common in Asians than they are in other races {27}. In Hong Kong, nasal NK/T-cell lymphoma is one of the more common subtypes, accounting for 8% of cases. By contrast, in Europe and North America, it accounts for less than 1% of all lymphomas. Other populations at increased risk for this disease are individuals of Native American descent in Central and South America, and Mexico {40, 341}, who are genetically related to Asians {892}. Finally, enteropathy-associated T-cell lymphoma is most common in individuals of Welsh and Irish descent, who share HLA haplotypes that confer an increased risk of gliadin allergy and susceptibility to gluten-sensitive enteropathy {548}. γδ PTCL occur with increased frequency

in the setting of immune suppression, especially following organ transplantation, a finding that is not well understood {758A, 1582A}. The combination of two factors, both immunosuppression and chronic antigenic stimulation, appear to increase risk. Hepatosplenic T-cell lymphomas are most common, but primary cutaneous and mucosa-associated T-cell lymphomas have been reported as well {331}. Recent data from the SEER program indicate a modest increase in the incidence of T-cell neoplasms in the United States to 2.6 cases per 100 000 persons per year, with the greatest increase occuring in the category of cutaneous T-cell lymphoma {492A, 1525A}.

Etiology

Infectious agents have been shown to contribute to the development of several types of mature B-cell, T-cell and NK-cell lymphomas. Epstein-Barr virus (EBV) is present in nearly 100% of endemic Burkitt lymphoma and in 15–35% of sporadic and HIV-associated cases {877, 1780A}, and it is involved in the pathogenesis of many B-cell lymphomas arising in immunosuppressed or elderly patients, including many post-transplant lymphoproliferative disorders, plasmablastic lymphoma and EBV+ large B-cell lymphoma of the elderly. EBV is also associated with extranodal NK/T-cell lymphoma and two paediatric T-cell lymphomas, systemic EBV+ T-cell LPD of childhood and hydroavacciniforme-like T-cell lymphoma. The exact cause of these EBV+ T-cell lymphomas of childhood is not clear. Risk factors may be either high viral load at presentation, or a defective immune response to the infection {1797}. Chronic active EBV infection may precede the development of some EBV+ T-cell lymphomas {1094, 1797}. In cases associated with chronic EBV infection, a polyclonal process may be seen early in the course, with progression to monoclonal EBV+ T-cell lymphoma {1094}.

Human herpesvirus-8 (HHV8) is found in primary effusion lymphoma and the lymphomas associated with multicentric Castleman disease, mainly seen in HIV-infected patients {372}. It is of interest that the same virus causes a number of B-cell lymphoproliferative disorders which differ in their clinical manifestations {617A}. Human T-cell leukaemia virus type I is the causative agent of adult T-cell lymphoma/ leukaemia, and is clonally integrated into

the genome of transformed T-cells {2148}. In this condition as in HHV8-associated disorders, a spectrum of clinical behaviours are seen, although most cases of ATLL are aggressive.

Hepatitis C virus has been implicated in some cases of lymphoplasmacytic lymphoma associated with type II cryoglobulinaemia, splenic marginal zone lymphoma, nodal marginal zone lymphoma and DLBCL {12A, 88A, 527A, 534A, 1073A, 1434, 1775A, 2506}. The role of the virus in tumour initiation is not clear. However, it does not directly infect neoplastic B-cells, and appears to influence lymphoma development through activation of a B-cell immune response.

Bacteria, or at least immune responses to bacterial antigens, have also been implicated in the pathogenesis of MALT lymphoma. These include *H. pylori* in gastric MALT lymphoma {998, 1587, 2444, 2445}, *B. burgdorferi* in cutaneous MALT lymphoma in Europe {192}, *Chlamydia psittaci*, *C. pneumoniae* and *C. trachomatis* in ocular adnexal MALT lymphomas in some geographic areas {394, 1898} and *Campylobacter jejuni* in intestinal MALT lymphoma associated with alpha heavy chain disease {1781, 1812}

Environmental exposures also have been linked to a risk of developing B-cell lymphoma. Epidemiological studies have implicated herbicide and pesticide use in the development of follicular lymphoma and DLBCL {460A, 903A}. Exposure to hair dyes had been identified as a risk factor in some older studies, but newer dye formations have removed potential carcinogens {2496A}.

Conclusion

The multiparameter approach to classification adopted by the WHO classification has been validated in international studies as being highly reproducible, and enhancing the interpretation of clinical and translational studies. In addition, accurate and precise classification of disease entities facilitates the discovery of the molecular basis of lymphoid neoplasms in the basic science laboratory {51, 1034, 1525A}.

CHAPTER 9

Precursor Lymphoid Neoplasms

B lymphoblastic leukaemia/lymphoma, not otherwise specified

B lymphoblastic leukaemia/lymphoma
with recurrent genetic abnormalities

T lymphoblastic leukaemia/lymphoma

B lymphoblastic leukaemia/lymphoma, not otherwise specified

M.J. Borowitz
J.K.C. Chan

Definition

B lymphoblastic leukaemia/lymphoblastic lymphoma is a neoplasm of precursor cells (lymphoblasts) committed to the B-cell lineage, typically composed of small to medium-sized blast cells with scant cytoplasm, moderately condensed to dispersed chromatin and inconspicuous nucleoli, involving bone marrow (BM) and blood (B acute lymphoblastic leukaemia/ALL) and occasionally presenting with primary involvement of nodal or extranodal sites (B lymphoblastic lymphoma/LBL). By convention, the term lymphoma is used when the process is confined to a mass lesion with no or minimal evidence of peripheral blood (PB) and BM involvement. With extensive BM and PB involvement, lymphoblastic leukaemia is the appropriate term. If the patient presents with a mass lesion and lymphoblasts in the BM, the distinction between leukaemia and lymphoma is arbitrary {1550}. For many treatment protocols, a figure of 25% BM blasts is used as the threshold for defining leukaemia. In contrast to myeloid leukaemias, there is no agreed-upon lower limit for the percentage of blasts required to establish a diagnosis of lymphoblastic leukaemias. In general, the diagnosis should be avoided when there are fewer than 20% blasts. Presentations with low blast counts can occur but are uncommon; currently there is no compelling evidence that failure to treat a patient when there are fewer than 20% BM lymphoblasts has an adverse effect on outcome.

The term B-ALL should not be used to indicate Burkitt leukaemia/lymphoma, in spite of its historical association with that lesion. Cases of B-ALL/LBL with recurrent genetic abnormalities are considered separately below.

ICD-O code

The provisional code proposed for the fourth edition of ICD-O is *9811/3*.

Epidemiology

Acute lymphoblastic leukaemia (ALL) is primarily a disease of children; 75% of cases occur in children under six years of age. The worldwide incidence is estimated at 1–4.75/100 000 persons per year {1827}. The estimated number of new cases in the United States in 2000 is approximately 3200, with approximately 80–85% being of precursor B-cell phenotype {1845, 2039}.

B-LBL constitutes ~10% of lymphoblastic lymphomas, and the remainder are of T lineage {242}. Approximately 64% of 98 cases reported in a literature review were less than 18 years of age {1367}. One report indicated a male predominance {1310}.

Etiology

Some translocations associated with B-ALL have been detected in neonatal specimens long before the onset of leukaemia, and monozygotic twins with concordant leukaemia frequently share genetic abnormalities {832, 1514}, suggesting a genetic component to at least some cases. Many of these translocations appear to be primary initiating events.

Sites of involvement

By definition, BM is involved in all cases classified as B-ALL, and PB is usually involved. Extramedullary involvement is frequent, with particular predilection for the central nervous system, lymph nodes, spleen, liver and testis in males. The most frequent sites of involvement in B-LBL are the skin, soft tissue, bone and lymph nodes {202, 1310, 1367}. Mediastinal masses are infrequent {202, 1367, 1928}.

Clinical features

Most patients with B-ALL present with evidence and consequences of BM failure: thrombocytopenia and/or anaemia and/or neutropenia. The leukocyte count may be decreased, normal or markedly elevated. Lymphadenopathy, hepatomegaly and splenomegaly are frequent. Bone pain and arthralgias may be prominent. Patients with B-LBL without leukaemia are usually asymptomatic, and most have limited stage disease. Head and neck presentations are particularly common, especially in children. Marrow and PB involvement may be present, but the

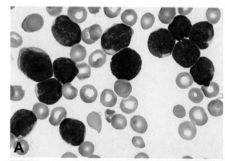

Fig. 9.01 B lymphoblastic leukaemia. Bone marrow smear. **A** Several lymphoblasts with a high nuclear/cytoplasmic ratio and variably condensed nuclear chromatin. **B** B lymphoblasts containing numerous coarse azurophilic granules.

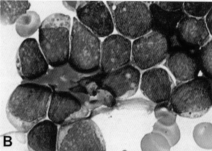

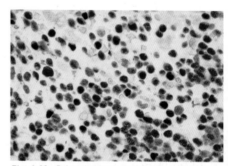

Fig. 9.02 B lymphoblastic leukaemia. Immunohistochemical demonstration of nuclear TdT in a bone marrow biopsy.

percentage of lymphoblasts in the BM is <25% {1310, 1367}.

Morphology

The lymphoblasts in B-ALL/LBL in smear and imprint preparations vary from small blasts with scant cytoplasm, condensed nuclear chromatin and indistinct nucleoli to larger cells with moderate amounts of light blue to blue-grey cytoplasm, occasionally vacuolated, dispersed nuclear chromatin and multiple variably prominent nucleoli. The nuclei are round, irregular or convoluted. Coarse azurophilic granules are present in some lymphoblasts in approximately 10% of cases. In some cases, the lymphoblasts have a cytoplasmic pseudopod (hand mirror cells). In most cases the morphology of the lymphoblasts differs from that of normal B-cell precursors (haematogones) with which they may be confused. The latter typically have even higher nucleus/cytoplasm (N/C) ratios, more homogeneous chromatin and no discernible nucleoli.

In BM biopsies, the lymphoblasts in B-ALL are relatively uniform in appearance with round to oval, indented or convoluted nuclei. Nucleoli range from inconspicuous to prominent. The chromatin is finely dispersed. The number of mitotic figures varies. Lymphoblastic lymphoma is generally characterized by a diffuse, or less commonly, paracortical pattern of involvement of lymph node or other tissue. A single-file pattern of infiltration of soft tissues is common. Mitotic figures are usually numerous and in some cases there may be a focal "starry sky" pattern. The morphologic features of B and T lymphoblastic proliferations are indistinguishable.

Cytochemistry

Cytochemistry seldom contributes to the diagnosis of ALL. Lymphoblasts are negative for myeloperoxidase. Granules, if present, may stain light grey with Sudan Black-B staining but are less intense than myeloblasts. Lymphoblasts may show PAS positivity, usually in the form of coarse granules. Lymphoblasts may react with non-specific esterase with a multifocal punctate or Golgi zone pattern that shows variable inhibition with sodium fluoride.

Immunophenotype

The lymphoblasts in B-ALL/LBL are almost always positive for the B-cell markers CD19, cytoplasmic CD79a and cytoplasmic CD22; while none of these by itself is specific, positivity in combination or at high intensity strongly supports the B lineage. The lymphoblasts are positive for CD10, surface CD22, CD24, PAX5 and TdT in most cases, while CD20 and CD34 expression is variable; CD45 may be absent. The myeloid-associated antigens CD13 and CD33 may be expressed, and the presence of these myeloid markers does not exclude the diagnosis of B-ALL. In tissue sections, CD79a and PAX5 are most frequently used to demonstrate B-cell differentiation, but the former reacts with some cases of T-ALL and is not specific {906}. PAX5 is generally considered the most sensitive and specific marker for B lineage in sections {2251} but it is also positive in cases of AML with t(8;21) and rarely in other AML {2285}. Myeloperoxidase expression in leukaemic cells detected with anti-MPO antibodies excludes this diagnosis and would indicate either acute myeloid leukaemia or B/myeloid leukaemia.

The degree of differentiation of B-lineage lymphoblasts has clinical and genetic correlates. In the earliest stage, so called early precursor B-ALL or pro-B-ALL, the blasts express CD19, cytoplasmic CD79a, cytoplasmic CD22 and nuclear TdT. In the intermediate stage, so called common ALL, the blasts express CD10. In the most mature precursor B differentiation stage, so called pre-B-ALL, the blasts express cytoplasmic μ chains (c-μ). Surface immunoglobulin is characteristically absent although its presence does not exclude the possibility of B-ALL/LBL {1584}, provided that other immunophenotypic features, morphology and cytogenetics are consistent with B-ALL. Although CD10-positivity is seen both in B-ALL and in normal haematogones, the immunophenotype of precursor B-ALL differs in almost all cases from that seen in normal B-cell precursors. The latter show a continuum of expression of markers of B-cell maturation, including surface Ig light chain, and display a reproducible pattern of acquisition and loss of normal antigens {1442}. In contrast, cases of B-ALL show patterns that differ from normal with either overexpression or underexpression of many markers including CD10, CD45, CD38, CD58 or TdT, among others {326, 401, 1342, 2372}. These differences can be very useful in evaluation of followup BM specimens for minimal residual disease.

Genetics

Antigen receptor genes

Nearly all cases of B-ALL have clonal DJ rearrangements of the *IGH@* gene. In addition, T-cell receptor gene rearrangements may be seen in a significant proportion of cases (up to 70%) {2294} so that these rearrangements are not helpful for lineage assignment.

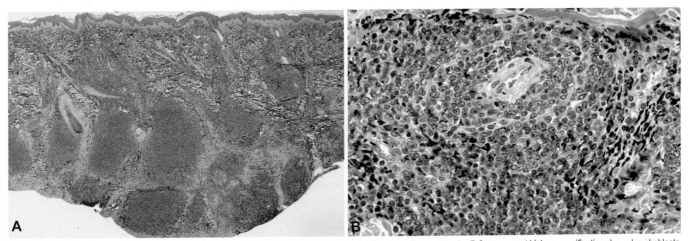

Fig. 9.03 B lymphoblastic lymphoma. **A** Skin. The neoplastic cells diffusely infiltrate the dermis with sparing of the epidermis. **B** Same case at higher magnification shows lymphoblasts surrounding a blood vessel.

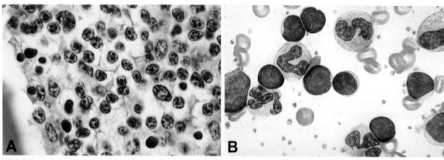
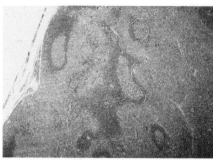

Fig. 9.04 Increased haematogones. **A** Bone marrow section. **B** Bone marrow smear from an eight year-old male, showing lymphoid cells with a high nuclear/cytoplasmic ratio and homogeneous nuclear chromatin; nucleoli are not observed or are indistinct. These cells resemble the lymphoblasts in ALL of childhood.

Fig. 9.05 B lymphoblastic leukaemia. Lymph node. The neoplastic cells infiltrate diffusely sparing normal follicles.

Cytogenetic abnormalities and oncogenes
Cytogenetic abnormalities are seen in the majority of cases of B-ALL/LBL; in many cases they define specific entities with unique phenotypic and prognostic features. These cases are considered separately. Additional genetic lesions that are not associated with these entities include del(6q), del(9p), del(12p), though these do not have an impact on prognosis. Some genetic lesions that may be associated with poor prognosis include the very rare t(17;19); *E2A-HLF* ALL and the intrachromosomal amplification of the *AML1* gene on chromosome 21 (iAMP21), which accounts for about 5% of cases of ALL {1510}. The latter is being recognized with increasing frequency with the increased

use of FISH studies to detect *TEL-AML1* translocations, because it can be detected with the same *AML1* probe.

Postulated normal counterpart
Depending upon the specific leukaemia, B-ALL arises in either a haematopoietic stem cell or a B-cell progenitor.

Prognosis and predictive factors
B-ALL has a good prognosis in children, but it is less favourable in adults. In children, the overall complete remission rate is >95% and in adults 60–85%. Approximately 80% of children with B-ALL appear to be cured, while this figure is less than 50% for adults. More intensive therapy makes a difference in cure rates, and

there is some evidence for younger adults at least, that therapy with more intensive "paediatric-type" regimens is associated with better outcome {233, 872}. Infancy, increasing age (>10 years), higher white blood cell count, slow response to initial therapy as assessed by morphologic examination of PB and/or BM, and the presence of minimal residual disease after therapy are all associated with adverse prognosis {488, 679, 1976, 2023, 2093, 2295}. The presence of CNS disease at diagnosis is associated with adverse outcome, and requires specific therapy {446}. The prognosis of B-LBL is also considered relatively favourable, and as with B-ALL appears better in children than adults {1367}.

B lymphoblastic leukaemia/lymphoma with recurrent genetic abnormalities

M.J. Borowitz
J.K.C. Chan

This group of diseases is characterized by recurrent genetic abnormalities, including balanced translocations and other chromosomal abnormalities. Many chromosomal abnormalities that are non-randomly associated with B acute lymphoblastic leukaemia (B-ALL) are not included as separate entities in this section. While inclusion or exclusion of a genetic "entity" is somewhat arbitrary, those lesions that are specifically mentioned are chosen because they are associated with distinctive clinical or phenotypic properties, have important prognostic implications, demonstrate other evidence that they are biologically distinct and are generally mutually exclusive with other entities.

B Lymphoblastic leukaemia/lymphoma with t(9;22)(q34;q11.2); BCR-ABL1

Definition
A neoplasm of lymphoblasts committed to the B-cell lineage in which the blasts harbour a translocation between the BCR gene on chromosome 22 and the ABL1 oncogene on chromosome 9.

ICD-O code
The provisional code proposed for the fourth edition of ICD-O is 9812/3.

Epidemiology and clinical features
Presenting features are generally similar to those of other patients with B-ALL. BCR-ABL1 associated ("Ph+") ALL is relatively more common in adults than children, accounting for about 25% of adult ALL but only 2–4% of childhood ALL. Most children with Ph+ B-ALL would be considered "high risk" by standard age and white blood cell (WBC) features, but there are otherwise no characteristic clinical findings. Though patients with t(9;22) B-ALL may have organ involvement, lymphomatous presentations are rare.

Morphology and cytochemistry
There are no unique morphologic or cytochemical features that distinguish this from other types of ALL.

Immunophenotype
B-ALL with t(9;22) is typically CD10+ CD19+ and TdT+. There is more frequent expression of myeloid-associated antigens CD13 and CD33 {985}; CD117 is typically not expressed. CD25 is highly associated with t(9;22) B-ALL, at least in adults {1679}. Rare cases of t(9;22) ALL have a T precursor phenotype.

Genetics
The t(9;22) results from fusion of BCR at 22q11.2 and the cytoplasmic tyrosine kinase gene ABL1 at 9q34, with production of a BCR-ABL1 fusion protein. In most childhood cases of ALL with the t(9;22), a p190 kd BCR-ABL1 fusion protein is produced. In adults, about one half of cases of ALL with the t(9,22) produce the p210 kd fusion protein that is present in chronic myelogenous leukaemia (CML), and the remainder produce the p190. No definite clinical differences have been attributed to these two different gene products. The t(9;22) may be associated with other genetic abnormalities, including rare cases that might otherwise cause a case to be placed in one of the other categories below. It is generally considered that clinical features in such cases are governed by the presence of the t(9;22).

Postulated normal counterpart
There is some suggestion that the cell of origin of t(9;22) ALL is more immature than that of other B-ALL cases {452}.

Prognosis and predictive factors
In both children and adults, t(9;22) ALL has the worst prognosis among patients with ALL. Its higher frequency in adult ALL explains in part but not completely the relatively poorer outcome of adults with ALL. In children, the presence of favourable clinical features including age, white count and response to therapy, is associated with somewhat better outcome {77}, although prognosis is still considered relatively poor. Treatment with imatinib in addition to high-dose chemotherapy has been reported to improve early event-free survival {1975}.

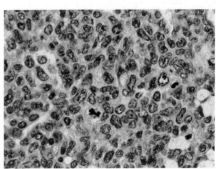

Fig. 9.06 This bone marrow from an adult with t(9;22) positive B-ALL is completely replaced by lymphoblasts. Mitotic figures are numerous.

B Lymphoblastic leukaemia/lymphoma with t(v;11q23); MLL rearranged

Definition
A neoplasm of lymphoblasts committed to the B lineage that harbours a translocation between the MLL gene at band 11q23 and any one of a large number of different fusion partners. Patients with leukaemias that have deletions of 11q23 without MLL rearrangements are not included in this group.

ICD-O code
The provisional code proposed for the fourth edition of ICD-O is 9813/3.

Etiology
While the specific etiology of leukaemia with MLL translocations is unknown, this translocation may occur in utero, with a short latency between the translocation and development of disease. Evidence for this includes the fact that these leukaemias are frequent in very young infants, as well as the fact that this translocation has been identified in neonatal blood spots of patients who subsequently develop leukaemia {745}.

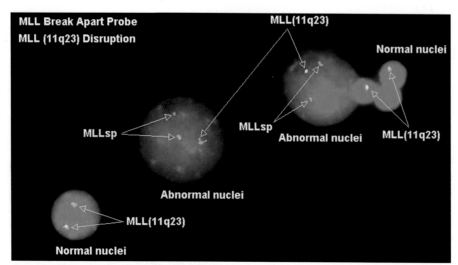

Fig. 9.07 B lymphoblastic leukaemia/lymphoma with *MLL* rearrangement. FISH study using an *MLL* breakapart probe. The normal *MLL* gene "MLL(11q23)" appears as a juxtaposed red and green, or sometimes yellow signal. The translocation is demonstrated by separation of the red and green probes ("MLLsp") (Courtesy of Dr. AJ Carroll).

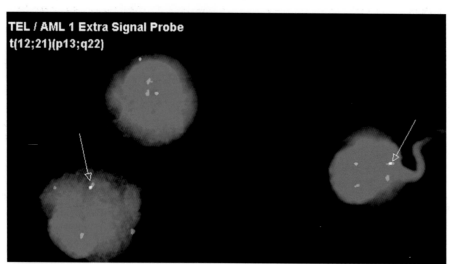

Fig. 9.08 B lymphoblastic leukaemia/lymphoma with t(12;21) (p13;q22); *TEL/AML1* (*ETV6-RUNX1*) FISH study using a red probe against *RUNX1* and a green probe against *ETV6*. The normal genes appear as isolated red or green signals, while evidence of the fusion gene (arrows) appears as a yellow signal. (Courtesy of Dr. AJ Carroll).

Epidemiology and clinical features

ALL with *MLL* rearrangements is the most common leukaemia in infants <1 year of age. It is less common in older children and increases with age into adulthood. Typically patients with this leukaemia present with very high white blood cell counts, frequently >100x10⁹/L. There is also a high frequency of CNS involvement at diagnosis. While organ involvement may be seen, pure lymphomatous presentations are not typical.

Morphology and cytochemistry

There are no unique morphologic or cytochemical features that distinguish this from other types of ALL. In some cases of leukaemias with *MLL* rearrangements it may be possible to recognize distinct lymphoblastic and monoblastic populations, which can be confirmed by immunophenotyping; such cases should be considered B/myeloid leukaemias.

Immunophenotype

ALL with *MLL* translocations, and most especially t(4;11) ALL typically have a CD19+, CD10-negative, CD24-negative pro-B immunophenotype, also positive for CD15 {985, 1691}. The chondroitin sulfate proteo-glycan neural-glial antigen 2 (NG2) is also characteristically expressed and is relatively, though not absolutely, specific.

Genetics

The *MLL* gene on chromosome 11q23 has many fusion partners. The most common partner gene is *AF4* on chromosome 4q21. Other common partner genes include *ENL* on chromosome 19p13 and *AF9* on chromosome 9p22. *MLL-ENL* fusions are also common in T-ALL, and fusions between *MLL* and *AF9* are more typically associated with myeloid leukaemia. Leukaemias with *MLL* translocations are frequently associated with overexpression of *FLT-3* {80}. Cases with deletions of 11q23 are not included in this group of leukaemias as they appear not to share the same clinical, phenotypic or prognostic features.

Prognosis and predictive factors

Leukaemias with the *MLL-AF4* translocation have a poor prognosis. There is some controversy as to whether leukaemias with translocations other than the *MLL-AF4* rearrangement have as poor a prognosis as those that do. Infants with *MLL* translocations, particularly those <6 months of age, have a particularly poor prognosis.

B Lymphoblastic leukaemia/lymphoma with t(12;21)(p13;q22); TEL-AML1 (ETV6-RUNX1)

Definition

A neoplasm of lymphoblasts committed to the B lineage with a translocation between the *TEL* (*ETV6*) gene on chromosome 12 with the *AML1* (*RUNX1*) gene on chromosome 12.

ICD-O code

The provisional code proposed for the fourth edition of ICD-O is *9814/3*.

Epidemiology and clinical features

This leukaemia is common in children, accounting for about 25% of cases of B-ALL. It is not seen in infants and decreases in frequency in older children to the point that it is rare in adulthood. Presenting features are generally similar to those of other patients with ALL.

Morphology and cytochemistry

There are no unique morphologic or cytochemical features that distinguish this from other types of ALL.

Immunophenotype

Blasts have a CD19+, CD10+ phenotype and are most often CD34+; other phenotypic features, including near or complete absence of CD9, CD20 and CD66c {245, 533, 985}, are relatively but not absolutely specific. Myeloid-associated antigens, especially CD13, are frequently expressed, but this does not indicate mixed phenotype acute leukaemia {155}.

Genetics

The t(12;21)(p13;q22); *ETV6-RUNX1* translocation results in the production of a fusion protein that likely acts in a dominant negative fashion to interfere with normal function of the transcription factor RUNX1. This leukaemia appears to possess a unique gene expression signature {2469}. The *ETV6-RUNX1* translocation is considered to be an early lesion in leukaemogenesis, as evidenced by studies of neonatal blood spots that have shown the presence of the translocation in children who develop leukaemia many years later {2400}. There is evidence that the translocation is necessary but not sufficient for the development of leukaemia {2400}.

Postulated normal counterpart

This leukaemia appears to derive from a B-cell progenitor rather than from a haematopoietic stem cell {344}.

Prognosis and predictive factors

B-ALL with the *TEL-AML1* translocation has a very favourable prognosis with cures seen in >90% of children, especially if they have other favourable risk factors. Relapses often occur much later than those of other types of ALL. Because this translocation appears to occur as an early event, it has been suggested that some late relapses in fact derive from persistent "preleukaemic" clones that harbour the translocation and undergo additional genetic events after the first leukaemic clone has been eliminated {719}. Children with this leukaemia who also harbour adverse prognostic factors, such as age over 10 years or high white count do not have as good a prognosis, but may still fare better as a group than other patients with these same adverse factors.

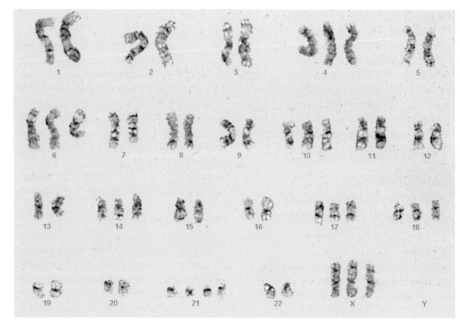

Fig. 9.09 Hyperdiploid ALL. G banded karyotype showing 55 chromosomes, including trisomies of 4, 10 and 17 and tetrasomy 21. There are no structural abnormalities. (Courtesy of Dr. AJ Carroll).

B Lymphoblastic leukaemia/ lymphoma with hyperdiploidy

Definition

A neoplasm of lymphoblasts committed to the B lineage whose blasts contain >50 and usually <66 chromosomes, typically without translocations or other structural alterations. There is controversy as to whether specific chromosomal additions, rather than the specific number of chromosomes, should be part of the definition {894, 1806, 2123}.

ICD-O code

The provisional code proposed for the fourth edition of ICD-O is *9815/3*.

Synonyms

Hyperdiploid ALL; high hyperdiploid ALL; ALL with favourable trisomies.

Epidemiology

This leukaemia is common in children, accounting for about 25% of cases of B-ALL. It is not seen in infants, and decreases in frequency in older children to the point that it is rare in adulthood.

Clinical features

Presenting features are generally similar to those of other patients with ALL.

Morphology and cytochemistry

There are no unique morphologic or cytochemical features that distinguish this from other types of ALL.

Immunophenotype

Blasts are CD19+, CD10+, and express other markers typical of B-ALL. Most cases are CD34+ and CD45 is often absent {985}. Patients with T-ALL with hyperdiploidy should not be considered part of this group, though most such patients have near tetraploid karyotypes.

Genetics

Hyperdiploid B-ALL contains a numerical increase in chromosomes, usually without structural abnormalities. Extra copies of chromosomes are non random, with chromosomes 21, X, 14 and 4 being the most common and chromosomes 1, 2 and 3 being the least often seen {915}. Hyperdiploid B-ALL may be detected by standard karyotyping, FISH or flow cytometric DNA index {1401}. Some cases that appear as hyperdiploid ALL by standard karyotyping may in fact represent hypodiploid ALL that has undergone endoreduplication, doubling the number of chromosomes. Specific chromosomes that appear as trisomies may be more important to prognosis than the actual number of chromosomes, with simultaneous trisomies of 4, 10 and 17 carrying the best prognosis {2123}.

Prognosis and predictive factors

Hyperdiploid B-ALL has a very favourable prognosis with cures seen in >90% of children, especially if their risk profile is favourable. Presence of adverse factors, such as advanced age or high white count may adversely affect the prognosis, but patients may not fare as badly as others without this favourable abnormality.

B Lymphoblastic leukaemia/lymphoma with hypodiploidy (Hypodiploid ALL)

Definition

A neoplasm of lymphoblasts committed to the B lineage whose blasts contain <46 chromosomes. A stricter definition of <45 chromosomes, and possibly even <44 chromosomes, more accurately reflects the clinical pathologic entity {1554}.

ICD-O code

The provisional code proposed for the fourth edition of ICD-O is 9816/3.

Epidemiology and clinical features

Hypodiploid ALL accounts for about 5% of ALL overall, but if the definition is restricted to those with <45 chromosomes the figure is closer to 1%. It is seen in both children and adults, although near haploid ALL (23–29 chromosomes) appears limited to childhood. Presenting features are generally similar to those of other patients with ALL.

Morphology and cytochemistry

There are no unique morphologic or cytochemical features that distinguish this from other types of ALL.

Immunophenotype

Blasts have a B-precursor phenotype, typically CD19+, CD10+ but there are no other distinctive phenotypic features.

Genetics

All patients by definition show loss of one or more chromosomes, having from 45 chromosomes to near haploid. Structural abnormalities may be seen in the remaining chromosomes though there are no specific abnormalities that are characteristically associated. Structural abnormalities are uncommon in near-haploid B-ALL. The diagnosis of near haploid or low hypodiploid B-ALL may be missed by standard karyotyping because the hypodiploid clone may undergo endoreduplication, doubling the number of chromosomes, resulting in a near diploid or hyperdiploid karyotype. Flow cytometry can generally detect a clone with a DNA index <1.0, though this may be a minor population. FISH may also detect cells hypodiploid for certain chromosomes, and this diagnosis should be suspected when there is a discrepancy between karyotype and FISH results with respect to the number of chromosomes present.

Prognosis and predictive features.

Hypodiploid B-ALL has a poor prognosis. The prognosis depends on the number of chromosomes: those with 44–45 chromosomes have the best prognosis{1554}, and those with near haploid B-ALL fare worst in some but not all studies {900, 1554}. There is some evidence that, in contrast to other types of B-ALL, patients may fare poorly even if they do not have minimal residual disease following therapy.

B Lymphoblastic leukaemia/lymphoma with t(5;14)(q31;q32); IL3-IGH

Definition

A neoplasm of lymphoblasts committed to the B lineage in which the blasts harbour a translocation between the IL3 gene and the IGH@ gene, resulting in a variable eosinophilia. This diagnosis may be made based on immunophenotypic and genetic findings even if the bone marrow (BM) blast count is low.

ICD-O code

The provisional code proposed for the fourth edition of ICD-O is 9817/3.

Epidemiology and clinical features

This is a rare disease, accounting for <1% of cases of ALL. It has been reported in both children and adults. Presenting clinical characteristics may be similar to other patients with ALL, or patients may present with an asymptomatic eosinophilia, and blasts may not even be present in the PB to raise the suspicion of leukaemia.

Morphology and cytochemistry

Blasts in this neoplasm have the typical morphology of lymphoblasts, but the striking finding is the presence of an increase in circulating eosinophils. This is a reactive population and not part of the leukaemic clone.

Immunophenotype

Blasts have a CD19+CD10+ phenotype. Finding even small numbers of blasts with this phenotype in a patient with eosinophilia should strongly suggest this diagnosis.

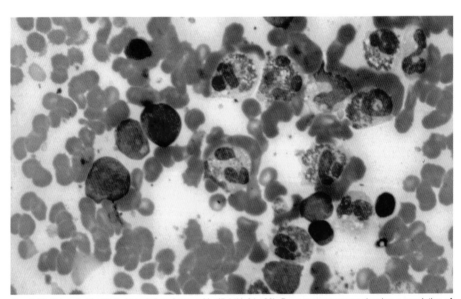

Fig. 9.10 B lymphoblastic leukaemia/lymphoma with t(5;14)(q31;q32). Bone marrow smear showing a population of typical lymphoblasts along with numerous mature eosinophils. The granule distribution in some of the eosinophils is unusual, but this is not a consistent factor.

Genetics

The unique characteristics of this neoplasm derive from a functional re-arrangement between the *IL3* gene on chromosome 5 and the *IGH@* gene on chromosome 14, resulting in constitutive overexpression of the *IL3* gene {846}. Functional consequences of this re-arrangement other than eosinophilia, if any, are not well understood. The abnormality is typically detected by standard karyotyping; it can also be detected by FISH, though appropriate probes are not widely available.

Prognosis and predictive features

The prognosis is not considered to be different from other cases of ALL, though there are too few cases to be certain. Blast percentage at diagnosis is not known to be a predictive factor.

B Lymphoblastic leukaemia/ lymphoma with t(1;19) (q23;p13.3); E2A-PBX1 (TCF3-PBX1)

Definition

This is a neoplasm of lymphoblasts committed to the B lineage with a t(1;19) translocation between the *E2A(TCF3)* gene on chromosome 19 and the *PBX1* gene on chromosome 1.

ICD-O code

The provisional code proposed for the fourth edition of ICD-O is *9818/3*.

Epidemiology and clinical features

This leukaemia is relatively common in children, accounting for about 6% of cases of B-ALL. It is also seen in adults, but not at as high a frequency. Presenting features are generally similar to those of other patients with ALL.

Morphology and cytochemistry

There are no unique morphologic or cytochemical features that distinguish this from other types of ALL.

Immunophenotype

Blasts typically have a CD19+,CD10+ cytoplasmic μ (cμ) heavy chain-positive pre-B-cell phenotype, although not all cases of pre-B-ALL have the t(1;19). This leukaemia can be suspected even when cμ is not determined as these leukaemias typically show strong expression of CD9 and lack CD34, or show very limited CD34 expression on only a minor subset of leukaemic cells {244}.

Genetics

The *E2A-PBX1* translocation results in the production of a fusion protein that has an oncogenic role as a transcriptional activator, and also likely interferes with the normal function of the transcription factors coded by *E2A* and *PBX1* {1262}. The functional fusion gene resides on chromosome 19, and there may be loss of the derivative chromosome 1 in some but not all cases, resulting in an unbalanced translocation. Gene expression profiling studies have shown a unique signature to this lesion {2469}. An alternative *E2A* translocation t(17;19) occurs in rare cases of ALL involving the *HLF* gene on chromosome 17 and is associated with a dismal prognosis. Thus demonstration of an *E2A* rearrangement by itself is not a diagnostic criterion for this leukaemia. A subset of B-ALL, usually hyperdiploid B-ALL, has a karyotypically identical t(1;19) translocation that involves neither *E2A* nor *PBX1* and should not be confused with this entity. Cases of B-ALL with t(1;19) that lack the expected phenotype probably do not represent *E2A-PBX1* B-ALL.

Prognosis and predictive features

In early studies, *E2A-PBX1* was associated with a poor prognosis, but this is now readily overcome with modern intensive therapy. Many treatment protocols no longer require identification of this genetic lesion, but the findings of unique immunophenotypic and genetic features supports its inclusion as a distinct entity.

T lymphoblastic leukaemia/lymphoma

M.J. Borowitz
J.K.C. Chan

Definition

T lymphoblastic leukaemia/ lymphoblastic lymphoma is a neoplasm of lymphoblasts committed to the T-cell lineage, typically composed of small to medium-sized blast cells with scant cytoplasm, moderately condensed to dispersed chromatin and inconspicuous nucleoli, involving bone marrow (BM) and blood (T-acute lymphoblastic leukaemia, T-ALL) or presenting with primary involvement of thymus, nodal or extranodal sites (T-acute lymphoblastic lymphoma, T-LBL). By convention, the term lymphoma is used when the process is confined to a mass lesion with no or minimal evidence of peripheral blood (PB) and BM involvement. With extensive BM and PB involvement, lymphoblastic leukaemia is the appropriate term. If the patient presents with a mass lesion and lymphoblasts in the BM, the distinction between leukaemia and lymphoma is arbitrary. For many treatment protocols, a figure of >25% BM blasts is used as the threshold for defining leukaemia. In contrast to myeloid leukaemias, there is no agreed-upon lower limit for the percentage of blasts required to establish a diagnosis of ALL. In general, the diagnosis should be avoided when there are <20% blasts.

ICD-O code

The provisional code proposed for the fourth edition of ICD-O is *9837/3*.

Epidemiology

T-ALL comprises about 15% of childhood ALL; it is more common in adolescents than in younger children and more common in males than in females. T-ALL comprises approximately 25% of cases of adult ALL. T-LBL comprises approximately 85–90% of all lymphoblastic lymphomas; similar to its leukaemic counterpart, it is most frequent in adolescent males but may be seen in any age group.

Etiology

One study reported T-ALL in monozygotic twins that share the same T-cell receptor gene rearrangement {720}, suggesting

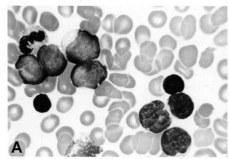 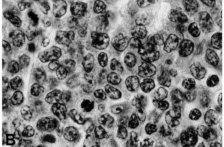

Fig. 9.11 T-lymphoblastic leukaemia. **A** Blood smear. The lymphoblasts vary in size from large cells to small cells with a very high nuclear/cytoplasmic ratio. **B** Bone marrow section.

an *in utero* origin of the earliest genetic lesions.

Sites of involvement

The BM is involved in all cases of T-ALL, and in contrast to B-ALL, aleukaemic presentations in the face of BM replacement are uncommon. T-LBL frequently shows mediastinal (thymic) involvement, though it may involve any lymph node or extranodal site. Skin, tonsil, liver, spleen, central nervous system and testis in males may be involved, although presentation at these sites without nodal or mediastinal involvement is uncommon.

Clinical features

T-ALL typically presents with a high leukocyte count, and often a large mediastinal mass or other tissue mass. Lymphadenopathy and hepatosplenomegaly are common. For a given leukocyte count and tumour burden, T-ALL patients often show relative sparing of normal BM haematopoiesis compared with B-ALL.

T-LBL frequently presents with a mass in the anterior mediastinum, often exhibiting rapid growth, and sometimes presenting as a respiratory emergency. Pleural effusions are common.

Morphology

The lymphoblasts in T-ALL/LBL are morphologically indistinguishable from those of B-ALL/LBL. In smears, the cells are of medium size with a high nuclear/ cytoplasmic ratio; there may be a considerable size range from small lymphoblasts

with very condensed nuclear chromatin and no evident nucleoli to larger blasts with finely dispersed chromatin and relatively prominent nucleoli. Nuclei range from round to irregular to convoluted. Cytoplasmic vacuoles may be present. Occasionally blasts of T-ALL may resemble more mature lymphocytes; in such cases immunophenotypic studies may be required to distinguish this disease from a mature (peripheral) T-cell leukaemia.

In BM sections the lymphoblasts have a high nuclear/cytoplasmic ratio, thin nuclear membrane, finely-stippled chromatin and inconspicuous nucleoli. The number of mitotic figures is reported to be higher in T-ALL than B-ALL. In T-LBL, the lymph node generally shows complete effacement of architecture and involvement of the capsule. Partial involvement in a paracortical location with sparing of germinal centres may occur. Sometimes, a multinodular pattern is produced due to stretching of the fibrous framework, mimicking follicular lymphoma. A starry-sky effect may be present, thus sometimes resembling Burkitt lymphoma, although typically the nucleoli and cytoplasm are less prominent. The blasts can have round or convoluted nuclei. Mitotic figures are often numerous. In the thymus, there is extensive replacement of the thymic parenchyma and permeative infiltration. Cases with histological findings of T-LBL with a significant infiltrate of eosinophils among the lymphoma cells may be associated with eosinophilia and myeloid hyperplasia and a 8p11.2 cytogenetic abnormality involving the *FGFR1* gene {3, 1006} (See Chapter 3).

Cytochemistry
T lymphoblasts frequently show focal acid phosphatase activity in smear and imprint preparations, though this is not specific.

Immunophenotype
The lymphoblasts in T-ALL/LBL are usually TdT positive and variably express CD1a, CD2, CD3, CD4, CD5, CD7 and CD8. Of these, CD7 and cytoplasmic CD3 (cCD3) are most often positive, but of these only CD3 is considered lineage specific. CD4 and CD8 are frequently co-expressed on the blasts, and CD10 may be positive. These latter phenotypes are not specific for T-ALL as CD4 and CD8 double positivity may be seen in T-PLL and CD10 in peripheral T-cell lymphomas, most commonly angioimmunoblastic T-cell lymphoma. In addition to TdT, the most specific markers to indicate the precursor nature of T lymphoblasts are CD99, CD34 and CD1a; the first of these is most useful {1852}. In 29–48% of cases, there is nuclear staining for TAL-1, but this does not necessarily correlate with presence of *TAL-1* gene alteration {407, 543}.

CD79a positivity has been observed in approximately 10% of cases {1750}. One or both of the myeloid associated antigens CD13 and CD33 are expressed in 19–32% of cases {1139, 2277}. CD117 (c-kit) is occasionally positive; such cases have been associated with activating mutations of *FLT3* {1677}. The presence of myeloid markers does not exclude the diagnosis of T-ALL/LBL, nor does it indicate

mixed phenotype T/myeloid leukaemia. Many markers characteristic of immature T-cells such as CD7 and CD2, and even CD5 and cCD3 may also be seen in natural killer cell precursors {2070}. Thus it may be very difficult to distinguish the rare true NK precursor ALL from T-ALL that expresses only immature markers. CD56 expression, while characteristic of NK-cells, does not exclude T-cell leukaemia. T-ALL/LBL can be stratified into different stages of intrathymic differentiation according to the antigens expressed: pro-T (cCD3 +, CD7+, CD2-, CD1a-, CD34+/-); pre-T (cCD3+, CD7+, CD2+, CD1a-, CD34+/-); cortical T (cCD3 +, CD7+, CD2+, CD1a+, CD34-) and medullary T (cCD3+, CD7+, CD2+, CD1a-, CD34-, surface CD3+). The pro-T and pre-T stages are double-negative for CD4 and CD8, and the cortical T stage shows a double-positive (CD4+ CD8+) phenotype. The medullary T stage expresses only either CD4 or CD8 {187, 879}. Some studies have shown a correlation between the stages of T-cell differentiation and survival {500}. T-ALL tends to show a more immature immunophenotype compared with T-LBL, but the groups overlap {2376}.

Genetics
Antigen receptor genes
T-ALL/LBL almost always shows clonal rearrangements of the T-cell receptor genes *(TCR)*, but there is simultaneous presence of *IGH@* gene rearrangements in approximately 20% of cases {1749, 2138}.

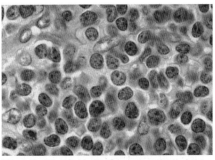

Fig. 9.13 T lymphoblastic leukaemia. In this example, the lymphoblasts lack nuclear convolutions. The chromatin is finely stippled.

Cytogenetic abnormalities and oncogenes
An abnormal karyotype is found in 50–70% of cases of T-ALL/LBL {830, 879}. The most common recurrent cytogenetic abnormality involves the alpha and delta *TCR* loci at 14q11.2, the beta locus at 7q35, and the gamma locus at 7p14-15, with a variety of partner genes {830, 879}. In most cases, these translocations lead to a dysregulation of transcription of the partner gene by juxtaposition with the regulatory region of one of the *TCR* loci. The most commonly involved genes include the transcription factors *HOX11* (*TLX1*) (10q24) occurring in 7% of childhood and 30% of adult T-ALL, and *HOX11L2* (*TLX3*) (5q35), occurring in 20% of childhood cases and 10–15% of adult {830}. Other transcription factors that may be involved in translocations include *MYC* (8q24.1), *TAL1* (1p32), *RBTN1* (*LMO1*) (11p15), *RBTN2* (*LMO2*) (11p13) and *LYL1* (19p13) {519, 830}. The cytoplasmic tyrosine kinase *LCK* (1p34.3-35) can also be

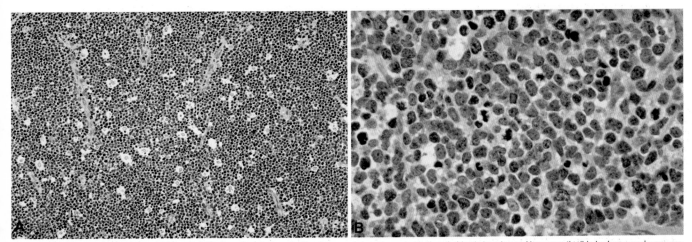

Fig. 9.12 T lymphoblastic lymphoma. **A** Low magnification of a lymph node showing complete replacement by lymphoblastic lymphoma. Numerous tingible body macrophages are scattered throughout the node. **B** High magnification of the specimen in (**A**) showing lymphoblasts with round to oval to irregularly-shaped nuclei with dispersed chromatin and distinct but not unusually prominent nucleoli. Several mitotic figures are present.

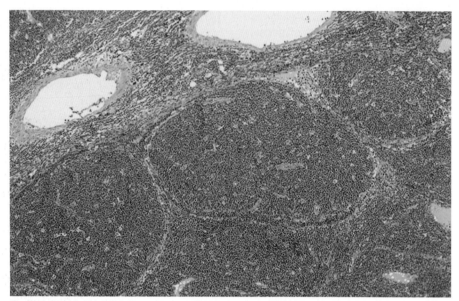

Fig. 9.14 T lymphoblastic lymphoma. Low magnification showing a multinodular or "pseudofollicular" pattern that can sometimes mimic follicular lymphoma.

involved in a translocation. In many cases translocations are not detected by karyotyping but only by molecular genetic studies. For example, the *TAL1* locus is altered by translocation in about 20–30% of cases of T-ALL. In only about 3% of cases can a t(1;14)(p32;q11) translocation be detected, but much more often it is fused to the *SIL* gene as a result of a cryptic interstitial deletion at chromosome 1p32 {281, 914, 1046}. Aberrant TAL1 expression interferes with differentiation and proliferation by inhibiting the transcriptional activity of E47/HEB {1615}. Other important translocations in T-ALL include *PICALM-MLLT10* [*CALM-AF10*; t(10;11)(p13;q14)], occurring in 10% of cases, and translocations involving *MLL* (8%), most often with the partner *ENL* at 19p13 {830}. Neither of these is T-ALL specific, as the first occurs in AML and the second in B-ALL. Aberrant expression of TAL1, LYL1, HOX11 and HOX11L2 appear to be mutually exclusive from each other and also from *PICALM* and *MLL* translocations, suggesting non-overlapping, patho-genetically distinct subgroups {519}.

Deletions also occur in T-ALL. The most important is del(9p), resulting in loss of the tumour suppressor gene *CDKN2A* (an inhibitor of the cyclin-dependent kinase *CDK4*), which occurs at a frequency of about 30% by cytogenetics, and a higher percentage by molecular testing. This leads to loss of G1 control of cell cycle.

About 50% of cases show activating mutations involving the extracellular heterodimerization domain and/or C-terminal PEST domain of the *NOTCH1* gene, which encodes a protein critical for early T-cell development {2385}. The direct downstream target of *NOTCH1* appears to be *MYC*, which contributes to the growth of the neoplastic cells {2386}. According to one study, *NOTCH1* mutation is associated with shorter survival in adult but not paediatric patients {2498}. In about 30% of cases, there are mutations in *FBXW7* gene, a negative regulator of *NOTCH1*, These missense mutations result in increased half-life of the Notch1 protein {1375}.

Gene expression profiling studies have identified several gene expression signatures, some of which correspond to specific stages of normal thymocyte development: LYL1+ signature corresponds to pro-T stage, HOX11+ to early cortical stage, and TAL1+ to late cortical thymocyte stage {689}. The HOX11+ group appears to have a relatively favourable prognosis.

Postulated normal counterpart
T-cell progenitor (T-ALL) or thymic lymphocyte (T-LBL).

Prognosis and predictive factors
T-ALL in childhood is generally considered a higher risk disease than B-ALL, though this is in part due to the frequent presence of high-risk clinical features (older age, higher white blood cell count). However, T-ALL patients without high-risk features do not fare as well as B-ALL standard risk patients unless intensive therapy is given. Compared to B-ALL patients, T-ALL patients have increased risk for induction failure, early relapse and isolated CNS relapse {809}. In contrast to B-ALL, white count does not appear to be a prognostic factor. The presence of minimal residual disease following therapy is a strong adverse prognostic factor {2406}. In adult protocols, T-ALL is treated similarly to other types of ALL. The prognosis of T-ALL may be better than B-ALL in adults, though this may reflect the lower incidence of adverse cytogenetic abnormalities. The prognosis of T-LBL, as with other lymphomas, depends on the age of the patient, stage and LDH levels {1512}.

Rare cases of indolent T lymphoblastic proliferation involving the upper aerodigestive tract, characterized by multiple local recurrences but no systemic dissemination, have been described {2106, 2323}. These cases are morphologically and immunophenotypically indistinguishable from T-LBL, but lack clonal rearrangements of the *TCR* genes.

CHAPTER 10

Mature B-cell Neoplasms

Chronic lymphocytic leukaemia /small lymphocytic lymphoma

B-cell prolymphocytic leukaemia

Splenic marginal zone lymphoma

Hairy cell leukaemia

Splenic lymphoma/leukaemia, unclassifiable

Lymphoplasmacytic lymphoma

Heavy chain diseases

Plasma cell neoplasms

Extranodal marginal zone lymphoma of mucosa-associated
lymphoid tissue (MALT lymphoma)

Nodal marginal zone lymphoma

Follicular lymphoma

Primary cutaneous follicle centre lymphoma

Mantle cell lymphoma

Diffuse large B-cell lymphoma (DLBCL), NOS

T-cell/histiocyte-rich large B-cell lymphoma

Primary DLBCL of the CNS

Primary cutaneous DLBCL, leg type

EBV positive DLBCL of the elderly

DLBCL associated with chronic inflammation

Lymphomatoid granulomatosis

Primary mediastinal (thymic) large B-cell lymphoma

Intravascular large B-cell lymphoma

ALK positive large B-cell lymphoma

Plasmablastic lymphoma

Large B-cell lymphoma arising in HHV8-associated multicentric
Castleman disease

Primary effusion lymphoma

Burkitt lymphoma

B-cell lymphoma, unclassifiable, with features intermediate between
DLBCL and Burkitt lymphoma

B-cell lymphoma, unclassifiable, with features intermediate between
DLBCL and classical Hodgkin lymphoma

Chronic lymphocytic leukaemia/small lymphocytic lymphoma

H.K. Müller-Hermelink
E. Montserrat
D. Catovsky
E. Campo
N.L. Harris
H. Stein

Definition

Chronic lymphocytic leukaemia/small lymphocytic lymphoma (CLL/SLL) is a neoplasm composed of monomorphic small, round to slightly irregular B lymphocytes in the peripheral blood (PB), bone marrow (BM), spleen and lymph nodes, admixed with prolymphocytes and paraimmunoblasts forming proliferation centres in tissue infiltrates.The CLL/SLL cells usually coexpress CD5 and CD23. In the absence of extramedullary tissue involvement, there must be ≥5x10^9/L monoclonal lymphocytes with a CLL phenotype in the PB. The International Workshop on Chronic Lymphocytic Leukemia (IWCLL) report requires that the lymphocytosis be present for at least 3 months and also allows for the diagnosis of CLL to be made with lower lymphocyte counts in patients with cytopenias or disease-related symptoms {873A}. Whether patients who would have fulfilled the criteria in the past for CLL but who fulfill the criteria only for monoclonal B lymphocytosis (MBL) are better considered to have low stage CLL or MBL remains to be determined. Some may prefer to still consider many of these cases more like CLL.

The term SLL is used for non-leukaemic cases with the tissue morphology and immunophenotype of CLL. The IWCLL definition of SLL requires lymphadenopathy, no cytopenias due to BM infiltration by CLL/SLL and <5x10^9/L PB B-cells {873A}.

ICD-O code 9823/3

Epidemiology

CLL is the most common leukaemia of adults in Western countries. The incidence rate is about 2–6 cases per 100,000 person per year, increasing with age reaching 12.8/100,000 at age 65, the mean age at diagnosis {1888}. It is now diagnosed more often in younger individuals {525}. CLL has a male:female ratio of 1.5–2:1. CLL/SLL accounts for 6.7% of non-Hodgkin lymphomas in biopsies {51}. It is very rare in far Eastern countries. This low incidence is maintained in migrant populations speaking in favour of a genetic predisposition.

Etiology

B-cell receptors (BCR) of CLL cells demonstrate highly selected immunoglobulin heavy chain variable *(IGHV)* gene usage or even very similar entire antigen-binding sites, coded by both heavy and light chain genes, and thus differ from the much broader diversity found in normal B lymphocytes. These findings argue in favour of a limited set of (auto-)antigens promoting division of precursor cells and clonal evolution {423, 1153, 2243}.

Sites of involvement

Peripheral blood and BM are usually involved. Lymph nodes, liver and spleen are also typically infiltrated, and other extranodal sites may occasionally be involved. Rarely, patients with CLL/SLL present with aleukaemic tissue involvement, but usually develop BM and PB involvement during the evolution of the disease.

Clinical features

Clinical features are very variable including presentation, course and outcome. Most patients are asymptomatic, but some present with fatigue, autoimmune haemolytic anaemia, infections, splenomegaly, hepatomegaly, lymphadenopathy or extranodal infiltrates {221, 1805}. A small M-component may be found in some patients.

Monoclonal B-cell lymphocytosis

Healthy individuals may show monoclonal or oligoclonal B-cell expansions with the characteristic phenotype of CLL in about 3.5% of tested subjects >40 years old {1395, 1823}. Monoclonal B-cell lymphocytosis with a non-CLL phenotype (CD5-) may correspond to similar phenomena in other B-cell neoplasms {30}. Whether MBL is a predisposing condition or even a precursor of overt CLL has to be elucidated.

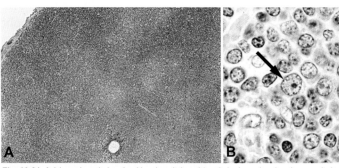

Fig. 10.01 A A Lymph node involved by chronic lymphocytic leukaemia, showing regularly-spaced proliferation centres in a dark background (Giemsa stain). **B** High magnification illustrating a mixture of small lymphocytes with scant cytoplasm and clumped chromatin, some sligtly larger prolymphocytes with more dispersed chromatin and small nucleoli, and single paraimmunoblasts (arrows), which are larger cells with round to oval nuclei, dispersed chromatin and a central nucleolus.

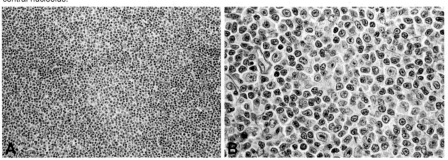

Fig. 10.02 Chronic lymphocytic leukaemia, lymph node. **A** A proliferation centre embedded in a darker background of small lymphocytes (PAS stain). **B** High magnification showing a clustering of larger lymphoid cells (prolymphocytes and paraimmunoblasts) in the proliferation centre.

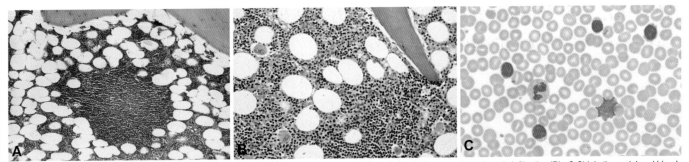

Fig. 10.03 CLL/SLL, bone marrow trephine section illustrating a nodular pattern of infiltration (**A**), an interstitial pattern of lymphocytic infiltration (**B**). **C** CLL in the peripheral blood, The CLL lymphocytes are small, round, with distinct clumped chromatin. Smudge cells are commonly seen (Courtesy of Dr M. Rozman).

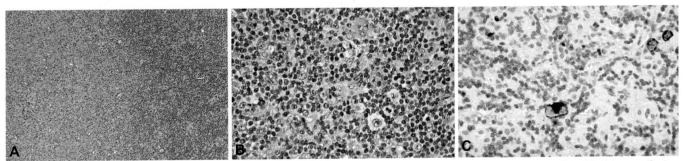

Fig. 10.04 Classical Hodgkin lymphoma (CHL) in a patient with CLL. **A** The dark area represents the infiltrate of CLL, while the pale area represents CHL. **B** At higher magnification, there are classical Reed-Sternberg (RS) cells in a background of lymphocytes and histiocytes. **C** Immunoperoxidase stain for CD15, showing typical membrane and Golgi region staining of the RS cells.

Morphology

Lymph nodes and spleen

Enlarged lymph nodes in patients with CLL/SLL show effacement of the architecture, with a pseudofollicular pattern of regularly-distributed pale areas corresponding to proliferation centres containing larger cells in a dark background of small cells {184, 1273}. Involvement may be limited to interfollicular areas. The predominant cell is a small lymphocyte, which may be slightly larger than a normal lymphocyte, with clumped chromatin, usually a round nucleus, and occasionally a small nucleolus. Mitotic activity is usually very low. Proliferation centres contain a continuum of small, medium and large cells. Prolymphocytes are small to medium-sized cells with relatively clumped chromatin and small nucleoli; paraimmunoblasts are larger cells with round to oval nuclei, dispersed chromatin, central eosinophilic nucleoli and slightly basophilic cytoplasm. The size of proliferation centres and number of paraimmunoblasts vary from case to case, but there is no correlation between lymph node histology and clinical course {184}. In the spleen, white pulp involvement is usually prominent, but the red pulp is also involved; proliferation centres may be seen but are less conspicuous than in lymph nodes. In some cases, the small lymphoid cells show moderate nuclear irregularity, which can lead to a differential diagnosis of mantle cell lymphoma {235}. Some cases show plasmacytoid differentiation.

Bone marrow and blood

On BM and PB smears, CLL cells are small lymphocytes with clumped chromatin and scanty cytoplasm {191}. Smudge or basket cells are typically seen in PB smears. The proportion of prolymphocytes (larger cells with prominent nucleoli) in PB films is usually <2%. Increasing numbers correlate with a more aggressive disease course. More than 55% prolymphocytes, however, would favour the diagnosis of B-cell prolymphocytic leukaemia (B-PLL). Atypical CLL shows less condensed nuclear chromatin and nuclear irregularities in PB lymphocytes. These findings are more frequent in cases with trisomy 12 and other chromosomal abnormalities {191}. Bone marrow involvement as seen in trephine biopsies may be interstitial, nodular and/or diffuse {1509, 1888}; proliferation centres are less common in the BM than in lymph nodes; paratrabecular aggregates are not typical. The definition of minimal BM involvement required to diagnose CLL/SLL in the absence of other defining features is not established, although the IWCLL describes >30% lymphoid cells as "characteristically" present {873A}.

Immunophenotype

Using flow cytometry, the tumour cells express dim surface IgM/IgD, CD20, CD22, CD5, CD19, CD79a, CD23, CD43 and CD11c (weak). CD10 is negative and FMC7 and CD79b are usually negative or weakly expressed in typical CLL. The immunophenotype of PB lymphocytes has been integrated into a scoring system that helps in the differential diagnosis between CLL and other B-cell leukaemias {1430, 1511}. In tissue sections, cytoplasmic Ig may be detectable, and cyclin D1 is negative {2508}; however cyclin D1 has been detected in cells of the proliferation centres {1614}. Some cases may have an atypical immunophenotype (e.g. CD5- or CD23-, FMC7+ or CD11c+, strong sIg, or CD79b+) {492, 1429}.

Genetic susceptibility

CLL has the highest genetic predisposition of all haematologic neoplasias. A family predisposition can be documented in 5–10% of patients with CLL based on finding 2 or more cases in the same family. The overall risk is 2–7 times increased in first degree relatives of CLL patients {810, 1990}. Family members of patients with CLL show an increased incidence of CLL-phenotype monoclonal B-cell lymphocytosis at all ages, but especially in those <40 years old {530}.

Genetics

Antigen receptor genes
IG genes are rearranged with 40–50% of cases unmutated (>98% homology with germline) and 50–60% showing somatic hypermutation {505, 876}. These two subtypes differ in many other biological and clinical parameters. IGHV gene usage in CLL is highly selective, and often associated with autoantibody reactivity {1658}. BCR signaling is most important in unmutated CLL {403, 538, 1252}.

Gene expression profiling
Mutated and unmutated CLL show a single distinctive signature, although there is a group of genes that distinguishes these two genetic subtypes {1160, 1867}. The tyrosine kinase ZAP-70 is among the genes whose expression is associated with an IGHV unmutated CLL genotype {2402}. Flow cytometry assays for ZAP-70 have been developed as a surrogate for CLL mutational status; however, in up to 20% of the cases the mutational status and ZAP-70 expression are discordant {490, 1653, 1822}.

Cytogenetic abnormalities and oncogenes
About 80% of the cases have cytogenetic abnormalities detected by FISH {601}. About 50% of CLL show del 13q14.3, about 20% trisomy 12 and, less commonly, deletions of 11q22-23, 17p13 and 6q21 {601, 1196, 1197, 1429}. The distribution of these abnormalities varies based on mutational status. The possible

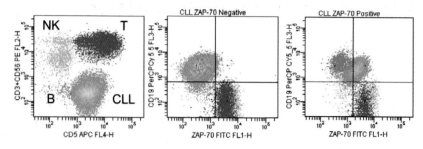

Fig. 10.05 Flow cytometry detection of ZAP-70 in CLL. The left plot shows the selection of the lymphocyte subpopulations according to the phenotype (T-cells in dark blue, NK-cells in light blue, CLL cells in orange and residual normal B-cells in grey). The CLL cells are CD5+ (see in left plot) and CD19+ (seen in other plots). The plot in the centre shows a CLL with no ZAP-70 expression (2% positive CLL cells) and the plot on the right a CLL with high ZAP-70 expression (65% positive CLL cells) . CLL cases with more than 20% ZAP-70 expression are usually considered as positive.

targets in the 13q14.3 region are two micro-RNA genes, miR-16-1 and miR-15a, ATM in the 11q22-23 region and TP53 in the 17p13 region {475, 601, 1957}. A specific micro-RNA expression signature that includes miR-16-1 and miR-15a has been reported to distinguish between mutated and unmutated CLL and ZAP-70 negative versus positive CLL {315}.

Postulated normal counterpart
Antigen experienced B-cell {424}.

Prognosis and predictive factors
The Rai and Binet clinical staging systems are used to define disease extent and prognosis {221, 1805}. New biological prognostic factors have become increasingly important especially in early stage CLL {222, 1129, 1986}. Patients with mutated CLL have a better prognosis than those with unmutated CLL, at least for those with a low stage (median survival 293 months versus 95 months for patients with Binet stage A) {876}. Expression of ZAP-70 and CD38 are both associated with an adverse prognosis {790}. Del11q22-23, del17p and del 6q are associated with a worse outcome and isolated del 13q14.3 is associated with a more favourable clinical course {475, 601}. Usage of VH3-21 independent of VH mutation status is an adverse prognostic marker {2244}. Additional adverse predictive factors include a rapid lymphocyte doubling time in the PB (<12 months) and serum markers of rapid cell turnover, including elevated thymidine kinase, sCD23 and β-2 microglobulin {222}.

Progression and transformation of CLL to high grade lymphoma
Over time, CLL may show an increase in cell size and proliferative activity as well as confluence of proliferation centres in lymph nodes and BM. Often, this may correlate with an increase in prolymphocytes in the PB. Progression of CLL to B-PLL is extremely rare.

2–8% of patients with CLL develop diffuse large B-cell lymphoma (DLBCL) and <1% develop classical Hodgkin lymphoma (HL) {269}. The median survival for patients with DLBCL (Richter's syndrome) is less than one year. The majority of the DLBCL have been reported to be clonally related to the previous CLL and are unmutated, whereas the clonally unrelated cases of DLBCL usually occurred in mutated CLL {1385, 2240}. The vast majority of HL cases occur in mutated CLL. Epstein-Barr virus (EBV)-associated Hodgkin or Reed-Sternberg (RS) cells frequently are unrelated to the CLL clone {1385}. Some CLL cases show scattered EBV-positive or sometimes negative Reed-Sternberg cells in the background of CLL. These cases should not be diagnosed as Hodgkin lymphoma. The diagnosis of Hodgkin lymphoma in the setting of CLL requires classical RS cells in an appropriate background. EBV-associated lymphoproliferative disorders including Hodgkin lymphomas may occur after fludarabine therapy {4, 2234}.

Table 10.01 Relation of VH mutation status and genomic aberrations in CLL {1197}.

Aberration	Mutated VH n=132 (44%)	Unmutated VH n=168 (56%)
Clonal aberrations	80%	84%
13q deletion*	65%	48%
Isolated 13q deletion*	50%	26%
Trisomy 12	15%	19%
11q deletion*	4%	27%
17p deletion*	3%	10%
17p or 11q deletion*	7%	35%

* Significant difference between cases with and without VH mutations.

B-cell prolymphocytic leukaemia

E. Campo
D. Catovsky
E. Montserrat
H.K. Müller-Hermelink
N.L. Harris
H. Stein

Definition
B-cell prolymphocytic leukaemia (B-PLL) is a neoplasm of B prolymphocytes affecting the peripheral blood (PB), bone marrow (BM) and spleen. Prolymphocytes must exceed 55% of lymphoid cells in the PB. Cases of transformed chronic lymphocytic leukaemia (CLL), CLL with increased prolymphocytes and lymphoid proliferations with relatively similar morphology but carrying the t(11;14)(q13;q32) translocation are excluded.

ICD-O code   9833/3

Epidemiology
B-PLL is an extremely rare disease, comprising approximately 1% of lymphocytic leukaemias. Most patients are over 60-year-old, with a median age of 65–69 and similar male:female distribution {1456}.

Sites of involvement
The leukaemic cells are found in the PB, BM and spleen.

Clinical features
Most patients present with B symptoms, massive splenomegaly with absent or minimal peripheral lymphadenopathy, and a rapidly rising lymphocyte count, usually over 100×10^9/L. Anaemia and thrombocytopenia are seen in 50% {1194}.

Morphology
Peripheral blood and bone marrow
The majority (>55% and usually >90%) of the circulating cells are prolymphocytes —medium-sized cells (twice the size of a lymphocyte) with a round nucleus, moderately condensed nuclear chromatin, a prominent central nucleolus and a relatively small amount of faintly basophilic cytoplasm {750, 1456}. Although the nucleus is typically round, there may be some indentation in some cases. The BM shows an interstitial or nodular infiltrate of nucleolated cells with an intertrabecular distribution.

Tissues other than bone marrow
The morphology of B-PLL in tissues is not well known since previous histological studies have included cases with the t(11;14) translocation that correspond to leukaemic variants of mantle cell lymphoma (MCL) {1892, 1963}. The spleen shows expanded white pulp nodules and red pulp infiltration by intermediate to large cells with abundant cytoplasm and irregular or round nuclei with the presence of a central eosinophilic nucleolus {1892}. Lymph nodes show diffuse or vaguely nodular infiltrates of similar cells. Proliferation centres (pseudofollicles) are not seen. Distinction from blastoid variants of MCL, splenic marginal zone lymphoma, and CLL with an increased number of prolymphocytes may be difficult on morphological grounds. The differential diagnosis requires immunophenotypic and genetic studies, in part to rule out the presence of the t(11;14) translocation or cyclin D1 overexpression.

Immunophenotype
The cells of B-PLL strongly express surface IgM+/- IgD as well as B-cell antigens (CD19, CD20, CD22, CD79a and b, FMC7); CD5 and CD23 are only positive in 20–30% and 10–20% of cases, respectively {542, 1194, 1892}. ZAP-70 and CD38 are expressed in 57% and 46% of the cases but they are not related to the mutational status of the immunoglobulin genes {542}.

Genetics
Antigen receptor genes
Immunoglobulin genes are clonally rearranged with an unmutated heavy chain gene in about half of the cases. All B–PLL

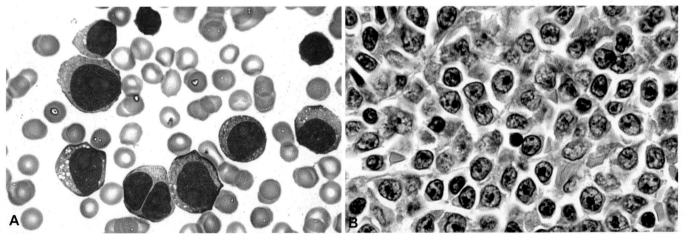

Fig. 10.06 **A** B-cell prolymphocytic leukaemia peripheral blood smear. The cells are medium to large, twice the size of small lymphocytes with moderately condensed nuclear chromatin and prominent vesicular nucleoli. The nuclear outline is usually regular and the cytoplasm weakly basophilic. **B** B-cell prolymphocytic leukaemia. Spleen, showing an infiltrate of prolymphocytes.

have been reported to use members of the *VH3* (68%) and *VH4* (32%) gene families {542}.

Cytogenetic abnormalities and oncogenes
Initial studies had demonstrated the t(11;14)(q13;q32) translocation in up to 20% of B-PLL {274}. However, these cases are now considered leukaemic variants of MCL {1892, 1963, 2439}. Complex karyotypes are common {1963}. Del(17p) is detected in 50% of the cases {542} and is associated with *TP53* gene mutations {1277}. This probably underlies the progressive course and relative treatment resistance of B-PLL. FISH analysis detects deletions at 13q14 in 27% of the cases {542}. Trisomy 12 is uncommon {542}.

Postulated normal counterpart
Unknown mature B-cell.

Prognosis and predictive factors
B-PLL responds poorly to therapies for CLL and median survival is 30–50 months {542, 1892}. Neither ZAP-70 expression, CD38 positivity, 17p deletions nor the mutational status of the immunoglobulin genes seem to correlate with survival {542}. Splenectomy may improve the patient's symptoms. Responses have been recorded with the combination CHOP (cyclophosphamide, doxorubicin, vincristine and prednisone), and the nucleoside analogs fludarabine and cladribine. A combination of chemotherapy and rituximab may be a reasonable approach to treat these patients {1194}.

Splenic marginal zone lymphoma

P. G. Isaacson   C. Thieblemont
M.A. Piris   S. Pittaluga
F. Berger   N.L. Harris
S.H. Swerdlow

Definition

Splenic marginal zone lymphoma (SMZL) is a B-cell neoplasm composed of small lymphocytes which surround and replace the splenic white pulp germinal centres, efface the follicle mantle and merge with a peripheral (marginal) zone of larger cells including scattered transformed blasts; both small and larger cells infiltrate the red pulp. Splenic hilar lymph nodes and bone marrow (BM) are often involved; lymphoma cells may be found in the peripheral blood (PB) as villous lymphocytes.

ICD-O code   9689/3

Synonym

Splenic lymphoma with circulating villous lymphocytes (SLVL).

Epidemiology

SMZL is a rare disorder, comprising less than 2% of lymphoid neoplasms {79}, but it may account for most cases of otherwise unclassifiable chronic lymphoid leukaemias that are CD5-. Most patients are over 50 and there is an equal sex incidence {195}.

Sites of involvement

The tumour involves the spleen and splenic hilar lymph nodes, BM and often the PB. The liver may be involved. Peripheral lymph nodes are not typically involved {195, 1497}.

Clinical features

Patients present with splenomegaly, sometimes accompanied by autoimmune thrombocytopenia or anaemia and a variable presence of PB villous lymphocytes. The BM is regularly involved, but peripheral lymphadenopathy and extranodal infiltration are extremely uncommon. About one third of the patients may have a small monoclonal serum protein, but marked hyperviscosity and hypergammaglobulinaemia are uncommon {195, 1497}. An association with hepatitis C virus has been described in southern Europe {72, 926}.

Morphology

In the splenic white pulp, a central zone of small round lymphocytes surrounds, or more commonly replaces reactive germinal centres with effacement of the normal follicle mantle {1014, 1497}. This zone merges with a peripheral zone of small to medium-sized cells with more dispersed

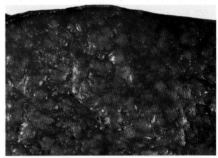

Fig. 10.08 Splenic marginal zone lymphoma. Gross photograph of spleen showing marked expansion of the white pulp, as well as infiltration of the red pulp.

chromatin and abundant pale cytoplasm, which resemble marginal zone cells and interspersed transformed blasts. The red pulp is always infiltrated, with both small nodules of the larger cells and sheets of the small lymphocytes, which often invade sinuses. Epithelioid histiocytes may be present in the lymphoid aggregates. Some cases may have a markedly predominant population of the larger marginal zone-like cells {878}. Plasmacytic differentiation may occur and in rare cases, clusters of plasma cells may be present in the centres of the white pulp nodules. In splenic hilar lymph nodes the sinuses are dilated and lymphoma

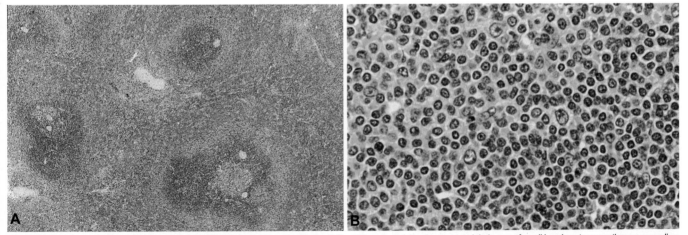

Fig. 10.07 Splenic marginal zone lymphoma showing infiltration of white and red pulp. **A** The white pulp nodules show a central dark zone of small lymphocytes sometimes surrounding a residual germinal centre giving way to a paler marginal zone. **B** High magnification of white pulp nodule showing the small lymphocytes merging with a marginal zone comprising larger cells with pale cytoplasm and occasional transformed blasts.

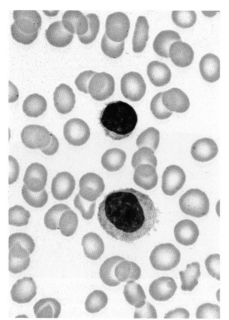

Fig. 10.09 Splenic marginal zone lymphoma. Peripheral blood containing tumour cells with polar villi (villous lymphocytes).

surrounds and replaces germinal centres, but the two cell types (small lymphocytes and marginal zone cells) are often more intimately admixed without the formation of a distinct "marginal" zone. This has given rise to doubts about suggestions that the tumour arises from splenic marginal zone cells. In the BM there is a nodular interstitial infiltrate cytologically similar to that in the lymph nodes. Occasionally, neoplastic cells surround reactive follicles. Intrasinusoidal lymphoma cells, better revealed after CD20 immunostaining, are a helpful feature although they are sometimes observed in other lymphomas {727}. When lymphoma cells are present

in the PB, they are usually, but not always, characterized by the presence of short polar villi. Some may appear plasma-cytoid {1457}. The differential diagnosis includes other small B-cell lymphomas/leukaemias, including chronic lymphocytic leukaemia, hairy cell leukaemia, mantle cell lymphoma, follicular lymphoma and lymphoplasmacytic lymphoma. The nodular pattern on BM biopsy excludes hairy cell leukaemia, but the morphologic features on BM examination may not be sufficient to distinguish between the other subtypes. This requires integration with the morphology and immunophenotype of the cells in the PB and BM.

Immunophenotype

Tumour cells express surface IgM and usually, but not always, IgD, are CD20+, CD79a+, CD5-, CD10-, CD23-, CD43- and annexin A1- {1014, 1428}. CD103 is usually, but not always, negative and cyclin D1 is absent {1945}. Staining for Ki67 shows a distinctive targetoid pattern based on the presence of an increased growth fraction in both the germinal centre (if present) and the marginal zone. The absence of cyclin D1 and the infrequent expression of CD5 are useful in excluding mantle cell lymphoma and chronic lymphocytic leukaemia respectively. Absence of annexin A1 excludes hairy cell leukaemia, and absence of CD10 and BCL6 helps to exclude follicular lymphoma {1945}.

Genetics

Antigen receptor genes

Immunoglobulin heavy and light chain genes are rearranged and approximately half of the cases have somatic hypermutation. Bias in *VH1-2* usage has been

found in both mutated and unmutated cases suggesting that this tumour derives from a highly selected B-cell population {23}. Other biased *VH* gene usage has also been reported {125}. In addition, intraclonal variation has been rarely detected, suggesting ongoing mutations {624, 2497}.

Cytogenetic abnormalities

Allelic loss of chromosome 7q31-32 has been described in up to 40% of SMZL {1416}. Dysregulation of the *CDK6* gene located at 7q21 has been reported in several cases of SLVL with translocations involving this region {474}. Trisomy 3q and a number of other cytogenetic abnormalities have been described {319, 766, 859, 929, 1669} while *BCL2* rearrangement and t(14;18) are absent. *CCND1* rearrangement, t(11;14) and cyclin D1 expression have been reported in a small proportion of the cases; however, the possibility that these cases represent examples of mantle cell lymphoma has not been excluded, since cyclin D1 expression is absent from well-characterized cases of SMZL {1945}. Translocation t(11;18), common in extranodal marginal zone lymphoma of mucosa-associated lymphoid tissue (MALT) type, is not a feature of SMZL {575, 1837}. Splenic marginal zone lymphoma has a specific transcriptional profile compared with other B-cell, especially small B-cell lymphomas. This specific molecular signature includes genes involved in the signaling cascade of the AKT1 pathway and B-cell receptor signaling {374, 2197}.

Postulated normal counterpart

B-cell of unknown differentiation stage. The presence of *IG* gene somatic hypermutations in 50% of cases suggests

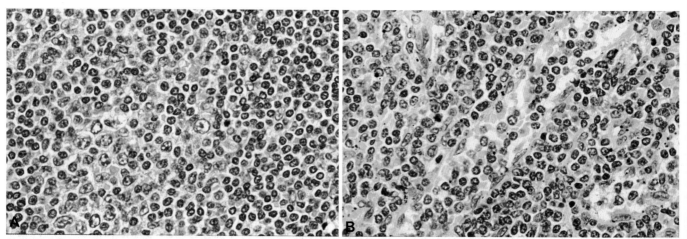

Fig.10.10 Splenic marginal zone lymphoma. **A** Small lymphocytes invading splenic red pulp with an ill-defined nodule of larger cells. **B** Infiltration of red pulp sinuses.

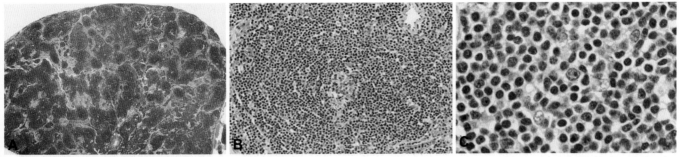

Fig. 10.11 Splenic marginal zone lymphoma. **A** Splenic hilar lymph node showing a nodular infiltrate. **B** Splenic hilar lymph node nodule showing a small residual germinal centre. **C** High magnification shows a mixture of small lymphocytes and larger cells.

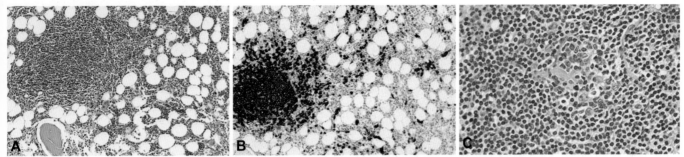

Fig. 10.12 Bone marrow involvement in splenic marginal zone lymphoma. **A** Large lymphoid aggregate is present in the intertrabecular region. **B** The lymphoid aggregate is CD20-positive and CD20-positive B-cells infiltrate the sinusoids of the marrow. **C** A lymphoid aggregate with a small residual germinal centre.

exposure to antigen in the germinal centre microenvironment.

Prognosis and predictive factors

The clinical course is indolent, even with BM involvement {72, 195, 1538, 2196, 2197}. Response to chemotherapy of the type that is typically effective in other chronic lymphoid leukaemias is often poor, but patients typically have haematologic responses to splenectomy, with long-term survival. Transformation to large B-cell lymphoma may occur, as in other indolent B-cell neoplasms {1538}. HCV-positive cases have been reported to respond to antiviral treatment using interferon γ with or without ribovarine {926, 2195}. Adverse clinical prognostic factors include a large tumour mass or poor general health status {374}. A clinical scoring system has been proposed {72} and cases with mutated *TP53* may show an aggressive course {858}. The presence of 7q deletion and unmutated *IGHV* genes may be associated with an unfavourable outcome {23, 2263}.

Hairy cell leukaemia

K. Foucar
B. Falini
D. Catovsky
H. Stein

Definition
Hairy cell leukaemia (HCL) is an indolent neoplasm of small mature B lymphoid cells with oval nuclei and abundant cytoplasm with "hairy" projections involving peripheral blood (PB) and diffusely infiltrating the bone marrow (BM) and splenic red pulp.

ICD-O code   9940/3

Epidemiology
Hairy cell leukaemia is a rare disease, comprising 2% of lymphoid leukaemias. Patients are predominantly middle-aged to elderly adults with a median age of 50 years; HCL has been diagnosed rarely in patients in their 20's, but is exceptionally uncommon in children. The male:female ratio is 5:1 {642}.

Etiology
Although the nature of the underlying oncogenic events in HCL is not known, several studies provide an explanation for many of the unique features of this entity {157, 348, 2235} (Table 10.02).

Sites of involvement
Tumour cells are found predominantly in the BM and spleen. Typically a small number of circulating cells are noted. Tumour infiltrates may occur in the liver and lymph nodes, and occasionally also in the skin. Rare patients demonstrate prominent abdominal lymphadenopathy, which is associated with large hairy cells; this may represent a form of transformation {1999}.

Clinical features
The most common presenting symptoms include weakness and fatigue, left upper quadrant pain, fever and bleeding. Most patients present with splenomegaly and pancytopenia with few circulating neoplastic cells. Monocytopenia is characteristic. Other common distinctive manifestations include hepatomegaly and recurrent opportunistic infections, while less common unique findings include vasculitis, bleeding disorders, neurologic disorders, skeletal involvement and other immune dysfunction {951}.

Morphology
Peripheral blood and bone marrow
Hairy cells are small to medium-sized lymphoid cells with an oval or indented (bean-shaped) nucleus with homogeneous, spongy, ground-glass chromatin that is slightly less clumped than that of a normal lymphocyte. Nucleoli are typically absent or inconspicuous. The cytoplasm is abundant and pale blue, with circumferential "hairy" projections on smears {212, 1999}. Occasionally the cytoplasm contains discrete vacuoles or rod-shaped inclusions that represent the ribosome lamellar complexes that have been identified by electron microscopy {1999}.

The diagnosis is best made on BM biopsy. The extent of BM effacement in HCL is variable. The primary pattern is interstitial or patchy with some preservation of fat and haematopoietic elements. The infiltrate is characterized by widely-spaced lymphoid cells with oval or indented nuclei,

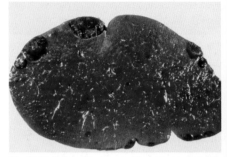

Fig. 10.14 Hairy cell leukaemia. The spleen is markedly enlarged with diffuse expansion of the red pulp. White pulp is not discernable. Numerous blood cell lakes of varying size are visible.

in contrast to the closely packed nuclei of most indolent lymphoid neoplasms involving the BM. The abundant cytoplasm and prominent cell borders may produce a "fried-egg" appearance {212, 1999}. Mitotic figures are virtually absent. When infiltration is minimal, the subtle clusters of hairy cells can be overlooked. In patients with advanced disease, a diffuse solid infiltrate may be evident. The obvious discrete aggregates that typify BM infiltrates of many other chronic lymphoproliferative disorders are not a feature of HCL. An increase in reticulin fibres is associated with all hairy cell infiltrates in BM and other sites, and often results in a "drytap". In a proportion of patients, the BM is hypocellular with a loss of haematopoietic elements, especially the granulocytic lineage, which can lead to an erroneous diagnosis of aplastic anaemia. In such cases, immunostaining for a B-cell antigen such

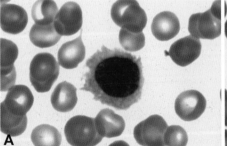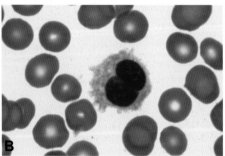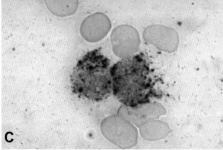

Fig. 10.13 Hairy cell leukaemia, smears. **A,B** Note the typical morphologic features of circulating hairy cells highlighting the range in nuclear morphology. **C** There is strong tartrate resistant acid phosphatase positivity characteristic of hairy cell leukaemia

as CD20 is essential for the identification of an abnormal B-cell infiltrate, prompting the performance of more specific immunohistochemical stains for HCL. The production of cytokines by the hairy cells is presumed to be the cause of this haematopoietic suppression {348}.

Other leukaemias/lymphomas such as splenic marginal zone lymphomas and some unclassifiable splenic lymphomas/leukaemias show morphologic and immunophenotypic overlap with hairy cell leukaemia.

Spleen and other tissues

In the spleen, HCL infiltrates are found in the red pulp. The white pulp is typically atrophic. The cells characteristically fill the red pulp cords. Red blood cell lakes, collections of pooled erythrocytes surrounded by elongated hairy cells, are the presumed consequence of disruption of normal blood flow in the red pulp {212, 1999}. The liver may show infiltrates of hairy cells, predominantly in the sinusoids. Lymph node infiltration may occur especially with advanced disease, and is variably interfollicular/paracortical, with sparing of follicles and intact sinuses.

Cytochemistry

The only cytochemical stain utilized in the diagnosis is tartrate-resistant acid phosphatase (TRAP), and this technically challenging cytochemical stain has been largely supplanted by immunophenotypic/immunohistochemical techniques. If appropriate air-dried unfixed slide preparations are available, virtually all cases of HCL will contain at least some cells with strong, granular cytoplasmic TRAP positivity, while weak staining is not of diagnostic utility {212, 1999}.

Immunophenotype

The assessment of an antigen profile that takes into account intensity of antigen expression and assessment of multiple antigens is very useful in the diagnosis of HCL. The classic immunophenotypic profile of HCL consists of bright monotypic surface immunoglobulin, bright coexpression of CD20, CD22 and CD11c, and expression of CD103, CD25, CD123, T-bet, Annexin A1 (ANXA1), DBA.44 (CD72), FMC-7 and cyclin D1 (usually weak) {348, 541, 670, 1062, 1423, 1999, 2392}. Most cases of HCL lack both CD10 and CD5, although immunophenotypic variants are well known {404, 1050}. Annexin A1 is

Table 10.02 Pathogenesis of hairy cell leukaemia.

Property	Proposed pathogenetic mechanism(s)
Clonal B-cell	Derived from mature memory B-cell. Leukaemic hairy cells differ from normal memory B-cells because of altered expression of chemokine and adhesion receptors.
Hairy cell morphology	Influenced by overexpression and constitutive activation of members of Rho family of small GTPases and up-regulation of the growth arrest-specific molecule Gas7.
Patchy, interstitial distribution of hairy cells	May relate to constitutive activation of adhesion/motility receptors, hairy cells interact spontaneously with extracellular matrix components; hairy cells adhere and bind firmly onto fibronectin in bone marrow microenvironment.
Reticulin fibrosis	HCL cells synthesize and bind to fibronectin in bone marrow microenvironment. Production rate of fibronectin is under control of autocrine basic fibroblast growth factor (bFGF) secreted by hairy cells. Transforming growth factor β1 (TGFβ1) also plays a role in reticulin fibrosis.
Homing to bone marrow, splenic red pulp and hepatic sinusoids	Hairy cells home to "blood-related" compartments via constitutively activated integrin receptors and over expression of matrix-metalloproteinase inhibitors. Down regulation of chemokine receptors such as CCR7 and CXCR5 explains absence of lymph node involvement.
Phagocytosis	Overexpression of Annexin 1 and actin possible mediators.
Pseudosinus formation in spleen	Interaction of hairy cells with endothelial cells resulting in replacement of endothelial cells by leukaemic hairy cells.
Tartrate-resistant acid phosphase positivity	Related to constitutive cell activation.
Prolonged cell survival	Constitutive production of tumour necrosis factor (TNF), interleukin -6 (IL-6) and overexpression of apoptosis inhibitor, BCL2.
Inhibition of normal haematopoiesis (hypocellular HCL)	Constitutive production of transforming growth factor-β (TGF-β) by hairy cells.
References {157, 348, 2235}.	

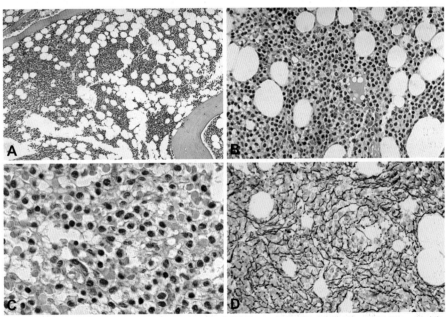

Fig. 10.15 Hairy cell leukaemia, bone marrow biopsy. **A** This low magnification photomicrograph shows a subtle diffuse, interstitial infiltrate of hairy cells. **B** Extensive diffuse interstitial infiltration by hairy cell leukaemia. Note widely spaced oval nuclei and paucity of mitotic activity. **C** A "fried egg" appearance of hairy cells is evident on high magnification. **D** Note the diffuse increase in reticulin fibres.

the most specific marker since it is not expressed in any B-cell lymphoma other than HCL {670}. Expression of Annexin A1 can be used to distinguish HCL from splenic marginal zone lymphoma and HCL variant which are both Annexin A1 negative {670}. Immunostaining for Annexin A1 must always be compared with that for a B-cell antigen (e.g. CD20), since Annexin A1 is also expressed by myeloid cells and a proportion of T-cells {670}. For this reason, Annexin A1 is not a suitable marker for monitoring minimal residual disease. More suitable approaches for assessment for residual disease after therapy include either multicolor flow cytometry targeting the distinctive HCL profile or immunohistochemical techniques including CD20, TRAP, DBA.44 (CD72) and T-bet. However, low numbers of TRAP positive or DBA.44 (CD72) positive cells may be seen in normal BM {1423}. Similarly, some T-cells may be T-bet positive, and weak staining for T-bet may be seen in other B-cell neoplasms {1062}. The clinical value of monitoring for residual disease is not yet established.

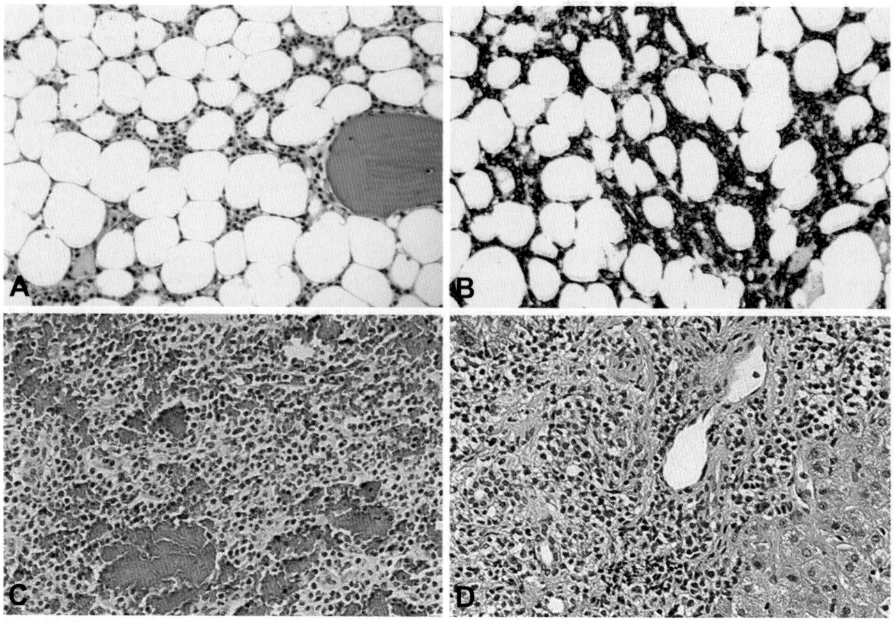

Genetics

Antigen receptor genes

Although exceptions have been reported, the majority (>85%) of cases of HCL demonstrate *VH* genes with somatic hypermutation indicative of a post germinal centre stage of maturation {83, 348, 2235}. A unique feature of HCL is the common co-expression of multiple clonally related Ig isotypes, suggesting arrest at some point during isotype switching {2235}.

Cytogenetic abnormalities

No cytogenetic abnormality is specific for HCL; numerical abnormalities of chromosomes 5 and 7 have been described, but translocations are distinctly uncommon {348}.

Postulated normal counterpart

Late, activated memory B-cell.

Prognosis and predictive factors

HCL is uniquely sensitive to either α-interferon or nucleosides (purine analogs) such as pentostatin and cladribine. Patients receiving purine analogs often achieve complete and durable remissions {2235}. Prolonged remission may also result from splenectomy, but this is uncommon {798}. The overall 10-year survival rate exceeds 90% {642, 798}. Rituximab

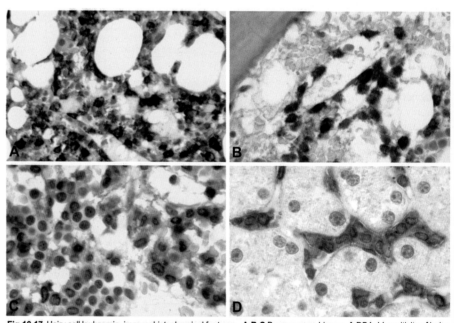

Fig.10.16 Hairy cell leukaemia. **A,B** Bone marrow biopsy. Hypocellular hairy cell leukaemia with subtle interstitial infiltrates (**A**). Immunoperoxidase for CD20 highlights subtle leukaemic infiltrates in hypocellular HCL (**B**). **C** Spleen. Red pulp infiltration with numerous red blood cell lakes. **D** Liver. Both portal and sinusoidal infiltration by hairy cells is present.

Fig.10.17 Hairy cell leukaemia, immunohistochemical features. **A,B,C** Bone marrow biopsy. **A** DBA.44 positivity of hairy cells accentuating hairy projections. **B** CD123 positivity of hairy cells. **C** Hairy cells express Annexin 1 while erythroid precursors are negative. **D** Liver. Sinusoidal infiltration by Annexin A1-positive leukaemic hairy cells.

offers therapeutic efficacy in combination with purine analogs in patients with refractory/relapsed HCL; experimental therapeutic agents include anti-CD22 antibody therapy or anti-CD25 immunotoxin therapy {1850}. Long term HCL survivors have an increased risk of second cancers compared to the general population with a cumulative probability of 30% for second neoplasms by 25 years after

HCL diagnosis {940}. Hodgkin and non-Hodgkin lymphomas as well as thyroid cancer predominate in these long term survivors {940}.

Splenic B-cell lymphoma/leukaemia, unclassifiable

M. Piris
K. Foucar
M. Mollejo
E. Campo
B. Falini

There are a number of variably well-defined entities that represent small B-cell clonal lymphoproliferations involving the spleen, but which do not fall into any of the other types of B-cell lymphoid neoplasms recognized in the WHO classification. This chapter reviews the two best defined of these relatively rare provisional entities, splenic diffuse red pulp small B-cell lymphoma and hairy cell leukaemia variant. The relationship of splenic diffuse red pulp small B-cell lymphoma to hairy cell leukaemia variant and other primary splenic B-cell lymphomas remains uncertain, their precise diagnostic criteria are not fully established and the most appropriate terminology is unsettled. Other splenic small B-cell lymphomas not fulfilling the criteria for either of these provisional entities or for other better established B-cell lymphomas should be diagnosed as splenic B-cell lymphoma/leukaemia, unclassifiable until more is known.

Splenic diffuse red pulp small B-cell lymphoma

Definition

Splenic diffuse red pulp small B-cell lymphoma is an uncommon lymphoma with a diffuse pattern of involvement of the splenic red pulp by small monomorphous B lymphocytes. The neoplasm also involves bone marrow (BM) sinusoids and peripheral blood (PB), commonly with a villous cytology. This is a provisional entity that needs additional molecular studies for defining its main features and

diagnostic markers. This diagnosis should be restricted to characteristic cases, fulfilling the major features described here and not applied to any lymphoma growing diffusely in the spleen. Chronic lymphocytic leukaemia (CLL), hairy cell leukaemia (HCL), lymphoplasmacytic lymphoma (LPL) and prolymphocytic leukaemia (PLL) should be excluded through appropriate studies. A certain diagnosis may require the examination of the spleen, but may be suggested for cases showing purely intrasinusoidal BM involvement and villous lymphocytes in the PB. In case of doubt, the use of the term splenic B-cell lymphoma/leukaemia, unclassifiable is warranted.

Some degree of overlap exists with cases that fulfil the criteria for hairy cell leukaemia variant {1913A, 1431}. The neoplastic cells in both entities are DBA.44 (CD72)+, frequently IgG+, IgD- and have frequent chromosomal alterations. Additional studies are required to confirm these findings and to further evaluate the extent of overlap between these entities, particularly as not all studies report the same phenotypic or cytogenetic findings. A rare subtype of large B-cell lymphoma involving the sinusoids, both in the spleen and the BM, has been described by two different groups {1495A, 1523}. Although these cases may be related to those described above, the diagnosis of splenic diffuse red pulp small B-cell lymphoma is restricted to an indolent lymphoma composed of small lymphocytes.

Synonyms

Splenic marginal zone lymphoma (SMZL)-diffuse variant {1496}, lymphocytic lymphoma simulating hairy cell leukaemia {1681}, splenic B-cell lymphoma with villous lymphocytes (also used for SMZL and HCL-variant), splenic red pulp lymphoma with numerous basophilic villous lymphocytes {2262}.

ICD-O code   9591/3

Epidemiology

Splenic diffuse red pulp small B-cell lymphoma is a rare disorder, accounting for <1% of non-Hodgkin lymphomas. It represents about 10% of the B-cell lymphomas diagnosed in splenectomy specimens. Most patients are over 40 and there is no gender bias.

Sites of involvement

All cases are diagnosed at clinical stage IV, with spleen, BM and PB involvement. Peripheral lymph node involvement is only rarely reported.

Clinical features

Splenic diffuse red pulp small B-cell lymphoma is a leukaemic neoplasm, usually with a relatively low lymphocytosis. Almost all patients have, frequently massive, splenomegaly. Although not consistent among all studies, thrombocytopenia and leukopenia are frequently present, while anaemia has been reported more rarely. B symptoms are infrequent. A small group of these patients show cutaneous infiltration

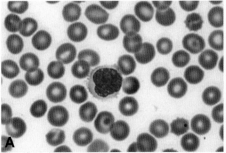
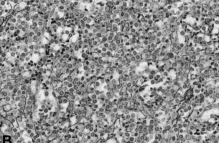
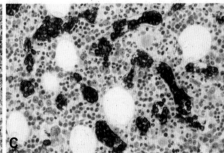

Fig. 10.18 Splenic diffuse red pulp small B-cell lymphoma. **A** Peripheral blood cytology with villous cell. **B** Reticulin staining outlines the mixed infiltration of both red pulp components: cords and sinusoids. **C** Bone marrow intrasinusoidal infiltration highlighted by CD20 staining.

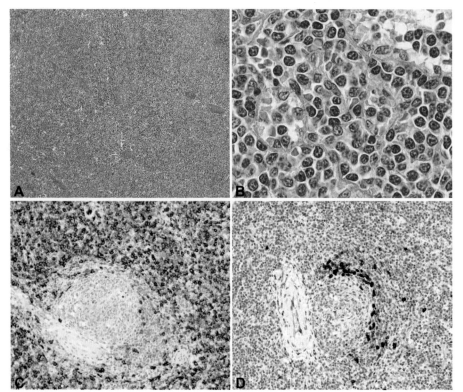

Fig.10.19 Splenic diffuse red pulp small B-cell lymphoma, spleen. **A** Diffuse infiltration of the red pulp. **B** Spleen high magnification showing the infiltration of both red pulp cord and sinusoids. **C** DBA.44 staining of the tumoural cells. **D** IgD staining is usually negative, outlining residual IgD+ mantle zone cells.

in the form of erythematous and pruritic papules at the time of the initial diagnosis. Presence of a paraprotein has not been reported.

Morphology
Peripheral blood: Villous lymphocytes similar to those reported in SMZL are present.

Bone marrow: Intrasinusoidal infiltration is the rule, occasionally as a sole finding. This can be accompanied by interstitial and nodular infiltration. Lymphoid follicles, as in SMZL, have not been reported.

Spleen: A diffuse pattern of involvement of the red pulp, with both cord and sinusoid infiltration is present. Characteristic intrasinusoidal aggregates with occasional pseudosinuses lined by tumoural cells may be seen. In contrast to SMZL, the tumour shows an absence of follicular replacement, biphasic cytology or marginal zone infiltration. The neoplastic infiltrate is composed of a monomorphous population of small to medium-sized lymphocytes, with round and regular nuclei, vesicular chromatin and occasional distinct small

nucleoli, with scattered nucleolated blast cells. Tumoural cells have a pale or lightly eosinophilic cytoplasm, with plasmacytoid features but lacking other features of plasmacytoid differentiation, such cytoplasmic Ig or CD38 expression.

Cytochemistry
Tartrate-resistant acid phospatase (TRAP) staining is not present.

Immunophenotype
The characteristic profile is CD20+, DBA.44 (CD72)+, IgG+, IgD-, Annexin A1-, CD25-, CD5-, CD103-, CD123-, CD11c-, CD10-, CD23- {1429A, 1496, 1922}. IgD+ cases can be seen with similar features. Others have reported cases with IgM+IgG±, CD103+ and CD11c+ with infrequent CD5 and CD123 expression {2262}.

Genetics
Most cases seem to harbour a relatively low load of somatic hypermutation in the *IGHV* genes. No bias for *VH1.2* gene has been seen, as in SMZL. Overrepresentation of *VH3-23* and *VH4-34*, as in HCL, has been reported {2262}. Complex cytogenetic alterations, including

translocation t(9;14)(p13;q32) involving *PAX5* and *IGH@* genes have been found in these cases {141} but they lack del 7q and t(11;14). Frequent *TP53* alterations have been described, with increased p53 expression {1496}. Others have reported a frequent absence of any cytogenetic abnormalities and occasional cases of del 7q {2262}.

Postulated normal counterpart
Unknown peripheral blood B-cell.

Prognosis and predictive factors
This is an indolent but incurable disease, with good responses after splenectomy.

Hairy cell leukaemia-variant (HCL-v)

Definition
The designation HCL-v encompasses cases of B chronic lymphoproliferative disorders that resemble classic HCL but exhibit variant "cytohaematologic" features (i.e. leukocytosis, presence of monocytes, cells with prominent nucleoli, cells with blastic or convoluted nuclei and/or absence of circumferential shaggy contours), variant immunophenotype (i.e. absence of CD25, annexin-A1, or TRAP) and resistance to conventional HCL therapy (i.e. lack of dramatic response to cladribine). These cases are no longer considered to be biologically related to HCL.

ICD-O code   9591/3

Synonym
Prolymphocytic variant of HCL.

Epidemiology
Cases of HCL-v account for about 10% of HCL with an incidence of approximately 0.03 per 100,000 persons per year {1850}. Middle-aged to elderly patients are affected and there is a slight male predominance {1431}. Cases of HCL-v have been described in Asian patients where HCL-v may be more common than HCL {1431}.

Sites of involvement
Spleen, BM and PB are involved but hepatomegaly and lymphadenopathy are relatively uncommon {1431}. Involvement of other solid tissues is rare.

Clinical features
Patients with HCL-v typically manifest

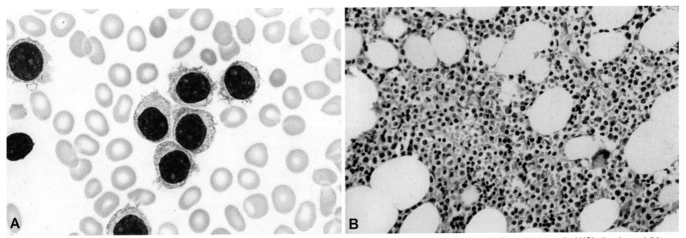

Fig. 10.20 Hairy cell variant. **A** Blood smear. The cells have abundant moderately basophilic cytoplasm with villous projections, but in contrast to typical HCL, they have visible nucleoli, resembling prolymphocytes. **B** The bone marrow biopsy shows a diffuse, interstitial pattern of infiltration similar to that of typical HCL.

signs and symptoms related to either splenomegaly or cytopenias. Leukocytosis is a consistent feature with an average white blood cell count of about 35x10⁹/L, while thrombocytopenia is present in about half of the patients and anaemia in one quarter {1431}. The absolute monocyte count is typically within normal range.

Morphology
Circulating HCL-v cells are readily apparent on the PB smear; commonly these cells exhibit the hybrid features of prolymphocytic leukaemia and classic HCL, although several other morphologic subtypes (blastic, convoluted) have also been described {1850}. Nuclear features range from condensed chromatin with prominent central nucleoli of a prolymphocytic cell to dispersed chromatin with highly irregular nuclear contours. Cytoplasmic features are similarly variable, although some degree of hairy projections is typically noted {373}. Transformation to large cells with convoluted nuclei has been described and cases of so-called convoluted HCL may be explained by this phenomenon {1431}. Unlike classic HCL, the BM is aspirable without significant reticulin fibrosis {373}. The infiltrates of HCL-v

may be subtle and very inconspicuous, often requiring immunohistochemical stains to highlight the pattern and extent of infiltration {373}. Recent publications note a distinct predilection for nearly exclusive sinusoidal infiltration {373, 1431, 2460}.
Similar to HCL and splenic diffuse red pulp small B-cell lymphoma, the red pulp of the spleen is diffusely involved and expanded in HCL-v, resulting in atretic or absent white pulp follicles. The leukaemic cells fill dilated sinusoids and red blood cell lakes may be noted {1431}. Liver involvement is characterized by both portal tract and sinusoidal infiltrates.

Cytochemistry
Unlike classic HCL, cytochemical staining for tartrate-resistant acid phospatase (TRAP) is weak to negative in HCL-v {541, 1431, 1850}.

Immunophenotype
Cases of HCL-v share many immunophenotypic and immunohistochemical (IHC) features with HCL, although HCL-v cells characteristically lack several key HCL antigens usually including CD25, Annexin A1, TRAP-IHC, CD123 and HC2 {670, 1431, 1850}. Positive "markers" in

HCL-v include DBA.44 (CD72), pan-B-cell antigens, CD11c, bright monotypic surface immunoglobulin (more frequently IgG), CD103 and FMC7 {1423, 1431}.

Genetics
There are no known specific genetic changes. Some cases demonstrate complex cytogenetic abnormalities involving 14q32 or 8q24 and *TP53* deletions {1431}.

Postulated normal counterpart
Activated B-cell at late stage of maturation.

Prognosis and predictive factors
These patients have an indolent course with a long survival time, even though patients with HCL-v do not typically respond to either IFN-α or purine nucleoside analogs (pentostatin and cladribine) {1850}. Recent preliminary studies suggest that monoclonal antibody therapy (rituximab and anti-CD22 immunotoxin) is highly effective {1850}. In addition, good clinical responses have been achieved with resolution of cytopenias after splenectomy {1850}.

Lymphoplasmacytic lymphoma

S.H. Swerdlow
F. Berger
S.A. Pileri
N.L. Harris
E.S. Jaffe
H. Stein

Definition

Lymphoplasmacytic lymphoma (LPL) is a neoplasm of small B lymphocytes, plasmacytoid lymphocytes, and plasma cells, usually involving bone marrow (BM) and sometimes lymph nodes and spleen, which does not fulfill the criteria for any of the other small B-cell lymphoid neoplasms that may also have plasmacytic differentiation. Because the distinction between LPL and one of these other lymphomas, especially some marginal zone lymphomas (MZL), is not always clear-cut, some cases may need to be diagnosed as a small B-cell lymphoma with plasmacytic differentiation and a differential diagnosis provided. Although often associated with a paraprotein usually of IgM type, it is not required for the diagnosis. Waldenström macroglobulinemia (WM) is found in a significant subset of patients with LPL and is defined as LPL with BM involvement and an IgM monoclonal gammopathy of any concentration {1673}.

ICD-O code   9671/3

Epidemiology

LPL occurs in adults with a median age in the 60s and a slight male predominance {581, 2337}.

Etiology

A familial predisposition may exist in up to 20% of patients with WM {29, 2267}. These patients are diagnosed at a younger age and with greater BM involvement.

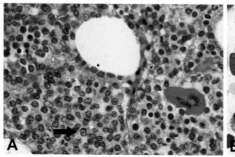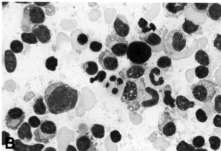

Fig. 10.22 Lymphoplasmacytic lymphoma. **A** Bone marrow biopsy shows a lymphoplasmacytic infiltrate with a PAS-positive Dutcher body (arrow). **B** The lymphoplasmacytic infiltrate is also seen in the aspirate smear.

Hepatitis C virus (HCV) is associated with type II cryoglobulinemia and with LPL in some but not all series, perhaps related to geographic differences {534, 1271, 1450A, 1597, 1680, 1791, 1932, 2166}. Some of the HCV-associated lymphoplasmacytic proliferations even if monotypic, are non-progressive and others may be more like chronic lymphocytic leukaemia (CLL) {1506, 2326}. Treatment of these patients with anti-viral agents may lead to regression of the lymphoplasmacytic proliferations {1434, 2166}. Apart from the role of HCV, mast cells may help drive the proliferation in LPL {2259}.

Sites of involvement

Most cases involve the BM and some, lymph nodes and other extranodal sites. About 15–30% of patients with WM also have splenomegaly, hepatomegaly and/or adenopathy {581}. Peripheral blood (PB) may also be involved.

Clinical features

Most patients present with weakness and fatigue, usually related to anaemia. The majority of patients have an IgM serum paraprotein although others may have a different paraprotein or no paraprotein at all. A minority have both IgM and IgG or other paraproteins. Hyperviscosity occurs in up to 30% of patients. The paraprotein may also have autoantibody or cryoglobulin activity, resulting in autoimmune phenomena or cryoglobulinemia (seen in up to ~20% of patients with WM). Neuropathies occur in a minority of patients and may result from reactivity of the IgM paraprotein with myelin sheath antigens, cryoglobulinemia or paraprotein deposition. Deposits of IgM may occur in the skin or the gastrointestinal tract, where they may cause diarrhoea. Coagulopathies may be caused by IgM binding to clotting factors, platelets and fibrin. IgM paraproteins are not diagnostic of either LPL or WM as they can occur in patients with other lymphoid

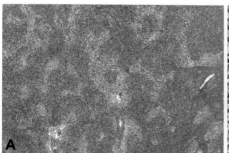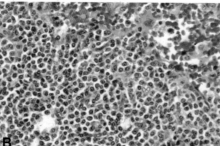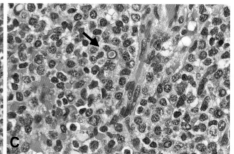

Fig. 10.21 Lymphoplasmacytic lymphoma. Lymph node. **A** Classical lymphoplasmacytic lymphoma in a patient with Waldenström macroglobulinemia. Note the widely patent sinuses and relatively monotonous lymphoplasmacytic infiltrate in the intersinus regions. **B** Typical relatively monotonous appearance of lymphocytes, plasmacytoid lymphocytes and plasma cells adjacent to an open sinus. **C** A Dutcher body (arrow) is seen in the H&E stain in this relatively plasma cell-rich case.

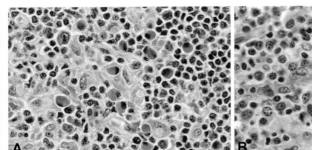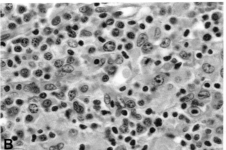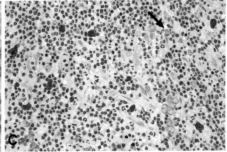

Fig. 10.23 Lymphoplasmacytic lymphoma. **A** In this somewhat polymorphic case, note the prominent cytoplasmic immunoglobulin accumulation and epithelioid histiocytes. **B** In this more polymorphic case that also has admixed epithelioid histiocytes, it is more controversial whether the best diagnosis is an LPL or some other type of lymphoma with plasmacytic differentiation, such as a marginal zone lymphoma. **C** Giemsa stain highlights the characteristic increased mast cells and haemosiderin (arrow).

neoplasms or without an overt neoplasm. A minority of patients initially present with an IgM-related disorder such as cryoglobulinemia or IgM-monoclonal gammopathy of undetermined significance and only later develop an overt LPL {370, 1230, 1524}.

Morphology

Bone marrow and peripheral blood
Bone marrow involvement is characterized by a nodular, diffuse and/or interstitial infiltrate usually composed predominantly of small lymphocytes admixed with variable numbers of plasma cells and plasmacytoid lymphocytes {1672, 1673}. Paratrabecular aggregates may also be present. Increased mast cells are often present. Similar cells may be present in the PB, but the white blood count is typically lower than in CLL.

Lymph nodes and other tissues
In the most classic cases that are usually associated with WM, lymph nodes show retention of normal architectural features with dilated sinuses with PAS+ material and sometimes small portions of residual germinal centres. There is a relatively monotonous proliferation of small lymphocytes, plasma cells and plasmacytoid lymphocytes with relatively few transformed cells. Dutcher bodies (PAS+ intranuclear pseudo-inclusions), increased mast cells and haemosiderin are other typical features. Other cases show greater architectural destruction, may have a vaguely follicular growth pattern, more prominent residual germinal centres, epithelioid histiocyte clusters and sometimes a much greater proportion of plasma cells or a more polymorphic appearance with more numerous transformed cells/immunoblasts {1934A}. Proliferation centres, as seen in CLL/small lymphocytic lymphoma (SLL) must be absent and the presence of paler-appearing

marginal zone type differentiation should suggest the diagnosis of one of the MZL. There may be associated amyloid, other immunoglobulin deposition or crystal storing histiocytes. Spleens demonstrate a lymphoplasmacytic infiltrate that may form small nodules in the red pulp or grow more diffusely.

Immunophenotype

Most cells express surface Ig and the plasmacytic cells express cytoplasmic Ig, usually IgM, sometimes IgG and rarely IgA. They are typically IgD-, express B-cell-associated antigens (CD19, CD20, CD22, CD79a) and are CD5-, CD10-, CD103- and CD23- with frequent but not invariable CD25 and CD38 expression. Some studies report more variation especially in CD22 and CD23 expression. The plasma cells are CD138 positive. Lack of CD5 in most but not all cases and the presence of strong cytoplasmic Ig are useful in the distinction from CLL/SLL.

Genetics

Antigen receptor genes
IG genes are rearranged usually with V regions that show somatic hypermutation but lack ongoing mutations {2349}. There may be biased VH usage {1026, 1193}.

Cytogenetic abnormalities and oncogenes
No specific chromosomal or oncogene abnormalities are recognized in LPL. The previously reported IGH@/PAX5 t(9;14) is rarely, if ever, found in LPL {463, 774, 1379}. Deletion 6q is reported in up to somewhat over half of BM-based cases but it is not a specific finding and appears at best to be infrequent in tissue based LPL {464, 1379, 1617, 1972}. Trisomy 3 and 18 are infrequent. Trisomy 4 has been reported in about 20% of WM {2183}. LPL do not demonstrate any of the other B-cell lymphoma-associated translocations such as those

involving the CCND1, MALT1, BCL10 or BCL2 genes with the possible rare exception of the latter. WM is reported to have a homogeneous gene expression profile, independent of 6q deletion, that is more similar to CLL and normal B-cells than to myeloma {429}. This study also suggested the importance of upregulated IL6 and its downstream MAPK signaling pathway.

Postulated normal counterpart
Probable post-follicular B-cell that differentiates to plasma cells.

Prognosis and predictive factors
The clinical course is typically indolent, with median survivals of 5–10 years {581, 2337}. Advanced age, PB cytopenias especially anaemia, performance status and high β-2 microglobulin levels have been reported to be associated with a worse prognosis {581, 2337}. Cases with increased transformed cells/immunoblasts may also be associated with an adverse prognosis; however, a validated grading system does not exist {43, 194}. Cases with del(6q) have been associated with features of adverse prognosis {1617}. Transformation to diffuse large B-cell lymphoma occurs in a small proportion of the cases and is associated with poor survival {1311}. Patients who have developed Hodgkin lymphoma are also reported {1863}.

Variant: gamma heavy chain disease
Gamma heavy chain disease results from secretion of a truncated gamma chain, which lacks light-chain binding sites. It is usually associated with a lymphoma that fulfills the criteria for LPL involving lymph nodes, BM, liver, spleen and PB but some cases resemble plasma cell myeloma. The clinical course is variable, but probably more aggressive than that of typical IgM-producing LPL.

Heavy chain diseases

N.L. Harris
P.G. Isaacson
T.M. Grogan
E.S. Jaffe

Definition
The heavy chain diseases (HCD) comprise 3 rare B-cell neoplasms that produce monoclonal heavy chains and typically no light chains. The monoclonal immunoglobulin component is composed of either IgG (gamma HCD), IgA (alpha HCD) or IgM (mu HCD). The heavy chain is usually incomplete and thus incapable of full assembly. Variably sized proteins are produced, that may not produce a characteristic serum protein electrophoresis peak, and require immunoelectrophoresis or immunofixation to detect. Alpha HCD is considered to be a variant of extranodal marginal zone lymphoma of mucosa-associated lymphoid tissue (MALT). Gamma HCD is characterized by a lymphoplasmacytic population resembling lymphoplasmacytic lymphoma and Mu HCD typically resembles CLL; however both are sufficiently distinctive to be considered separate entities.

ICD-O code   9762/3

Gamma heavy chain disease

Definition
Gamma heavy chain disease (gamma HCD) is a neoplasm of lymphocytes, plasmacytoid lymphocytes and plasma cells that produces a truncated gamma immunoglobulin heavy chain, which lacks light chain binding sites and does not bind to light chains to form a complete immunoglobulin molecule.

Synonym
Franklin disease.

Epidemiology
This is a rare disease of adults with a median age of 60; approximately 130 cases have been described {687, 2352}. There is no particular geographic distribution, and a slight male predominance in most but not all series {2352}.

Sites of involvement
The tumour may involve the lymph nodes, Waldeyer ring, gastrointestinal tract and other extranodal sites, bone marrow (BM), liver, spleen and peripheral blood (PB).

Clinical features
Most patients have systemic symptoms such as anorexia, weakness, fever, weight loss or recurrent bacterial infections. Autoimmune manifestations are found in about 25% of the cases, most frequently rheumatoid arthritis, but also autoimmune haemolytic anaemia or thrombocytopenia or both, vasculitis, Sjögren syndrome, systemic or cutaneous lupus erythematosus, myasthenia gravis or thyroiditis {687, 997, 2352}. Autoimmune disease may precede the diagnosis of lymphoma by several years. Most patients have generalized disease, including lymphadenopathy, splenomegaly and hepatomegaly; involvement of Waldeyer ring, skin and subcutaneous tissues, thyroid, salivary glands or gastrointestinal tract may occur, and PB eosinophilia may be present {687}. Circulating plasma cells or lymphocytes may occasionally be present. The patients generally do not have lytic bone lesions or amyloid deposition. The BM is involved in 30–60% of the cases {687, 997, 2352}. Clinical and laboratory distinction from an infection or inflammatory process may be difficult in view of this constellation of symptoms and the sometimes broad band or near-normal serum protein electrophoresis.

The diagnosis is made by demonstration of IgG without light chains by immunofixation in the PB, urine or both.

Morphology
Lymph nodes typically show a polymorphous proliferation with admixed lymphocytes, plasmacytoid lymphocytes, plasma cells, immunoblasts, histiocytes and eosinophils {1540A}. The presence of eosinophils, histiocytes and immunoblasts may cause a resemblance to angioimmunoblastic T-cell lymphoma (AITL) or Hodgkin lymphoma (HL); it is not clear whether rare reported cases of gamma HCD associated with AITL or HL represent a true association or a resemblance of the infiltrate of gamma HCD to HL {565, 992}. In some cases plasma cells predominate and may resemble plasmacytoma. The PB may show lymphocytosis with or without plasmacytoid lymphocytes, resembling chronic lymphocytic leukaemia (CLL) or lymphoplasmacytic lymphoma. Transformation to diffuse large B-cell lymphoma (DLBCL) is rare {687}. The BM may show lymphoplasmacytic aggregates or only a subtle increase in plasma cells with monotypic gamma heavy chains without light chains.

Immunophenotype
The cells contain monoclonal cytoplasmic gamma chain without light chains, express CD79a, CD20 on the lymphocytic

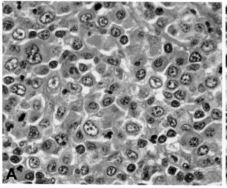
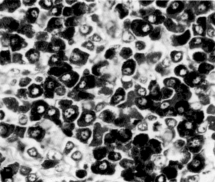

Fig. 10.24 Gamma heavy chain disease. **A** This polymorphous lymphoplasmacytic proliferation is comprised of admixed plasma cells, plasmacytoid lymphocytes and lymphoid cells. **B** Immunohistochemistry shows monotypic staining for gamma heavy chain.

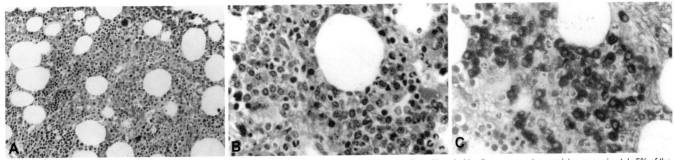

Fig. 10.25 Gamma heavy chain disease. Bone marrow biopsy. **A** Small aggregates composed of plasma cells and lymphoid cells are present, comprising approximately 5% of the overall marrow cellularity. Some plasma cells appear mature, while others are atypical with open chromatin (**B**). **C** Immunohistochemical stain shows cytoplasmic IgG Images courtesy of Dr. Aliyah Rahemtullah {1540A}.

component, CD138 on the plasma cell component, and are CD5 and CD10 negative {1540A}.

Genetics
Immunoglobulin genes are clonally rearranged and contain high levels of somatic hypermutation {686}. Deletions in the gamma heavy chain gene are present that result in expression of a defective heavy chain protein that cannot bind light chain to form a complete immunoglobulin molecule {21, 658, 686, 728, 732, 1989, 2351}. These deletions involve the *VH* region and variable amounts of the *CH1* region, and there may be insertions of large amounts of DNA of unknown origin {686}. Abnormal karyotypes have been present in about half of the reported cases, but no specific or recurring genetic abnormality has been reported {2352}.

Postulated normal counterpart
Post-germinal centre B cell with the ability to differentiate to a plasma cell, with a defective gamma heavy chain gene.

Prognosis and predictive factors
The clinical outcome is variable, ranging from indolent to rapidly progressive; the

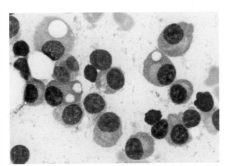

Fig. 10.26 Mu heavy chain disease. Bone marrow aspirate shows predominantly plasma cells with prominent cytoplasmic vacuolation.

median survival has been reported to be 12 months {686}; but a recent study of 23 cases reported a median of 7.4 years, with over half the deaths not related to the lymphoproliferative disorder {2352}. Most patients with low-grade appearing lympho-plasmacytic infiltrates appear to respond to non-anthracycline-containing chemotherapy, and responses to rituximab have been reported {2352}.

Mu heavy chain disease

Definition
Mu heavy chain disease (mu HCD) is a B-cell neoplasm resembling chronic lymphocytic leukaemia (CLL), in which a defective mu heavy chain lacking a variable region is produced. The BM contains an infiltrate of characteristic vacuolated plasma cells, admixed with small, round lymphocytes.

Epidemiology
This is an extremely rare disease of adults, with between 30 and 40 cases reported; a median age of 60 and an approximately equal frequency in males and females {686}.

Sites of involvement
Spleen, liver, BM and PB are involved; peripheral lymphadenopathy is usually not present.

Clinical features
Most patients present with a slowly progressive disease resembling chronic lymphocytic leukaemia. Mu HCD differs from most cases of CLL in the high frequency of hepatosplenomegaly and the absence of peripheral lymphadenopathy. Routine serum protein electrophoresis is frequently

normal. Immunoelectrophoresis reveals reactivity to anti-mu in polymers of diverse sizes. Although mu chain is not found in the urine, Bence Jones light chains are commonly found (50%) in the urine, particularly kappa chains. The latter, while still produced in mu HCD, are not assembled into a complete immunoglobulin protein because of heavy chain gene aberrancies leading to truncated forms {136, 2350}.

Morphology
The BM contains vacuolated plasma cells, which are typically admixed with small, round lymphocytes similar to chronic lymphocytic leukaemia cells.

Immunophenotype
The cells contain monoclonal cytoplasmic mu heavy chain, with or without monotypic light chain, express B-cell antigens, and are CD5 and CD10 negative.

Genetics
Immunoglobulin genes are clonally rearranged and contain high levels of somatic hypermutation {686}. Deletions in the mu heavy chain gene are present that result in expression of a defective heavy chain protein that cannot bind light chain to form a complete immunoglobulin molecule {686, 729}. These deletions involve the *VH* region and variable amounts of the *CH1* region, and there may be insertions of large amounts of DNA of unknown origin {686}.

Postulated normal counterpart
Post-germinal centre B cell which is able to differentiate to a plasma cell, with an abnormal mu heavy chain gene.

Prognosis
The clinical course is slowly progressive in most cases {136, 686, 729, 2350}.

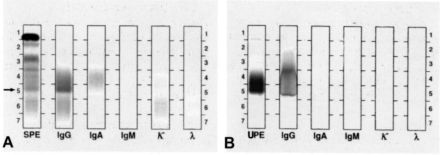

Fig. 10.27 Serum protein electrophoresis (SPE) and urine protein electrophoresis (UPE) in gamma heavy chain disease. A distinct band was identified by SPE in the immunoglobulin region anodal to the point of origin (**A**, arrow). The M-component typed as IgG (denoted by the band seen in the IgG lane), but without a corresponding light chain (only faint polyclonal patterns were seen in the kappa and lambda lanes) (**A**). UPE performed revealed similar results, with a broad monoclonal band corresponding to IgG without a corresponding light chain (**B**). Reprinted from {1540A}. (Images courtesy of Dr. M. Murali)

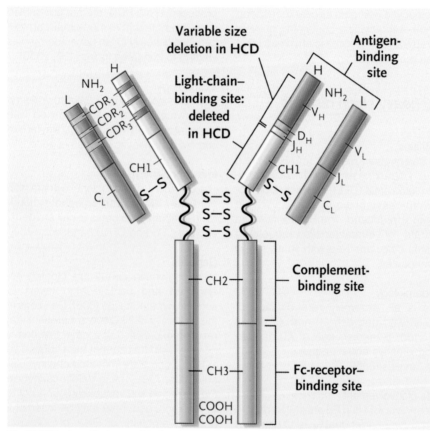

Fig. 10.28 Structure of the immunoglobulin molecule in heavy chain disease. An immunoglobulin molecule is composed of two heavy chains (H) and two light chains (L), which are joined by disulfide bonds (S–S). The normal heavy chain constant region has 3 constant domains: CH1 is responsible for binding to the light chain, CH2 for binding to complement and CH3 for binding to Fc receptors. In the absence of an associated light chain, the CH1 domain binds to heat-shock protein 78 and undergoes proteasomal degradation; thus, normal free heavy chains are not secreted. In heavy chain diseases (HCD), non-contiguous deletions in the CH1 domain prevent both binding of the heavy chain to the light chain and degradation in the proteasome, and free heavy chains are secreted. Variable-sized deletions also occur in the heavy chain diversity region (DH), the heavy chain joining region (JH) and the heavy chain variable region (VH). CDR denotes complementarity-determining region, CL light chain constant region, COOH carboxyl terminal, JL light chain joining region, NH2 amino terminal and VL light chain variable region. Reprinted with permission from {1540A}. (Figure courtesy of Dr N. Munshi)

Alpha heavy chain disease

Definition
The term alpha heavy chain disease (alpha HCD) has been extensively used in the literature, since many cases are initially recognized by the presence of an abnormal alpha chain in the serum. However, the term immunoproliferative small intestinal disease (IPSID) was adopted by the WHO in 1978 and will be used here. IPSID is a variant of extranodal marginal zone lymphoma of mucosa associated lymphoid tissue (MALT), in which defective alpha heavy chains are secreted; it is also discussed in the chapter on MALT lymphoma. It occurs in young adults and involves the gastrointestinal tract, resulting in malabsorption and diarrhoea. IPSID begins as a process sometimes reversible by antibiotics but may progress to diffuse large B-cell lymphoma (DLBCL).

Epidemiology
This is the most common of the heavy chain diseases. Unlike the other HCD, IPSID involves a young age group with a peak incidence in the second and third decades; it is rare in young children and older adults, and there is an equal incidence in males and females. It is most common in areas bordering the Mediterranean including Israel, Egypt, Saudi Arabia and North Africa. It is associated with low socioeconomic status including poor hygiene, malnutrition and frequent intestinal infections {1781, 1812, 1988}.

Etiology
Chronic intestinal infection, with Campylobacter jejuni in some cases, is believed to result in chronic inflammation, a setting in which neoplastic transformation of a clone of abnormal B cells develops {1264}.

Sites of involvement
This disorder involves the gastrointestinal tract, mainly the small intestine and mesenteric lymph nodes; gastric and colonic mucosa may be involved {686}. The BM and other organs are usually not involved, although rare respiratory tract involvement is described {1988}.

Clinical features at presentation
Patients typically present with malabsorption, diarrhoea, hypocalcemia, abdominal pain, wasting, fever and steatorrhoea. Because of defective heavy chain assembly and consequent diversity of IgA molecular

forms, the serum protein electrophoresis (SPE) is usually normal or shows hypogammaglobulinemia. Typically, specific anti-IgA antibody is required to detect aberrant IgA by immunofixation {1988}.

Morphology
The lamina propria of the bowel is heavily infiltrated with plasma cells and admixed small lymphocytes; marginal zone B-cells may be present with formation of lymphoepithelial lesions. The lymphoplasmacytic infiltrate separates the crypts, and villous atrophy may be present {1012, 1781, 1812}. Sheets of large plasmacytoid cells and immunoblasts that form solid, destructive aggregates with ulceration characterize progression to DLBCL {686}.

Immunophenotype
The plasma cells and marginal zone cells express monoclonal cytoplasmic alpha chain without light chain. Marginal zone cells express CD20 and are CD5 and CD10 negative; plasma cells are typically CD20 negative and CD138 positive {1012}.

Genetics
Immunoglobulin heavy and light chain genes are clonally rearranged and contain high levels of somatic hypermutation {686}. Deletions in the alpha heavy chain gene are present that result in expression of a defective heavy chain protein that cannot bind light chain to form a complete immunoglobulin molecule. These deletions involve the *VH* region and *CH1* region, and there may be insertions of DNA of unknown origin {686}.

Cytogenetic abnormalities have been reported in rare single cases. The t(11;18) associated with gastric and pulmonary MALT lymphomas has not been described {1721}. One reported case had t(9;14)(p11;q32) {1721}.

Prognosis and predictive factors
In the early phase, IPSID may completely remit with antibiotic therapy. Many patients, however, experience transformation to diffuse large B-cell lymphoma, and a fatal outcome is frequent {182, 1988}. Treatment with anthracycline-containing regimens has been reported to result in remission and long-term survival in some patients {16}.

Plasma cell neoplasms

R.W. McKenna
R.A. Kyle
W.M. Kuehl
T.M. Grogan
N.L. Harris
R.W. Coupland

The plasma cell neoplasms result from the expansion of a clone of immunoglobulin (Ig)-secreting, heavy-chain class-switched, terminally differentiated B cells that typically secrete a single homogeneous (monoclonal) immunoglobulin called a paraprotein or M-protein; the presence of such a protein is known as monoclonal gammopathy. The true plasma cell neoplasms, discussed in this chapter, include plasma cell myeloma, plasmactyoma and the syndromes defined by the consequence of tissue immunoglobulin deposition, primary amyloidosis (AL) and light and heavy chain deposition diseases. The presence in the peripheral blood (PB) of a low level of paraprotein that is below the usual threshold for the diagnosis of plasma cell myeloma may precede the development of overt myeloma for a varying time; this phenomenon, known as monoclonal gammopathy of undetermined significance (MGUS), is also included in this chapter as a precursor lesion. Other immunoglobulin-secreting neoplasms that comprise both lymphocytes and plasma cells, including lymphoplasmacytic lymphoma, Waldenström macroglobulinemia and the heavy chain diseases, are discussed in other chapters.

Table 10.03 Plasma cell neoplasms.

Monoclonal gammopathy of undetermined significance (MGUS)

Plasma cell myeloma
    Variants:
        Asymptomatic (smoldering) myeloma
        Non-secretory myeloma
        Plasma cell leukaemia

Plasmacytoma
    Solitary plasmacytoma of bone
    Extraosseous (extramedullary) plasmacytoma

Immunoglobulin deposition diseases
    Primary amyloidosis
    Systemic light and heavy chain
      deposition diseases

Osteosclerotic myeloma (POEMS syndrome)

Monoclonal gammopathy of undetermined significance (MGUS)

Definition
MGUS is defined as the presence in the serum of an M-protein <30 g/L, bone marrow (BM) clonal plasma cells <10%, no end organ damage (CRAB: hypercalcemia, renal insufficiency, anaemia, bone lesions) and no evidence of B-cell lymphoma or other disease known to produce an M-protein. Although it reflects the presence of an expanded clone of immunoglobulin-secreting cells, this process is not considered neoplastic since it does not always progress to overt malignancy. The presence of a small IgM paraprotein (IgM MGUS) is associated with a clone of lymphoplasmacytic cells that may progress to a lymphoplasmacytic lymphoma, and/ or Waldenström macroglobulinemia (WM). Non-IgM MGUS (IgG, IgA) is associated with the presence of clonal plasma cells, and may progress to a malignant plasma cell neoplasm. Although the two forms of MGUS may be identical in their clinical presentation, they have a different genetic basis and different outcomes in terms of malignant progression.

ICD-O code   9765/1

Synonyms
Monoclonal gammopathy, unattributed/ unassociated; Benign monoclonal gammopathy; Idiopathic paraproteinemia; Non-myelomatous gammopathy.

Epidemiology
When sensitive techniques of detection are used, MGUS is found in approximately 3% of persons over age 50 and in more than 5% of individuals past 70 {1232}. MGUS is more common in men than women (~1.5:1) and more than twice as frequent in African Americans as in Caucasians {1229, 1249}.

Etiology
No specific cause of MGUS has been

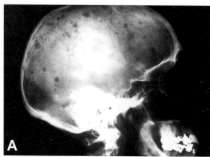

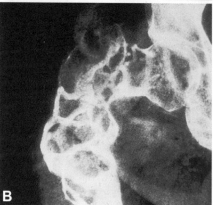

Fig. 10.29 Radiographs of (**A**) skull and (**B**) femoral head demonstrate multiple lytic bone lesions.

identified. It may be associated with connective tissue disorders, peripheral neuropathies, dermatological, endocrine and liver diseases {1229}. Transient oligoclonal and monoclonal gammopathies have been described in patients following solid organ and BM/stem cell transplantation {1229, 1491}.

Sites of involvement
The clonal plasma cells producing non-IgM MGUS are in the BM; lymphoplasmacytic cells that produce IgM MGUS may be in BM and other sites, such as spleen and lymph nodes.

Clinical features
Patients exhibit no symptoms or physical findings related to MGUS. The typical laboratory and radiographic abnormalities associated with plasma cell myeloma are lacking. The M-protein is usually discovered unexpectedly on serum protein electrophoresis. Approximately 70% are IgG,

Table 10.04 Diagnostic criteria for MGUS.

M-protein in serum <30 g/L
Bone marrow clonal plasma cells <10% and low level of plasma cell infiltration in a trephine biopsy
No lytic bone lesions
No myeloma-related organ or tissue impairment (CRAB: hypercalcemia, renal insufficiency, anaemia, bone lesions)
No evidence of other B-cell proliferative disorder

Modified from {56}.

15% IgM, 12% IgA and 3% are biclonal {1229}. Up to 20% of MGUS may consist only of an Ig light chain that may be detected only with the serum free light chain assay {1124, 1374}. Reduction of uninvolved immunoglobulins is found in 30–40% of patients with MGUS and monoclonal light chain in urine in nearly a third {1233}.

Morphology
Marrow aspirates contain a median of 3% plasma cells and trephine biopsies show no or a minimal increase in plasma cells that are interstitial and evenly scattered throughout the BM, or occasionally in small clusters {56}. They are usually mature appearing but mild changes, including cytoplasmic inclusions and nucleoli, are occasionally observed.

Immunophenotype
Staining for CD138 facilitates enumeration of plasma cells on BM trephine biopsies. Detection of the plasma cells that express monotypic cytoplasmic Ig of the same isotype as the M-protein is often difficult, because the clone may be small and in a background of normal plasma cells; monotypic light chain staining is not always detectable by immunohistochemistry {1731}. Immunophenotyping by flow cytometry frequently shows two populations of plasma cells, one with a normal immunophenotype (CD38 bright+, CD19+, CD56-) that is polyclonal and a monoclonal population with an aberrant phenotype, most often either CD19-/CD56+ or CD19-/CD56- {1726}. The monoclonal population may exhibit weaker expression of CD38 and other aberrant antigen expression {1618, 1643, 1726}.

Genetics
Abnormal karyotypes are rarely seen in MGUS. FISH studies have demonstrated both numerical and structural abnormalities in most patients {113, 430, 717, 718}. The abnormalities in non-IgM MGUS are the same as those found in myeloma although the prevalence may differ. Translocations involving the *IGH@* gene (14q32) are found in nearly half of the cases with different studies showing that t(11;14) (q23;q32) is present in 15–25%, t(4;14) (p16.3;q32) in 2–9% and t(14;16)(q32;q23) in 1–5% {113, 717}. Deletions of 13q are present in 40–50% of cases of MGUS compared to 50% of those with myeloma {717, 718, 1180}. It is not clear if 13q deletions sometimes are associated with progression of MGUS {1125, 1229}. Hyperdiploidy is observed in about 40% of MGUS with chromosomal trisomies similar to those in myeloma {430}. No obvious clinical correlations are associated with chromosome abnormalities in MGUS but this may reflect lack of sufficient data {717}. Activating *K-* and *NRAS* mutations are much less frequent in MGUS (~5%) compared to myeloma (30–40%) {1821}. Although genetic alterations and gene expression patterns probably can distinguish advanced myeloma from MGUS there are no unequivocal intrinsic differences that distinguish MGUS from myeloma.

Postulated normal counterpart
IgG and IgA MGUS are produced by post-germinal centre plasma cells with immunoglobulin genes that have somatic hypermutation of the variable regions and are class-switched. IgM MGUS is produced by B lymphocytes with somatic hypermutation of the *IGV* genes but without class switch {1234}.

Prognosis and predictive factors
The clinical course in most persons with MGUS is stable with no increase in M-protein or other evidence of progression. However, there can be evolution to an overt plasma cell myeloma, amyloidosis (in non-IgM MGUS), WM or other lymphoproliferative disorder (in IgM MGUS) {56, 1229}. The risk of progression is about 1% per year and indefinite, persisting even after 30 years {1233}. Thus, MGUS should be considered a pre-neoplastic condition {1697}. Size and type of M-protein and serum free light chain ratio are significant clinical risk factors {56, 1233, 1697}. Risk of progression for patients with an M-protein of 25 g/L is >4 times that of one with <5 g/L. Patients with an IgM or IgA MGUS are at greater risk of progression (~1.5% per year) to a malignant disorder than

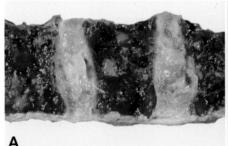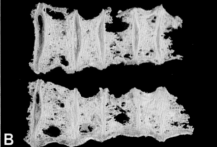

Fig. 10.30 Plasma cell myeloma. **A** Gross photograph of the vertebral column, showing multiple lytic lesions, filled with grey, fleshy tumour. **B** Vertebral column after maceration, showing multiple lytic lesions.

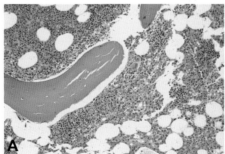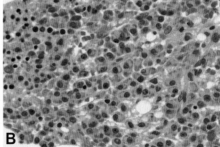

Fig. 10.31 Plasma cell myeloma. Low (**A**) and high (**B**) magnifications of a bone marrow biopsy. There is extensive marrow replacement with neoplastic plasma cells. The pattern of involvement is mixed, interstitial and focal. The plasma cells exhibit mature features with abundant cytoplasm, eccentric nuclei with coarse chromatin; most lack visible nucleoli.

those with IgG {1229, 1234}. In addition, the fraction of BM plasma cells with an abnormal immunophenotype, the detection of DNA aneuploidy and subnormal levels of polyclonal Ig also appear to be significant clinical risk factors {1726}.

Plasma cell myeloma

Definition
Plasma cell myeloma is a BM-based, multifocal plasma cell neoplasm associated with an M-protein in serum and/or urine. In most cases there is disseminated BM involvement. The disease spans a clinical spectrum from asymptomatic to aggressive forms and disorders due to deposition of abnormal immunoglobulin chains in tissues {1374}. The diagnosis is based on a combination of pathological, radiological and clinical features.

ICD-O code   9732/3

Synonyms
Multiple myeloma; Myelomatosis; medullary plasmacytoma; Kahler's disease.

Epidemiology
Plasma cell myeloma comprises about 1% of malignant tumours, 10–15% of haematopoietic neoplasms and causes 20% of deaths from haematologic malignancies {1052, 1844}. An estimated 20,000 cases were diagnosed and more than 10,000 patients died of myeloma in the United States in 2007 {1052}. Plasma cell myeloma is more common in men than women (1.4:1) and occurs twice as frequently in African Americans as in Caucasians {1844}. Myeloma is not found in children and only rarely in adults less than 30 years of age; the incidence increases progressively with age thereafter, with approximately 90% of cases occurring over age 50 and a median age at diagnosis of about 70 years. The risk of plasma cell myeloma is 3.7 fold higher for individuals with a first degree relative with the disease {282}.

Etiology
Chronic antigenic stimulation from infection or other chronic disease and exposure to specific toxic substances or radiation has been associated with an increased incidence of plasma cell myeloma {1289, 1315}. An antigenic stimulus giving rise to multiple benign clones

could be followed by a mutagenic event initiating malignant transformation {873}. Most patients have no identifiable toxic exposure or known chronic antigenic stimulation {1315}.

Sites of involvement
Generalized BM involvement is typically present. Lytic bone lesions and focal tumoural masses of plasma cells also occur. The most common sites are in BM areas of most active haematopoiesis. Extramedullary involvement is generally a manifestation of advanced disease.

Clinical features
Symptomatic plasma cell myeloma is defined by the presence of end-organ damage (CRAB: hypercalcemia, renal insufficiency, anaemia, bone lesions) in a patient with an M component and clonal BM plasma cells. In most patients there is a constellation of clinical, laboratory, radiological and pathological findings {1374}. Radiographic studies reveal lytic lesions, osteoporosis or fractures in 70% of cases of myeloma at diagnosis, often associated with bone pain and hypercalcemia {56, 1224, 1840}. Renal failure is due to tubular damage resulting from monoclonal light chain proteinuria; recurrent infections may be partly a consequence of depressed normal immunoglobulin

production; and anaemia (67%) results from BM replacement and renal damage with resultant loss of erythropoietin. An M-protein is found in the serum or urine in about 97% of patients {1226} (IgG 50%, IgA 20%, light chain 20% {56}, IgD, IgE, IgM and biclonal <10%); ~3% of cases are non-secretory. The serum M-protein is usually >30g/L of IgG and >20g/L of IgA. In 90% of patients there is a decrease in polyclonal Ig (<50% of normal). Other laboratory findings include hypercalcemia (20%), elevated creatinine (20-30%) {1226}, hyperuricemia (>50%) and hypoalbuminemia (~15%) {842, 1226}.

Clinical variants
Asymptomatic (smoldering) plasma cell myeloma
In asymptomatic plasma cell myeloma, the diagnostic criteria for myeloma are met but no related organ or tissue impairment (end-organ damage) is present {56, 1227}. Asymptomatic plasma cell myeloma is similar to MGUS in its lack of clinical manifestations, but is much more likely to progress to symptomatic myeloma {582, 1231, 1233}. Patients with Durie-Salmon stage I disease are included in this category and in some series so are asymptomatic patients with an apparent solitary plasmacytoma but with additional bone abnormalities detected only by MRI {56,

Table 10.05 Diagnostic criteria for plasma cell myeloma.

Symptomatic plasma cell myeloma
M-protein in serum or urine*
Bone marrow clonal plasma cells or plasmacytoma#
Related organ or tissue impairment^ (CRAB: hypercalcemia, renal insufficiency, anaemia, bone lesions)
Asymptomatic (smoldering) myeloma
M-protein in serum at myeloma levels (>30g/L)
AND/OR
10% or more clonal plasma cells in bone marrow
No related organ or tissue impairment [end organ damage or bone lesions (CRAB: hypercalcemia, renal insufficiency, anaemia, bone lesions)] or myeloma-related symptoms

* No level of serum or urine M-protein is included. M-protein in most cases is >30g/L of IgG or >25g/L of IgA or >1g/24 hr of urine light chain but some patients with symptomatic myeloma have levels lower than these.

\# Monoclonal plasma cells usually exceed 10% of nucleated cells in the marrow but no minimal level is designated because about 5% of patients with symptomatic myeloma have <10% marrow plasma cells.

^ The most important criteria for symptomatic myeloma are manifestations of end organ damage including anaemia, hypercalcemia, lytic bone lesions, renal insufficiency, hyperviscosity, amyloidosis or recurrent infections.

Modified from {56}.

582}. About 8% of patients with myeloma are initially asymptomatic {1231}. The majority have between 10 and 20% BM plasma cells and the median level of serum M-protein is nearly 30g/L. Normal polyclonal immunoglobulins are reduced in >90% of patients and ~70% have monoclonal light chains in urine {1226}. Patients may have stable disease for long periods but the cumulative probability of progression to symptomatic myeloma or amyloidosis is 10% per year for the first 5 years, 3% per year for the next 5 years and approximately 1% for the subsequent 10 years {1231}.

Non-secretory myeloma

In approximately 3% of plasma cell myelomas there is absence of an M-protein on immunofixation electrophoresis {56, 1226}. Cytoplasmic M-protein is present in the neoplastic plasma cells in about 85% of these when evaluated by immunohistochemistry, consistent with impaired secretion of Ig {56}. In about 15% of these patients, no cytoplasmic Ig synthesis is detected (non-producer myeloma). Acquired mutations of the Ig light chain variable genes or alteration in the light chain constant region have been implicated in the pathogenesis of the non-secretory state {477, 622}. In up to two-thirds of cases, however, elevated serum free light chains and/or an abnormal free light chain ratio are detectable, suggesting that many are at least minimally secretory {610}. The clinical features of non-secretory myeloma are similar to other plasma cell myelomas except for a lower incidence of renal insufficiency and hypercalcemia and less depression of normal Ig {56, 2037}.

Plasma cell leukaemia (PCL)

In PCL, the number of clonal plasma cells in the PB exceeds 2×10^9/L or is 20% of the leukocyte differential count {56}. In addition to PB and BM, the neoplastic plasma cells may be found in extramedullary tissues, such as spleen and liver and in pleural effusions, ascites and cerebrospinal fluid. PCL may be present at the time of diagnosis (primary PCL) or evolve as a late feature in the course of plasma cell myeloma (secondary PCL) {757}. Primary PCL is found in 2–5% of cases of myeloma {112, 583, 757}. Compared to IgG or IgA myeloma, a higher proportion of light chain only, IgD, or IgE myeloma present as PCL {757, 916}. The cytologic

characteristics of the leukaemic plasma cells span much of the morphologic spectrum found in other myelomas but often, many of the plasma cells are small with relatively little cytoplasm and may resemble plasmacytoid lymphocytes {288}. Typically, the immunophenotype of PCL differs from that of most other myelomas by the lack of aberrant CD56 expression {1719}. An abnormal karyotype is more frequently found and there is a higher incidence of unfavourable cytogenetics

{112}. Most clinical signs of myeloma are observed in PCL, although osteolytic lesions and bone pain are less frequent and lymphadenopathy, organomegaly and renal failure are more often present {757}. PCL is an aggressive disease with short survival {112, 583, 757}.

Macroscopy

In plasma cell myeloma, the bone defects on gross examination are filled with a soft gelatinous, fish-flesh, haemorrhagic tissue.

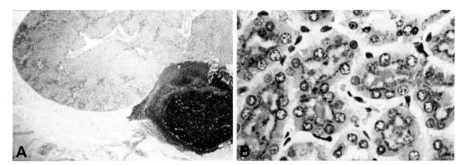

Fig.10.32 Plasma cell myeloma. **A** Perirenal involvement (extramedullary plasmacytoma). Immunohistochemical assay reveals lambda light chain-bearing perirenal plasmacytoma. **B** Section of kidney showing renal tubular lambda deposition with casts reflecting renal tubular Bence Jones protein reabsorption (Immunoperoxidase, anti-lambda light chain).

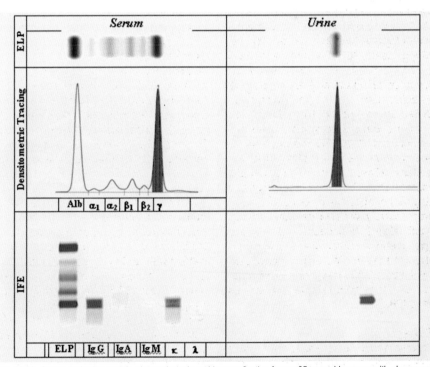

Fig. 10.33 Serum and urine protein electrophoresis and immunofixation from a 65-year-old woman with plasma cell myeloma who presented with back, neck, and pelvic pain and generalized weakness. There was no hypercalcemia, renal failure or anaemia; however, a skeletal survey revealed multiple lytic lesions in the skull, ribs, pelvis, clavicles, scapula and spine. A bone marrow biopsy showed 13% plasma cells. Protein electrophoresis (ELP) revealed a 31 g/L, serum IgGk M-protein and a 347.4 mg/24 h, urine M-protein. The M-protein was identified by immunofixation electrophoresis (IFE) as IgG kappa. (Courtesy of Drs Frank H. Wians, Jr. and Dennis C. Wooten).

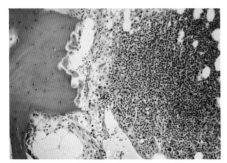

Fig. 10.34 Plasma cell myeloma in a bone marrow biopsy. A discrete plasma cell mass displaces normal marrow fat cells and haematopoietic elements. Near the myeloma mass note prominent osteoclastic activity in the trabecular bone.

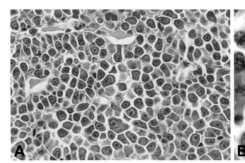

Fig. 10.35 Plasma cell myeloma bone marrow biopsies. This composite illustrates the histological features of two immature myelomas. **A** The plasma cells are relatively uniform and most have eccentrically located nuclei. The nuclear chromatin is dispersed and nearly every nucleus contains a prominent centrally located brightly eosinophilic nucleolus. **B** The plasma cells are profoundly pleomorphic with frequent multinucleated cells consistent with the term "anaplastic plasma cell myeloma".

Morphology

Bone marrow biopsy

In contrast to normal plasma cells, which are typically found in small clusters around BM arterioles, myeloma plasma cells usually occur in interstitial clusters, focal nodules or diffuse sheets {152, 288}. There is often considerable BM sparing and preservation of normal haematopoiesis, with interstitial and focal patterns of involvement. With diffuse involvement, expansive areas of the BM are replaced and haematopoiesis may be markedly suppressed. There is typically progression from interstitial and focal disease in early myeloma to diffuse involvement in advanced stages of disease {152}. Generally, when 30% of the BM volume is comprised of plasma cells, a diagnosis of myeloma is likely, although rare cases of reactive plasmacytosis may reach that level. A tumoural mass of plasma cells displacing normal BM elements strongly favours a diagnosis of plasma cell myeloma, even if the overall percentage of plasma cells is <30. Occasionally prominent osteoclastic activity is observed in biopsy sections, resulting in the bone lesions on radiographs.

Immunohistochemistry is useful in quantifying plasma cells on biopsies, in confirming a monoclonal plasma cell proliferation and in distinguishing myeloma from other neoplasms. A CD138 stain is useful for quantifying plasma cells, and clonality can usually be established with stains for kappa and lambda light chains {56, 1731}.

Bone marrow aspiration

The number of plasma cells seen on aspirate smears varies from barely increased to upwards of 90% {1226}. Myeloma plasma cells vary from mature forms indistinguishable from normal to immature, plasmablastic, and pleomorphic {152, 288, 840}. Mature plasma cells are usually oval, with a round eccentric

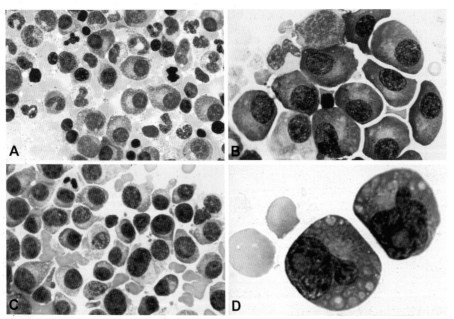

Fig. 10.36 Plasma cell myeloma, cytologic features in marrow aspirations showing variation from mature (**A,B**) to immature (**C,D**) plasma cells. The more mature cells have clumped nuclear chromatin, abundant cytoplasm, low nuclear-cytoplasmic ratio and only rare nucleoli compared to the less mature cells, which have more prominent nucleoli, loose reticular chromatin and a higher nuclear-cytoplasmic ratio. **D** Plasmablasts from a plasmablastic myeloma with prominent nucleoli, reticular chromatin and high nuclear-cytoplasmic ratio.

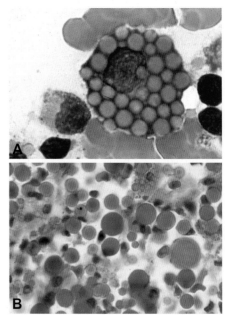

Fig. 10.37 Plasma cell myeloma, morphologic variants based on cytoplasmic features. **A** So-called Mott cell with abundant "grape-like" cytoplasmic inclusions of immunoglobulin. **B** Numerous Russell bodies.

nucleus and "spoke wheel" or "clock-face" chromatin without nucleoli. There is generally abundant basophilic cytoplasm and a perinuclear hof. In contrast, immature forms have more dispersed nuclear chromatin, a higher nuclear/cytoplasmic ratio, and often, prominent nucleoli. In almost 10% of cases there is plasmablastic morphology {840}. Multinucleated, polylobated, pleomorphic plasma cells are prominent in some cases {152, 288}. Because nuclear immaturity and pleomorphism rarely occur in reactive plasma cells, they are reliable indicators of neoplastic plasma cells. The cytoplasm of myeloma cells has abundant endoplasmic reticulum (ER), which may contain, condensed or crystallized cytoplasmic Ig producing a variety of morphologically distinctive findings, including: multiple pale bluish-white, grape-like accumulation (Mott cells, Morula cells), cherry-red refractive round bodies (Russell bodies), vermilion staining glycogen-rich IgA (flame cells), overstuffed fibrils (Gaucher-like cells, thesaurocytes) and crystalline rods {288}. Other than the presence of crystalline rods, these changes are not pathognomonic of myeloma since they may be found in reactive plasma cells.

In about 5% of cases of symptomatic myeloma there are <10% plasma cells in the BM aspirate smears {56}. This may be due to a sub-optimal BM aspirate or the frequent focal distribution of myeloma in the BM. In such instances, larger numbers of plasma cells and focal clusters are sometimes observed in the trephine biopsy sections. Biopsies directed at radiographic lesions may be necessary to establish the diagnosis in some patients.

Peripheral blood
Rouleaux formation is usually the most striking feature on PB smears and is related to the quantity and type of M-protein. A leukoerythroblastic reaction is observed in some cases. Plasma cells are found on PB smears in approximately 15% of cases, usually in small numbers. Marked plasmacytosis accompanies plasma cell leukaemia.

Kidney
Bence Jones protein accumulates as aggregates of eosinophilic material in the lumina of the renal tubules. Renal tubular reabsorption of Bence Jones protein is largely responsible for renal damage in plasma cell myeloma.

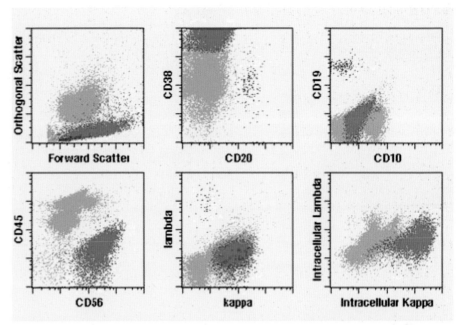

Fig.10.38 Flow cytometry histograms of a bone marrow from a patient with plasma cell myeloma. The neoplastic plasma cells are painted red; normal B lymphocytes are blue. The myeloma cells express bright CD38 and are negative for CD20, CD19 and CD10. They express CD56 and partial CD45, are negative for surface light chains and express cytoplasmic kappa.

Immunophenotype
Plasma cell myelomas typically have monotypic cytoplasmic Ig and lack surface Ig. They usually express CD79a, VS38c, CD138 and strong CD38, similarly to normal plasma cells but in contrast to normal plasma cells, they are nearly always CD19 negative; CD56 is aberrantly expressed in 67–79% of cases {1312, 1719, 1908}. In addition to CD56, myeloma plasma cells may aberrantly express CD117, CD20, CD52 and CD10, in decreasing order of frequency, and occasionally, myeloid and monocytic antigens are found {26, 850, 1312}. Unlike most myelomas, about 80% of plasma cell leukaemias are CD56 negative {757, 1719, 1908}. Some cases are cyclin D1 positive. This finding correlates with the presence of t(11;14)(q13;q32) involving the *CCND1* gene and has been associated with a lymphoplasmacytic morphologic appearance.

Genetics
Antigen receptor genes
Immunoglobulin heavy and light chain genes are clonally rearranged. There is a high load of *IGHV* gene somatic hypermutation consistent with derivation from a post-germinal centre, antigen-driven B-cell {134}. Immunoglobulin gene deletion is sometimes found; in patients with

light chain only disease or Bence Jones proteinuria, *JH* segments and/or parts or all of chromosome 14 may be lost {140}.
Genetic abnormalities and oncogenes
Abnormalities are detected by conventional cytogenetics in about one third of myelomas {561, 1947}. Fluorescence *in situ* hybridization (FISH) increases the proportion with chromosomal abnormalities to >90% {111, 430, 718, 1181, 1947}. Both numerical and structural abnormalities are found and include trisomies, whole or partial chromosome deletions and translocations; complex cytogenetic abnormalities are common {561}. The most frequent chromosome translocations involve the heavy chain locus *(IGH@)* on chromosome 14q32 and are present in 55–70% of tumours {113, 718}. Five major recurrent oncogenes are involved in 14q32 translocations: *cyclin D1* (11q13) (15–18%); *C-MAF* (16q23) (5%); *FGFR3/MMSET* (4p16.3) (15%); *cyclin D3* (6p21) (3%); and *MAFB* (20q11) (2%) {111, 199, 200, 1201}. Together these 5 translocations are found in about 40% of cases of myeloma, most of which are non-hyperdiploid (<48 and/or >75 chromosomes). The remaining tumours, which only infrequently have one of the five recurrent *IGH@* translocations, are mostly hyperdiploid, usually with gains in the odd numbered chromosomes, 3, 5, 7, 9, 11,

Table 10.06 Translocation and Cyclin D groups in plasma cell myelomas.

Group	Primary translocation	Gene	D-Cyclin	Ploidy	Frequency	Prognosis
6p21	6p21	CCND3	D3	NH	3%	Good
11q13	11q13	CCND1	D1	D, NH	16%	Good
D1	None	None	D1	H	34%	Good
D1+D2	None	None	D1+D2	H	6%	? Poor
D2	None	None	D2	H, NH	17%	?
None	None	None	None	NH	2%	? Good
4p16	4p16	FGFR3/MMSET	D2	NH>H	15%	Poor
maf	16q23	c-maf	D2	NH	5%	Poor
	20q11	mafB	D2	NH	2%	Poor

*D, diploid; H, hyperdiploid; NH, non-hyperdiploid. Modified from {200}.

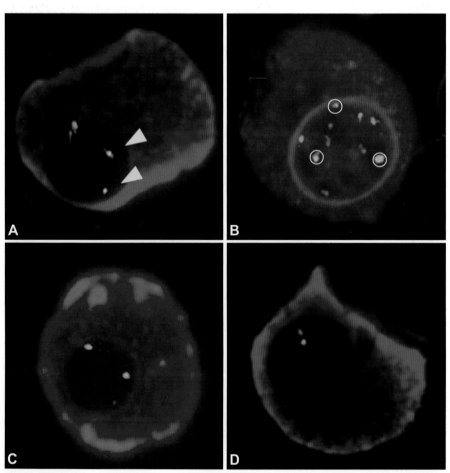

Fig. 10.39 Interphase FISH analyses of recurrent abnormalities in plasma cell myeloma. **A** Fusion signals for t(4;14)(p16;q32). *IgH* probes-green; *MMSET/FGFR3* probes-red. Two fusion signals indicated by yellow arrowheads most likely identify der(4) and der(14) but could represent two copies of der(4). **B** Extra copies of three chromosomes in a hyperdiploid tumour. Three copies of chromosome 5 (LSI D5S23/D5S721-green) and chromosome 9 (*CEP* 9-aqua [circled] and four copies of chromosome 15 (*CEP* 15-red). **C** Two copies of chromosome 17 and deletion of one copy of *TP53*. *TP53*-red, *CEP* 17-green. **D** Loss of one copy of chromosome 13/13q. LSI 13[containing *RB1*]-green, D13S319-red. In all four panels, the cytoplasm is blue due to immunostaining of Ig-kappa or Ig-lambda expressed by the tumour plasma cells, and the probes are from Vysis. Courtesy of Dr Scott Van Wier and Dr Rafael Fonseca.

15, 19 and 21 {430, 431, 718, 2099}. Both *IGH@* translocations and hyperdiploidy, appear to be early events in the genesis of plasma cell neoplasms, unified by associated upregulation of one of the *cyclin D* genes (D1, D2, D3) {199, 201, 405, 2099}. Gene expression profiling can determine the expression levels of *cyclin D1*, D2 and D3 and identify myeloma that overexpress oncogenes dysregulated by the five recurrent *IGH@* translocations. Using patterns of translocations (T) and cyclin (C) D expression (TC groups) plasma cell myelomas can be classified into 8 groups that are based mostly on initiating or early pathogenic events {200}. Some or all of these groups may represent distinct disease entities that require different therapeutic approaches {200}. Another molecular classification is based on unsupervised clustering of tumours by gene expression profiles {2495}. This identifies seven molecular groups that are similar although not identical to the TC groups, with one of the seven molecular groups being defined by progression events that lead to increased proliferation.

Monosomy or partial deletion of chromosome 13 (13q14), which is found in nearly half of tumours by FISH, is another early event in pathogenesis, although the precise timing of these various early events is poorly understood {111, 718}. Activating mutations of *K*- or *NRAS* are present in about 30–40% of tumours, and are thought to represent an early event in progression, perhaps mediating the MGUS to myeloma transition in some patients {718, 1821}. Some other recurrent genetic changes associated with disease progression in both non-hyperdiploid and hyperdiploid tumours include the following: secondary *IGH@* or *IGL* translocations, deletion and/or mutation of *TP53* (17p13), translocations involving *MYC* or less often *N-MYC*, gains of chromosome 1q and loss of 1p, mutations of genes that result in activation of the NF-kappa B pathway, mutations of *FGFR3* in tumours with t(4;14), and inactivation of *p18INK4c* or *RB1* {45, 111, 200, 571, 880, 1131, 1201, 2017, 2099}. Epigenetic changes manifested by DNA methylation also are associated with tumour progression.

Although genetic events appear to play the key role in initiation and progression of plasma cell myeloma, the BM microenvironment is also important in pathogenesis and progression {1489}.

Extracellular matrix proteins, secreted cytokines and growth factors, and/or the functional consequences of direct interaction of the BM stromal cells with neoplastic plasma cells are major constituents that influence the pathophysiology of myeloma {1489}.

Postulated normal counterpart
Post-germinal centre long-lived plasma cells in which the immunoglobulin genes have undergone class switch and somatic hypermutation.

Prognosis and predictive factors
Plasma cell myeloma is usually incurable, with a median survival of 3–4 years, but the range varies from <6 months to >10 years {842}. The Durie and Salmon (DS) staging system applies commonly available clinical parameters to predict myeloma cell tumour burden —low, intermediate and high tumour cell burden {160, 633} (Table 10.07). There is a significant difference in survival between each of three tumour mass stages; normal renal function versus renal insufficiency further defines lower versus higher risk patients in each stage {633, 842, 1808}. Additional indicators of higher risk patients include elevated serum ß-2-microglobulin (ß2M), low serum albumin, elevated lactate dehydrogenase, high C-reactive protein, increased plasma cell proliferative activity, high degree of BM replacement, plasmablastic morphology and genetics {159, 160, 841, 1808}. An international staging system (ISS) for plasma cell myeloma provides highly significant prognostic correlations, using a combination of serum ß2M and albumin level to define 3 stages {842} (Table 10.08).
Patients with abnormalities by conventional (metaphase) cytogenetics have a significantly shorter median survival than those without {111, 416, 428, 787, 842, 880, 912, 1132, 1181, 2000, 2099}. The most important independent negative prognostic indicators include: high risk t(4;14) and the *MAF* translocations t(14;16) and t(14;20), deletion of 17p/*TP53* sequences and increased serum ß2M. A high-risk molecular signature based on the expression of either 70 or 17 genes provides perhaps the most robust, independent prognostic indicator {2001}.

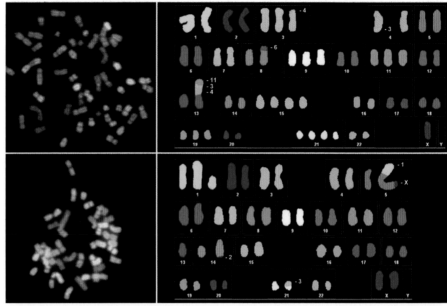

Fig. 10.40 Spectral karyotypic (SKY) analysis of hyperdiploid and non-hyperdiploid plasma cell myeloma. **A,C** Metaphase spreads in display colors. **B,D** Classification of chromosomes; **A, B** Hyperdiploid tumour with 53 chromosomes, including four rearranged chromosomes involving two or more different chromosomes, trisomies of chromosomes 3, 9, 11, 19 and tetrasomies of chromomes 15 and 21. From FISH analyses (not shown), there is no *IGH* or *IGL* translocation, but *MYC* is inserted on chromosome 6p23. **C,D** Non-hyperdiploid tumour with 46 chromosomes, including at least three rearranged chromosomes involving two or more different chromosomes, an internally deleted chromosome 14, and loss of one copy of chromosome 13. FISH analyses (not shown) confirm the presence of a t(2;14)(p23;q32) involving *N-MYC* and a karyotypically silent t(4;14)(p16;q32). Courtesy of Dr Anna Roschke and Dr Ana Gabrea.

Table 10.07 Myeloma staging system. Modified from Durie and Salmon {633}.

Stage I:
- Low M-protein levels: IgG <50g/L, IgA <30g/L; Urine BJ <4g/24hr
- Absent or solitary bone lesions.
- Normal haemoglobin, serum calcium, Ig levels (non-M protein).

Stage II: Overall values between I and III

Stage III: Any one or more of the following:
- High M-protein: IgG >70g/L, IgA > 50g/L; Urine light chain >12g/24hr
- Advanced, multiple lytic bone lesions.
- Haemoglobin <8.5g/dL, serum calcium >12mg/dL.

Subclassification: Based on renal function
  A = serum creatinine <2 mg/dL
  B = serum creatinine ≥2 mg/dL

Table 10.08 International staging system for plasma cell myeloma.

Stage	Criteria	Median survival
I	Serum ß₂-microglobulin <3.5 mg/L Serum albumin >3.5 g/dL	62 months
II	Not stage I or III*	44 months
III	Serum ß₂-microglobulin >5.5 mg/L	29 months

*There are two categories for stage II: serum ß₂-microglobulin <3.5 mg/L but serum albumin <3.5 g/dL; or serum ß₂-microglobulin 3.5 to <5.5 mg/L irrespective of the serum albumin level.
Modified from {842}.

Table 10.09
Cytogenetic prognostic groups in plasma cell myeloma.

Unfavourable risk:
Deletion 13 or aneuploidy by metaphase analysis
t(4;14) or t(14;16) or t(14;20) by FISH
Deletion 17p13 by FISH
Hypodiploidy
Favourable risk:
Absence of unfavourable risk genetics and presence of hyperdiploidy, t(11;14) or t(6;14) by FISH
Modified from {2099}.

Solitary plasmacytoma of bone

Definition
Solitary plasmacytoma of bone (osseous plasmacytoma) is a localized bone tumour consisting of monoclonal plasma cells. Complete skeletal radiographs show no other lesions. There are no clinical features of plasma cell myeloma and no evidence of BM plasmacytosis except for the solitary lesion {56, 2061}.

ICD-O code   9731/3

Epidemiology
Solitary plasmacytoma of bone comprises 3–5% of plasma cell neoplasms {56}. It is more common in men (65%); median age at diagnosis is 55 years {56, 582}.

Sites of involvement
The most common sites are bones with active BM haematopoiesis; in order of frequency, the vertebrae, ribs, skull, pelvis, femur, clavicle and scapula {582}. Thoracic vertebrae are more commonly involved than cervical or lumbar, and long bone involvement below the elbow or knee is rare {56, 545}.

Clinical features
Patients most frequently present with bone pain at the site of the lesion or with a pathological fracture. Vertebral lesions may be associated with symptomatic cord compression {545}. Soft tissue extension may produce a palpable mass {56}. An M-protein is found in serum or urine in 24–72% of patients {56, 582, 2061, 2403}. In most cases polyclonal immunoglobulins are at normal levels {582, 2061}. There is no anaemia, hypercalcemia or renal failure related to the plasmacytoma {56}. MRI is useful to exclude

additional lesions and is considered a prerequisite for diagnosis by some investigators {1296, 2061}.

Morphology, immunophenotype and genetics
Plasmacytomas are usually easily recognizable in tissue sections unless the plasma cells are very poorly differentiated, e.g. plasmablastic or anaplastic. Confirmation of a clonal plasma cell lesion can be accomplished by immunohistochemistry. Even when the diagnosis is apparent, determination of light chain type is suggested. The immunophenotype and genetics are similar to those of plasma cell myeloma

Prognosis and predictive factors
Local control is achieved by radiotherapy in most cases, but up to two thirds of patients eventually evolve to generalized myeloma or additional solitary or multiple plasmacytomas {56, 545, 955}. Approximately one-third of patients remain disease free for >10 years; median overall survival is ~10 years {56}. Older patients and those with a solitary plasmacytoma larger than 5 cm or persistence of an M-protein following local radiotherapy reportedly have a higher incidence of progression {56, 582, 1296, 2272, 2403}. However, these unfavourable features have not been consistent between series {2061}. Osteopenia and low levels of uninvolved immunoglobulins, both of which suggest occult plasma cell myeloma, are also reported as adverse prognostic factors {582, 1030}. Measurement of the free light chain ratio is useful for predicting progression {587}.

Extraosseous plasmacytoma

Definition
Extraosseous (extramedullary) plasmacytomas are localized plasma cell neoplasms that arise in tissues other than bone. Lymphomas with prominent plasmacytic differentiation, particularly extranodal marginal zone (MALT) lymphoma, must be excluded.

ICD-O code   9734/3

Synonym
Plasmacytoma, extramedullary.

Epidemiology
Extraosseous (extramedullary) plasmacytomas constitute 3–5% of all plasma cell neoplasms {22}. Two thirds of patients are male; the median age at diagnosis is about 55 years.

Sites of involvement
Approximately 80% of extraosseous plasmacytomas occur in the upper respiratory tract, including the oropharynx, nasopharynx, sinuses and larynx, but they may occur in numerous other sites, including the gastrointestinal tract (GI), lymph nodes, bladder, CNS, breast, thyroid, testis, parotid and skin {22}. Plasmacytomas of the upper respiratory track spread to cervical lymph nodes in ~15% of cases {1460}.

Clinical features
Symptoms are generally related to the tumour mass and include rhinorrhoea, epistaxis and nasal obstruction. Radiographic and morphologic assessments show no evidence of BM involvement. Approximately 20% of patients have a small M-protein, most commonly IgA {56, 2061}. There are no clinical features of plasma cell myeloma.

Morphology
The morphologic features are similar to those of solitary plasmacytoma of bone. However, in extraosseous sites, distinction between lymphomas that exhibit extreme plasma cell differentiation and plasmacytoma may be difficult {580}. Marginal zone lymphoma of MALT type, lymphoplasmacytic lymphoma and occasionally, immunoblastic or plasmablastic large cell lymphomas may be misdiagnosed as plasmacytoma {580, 999}. Distinction from a marginal zone lymphoma with marked plasma cell differentiation is especially problematic, particularly in skin and GI, and may not be possible in some instances. Areas with features of marginal zone lymphoma may be identified in tissue sections in some cases and in others a clonally related lymphocyte population may be identified by flow cytometry.

Immunophenotype and genetic features
The immunophenotype and genetic features are not extensively studied, but appear to be similar to those of plasma cell myeloma. Immunohistochemistry or *in situ* hybridization for Ig light chains can be useful in distinguishing neoplastic from

reactive plasma cell infiltrates. Expression of CD20 by lymphocytes within the lesion or by the plasmacytoid cells or expression of μ rather than γ heavy chain favours a diagnosis of lymphoma over plasmacytoma.

Prognosis and predictive factors
In most cases the lesions are eradicated with local radiation therapy. Regional recurrences develop in up to 25% of patients and occasionally there is metastasis to distant extraosseous sites. Progression to plasma cell myeloma is infrequent, occurring in ~15% of cases {22}. About 70% of patients remain disease free at 10 years {579}. This indolent course may suggest that many cases are more closely related to MALT lymphoma than to myeloma.

Monoclonal immunoglobulin deposition diseases

The monoclonal immunoglobulin deposition diseases (MIDD) are closely-related disorders that are characterized by visceral and soft tissue deposition of immunoglobulin, resulting in compromised organ function {106, 304, 934, 1085, 1225, 1779, 1814, 1994, 2433}. The underlying disorder is typically a plasma cell neoplasm, or

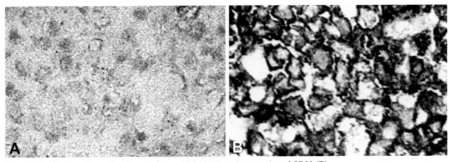

Fig. 10.41 Plasmacytoma showing absence of CD20 (**A**) and expression of CD38 (**B**).

rarely a lymphoplasmacytic neoplasm {785, 786}; however, the immunoglobulin molecule accumulates in tissue before the development of a large tumour burden. Thus, these patients typically do not have overt myeloma, or lymphoplasmacytic lymphoma at the time of the diagnosis. The MIDD appear to be chemically different manifestations of similar pathological processes, resulting in clinically similar but not identical conditions. There are two major categories of MIDD: primary amyloidosis and light chain deposition disease (LCDD); rarely light and heavy chain deposition disease (LHCDD) and heavy chain deposition disease (HCDD) may be seen.

Primary amyloidosis

Definition
Primary amyloidosis is caused by a plasma cell, or rarely, a lymphoplasmacytic neoplasm that secretes intact or fragments of abnormal immunoglobulin light chains, or rarely, heavy chains, which deposit in various tissues and form a ß-pleated sheet structure (AL amyloid) that binds Congo red dye with characteristic birefringence {785, 786, 813, 1157, 1225, 1994}.

ICD-O code   9769/1

Epidemiology
The median age at diagnosis of primary amyloidosis is 64 years and >95% of patients are over 40; 65–70% are male {1225, 1228}.

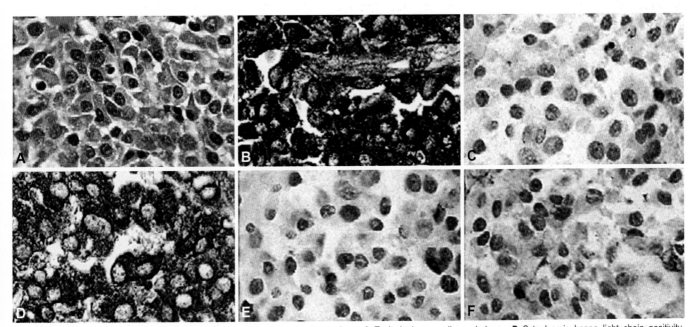

Fig. 10.42 Plasmacytoma. Composite figure illustrates immunoglobulin expression. **A** Typical plasma cell morphology. **B** Cytoplasmic kappa light chain positivity. **C** Absence of lambda light chain disease expression. **D** Expression of cytoplasmic gamma heavy chain. **E,F** Absence of mu and alpha heavy chains.

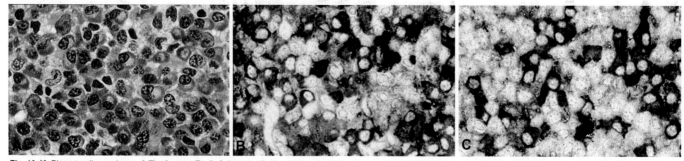

Fig. 10.43 Plasma cell granuloma. **A** The "mass effect" of plasma cells simulates a neoplasm. Immunoperoxidase stains show polytypic cytoplasmic immunoglobulin with some plasma cells expressing (**B**) kappa light chains and some expressing (**C**) lambda light chains.

Approximately 20% of patients have plasma cell myeloma but most have criteria for MGUS with production of a M-protein that results in pathological deposition of Ig light chains in various tissues. Among patients with myeloma, up to 10% have or will develop amyloidosis {56, 1225, 1226, 1994}.

Sites of involvement

AL amyloid accumulates in many tissues and organs including subcutaneous fat, kidney, heart, liver, GI, peripheral nerves and BM. The diagnostic biopsy site generally is the abdominal subcutaneous fat-pad, BM or the rectum {1225, 1994}.

Clinical features

Clinical findings are usually related to deposition of amyloid in organs, resulting in organomegaly. Purpura (15%) (particularly periorbital or facial), bone pain (5%), peripheral neuropathy (17%) and carpal tunnel syndrome (21%) are early signs of disease. Haemorrhagic manifestations are found in approximately one-fifth of cases. Bleeding may occur due to increased fragility of blood vessels from amyloid deposits, binding of coagulation factor X and/or vascular structures to amyloid proteins. Symptoms referable to congestive heart failure (17%), nephrotic syndrome (28%) or malabsorption (5%) are all relatively common {1225}. Hepatomegaly is found in 25–30% of patients and macroglossia in about 10% {1225}. Edema is often present in patients with congestive heart failure or nephrotic syndrome {1225}. An M-protein is found in the serum and/or urine by immunofixation in >90% of patients with primary amyloidosis and with a combination of immunofixation and serum free light chain ratio analysis in 99% {57, 1123, 1225}. The light chain is lambda in 70% of patients {1225}.

Pathophysiology

AL amyloid is composed of intact immunoglobulin light chains or rarely, heavy chains that are secreted by monoclonal plasma cells and then ingested, processed and discharged by macrophages into the extracellular matrix. The accumulated amyloid includes both intact light chain and fragments of the variable (V) NH2-terminus region. All light chain V region fragments are potentially amyloidogenic, and all plasma cell neoplasms that produce VλVI have AL {1225, 1994}.

Macroscopy

On gross inspection amyloid has a dense "porcelain-like" or waxy appearance.

Morphology

Biopsy sections of BM vary from no pathologic findings to extensive replacement with amyloid, overt myeloma, or rarely, lymphoplasmacytic lymphoma. The most common finding is a mild increase in plasma cells that may appear normal or exhibit any of the changes found in plasma cell myeloma {1225}. Amyloid is present in many other tissues and organs. In H&E stained sections, it is a pink, amorphous, waxy-appearing substance, with a characteristic cracking artifact. Typically, it is found focally in thickened blood vessel walls, on basement membranes, and in the interstitium of tissues such as fat or BM {2433}. Macrophages and foreign-body giant cells may be found around deposits. Organ parenchyma may be massively replaced by amyloid (amyloidoma). Plasma

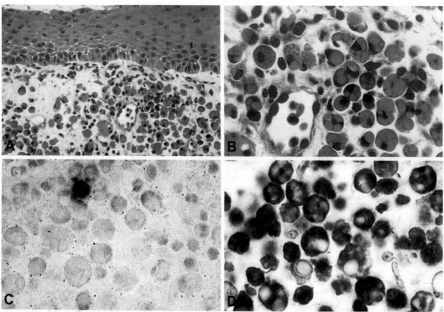

Fig. 10.44 Extramedullary plasmacytoma of the skin with abundant Russell body formation (**A,B**) which can produce non-specific staining by immunohistochemistry. Monoclonality is demonstrated by non-radioactive *in situ* hybridization showing absence of kappa (**C**) and presence of lambda mRNA transcripts (**D**).

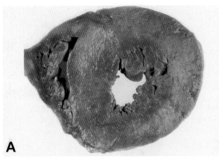
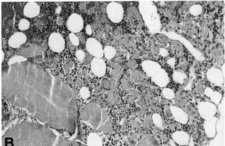
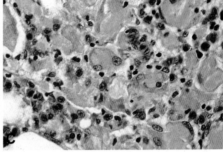

Fig. 10.45 A Primary amyloidosis in a patient with plasma cell myeloma. Gross photograph of a section of heart shows the diffuse enlargement characteristic of amyloid deposition, especially in the left ventricle. Bone marrow biopsy of primary amyloidosis showing characteristic pale, waxy amorphous deposits (**B**) and associated histiocytes, often multinucleated, and neoplastic plasma cells (**C**).

cells may be increased in the adjacent tissues. Congo red stains amyloid pink to red by standard light microscopy and under polarized light produces a characteristic "apple-green" birefringence. Electron microscopic studies will differentiate AL amyloid from LCDD.

Immunophenotype

The immunophenotypic features of the plasma cells are similar to those of myeloma. Immunohistochemical staining of BM sections for kappa and lambda light chains shows a monoclonal plasma cell staining pattern unless the clone is unusually small and masked by normal polyclonal plasma cells {675, 2433, 2452}. Staining for amyloid P component is positive. Immunohistochemical techniques using anti-amyloid fibril antibodies to AL kappa and lambda are useful in distinguishing primary and secondary amyloidosis (AA) in some cases but are definitive less than half the time {675}. AA amyloid, however, can be recognized by immunohistochemistry in essentially all cases {57}.

Genetics

The genetic abnormalities reported in primary amyloidosis are similar to those in non-IgM MGUS and plasma cell myeloma. One exception is the unexplained observation that the t(11;14) is present in >40% of individuals with amyloidosis but only 15–20% of those with a diagnosis of non-IgM MGUS or myeloma {718, 912}.

Prognosis

The median survival for patients with primary amyloidosis is approximately 2 years from diagnosis {1228}. Patients with amyloidosis and plasma cell myeloma have a shorter survival than those with amyloidosis or myeloma alone {1225}.

Parameters that have been associated with poor prognosis include elevated serum creatinine, hepatomegaly, major weight loss, excretion of lambda light chains in the urine (vs kappa light chains or no M-protein), elevated ß2 microglobulin levels and a large whole body amyloid load {57, 784, 1228}. The single most frequent cause of death is amyloid related cardiac disease (~40%) {1228}.

Monoclonal light and heavy chain deposition diseases

Definition

Monoclonal light and heavy chain deposition diseases are plasma cell or rarely lymphoplasmacytic neoplasms that secrete an abnormal light or, less often, heavy chain or both, which deposit in tissues causing organ dysfunction but do not form amyloid ß-pleated sheets, bind Congo red or contain amyloid P-component {106, 304, 580, 934, 1085, 1779, 1814}. These disorders include light chain deposition disease (LCDD) {304, 1776, 1779, 1814}, heavy chain deposition disease (HCDD) {106, 934, 1085} and light and heavy chain deposition disease (LHCDD) {304, 580}.

Synonym

Randall disease {1814}.

Epidemiology

These are rare diseases of adults (median age 56 years, range 33–79) which occur in association with either myeloma (65% of cases) or MGUS {304, 1085, 1776, 1779}. There is no evidence of an ethnicity effect and the male:female incidence is nearly equal {304, 1085, 1779}.

Sites of involvement

LCDD and HCDD may involve many organs, most commonly the kidneys {1776}. The liver, heart, nerves, blood vessels and occasionally joints may be involved {106, 304, 934, 1085, 1779, 1814, 2433}. There is prominent deposition of the aberrant Ig on basement membranes, elastic and collagen fibres. Pulmonary involvement, either diffuse or nodular, has been reported {214, 1875}

Clinical features

Patients present with symptoms of organ dysfunction as a result of diffuse, systemic immunoglobulin deposits, usually manifested by nephrotic syndrome and/or renal failure {564, 1776}. Symptomatic extrarenal deposition in LCDD is uncommon and involves the heart (21%), liver (19%)

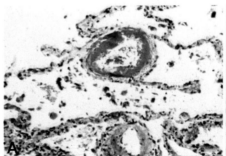
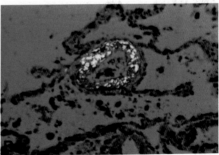

Fig. 10.46 Primary amyloidosis. Pulmonary blood vessel with amyloid deposition, showing Congo red staining (**A**) and apple-green birefringence in polarized light (**B**).

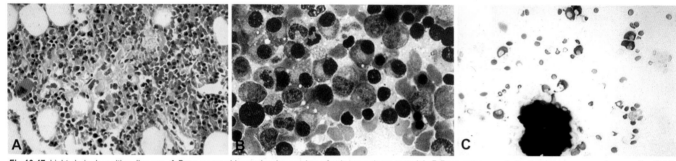

Fig.10.47 Light chain deposition disease. **A** Bone marrow biopsy showing patches of pale amorphous material. **B** Bone marrow aspirate showing numerous plasma cells. **C** Joint fluid aspirate showing clumps of amorphous material and plasma cells, both staining for kappa light chain by immunoperoxidase.

and peripheral nervous system (8%) {304, 1462, 1776}. HCDD of IgG3 or IgG1 isotypes result in hypocomplementemia since the IgG3 and IgG1 subclasses most readily fix complement {934}. There is an M-protein in 85% of cases.

Pathophysiology

The M-protein in non-amyloid MIDD has undergone structural change due to deletional and mutational events {304, 580, 1085, 1779}. In LCDD the primary defect involves multiple mutations of the *Ig* light chain variable region with kappa light chain of VκIV type notably overrepresented {304, 580, 1779}. In HCDD the critical event is deletion of the CH1 constant domain which causes failure to associate with heavy chain binding protein, resulting in premature secretion {106, 934, 1085, 1779}. In HCDD the variable regions also contain amino acid substitutions that cause an increased propensity for tissue deposition and for binding blood elements {106, 304, 1085}.

Morphology

There are prominent tissue deposits of a non-amyloid, nonfibrillary, amorphous eosinophilic material, which do not stain with Congo red. They are often seen as refractile eosinophilic material in the glomerular and tubular basement membranes, but may also be seen in BM and other tissues. LCDD is usually diagnosed by renal biopsy using fluorescent anti-light chain antibodies and electron microscopy {1776}. Kappa chains are observed by immunoflourescence in the renal glomerular and tubular basement membrane. The hallmark of the disease is the prominent, smooth, ribbon-like linear peritubular deposits of monotypic immunoglobulin along the outer edge of the tubular basement membrane. These deposits by electron microscopy are typically discrete, dense punctate, granular, nonfibrillary deposits, with an absence of the ß-pleated sheet structure by X-ray diffraction. Although in some cases plasma cells are found in the vicinity of deposits, it is more common to find Ig deposition in visceral organs with few, if any, plasma cells. Bone marrow plasmacytosis is present in most cases; rarely, a lymphoplasmacytic or marginal zone lymphoma has been reported {214, 305, 2391}.

Immunophenotype

In contrast with primary amyloidosis, which has a predominance of lambda light chain with overrepresentation of the VλVI variable region, LCDD has a prevalence of kappa light chains (80%) with overrepresentation of the VκIV variable region {304}. Immunohistochemistry on BM sections may reveal an aberrant kappa/lambda ratio {2433}.

Prognosis

The median overall survival for patients with LCDD is approximately 4 years. Prognosis is correlated with age, the presence of plasma cell myeloma and extrarenal light chain deposition {1462, 1776}.

Osteosclerotic myeloma (POEMS syndrome)

Definition

Osteosclerotic myeloma is a plasma cell neoplasm characterized by fibrosis and osteosclerotic changes in bone trabeculae, and often with lymph node changes resembling the plasma cell variant of Castleman disease. This disorder is often a component of a rare syndrome that includes polyneuropathy, organomegaly, endocrinopathy, monoclonal gammopathy, and skin changes (POEMS) {1483}. The relationship of this disease to typical plasma cell myeloma is not known.

Synonym

Crow-Fukase syndrome.

Epidemiology

This is a rare disease, occurring predominantly in adults, and estimated to comprise 1–2% of plasma cell dyscrasias {1483}. Many cases have been reported from Japan. Men are affected slightly more often than women (M:F ratio 1.4:1) and the median age is about 50 years {590}.

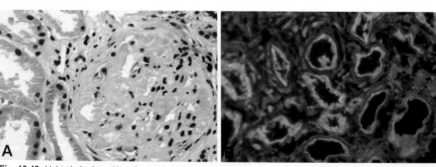

Fig. 10.48 Light chain deposition disease in kidney showing (**A**) pale amorphous patches within glomeruli (nodular glomerulosclerosis) and (**B**) immunofluorescence stain showing renal tubular and extratubular deposition of kappa light chain in a smooth linear pattern.

Etiology

An imbalance of pro-inflammatory cytokines is common in POEMS syndrome. Vascular endothelial growth factor (VEGF) produced by the tumour cells may be responsible for some of the symptoms of the disease {634, 2363}. Some cases of POEMS syndrome, especially those associated with Castleman disease, have been reported to be associated with human herpesvirus 8 (HHV8) {175, 1483}.

Clinical features

Most patients do not present with all of the manifestations of POEMS syndrome and not all are required for diagnosis. The major clinical feature is a chronic progressive polyneuropathy {590}. Organomegaly is present in at least 50% of patients and endocrinopathy and skin changes each in two-thirds {590}. In 75–85% of patients there is a serum M-protein that is either IgG lambda or IgA lambda; the quantity is typically low (median 1.1 g/dL) {590}. An M-protein is found in urine in <50% of patients. Relatively common clinical findings include edema and serous cavity effusions, papilledema, thrombocytosis, weight loss, fatigue, clubbing, bone pain and arthralgias. Hypercalcemia, renal insufficiency, and pathological fractures are rare. Radiographic bone abnormalities are found in nearly all cases. These vary from single sclerotic lesions in about half to more than three lesions in one-third of cases {590}.

Morphology

The characteristic lesion is an osteosclerotic plasmacytoma, which may be single or multiple. The lesion is comprised of focally thickened trabecular bone with closely associated paratrabecular fibrosis with entrapped plasma cells. The plasma cells may appear elongated due to distortion by small bands of connective tissue. The BM away from the osteosclerotic lesion usually contains <5% plasma cells, which are typically normal appearing. In a minority of patients with more generalized osteosclerotic myeloma, >10% plasma cells may be found in random BM biopsies {2058}. Two-thirds of patients with lymphadenopathy have changes consistent with the plasma cell variant of Castleman's disease {590}.

Immunophenotype

The plasma cells contain monoclonal cytoplasmic Ig which may be IgG or IgA. The light chain is lambda in almost all patients.

Prognosis

The median overall survival is 14.7 years {590, 1483}. The most common causes of death are cardiorespiratory failure and infection.

Extranodal marginal zone lymphoma of mucosa-associated lymphoid tissue (MALT lymphoma)

P.G. Isaacson
A. Chott
S. Nakamura
H.K. Müller-Hermelink
N.L. Harris
S.H. Swerdlow

Definition

Extranodal marginal zone lymphoma of mucosa-associated lymphoid tissue (MALT lymphoma) is an extranodal lymphoma composed of morphologically hetero-geneous small B-cells including marginal zone (centrocyte-like) cells, cells resem-bling monocytoid cells, small lymphocytes, and scattered immunoblasts and centro-blast-like cells. There is plasma cell dif-ferentiation in a proportion of the cases. The infiltrate is in the marginal zone of re-active B-cell follicles and extends into the interfollicular region. In epithelial tissues, the neoplastic cells typically infiltrate the epithe-lium forming lymphoepithelial lesions {1013}.

ICD-O code	9699/3

Synonym

Extranodal marginal zone B-cell lymphoma of mucosa-associated lymphoid tissue.

Epidemiology

MALT lymphoma comprises 7–8% of all B-cell lymphomas {51}, and up to 50% of primary gastric lymphoma {600, 1801}. Most cases occur in adults with a median age of 61 and a slight female preponder-ance (male:female ratio 1:1.2) {51}. There appears to be a higher incidence of gas-tric MALT lymphomas in north-east Italy {600} and a special subtype previously known as alpha heavy chain disease and now called immunoproliferative small in-testinal disease (IPSID) occurs in the Middle East {1751}, the Cape region of South Africa {1781} and a variety of other tropical and subtropical locations.

Etiology

Hussell and colleagues {998} have shown that continued proliferation of gastric MALT lymphoma cells from patients in-fected with Helicobacter (H.) pylori depends on the presence of T-cells specifically ac-tivated by H. pylori antigens. The impor-tance of this stimulation in vivo has been clearly demonstrated by the induction of remissions in gastric MALT lymphomas with antibiotic therapy to eradicate H. pylori {2444}. A role for antigenic stimulation

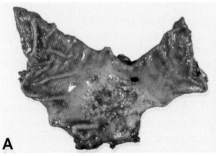
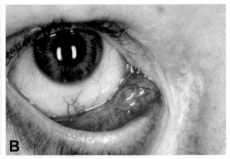

Fig. 10.49 Extranodal marginal zone lymphoma of mucosa-associated lymphoid tissue. **A** Resection specimen of a gastric MALT lymphoma. **B** MALT lymphoma of the conjunctiva.

by Chlamydia psittaci, Campylobacter jejuni and Borrelia burgdorferi has been proposed for some cases of ocular ad-nexal MALT lymphoma, IPSID and cuta-neous MALT lymphoma respectively {364, 695, 1264}. Isaacson has suggested that "acquired MALT" secondary to autoimmune disease or infection in these sites may form the substrate for lymphoma devel-opment {1011}.

Precursor lesions

In many cases of MALT lymphoma, there is a history of a chronic inflammatory disorder that results in accumulation of extranodal lymphoid tissue. The chronic inflammation may be the result of infec-tion, autoimmunity or other unknown stim-ulus. Examples of infectious organisms that may cause accumulation of MALT that precedes MALT lymphoma include H. pylori (gastric MALT lymphoma) {2445}, Chlamydia psittaci (ocular adnexal MALT

lymphoma) {394, 695}, Campylobacter jejuni (IPSID) {1264, 1781, 1812} and Bor-relia burgdoferi (cutaneous MALT lym-phoma) {364}. At least in ocular and cutaneous MALT lymphomas, there is great variation in the strength of these associations that might relate in part to geographic diversity {394, 1290, 1898}. In the first study in which the association of gastric MALT lymphoma with H. pylori infection was examined, the organism was present in over 90% of cases {2445}. Subsequent studies have shown a lower incidence {1566} but also that the density and detectability of H. pylori decreases as lymphoma evolves from chronic gastritis {1562}. The organism may be unde-tectable using histopathological tech-niques in patients who are seropositive {636}. Autoimmune based chronic inflam-mation in the form of Sjögren syndrome and Hashimoto thyroiditis is known respectively to precede salivary gland

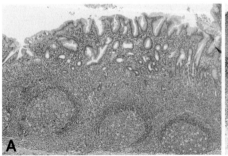
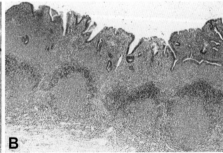

Fig. 10.50 Gastric MALT lymphoma. **A** The tumour cells surround reactive follicles and infiltrate the mucosa. The fol-licles have a typical starry-sky appearance. **B** The marginal zone cells infiltrate the lamina propria in a diffuse pattern and have colonized the germinal centres of reactive B-cell follicles. The colonized follicles do not show a starry-sky pattern.

and thyroid MALT lymphoma. Patients with Sjögren syndrome (SS) or lympho-epithelial sialadenitis (LESA) have a 44-fold increased risk of developing overt lymphoma, comprising about 4–7% of patients {1114, 2150}. Approximately 85% of lymphomas in patients with SS/LESA are MALT lymphomas. Patients with Hashimoto thyroiditis have a 3-fold excess risk of developing lymphoma and a 70-fold increased risk of thyroid lymphoma, for an overall lymphoma risk of 0.5–1.5% {60, 958, 1116}. 94% of thyroid lymphomas have evidence of lymphocytic thyroiditis {558}.

Sites of involvement
The gastrointestinal (GI) tract is the most common site of MALT lymphoma, comprising 50% of all cases, and within the GI tract, the stomach is the most common location (85%) {1801}. The small intestine is typically involved in patients with IPSID. Other common sites include salivary gland, lung (14%), head and neck (14%), ocular adnexa (12%), skin (11%), thyroid (4%) and breast (4%) {2193}.

Clinical features
The majority of patients present with stage I or II disease. A minority of patients (2–20%) have bone marrow (BM) involvement {79, 1802, 2194}. The frequency of BM involvement is lower in gastric cases and higher in MALT lymphomas arising in the lung and ocular adnexa {2193, 2194}. Multiple extranodal sites may be involved in up to 25% of gastric cases and 46% of extragastric cases at the time of presentation {1802}. Multifocal nodal involvement is rare (7.5% of the cases) {2193}. Application of staging systems for nodal lymphomas can be misleading in MALT lymphomas, since involvement of multiple extranodal sites, particularly of paired organs (e.g. salivary glands) or organ systems (e.g. gastrointestinal tract, skin) may not reflect truly disseminated disease. Plasmacytic differentiation is a feature of many of the cases and a serum paraprotein (M-component) can be detected in a third of patients with MALT lymphoma {2429}. The major exception is IPSID, in which an aberrant alpha heavy chain can usually be found in the peripheral blood {1781}.

Morphology
The lymphoma cells infiltrate around reactive B-cell follicles, external to a preserved follicle mantle, in a marginal zone distribution and spread out to form larger confluent areas which eventually overrun some or most of the follicles {1018, 1019}. The characteristic marginal zone B-cells have small to medium-sized, slightly irregular nuclei with moderately dispersed chromatin and inconspicuous nucleoli, resembling those of centrocytes; they have relatively abundant, pale cytoplasm. The accumulation of more pale-staining cytoplasm may lead to a monocytoid appearance. Alternatively, the marginal zone

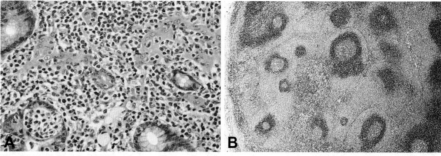

Fig. 10.51 A Gastric MALT lymphoma with prominent lymphoepithelial lesions. **B** Gastric lymph node involved by MALT lymphoma. The tumour cells infiltrate the marginal zones and spread into the interfollicular areas.

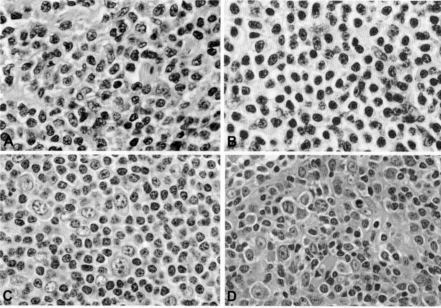

Fig. 10.52 Morphologic spectum of MALT lymphoma cells. **A** Neoplastic marginal zone B-cells with nuclei resembling those of centrocytes, but with more abundant cytoplasm. **B** The cells of this MALT lymphoma have abundant pale staining cytoplasm leading to a monocytoid appearance. **C** Lymphoma cells resembling small lymphocytes. There are scattered transformed blasts. **D** Increased number of large cells.

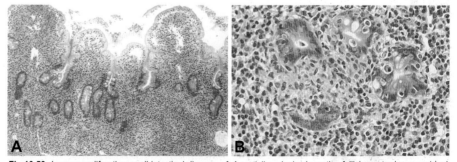

Fig. 10.53 Immunoproliferative small intestinal disease. **A** A partially colonized reactive follicle centre is present just above the muscularis mucosae at the right. Clusters of pale staining marginal zone cells are present adjacent to the follicle and elsewhere in the biopsy. The lamina propria and small intestinal villi are expanded by plasma cells. **B** A lymphoepithelial lesion in a case of IPSID showing destruction of intestinal crypts by marginal zone cells with surrounding plasma cells.

cells may more closely resemble small lymphocytes. Plasmacytic differentiation is present in approximately one third of gastric MALT lymphomas, is frequently found in cutaneous MALT lymphomas and is a constant and often striking feature in thyroid MALT lymphomas. The histological features of IPSID are similar to those of other cases of MALT lymphoma, but typically show striking plasmacytic differentiation {182, 1012, 1781}. Large cells resembling centroblasts or immunoblasts are usually present, but are in the minority. In glandular tissues, epithelium is often invaded and destroyed by discrete aggregates of lymphoma cells resulting in the so-called lymphoepithelial lesions. Lymphoepithelial lesions are aggregates of three or more marginal zone cells with distortion or destruction of the epithelium, often together with eosinophilic degeneration of epithelial cells. The lymphoma cells sometimes specifically colonize the germinal centres of the reactive follicles and in extreme examples, this can lead to a close resemblance to follicular lymphoma. In lymph nodes, MALT lymphoma invades the marginal zone with subsequent interfollicular expansion. Discrete aggregates of monocytoid B-cells may be present in a parafollicular and perisinusoidal distribution. Cytological heterogeneity is still present and both plasma cell differentiation and follicular colonization may be seen.

MALT lymphoma as defined is a lymphoma composed predominantly of small cells. Transformed centroblast- or immunoblast-like cells may be present in variable numbers in MALT lymphoma but, when solid or sheet-like proliferations of

transformed cells are present, the tumour should be diagnosed as diffuse large B-cell lymphoma and the presence of accompanying MALT lymphoma noted. The term "high-grade MALT lymphoma" should not be used, and the term "MALT lymphoma" should not be applied to a large B-cell lymphoma even if it has arisen in a MALT site or is associated with lymphoepithelial lesions.

Differential diagnosis

The differential diagnosis of MALT lymphoma includes the reactive inflammatory processes that typically precede the lymphoma including *Helicobacter pylori* gastritis, lymphoepithelial sialadenitis, Hashimoto thyroiditis and other small B-cell lymphomas (follicular lymphoma, mantle cell lymphoma, small lymphocytic lymphoma). Distinction from reactive processes is based mainly on the presence of destructive infiltrates of extra-follicular B-cells, typically with the morphology of marginal zone cells {2444}. In borderline cases, immunophenotyping or molecular genetic analysis to assess B-cell clonality is necessary to help establish or exclude a diagnosis of MALT lymphoma, although molecular studies may also demonstrate clonal B-cells in some non-neoplastic MALT proliferations or persistent clonal populations in gastric MALT lymphomas even after histologic complete remissions {1502, 1792, 2457}. Distinction from other small B-cell lymphomas is based on a combination of the characteristic morphologic and immunophenotypic features.

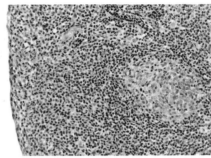

Fig.10.54 Conjunctival MALT lymphoma. Neoplastic marginal zone cells infiltrate around a reactive follicle and infiltrate overlying epithelium.

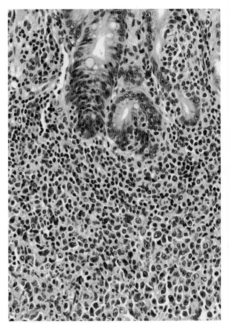

Fig.10.55 Diffuse large B-cell lymphoma (bottom of field) with residual MALT lymphoma in the superficial mucosa.

Immunophenotype

Tumour cells typically express IgM, and less often IgA or IgG, and show light chain restriction. In IPSID, both the plasma cells and marginal zone cells express alpha heavy chain without any light chain {1012}. The tumour cells of MALT lymphoma are CD20+, CD79a+, CD5-, CD10-, CD23-, CD43+/-, CD11c+/- (weak). Infrequent cases are CD5+. The lymphoma cells express the marginal zone cell-associated antigens CD21 and CD35. Staining for CD21 and CD35 also typically reveals expanded meshworks of follicular dendritic cells corresponding to colonized follicles. There is no specific marker for MALT lymphoma at present. The demonstration of immunoglobulin light chain restriction is important in the differential diagnosis with benign lymphoid

Table 10.10
Anatomic site distribution and frequency (%) of chromosomal translocations and trisomies 3 and 18 in MALT lymphomas[1].

Site	t(11;18) (q21;q21)	t(14;18) (q32;q21)	t(3;14) (p14.1;q32)	t(1;14) (p22;q32)	+3	+18
Stomach	6–26	1–5	0	0	11	6
Intestine	12–56	0	0	0–13	75	25
Ocular adnexa/orbit	0–10	0–25	0–20	0	38	13
Salivary glands	0–5	0–16	0	0–2	55	19
Lung	31–53	6–10	0	2–7	20	7
Skin	0–8	0–14	0–10	0	20	4
Thyroid	0–17	0	0–50	0	17	0

[1]Data summarized according to Streubel *et al.* {2109A} and Remstein *et al.* {1836}.

infiltrates. In the differential diagnosis with other small B-cell lymphomas, absence of the characteristic markers for those neoplasms is important: lack of CD5 is useful in distinction from most mantle cell and small lymphocytic lymphomas, cyclin D1 in distinction from mantle cell lymphomas and CD10 in the differential diagnosis with many follicular lymphomas.

Genetics
Antigen receptor genes
Immunoglobulin heavy and light chain genes are rearranged and show somatic hypermutation of variable regions, consistent with derivation from a post-germinal centre, memory B-cell {618, 1789}.

Cytogenetic abnormalities and oncogenes
Chromosomal translocations associated with MALT lymphomas include t(11;18)(q21;q21), t(1;14)(p22;q32), t(14;18)(q32;q21) and t(3;14)(p14.1;q32), resulting in the production of a chimeric protein (API2-MALT1) or in transcriptional deregulation (BCL10, MALT1, FOXP1) respectively {574, 1285, 1667, 2110, 2111, 2416, 2446}. Trisomy 3, 18 or less commonly of other chromosomes is a non-specific but also not infrequent finding in MALT lymphomas. The frequencies at which the translocations or trisomies occur vary markedly with the primary site of disease. The t(11;18)(q21;q21) is mainly detected in pulmonary and gastric tumours, the t(14;18)(q32;q21) in ocular adnexae/orbit and salivary gland lesions and the t(3;14)(p14.1;q32) in MALT lymphomas arising in the thyroid, ocular adnexae/orbit and skin. Similarly, geographic variability in incidence and anatomic site specificity

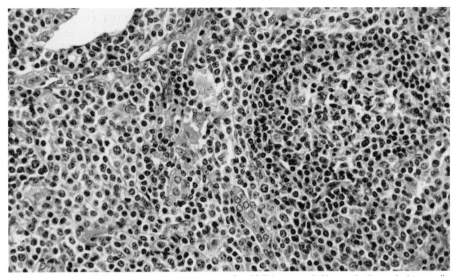

Fig. 10.56 Pulmonary MALT lymphoma showing a reactive B-cell follicle surrounded by neoplastic marginal zone cells that infiltrate bronchiolar epithelium (upper left).

of the translocations has been noted, suggesting different environmental influences such as infectious or other etiologic factors {1836, 2110}.

Postulated normal counterpart
Post germinal centre, marginal zone B-cell.

Prognosis and predictive factors
MALT lymphomas have an indolent natural course and are slow to disseminate. Recurrences, that can occur after many years, may involve other extranodal sites and occur more often in patients with extragastric MALT lymphomas than in patients with primary gastric disease {1802}. The tumours are sensitive to radiation therapy, and local treatment may be followed by prolonged disease-free intervals.

Involvement of multiple extranodal sites and even BM involvement do not appear to confer a worse prognosis {2194}. Protracted remissions may be induced in H. pylori-associated gastric MALT lymphoma by antibiotic therapy for H. pylori {1587, 2444}. Cases with the t(11;18)(q21;q21) appear to be resistant to H. pylori eradication therapy {1321}. In IPSID, remissions have followed therapy with broad-spectrum antibiotics {182, 1264}. Antibiotics have also been used to successfully treat selected other MALT lymphomas. Transformation to diffuse large B-cell lymphoma may occur.

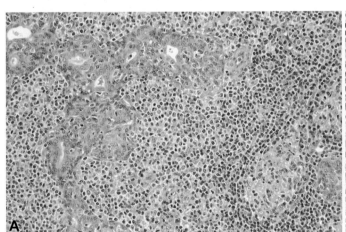
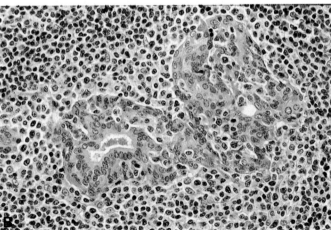

Fig. 10.57 MALT lymphoma of salivary gland. **A** A reactive B-cell follicle is surrounded by neoplastic marginal zone cells that invade salivary duct remnants. **B** Lymphoid cells with pale cytoplasm are present in and around the lymphoepithelial lesions.

Nodal marginal zone lymphoma

E. Campo
S.A. Pileri
E.S. Jaffe
H.K. Müller-Hermelink
B.N. Nathwani

Definition
Nodal marginal zone lymphoma (NMZL) is a primary nodal B-cell neoplasm that morphologically resembles lymph nodes involved by MZL of extranodal or splenic types, but without evidence of extranodal or splenic disease.

ICD-O code   9699/3

Synonyms
Monocytoid B-cell lymphoma; parafollicular B-cell lymphoma; Nodal marginal zone B-cell lymphoma.

Epidemiology
Nodal MZL comprises only 1.5–1.8% of all lymphoid neoplasms {195, 1578}. Most cases occur in adults with a median age around 60 years and a similar proportion in males and females {73}. This lymphoma may occur in children {2140}. Hepatitis C virus has been detected in

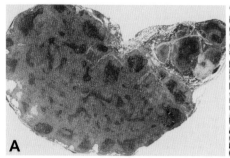
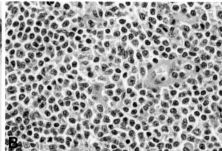

Fig. 10.58 Nodal marginal zone lymphoma. **A** Reactive follicles are separated by an interfollicular infiltrate of paler staining cells. **B** The neoplastic cells in nodal marginal zone lymphoma have irregularly-shaped nuclei and moderately abundant pale cytoplasm. Occasional plasma cells and transformed blasts are present.

20–24% of the patients in some studies {73, 2506}, but has not been observed in other series {2264}.

Sites of involvement
Peripheral lymph nodes, occasionally bone marrow and peripheral blood {195, 1578}.

Clinical features
Most patients present with asymptomatic, localized or generalized peripheral lymphadenopathy {73, 195}. Presence of a primary extranodal marginal zone lymphoma should be ruled out since approximately one third of the cases presenting as nodal MZL represent nodal dissemination

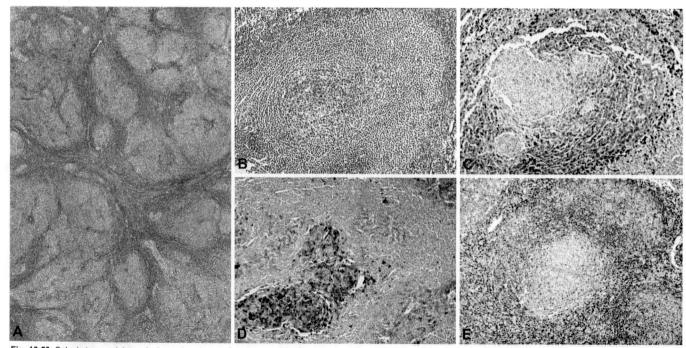

Fig. 10.59 Splenic type nodal marginal zone lymphoma. **A** At low magnification, note the follicular growth pattern with pale cells that focally surround portions of reactive germinal centres. **B** The tumour is composed of a proliferation of small cells expanding between a reactive germinal centre and an attenuated mantle cell cuff. **C** IgD staining shows the weak positivity of the tumour cells that surround the negative germinal centre whereas the residual mantle cells are strongly positive. **D** CD10 staining. The tumour cells are negative whereas the residual germinal centre is positive. **E** BCL2 staining. The tumour cells are positive whereas the reactive germinal centre is negative.

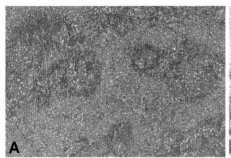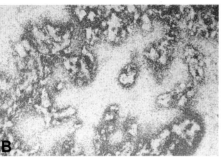

Fig. 10.60 Nodal marginal zone lymphoma, paediatric type commonly exhibits progressive transformation of germinal centres (**A**). The atypical cells are found primarily in the interfollicular areas and may disrupt the follicles. **B** IgD staining highlights the disrupted and expanded mantle cuff; the tumour cells are IgD negative.

of a MALT lymphoma, particularly in patients with Hashimoto thyroiditis or Sjögren syndrome {328,1601}.

Morphology

The tumour cells surround reactive follicles and expand into the interfollicular areas. Follicular colonization may be present. In cases with a diffuse pattern, follicle remnants may be detected with stains for follicular dendritic cells and germinal centre markers. The tumour cells are composed of variable numbers of marginal zone (centrocyte-like and monocytoid) B-cells, plasma cells and scattered transformed B-cells {321, 1578, 1601, 2264}. Cases with a predominant monocytoid B-cell population are uncommon. Plasma cell differentiation may be prominent and the differential diagnosis with lymphoplasmacytic lymphoma or even nodal plasmacytoma may be difficult. Some of these cases may have prominent eosinophilia. The presence of remnants of follicular dendritic meshworks suggestive of colonized follicles would favour the diagnosis of nodal MZL. Some cases have more numerous large transformed cells (sometimes >20%). However, these cells are usually mixed with small cells and may be more common in the colonized germinal centres

{1578, 2264}. Some cases mimic splenic MZL with the tumour cells composed of small to medium size lymphocytes with pale cytoplasm and occasional transformed cells growing inside an attenuated mantle zone and often around a residual germinal centre {328}. Composite nodal MZL and HL have been reported {2493}.

Immunophenotype

Most nodal MZL express pan-B-cell markers with CD43 coexpression in 50% of the cases. CD5, CD23, CD10, BCL6 and cyclin D1 are negative and BCL2 is positive in most cases. IgD is positive in a minority of the cases. Tumours mimicking splenic MZL have a similar phenotype but are usually IgD positive {328}.

Genetics

The immunoglobulin genes are clonally rearranged with a predominance of mutated *VH3* and *VH4* families {321, 2263}. Trisomies 3, 18 and 7 have been observed. The translocations associated with extranodal MZL are not detected {575, 2264}.

Postulated normal counterpart

Post-germinal centre marginal zone B-cell.

Prognosis and predictive factors

60–80% of the patients survive longer than 5 years {73}. The prognosis of these patients may be predicted using the follicular lymphoma international prognostic index (FLIPI) {73}. The number of isolated large cells does not seem to be of prognostic significance {2264}. Transformation to a large B-cell lymphoma may occur. Diagnosis of transformation requires the identification of sheets of large cells.

Paediatric nodal marginal zone lymphomas

Nodal MZL in the paediatric age have distinctive clinical and morphological characteristics {2140}. They present predominantly in males (ratio 20:1) with asymptomatic and localized (90% stage I) disease, mainly in the head and neck lymph nodes. Histologically the tumour is similar to that seen in adults except that there are often progressively transformed germinal centres in which the outer border of the follicles is disrupted and infiltrated by neoplastic cells. The immunophenotype is similar to adult NMZL {2140}. The differential diagnosis with atypical marginal zone hyperplasia with monotypic Ig expression may be difficult because the large cells in this condition also express CD43 {100}. Although this latter process has been reported in extranodal sites, some caution is advised as a similar process might also occur in the lymph nodes. Particularly for these reasons, studies for clonal rearrangements of the *IGH@* chain are necessary to help distinguish paediatric NMZL from reactive conditions {2140}. The prognosis of paediatric nodal MZL is excellent with a very low relapse rate and long survival after conservative treatment.

Follicular lymphoma

N.L. Harris
S.H. Swerdlow
E.S. Jaffe
G. Ott

B.N. Nathwani
D. de Jong
T. Yoshino
D. Spagnolo

Definition

Follicular lymphoma (FL) is a neoplasm composed of follicle centre (germinal centre) B-cells (typically both centrocytes and centroblasts/large transformed cells), which usually has at least a partially follicular pattern. If diffuse areas of any size comprised predominantly or entirely of blastic cells are present in any case of follicular lymphoma, a diagnosis of diffuse large B-cell lymphoma is also made. Lymphomas composed of centrocytes and centroblasts with an entirely diffuse pattern in the sampled tissue may be included in this category. Primary cutaneous lymphomas of germinal centre cells are separately classified.

Table 10.11 Follicular lymphoma grading.

Grading	Definition
Grade 1-2 (low grade)	0–15 centroblasts per hpf
1	0–5 centroblasts per hpf
2	6–15 centroblasts per hpf
Grade 3	>15 centroblasts per hpf
3A	Centrocytes present
3B	Solid sheets of centroblasts

Reporting of pattern	Proportion follicular
Follicular	>75%
Follicular and diffuse	25–75% *
Focally follicular	<25% *
Diffuse	0%**

Diffuse areas containing >15 centroblasts per hpf are reported as diffuse large B-cell lymphoma with follicular lymphoma (Grade 1–2, Grade 3A or Grade 3B)*.

hpf, high-power field of 0.159 mm² (40x objective, 18 mm field of view ocular; count 10 hpf and divide by 10).
If using a 20 mm field of view ocular, count 8 hpf and divide by 10 or count 10 hpf and divide by 12 to get the number of centroblasts/0.159 mm² hpf.
If using a 22 mm field of view ocular, count 7 hpf and divide by 10 or count 10 hpf and divide by 15 to get the number of centroblasts/0.159 mm² hpf.
*Give approximate % of each in report.
** If the biopsy specimen is small, a note should be added that the absence of follicles may reflect sampling error.

ICD-O codes

Follicular lymphoma	9690/3
Grade 1	9695/3
Grade 2	9691/3
Grade 3A	9698/3
Grade 3B	9698/3

Epidemiology

FL accounts for about 20% of all lymphomas with the highest incidence in the USA and Western Europe. In Eastern Europe, Asia and in developing countries the incidence is much lower {37}. It affects predominantly adults, with a median age in the 6th decade and a male:female ratio of 1:1.7 {51}. FL rarely occurs in individuals under the age of 20 years; paediatric patients are predominantly males {707, 1337, 1754, 2132}.

Sites of involvement

FL predominantly involves lymph nodes, but also spleen, bone marrow (BM), peripheral blood (PB) and Waldeyer ring. Involvement of non-haematopoietic extranodal sites, such as the gastrointestinal tract (GI) or soft tissue may occur in a setting of widespread nodal disease. FL may occasionally be primary in extranodal sites, including skin, GI tract, particularly the duodenum, ocular adnexa, breast and testis.

Clinical features

Most patients have widespread disease at diagnosis, including peripheral and central (abdominal and thoracic) lymphadenopathy and splenomegaly. The BM is involved in 40–70%. Only one third of patients are in Stage I or II at the time of the diagnosis {51}. Despite widespread disease, patients are usually otherwise asymptomatic.

Morphology
Pattern

Most cases of FL have a predominantly follicular pattern with closely-packed follicles that efface the nodal architecture. Neoplastic follicles are often poorly defined and usually have attenuated or absent mantle zones. In contrast to reactive

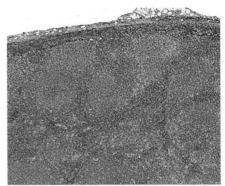

Fig. 10.61 Follicular lymphoma. The neoplastic follicles are closely packed, focally show an almost back-to-back pattern, and lack mantle zones.

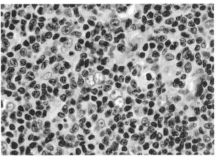

Fig. 10.62 Follicular lymphoma, illustrating follicular dendritic cells (FDC). Four FDC, arranged in the form of two pairs, are present in the centre of the field. The nuclei are round, but with flattening of adjacent nuclear membranes, and have bland, dispersed chromatin with one small, centrally located nucleolus. The cytoplasm is not seen in H&E or Giemsa-stained sections. Centroblasts, in contrast to FDC, have vesicular chromatin and multiple distinct nucleoli that are usually located adjacent to the nuclear membranes.

germinal centres where centroblasts and centrocytes occupy different zones (polarization), in FL the two types of cells are randomly distributed. Similarly, tingible body macrophages, characteristic of reactive germinal centres, are usually absent in FL. In some cases, follicles may be large, irregular, and serpiginous, resembling diffuse areas. Staining for follicular dendritic cells (FDC) (CD21/CD23) may be necessary to distinguish between large follicles and diffuse areas. Interfollicular spread by neoplastic cells is common and this does not constitute a diffuse pattern.

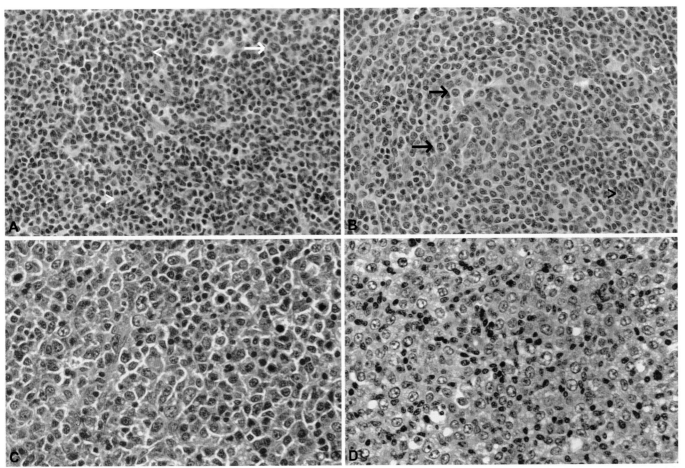

Fig. 10.63 Follicular lymphoma grading. **A** Grade 1-2 of 3. There is a monotonous population of small cells with irregular nuclei (centrocytes) with only rare large cells (centroblasts) with 1 or more basophilic nucleoli and a moderate amount of cytoplasm (arrow). Most of the large nuclei present in this field are those of follicular dendritic cells (FDC) (arrowhead); these cells have more delicate nuclear membranes and violet-coloured nucleoli, and are often binucleate. **B** Grade 1-2 of 3. The majority of the cells are centrocytes, but more numerous centroblasts are present (arrows); several FDC with double nuclei are present (arrowhead). **C** Grade 3A. There are more than 15 centroblasts per high power field, but centrocytes are still present. **D** Grade 3B. The majority of the cells are centroblasts.

The interfollicular neoplastic cells are often centrocytes that are smaller than those in the germinal centres, with a less irregular nuclear contour, and they may show immunophenotypic differences from the cells in the germinal centres {599}.

Diffuse areas may be present, often with sclerosis, particularly in mesenteric and retroperitoneal infiltrates. A diffuse area is defined as an area of the tissue completely lacking follicles defined by CD21+/CD23+ FDC. Distinction between an extensive interfollicular component and a diffuse component may sometimes be arbitrary.

Diffuse areas comprised predominantly of centrocytes are not thought to be clinically significant. However, the presence of diffuse areas comprised entirely or predominantly of large blastic/transformed cells (that would fulfill criteria for Grade 3 follicular lymphoma) in a FL of any grade

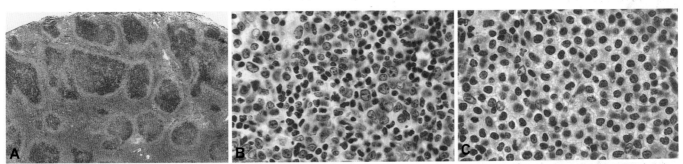

Fig.10.64 Follicular lymphoma, Grade 1-2, with marginal zone differentiation. **A** At the periphery of the follicles, there is a pale rim corresponding to marginal zone differentiation. **B** The centres of the follicles contain the typical mixture of centrocytes and centroblasts. **C** The cells at the periphery of the follicles are medium-sized cells with slightly irregular nuclei and abundant lightly eosinophilic to pale staining cytoplasm, consistent with marginal zone or monocytoid B-cells.

is equivalent to diffuse large B-cell lymphoma, and a separate diagnosis of diffuse large B-cell lymphoma should be made {897} (See grading of follicular lymphoma below). Despite the unclear clinical significance of diffuse areas comprised predominantly of centrocytes with only rare centroblasts (Grade 1-2), it is recommended that the relative proportions of follicular and diffuse areas be noted in the pathology report as follicular (>75% follicular), follicular and diffuse (25–75% follicular), or focally follicular/predominantly diffuse (<25% follicular) {897}.

Diffuse follicular lymphoma

Rare lymphomas with the morphology and immunophenotype of FL have an entirely diffuse growth pattern. This phenomenon is usually seen on small biopsy specimens, and likely represents a diffuse area in a FL that is not adequately sampled. In these cases, the pathologist should suggest that more tissue be obtained if possible. A diagnosis of diffuse FL may be made when the lymphoma is composed of cells resembling centrocytes, with a minor component of centroblasts and an entirely diffuse pattern; both the small and large cells must have the immunophenotype of germinal centre cells or presence of a classical t(14;18) translocation should be demonstrated. Thus, a diagnosis of diffuse FL cannot be made without these ancillary studies.

Partial nodal involvement and "in situ" follicular lymphoma

Non-neoplastic follicles may be present in lymph nodes involved by otherwise typical FL, and their presence has been reported to predict for lower stage at diagnosis {8}. Non-neoplastic follicles may also be partially colonized by FL cells, both in lymph nodes with areas of obvious FL, in lymph nodes adjacent to those involved by FL or occasionally in isolated lymph nodes in patients with or without FL elsewhere. The latter pattern has been called "in situ" follicular lymphoma (see below) {462}.

Bone marrow and blood

In BM, FL characteristically localizes to the paratrabecular region and may spread into the interstitial areas. A follicular growth pattern with a meshwork of follicular dendritic cells is rare but can be seen. The morphology of the tumour cells most commonly resembles that of the neoplastic interfollicular cells in lymph nodes. The same cells may be seen in the PB.

Cytology

FL is typically composed of the two types of B-cells normally found in germinal centres. Small to medium-sized cells with angulated, elongated, twisted or cleaved nuclei, inconspicuous nucleoli and scant pale cytoplasm are called centrocytes. Large cells with usually round or oval, but occasionally indented or multilobated nuclei, vesicular chromatin, 1 to 3 peripheral nucleoli and a narrow rim of cytoplasm are called centroblasts. Typically, they are at least 3 times the size of lymphocytes, but they may be smaller in some cases. Centrocytes predominate in most cases; centroblasts are always present, but are usually in the minority, so that most cases have a monomorphic appearance, in contrast to reactive follicles. The number of centroblasts varies from case to case and is the basis of grading. In some cases, neoplastic centroblasts may have irregular or lobulated nuclei resembling large centrocytes, and infrequent cases show nuclei with very dispersed chromatin and a lymphoblast-like appearance.

In about 10% of FL there may be discrete foci of marginal zone or monocytoid-appearing B-cells, typically at the periphery of the neoplastic follicles {816, 1577, 2252}. These cells are part of the neoplastic clone {1853}. Plasmacytic differentiation may be marked and signet ring cells may also occur.

Grading of follicular lymphoma

FL has been graded in many classifications (Rappaport {1820}, Working formulation {47}, R.E.A.L. {898}, WHO 3rd edition {1039}) according to the proportion of large cells (centroblasts), and a number of studies suggest that this histological grading predicts clinical outcome, with cases with more large cells behaving more aggressively and having a higher likelihood of progression to a diffuse large cell lymphoma than those with fewer large cells {38, 47, 153, 748, 806, 807, 1070, 1102, 1335, 1400, 1820}. However, the optimal method and clinical significance of grading have been debated, and no method has shown high reproducibility {51, 1468, 1579}. The 3rd edition of this series used the method of counting large transformed cells (centroblasts) described by Mann and Berard {1039, 1378, 1579}, to define 3 grades. It has been suggested that the number of grades could be reduced, since there are no important clinical

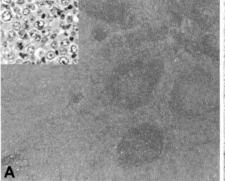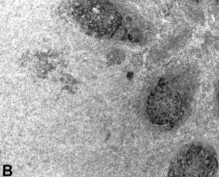

Fig. 10.65 Follicular lymphoma associated with DLBCL. **A** Neoplastic follicles are present on the right, with a diffuse area on the left. The diffuse area is comprised predominantly of large cells (inset), so a separate diagnosis of DLBCL is made. **B** Staining for CD21 shows FDC meshworks in the follicles, but not in the areas of DLBCL.

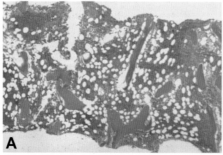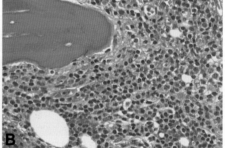

Fig. 10.66 Bone marrow involvement by follicular lymphoma. **A** At low magnification, there are paratrabecular lymphoid aggregates. **B** The cells are small centrocytes.

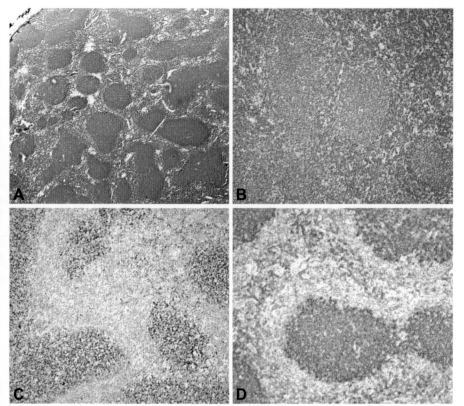

Fig. 10.67 Immunophenotype of follicular lymphoma. **A** The follicles and interfollicular regions contain CD20+ B-cells. **B** The follicles are uniformly BCL2+. **C** BCL6 is expressed by the follicles, but to a lesser degree by interfollicular neoplastic cells. **D** CD10 expression is similar to that of BCL6.

differences between grades 1 and 2. Distinction of grade 3 cases from low-grade (grades 1 and 2) cases is clinically relevant. Although it is still controversial, there is evidence that there may be important clinical and biological differences between grade 3A and grade 3B cases {248, 249, 1119, 1668}. There is insufficient evidence at this time to recommend an alternative method or to recommend eliminating grading altogether.

Follicular lymphoma is graded by counting or estimating the absolute number of centroblasts (large or small) in ten neoplastic follicles, expressed per 40x high-power microscopic field (hpf) {1039, 1378, 1579}. At least 10 high power fields within different follicles are evaluated; these should be representative follicles, not selected for those with the most numerous large cells. Grade 1 and grade 2 cases have a marked predominance of centrocytes and only few centroblasts (grade 1 = 0–5 centroblasts/hpf; grade 2 = 6–15 centroblasts/hpf). Since grades 1 and 2 represent a continuum and are both clinically indolent, distinction between them is not encouraged, and a grade of "1-2 of 3" can be reported. Grade 3 cases have

>15 centroblasts/hpf. Grade 3 is further subdivided according to the proportion of centrocytes. In grade 3A, centrocytes are still present, while grade 3B follicles are composed entirely of large blastic cells (centroblasts or immunoblasts).

If distinct areas of grade 3 FL are present in a biopsy of an otherwise grade 1-2 FL, a separate diagnosis of grade 3 FL should also be made, and the approximate amount of each grade reported. Since both pattern and cytology vary among follicles, lymph nodes must be adequately sampled.

Any area of diffuse large B-cell lymphoma (DLBCL) in a FL should be reported as the primary diagnosis, with an estimate of the proportion of DLBCL and FL present. Thus, in grade 3 follicular lymphoma, the presence of a diffuse component warrants a separate diagnosis of diffuse large B-cell lymphoma. In other words, it is never correct to make a diagnosis of "follicular lymphoma, grade 3 (A or B) with diffuse areas"; the diagnosis is: "1. Diffuse large B-cell lymphoma (_%) 2. Follicular lymphoma, grade 3 (A or B) (_%). To distinguish large, confluent follicles or interfollicular involvement from areas of DLBCL, staining

for follicular dendritic cells (FDC) may be essential.

The vast majority of follicular lymphomas are grade 1-2 (80–90% in most unselected series). Paediatric cases are more likely to be grade 3 {707, 1337, 1754, 2132}. Only a few studies have compared the frequency of grade 3A vs 3B cases. In published studies {883, 1119, 1668}, among purely follicular cases of grade 3 FL, the proportion of grade 3B cases is 20–25%. Areas of diffuse large B-cell lymphoma are present in 60–80% of grade 3B cases and less frequently in grade 3A {883, 1119}.

Immunophenotype

The tumour cells are usually SIg+ (IgM+/-IgD, IgG or rarely IgA), express B-cell associated antigens (CD19, CD20, CD22, CD79a) and are BCL2+, BCL6+, CD10+, CD5- and CD43-. Some cases, especially grade 3B, may lack CD10, but retain BCL6 expression {248, 346, 1111, 1239, 1668, 1760}. CD10 expression is often stronger in the follicles than in interfollicular neoplastic cells, and may be absent in the interfollicular component, as well as in areas of marginal zone differentiation, PB and BM {599, 899}. BCL6 is frequently downregulated in the interfollicular areas. IRF4/MUM1 is typically absent in FL. Rare cases of predominantly Grade 3B, CD10-FL have been described that express IRF4/MUM1 and lacked BCL2 rearrangement; 59% were associated with DLBCL {1111}. Meshworks of FDC are present in follicular areas {2508}; these may be sparser than in normal follicles, and may variably express CD21 and CD23, so that antibodies to both antigens may be needed to detect FDC meshworks.

BCL2 protein is expressed by a variable proportion of the neoplastic cells in 85–90% of cases of grade 1 and grade 2 FL, but only 50% of grade 3 FL using standard antibodies {1238}. In a proportion of the cases, absence of BCL2 protein is due to mutations in the BCL2 gene that eliminate the epitopes recognized by the most commonly used antibody, and BCL2 can be detected using antibodies to other BCL2 epitopes {1973}. BCL2 protein can be useful in distinguishing neoplastic from reactive follicles, although absence of BCL2 protein does not exclude the diagnosis. It is essential for the diagnosis of "in situ" FL; in these cases and in partially involved follicles, the expression of BCL2 is often much stronger than in more typical neoplastic follicles. BCL2 protein is

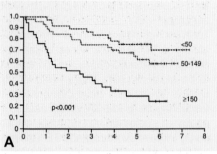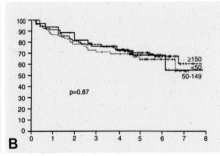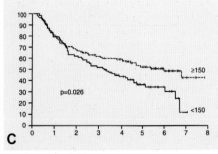

Fig.10.68 Survival curves for patients with follicular lymphoma, graded according to the WHO criteria {2374}. **A** Overall survival of patients treated with regimens not containing doxorubicin (palliative therapy): there is no difference in survival for patients with grade 1 vs grade 2 follicular lymphoma (0–50 and 51–150 centroblasts/10 hpf), while those with grade 3 (>150 centroblasts/10 hpf) had a significantly worse overall survival. **B** Overall survival of patients treated with doxorubicin-containing regimens (curative intent): the 3 survival curves are identical, indicating that there is no survival benefit for patients with grade 1 and grade 2 FL treated with doxorubicin, but that the adverse prognosis of grade 3 FL is eliminated by aggressive therapy. **C** Failure-free survival of patients treated with doxorubicin: there is a suggestion of a plateau in the curve for grade 3 FL (>150 centroblasts/10 hpf), suggesting the possibility of cure for some of these patients; in contrast, patients with grade 1 and grade 2 FL continue to experience relapses.

not useful in distinguishing follicular from other types of low-grade B-cell lymphoma, most of which also express BCL2 protein. The interpretation of BCL2 immunostaining in germinal centre cells requires caution as T-cells, primary follicles and mantle zones normally express this protein. Occasional cases of grade 3 follicular lymphoma are CD43+.

In addition to FDC, neoplastic follicles contain numerous other non-neoplastic cells normally found in germinal centres, including follicular T-cells (CD3+, CD4+, CD57+, PD1+, CXCL13+) and varying numbers of histiocytes.

The proliferation index in FL generally correlates with histologic grade; most grade 1-2 cases have a proliferation fraction <20%, while most grade 3 cases have a proliferation fraction >20%, although there is considerable variation among studies, probably due to technical differences in immunostaining {1183, 1400, 1668, 2358B}. A subgroup of morphologically low-grade FL with a high

Table 10.12 Genetic abnormalities in follicular lymphoma.

Cytogenetic abnormalities	
t(14;18)(q32;q21)	80%
+7	20%
+18	20%
3q27-28	15%
6q23-26*	15%
17p*	15%
Oncogene abnormalities	
BCL2 rearranged	80%
BCL6 rearranged	15%
BCL6 5' mutations	40%

*Associated with a worse prognosis {2239}.

proliferative index has been described {1183, 2358B}, which behaved more aggressively than those with a low proliferative index, and similarly to grade 3 FL {2358B}. Thus, Ki67 staining should be considered as an adjunct to histologic grading and its use is clinically justified, although not formally required at this time.

Genetics

Antigen receptor genes
Immunoglobulin heavy and light chains are rearranged; variable region genes show extensive and ongoing somatic hypermutation {448, 1670}. As a result of these mutations in the CDR-regions, PCR primer annealing may be hampered and depending on the primers used, immunoglobulin-PCR may not yield monoclonal products in a proportion of FL cases (10–40%). Multiplex PCR reactions using BIOMED-2 expanded primer sets detect closer to 90% of IGH(V-D-J) gene rearrangements, and clonality detection approximates 100% when primers detecting IGH(D-J) and light chain gene rearrangements are included {652}.

Cytogenetic abnormalities and oncogenes
FL is genetically characterized by the translocation t(14;18)(q32;q21) and BCL2 gene rearrangements. Alternative BCL2 translocations to immunoglobulin light chain genes have been reported. The t(14;18) is present in up to 90% of the grade 1-2 FL {979, 1885} but the proportion depends on the technique used {18, 93, 1508, 2280}. FISH seems to be the most sensitive and specific method {2280}. BCL2 rearrangements are much less frequent in grade 3B FL {1668}. Geographic variation in the detection of

BCL2 translocations in FL between Western and Asian populations has been reported {215}. The BCL2/IGH@ rearrangement is found in the PB of 25–75% of healthy donors, and also in reactive nodes, particularly if using sensitive nested or RT-PCR assays {1876, 1967, 2121}. A recent study suggests that rather than being naïve B-cells, these BCL2-rearranged cells are memory B-cells {1877}. Abnormalities of 3q27 and/or BCL6 rearrangement are found in 5–15% of FL, most commonly in grade 3B cases {1119, 1668}. FL grade 3B associated with DLBCL have been reported to have a frequency of BCL6 rearrangements similar to that seen in DLBCL {248, 249, 1119, 1668}.

In addition to the t(14;18), other genetic alterations are found in 90% of FL and most commonly include loss of 1p, 6q, 10q and 17p and gains of chromosomes 1, 6p, 7, 8, 12q, X and 18q/dup {954, 1621, 2239}. The number of additional alterations increases with histological grade and transformation {1930}. Rare cases of FL carry the t(8;14) or variants together with the t(14;18) {102, 2343}.

Gene expression profile studies have shown the importance of the microenvironment in the pathogenesis, evolution and prognosis of FL {510, 804}.

Transformation to DLBCL may follow different genetic pathways including inactivation of TP53, $p16^{INK4a}$, and activation of MYC {513, 637, 1338, 1756, 1930}.

Postulated normal counterpart
Germinal centre B-cell.

Prognosis and predictive factors
Prognosis is closely related to the extent of the disease at diagnosis. The International

Prognostic Index (IPI) and especially the International Prognostic Index for FL (FLIPI) are strong predictors of outcome {49, 51, 2048}.

Histological grade correlates with prognosis in follicular lymphoma, with grade 1-2 cases being indolent and not usually curable, except for the infrequent localized cases {40, 806, 1070, 1335}. The majority of published studies show a significantly more aggressive clinical course for follicular lymphomas classified as large cell or Grade 3 {40, 153, 1400, 1443}; but the use of regimens containing doxorubicin and/or rituximab may obviate these differences and requires further study {38, 153, 752, 807, 883, 1102, 1860, 2374, 2384}.

Many studies have indicated {47, 1273, 1820, 2360} that the presence of even very large diffuse areas in follicular lymphoma classified as grade 1-2 ("small cleaved" or "mixed small and large cell") does not significantly alter the prognosis. In most reported studies, cases of grade 3 FL with diffuse areas >25% (now recognized as areas of DLBCL) have a worse prognosis than purely follicular cases {38, 153, 752, 807, 883, 1860, 2346, 2384}.

The presence of more than 6 chromosomal breaks and a complex karyotype has been shown to be associated with a poor outcome; in addition, del 6q23-26, del17p and mutations in *TP53* as well as −1p, +12, +18p, +Xp confer a worse prognosis and a shorter time to transformation {1284, 2239}. Rare cases with both t(14;18) and t(8;14) have a poor prognosis {102, 2343}. Recent gene expression data have suggested a role of the microenvironment, including T-cells and accessory cells including FDC and macrophages in determining the clinical behaviour of FL {510, 804, 893}. Currently, no specific markers are available other than histologic grade and proliferation fraction that can be used in clinical practice to predict outcome or direct therapy.

In 25–35% of patients with FL, transformation or "progression" to a high grade lymphoma occurs, usually DLBCL, but occasionally resembling Burkitt lymphoma or with features intermediate between DLBCL and Burkitt lymphoma {28A, 748, 964A, 1803A}. This occurrence is usually associated with a rapidly progressive clinical course and death from tumour that is refractory to treatment {88B, 748}. Rare patients develop acute B-cell lymphoblastic leukaemia, which in most cases appears to represent blast transformation of the original B cell tumour {518A, 764A, 1197A}. Transformation typically involves additional genetic abnormalities, particularly *MYC* translocations; the combination of a *BCL2* and a *MYC* rearrangement is associated with a particularly aggressive course {702A, 1266A, 2468A}. Recently, the occurrence of histiocytic/dendritic cell sarcomas has been described in patients with FL, in which the sarcomas shared both *IGH@* and *BCL2* rearrangements with the FL. This phenomenon may represent de-differentiation of a B cell due to loss of PAX5 activity {675A}.

Variants

Paediatric follicular lymphoma

This variant often involves cervical lymph nodes, other peripheral lymph nodes or Waldeyer ring; however, other extranodal involvement also occurs, with FL of the testis well described {707, 1337, 1754, 2132}. Children with FL typically have early-stage disease {707, 1337, 1754, 2132}. Paediatric follicular lymphomas have many features indistinguishable from those seen in adults, but demonstrate an increased proportion that are localized, lack BCL2 protein expression and t(14;18) and are grade 3 {1337, 2132}. They also tend to have large expansile follicles. Rare cases of florid follicular hyperplasia, particularly in young males, may have clonal populations of CD10+ B-cells detected by flow cytometry and molecular analysis. A diagnosis of lymphoma should not be made in the absence of morphologic features of malignancy {1211}. The prognosis of paediatric patients appears to be good, with the majority of reported cases disease free at the time of last follow-up {707, 1337, 1754}. Expression of BCL2 protein in paediatric FL was associated in one report with higher stage at diagnosis and a worse outcome than BCL2 negative cases {1337}.

Primary intestinal follicular lymphoma

The majority of cases of primary follicular lymphoma in the GI tract occur in the small intestine, and involvement of the duodenum is a frequent feature {1486, 1939, 2005, 2472}. Duodenal follicular lymphoma is predominantly found in the second portion of the duodenum, presenting as multiple small polyps, often as an incidental finding on endoscopy performed for other reasons. The morphology, immunophenotype and genetic features are similar to those of nodal follicular lymphomas. Most patients have localized disease (stage IE or IIE), and survival appears to be excellent even without treatment.

Other extranodal follicular lymphomas

Follicular lymphomas can occur in almost any extranodal site {697}. In many of these sites, the morphology, immunophenotype and genetic features appear to be similar to those of nodal FL, although data are sparse. Despite this, patients usually have localized extranodal disease, and systemic relapses are uncommon. Testicular follicular lymphomas are reported with increased frequency in children but also are reported in adults {119}.

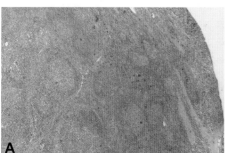 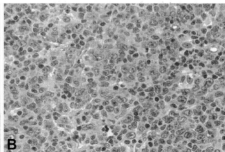 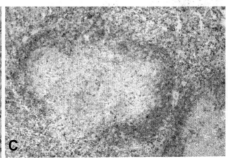

Fig. 10.69 Paediatric follicular lymphoma. **A** Follicles of varying size and shape, many with preserved mantle zones, extending beyond the lymph node capsule. **B** There is a predominance of centroblasts (Grade 3). **C** The follicles are negative for BCL2.

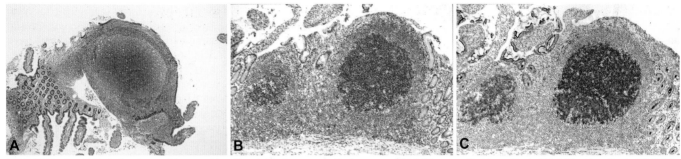

Fig.10.70 Duodenal follicular lymphoma. **A** Large nodules of lymphoid cells are present in the mucosa. The follicles are uniformly positive for BCL2 (**B**) and positive for CD10 (**C**).

Intrafollicular neoplasia/ *"In situ"* follicular lymphoma

Cases occur in which architecturally normal-appearing lymph nodes and other lymphoid tissues have one or more follicles that demonstrate BCL2-overexpressing centrocytes and centroblasts, with or without a monomorphic cytologic appearance suggestive of follicular lymphoma {462}. Some of these patients are found to have follicular lymphoma elsewhere, either before or simultaneously,

some develop overt FL later, and others have remained without evidence of FL. In patients with overt FL elsewhere, this phenomenon likely represents colonization of pre-existing follicles by neoplastic follicle centre cells. In patients without known FL, the significance of this phenomenon is difficult to ascertain. It may represent the tissue counterpart of circulating clonal B-cells with *BCL2* rearrangement —that is, a clone of cells that have the translocation but not the other genetic abnormalities to

result in overt progressive malignancy, or in some cases it may represent the earliest evidence of a true follicular lymphoma that will progress to overt lymphoma.

This phenomenon cannot be recognized without BCL2 staining. The pathology report should indicate that the significance of the finding is unknown, and that clinical evaluation for evidence of overt FL elsewhere is suggested.

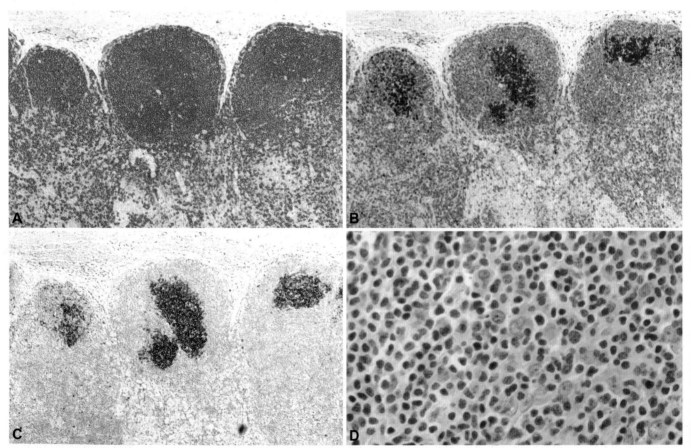

Fig. 10.71 Intrafollicular involvement by BCL2+ germinal centre cells (*in situ* follicular lymphoma or intrafollicular neoplasia). **A** The lymph node architecture is preserved, with CD20+ cells present in follicles. **B** Several germinal centres contain strongly BCL2+ cells. **C** The BCL2+ follicles are strongly CD10+. **D** The follicle appears more monotonous than a typical germinal centre, with a predominance of centrocytes. The patient had no evidence of follicular lymphoma elsewhere.

Primary cutaneous follicle centre lymphoma

R. Willemze
S.H. Swerdlow
N.L. Harris
B. Vergier

Definition

Primary cutaneous follicle centre lymphoma (PCFCL) is a tumour of neoplastic follicle centre cells, including centrocytes and variable numbers of centroblasts, with a follicular, follicular and diffuse or diffuse growth pattern, that generally presents on the head or trunk {2407}. Lymphomas with a diffuse growth pattern and a monotonous proliferation of centroblasts and immunoblasts are, irrespective of site, classified as primary cutaneous diffuse large B-cell lymphoma (PCLBCL), leg type {2407}.

ICD-O code

The provisional code proposed for the fourth edtion of ICD-O is *9597/3*.

Synonym

Reticulohistiocytoma of the dorsum (Crosti's disease) {206}.

Epidemiology

Primary cutaneous follicle centre lymphoma is the most common type of primary cutaneous B-cell lymphoma, accounting for approximately 60% of all cases. It mainly affects adults with a median age of onset of 51 years and a male:female ratio of approximately 1.5:1 {1993, 2502}.

Sites of involvement

Primary cutaneous follicle centre lymphoma characteristically present with solitary or localized skin lesions on the scalp, the forehead or on the trunk. Approximately 5% present with skin lesions on the legs, and 15% with multifocal skin lesions {1170, 1993, 2502}.

Clinical features

The clinical presentation consists of firm erythematous to violaceous plaques, nodules or tumours of variable size. Particularly on the trunk, tumours may be surrounded by erythematous papules and slightly infiltrated, sometimes figurate plaques, which may precede the development of tumourous lesions by months or years {206, 1933, 2409}. In the past PCFCL with such a typical presentation on the back were referred to as "reticulohistiocytoma

of the dorsum" or "Crosti's lymphoma" {206}. The skin surface is smooth and ulceration is rarely observed. Presentation with multifocal skin lesions is observed in a small minority of patients, but is not associated with a more unfavourable prognosis {824, 1993}. If left untreated, the skin lesions gradually increase in size over years, but dissemination to extracutaneous sites is uncommon (~10% of patients) {1993, 2502}. Recurrences tend to be proximate to the initial site of cutaneous presentation.

Morphology

Primary cutaneous follicle centre lymphoma show perivascular and periadnexal to diffuse infiltrates with almost constant sparing of the epidermis. The infiltrates show a spectrum of growth patterns with a morphologic continuum from follicular to follicular and diffuse to diffuse {1933, 2407, 2409}. The lesions are composed predominantly of medium-sized and large centrocytes and variable proportions of centroblasts. In small and/or early lesions a clear-cut follicular growth pattern or more often remnants of a follicular growth pattern may be observed. In contrast to cutaneous follicular hyperplasias, the follicles in these PCFCL are ill-defined, show a monotonous proliferation of BCL6+ follicle centre cells enmeshed in a network of CD21+ or CD35+ follicular dendritic cells, lack tingible body macrophages and generally have an attenuated or absent mantle zone {360, 818}. Reactive T-cells may be numerous and a prominent stromal component is usually present.

Advanced tumours usually show a monotonous population of large centrocytes and multilobated cells and in rare cases spindle-shaped cells, with a variable admixture of centroblasts {206, 362, 824, 1933, 2409}. Reactive T-cells are less pronounced and follicular structures, if present before, are no longer visible except for occasional scattered CD21+ or CD35+ follicular dendritic cells.

Immunophenotype

The neoplastic cells express CD20 and CD79a, but are usually Ig negative.

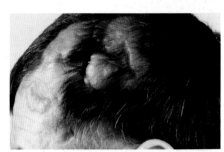

Fig. 10.72 Primary cutaneous follicle centre lymphoma. Characteristic clinical presentation with localized skin lesions on the scalp.

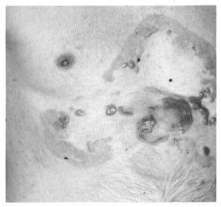

Fig. 10.73 Primary cutaneous follicle centre lymphoma. Characteristic clinical presentation with localized skin lesions on the chest.

Primary cutaneous follicle centre lymphoma consistently express BCL6, while CD10 is often positive in cases with a follicular growth pattern and generally negative in cases with a diffuse growth pattern {522, 819, 949, 1146, 1170, 1485, 1993}. Most cases do not express BCL2 or show faint BCL2 staining (weaker than admixed T-cells) in a minority of neoplastic B-cells {360, 363, 419, 768, 949, 1170, 1993}. However, several studies report BCL2 expression in a significant proportion of PCFCL with at least a partially follicular growth pattern {13, 819, 1146, 1485}. Notwithstanding, strong expression of both BCL2 and CD10 by the neoplastic B-cells should always raise suspicion of a nodal follicular lymphoma involving the skin secondarily. Staining for IRF4/MUM1 and Fox-P1 is negative in most cases {1170, 1993}. Similarly for CD5 and CD43 is negative in the tumour cells.

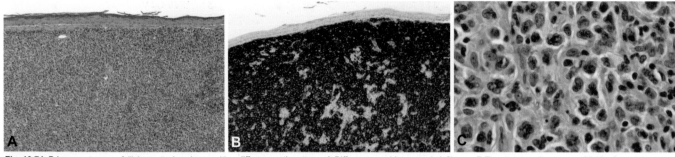

Fig. 10.74 Primary cutaneous follicle centre lymphoma with a diffuse growth pattern. **A** Diffuse non-epidermotropic infiltrate. **B** The tumour cells express CD20. **C** At higher magnification, cellular infiltrate contains many multilobated cells.

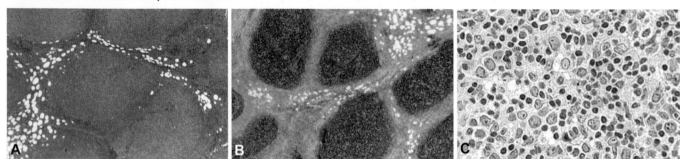

Fig. 10.75 Primary cutaneous follicle centre lymphoma with a follicular growth pattern. **A** Closely packed follicles without mantle zones. **B** Networks of CD35-positive follicular dendritic cells. **C** Detail of neoplastic follicle showing a mixture of small, medium-sized and large follicle centre cells.

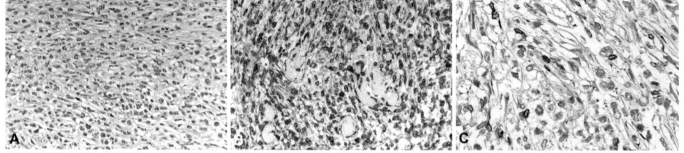

Fig. 10.76 Primary cutaneous follicle centre lymphoma with a diffuse population of spindle-shaped cells (**A**), which are strongly positive for CD79a (**B**), but negative for BCL2 (**C**).

Genetics

Antigen receptor genes
Clonally rearranged immunoglobulin genes, with somatic hypermutation are present, but may be not detectable by PCR.

Cytogenetic analyis and oncogenes
In many studies, PCFCL, including cases with a follicular growth pattern, do not show *BCL2* rearrangements {363, 419, 768, 818, 819, 2329}. However, other studies report *BCL2* rearrangements in about 10–40% of PCFCL with a follicular growth pattern using PCR and/or FISH {13, 1146, 1485}. Primary cutaneous follicle centre lymphoma show the gene expression profile of germinal centre-like large B-cell lymphomas, and often show amplification of the *REL* gene {1, 577, 948}. Deletion of chromosome 14q32.33 has been reported {577}. In contrast to PCLBCL, leg type,

deletions of a small region on chromosome 9p21.3 containing the *CDKN2A* and *CDKN2B* gene loci are either absent or only rarely found in PCFCL {577}.

Postulated normal counterpart
Mature germinal centre derived B lymphocyte.

Prognosis and predictive factors
Irrespective of the growth pattern (follicular or diffuse), the number of blast cells, the presence of t(14;18) and/or BCL2 expression or the presence of either localized or multifocal skin disease, PCFCL have an excellent prognosis with a 5-year-survival over 95% {818, 824, 1485, 1933, 1993, 2502}. Primary cutaneous follicle centre lymphoma presenting on the leg are reported to have a more unfavourable prognosis {1170, 1993}. Cutaneous relapses,

observed in ~30% of patients, do not indicate progressive disease. Systemic therapy is only required in patients with very extensive cutaneous disease, extremely thick skin tumours or with extracutaneous disease {611, 1993}.

Mantle cell lymphoma

S.H. Swerdlow
E. Campo
M. Seto
H.K. Müller-Hermelink

Definition

Mantle cell lymphoma (MCL) is a B-cell neoplasm generally composed of monomorphic small to medium-sized lymphoid cells with irregular nuclear contours and a *CCND1* translocation {139, 329, 1253, 1276, 1693, 2134, 2246}. Neoplastic transformed cells (centroblasts), paraimmunoblasts and proliferation centres are absent.

ICD-O code   9673/3

Epidemiology

MCL comprises approximately 3–10% of non-Hodgkin lymphomas {51}. It occurs in middle-aged to older individuals with a median age of about 60 and a variably marked male predominance (about 2:1 or greater) {74, 247, 329, 1253, 2134, 2136}. Familial aggregation of MCL or MCL with other B-cell neoplasms has been reported {2255}.

Sites of involvement

Lymph nodes are the most commonly involved site; the spleen and bone marrow (BM), with or without peripheral blood (PB) involvement, are other important sites of disease {74, 247, 1605, 2134}. Other extranodal sites are frequently involved, including the gastrointestinal tract and Waldeyer ring {772, 1916}. Most cases of multiple lymphomatous polyposis represent mantle cell lymphoma {1203, 1611, 1900}.

Clinical features

Most patients present with stage III or IV disease with lymphadenopathy, hepatosplenomegaly and BM involvement {247, 329, 1605, 2136}. Peripheral blood involvement is common and present in almost all patients by flow cytometry {691}. Some patients have a marked lymphocytosis mimicking prolymphocytic leukaemia {74, 247, 1605}.

Morphology

Classical MCL is a monomorphic lymphoid proliferation with a vaguely nodular, diffuse, mantle zone or rarely follicular growth pattern {139, 1253, 1276, 2134, 2246}. Infrequent cases may show involvement almost exclusively restricted to the inner mantle zones or to narrow mantles ("*in situ*" MCL) {1602, 1842}. Most cases are composed of small to medium-sized lymphoid cells with slightly to markedly irregular nuclear contours, most closely resembling centrocytes. The nuclei have at least somewhat dispersed chromatin but inconspicuous nucleoli. Neoplastic transformed cells resembling centroblasts, immunoblasts or paraimmunoblasts and proliferation centres are absent. Hyalinized small vessels are commonly seen. Many cases have scattered single epithelioid histiocytes which in occasional cases can create a "starry sky" appearance. Plasma cells may be present but are almost always non-neoplastic {2475}.

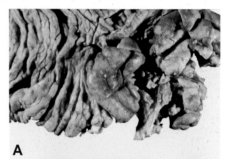

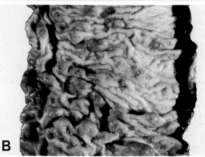

Fig. 10.77 Mantle cell lymphoma involving the colon (multiple lymphomatous polyposis), gross photograph. **A** Overview showing one large and multiple small polypoid mucosal lesions. **B** Closeup showing tiny polypoid mucosal lesions.

Histological transformation to typical large cell lymphoma does not occur; however, loss of a mantle zone growth pattern, increase in nuclear size, pleomorphism and chromatin dispersal, and increase in mitotic activity may be seen in some cases at relapse {74, 1253, 1605, 2134}. Some of the latter cases will fulfil the criteria for a blastoid or pleomorphic mantle cell lymphoma.

A spectrum of morphologic variants is recognized. The blastoid and pleomorphic variants are considered to be of important clinical significance (Table 10.13). Although MCL is not graded, evaluation of the proliferation fraction either by counting mitotic figures or estimating the proportion of Ki67 positive nuclei is important because of its prognostic impact.

Immunophenotype

The cells express relatively intense surface IgM/IgD, more frequently with lambda than kappa restriction {329, 2134, 2246}. They are usually positive for CD5,

Table 10.13 Morphologic variants of mantle cell lymphoma.

Aggressive variants

- Blastoid: cells resemble lymphoblasts with dispersed chromatin and a high mitotic rate (usually at least 20–30/10 hpf).

- Pleomorphic: cells are pleomorphic but many are large with oval to irregular nuclear contours, generally pale cytoplasm and often prominent nucleoli in at least some of the cells.

Other variants

- Small cell: small round lymphocytes with more clumped chromatin, either admixed or predominant, mimicking a small lymphocytic lymphoma.

- Marginal zone-like: prominent foci of cells with abundant pale cytoplasm resembling marginal zone or monocytoid B-cells mimicking a marginal zone lymphoma; sometimes these paler foci may also resemble proliferation centres of chronic lymphocytic leukaemia/small lymphocytic lymphoma.

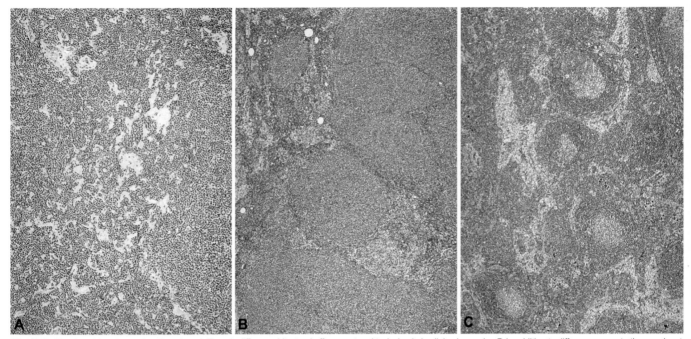

Fig. 10.78 Mantle cell lymphoma, lymph nodes. **A** There is diffuse architectural effacement and typical pale hyalinized vessels. **B** In addition to diffuse areas, note the prominent vague neoplastic nodules. **C** A mantle zone growth pattern is seen in this lymph node with an intact architecture.

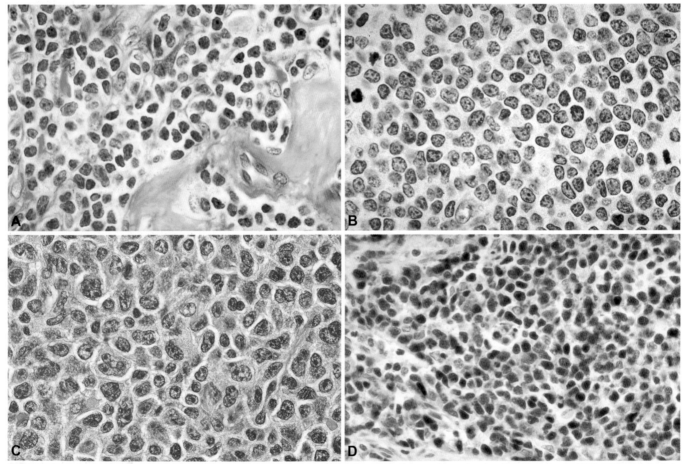

Fig.10.79 Mantle cell lymphoma. **A** This typical MCL demonstrates a homogeneous population of cells that resemble centrocytes of a germinal centre (PAS stain). **B** The cells in the blastoid variant resemble lymphoblasts and have a high mitotic rate. **C** Note the large and pleomorphic cells including cells with prominent nucleoli in the pleomorphic variant. **D** The cyclin D1 immunostain shows nuclear positivity.

FMC-7 and CD43, but negative for CD10 and BCL6. CD23 is negative or weakly positive. Aberrant phenotypes have been described, sometimes in association with blastoid/pleomorphic variants, including absence of CD5 and expression of CD10 and BCL6 {323, 1518, 2470}. Immunohistological stains demonstrate loose meshworks of follicular dendritic cells. All cases are BCL2 protein positive and almost all express cyclin D1, including the minority of cases that are CD5 negative {412, 2135, 2137, 2250, 2467, 2509}. Cyclin D1 staining may be required to recognize the cases of "*in situ*" MCL.

Genetics

Antigen receptor genes

Immunoglobulin genes are rearranged. Variable region genes are unmutated in the majority of the cases, but in 15–40% of the cases, *IG* genes show somatic hypermutation although the load of mutations is usually lower than in mutated CLL {322, 1143, 1652, 2192}. A biased use of the *VH* genes is reported in MCL, suggesting that these tumours may originate from specific subsets of B-cells {322, 1143, 1652, 2192}. In contrast to CLL, *VH3-21* gene usage in MCL occurs mainly in cases that are unmutated, have fewer genomic imbalances and a better prognosis {2192}. Also in contrast to CLL, the *VH* gene mutational status in MCL does not correlate with survival or ZAP-70 expression {322, 340, 1143}.

Cytogenetic abnormalities and oncogenes

The t(11;14)(q13;q32) between *IGH@* and cyclin D1 *(CCND1)* genes is present in almost all cases and considered the primary genetic event {1291, 1866, 2281, 2308, 2410, 2411}. Variant *CCND1* translocations with the immunoglobulin light chains have also been reported {1179}. The translocation results in deregulated overexpression of *CCND1* mRNA and protein {246, 515, 1995}. Some MCL express aberrant transcripts resulting in an increased half-life of cyclin D1. Tumours with these truncated transcripts have very high levels of cyclin D1 expression {246, 515, 1995}, high proliferation and more aggressive clinical behaviour {1871}. Deregulated expression of cyclin D1 is assumed to overcome the cell cycle suppressive effect of RB1 and p27kip1, leading to the development of MCL {1048, 1793}. MCL carries a high number of non-random secondary chromosomal aberrations

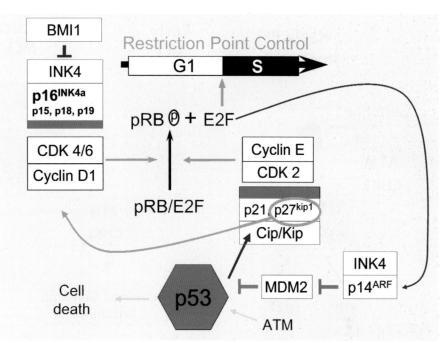

Fig. 10.80 Cell cycle and DNA damage repair pathways altered in mantle cell lymphoma. The cyclin D1/cyclin dependent kinase (CDK) 4/6 complex promotes phosphorylation of the retinoblastoma protein (pRB). This leads to release of the E2F transcription factors which then lead to progression of the cell cycle into the S phase. The cyclin D1/CDK 4/6 complex is inhibited by p16INK4a. BMI1 is a transcriptional repressor of the *INK4a/ARF* locus. Abnormalities in MCL that lead to progression of cells from G1 to S phase include increased cyclin D1 in almost all cases and loss of p16INK4a, *RB* deletions, increased CDK4 and increased BMI1 in a minority of cases especially those that are more aggressive. Deregulated E2F also induces p14ARF transcription. p14ARF leads to stabilization of p53 by inhibiting the activity of MDM2 which leads to the degradation of p53. The tumour suppressor p53 leads to increased expression of p21 in addition to leading to cell cycle arrest or apoptosis. The *ATM* gene is required for activation of p53 after DNA damage. Many MCL have *ATM* abnormalities and some patients have germline mutations of this gene. Some MCL have loss or transcriptional repression of the *INK4a/ARF* locus lacking p16INK4a/p14ARF, loss or mutation of *TP53* or high levels of MDM2. Finally, cyclin E/CDK2 complexes also lead to cell cycle progression and are inhibited by p21/p27kip1. In MCL, increased levels of cyclin D1 lead to sequestration of these cell cycle inhibitors and, in addition, they may increase p27 degradation.

including gains of 3q26 (31–50%), 7p21 (16–34%) and 8q24 (16–36%: *MYC*), and losses of 1p13-p31 (29–52%), 6q23-q27 (23–38%), 9p21 (18–31%), 11q22-q23 (21–59%), 13q11-q13 (22–55%), 13q14-q34 (43–51%) and 17p13-pter (21–45%) {165, 1890, 1995}. Trisomy 12 has been reported in 25% of cases {496}. In addition to chromosomal imbalances, MCL may demonstrate tetraploid clones that are more common in pleomorphic (80%) and blastoid variants (36%) than in cases with typical morphology (8%) {1666}. The presence of a t(8;14)(q24;q32) with *MYC* translocation occurs rarely and is associated with an aggressive clinical course {2283}. *BCL6/3q27* translocations also occur uncommonly and are reportedly associated with BCL6 protein expression {323}. Some cytogenetic abnormalities may also have associations with various clinical parameters including a leukaemic presentation {691, 1693}.

Oncogenic alterations have been found in several genes targeting the DNA damage response pathway and cell cycle regulatory elements {688}. Inactivating mutations of the *ATM* gene at 11q22-23 have been detected in 40–75% of MCL {320, 1956}. *ATM* mutations have been also detected in the germline of some patients with MCL {320}. Highly proliferative variants of MCL have frequent *TP53* mutations, homozygous deletions of *INK4a/ARF*, the CDK inhibitor *p18INK4c*, amplifications and overexpression of the *BMI1* polycomb and *CDK4* genes and occasional microdeletions of the *RB1* gene {165, 166, 329, 839, 930, 1341, 1755, 1757, 2412, 2413}.

Cyclin D1 negative MCL

Rare MCL are negative for cyclin D1 and the t(11,14) but have an expression profile and other features indistinguishable from conventional MCL {738, 1871, 1918}. These cases have a high expression of

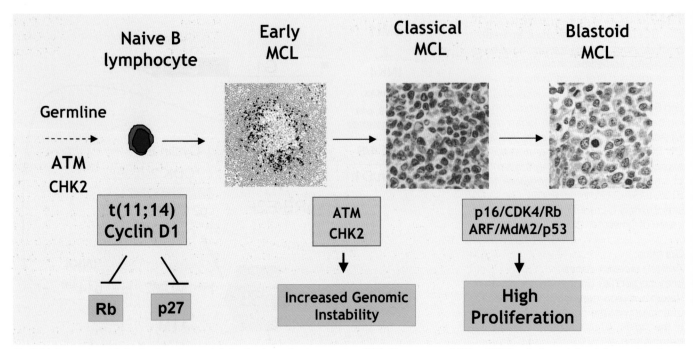

Fig.10.81 Proposed model of molecular pathogenesis in the development and progression of MCL. The presence of *ATM* or *CHK2* inactivating mutations in the germline of some patients suggests that they may facilitate the development of the tumour. The t(11;14) translocation occurs in an immature B-cell and leads to the constitutive deregulation of cyclin D1 and early expansions of tumour B-cells in the mantle zone areas of lymphoid follicles. Acquired inactivation of DNA damage response pathways may facilitate the development of additional genetic alterations and expansion of MCL cells with a classical morphology. Increased genomic instability may target genes in the cell cycle and senescence regulatory pathways that would lead to more aggressive variants of MCL. Modified with permission from Jares P. *et al.* {1048A}.

cyclin D2 or cyclin D3. Some of these cases carry a t(2;12)(p12;p13) translocation fusing cyclin D2 to the kappa light chain gene locus {789}. This diagnosis must be made only with great caution due to the many lymphomas that may mimic MCL.

Postulated normal counterpart
Peripheral B-cell of inner mantle zone, mostly of naïve pre-germinal centre type.

Prognosis and predictive factors
Mantle cell lymphoma has a median survival of 3–5 years, but the vast majority of patients cannot be cured {329, 2136}. The impact of some of the newer therapeutic approaches remains to be established {1917, 2487A}. The most consistently reported adverse histopathological prognostic parameter is a high mitotic rate

(>10–37.5/15 hpf, >50/mm^2) {74, 247, 2134, 2237}. A high proportion of Ki67 positive cells, e.g. >40% or >60%, is also an adverse prognostic indicator {1120, 2237}. The most significant prognostic indicator identified in a major gene expression profiling study was the proliferation signature score {1871}. Although not necessarily all independent of the proliferation fraction, the following have been reported in at least some studies to be adverse prognostic features: blastoid/ pleomorphic morphology, trisomy 12, karyotypic complexity, *TP53* mutation/ overexpression/loss and a variety of clinical parameters including overt PB involvement (at least in patients with adenopathy) {165, 247, 329, 496, 839, 1341, 1761, 1918, 2134}. Gains of chromosome 3q and deletions of 9q are associated with a poor prognosis independent

of the proliferation fraction {1918}. The small cell variant appears to have a more indolent course with the impact of a mantle zone or nodular pattern less settled {247, 1253, 1368, 1605, 1871, 2134, 2237}. Patients presenting with PB, BM and sometimes splenic involvement but without adenopathy have been reported to have a better prognosis (median survival, 79 months) {1652}. Although not a prognostic indicator, mutated *IG* genes were associated with the long-term survivors in the latter study. Patients with *in situ* MCL also may have a better prognosis with long term survival even without therapy, although caution is advised as this morphologic pattern may be associated with more overt disease and a rapid course {1602, 1842}.

Diffuse large B-cell lymphoma, not otherwise specified

H. Stein
R.A. Warnke
W.C. Chan
E.S. Jaffe

J.K.C. Chan
K.C. Gatter
E. Campo

Definition

Diffuse large B-cell lymphoma (DLBCL) is a neoplasm of large B lymphoid cells with nuclear size equal to or exceeding normal macrophage nuclei or more than twice the size of a normal lymphocyte, that has a diffuse growth pattern.

Morphological, biological and clinical studies have subdivided diffuse large B-cell lymphomas into morphological variants, molecular and immunophenotypical subgroups and distinct disease entities (Table 10.14). However, a large number of cases remain that may be biologically heterogeneous, but for which there are no clear and accepted criteria for subdivision. These are classified as DLBCL, not otherwise specified (NOS). DLBCL, NOS comprises all DLBCL cases that do not belong to specific subtypes or disease entities mentioned in Table 10.14

ICD-O code   9680/3

Epidemiology

DLBCL, NOS constitutes 25–30% of adult non-Hodgkin lymphomas in western countries and a higher percentage in developing countries. It is more common in the elderly. The median age is in the 7th decade but it may also occur in children and young adults. It is slightly more common in males than in females {51, 79}.

Etiology

The etiology of DLBCL, NOS remains unknown. It usually arises *de novo* (referred to as primary) but can represent progression or transformation (referred to as secondary) of a less aggressive lymphoma, e.g. chronic lymphocytic leukaemia/ small lymphocytic lymphoma (CLL/SLL), follicular lymphoma, marginal zone lymphoma or nodular lymphocyte predominant Hodgkin lymphoma (NLPHL). Underlying immunodeficiency is a significant risk factor. DLBCL, NOS occurring in the setting of immunodeficiency are more often Epstein-Barr virus (EBV)-positive than sporadic DLBCL, NOS. In DLBCL cases without an overt immunodeficiency, the EBV infection rate is approximately 10% {993, 1690}.

Sites of involvement

Patients may present with nodal or extranodal disease with up to 40% being at least initially confined to extranodal sites {898}. The most common extranodal site is the gastrointestinal tract (stomach and ileocoecal region) but virtually any extranodal location may be a primary site. Other common sites of extranodal presentation include bone, testis, spleen, Waldeyer ring, salivary gland, thyroid, liver, kidney and adrenal gland. Cutaneous lymphomas composed of large B lymphocytes are dealt with separately in this volume. Bone marrow (BM) involvement is reported in 11–27% of cases {327, 442}. The detection rate of minimal involvement may be increased if ancillary studies like immunohistochemistry or PCR are added to the morphological evaluation of the BM specimen {2151}. Bone marrow involvement may be with DLBCL (concordant), but more commonly discordant {442}, with the presence of a low-grade B-cell lymphoma in the BM. The frequency of discordant BM involvement varies in different reports from rare to 70% of the positive cases {67, 945, 1190}. Morphologic examination of peripheral blood (PB) smears revealed that approximately one third of DLBCL patients with BM involvement also had malignant cells in the PB {67}.

Clinical features

Patients usually present with a rapidly enlarging tumour mass at single or multiple nodal or extranodal sites. Almost half of the patients have stage I or II disease. Most patients are asymptomatic but when symptoms are present they are highly dependent on the site of involvement {51, 79}.

Morphology

Lymph nodes demonstrate a diffuse proliferation of large lymphoid cells that have totally (more common pattern) or partially effaced the architecture. Partial nodal involvement may be interfollicular and/or less commonly sinusoidal. The perinodal tissue is often infiltrated. Broad or fine bands of sclerosis may be observed. Cytomorphologically, DLBCL, NOS is diverse and can be divided into common and rare morphologic variants. Cases predominated by medium-sized cells may require special studies to exclude extramedullary leukaemias, Burkitt lymphoma variants and blastoid mantle cell lymphomas.

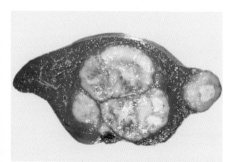

Fig. 10.82 Spleen involved by diffuse large B-cell lymphoma contains large tumour nodules.

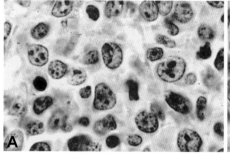
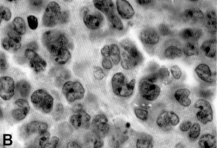

Fig. 10.83 Diffuse large B-cell lymphoma. Centroblastic variant. **A** Typical appearance. **B** In this example, the tumour cells have a polymorphic and polylobated appearance.

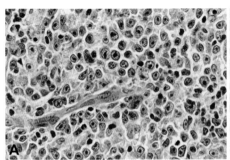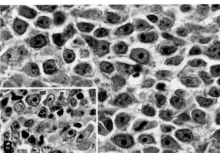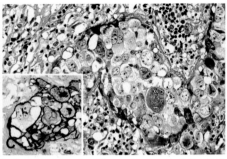

Fig. 10.84 Diffuse large B-cell lymphoma. **A** Immunoblastic variant. A uniform cytologic appearance can be appreciated in the neoplastic cells. **B** Immunoblastic variant. Nearly all of the lymphoma cells have prominent central nucleoli. **C** Anaplastic variant. Large lymphoma cells with pleomorphic nuclei infiltrate the sinus. The inset shows strong membranous and paranuclear labeling of the lymphoma cells for CD20.

Common morphologic variants

Three common and additional minor morphological variants have been recognized. All variants may be admixed with a high number of T-cells and/or histiocytes. These cases should not be categorized as T-cell/histiocyte-rich large B-cell lymphoma (TCRBCL) as long they do not fulfil all the criteria of this DLBCL subtype.

Centroblastic variant: This is the most common variant. Centroblasts are medium-sized to large lymphoid cells with oval to round, vesicular nuclei containing fine chromatin. There are two to four nuclear membrane-bound nucleoli. The cytoplasm is usually scanty and amphophilic to basophilic. In some cases, the tumour is monomorphic, i.e. it is composed entirely (>90%) of centroblasts. In most cases, however, the tumour is polymorphic with an admixture of centroblasts and immunoblasts (<90%) {645, 1274}. The tumour cells may have multilobated nuclei which predominate in rare instances, especially in manifestations of the bone and other extranodal sites.

Immunoblastic variant: Greater than 90% of the cells in this variant are immunoblasts with a single centrally located nucleolus and an appreciable amount of basophilic cytoplasm. Immunoblasts with plasmacytoid differentiation may also be present. Clinical and/or immunophenotypic findings may be essential in differentiating this variant from extramedullary involvement by a plasmablastic lymphoma or an immature plasma cell myeloma. The distinction of the immunoblastic variant from the common centroblastic variant has generally met with poor intraobserver and interobserver reproducibility {898}.

Anaplastic variant: This variant is characterized by large to very large round, oval or polygonal cells with bizarre pleomorphic nuclei that may resemble, at least in part, Hodgkin and/or Reed-Sternberg cells, and may resemble tumour cells of anaplastic large cell lymphoma. The cells may show a sinusoidal and/or a cohesive growth pattern and may mimic undifferentiated carcinoma {891}. They are biologically and clinically unrelated to anaplastic large cell lymphoma which is

Table 10.14 Diffuse large B-cell lymphoma: variants, subgroups and subtypes/entities.

Diffuse large B-cell lymphoma, not otherwise specified (NOS)
Common morphologic variants
Centroblastic
Immunoblastic
Anaplastic
Rare morphologic variants
Molecular subgroups
Germinal centre B-cell-like (GCB)
Activated B-cell-like (ABC)
Immunohistochemical subgroups
CD5-positive DLBCL
Germinal centre B-cell-like (GCB)
Non-germinal centre B-cell-like (non-GCB)
Diffuse large B-cell lymphoma subtypes
T-cell/histiocyte-rich large B-cell lymphoma
Primary DLBCL of the CNS
Primary cutaneous DLBCL, leg type
EBV positive DLBCL of the elderly
Other lymphomas of large B cells
Primary mediastinal (thymic) large B-cell lymphoma
Intravascular large B-cell lymphoma
DLBCL associated with chronic inflammation
Lymphomatoid granulomatosis
ALK-positive LBCL
Plasmablastic lymphoma
Large B-cell lymphoma arising in HHV8-associated multicentric Castleman disease
Primary effusion lymphoma
Borderline cases
B-cell lymphoma, unclassifiable, with features intermediate between diffuse large B-cell lymphoma and Burkitt lymphoma
B-cell lymphoma, unclassifiable, with features intermediate between diffuse large B-cell lymphoma and classical Hodgkin lymphoma

of cytotoxic T-cell derivation and unrelated to ALK-positive LBCL.

Rare morphologic variants: Rare cases of DLBCL, NOS have a myxoid stroma or a fibrillary matrix. A few cases show pseudo-rosette formation. Occasionally the neoplastic cells are spindle-shaped or display features of signet ring cells. Cytoplasmic granules, microvillous projections and intercellular junctions can also be seen.

Immunophenotype

The neoplastic cells express pan B-cell markers such as CD19, CD20, CD22 and CD79a, but may lack one or more of these. Surface and/or cytoplasmic immunoglobulin (IgM>IgG>IgA) can be demonstrated in 50–75% of the cases {1328}. The presence of cytoplasmic immunoglobulin does not correlate with the expression of plasma cell markers such as CD38 and CD138. Both markers are rarely co-expressed in CD20 positive cells. CD30 may be expressed especially in the anaplastic variant {1758}. The neoplastic cells express CD5 in 10% of the cases {2142}. These CD5 positive DLBCL cases usually represent *de novo* DLBCL and only rarely arising from CLL/SLL. CD5 positive DLBCL can be distinguished from the blastoid variant of mantle cell lymphoma by the absence of cyclin D1 expression {1418, 2463}.

The reported incidence of CD10, BCL6 and IRF4/MUM1 expression varies. Expression of CD10 is found in 30–60%, BCL6 in 60–90% and IRF4/MUM1 in 35–65% of the cases {31, 196, 460, 521, 994, 1547}. Unlike normal germinal centre B-cells, in which the expression of IRF4/MUM1 and BCL6 is mutually exclusive, co-expression of both markers was found in 50% of DLBCL in one study {661}. A uniform high expression of FOXP1 has been reported in DLBCL cases that lack the germinal centre phenotype and express IRF4/MUM1 and BCL6 in the absence of t(14;18) {146}. Expression of BCL6 varies in different reports, ranging from 47–84% {460, 759, 925, 994}.

The proliferation fraction as detected by Ki67 staining is high (usually much more than 40%) and may be greater than 90% in some cases {1478}. p53 is expressed in 20–60% of cases {420, 1171, 1281, 2476}.

Subgrouping DLBCL, NOS by immunophenotyping

An immunophenotypical subdivision of DLBCL, NOS into germinal centre-like (GCB) and non-germinal centre-like (non-GCB) subgroups has been proposed by different groups using a combination of antibodies to CD10, BCL6 and IRF4/MUM1 {460, 882}. Cases with CD10 expression by >30% of cells are regarded as GC type as well as cases that are CD10-, BCL6+, IRF4/MUM1-. All other cases are regarded as of non-GC type {882}. However, this immunophenotypic subdivision does not correlate exactly with gene expression-based subgrouping of DLBCL {994, 1869}. The addition of other markers such as BCL2 and Cyclin D2 may lead to an improvement in the immunophenotypic subgrouping of DLBCL {31}. This immunophenotypic subgrouping does not currently determine therapy.

Genetics

Antigen receptor genes

Clonally rearranged immunoglobulin heavy and light chain genes are detectable. They show somatic hypermutations in the variable regions.

Aberrant somatic hypermutations

Aberrant somatic hypermutations targeting multiple genetic loci, including the genes *PIMI, MYC, RHOH/TTF (ARHH)* and *PAX5* are encountered in more than 50% of DLBCL cases. These genetic alterations may contribute to the oncogenesis of this lymphoma group {1699}.

Chromosomal translocations

Up to 30% of cases show abnormalities of the 3q27 region involving the *BCL6* gene, which is the commonest translocation in DLBCL {158, 1620, 1626}. Translocation of the *BCL2* gene, i.e. t(14;18), a hallmark of follicular lymphoma, occurs in 20–30% of cases {994, 1316, 2379}. A *MYC* rearrangement was observed in up to 10% of an unselected series of cases {2481} and is usually associated with a complex pattern of genetic alterations {994}. The *MYC* break partner is an *IG* gene in 60% and a non-*IG* gene in 40% of cases {994}. Approximately 20% of cases with a *MYC* break have a concurrent *IGH-BCL2* translocation and/or *BCL6* break or both {994, 2278}. These cases usually have a high proliferation (>90% Ki67+) and may be better categorized as "B-cell lymphomas, unclassified with features intermediate

between diffuse large B-cell lymphoma and Burkitt lymphoma".

Gene expression profiling

Alizadeh *et al.* {24} identified two subgroups of DLBCL. One subgroup (termed GCB-like) has the gene expression profile of germinal centre B-cells (45–50% of cases) and the other (termed ABC-like) has the profile of activated peripheral B-cells. This was confirmed by a subsequent study {1869}. Initially, a third subgroup (termed type 3) was defined. This proved to be a collection of cases that cannot be classified as the GCB- and the ABC-subgroup and does not represent a distinct subgroup {994, 2449}. The two established subgroups are associated with different chromosomal aberrations. The ABC-DLBCL subgroup has frequent gains of 3q, 18q21-q22 and losses of 6q21-q22, whereas the GCB-DLBCL subgroup displays frequent gains at 12q12 {167, 2142}. A number of the GCB-like cases carry a *BCL2* rearrangement {526, 988}.

The immunoblastic variant and the centroblastic variant cases with a polymorphic centroblast-like cells and/or a higher content of immunoblasts are more common in the ABC-subgroup but were also observed in the GCB-subgroup. This indicates that the GCB-like and ABC-like subgroups cannot reliably be recognized by morphology. The correlation between the gene expression subtypes of DLBCL and those defined as GC and non-GC DLBCL by immunohistochemistry is variable {882, 994}.

Table 10.15
International Prognostic Index for aggressive lymphomas.

Unfavourable variables
Age >60 years
Poor performance status (ECOG≥2)
Advanced Ann Arbor stage (III-IV)
Extranodal involvement ≥2 sites
High serum LDH (>normal)

Risk group	Unfavourable variables	
	All patients	Patients ≤60*
Low	0 or 1	0
Low/intermediate	2	1
High/intermediate	3	2
High	4 or 5	3

* In patients ≤60 year-old the age-adjusted international prognostic index (aaIPI) is calculated with three unfavourable variables that include poor performance status, advanced Ann Arbor stage and high serum LDH.

Postulated normal counterpart

Peripheral B-cells of either germinal centre or post germinal centre (activated B-cell) origin.

Prognosis and predictive factors

In the pre-rituximab era the long-term remission rate was between 50–60%. Although individual prognosis varies widely, the International Prognostic Index (IPI) based on clinical parameters has proved to be highly valuable {79}. However, the IPI seems to lose some of its predictive value in patients treated with rituximab {1985} which has improved prognosis significantly {455}.

Concordant BM involvement is associated with a very poor prognosis (5-year overall survival, 10%) while discordant involvement does not influence the clinical outcome significantly (5-year overall survival, 62%). The poor survival associated with concordant involvement was independent of the IPI score {327, 442, 1851}.

Morphology

There are many conflicting reports on the prognostic impact of immunoblastic features {79, 275, 645, 1453, 1915}. Some studies found an adverse prognostic impact of immunoblastic morphology whereas others did not.

Immunophenotype

A large number of immunohistochemical markers have been reported to be associated with prognostic effects: the expression of BCL2, X-linked inhibitor of apoptosis (XIAP), IRF4/MUM1, cyclin D2, cyclin D3, p53, CD5, FOXP1, PKC-β, ICAM1, HLA-DR, c-FLIP have been associated with an adverse prognosis and the expression of BCL6, CD10, LMO2 with a favourable outcome {10, 146, 196, 460, 526, 759, 881, 925, 1009, 1479, 1546, 2318, 2463}. However, the results obtained in these different studies are often conflicting and their interpretation is thus controversial. Finally, the addition of the anti-CD20 antibody rituximab has improved the survival of patients with DLBCL considerably {455} and was reported to have eliminated the negative impact of the expression of BCL2 and the positive impact of BCL6 on clinical outcome {455, 1528, 1529, 2423}. Patients with EBV-infected DLBCL, as revealed by EBER *in situ* hybridization, have been found in one study to have a worse clinical outcome than patients with an EBV-negative DLBCL {1690}.

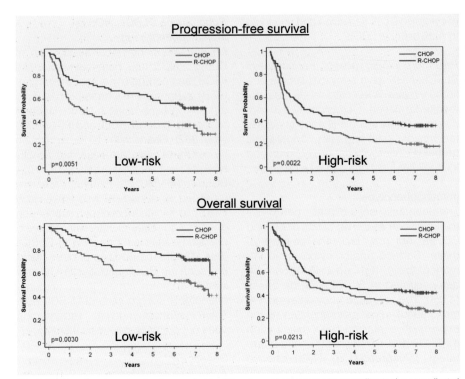

Fig.10.85 Overall and progression-free survival in diffuse large B-cell lymphoma according to the age-adjusted International Prognostic Index in patients treated with CHOP with and without rituximab according to the study conducted by the GELA (courtesy of Dr B. Coiffier).

Immunohistochemical panels

Hans *et al.* {882} reported that a combination of CD10, BCL6 and IRF4/MUM1 expression, the so-called "Hans classifier", could subdivide DLBCL patients into long- and short-term survivors; this result has been confirmed by some studies but not by others {31, 460, 1339, 1526, 1610, 2301}. Whether the addition of rituximab to

CHOP will eliminate its prognostic value needs to be further investigated {1610}. The study of other immunohistochemical panels including markers such as cyclin D2, BCL2 and LMO2 may improve the prognostic prediction {31, 1580}. However, the use of immunohistochemical panels to assign prognostic groups does not currently have a role in routine clinical

Table 10.16
Genetic, molecular and clinical characteristics of the DLBCL subgroups and PMBL recognized by expression profiling.

Characteristic	ABC	GCB	PMBL
t(14;18)	0	35%	0
3q gain/amplification	26%	0	5%
9p gain/amplification	6%	0	35%
12q12	5%	20%	5%
Ongoing *IG* mutations	No	Yes	No
BCL2 rearrangement	0	20–25%	0
REL amplification	0	15%	
SOCS1 inactivation			45%
NFkB activation	Yes	No	Yes
5 year survival	15–30%	50–60%	65%
Disease hallmarks		Late relapses	Predominantly women <35 years Mediastinal

ABC, activated B-cell-like; GCB, germinal centre B-cell-like; PMBL, primary mediastinal large B-cell lymphoma.

practice. One of the major limitations is the well-documented problems with reproducibility in the performance and interpretation of some immunohistochemical stains {518, 2505}.

Proliferation

A high proliferation fraction, as assessed by the Ki67 index, has been associated with worse survival in some series {1478}. This is supported by one gene expression study in which the proliferation signature proved to be a strong predictor of an adverse outcome {1869}. However other studies have failed to confirm a prognostic value for the Ki67 index {460, 1904, 2423, 2496}

Genetics

In some studies, *BCL6* translocation has been reported to be associated with a better prognosis, but not in others {158, 1056, 1188, 1543, 1598, 1620, 1728, 2339}. In contrast, the presence of a *MYC* break is linked with a very unfavourable outcome {994}. *TP53* mutations have been associated with poor survival in some series of DLBCL including one study in which mutations in the DNA binding domain proved to be the most important predictor {420, 1000, 1171, 1281, 2421, 2476}. p53 protein expression does not seem to be of prognostic value in DLBCL patients {1187, 1353, 2043}. Patients with a molecularly defined GCB-subtype of DLBCL have been shown to have a significantly better clinical outcome than those with the ABC subtype {24, 994, 1869}. Whether this difference persists in patients treated with rituximab remains to be seen. Other subgroups, i.e. "oxidative phosphorylation", "BCR/proliferation" and "host response" identified by gene arrays, did not predict survival, but may suggest targets for therapy {1507}.

Microenvironment

The immune response appears to have a strong impact on the clinical outcome after chemotherapy. The MHC class II gene expression signature correlates with a favourable outcome {1479, 1869, 2318}. The loss of *MHC* class II gene and protein expression in patients with DLBCL was found to correlate with reduced numbers of tumour-infiltrating CD8+ T-cells and a poor outcome {1846}. The lymph node signature as identified by gene expression profiling is associated with a good clinical outcome {1869}. This signature is characterized by genes that encode components of extracellular matrix and connective tissue growth factor.

Therapy

DLBCL are aggressive but potentially curable with multi-agent chemotherapy. The CHOP regimen has been the mainstay of therapy for several decades. Whereas attempts to improve outcome with more intensive chemotherapy failed to show additional benefit. The addition of the anti-CD20 monoclonal antibody rituximab to CHOP (R-CHOP) has led to a marked improvement in survival {455}.

T cell/histiocyte-rich large B-cell lymphoma

C. De Wolf-Peeters
J. Delabie
E. Campo
E.S. Jaffe
G. Delsol

Definition

T-cell/histiocyte-rich large B-cell lymphoma (THRLBCL) is characterized by a limited number of scattered, large, atypical B cells embedded in a background of abundant T cells and frequently histiocytes.

ICD-O code   9688/3

Synonyms

T-cell-rich B-cell lymphoma {1813}, large B-cell lymphoma rich in T-cells and simulating Hodgkin disease {426}, histiocyte rich/T-cell-rich large B-cell lymphoma {544}.

Epidemiology

THRLBCL affects mainly middle-aged man. It accounts for <10% of all diffuse large B-cell lymphomas (DLBCL).

Sites of involvement

THRLBCL mainly affects the lymph nodes but bone marrow (BM), liver and spleen involvement are frequently found at diagnosis.

Clinical features

Patients present with fever, malaise, splenomegaly and/or hepatomegaly. Almost half of them are at advanced Ann Arbor stage with an intermediate to high risk International Prognostic Index (IPI) score. The disease is often refractory to chemotherapy presently in use.

Table 10.17 T-cell/histiocyte-rich large B-cell lymphoma.

Median age	12-61 years
Male	75%
Stage III-IV	64%
Liver involvement	13-70%
Spleen involvement	33-67%
Bone marrow involvement	17-60%

Data based on 277 cases of patients with T-cell/histiocyte-rich large B-cell lymphoma in the literature {13A, 251, 252, 725, 1329A, 1361A, 1847A, 2236A, 2273A, 2358A}.

Morphology

THRLBCL has a diffuse or less commonly vaguely nodular growth pattern replacing most of the normal lymph node parenchyma. It is comprised of scattered, single, large B cells embedded in a background of small lymphocytes that represent T cells, and variable numbers of histiocytes. The tumour cells are always dispersed and do not form aggregates or sheets. These cells may mimic the neoplastic lymphocyte predominant (LP) cells of nodular lymphocyte-predominant Hodgkin lymphoma (NLPHL), but usually show a more pronounced variation in size and in some cases may resemble centroblasts or more pleomorphic cells mimicking Reed-Sternberg or Hodgkin cells {598, 1299}. They are typically found within clusters of bland-looking non-epithelioid histiocytes that may not be obvious on conventional examination. These histiocytes represent a main and distinctive component of THRLBCL and are useful for the diagnosis {6}. The background lymphocytes are nearly all of T-cell lineage. Eosinophils or plasma cells are not found. The histology resembles cases of NLPHL with a diffuse component, in which the LP cells have infiltrate the extrafollicular compartment but these THRLBCL-like areas in NLPHL do not represent a transition towards THRLBCL and do not carry a bad prognostic significance {252}. Nevertheless, there are some cases of histological progression in NLPHL, in which the process is entirely diffuse and the histological appearance is virtually indistinguishable from *de novo* THRLBCL. The relationship between secondary THRLBCL and primary cases remains controversial. They may represent distinct, but morphologically and immunophenotypically similar entities.

In the spleen, a multifocal or micronodular involvement of the white pulp is found and in the liver the lymphomatous foci are localized in the portal tracts {598}. In these extranodal locations as well as in the BM, the lymphoma is characterized by the same composition as in the lymph node.

On recurrence, the number of atypical cells may increase, resulting in a picture of DLBCL. The latter heralds a bad outcome within a short time {7}.

Several studies have recognized cases with similar morphology but without histiocytes. Whether these cases represent the same entity as typical THRLBCL is not still clear. Studies including cases rich in T cells with and without histiocytes have defined a more heterogeneous group of large B-cell lymphomas, which probably include more than one entity {2, 836, 1195, 1299, 1813, 1861}. Further studies should clarify the relationship between these lymphomas. At present, while cases lacking significant numbers of histiocytes may be included in THRLBCL, the absence of histiocytes should be noted. Lymphomas containing B cells with a spectrum of cell size, morphology and distribution (clusters or sheets of medium to large B cells), should not be included within the category of THRLBCL, and may be considered a subtype of DLBCL, NOS.

Immunophenotype

The large atypical cells express pan B-cell markers and BCL6; a variable number stain for BCL2 and EMA and no expression of CD15, CD30 and CD138 is found. The background is composed of variable number of CD68-positive histiocytes and CD3, CD5, positive T cells. T-cell rosettes around the tumour cells and remnants of B follicles or clusters of small B lymphocytes are absent. Lack of residual IgD positive mantle cells and follicular dendritic cell meshwork are of further diagnostic help differentiating THRLBCL from NLPHL {6, 725}. There are aggressive B-cell lymphomas, rich in reactive T-cells, in which the neoplastic cells are sparse, and are EBV-positive. In such cases, the neoplastic cells may exhibit a Hodgkin-like morphology. Such cases should not be classified as THRLBCL, and should be considered within the spectrum of EBV-positive DLBCL {1299}.

Genetics

The tumour B cells have the same clonal rearranged *IG* genes carrying high number

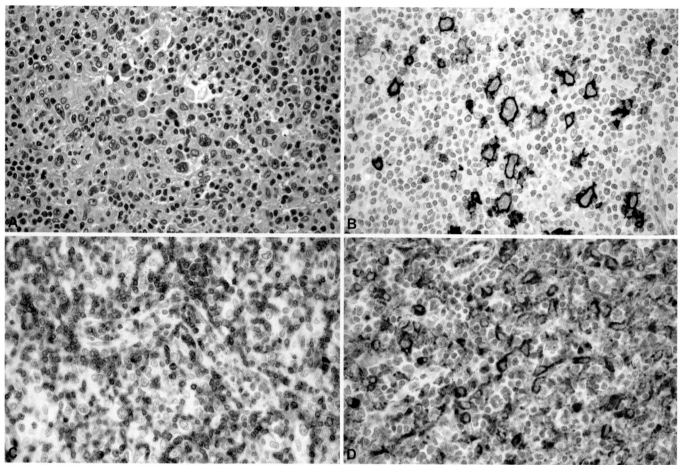

Fig. 10.86 T-cell/histiocyte-rich large B-cell lymphoma. **A** A small number of large atypical cells surrounded by bland looking histiocytes and small lymphocytes. **B** Immunohistochemistry for the B-cell marker CD20 shows the B-cell phenotype of the scattered atypical cells. **C** Small lymphocytes correspond to CD3 positive T-cells. **D** A large number of histiocytes stained for CD68.

of somatic mutations and intraclonal diversity {263} as germinal centres cells. Limited karyotypic studies have not shown recurrent abnormalities. Comparative genomic hybridization on microdissected tumour cells demonstrated more imbalances in NLPHL than in THRLBCL with common anomalies involving 4q and 19p {731}. Gene expression profiling has identified a subgroup of DLBCL characterized by a host immune response and a very bad prognosis {1507} and includes most of the cases diagnosed as THRL-BCL.

Postulated normal counterpart
Germinal centre B cell {263}.

Prognosis and predictive factors
THRLBCL is considered an aggressive lymphoma although clinical heterogeneity is described. Cases with histiocytes are reported to represent a more homogeneous group of patients with a very aggressive lymphoma, frequent failure of current therapies and with the IPI score being the only parameter of prognostic significance {7, 251}.

Primary diffuse large B-cell lymphoma of the CNS

P.M. Kluin
M. Deckert
J.A. Ferry

Definition
Diffuse large B-cell lymphoma of the central nervous system (CNS DLBCL) represents all primary intracerebral or intraocular lymphomas. Excluded are lymphomas of the dura, intravascular large B-cell lymphoma, lymphomas with evidence of systemic disease or secondary lymphomas, as well as all immunodeficiency-associated lymphomas.

ICD-O code   9680/3

Synonyms
These cases are also diagnosed as primary CNS lymphoma (PCNSL) or primary intraocular lymphoma (PIOL).

Epidemiology
CNS DLBCL represents <1% of all non-Hodgkin lymphomas (NHL) and approximately 2–3% of all brain tumours. The median age is approximately 60 years, and there is a slight preponderance of male patients. Some studies suggest an increase in the incidence of CNS DLBCL {485}, but it is unknown whether this is due to improved diagnostic tools or reflects a real increase.

Etiology
Epstein-Barr virus is generally absent from CNS DLBCL in immunocompetent patients. Expression or absence of chemokines and chemokine receptors or cytokines may contribute to the specific localization {2038}. Tumour cells and endothelial cells may interact via activation of IL4 to create

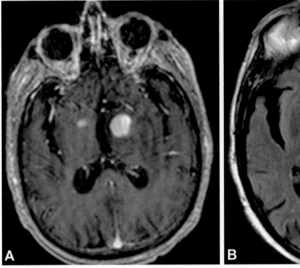

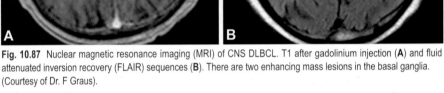

Fig. 10.87 Nuclear magnetic resonance imaging (MRI) of CNS DLBCL. T1 after gadolinium injection (**A**) and fluid attenuated inversion recovery (FLAIR) sequences (**B**). There are two enhancing mass lesions in the basal ganglia. (Courtesy of Dr. F Graus).

a favourable microenvironment for tumour growth {1889}. CNS DLBCL show a restricted homing to the main immune sanctuaries (brain, eyes and testis). Many DLBCL of the CNS and testis show decreased or absent expression of HLA class I and II proteins allowing the tumour cells to further escape from immune attack {240, 1843}.

Sites of involvement
Approximately 60% of all CNS DLBCL are located supratentorially. In 20–40%, multiple lesions are present. Using NMRI, CNS DLBCL may show a homogeneous lesion but also signs of central necrosis. The leptomeninges are affected in 5%.

Approximately 20% of the patients develop intraocular lesions, and 80–90% of patients with intraocular DLBCL develop contralateral tumours and parenchymal CNS lesions. Dissemination to extraneural sites including the bone marrow is very rare.

Clinical features
Focal neurological deficits are observed in 50–80% of the patients. Neuropsychiatric symptoms (20–30%) and symptoms due to increased intracranial pressure are also seen. Leptomeningeal involvement presents with headache and asymmetric cranial neuropathies. Intraocular disease presents with a blurred vision and floaters.

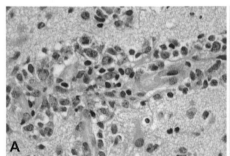
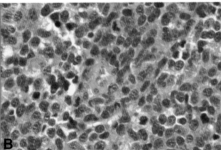
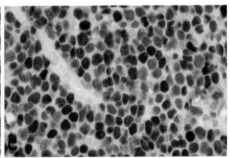

Fig. 10.88 Primary diffuse large B-cell lymphoma of the CNS. **A** Accumulation of tumour cells within the perivascular space. **B** More solid pattern, with still some accumulation in the perivascular space. **C** Strong IRF4/MUM1 staining in more than 70% of the tumour cells in CNS DLBCL.

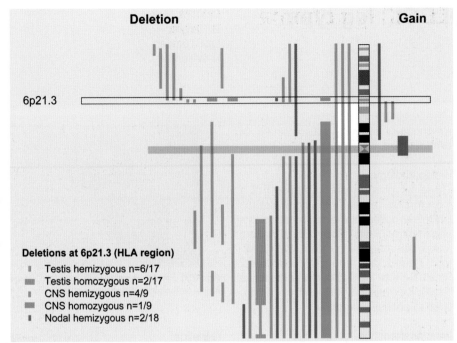

Deletion   **Gain**

6p21.3

Deletions at 6p21.3 (HLA region)
- Testis hemizygous n=6/17
- Testis homozygous n=2/17
- CNS hemizygous n=4/9
- CNS homozygous n=1/9
- Nodal hemizygous n=2/18

Fig. 10.89 Array CGH analysis of 9 primary CNS DLBCL, 17 primary testicular DLBCL and 18 primary nodal (stage I/II) DLBCL, showing (sometimes very small) deletions at 6p21.3.

Morphology

Most intraparenchymal lymphomas show a diffuse growth pattern; characteristically, tumour cells are present in the perivascular space, which is best appreciated at the periphery of the tumour or areas where the tumour cells dissociate. The tumour cells mostly resemble centroblasts, but shrinkage artefacts may hinder assessment of the exact nuclear size. Tumour cells may be intermingled with reactive small lymphocytes, macrophages, activated microglial cells and reactive astrocytes. Large areas of necrosis or foamy histiocytes may be present, particularly in patients treated with high dose corticosteroids. This may result in so-called "vanishing tumours".

Immunophenotype

All tumours are positive for B-cell markers CD20, CD22 or CD79a. CD10 expression is present in approximately 10–20%, BCL6 in 60–80% and strong IRF4/MUM1 in approximately 90% {261, 324, 1305}; BCL2 expression, not related to the t(14;18)(q32;q21), is frequent {453}.

Genetics

Antigen receptor genes

CNS DLBCL contain a very high load of (ongoing) somatic hypermutations (up to 27%) and a striking maintenance of the open reading frame {1503}. A biased use of *VH* genes, in particular *VH4/34*, suggests an antigen dependent proliferation. Mutations also affect *BCL6*, *PIM1*, *MYC*, *RhoH/TTFn* and *PAX5* {1505}.

Cytogenetic abnormalities and oncogenes

Approximately 30–40% of CNS DLBCL have *BCL6* translocations but t(14;18)(q32;q21) and t(8;14)(q24;q32) are extremely rare {453}. There are common deletions at 6q and gains at 12q, 22q and 18q21 with copy number increase or amplification of *BCL2* and *MALT1* {2368}. Homozygous or hemizygous deletions at 9p21 frequently affect *CDKN2A/p16^{INK4a}* {453}. Small deletions, not visible by conventional comparative genomic hybridization (CGH), affect 6p21.3 (*HLA* region) and contribute to loss of HLA class II and I expression {240,1843}.

Postulated normal counterpart

Activated (late germinal centre) B-cell.

Prognosis and predictive factors

The formerly poor prognosis has been remarkably ameliorated by novel chemotherapeutic protocols that include methotrexate. Most relapses affect the CNS. The sporadic systemic relapses may involve any organ but relatively frequently the testis and breast {1043}. Individual biological prognostic factors have been described, but so far they have not been validated in independent studies {261, 324, 1767}.

Primary cutaneous DLBCL, leg type

C.J.L.M. Meijer
B. Vergier
L.M. Duncan
R. Willemze

Definition
A primary cutaneous diffuse large B-cell lymphoma composed exclusively of large transformed B-cells, most commonly arising in the leg.

ICD-O code   9680/3

Epidemiology
Primary cutaneous diffuse large B-cell lymphoma (PCLBCL, leg type) constitute 4% of all primary cutaneous lymphomas and 20% of all primary cutaneous B-cell lymphomas {2407} and typically occur in elderly patients, in particular in women, with a M:F ratio of 1:3–4. The median age is in the 7th decade {2334}.

Sites of involvement
These lymphomas preferentially affect the lower legs, but 10–15% arise at other sites {1170, 1993, 2502}.

Clinical features
PCLBCL, leg type presents with red or bluish-red tumours on one or both of the lower legs {824, 1170, 2334, 2502}. These lymphomas frequently disseminate to extracutaneous sites.

Histopathology
These lymphomas are comprised of a monotonous, diffuse, non-epidermotropic infiltrate of confluent sheets of centroblasts and immunoblasts, many with a striking round cell morphology {824, 2334}. Mitotic figures are frequently observed. Small B-cells are lacking and reactive T-cells are relatively few and often confined to perivascular areas.

Immunophenotype
The neoplastic B-cells express monotypic Ig, CD20 and CD79a. In contrast to primary cutaneous follicle centre lymphomas (PCFCL), PCLBCL, leg-type nearly always strongly express BCL2, IRF4/MUM1, and FOX-P1 {768, 819, 826, 948, 950, 1170}. However, approximately 10% of cases do not express either BCL2 or IRF4/MUM1 {1170, 1993}. BCL6 is expressed by most cases, whereas CD10 staining is usually negative {950}.

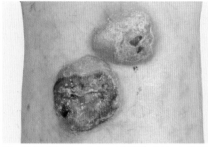

Fig. 10.91 Primary cutaneous DLBCL, leg type. Typical clinical presentation with tumours on a leg.

Genetics
PCLBCL, leg-type show many genetic similarities with diffuse large B-cell lymphomas (DLBCL) arising at other sites but marked differences with PCFCL. Interphase FISH analysis {874} frequently shows translocations involving MYC, BCL6 and IGH@ genes in PCLBCL, leg-type. Using array-based CGH and FISH analyses, high-level DNA amplifications of 18q21.31-q21.33, including the BCL2 and MALT1 genes, were detected in 67% of the cases {577}. Amplification of the BCL2 gene may well explain the strong BCL2 expression in these cases, particularly because the t(14;18) is not found in these lymphomas {577, 875}. Deletion of a small region on chromosome 9p21.3 containing the CDKN2A and CDKN2B gene loci has been reported in 67% of PCLBCL, leg-type.
PCLBCL, leg-type has the gene expression profile of activated B-cell-like DLBCL {948}.

Postulated normal counterpart
Peripheral B-cells of post-germinal centre origin.

Prognosis and predictive factors
These lymphomas have a 5-year survival of approximately 50% {824, 2334}. The presence of multiple skin lesions at diagnosis is a significant adverse risk factor {824}. BCL2-negative cases have the same prognosis. Inactivation of CDKN2A, either by deletion or promoter hypermethylation, has been found to be an unfavourable prognostic factor {577}.

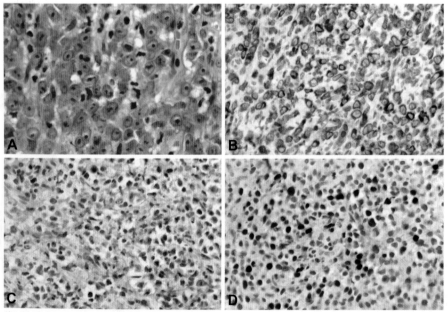

Fig.10.90 Primary cutaneous DLBCL, leg type. **A** H&E. Note large transformed cells with prominent nucleoli. **B** BCL2 staining shows strong cytoplasmic staining. Neoplastic cells show nuclear staining for both BCL6 (**C**) and IRF4/MUM1 (**D**).

EBV positive diffuse large B-cell lymphoma of the elderly

S. Nakamura
E.S. Jaffe
S.H. Swerdlow

Definition

EBV-positive diffuse large B-cell lymphoma (DLBCL) of the elderly is an EBV+ clonal B-cell lymphoid proliferation that occurs in patients >50 years and without any known immunodeficiency or prior lymphoma {1674, 1675, 2011}. Rare cases of a similar lymphoma may occur in younger individuals; however, the possibility of an undiagnosed underlying immunodeficiency must be very strongly considered in these circumstances. Cases of lymphomatoid granulomatosis, infectious mononucleosis or other well-defined disorders (such as plasmablastic lymphoma, primary effusion lymphoma and DLBCL associated with chronic inflammation) that may be EBV+ are excluded from this category.

ICD-O code   9680/3

Synonyms

Senile EBV-associated B-cell lymphoproliferative disorder; age-related EBV+ lymphoproliferative disorder; EBV-associated B-cell lymphoproliferative disorder of the elderly.

Epidemiology

In Asian countries, EBV+ DLBCL of the elderly accounts for 8–10% of DLBCL among patients without a documented predisposing immunodeficiency {1675, 1690}, with little data for Western countries. Among DLBCL, the proportion of EBV+ cases increases with increasing patient age with the highest proportion seen in those >90 years of age (20–25%) {1675}. The median age is 71 years (range: 45–92 years), with a male:female ratio of 1.4:1.

Etiology

EBV-positive DLBCL of the elderly is an EBV-driven B-cell lymphoma believed to be related to immunological deterioration or senescence in immunity that is a part of the aging process {1674, 1675, 2011}.

Sites of involvement

70% of patients present with extranodal disease (most commonly skin, lung, tonsil and stomach) with or without simultaneous lymph node involvement; 30% of patients have lymph node disease alone {1213, 1675}.

Clinical features

The clinical features at presentation are variable. More than half of the patients have high or high-intermediate International Prognostic Index (IPI) scores {1213, 1675, 1690, 2473}.

Morphology

The architecture of the involved tissues is effaced in contrast to infectious mononucleosis. Although no longer considered to be of clinical importance {1675}, cases were initially divided morphologically into polymorphous and large-cell lymphoma subtypes, both of which include many large transformed cells/immunoblasts and Hodgkin and Reed-Sternberg (HRS)-like

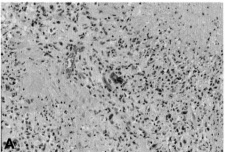
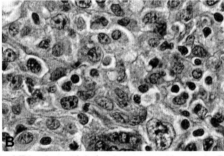
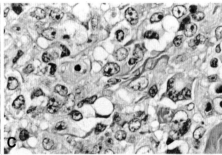

Fig. 10.92 EBV+ diffuse large B-cell lymphoma of the elderly. **A** This polymorphic lesion shows geographic necrosis. **B** There is a mixed proliferation of immunoblasts and medium-sized lymphoid cells as well as small reactive lymphocytes. **C** Monotonous proliferation of immunoblast-like or Hodgkin and Reed-Sternberg-like cells with prominent central nucleoli.

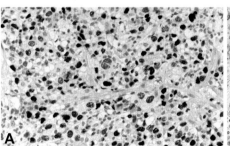
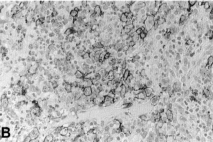
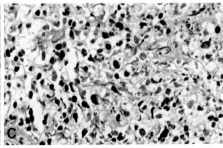

Fig. 10.93 EBV+ diffuse large B-cell lymphoma of the elderly. **A** The nuclei of the large lymphoid cells are EBNA-2 positive. **B** More than 50% of the large lymphoid cells are CD20-positive. **C** *In situ* hybridization (ISH) for Epstein-Barr virus latency-associated RNA (EBER) shows many positive cells.

giant cells. The polymorphous subtype shows a broad range of B-cell maturation and a variable component of reactive elements such as small lymphocytes, plasma cells, histiocytes and epithelioid cells. In the large-cell lymphoma subtype, most of the cells appear to be transformed. Both subtypes may demonstrate large areas of geographical necrosis and the histology is often variable from area to area, indicating a continuous spectrum between the two subtypes.

Immunophenotype
The neoplastic cells are usually positive for CD20 and/or CD79a, and light chain restriction may be difficult to demonstrate. CD10 and BCL6 are usually negative, while IRF4/MUM1 is commonly positive. Cases with immunoblastic or plasmablastic features may lack CD20 expression and have detectable cytoplasmic immunoglobulin. The large atypical cells are LMP1 and EBNA-2 positive in 94% and 28% of cases, respectively {1674, 1675}. The cells are variably CD30-positive, but are CD15-negative.

Genetics
Clonality of the immunoglobulin genes and EBV can usually be detected by molecular techniques. These studies are helpful for distinguishing the polymorphous cases from infectious mononucleosis of the elderly.

Postulated normal couterpart
Mature B lymphocyte, transformed by EBV.

Prognosis and predictive factors
The clinical course is aggressive, with a median survival of about two years {1675, 1690}. Neither IPI score nor histopathologic subtype affects prognosis. The presence of B symptoms and age >70 years appear to be reliable prognostic factors. Patients with 0, 1 or 2 of these factors have median overall survival times of 56, 25 and 9 months, respectively {1675}.

DLBCL associated with chronic inflammation

J.K.C. Chan
K. Aozasa
P. Gaulard

Definition
Diffuse large B-cell lymphoma (DLBCL) associated with chronic inflammation is a lymphoid neoplasm occurring in the context of long-standing chronic inflammation, and showing association with Epstein-Barr virus (EBV). Most cases involve body cavities or narrow spaces. Pyothorax-associated lymphoma (PAL) is a prototypic form, and develops in the pleural cavity of patients with long-standing pyothorax.

ICD-O code   9680/3

Epidemiology
The interval between the onset of chronic inflammation and malignant lymphoma is usually over 10 years {408, 1024, 1025}. PAL develops in patients with a 20–64 (median 37) year history of pyothorax resulting from artificial pneumothorax for treatment of pulmonary or pleural tuberculosis {63, 1024, 1568, 1734}. Age at diagnosis ranges from 5th to 8th decade, with a median age around 65–70 years {1568}. The male to female ratio is 12.3 {1024} versus near unity for chronic pyothorax, suggesting that males are more susceptible to this type of lymphoma than females. Although most cases of PAL have been reported in Japan, this lymphoma has also been described in the West {88, 1398, 1734}.

Etiology
Artificial pneumothorax, used in the past as a form of surgical therapy for pulmonary tuberculosis, is the only significant risk factor for development of PAL among chronic pyothorax patients {62, 960}. PAL is strongly associated with EBV, with expression of EBNA-2 and/or LMP1 together with EBNA-1 {739, 1629, 1936, 2147}. The EBV latency pattern is type III in more than 60% of cases {1734, 2146}. There is probably a role for chronic inflammation at the local site in the proliferation of EBV-transformed B cells by enabling them to escape from the host immune surveillance through production of IL-10, an immunosuppressive cytokine, and providing autocrine to paracrine growth

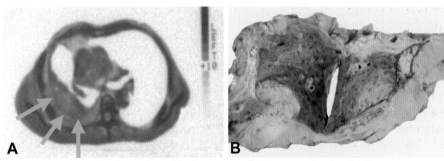

Fig. 10.94 Pyothorax-associated lymphoma. Massive tumour proliferation surrounding the whole lung.

via IL-6 and IL-6 receptor {1095, 1098}. For DLBCL occurring in other settings of long standing chronic suppuration/inflammation, such as chronic osteomyelitis, metallic implant or chronic skin ulcer, the tested cases have been EBV-positive {408, 471}.

Sites of involvement
The commonest sites of involvement are the pleural cavity (PAL), bone (especially femur), joint and periarticular soft tissue {408}. In PAL, the tumour mass is larger than 10 cm in more than half of the cases {63}. There is direct invasion of adjacent structures, but tumour is often confined to the thoracic cavity at the time of diagnosis, with about 70% of patients presenting with clinical stage I/II disease {1568}.

PAL thus differs from primary effusion lymphoma, which is characterized by lymphomatous serous effusions in the absence of tumour mass formation.
Patients with rheumatoid arthritis may develop large B-cell lymphoma around chronically inflamed joints, but these cases are EBV-negative, and probably best not classified into this category {817}.

Clinical features
Patients with PAL present with chest pain, back pain, fever, tumourous swelling in the chest wall, or respiratory symptoms such as productive cough, haemoptysis or dyspnea. Radiologic examination reveals a tumour mass in the pleura (80%), pleura and lung (10%), and lung near the pleura (7%). The serum lactate

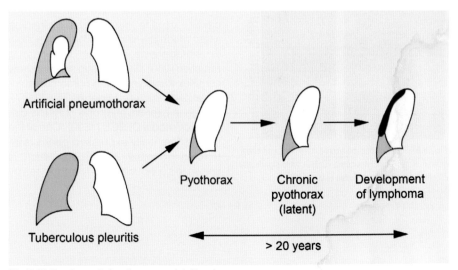

Fig.10.95 Development of pyothorax-associated lymphoma.

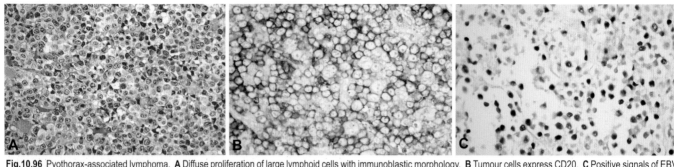

Fig.10.96 Pyothorax-associated lymphoma. **A** Diffuse proliferation of large lymphoid cells with immunoblastic morphology. **B** Tumour cells express CD20. **C** Positive signals of EBV in the nucleus of tumour cells by *in situ* hybridization with EBER probe.

dehydrogenase level is commonly elevated {1568, 1734}.

Patients who develop lymphoma in the bone, joint, periarticular soft tissue or skin many years after the onset of chronic osteomyelitis, insertion of metallic implant in a joint or bone, or chronic venous ulcer usually present with pain or mass lesion. The involved bone typically shows lytic lesions on radiologic examination.

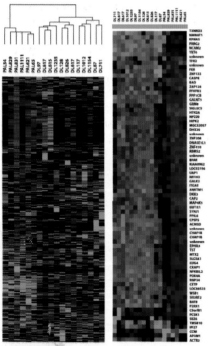

Fig.10.97 Patterns of gene expression in PAL and nodal diffuse large B-cell lymphoma (DLBCL) are significantly different. Modified from Nishiu *et al.* {1599}.

Morphology

The morphologic features are not different from DLBCL, NOS. Most cases show centroblastic/immunoblastic morphology, with round nuclei and large single or multiple nucleoli. Massive necrosis and angiocentric growth may be present.

Immunophenotype

Most cases express CD20 and CD79a. However, a proportion of cases may show plasmacytic differentiation, with loss of CD20 and/or CD79a, and expression of IRF4/MUM1 and CD138. CD30 can be expressed. Occasional cases may express in addition one or more T-cell markers (CD2, CD3, CD4 and/or CD7), causing problems in lineage assignment {1516, 1568, 1734, 2247}.

In most cases, ISH for EBV discloses EBER expression, and a type III LMP1+/EBNA-2+ latency profile {1734}.

Genetics

Immunoglobulin genes are clonally rearranged and hypermutated {1492}. *TP53* mutations are found in about 70% of cases, usually involving dipyrimidine sites, which are known to be susceptible to mutagenesis induced by ionizing radiation {960}. Cytogenetic studies show complex karyotypes with numerous numerical and structural abnormalities {2147}. The gene expression profile of PAL is distinct from nodal DLBCL {1599}. One of the most differentially expressed genes is interferon-inducible 27 *(IFI27)*, which is known to be induced in B lymphocytes by

stimulation of interferon-α, in keeping with the role of chronic inflammation in this condition. Down-regulation of HLA class I expression, which is essential for efficient induction of host cytotoxic T lymphocytes (CTL), and mutations of CTL epitopes in *EBNA-3B*, an immunodominant antigen for CTL responses, might also contribute to escape of PAL cells from host CTL {1096, 1097}.

Postulated normal counterpart

EBV-transformed late germinal centre/post-germinal centre B-cell.

Prognosis and predictive factors

DLBCL associated with chronic inflammation is an aggressive lymphoma. For PAL, the 5-year overall survival ranges from 20–35% {1568, 1572}. For those achieving complete remission with chemotherapy and/or radiotherapy, the 5-year survival is 50% {1568}. Complete tumour resection (pleuropneumonectomy with or without resection of adjacent involved tissues) has also been reported to give good results {1560}. Poor performance status, high serum levels of lactate dehydrogenase, glutamyl pyruvic transaminase or urea, and advanced clinical stage are unfavourable prognostic factors {61, 1572}.

Lymphomatoid granulomatosis

S. Pittaluga
W.H. Wilson
E.S. Jaffe

Definition

Lymphomatoid granulomatosis (LYG) is an angiocentric and angiodestructive lymphoproliferative disease involving extranodal sites, composed of Epstein-Barr virus (EBV)-positive B cells admixed with reactive T cells, which usually predominate. The lesion has a spectrum of histological grade and clinical aggressiveness, which is related to the proportion of large B cells.

ICD-O code   9766/1

Epidemiology

Lymphomatoid granulomatosis is a rare condition. It usually presents in adult life, but may be seen in children with immunodeficiency disorders. It affects males more often than females (M:F ratio ≥2:1) {1121}. It appears to be more common in western countries than in Asia.

Etiology

Lymphomatoid granulomatosis is an EBV-driven lymphoproliferative disorder. Patients with underlying immunodeficiency are at increased risk {861, 888}. Predisposing conditions include allogeneic organ transplantation, Wiskott-Aldrich syndrome, human immunodeficiency virus (HIV) infection and X-linked lymphoproliferative syndrome. Moreover, patients presenting without evidence of underlying immunodeficiency usually manifest reduced immune function upon careful clinical or laboratory analysis {2053, 2420}.

Sites of involvement

Pulmonary involvement occurs in over 90% of patients and is usually present at initial diagnosis. Other common sites of involvement include brain (26%), kidney (32%), liver (29%) and skin (25–50%). Upper respiratory tract and the gastrointestinal tract may be affected, but are relatively uncommon {493}. Lymph nodes and spleen are very rarely involved {1042, 1121, 1182, 1446}.

Clinical features

Patients frequently present with signs and symptoms related to the respiratory tract, such as cough (58%), dyspnoea (29%) and chest pain (13%). Other constitutional symptoms are common, including fever, malaise, weight loss, neurological symptoms, arthralgias, myalgias and gastrointestinal symptoms. Patients with central nervous system disease may be asymptomatic or have varied presentations depending on the site of involvement such as hearing loss, diplopia, dysarthria, ataxia and/or altered mental status {1707}. Few patients present with asymptomatic disease (<5%) {1042}.

Macroscopy

Lymphomatoid granulomatosis most commonly presents as pulmonary nodules that vary in size. The lesions are most often bilateral in distribution, involving the mid and lower lung fields. Larger nodules frequently exhibit central necrosis, and may cavitate. Nodular lesions are found in the kidney and brain, usually associated with central necrosis. Skin lesions are extremely diverse in appearance.

Nodular lesions are found in the subcutaneous tissue. Dermal involvement may also be seen, sometimes with necrosis and ulceration. Cutaneous plaques or a maculopapular rash are less common cutaneous manifestations {170, 1042, 1121, 1446}.

Morphology

Lymphomatoid granulomatosis is characterized by an angiocentric and angiodestructive polymorphous lymphoid infiltrate {1121, 1182}. Lymphocytes predominate, and are admixed with plasma cells, immunoblasts and histiocytes. Neutrophils and eosinophils are usually inconspicuous. The background small lymphocytes may show some atypia or irregularity, but do not appear overtly neoplastic. Lymphomatoid granulomatosis is composed of a variable, but usually small, number of EBV-positive B cells admixed with a prominent inflammatory background {861, 1122}. The EBV-positive cells usually show some atypia. They may resemble immunoblasts or, less commonly, have a more pleomorphic appearance reminiscent of Hodgkin cells. Multinucleated forms may be seen. Classical Reed-Sternberg

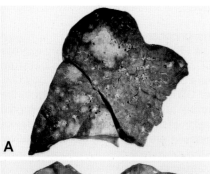

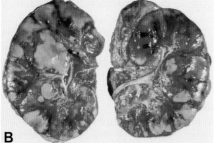

Fig. 10.98 Lymphomatoid granulomatosis. **A** Lung involved by lymphomatoid granulomatosis. Large nodules show central cavitation. **B** Large necrotic nodules are also found in the kidney.

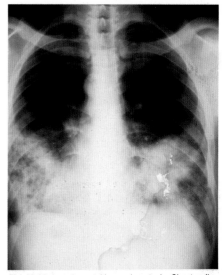

Fig. 10.99 Lymphomatoid granulomatosis. Chest radiograph identifies multiple nodules, mainly affecting the lower lung fields.

cells are generally not present, and if seen, should raise the possibility of Hodgkin lymphoma. Well-formed granulomas are typically absent in lung and most other extranodal sites {1317}. However, skin lesions often exhibit a prominent granulomatous reaction in subcutaneous tissue {170}.

Vascular changes are prominent in lymphomatoid granulomatosis. Lymphocytic vasculitis, with infiltration of the vascular wall is seen in most cases. The vascular infiltration may compromise the vascular integrity, leading to infarct-like tissue necrosis. More direct vascular damage in the form of fibrinoid necrosis is also common, and is mediated by chemokines induced by EBV {2185}. Lymphomatoid granulomatosis must be distinguished from extranodal NK/T-cell lymphoma, nasal type, which often has an angiodestructive growth pattern, and is also associated with EBV {1037}.

Grading

The grading of lymphomatoid granulomatosis relates to the proportion of EBV-positive B cells relative to the reactive lymphocyte background {862, 1317}. It is most important to distinguish grade 3 from grade 1 or 2. A uniform population of large atypical EBV-positive B cells without a polymorphous background should be classified as diffuse large B-cell lymphoma, and is beyond the spectrum of lymphomatoid granulomatosis as currently defined.

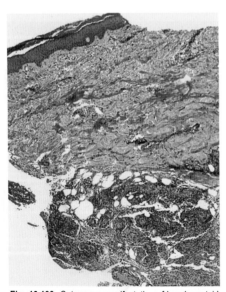

Fig. 10.100 Cutaneous manifestation of lymphomatoid granulomatosis, showing subcutaneous infiltration, with fat necrosis and a granulomatous response.

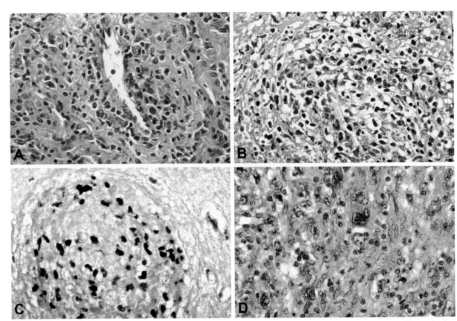

Fig. 10.101 Lymphomatoid granulomatosis. **A** Grade I lesion of the lung shows a polymorphous infiltrate in the vascular wall. **B** A Grade III lesion of the brain contains numerous large transformed lymphoid cells. **C** These cells are positive for Epstein-Barr virus by *in situ* hybridization with the EBER probe. **D** Large pleomorphic cells may be seen, most commonly in Grade III lesions, rarely in Grade II.

Grade 1 lesions contain a polymorphous lymphoid infiltrate without cytologic atypia. Large transformed lymphoid cells are absent or rare, and are better appreciated by immunohistochemistry. Necrosis is usually focal, when present. By *in situ* hybridization with EBER probe only infrequent EBV-positive cells are identified (<5 per high power field) {2420}. In some cases, EBV-positive cells may be absent, but in this setting the diagnosis should be made with caution, with studies to rule out other inflammatory or neoplastic conditions.

Grade 2 lesions contain occasional large lymphoid cells or immunoblasts in a polymorphous background. Small clusters can be seen especially by CD20 stain. Necrosis is more commonly seen. *In situ* hybridization for EBV readily identifies EBV-positive cells, which usually number 5–20/high power field. A variation in the number and distribution of EBV-positive cells can be seen within a nodule or among nodules, and occasionally up to 50 EBV-positive cells/high power field can be observed.

Grade 3 lesions still show an inflammatory background, but contain large atypical B cells which are readily identified by CD20 and can form larger aggregates. Markedly pleomorphic and Hodgkin-like cells are often present, and necrosis is usually

extensive. By *in situ* hybridization, EBV-positive cells are extremely numerous (>50/high power field), and focally may form small confluent sheets. It is important to take into consideration that *in situ* hybridization for EBV can be unreliable when large areas of necrosis are present due to poor RNA preservation; additional molecular studies for EBV may be helpful.

Immunophenotype

The EBV-positive B cells usually express CD20 {862, 2159, 2420}. The cells are variably positive for CD30, but negative for CD15. LMP1 may be positive in the larger atypical and more pleomorphic cells. Stains for cytoplasmic immunoglobulin are frequently non-informative, although in rare cases monoclonal cytoplasmic immunoglobulin expression may be seen, particularly in cells showing plasmacytoid differentiation {2420}. The background lymphocytes are CD3-positive T cells, with CD4+ cells more frequent than CD8+ cells.

Genetics

In most cases of Grade 2 or Grade 3 disease, clonality of the immunoglobulin genes can be demonstrated by molecular genetic techniques {861, 1446}. In some cases different clonal populations may be identified in different anatomic sites

{1490, 2420}. Southern blot analysis also may show clonality of EBV {1448}. Demonstration of clonality in Grade 1 cases is more inconsistent, an observation which may be related to the relative rarity of the EBV-positive cells in these cases. Alternatively, some cases of lymphomatoid granulomatosis may be polyclonal. T-cell receptor gene analysis shows no evidence of monoclonality {1446, 1448}. Alterations of oncogenes have not been identified.

Postulated normal counterpart
Mature B lymphocyte, transformed by EBV.

Prognosis and predictive factors
Some patients follow a waxing and waning clinical course with rare spontaneous remissions without therapy. However, in most patients the disease is more aggressive, with a median survival of under two years based on historical series {1121}. More recent series have shown responses to aggressive chemotherapy with rituximab for grade 3 lesions. Grade 1 and 2 lesions usually achieve durable responses to interferon-α 2b {2420}. Lymphomatoid granulomatosis may progress to an EBV+ diffuse large B-cell lymphoma (DLBCL).

Although some patients with grade 3 lymphomatoid granulomatosis may show spontaneous regression with immunotherapy or modification of the immune state, for clinical purposes these patients should be approached as diffuse large B-cell lymphoma {2420}.

Primary mediastinal (thymic) large B-cell lymphoma

P. Gaulard
N.L. Harris
S.A. Pileri
J.L. Kutok

H. Stein
A.M. Kovrigina
E.S. Jaffe
P. Möller

Definition

A diffuse large B-cell lymphoma arising in the mediastinum from putative thymic B-cell origin with distinctive clinical, immuno-phenotypic and genotypic features.

ICD-O code   9679/3

Synonym

Mediastinal large B-cell lymphoma.

Epidemiology

Primary mediastinal large B-cell lymphoma (PMBL) accounts for 2–4% of non-Hodgkin lymphomas (NHL) {150, 350} and occurs predominantly in young adults (median age, ~35 years) with a female predominance (M:F ratio, about 1:2) {350, 1257, 1943, 2500}.

Sites of involvement

PMBL most likely arises within the thymus. Patients present with a localized antero-superior mediastinal mass. The mass is often "bulky" and frequently invades adjacent structures such as lungs, pleura or pericardium. Spread to supraclavicular and cervical lymph nodes can occur {150, 350, 1257}. Absence of other lymph node or bone marrow (BM) involvement is a prerequisite to exclude a systemic DLBCL with secondary mediastinal involvement.

Clinical features

Symptoms are related to the mediastinal mass, frequently with superior vena cava syndrome. B symptoms may be present.

At progression, dissemination to distant extranodal sites including kidney, adrenal, liver or central nervous system is relatively common but BM involvement is usually absent.

Morphology

PMBL shows a wide morphological/cytological spectrum from case to case {1712}. It is commonly associated with compartmentalizing alveolar fibrosis {150, 350, 1499, 1712, 1744}. Tumour cells are medium-sized to large cells with abundant pale cytoplasm and more or less regular round or ovoid nuclei. In some cases, lymphoma cells have pleomorphic and/or multilobated nuclei which may resemble Reed-Sternberg cells and raise suspicion of Hodgkin lymphoma (HL) {1712, 2265}. Rarely, there are "grey zone" borderline cases combining features of PMBL and classical Hodgkin lymphoma (CHL) or cases of composite PMBL and CHL {2265}.

Immunophenotype

PMBL expresses B-cell antigens such as CD19, CD20, CD22 and CD79a, but, as a rule, lacks immunoglobulin (Ig) {150, 1092, 1328, 1744}. CD30 is present in more than 80% of the cases, however, usually weak and heterogeneous, compared to Hodgkin lymphoma {938, 1744}. CD15 is occasionally present {1500}. Tumour cells are frequently positive for IRF4/MUM1 (75%) and CD23 (70%), have variable expression of BCL2 (55–80%) and BCL6 (45–100%) and CD10 is less common

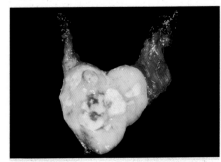

Fig. 10.103 Primary mediastinal large B-cell lymphoma. Cut surface showing fleshy tumour with necrosis.

(8–32%) {311, 520, 1744}. Tumour cells are also positive for MAL antigen, CD54 and CD95, coexpress TRAF1 and nuclear REL {470, 472, 1857}. Variable defects in the expression of HLA class I and/or class II molecules have been found in most of the cases {1498, 1500}.

Genetics

Antigen receptor genes

Immunoglobulin genes are clonally rearranged with a high load of somatic hypermutations without ongoing mutational activity {1270}.

Cytogenetic and oncogene abnormalities

Comparative genomic hybridization (CGH) demonstrated gains in chromosome 9p24 (up to 75%) and 2p15 (~50%), but also in chromosomes Xp11.4-21 (33%) and Xq24-26 (33%) {192, 1072, 2393}. Candidate genes include *REL* and *BCL11A* (at 2p), which are amplified in a proportion of PMBL {2387,

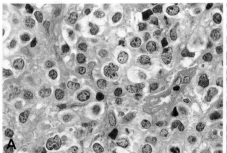
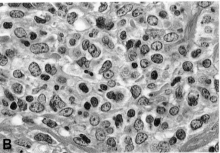
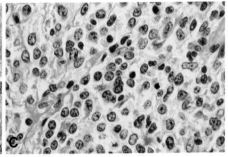

Fig. 10.102 Primary mediastinal large B-cell lymphoma. **A** Nuclei are round (centroblast-like) or sometimes multilobated. **B** Sheets of large cells with abundant pale cytoplasm, separated by collagenous fibrosis. **C** Medium-sized cells with large pale cytoplasm.

2389}, and *JAK2*, *PDL1* and *PDL2* (at 9p) {1072, 1459, 1870}. Nuclear accumulation of REL protein is common {1857, 2387} with an imperfect correlation with *REL* amplification and REL transcript abundance {701, 2387}.

PMBL has a unique transcriptional signature, but shares features with CHL {1870, 1944}. PMBL has constitutively activated NFκB {701} and JAK-STAT signaling pathways {864, 1459}, frequently related to inactivating mutations of *SOCS1* {1459, 2388}.

Rearrangements of *BCL2*, *BCL6* and *MYC* genes are absent or rare {1944, 1953, 2271} whereas inactivation of $p16^{INK4a}$ and *TP53* genes have been reported {1953}. The discordant expression of components of the B-cell receptor (BCR) (CD79a+, sIg-) is characteristic of PMBL {1092, 1328, 1744}. It cannot be ascribed to a lack of functional *IG* gene rearrangements nor to a defect in the transcription factors BOB.1, OCT-2 and PU.1 {1328, 1744} but, rather, to a downregulation of the intronic heavy chain enhancer {1848} or post-transcriptionnal blockage {1328}.

Postulated normal counterpart
Thymic medullary, asteroid, (AID-positive), B-cell {953, 1016, 1494}.

Prognosis and predictive factors
Variations in microscopic appearance do not predict differences in survival {1712}. Response to intensive chemotherapy, with or without radiotherapy, is usually good. Extension into adjacent thoracic viscera, pleural or pericardial effusion and poor performance status {350, 1257, 1943} has been associated with a poor prognosis. According to recent studies, outcome of PMBL patients is at least equivalent to or superior to that of other DLBCL patients {350, 1943, 2500} with a plateau seen in the survival curves beyond 2 years {1943}. In addition, the PMBL molecular signature was associated with a more favourable survival (compared to GCB and ABC DLBCL) {1870}, supporting a distinct natural history for PMBL.

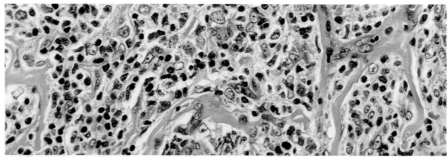

Fig. 10.104 Primary mediastinal large B-cell lymphoma. Classic clear-cell appearance of the tumour cells with associated delicate interstitial fibrosis.

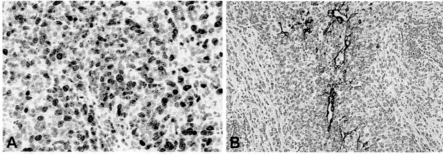

Fig.10.105 Primary mediastinal large B-cell lymphoma. **A** All large cells express CD20 on the membrane. **B** Nests of CD3-positive lymphocytes are present with a perivascular distribution.

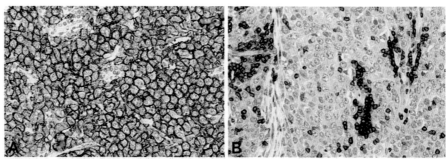

Fig. 10.106 Primary mediastinal large B-cell lymphoma. **A** More than 60% of the large cells express nuclear Ki67. **B** Thymic remnants infiltrated by tumour cells, the epithelial component is positive for cytokeratin.

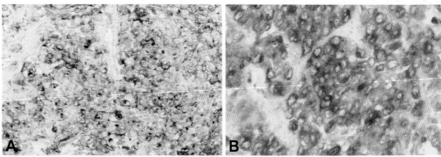

Fig. 10.107 Primary mediastinal large B-cell lymphoma. **A** Most tumour cells express CD23. **B** Tumour cells also express MAL with a cytoplasmic reinforcement in the Golgi area.

Intravascular large B-cell lymphoma

S. Nakamura
M. Ponzoni
E. Campo

Definition

Intravascular large B-cell lymphoma (IVLBCL) is a rare type of extranodal large B-cell lymphoma characterized by the selective growth of lymphoma cells within the lumina of vessels, particularly capillaries, with exception of larger arteries and veins.

ICD-O code   9712/3

Synonym

Angiotropic large cell lymphoma.

Epidemiology

This tumour occurs in adults (median, 67 years; range, 13–85 years) and with a M:F ratio of 1.1:1. The frequency and clinical presentation differ according to the geographical origin of the patients between the West and the Far East {621, 694, 1545}.

Sites of involvement

This lymphoma is usually widely disseminated in extranodal sites including bone marrow (BM) and may present virtually in any organ. However, lymph nodes are usually spared.

Clinical features

Two major patterns of clinical presentation have been recognized, a Western form characterized by symptoms related to the main organ involved, predominantly neurological or cutaneous, and an Asian variant in which the patients present with multi-organ failure, hepatosplenomegaly, pancytopenia and haemophagocytic syndrome. These presentations are seen more frequently, although not exclusively, in Western and Far East countries, respectively {621, 694, 1544, 1545, 1768}. B symptoms are very common (55–76% of patients) in both types of presentation. An isolated cutaneous variant has been identified invariably in Western females; it is characterized by limitation of the tumour to the skin and is associated with a better prognosis {693}. Conventional staging

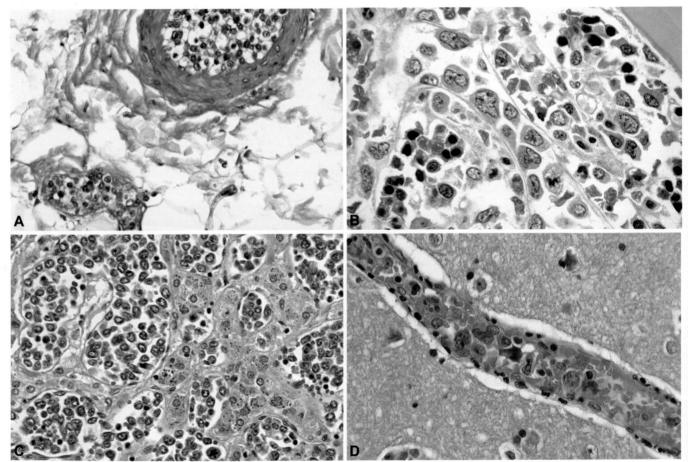

Fig.10.108 Intravascular large B-cell lymphoma. **A** The large lymphoma cells fill the vein (right upper) and capillary (left lower). **B** The large tumour cells are present in the sinuses of the bone marrow, having abundant cytoplasm surrounding a more or less irregular nucleus. **C** The large lymphoma cells fill the sinuses in the adrenal gland. **D** The large tumour cells are present in the lumen of small vessels in the central nervous system.

procedures are generally associated with a high proportion of false negatives because of the lack of detectable tumour masses.

Morphology

The neoplastic lymphoid cells are mainly lodged in the lumina of small or intermediate vessels in many organs. Fibrin thrombi, haemorrage and necrosis may be observed in some cases. The tumour cells are large with prominent nucleoli and frequent mitotic figures. Rare cases have cells with anaplastic features or smaller size {1769}. Minimal extravascular location of neoplastic cells may be seen. Sinusoidal involvement occurs in the liver, spleen and BM {1769}. Malignant cells are occasionally detected in peripheral blood.

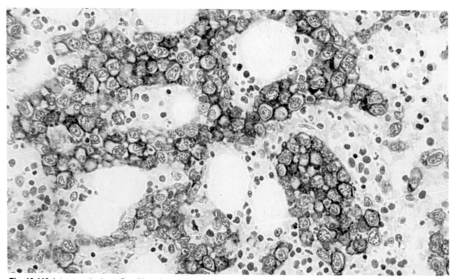

Fig. 10.110 Intravascular large B-cell lymphoma. Bone marrow biopsy. The tumour cells are highlighted by staining for CD20.

Immunophenotype

Tumour cells express B-cell-associated antigens. CD5 and CD10 coexpression is seen in 38% and 13% of the cases, respectively. Almost all of CD10-negative

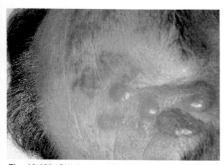

Fig. 10.109 Skin involved by intravascular large B-cell lymphoma.

cases are IRF4/MUM1 positive. Anecdotal cases of intravascular T-cell or NK-cell lymphoma have been reported {2145}, but they should be considered a different entity.

The intravascular growth pattern has been hypothesized to be secondary to a defect in homing receptors on the neoplastic cells {698}, such as the lack of CD29 (β1 integrin) and CD54 (ICAM-1) adhesion β-molecules {1766}.

Genetics

Immunoglobulin genes are clonally rearranged. Karyotypic abnormalities have been described but too few cases have been studied {1495}.

Postulated normal counterpart

Transformed peripheral B-cell.

Prognosis and predictive factors

This is an aggressive lymphoma which responds poorly to chemotherapy {692}. The poor prognosis reflects in part frequent delays in diagnosis due to the protean presentation. Neither clinical types of presentation nor clinical parameters predicts patient survival, with the exception of the better prognosis for the cases with disease limited to the skin {693, 1768}.

ALK-positive large B-cell lymphoma

G. Delsol
E. Campo
R.D. Gascoyne

Definition

ALK positive large B-cell lymphoma (ALK-positive LBCL) is a neoplasm of ALK-positive monomorphic large immunoblast-like B cells, sometimes with plasmablastic differentiation.

ICD-O code

9737/3

Synonyms

Large B-cell lymphoma expressing the ALK kinase and lacking the t(2;5) translocation; ALK-positive plasmablastic B-cell lymphoma.

Epidemiology

This lymphoma is very rare (<1% of DLBCL), with less than 40 cases so far been reported {1831}. It seems to occur more frequently in male adults (M:F ratio, 3:1) and spans all age groups (9–70 years) (median, 36 years) {1831}.

Sites of involvement

The tumour mainly involves lymph nodes {9, 553, 761, 1023, 1831, 2075} or presents as a mediastinal mass {527, 788}. Involvement of extranodal sites have been also reported including nasopharynx {1644}, tongue {527}, stomach {1444}, bone {1644} and soft tissues {417}.

Clinical features

Most patients present with advanced stage III/IV.

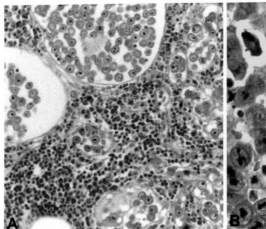
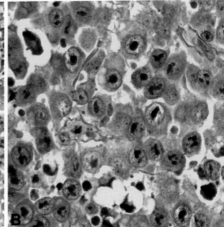

Fig. 10.112 ALK-positive large B-cell lymphoma, morphologic features. **A** There is massive invasion of lymphatic sinuses. **B** Neoplastic cells show immunoblastic and plasmablastic features.

Morphology

This lymphoma shows a sinusoidal growth pattern and is composed of monomorphic large immunoblast-like cells with round pale nuclei containing large central nucleoli and abundant cytoplasm. Some cases show plasmablastic differentiation {553, 761}. Atypical multinucleated neoplastic giant cells may be seen.

Immunophenotype

Lymphoma cells are strongly positive for ALK protein with a restricted granular cytoplasmic staining pattern highly indicative of the expression of CLTC-ALK protein. Few cases may show cytoplasmic, nuclear and nucleolar ALK staining associated with the NPM-ALK protein. In addition, they also characteristically strongly express EMA and plasma cell markers such as CD138 and VS38, being negative for lineage-associated leukocyte antigens (CD3, CD20, CD79a) {283, 553, 1962, 1963, 2075}. CD45 is weak or negative {553, 761}. CD30 is negative {553}, although focal and weak staining has been reported in few cases {2075}. Most tumours express cytoplasmic Ig (usually IgA, more rarely IgG) with light chain restriction {553}. As described in some plasma cell tumours,

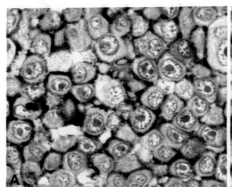
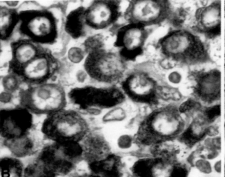
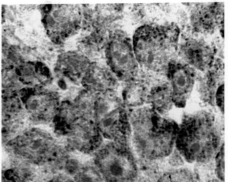

Fig. 10.111 Immunophenotype of ALK-positive large B-cell lymphoma. The tumour cells are positive for EMA (**A**) with a cytoplasmic membranous pattern, IgA (**B**), and ALK (**C**) with a restricted cytoplasmic granular pattern highly indicative of the expression of the CLTC-ALK fusion protein.

occasional cases are positive for cyto-keratin which, in addition to EMA positivity and weak/negative staining for CD45, may lead to the mistaken diagnosis of carcinoma {2075}. The tumours may be also positive for CD4, CD57, IRF4/MUM1 {2075}, focally for CD43 {2075} and perforin {2075}.

These tumours should be distinguished from CD30-positive ALK-positive T/null anaplastic large cell lymphoma and other large B-cell lymphomas with a sinusoidal growth pattern, and ALK-negative immunoblastic/plasmablastic lymphomas, such as those involving the oral cavity in HIV+ patients {459}.

Genetics

The immunoglobulin genes are clonally rearranged {417, 761}. This tumour may express full-length ALK {553} but the key oncogenic factor is the ALK fusion protein due to genetic alteration of the *ALK* locus on chromosome 2. The most frequent abnormality is the t(2;17)(p23;q23) responsible for Clathrin-ALK (CLTC-ALK) fusion protein {417, 527, 761, 788, 1023, 1444, 1831}. Few cases are associated with the t(2;5)(p23;35) as described in ALK-positive T/Null anaplastic large cell lymphoma (ALCL) {9, 1644}. A cryptic insertion of 3'*ALK* gene sequences into chromosome 4q22-24 has also been reported {2075}.

Postulated normal counterpart

Post-germinal centre B cell with plasma cell differentiation.

Prognosis and predictive factors

The overall median survival of high stage III/IV patients was 11 months {1831}. Long survival (>156 months) has been reported in children {553, 1644}. These tumours are usually negative for CD20 antigen and are thus insensitive to rituximab.

Plasmablastic lymphoma

H. Stein
N.L. Harris
E. Campo

Definition

Plasmablastic lymphoma (PBL) is a diffuse proliferation of large neoplastic cells most of which resemble B immunoblasts, but in which all tumour cells have the immunophenotype of plasma cells. It was originally described in the oral cavity but may occur in other, predominantly extranodal sites.

ICD-O code   9735/3

Epidemiology

PBL is uncommon. It has its highest incidence in HIV-positive individuals, predominantly males. It may also be associated with other immunodeficiency states, including advanced age. The median age at presentation is around 50 years, with a broad distribution, but mainly affecting adults. Rare cases are seen in children with immunodeficiency {459, 547}.

Etiology

Immunodeficiency, caused in the majority of cases by HIV, predisposes to the development of PBL. Other causes of immunodeficiency such as iatrogenic immunosuppression for autoimmune disease or prevention of post-transplant therapy allograft rejection may also be implicated. There are also cases without any history of immunodeficiency, but those patients tend to be elderly. The tumour cells are EBV-infected in the majority of patients {241, 459, 547, 604}.

Sites of involvement

PBL presents most frequently as a mass in the oral cavity, but it is also encountered in other extranodal sites —particularly mucosal sites— including the sinonasal cavity, orbit, skin, bone, soft tissues and gastrointestinal tract. Nodal involvement is seen but it is not common {459, 547, 604}. Plasmablastic lymphomas not associated with HIV-infection present more commonly in lymph nodes.

Clinical features

Most patients are at an advanced stage (III or IV) at presentation {459, 547, 604}. The international prognostic index (IPI) is of intermediate or high risk score. Computed tomography and positron emission tomography may show disseminated bone involvement {2184}. Tumours with features of PBL may occur in patients with prior plasma cell neoplasms, including plasma cell myeloma. Such cases should be considered plasmablastic transformation of myeloma and distinguished from primary plasmablastic lymphoma.

Morphology

PBL show a morphological spectrum varying from a diffuse and cohesive proliferation of cells resembling immunoblasts to cells with more obvious plasmacytic differentiation, which may resemble cases of plasmablastic plasma cell myeloma. Mitotic figures are frequent. Apoptotic cells and tingible body macrophages may be present, but are generally less prominent than in diffuse large B-cell lymphoma. Cases with monomorphic plasmablastic cytology are most commonly seen in the setting of HIV-infection and in the oral, nasal and paranasal area (oral mucosal type). Conversely, cases with plasmacytic differentiation tend to occur more commonly in other extranodal sites as well as lymph nodes {459, 547}. The differential diagnosis in the cases with plasmacytic differentiation may include anaplastic or plasmablastic plasma cell myeloma. The presence of a high proliferation fraction, extranodal localization, a history of immune deficiency, and the presence of EBV by *in situ* hybridization for EBER are useful in establishing the diagnosis of plasmablastic lymphoma.

Immunophenotype

The neoplastic cells express a plasma-cell phenotype including positivity for CD138, CD38, Vs38c and IRF4/MUM1 and are negative or only weakly positive for CD45, CD20 and PAX5. CD79a is positive in appoximately 50–85% of the cases.

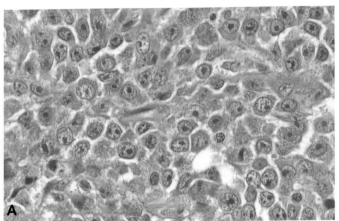
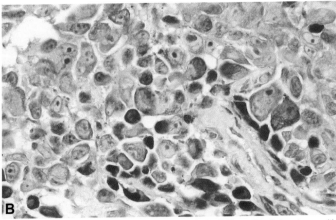

Fig. 10.113 A Plasmablastic lymphoma of the oral mucosa with a monomorphic proliferation of large, immunoblastic cells with prominent nucleoli. **B** Plasmablastic lymphoma with plasmacytic differentiation. The tumour cells are large with round nuclei and showing coarse chromatin and smaller or unapparent nucleoli. Smaller cells with plasmacytic differentiation are present.

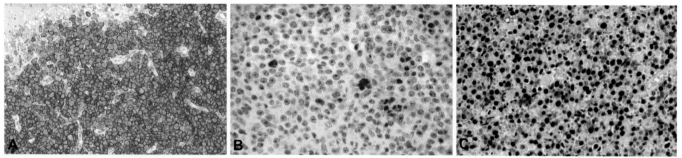

Fig. 10.114 The plasmablastic lymphoma cells are strongly positive for CD138 (**A**) but negative for CD20 (**B**). The EBER *in situ* hybridization reveals an infection of all plasmablastic lymphoma cells by EBV (**C**).

Cytoplasmic immunoglobulins are expressed in 50–70% of the cases, most frequently IgG and either kappa or lambda light chain. CD56 is usually negative in the oral mucosal type of PBL, but may be seen in cases with plasmacytic differentiation. The expression of CD56 should raise suspicion for underlying plasma cell myeloma. EMA and CD30 are frequently expressed. Ki67 index is usually very high (>90%). EBV EBER *in situ* hybridization is positive in 60–75% of the cases but LMP1 is rarely expressed. The rate of EBV-positivity is nearly 100% in the oral mucosal type of PBL, in association with HIV-infection. HHV8 is consistently absent {459, 547, 604, 2319}.

Genetics

Clonal *IgH* chain gene rearrangement is demonstrable, even when immunoglobulin expression is not detectable, and the *IgH* genes may show evidence of somatic hypermutation or be in an unmutated configuration {744}.

Postulated normal counterpart

Plasmablast, i.e. a blastic proliferating B-cell that has switched its phenotype to the plasma cell gene expression program.

Prognosis and predictive factors

The clinical course is very aggressive with most of the patients dying in the first year after diagnosis {459, 547, 604}, although the outcome may have improved more recently possibly due to a better management of HIV infection {2184}.

Large B-cell lymphoma arising in HHV8-associated multicentric Castleman disease

P.G. Isaacson
E. Campo
N.L. Harris

Definition

Large B-cell lymphoma arising in human herpes virus 8 (HHV8)-associated multi-centric Castleman disease (HHV8 MCD) is composed of a monoclonal proliferation of HHV8-infected lymphoid cells resembling plasmablasts expressing IgM and arising in the setting of multicentric Castleman disease (MCD). It is usually associated with human immunodeficiency virus (HIV) infection. The term plasmablastic is used for this lymphoma because the cells morphologically resemble plasma cells and have abundant cytoplasmic immunoglobulin; however it corresponds to a naïve, IgM-producing plasma cell without *IG* somatic hypermutation. This lymphoma must be distinguished from plasmablastic lymphomas presenting in the oral cavity or other extranodal sites that frequently show class-switched and hypermutated *IG* genes.

ICD-O code

The provisional code proposed for the fourth edition of ICD-O is *9738/3*.

Synonyms

HHV8-positive plasmablastic lymphoma (HHV8 PL), Kaposi sarcoma herpes virus (KSHV)-positive plasmablastic lymphoma.

Epidemiology

HHV8 PL occurs worldwide in HIV-positive patients who have developed HHV8 MCD. It less commonly occurs in HIV-negative patients who have developed HHV8 MCD usually in regions where HHV8 is endemic (Africa and Mediterranean countries) {250}.

Etiology

The neoplastic cells are positive for HHV8 in all cases. HHV8 encodes more than ten homologues to cellular genes that provide proliferative and anti-apoptotic signals {59, 84, 91, 1049}.

Sites of involvement

The lymphoma characteristically involves lymph nodes and spleen but can disseminate to other viscera via the blood stream

in which rarely it manifests as a leukaemia {627, 1638}.

Clinical features

On a background of the clinical features of HHV8 CD, patients who are developing HHV8 PL present with profound immuno-deficiency, enlarging lymph nodes and massive splenomegaly often accompanied by manifestations of Kaposi sarcoma {627, 1638}.

Morphology

HHV8-positive multicentric Castleman disease

The B-cell follicles of lymph nodes and spleen show varied degrees of involution and hyalinization of their germinal centres with a prominent mantle zone that may intrude into the germinal centres and completely efface them. Among these mantle zone cells, there are variable numbers of larger plasmablastic cells with dense amphophilic cytoplasm and vesicular, often eccentrically placed, nuclei

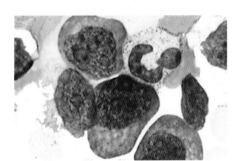

Fig. 10.115 HHV8-positive plasmablastic lymphoma. Wright-Giemsa stained tumour cells in peripheral blood.

containing one or two prominent nucleoli. Similar cells may be scattered in the interfollicular area which, in addition, is heavily infiltrated by mature plasma cells. As the disease progresses, the plasmablasts coalesce to form confluent microscopic clusters (so-called micro-lymphomas) and sheets both within and outside the germinal centres {627}.

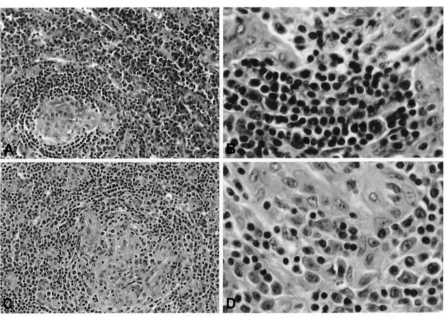

Fig. 10.116 HHV8-positive multicentric Castleman disease. **A** The B-cell follicle with a normal germinal centre is surrounded by a broad mantle zone. **B** Mantle zone contains scattered plasmablasts. **C** This B-cell follicle shows partial hyalinization of the germinal centre with an attenuated mantle zone. **D** Germinal centre containing numerous plasmablasts.

HHV8-positive plasmablastic lymphoma

The emergence of frank lymphoma is heralded by expansion of the small confluent sheets of HHV8 latent nuclear antigen 1 (LANA-1)-positive plasmablasts to completely efface the lymph node and splenic architecture, with massive splenomegaly. Infiltrates may also be present in the liver, lung, gastrointestinal tract and in some cases there is leukaemic involvement of the peripheral blood {627, 1638}.

Immunophenotype

The plasmablasts described above {1638} show stippled nuclear staining for LANA-1, viral interleukin-6 and strongly express cIgM with λ light chain restriction. They are CD20+ or -, CD79a-, CD138-, CD38-/+, CD27- and Epstein-Barr encoded RNA (EBER)-negative. The interfollicular plasma cells are typically cIgM negative, cIgA positive, express polytypic light chains and do not show nuclear expression of LANA-1 antigen.

Genetics

Antigen receptor genes

Despite constant expression of monotypic IgM by the plasmablasts in HHV8 MCD, careful molecular studies have shown that they constitute a polyclonal population {619}. The microlymphomas that develop as the disease progresses may be mono- or polyclonal and the frank HHV8 PL are monoclonal. In both disorders, the *IG* genes are unmutated.

Genetic abnormalities and oncogenes

Activation of the IL-6 receptor signaling pathway has been proposed to play a role in the development of HHV8-infected naïve B lymphoproliferative lesions {619}. There is no information about cytogenetic abnormalities in the tumours

Postulated normal counterpart

Naïve B-cell.

Prognosis and predictive factors

Both HHV8 MCD and PL are highly aggressive disorders with a median survival of a few months.

Associated conditions

Kaposi sarcoma is frequently present in patients with HHV8 PL and MCD. Primary effusion lymphoma (PEL) and its extracavitary counterpart may complicate HHV8 MCD but unlike HHV8 PL, the neoplastic cells do not express Ig and are

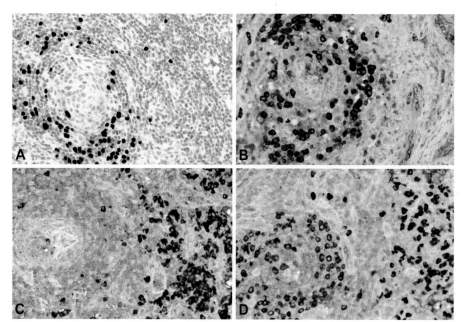

Fig. 10.117 HHV8 positive multicentric Castleman disease immunostained for HHV8 (**A**), IgM (**B**), κ light chain (**C**) and λ light chain (**D**). The plasmablasts express intranuclear HHV8 LANA, cIgM and show λ light chain restriction. Interfollicular plasma cells express polytypic Ig light chains.

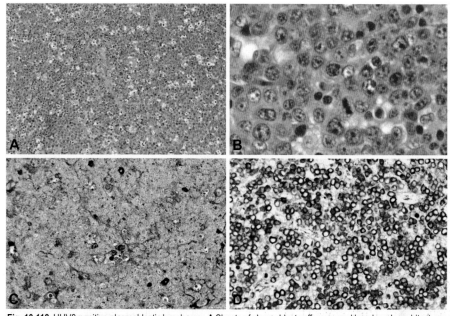

Fig. 10.118 HHV8-positive plasmablastic lymphoma. **A** Sheets of plasmablasts efface normal lymph node architecture. **B** High magnification of plasmablasts in (**A**). Tumour cells immunostained for κ Ig light chain (**C**) and λ chain (**D**) show λ light chain restriction.

usually co-infected with EBV.

In the germinotropic lymphoproliferative disorder, another monotypic HHV8-positive lymphoproliferative lesion that occurs in HIV negative individuals, HHV8-positive plasmablasts infiltrate germinal centres {618A}. The plasmablasts show either κ or λ light chain restriction but, like HHV8 MCD, these cells are polyclonal. Co-infection with EBV is also characteristic.

Primary effusion lymphoma

J. Said
E. Cesarman

Definition

Primary effusion lymphoma (PEL) is a large B-cell neoplasm usually presenting as serous effusions without detectable tumour masses. It is universally associated with human herpesvirus 8 (HHV8), also named Kaposi sarcoma herpesvirus (KSHV). It most often occurs in the setting of immunodeficiency. Some patients with PEL secondarily develop solid tumours in adjacent structures such as the pleura. Rare HHV8-positive lymphomas indistinguishable from PEL present as solid tumour masses, and have been termed extracavitary PEL.

ICD-O code   9678/3

Synonym

Body cavity based lymphoma.

Epidemiology

The majority of cases arise in young or middle-aged homosexual or bisexual males with human immunodeficiency virus (HIV) infection and severe immunodeficiency {1555, 1912}. There is co-infection with monoclonal Epstein-Barr virus (EBV) {372, 1555, 1912}. PEL has been reported in recipients of solid organ transplants {606, 1066, 1349}. The disease also occurs in the absence of immunodeficiency, usually in elderly patients (both men and women), mostly from areas with high prevalence for HHV8 infection such as the Mediterranean {2188}. In these latter patients the lymphoma cells contain HHV8 and may lack EBV {454, 1911}.

Etiology

The neoplastic cells are positive for HHV8 in all cases. Most cases are co-infected with EBV {58, 85, 963, 1912}, but EBV has restricted gene expression and may be not required for the pathogenesis. HHV8 encodes more than ten homologues to cellular genes that provide proliferative and anti-apoptotic signals {59, 84, 91, 1049}.

Sites of involvement

The most common sites are the pleural, pericardial and peritoneal cavities. Typically only one body cavity is involved {169, 556, 1665}. Extracavitary tumours with morphologic and phenotypic characteristics similar to PEL occur in extranodal sites including the gastrointestinal tract, skin, lung and CNS, or may involve lymph nodes {377, 487, 556}.

Clinical features

Patients typically present with effusions in the absence of lymphadenopathy or organomegaly. Approximately half of the

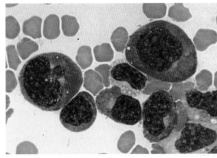

Fig. 10.120 Primary effusion lymphoma (PEL). Pleural fluid cytology. There is marked pleomorphism with prominent nucleoli and a plasmacytoid appearance in the cytoplasm. Wright stain.

patients have pre-existent or develop Kaposi sarcoma {58}. Occasional cases are associated with multicentric Castleman disease {2188}. PEL cases should be distinguished from rare cases of HHV8-negative effusion based lymphoma morphologically similar to PEL that have been described in ascites from patients with liver disease {1001, 1604, 1862}; and the EBV associated HHV8-negative large B-cell lymphomas also occurring with chronic suppurative inflammation, such as pyothorax associated lymphoma {63, 471}.

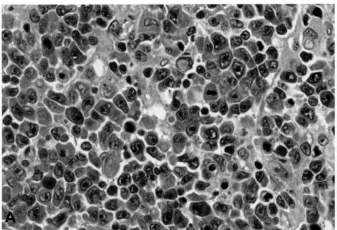
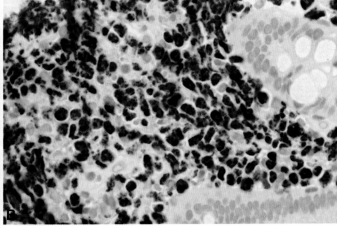

Fig. 10.119 Primary effusion lymphoma (PEL). **A** Solid tissue mass from the mediastinum of an HIV+ patient with PEL presenting with pleural effusions. The cells are large and pleomorphic with eosinophilic macronucleoli and abundant cytoplasm. Many have an anaplastic or plasmacytoid appearance. **B** Extracavitary PEL presenting initially as a mass in the large bowel of an HIV+ patient. The nuclei are strongly positive for latent HHV8 infection with antibody to ORF73 LNA-1 (LANA).

Morphology

In cytocentrifuge preparations, the cells exhibit a range of appearances, from large immunoblastic or plasmablastic cells to cells with more anaplastic morphology. Nuclei are large, round to more irregular in shape, with prominent nucleoli. The cytoplasm can be abundant and is deeply basophilic with vacuoles in occasional cells. A perinuclear hof consistent with plasmacytoid differentiation may be seen. Some cells resemble Reed-Sternberg cells. The cells often appear more uniform in histological sections than in cytospin preparations {58, 556, 1555}.

Immunophenotype

Lymphoma cells usually express CD45, but lack pan-B-cell markers such as CD19, CD20 and CD79a {1167, 1555}. Surface and cytoplasmic immunoglobulin is absent. Usually, BCL6 is absent. Activation and plasma cell-related markers and a variety of non lineage-associated antigens such as HLA-DR, CD30, CD38, Vs38c, CD138 and EMA are often demonstrable. The cells usually lack T/NK-cell antigens, although aberrant expression of T-cell markers may occur {169, 254, 1910}. The aberrant phenotype frequently makes it difficult to assign a lineage with immunophenotyping. The nuclei of the neoplastic cells are positive for the HHV8-associated latent protein LANA (ORF 73) {628}. This is very useful in establishing a diagnosis. Despite the usual presence of EBV with EBER *in situ* hybridization, EBV LMP1 is absent {58, 454, 963, 2188}. Solid tumours representing the extracavitary variant of PEL have a phenotype similar to PEL but express B-cell associated antigens and immunoglobulins slightly more often than cases of PEL {377}.

Genetics

Immunoglobulin genes are clonally rearranged and hypermutated {1419, 2353}. Some cases also have rearrangement of T-cell receptor genes (so-called genotypic infidelity) {956, 1910}. Rare cases diagnosed as T-PEL have been reported {487, 1263}. No recurrent chromosomal abnormalities have been identified. Comparative genomic analysis has revealed gains in chromosomes 12 and X {1537}. HHV8 viral genomes are present in all cases. Gene expression profiling of AIDS-related PEL shows a distinct profile with features of both plasma cells and EBV-transformed lymphoblastoid cell lines {1159}.

Postulated normal counterpart

Post-germinal centre B-cell.

Prognosis and predictive factors

The clinical outlook is extremely unfavourable, and median survival is less than six months. Rare cases have responded to chemotherapy and/or immune modulation {793}.

Burkitt lymphoma

L. Leoncini
M. Raphaël
H. Stein
N.L. Harris
E.S. Jaffe
P.M. Kluin

Definition

Burkitt lymphoma (BL) is a B-cell lymphoma with an extremely short doubling time that often presents in extranodal sites or as an acute leukaemia. It is composed of monomorphic medium-sized transformed cells. Translocation involving *MYC* is highly characteristic but not specific. No single parameter (such as morphology, genetic analysis or immunophenotyping) can be used as the gold standard for the diagnosis of BL, but a combination of several diagnostic techniques is necessary.

ICD-O code

Burkitt lymphoma, NOS   9687/3

Epidemiology

Three clinical variants of Burkitt lymphoma are recognized, each manifesting differences in clinical presentation, morphology and biology.

Endemic BL: This variant occurs in equatorial Africa, representing the most common childhood malignancy in this area with an incidence peak at 4 to 7 years and a male:female ratio of 2:1 {301, 2447}. BL is also endemic in Papua, New Guinea. In endemic regions there is a correlation between the geographical occurrence and some climatic factors (rainfall, altitude, etc.) which correspond to the geographical distribution of endemic malaria {301, 656, 2447}.

Sporadic BL: This variant is seen throughout the world, mainly in children and young adults {301, 1364, 2447}. The incidence is low, representing only 1–2% of all lymphomas in Western Europe and in the USA. BL accounts for 30–50% of all childhood lymphomas. The median age of the adult patients is 30 years {898}. The male:female ratio is 2 or 3:1, and in children it is even more common among males {230}. In some parts of the world, for example, in South America and North Africa, both true sporadic and endemic variants are seen.

Immunodeficiency-associated BL: This variant is primarily seen in association with the human immunodeficiency virus (HIV) infection, often occurring as the initial manifestation of the acquired immuno-deficiency syndrome (AIDS) {1818}.

Etiology

In endemic BL, the EBV genome is present in the majority of the neoplastic cells in all patients {2161, 2447} and there is strong epidemiological link with holoendemic malaria {528}. Recent data provide insights into the emerging concepts of polymicrobial disease pathogenesis {1855}. In particular, the potential mechanisms, by which Plasmodium falciparum infections could impact on immunity and viral persistence, include the exhaustion of Epstein-Barr virus (EBV)-specific T-cell response and Toll-like receptor (TLR) 9-mediated reactivation of latently infected memory B cells {203, 1855}. This is in line with evidence that EBV-positive tumours may derive from memory B cells {180, 2232}. However, epidemiological studies suggest that malaria and EBV alone cannot account for the distribution of endemic BL in high risk regions {1807, 2291}. Arboviruses and plant tumour promoters are other possible local cofactors that could explain such characteristics {2291}.

EBV may be detected in approximately 30% of sporadic BL cases, however, a low socio-economic status and early EBV infection are associated with a higher prevalence of EBV-positive sporadic BL. In immunodeficiency-associated cases, EBV is identified in only 25–40% of the cases {877, 1818}. BL is more common in HIV than in other forms of immunosuppression and BL appears early in the progression of HIV infection when CD4+ T-cell counts are still high {1301}. This suggests that immunosuppression *per se* does not explain the increased risk of BL. A potential mechanistic link between endemic and HIV-associated BL lies in the polyclonal B-cell activation that occurs after malaria and HIV infection. However, the oncogenic role of HIV itself cannot be

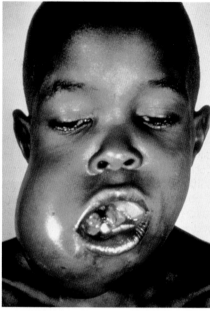

Fig. 10.121 Endemic Burkitt lymphoma. This African patient presented with a large jaw tumour.

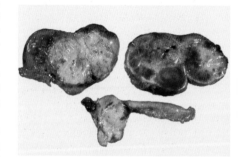

Fig. 10.122 Sporadic Burkitt lymphoma with bilateral ovarian tumours.

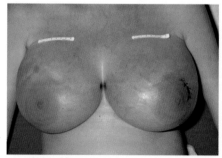

Fig. 10.123 Bilateral breast involvement may be the presenting manifestation during pregancy, and puberty. BL cells have prolactin receptors.

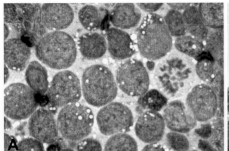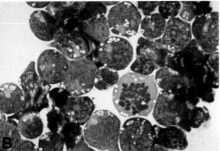

Fig.10.124 Burkitt lymphoma, touch imprint. **A** The deeply basophilic cytoplasm can be appreciated as well as abundant lipid vacuoles in the cytoplasm. **B** The cells in this case are relatively similar to (**A**), except they have more irregular nuclei.

ruled out {178}. In conclusion, one of the paradoxes in explaining the etiology of BL is the occurrence of this tumour in many different populations and settings. It is possible that distinct pathogenetic mechanisms exist among BL subtypes {179}. On the other hand, different and multiple environmental exposures may converge in a common pathogenetic mechanism involving the *MYC* gene at chromosome 8q24 {2014}.

Sites of involvement

Extranodal sites are most often involved with some variation according to the clinical variants. However, in all three clinical variants, patients are at risk for central nervous system involvement. In endemic BL, the jaws and other facial bones (orbit) are the site of presentation in about 50% of the cases {301, 2447}. The distal ileum, caecum and/or omentum, gonads, kidneys, long bones, thyroid, salivary glands and breasts may also be affected either with or without jaw involvement {302, 2447}. Although localization may sometimes be found in the bone marrow (BM), manifestation of leukaemia in the peripheral blood (PB) is not present {302, 2447}. In sporadic BL, jaw tumours are very rare {1612}. The majority of the cases presents with abdominal masses {1364}. The ileo-caecal region represents the most frequent site of involvement. Similarly to endemic BL, ovaries, kidneys and breasts are also frequently involved. Breast involvement (often bilateral and massive) has been associated with onset during puberty, pregnancy or lactation. Retroperitoneal masses may result in spinal cord compression with paraplegia. Lymph node presentation is seen more commonly in adults than in children. Waldeyer ring and mediastinal involvement are rare. In immunodeficiency-associated

BL, nodal localization is frequent as well as BM involvement {877, 1818}.

Clinical features

Clinical presentation varies according to the epidemiologic subtype and the site of involvement. Patients often present with bulky disease,and a high tumour burden due to the short doubling time of the tumour. In the typical paediatric cases, the parents of affected children will report symptoms for only a few weeks. Paediatric BL patients are staged according to the system of Murphy *et al.* {1551}. 70% of patients present at advanced stages (III and IV). Upon institution of therapy a tumour lysis syndrome can occur due to rapid tumour cell death {2381}.

Burkitt leukaemia variant

A leukaemic phase can be observed in patients with bulky disease, but only rare cases (mainly males) present purely as acute leukaemia with PB and BM involvement {1363, 1364, 2060}. This Burkitt leukaemia, or acute lymphocytic leukaemia-L3, according to the former FAB classification, tends to involve the CNS at diagnosis or early during the disease course. Its rapid chemosensitivity easily leads to an acute tumour lysis syndrome.

Morphology

The prototype of BL is observed in endemic BL and in a high percentage of sporadic BL cases, particularly in children {898, 2447}. The tumour cells of BL are medium-sized cells (nuclei similar or smaller to those of histiocytes) and show a diffuse monotonous pattern of growth. Some tumours surround and invade otherwise uninvolved lymph nodes. The cells appear to be cohesive but sometimes exhibit squared-off borders of retracted cytoplasm. The nuclei are round with finely clumped and dispersed chromatin, with multiple basophilic medium-sized, paracentrally situated nucleoli. The cytoplasm is deeply basophilic and usually contains lipid vacuoles. These cellular details are better perceived in imprints. The tumour has an extremely high proliferation fraction (many mitotic figures) as

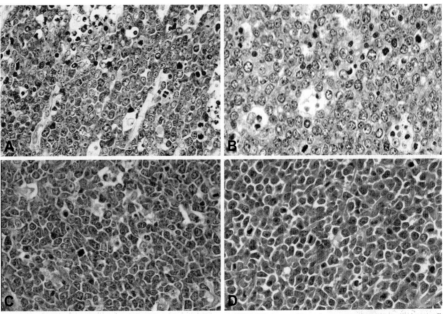

Fig.10.125 Burkitt lymphoma stained for Giemsa (**A**) and H&E (**B**) has uniform tumour cells with multiple small nucleoli and finely dispersed chromatin in their nuclei. In this Burkitt lymphoma stained for Giemsa (**C**) and H&E (**D**), there is greater nuclear irregularity.

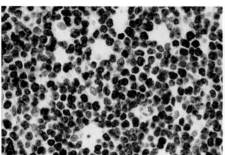
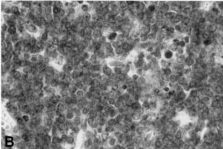
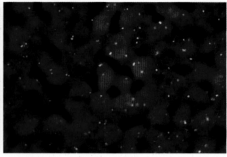

Fig. 10.126 Burkitt lymphoma. Immunohistochemistry shows a strong and homogeneous staining for Ki67/MIB1 (**A**) and CD10 (**B**). **C** FISH for *MYC* flanking probes {891A}, showing one allele with colocalization of both probes (red and green) and one allele with segregation of both probes.

well as a high fraction of apoptosis. A "starry sky" pattern is usually present, which is imparted by numerous benign macrophages that have ingested apoptotic tumour cells. Some cases may have a florid granulomatous reaction that may cause difficulties in the recognition of the tumour {891B}. These cases typically present with limited stage disease and have an especially good prognosis {1973A}. In some cases, tumour cells exhibit eccentric basophilic cytoplasm often with a single central nucleolus. Such cases, defined as BL with plasmacytoid differentiation, can occasionally be observed in children but are more common in immunodeficiency states {1818}. Other cases of BL may show greater nuclear pleomorphism and the nucleoli may be more prominent and fewer in number {898}. In the past, these cases have been referred to as atypical BL. However, these morphological variants share a similar gene expression profile, which supports the evidence that the morphological spectrum of BL is relatively wide {509, 994}.

Immunophenotype

In Burkitt lymphoma, including cases presenting with leukaemia, the tumour cells express moderate to strong levels of membrane IgM with light chain restriction and B-cell-associated antigens (e.g. CD19, CD20, CD22), CD10, BCL6, CD38, CD77 and CD43 {151, 898, 2447}. The neoplastic cells are usually negative or only weakly positive (in ~20% of the cases) for BCL2 and are uniformly TdT negative {264, 890, 1104, 1307, 1438}. Nearly 100% of the cells are positive for Ki67 {898}. There are very few admixed T-cells. Cases with a more atypical phenotype such as BCL2-positive, as seen in some adult patients, requires that the case otherwise has all the characteristic features of Burkitt lymphoma, including

IG;MYC translocation without *BCL2* or *BCL6* translocation.

Genetics
Antigen receptor genes
The tumour cells show clonal *IG* rearrangements with somatic hypermutation.

Cytogenetic abnormalities and oncogenes
Most of the cases have *MYC* translocation at band 8q24 to the *IG* heavy chain region, 14q32 or, less commonly, at the lambda, 22q11 or kappa, 2p12 light chain loci. Up to 10% of the cases may lack a demonstrable *MYC* translocation by FISH, the explanation for which is uncertain {890, 994}. These cases may have *MYC* translocation demonstrated using other techniques and must be otherwise completely typical to make a diagnosis of BL. Furthermore, *MYC* translocations are not specific for BL. Most *MYC/IG* breakpoints in endemic BL originate from aberrant somatic hypermutation. In sporadic cases, on the other hand, the translocation mostly involves the *IG* switch regions of the *IgH* locus at 14q32 {860, 2014}. These differences in *MYC* breakpoint may well be accounted for by the different maturational stage of the of EBV positive (mainly endemic) and EBV-negative (mainly sporadic) BL {180}. Mutations in *MYC* may enhance its tumourigenicity and some of these mutations may lead to decreased expression of BIM which binds and inactivates BCL2 {917, 2468}. Other genetic and epigenetic alterations occurring in a subset of BL, involving *p16^INK4a*, *TP53*, *p73*, *BAX*, *p130/RB2* and *BCL6*, may promote cell growth and/or inhibit apoptosis {179, 517, 1158, 1314, 1925}.

Gene profiling studies have demonstrated a consistent gene expression signature for BL, which is clearly distinct from that of DLBCL {509, 994}. However, intermediate cases were also found {509, 994}.

Postulated normal counterpart
Germinal centre or post germinal centre B cells.

Prognosis and predictive factors
In endemic and sporadic BL, the tumour is highly aggressive but potentially curable. Staging is performed according to the scheme proposed by Murphy and Hustu {1551} and modified by Magrath {1363}. Staging is largely related to tumour burden, and identifies patients with limited stage disease and patients with extensive intraabdominal or intrathoracic tumour {2381}. Bone marrow and central nervous system involvement, unresected tumour >10 cm in diameter, and a high LDH serum level are recognized as poor prognostic factors, particularly in sporadic BL. Intensive combination chemotherapy regimens result in cure rates of up to 90% in patients with low stage disease {1708} and 60–80% in patients with advanced stage disease {1363, 2060}. The results are better in children than in adults {591}. However, even patients with advanced stage disease, including BM and central nervous system involvement, may be cured with a high dose treatment program {310}. With high intensity treatment, most patients presenting with leukaemia also have a very good prognosis with 80–90% survival {2060, 2381}.

Relapse, if it occurs, is usually seen within the first year after diagnosis {1363, 2381}. Recently it has been reported that rituximab may be a useful additional therapeutic agent {531, 2229}. Although BL is curable, many patients still die of the disease mainly in Africa {892}.

B-cell lymphoma, unclassifiable, with features intermediate between diffuse large B-cell lymphoma and Burkitt lymphoma

P.M. Kluin
N.L. Harris
H. Stein
L. Leoncini

M. Raphaël
E. Campo
E.S. Jaffe

Definition

B-cell lymphomas with features intermediate between diffuse large B-cell lymphoma (DLBCL) and Burkitt lymphoma (BL) are aggressive lymphomas that have morphological and genetic features of both DLBCL and BL, but for biological and clinical reasons should not be included in these categories. Some of these cases were previously classified as Burkitt-like lymphoma (BLL).

The majority of the cases in this category have morphological features that are intermediate between DLBCL and BL, with some cells that are smaller than typical DLBCL, resembling BL, and some cells that are larger than typical BL, resembling DLBCL, as well as a high proliferation fraction, starry-sky pattern, and an immunophenotype consistent with BL. Some cases may be morphologically more typical of BL but have an atypical immunophenotype or genetic features that preclude a diagnosis of BL. The diagnosis of this type of unclassifiable B-cell lymphoma category should not be made in cases of morphologically typical DLBCL that have a MYC rearrangement, or in otherwise typical BL in which a MYC rearrangement cannot be demonstrated. Some transformed follicular lymphomas may fall into this category. This is a heterogeneous category that is not considered a distinct disease entity, but is useful in allowing the classification of cases not meeting criteria for classical BL or DLBCL.

ICD-O code   9680/3

Epidemiology

These lymphomas are relatively infrequent and mainly diagnosed in adults.

Sites of involvement

More than half of the patients present with widespread, often extranodal disease. Unlike BL, there is no preferential localization in the ileocaecal region or jaws. The bone marrow (BM) and peripheral blood (PB) may be involved as well.

Clinical features

Patients present with lymphadenopathy or mass lesions in extranodal sites. Some patients have a leukaemic presentation.

Morphology

These lymphomas are typically composed of a diffuse proliferation of medium- to large-sized transformed cells with few admixed small lymphocytes and no stromal reaction of fibrosis. Starry sky macrophages are typically present, as well as many mitotic figures and prominent apoptosis, causing a resemblance to BL. The cellular morphology is variable. In some cases, the cells resemble those of BL, but with more variation in nuclear size and contour than is considered acceptable for BL; some cases are consistent with BL morphologically but have an atypical immunophenotype and/or genetic features; other cases with an immunophenotype that is consistent with BL have a variable nuclear size that is intermediate between BL and DLBCL, often with either irregular nuclear contours or relatively large nucleoli. In rare cases the nuclei are relatively small and the chromatin is finely granular, resembling lymphoblastic lymphoma. Some of these latter cases have been classified as "blastic" or "blastoid". Immunohistochemistry for TdT is required to exclude lymphoblastic lymphoma. Cases of morphologically typical DLBCL with a very high proliferation index should not be included in this category {441}.

Immunophenotype

These lymphomas express B-cell markers, CD19, CD20, CD22 and CD79a and

Table 10.18 Morphologic, immunophenotypic, and genetic features that may be useful in distinguishing BL from DLBCL.

Characteristic	BL	Intermediate BL/DLBCL	DLBCL
Morphology			
Only small/medium-size cells	Yes	Common	No
Only large cells	No	No	Common
Mixture	No	Sometimes	Rare
Proliferation (Ki67/MIB1)			
>90% and homogeneous	Yes	Common	Rare
<90% or heterogeneous	No	Sometimes	Common
BCL2 expression			
Negative / weak	Yes	Sometimes	Sometimes
Strong	No	Sometimes	Sometimes
Genetic features			
MYC rearrangement	Yes*	Common	Rare
IG-MYC**	Yes	Sometimes	Rare
Non IG-MYC**	No	Sometimes	Rare
BCL2 but no MYC rearrangement	No	Rare	Sometimes
BCL6 but no MYC rearrangement	No	Rare	Sometimes
Double hit#	No	Sometimes	Rare
MYC-Simple karyotype***	Yes	Rare	Rare
MYC-Complex karyotype***	Rare	Common	Rare

* Approximately 5% of otherwise classical BL lack a detectable MYC rearrangement {891A, 994}.

**IG-MYC: juxtaposition of MYC to one of the IG loci: IGH@ at 14q32, IGL@ at 22q11 or IGK@ at 2p12. Non IG-MYC tumours contain a MYC rearrangement but no juxtaposition to one of the IG loci.

\# Double hit lymphomas contain a MYC/8q24 breakpoint in combination with a BCL2/18q21 (by far most frequent) and/or BCL6/3q27 breakpoint. The partner of BCL2/18q21 breakpoint mostly is the IGH locus at 14q32. In some cases a t(8;14;18) is present {1320A}.

***Simple karyotype: no or only few cytogenetic or (array) CGH abnormalities other than the MYC rearrangement. For array CGH a lymphoma with 6 or more abnormalities has been assigned as "MYC-complex" {994}.

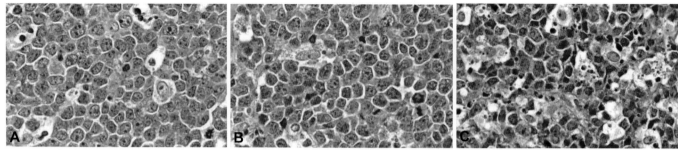

Fig. 10.127 Three lymphomas with t(8;14). **A** Typical BL composed of medium-sized, monomorphous cells with round nuclei, multiple nucleoli, and a moderate amount of cytoplasm, which has a mosaic-like appearance. Prominent apoptosis is evidenced by the presence of macrophages engulfing nuclear debris, creating the "starry-sky" pattern. Nine of 11 experts who reviewed this case independently made a diagnosis of BL; 1 made a diagnosis of atypical BL. **B** Another case with similar overall appearance, but with slightly more variation in size and shape of the cells. Six reviewers called this BL and 5 called it atypical BL. **C** DLBCL with a t(8;14) has a prominent starry-sky pattern. The cells are larger and more pleomorphic than the Burkitt and atypical Burkitt cases. Nine experts called this DLBCL and 2 called it atypical BL. Reproduced from from Harris NL and Horning SJ {896A}.

typically sIg, but so-called double hit cases may be sIg negative. In general, cases will be placed in this category when the immunophenotype is suggestive of BL (CD10+, BCL6+, BCL2- and IRF4/MUM1- or very weakly positive). Cases that morphologically resemble BL may be placed in this category when BCL2 is moderately to strongly positive. BCL2 positivity in a case that otherwise might be classified as BL should suggest the possibility of a double hit lymphoma with both *MYC* and *BCL2* translocations. The Ki67 labeling index is usually high, again raising the differential diagnosis of BL, but in reported cases it varies between 50 and 100% {264, 890, 1438}. Rare tumours with a *MYC* with or without *BCL2* rearrangement are TdT positive; classification of these cases is controversial, and the diagnosis of lymphoblastic lymphoma may be preferred {1561, 2191}.The usefulness of other markers remains to be established {922, 1858, 2179}.

Genetics

IG genes are clonally rearranged. Approximately 35–50% of the cases have 8q24/*MYC* translocations {890, 994, 1438}. However, whereas *MYC* in BL is juxtaposed to the one of the immunoglobulin genes *(IG-MYC)*, many of these cases have other translocations (non *IG-MYC*). Approximately 15% of the cases have a *BCL2* translocation, sometimes together with a *MYC* translocation ("double hit lymphoma"). Cases previously classified as Burkitt-like lymphoma may have a higher frequency of *MYC* and *BCL2* translocations as well as double hits {1104, 1359}. Less frequently, *BCL6* translocations are seen, sometimes together with *MYC* and/or *BCL2*. The relative incidence of double and triple hit lymphomas increases with age,

up to more than 30% in elderly patients (http://cgap.nci.nih.gov/Chromosomes/Mitelman). Cytogenetic analysis of both the non-*IG-MYC* and double hit cases often shows a complex karyotype with multiple abnormalities, in contrast to classical Burkitt lymphoma {1259}. Dependent on the algorithm used, gene profiling studies have shown that some double-hit cases have a profile intermediate between BL and DLBCL {994} or more similar to BL {509}. Cases of otherwise typical DLBCL with a *MYC* translocation should not be placed in this category. Conversely, lymphomas with a *IG-MYC* rearrangement as the only abnormality likely represent BL even if they are morphologically atypical.

Postulated normal counterpart

B-cell, most cases related to a germinal centre stage of differentiation.

Prognosis and predictive factors

These are aggressive lymphomas, for which the most appropriate therapeutic approach is not established. The double hit lymphomas show frequent involvement of the BM, PB and CNS; most cases are resistant to current therapies, which seems to be independent of the complexity of the other cytogenetic abnormalities {501, 994, 1259, 1438}.

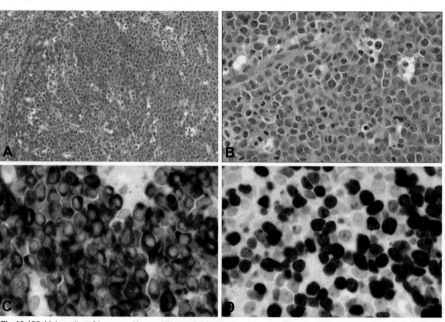

Fig.10.128 Male patient, 61 years, with a rapidly growing cervical nodal mass. "Double hit" lymphoma with both 8q24/*MYC* and 18q21/*BCL2* breakpoints. **A** Starry sky pattern. **B** Higher magnification showing a mixture of medium/large-sized nuclei with little pleomorphism but prominent nucleoli, absence of granular chromatin and many mitotic figures. **C** Strong BCL2 staining is very unusual for BL. **D** Ki67 staining was heterogeneous but elsewhere there were close to 100% positive cells.

B-cell lymphoma, unclassifiable, with features intermediate between diffuse large B-cell lymphoma and classical Hodgkin lymphoma

E.S. Jaffe
H. Stein
S.H. Swerdlow
E. Campo
S.A. Pileri
N.L. Harris

Definition
A B lineage lymphoma that demonstrates overlapping clinical, morphological and/or immunophenotypic features, between classical Hodgkin lymphoma (CHL) and diffuse large B-cell lymphoma (DLBCL), especially primary mediastinal large B-cell lymphoma (PMBL). While these lymphomas are most commonly associated with mediastinal disease, similar cases have been reported in peripheral lymph node groups as a primary site.

ICD-O code   9596/3

Synonyms
Grey zone lymphoma {1895, 2265}, large B-cell lymphoma with Hodgkin features {758}, Hodgkin-like anaplastic large cell lymphoma {2499, 2501}.

Epidemiology
These lymphomas are most common in young men, usually presenting between the ages of 20–40 years of age {758, 2265}. However, they have been reported in individuals as young as 13 years of age, and in older adults beyond the age of 70. Most cases have been reported from Western countries. Like CHL, they are less common in Blacks and Asians.

Etiology
The etiology is unknown. Epstein-Barr viral sequences have been identified in 20% or fewer cases.

Sites of involvement
The most common presentation is with a large anterior mediastinal mass, with or without involvement of supraclavicular lymph nodes {758, 2265}. Other peripheral lymph node groups are less commonly involved. There may be spread to lung by direct extension, as well as spread to liver, spleen and bone marrow. Non-lymphoid organs are rarely involved, in contrast to PMBL.

Clinical features
A large mediastinal mass may be associated with a superior vena caval syndrome,

or respiratory distress. Another phenomenon which may or may not be related to "grey zone lymphomas" is the occurrence of CHL and PMBL as composite lymphoma {815}, or sequentially, at different points in time {1727}. While either lymphoma subtype may present first, it is somewhat more common for the initial presentation to be CHL with relapse as PMBL, often within the first few years {2487}.

Morphology
The lymphoma is typically composed of a confluent, sheet-like growth of pleomorphic tumour cells in a diffusely fibrotic stroma {758, 2265}. Focal fibrous bands may be seen in some cases. The cells are larger and more pleomorphic than in the typical case of PMBL, although some centroblast-like cells may be present. Pleomorphic cells resembling lacunar cells and Hodgkin cells comprise the majority of the infiltrate. A characteristic feature is the broad spectrum of cytological appearances with different areas of the tumour showing variations in cytological appearance, i.e. some areas may more closely resemble CHL and others appear more like diffuse large B-cell lymphoma. There is usually a sparse inflammatory infiltrate, although scattered eosinophils, lymphocytes and histocytes may be present. Necrosis is frequent, but unlike CHL, the necrotic areas do not contain neutrophilic infiltrates.

Immunophenotype
The lymphoma cells exhibit an immunophenotype with transitional features between CHL and PMBL {758, 2265}. Neoplastic cells typically express CD45. In contrast to CHL, the B-cell programme is often preserved, but is aberrantly expressed in concert with Hodgkin markers, such as CD30 and CD15. CD20 and CD79a are frequently positive, and may be strongly expressed on the majority of the tumour cells. CD30 is positive and CD15 is positive in the majority of cases. Surface or cytoplasmic immunoglobulin (Ig) is absent. The transcription factors PAX5, OCT-2 and BOB.1 are usually expressed. BCL6 is variably positive but CD10 is generally negative. ALK is consistently negative. The background lymphocytes are predominantly CD3+, CD4+, as seen in CHL. In cases that morphologically resemble nodular sclerosis classical Hodgkin lymphoma (NSCHL), uniform strong expression of CD20 and other B-cell markers and absence of CD15 would favour the diagnosis of grey zone lymphoma. In cases that resemble PMBL, absence of CD20, expression of CD15 or presence of EBV would favour this diagnosis as well.

MAL, a marker associated with PMBL, is expressed in at least a subset of the cases presenting with mediastinal disease {472, 2265}. Supporting a relationship to PMBL, nuclear REL/p65 protein has been identified in those cases tested {758, 1857}. In one series, p53 was expressed in the

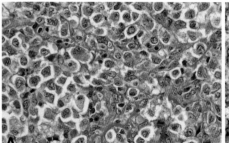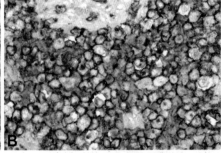

Fig. 10.129 B-cell lymphoma with features intermediate between diffuse large B-cell lymphoma and classical Hodgkin lymphoma. Mediastinal mass. **A** Lymphoma is composed of sheets of cells with clear cytoplasm and fine sclerosis. The appearance resembles that of primary mediastinal large B-cell lymphoma (PMBL). **B** Tumour cells were strongly CD15 positive and also CD30 positive (not shown).

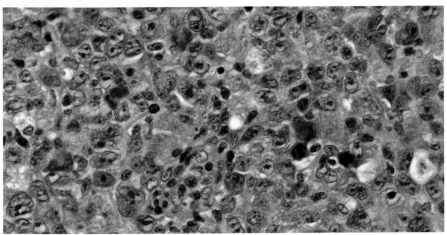

Fig. 10.130 B-cell lymphoma with features intermediate between diffuse large B-cell lymphoma and classical Hodgkin lymphoma. Mediastinal mass. The lymphoma is composed of a sheet-like growth of cells with amphophilic cytoplasm. The inflammatory background is minimal. The phenotype resembled that of CHL, with expression of CD30 and CD15, but transcription factors OCT-2 and BOB.1 were positive.

majority of cases {758}.

In instances of composite or metachronous lymphomas, the various components exhibit a phenotype characteristic of that entity, either CHL or PMBL.

Genetics

Only a few cases of metachronous CHL and PMBL have been studied at the genetic level; a clonal relationship has been shown between the two components {2265}. Specific genetic changes have not been associated with transformation of the lymphoma or its components to either CHL or PMBL. Because the morphological and phenotypic changes are reversible, it is likely that epigenetic rather than genetic alterations are responsible for the change in morphology and immunophenotype {933}. A close

relationship between CHL and PMBL has been shown by gene expression profiling studies, but specific genomic studies of "grey zone" or transitional lymphomas have not been performed {1870, 1944}.

Postulated normal counterpart

A thymic B-cell is the likely   for those cases arising in the mediastinum {2265}. For cases arising in the peripheral lymph nodes, an alternative B-cell origin is proposed.

Prognosis and predictive factors

These lymphomas generally have a more aggressive clinical course and poorer outcome than either CHL or PMBL. There is no consensus on the optimum treatment, although in some series therapy for an aggressive large B-cell lymphoma has been proposed as effective {2265, 2501} Others have proposed use of a Hodgkin type regimen {349}. Among CHL patients, strong expression of CD20, as seen in this transitional lymphoma, has been proposed as a poor prognostic indicator in Hodgkin lymphoma trials {1774}. However, other studies have reached an opposite conclusion {2275}.

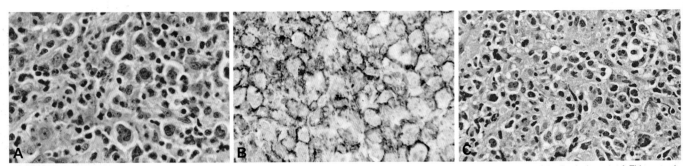

Fig. 10.131 B-cell lymphoma with features intermediate between diffuse large B-cell lymphoma and classical Hodgkin lymphoma. Biopsy of mediastinal mass. **A** This example resembles CHL. **B** CD20 is strongly and uniformly expressed in the tumour cells, a feature unusual for CHL. **C** The same case in different portions of the biopsy specimen more closely resembled a PMBL.

CHAPTER 11

Mature T- and NK-cell Neoplasms

T-cell prolymphocytic leukaemia

T-cell large granular lymphocytic leukaemia

Chronic lymphoproliferative disorders of NK cells

Aggressive NK cell leukaemia

EBV-positive T-cell lymphoproliferative disorders of childhood

Adult T-cell leukaemia/lymphoma

Extranodal NK/T cell lymphoma, nasal type

Enteropathy-associated T-cell lymphoma

Hepatosplenic T-cell lymphoma

Subcutaneous panniculitis-like T-cell lymphoma

Mycosis fungoides

Sézary syndrome

Primary cutaneous CD30 positive T-cell lymphoproliferative disorders

Primary cutaneous gamma-delta T-cell lymphomas

Peripheral T-cell lymphoma, NOS

Angioimmunoblastic T-cell lymphoma

Anaplastic large cell lymphoma (ALCL), ALK positive

Anaplastic large cell lymphoma (ALCL), ALK negative

T-cell prolymphocytic leukaemia

D. Catovsky
H.K. Müller-Hermelink
E. Ralfkiaer

Definition
T-cell prolymphocytic leukaemia (T-PLL) is an aggressive T-cell leukaemia characterized by the proliferation of small to medium-sized prolymphocytes with a mature post-thymic T-cell phenotype involving the peripheral blood (PB), bone marrow (BM), lymph nodes, liver, spleen and skin.

ICD-O code   9834/3

Synonym
T-cell chronic lymphocytic leukaemia was used historically as a synonym for some small cell variants.

Epidemiology
T-PLL is rare, representing approximately 2% of cases of mature lymphocytic leukaemias in adults over the age of 30 {1424}; median age is 65 years (range, 30–94 years).

Sites of involvement
Leukaemic T-cells are found in the PB, BM, lymph nodes, spleen, liver and sometimes skin.

Clinical features
Most patients present with hepatosplenomegaly and generalized lymphadenopathy. Skin infiltration is seen in 20% of patients, and serous effusions, chiefly pleural, in a minority {1424}. Anaemia and thrombocytopenia are common and the lymphocyte count is usually >100x10^9/L and >200x10^9/L in half of the patients. Serum immunoglobulins are normal. Serology for HTLV-I is negative.

Morphology
Peripheral blood and bone marrow
The diagnosis is made on PB films which show a predominance of small to medium-sized lymphoid cells with non-granular basophilic cytoplasm, round, oval or markedly irregular nuclei and a visible nucleolus. In 25% of cases the cell size is small and the nucleolus may not be visible by light microscopy (small cell variant) {1426}. In 5% of patients the nuclear

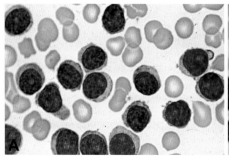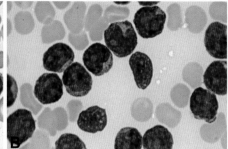

Fig. 11.01 A, B Peripheral blood films from typical cases of T-cell prolymphocytic leukaemia.

outline is very irregular and can even be cerebriform {1713}. Irrespective of the nuclear features, a common morphological feature is the presence of cytoplasmic protrusions or blebs. The BM is diffusely infiltrated, but the diagnosis is difficult to make by BM histology alone.

Other tissues
Cutaneous involvement consists of perivascular or more diffuse dermal infiltrates without epidermotropism {1373, 1424}. The spleen contains a dense red pulp infiltrate, which invades the spleen capsule, blood vessels and atrophied white pulp {1663}. In lymph nodes, the involvement is diffuse and tends to predominate in the paracortical areas, sometimes with sparing of follicles. Prominent high-endothelial venules may be numerous and are often infiltrated by neoplastic cells.

Cytochemistry
T prolymphocytes stain strongly with α-naphthyl acetate esterase and acid phosphatase with dot-like staining in the Golgi region {1425}. However, cytochemistry is rarely used for routine diagnosis currently.

Immunophenotype
T-prolymphocytes are peripheral T-cells which are TdT and CD1a negative while CD2, CD3 and CD7 are positive; the membrane expression of CD3 may be weak. CD52 is usually expressed at high density, and can be used as a target of therapy {535}.
In 60% of patients the cells are CD4+, CD8-, and in 25% they coexpress CD4 and

CD8, a feature almost unique to T-PLL; 15% are CD4-, CD8+ {1424}. The overexpression of the oncogene *TCL1* can be demonstrated by immunohistochemistry {921} and this method is useful for detecting residual T-PLL on BM sections after therapy.

Genetics
Antigen receptor genes
T-cell receptor *(TCR)* genes, *TRB@* and *TRG@*, are clonally rearranged.

Cytogenetic abnormalities and oncogenes
The most frequent chromosome abnormality in T-PLL involves inversion of chromosome 14 with breakpoints in the long arm at q11 and q32, seen in 80% of patients. In 10% there is a reciprocal tandem translocation t(14;14)(q11;q32) {272, 1372}. These translocations juxtapose the *TRA@* locus with the oncogenes *TCL1A and TCL1B* at 14q32.1 which are activated through the translocation {1718}. The translocation t(X;14)(q28;q11) is less common,

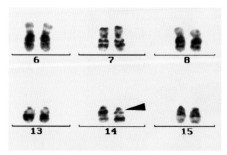

Fig. 11.02 T-cell prolymphocytic leukaemia. Partial karyotype showing inv14(q11;q32)

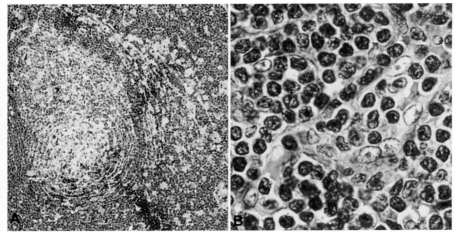

Fig. 11.03 T-cell prolymphocytic leukaemia. **A** Lymph node is diffusely infiltrated, but a follicle is unaffected. Giemsa stain. **B** Prominent high endothelial venule showing tumour cells in the lumen, in the wall and the adjacent paracortex. Giemsa stain.

but it also involves the *TCA@* locus at 14q11 with the *MTCP1* gene, which is homologous to *TCL1*, at Xq28 {2097}. Both *TCL1* and *MTCP1* have oncogenic properties as both can induce a T-cell leukaemia (CD4-/CD8+) in transgenic mice {849, 2338}. *TCL1* inhibits activation-induced death in the neoplastic T-cells, further contributing to the neoplastic process {560}.
Abnormalities of chromosome 8, idic (8p11), t(8;8)(p11-12;q12) and trisomy 8q are seen in 70–80% of cases {1718}. Deletions at 12p13 are also a feature of T-PLL when studied by FISH {937}.

Molecular and FISH studies also show deletions at 11q23, the locus for the Ataxia Telangiectasia Mutated *(ATM)* gene, and mutational analysis has shown missense mutations at the *ATM* locus in T-PLL {2100, 2344}. T-PLL is not an uncommon secondary neoplasm in patients with ataxia telangiectasia {272}. Abnormalities of chromosome 6 (33%) and 17 (26%) have also been described in T-PLL using conventional karyotyping and CGH studies {272, 483}. The *TP53* gene (at 17p13.1) is deleted with overexpression of p53 protein in a number of cases {273}.

Postulated normal counterpart

Unknown T-cell with a mature (post-thymic) immunophenotype. Strong CD7 and coexpression of CD4 and CD8 and weak membrane CD3 may suggest that T-PLL arises from a T-cell at an intermediate stage of differentiation between cortical thymocytes and mature T lymphocytes.

Prognosis and predictive factors

The course of the disease is aggressive with a median survival of usually less than one year. Cases with a more chronic course have also been reported {754}. Such cases may show an accelerated course after 2–3 years. The best responses have been reported with the monoclonal antibody alemtuzumab (anti-CD52) {536, 1130}. Both autologous and allogeneic stem cell transplants for patients who achieve remission are being explored, in conjunction with immunotherapy. Recent studies have identified both high expression of TCL1 and AKT1 as poor prognostic markers {923}.

T-cell large granular lymphocytic leukaemia

W.C. Chan
K. Foucar
W.G. Morice
D. Catovsky

Definition

T-cell large granular lymphocytic leukaemia (T-LGL) is a heterogeneous disorder characterized by a persistent (>6 months) increase in the number of peripheral blood (PB) large granular lymphocytes (LGL), usually between 2–20x10⁹/L, without a clearly identified cause.

ICD-O code   9831/3

Epidemiology

T-LGL leukaemia represents 2–3% of cases of mature lymphocytic leukaemias. There is an approximately equal male:female ratio with no clearly defined age peak. The disease is rare (<3%) before 25 years and the majority of cases (73%) occur in the 45–75 years age group.

Etiology

The underlying pathophysiologic mechanisms for T-LGL leukaemia are not well understood. This disorder is fairly unique in that the clonal T-LGL cells retain many phenotypic and functional properties of normal cytotoxic effector T-cells {220}. One theory postulates that T-LGL leukaemia arises in a setting of sustained immune stimulation. The frequent association of T-LGL leukaemia with autoimmune disorders supports this hypothesis {220, 2428}. Absence of homeostatic apoptosis is also a feature of the T-LGL, as these cells express high levels of FAS and FASL, leading investigators to propose activation of pro-survival pathways in T-LGL which prevents FAS signaling {648, 1954}. FASL levels are elevated *in sera* of many patients, which may be important in the pathogenesis of neutropenia {1323}.

Clonal expansions of T-LGL can be observed following allogeneic bone marrow (BM) transplantation, usually reflecting a restricted T-cell repertoire. However, rare cases of T-LGL leukaemia have also been observed as a form of post-transplant lymphoproliferative disorder {103, 1573}. A pitfall in diagnosis is the frequent development of oligoclonal T-cell populations following allogeneic BM transplantation

as lymphocyte reconstitution occurs {732A, 1414A}. Clonal populations of T-LGL are also often seen in association with low grade B-cell malignancies, including hairy cell leukaemia and chronic lymphocytic leukaemia. These are usually stable and do not progress to clinically significant disease. They appear to represent a type of host response {82, 1403}.

Sites of involvement

T-LGL leukaemia involves the PB, BM, liver and spleen. Lymphadenopathy is very rare.

Clinical features

Most cases have an indolent clinical course {390, 563, 1247, 1683}. Severe neutropenia with or without anaemia is frequent while thrombocytopenia is not; Lymphocytosis is usually between 2–20x10⁹/L. Severe anaemia due to red cell aplasia has been reported in association with T-LGL leukaemia {1247}. Moderate splenomegaly is the main physical finding. Rheumatoid arthritis, the presence

of autoantibodies, circulating immune complexes and hypergammaglobulinemia are also common {390, 1247}. Cases that are CD4+ have been reported to be frequently (30%) associated with an underlying malignancy {1303}. Morbidity and mortality are mostly due to the accompanying cytopenias or other accompanying diseases.

Morphology

The predominant lymphocytes in PB and BM films are LGL with moderate to abundant cytoplasm and fine or coarse azurophilic granules {278, 390, 1441}. The granules in the LGL often exhibit a characteristic ultrastructural appearance described as parallel tubular arrays {1441} and contain a number of proteins that play a role in cytolysis such as perforin and granzyme B. There is no agreement on the level of lymphocytosis required for diagnosis of T-LGL leukaemia {1992}, but a LGL count of >2x10⁹/L is frequently associated with a clonal proliferation. However, cases with LGL lower than 2x10⁹/L

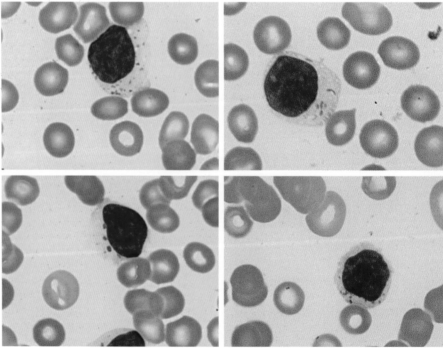

Fig.11.04 The various morphologic variants of LGL in the peripheral blood (Wright's stain).

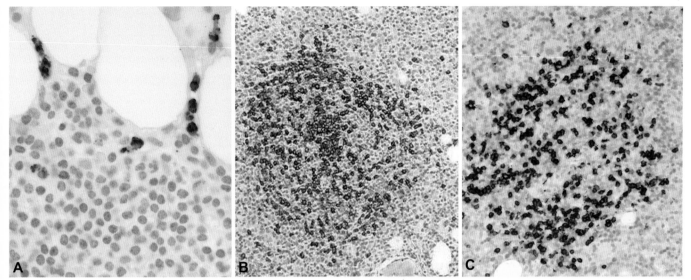

Fig. 11.05 Bone marrow findings in T-LGL leukaemia. **A** Neoplastic cells infiltrate interstitially, as demonstrated by stain for TIA1. **B,C** Reactive lymphoid aggregates. Lymphoid nodules in the bone marrow immunostained with anti-CD20 (**B**) and anti-CD3 (**C**). B-cells in the nodule are admixed with CD3 positive T-cells that predominate at the periphery.

but which meet all other appropriate criteria, are consistent with this diagnosis. Despite the cytopenias, the BM is normocellular or hypocellular in about 50% of cases; in the remainder, the BM is typically slightly hypercellular {1521, 1662}. The granulocytic series often show left shifted maturation and mild to moderate reticulin fibrosis is present {390}. The extent of BM involvement is variable and LGL usually comprise less than 50% of the cellular elements with interstitial/intrasinusoidal infiltrates which are difficult to identify by morphologic review {1521}. Non-neoplastic nodular lymphoid aggregates containing many B-cells surrounded by a rim of CD4+ T-cells are also frequently present {1662}. Splenic involvement is characterized by infiltration and expansion of the red pulp cords and sinusoids by T-LGL with sparing of the often hyperplastic white pulp {1663}.

Cytochemistry
The granules are acid phosphatase and β glucuronidase positive. However, enzyme cytochemical stains are rarely used for routine diagnosis.

Immunophenotype
T-LGL leukaemia is typically a disorder of mature CD3, CD8 and T-cell receptor (TCR) αβ-positive cytotoxic T-cells {390, 1683}. Uncommon variants include CD4 TCRαβ–positive cases and TCRγδ–positive cases; approximately 60% of the latter express CD8, the remainder are CD4/CD8-negative {1303, 1926, 1992}. Abnormally diminished or lost expression of CD5 and/or CD7 is common in T-LGL leukaemia {1348, 1520}. CD57 and CD16 are expressed in over 80% of the cases {1247, 1520}. Expression of the CD94/NKG2 and KIR families of NK-associated MHC-class I receptors can be detected in 50% or more of T-LGL leukaemias. KIR positive cases usually show uniform expression of a single isoform and this finding can serve as a surrogate indicator of clonality {1348, 1520}. The T-LGL express the cytotoxic effector proteins TIA1, granzyme B and granzyme M. Bone marrow core biopsy immunohistochemistry using antibodies to these antigens and CD8 can be used for confirmation of the diagnosis by revealing the mainly interstitial or intrasinusoidal T-LGL infiltrates {1519, 1521, 1662}.

Genetics
Antigen receptor genes
Cases classified as T-LGL leukaemia are, as a rule, clonal, as documented by *TCR* gene rearrangement studies {1247}. The *TRG@* gene is rearranged in all cases regardless of the type of receptors expressed. The *TRG@* gene is rearranged in cases expressing the *TCRαβ* receptor, but the *TRB@* gene may be in germline configuration in cases expressing the TCRγδ receptor {2336}.

Cytogenetic abnormalities
There is no unique karyotypic abnormality, but numeric and structural chromosomal abnormalities have been described in a small number of cases {1247}.

Postulated normal counterpart
CD8-positive T-cell subset for the common type and a subset and T lymphocytes for the rare type expressing the γδ TCR.

Prognosis and predictive factors
The lymphoproliferation is typically indolent and non-progressive and some investigators feel that it is better regarded as a clonal disorder of uncertain significance rather than a leukaemia. Morbidity is associated with the cytopenias especially neutropenia, but mortality due to this cause is uncommon. In a series of 68 patients, median survival was about 13 years {563}. Rare cases with an aggressive course have been described {773, 2249}. Patients who require treatment may benefit from cyclosporine A, cyclophosphamide and corticosteroids, low dose methotrexate or pentostatin {1247, 1664}.

Chronic lymphoproliferative disorders of NK cells

N. Villamor
W.G. Morice
W.C. Chan
K. Foucar

Definition

Chronic lymphoproliferative disorders of NK cells are rare and heterogeneous. They are characterized by a persistent (>6 months) increase in peripheral blood (PB) NK cells (usually ≥2x10^9/L) without a clearly identified cause. It is difficult to distinguish between reactive and neoplastic conditions, without highly specialized techniques. Chronic NK-cell lymphoproliferative disorder (CLPD-NK) represents a proliferation of NK cells associated with a chronic clinical course, and is considered a provisional entity.

ICD-O code   9831/3

Synonyms

Chronic NK-cell lymphocytosis, chronic NK-large granular lymphocyte (LGL) lymphoproliferative disorder, NK-cell lineage granular lymphocyte proliferative disorder, NK-cell LGL lymphocytosis, indolent large granular NK-cell lymphoproliferative disorder.

Epidemiology

CLPD-NK occurs predominantly in adults with a median age of 60 years without sex predominance {1248, 1304, 1799}. Unlike Epstein-Barr virus (EBV)-associated aggressive NK-cell leukaemia, there is no racial or genetic predisposition.

Etiology

A transient increase in circulating NK cells may be encountered in many conditions such as autoimmune disorders or viral infections {1248, 1799}. NK-cell activation due to an unknown stimulus, presumably viral, is postulated to play a role in the early pathogenesis of chronic lymphoproliferative disorders of NK cells by selecting NK-cell clones, although no evidence of direct NK-cell infection has been observed {1304, 1340, 1799, 2483}. A genetic susceptibility may be linked to haplotypes containing higher numbers of activating killer immunoglobulin-like receptor (*KIR*) genes {649, 1982, 2482}.

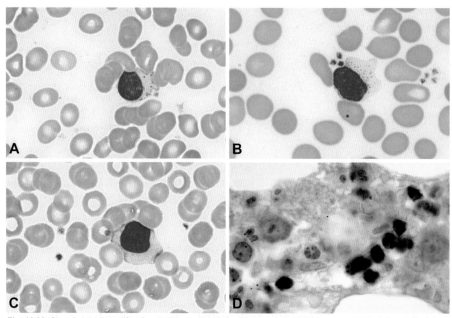

Fig. 11.06 Chronic lymphoproliferative disorders of NK cells. Peripheral blood films show the lymphocyte with coarse azurophilic granulation (**A**), lymphocyte with numerous fine granulations (**B**), lymphocyte with scarce granulation in the limit of visibility (**C**). **D** Intrasinusoidal marrow infiltration by granzyme B positive cells. Note the bland nuclear cytology of the antigen positive cells.

Sites of involvement

Predominantly PB and bone marrow (BM).

Clinical features

The majority of patients are asymptomatic, but some may present with systemic symptoms and/or cytopenia(s) (mainly neutropenia and anaemia). Lymphadenopathy, hepatomegaly, splenomegaly and cutaneous lesions are infrequent {1304, 1661, 1799}. Chronic lymphoproliferative disorders of NK cells may occur in association with other medical conditions such as solid and haematologic tumours, vasculitis, splenectomy, neuropathy and autoimmune disorders {1304, 1661, 1695, 1799}.

Morphology

The circulating NK cells are typically intermediate in size with round nuclei with condensed chromatin and moderate amounts of slightly basophilic cytoplasm containing fine or coarse azurophilic granules. The BM biopsy is characterized by intrasinusoidal and interstitial infiltration by cells with small, minimally irregular nuclei and modest amounts of pale cytoplasm. These infiltrates are difficult to detect without the aid of immunohistochemistry.

Immunophenotype

Surface CD3 is negative, while cytoplasmic CD3ε is often positive. CD16 is positive, while weak CD56 expression is frequently observed {1304, 1519, 1520, 1695, 2361}. Cytotoxic markers including TIA1, granzyme B and granzyme M are positive. There may be diminished or lost expression of CD2, CD7 and CD57; also seen are aberrant coexpression of CD5 and abnormal uniform expression of CD8 {1517, 1520}. Expression of the KIR family of NK-cell receptors (NKR) is abnormal in CLPD-NK; either restricted KIR isoform expression or a complete lack of detectable KIR may be seen {649, 952, 1520, 1695, 2482, 2485}. KIR-positive cases preferentially express activating receptor isoforms {649, 2482}. Other abnormalities of NKR include uniform, bright CD94/NKG2A heterodimer expression and diminished CD161 expression {1304, 1520, 1982, 2361}.

Genetics
Karyotype is normal in most cases {1661, 1799, 2173}. There are no rearrangements of the immunoglobulin and T-cell receptor genes, as expected for NK cells. In female patients, it is possible to exploit X-chromosome inactivation as an indirect marker of clonality. A skewed ratio of X-chromosome inactivation restricted to NK cells is indicative of the presence of a clonal population. With such methodologies, clonality is confirmed in some but not in all patients {1135, 1304, 1575}. Unlike aggressive NK-cell leukaemia, EBV is negative {1248, 1340, 2483}.

Postulated normal counterpart
Mature NK-cell.

Prognosis and predictive factors
In the majority of patients the clinical course is indolent over a prolonged period. Disease progression with increasing lymphocytosis and worsening of cytopenias is observed in some cases. The presence of cytopenias, recurrent infections and comorbidity may be harbingers of a worse prognosis. Rare cases with either spontaneous complete remission {1304, 1661, 1799, 2484} or transformation to an aggressive NK-cell disorder have been described {990, 1628, 1878}. The presence of cytogenetic abnormalities may imply a worse prognosis and could be related to rare transformations reported in the literature {1628}.

Aggressive NK-cell leukaemia

J.K.C. Chan
E.S. Jaffe
E. Ralfkiaer
Y.-H. Ko

Definition

A systemic neoplastic proliferation of NK-cells almost always associated with Epstein-Barr virus (EBV) and an aggressive clinical course.

ICD-O code   9948/3

Synonym

Aggressive NK-cell leukaemia/lymphoma.

Epidemiology

This is a rare form of leukaemia which is much more prevalent among Asians than other ethnic populations {1901}. Patients are most commonly young to middle-aged adults, with a median age of 42 years {2052, 2128}. There is no sex predilection or a slight male predominance {381, 386, 1004, 1221, 1223, 1659, 1901, 1902, 2052, 2128}.

Etiology

Little is known about the etiology of aggressive NK-cell leukaemia, but the strong association with EBV suggests a pathogenetic role of the virus. Rare patients may manifest features of hypersensitivity to mosquito bites or chronic active EBV infection {1020, 1021}, leading to overlap with EBV+ T-cell lymphoproliferative disorders of childhood.

Sites of involvement

The most commonly involved sites are peripheral blood (PB), bone marrow (BM), liver and spleen, but any organ can show involvement in addition. Since the number of neoplastic cells in the PB and BM can be limited, the disease is different from the usual leukaemias and thus also has been called "aggressive NK-cell leukaemia/lymphoma". There can be overlap with extranodal NK/T-cell lymphoma showing multiorgan involvement; it is unclear whether aggressive NK-cell leukaemia represents the leukaemic counterpart of extranodal NK/T-cell lymphoma {381}.

Clinical features

The patients usually present with fever, constitutional symptoms and a leukaemic

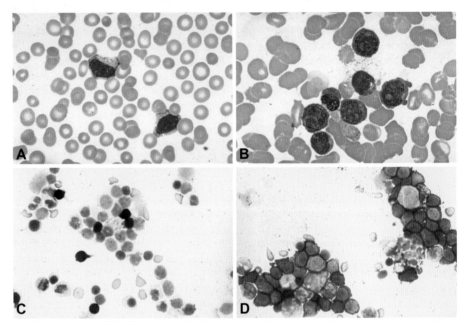

Fig. 11.07 Aggressive NK-cell leukaemia. **A** In this blood smear, the neoplastic cells are very similar to normal large granular lymphocytes. **B** In this case, the neoplastic cells have basophilic cytoplasm, and nuclei with more open chromatin and distinct nucleoli. Azurophilic granules can be observed in the cytoplasm. **C** The neoplastic cells are negative for surface CD3 (Leu4), while the normal T lymphocytes are stained. **D** The neoplastic cells show strong immunoreactivity for CD56.

blood picture. The number of circulating leukaemic cells may be low or high (a few percent to >80% of all leukocytes); anaemia, neutropenia and thrombocytopenia are common. Serum lactate dehydrogenase level is often markedly elevated. Hepatosplenomegaly is common, sometimes accompanied by lymphadenopathy, but skin lesions are uncommon. The disease may be complicated by coagulopathy, haemophagocytic syndrome or multiorgan failure {386, 1004, 1223, 1515, 1639, 2052, 2128}. Rare cases may evolve from extranodal NK/T-cell lymphoma or chronic lymphoproliferative disorders of NK cells {911, 1628, 1661, 2049}.

While it has been suggested that aggressive NK-cell leukaemia may merely represent the leukaemic manifestation of extranodal NK/T-cell lymphoma, the following features are distinctive for the former: younger median age by more than a decade; high frequency of hepatosplenic and BM involvement; low frequency of cutaneous involvement; disseminated disease with uniformly fatal outcome irrespective of treatment; and frequent expression of CD16 {1582, 2128}.

Morphology

Circulating leukaemic cells can show a range of appearances from cells indistinguishable from normal large granular lymphocytes to cells with atypical nuclei featuring enlargement, irregular foldings, open chromatin or distinct nucleoli. There is an ample amount of pale or lightly basophilic cytoplasm containing fine or coarse azurophilic granules. The BM shows massive, focal or subtle infiltration by the neoplastic cells and there can be intermingled reactive histiocytes with haemophagocytosis. In tissue sections, the leukaemic cells show diffuse or patchy destructive infiltrates. They often appear monotonous, with round or irregular nuclei, condensed chromatin and small nucleoli, but they can sometimes show significant nuclear pleomorphism. There are frequently admixed apoptotic

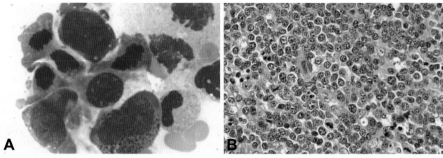

Fig. 11.08 Aggressive NK-cell leukaemia. **A** Giemsa-stained marrow aspirate. The neoplastic cells show pleomorphic irregularly folded nuclei, prominent nucleoli and cytoplasmic azurophilic granules in the basophilic cytoplasm. **B** Lymph node. The neoplastic cells appear monotonous, and possess round nuclei. There are many interspersed apoptotic bodies.

bodies. Necrosis is common, and there may or may not be angioinvasion.

Immunophenotype

The neoplastic cells are CD2+, surface CD3-, CD3ε+, CD56+ and positive for cytotoxic molecules. Thus, the immunophenotype is identical to that of extranodal NK/T-cell lymphoma, except that CD16 is frequently positive (75%) {2128}. CD11b may be expressed, while CD57 is usually negative {381, 1659}. The neoplastic cells express FAS ligand, and high levels of FAS ligand can be found in the serum of affected patients {1117, 1369, 2156}.

Genetics

T-cell receptor *(TCR)* genes are in germline configuration. Clonality therefore has to be established by other methods, such as cytogenetic studies and pattern of X chromosome inactivation in female patients.

More than 90% of cases harbour EBV, which occurs in a clonal episomal form {386, 903, 1126}.

A variety of clonal cytogenetic abnormalities have been reported, such as del(6)(q21q25) and 11q deletion {1902}. An array-based comparative genomic hybridization study has shown significant differences in genetic changes between aggressive NK-cell leukaemia and extranodal NK/T-cell lymphoma: 7p-, 17p- and 1q+ are frequent in the former but not the latter, while 6q- is common in the latter but rare in the former {1567}.

Postulated normal counterpart

NK cells.

Prognosis and predictive factors

Most cases pursue a fulminant clinical course frequently complicated by multiorgan failure, coagulopathy and haemophagocytic syndrome. The median survival is less than 2 months {381, 1902, 2052, 2128}. Response to chemotherapy is usually poor, and relapse is almost the rule in patients achieving remission with or without BM transplantation {2128}.

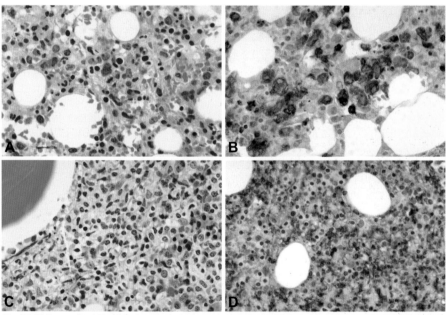

Fig. 11.09 Aggressive NK-cell leukaemia, bone marrow biopsy. **A** Patchy involvement by neoplastic cells with significant nuclear pleomorphism. **B** Immunostaining for CD3 highlights the neoplastic population, and further accentuates the nuclear irregularities. **C** Extensive involvement by a monotonous population of uniform-appearing cells. **D** The neoplastic cells show positive staining for CD56.

EBV-positive T-cell lymphoproliferative disorders of childhood

L. Quintanilla-Martinez
H. Kimura
E.S. Jaffe

Two major types of Epstein-Barr (EBV)-associated T-cell lymphoproliferative disorders have been reported in the paediatric age group. Both occur with increased frequency in Asians, and in Native Americans from Central and South America and Mexico. Hydroa vacciniforme-like lymphoma is a cutaneous malignancy with an indolent clinical course, but it usually progresses over time. Systemic EBV+ T-cell lymphoproliferative disease (LPD) of childhood has a very fulminant clinical course. It may be associated with chronic active EBV-infection (CAEBV), and in these patients is preceded by a prodromal phase of polyclonal or oligoclonal expansion of EBV-infected T-cells.

Systemic EBV-positive T-cell lymphoproliferative disease of childhood

Definition
Systemic EBV+ T-cell LPD of childhood is a life-threatening illness of children and young adults characterized by a clonal proliferation of EBV-infected T-cells with an activated cytotoxic phenotype. It can occur shortly after primary acute EBV infection or in the setting of chronic active EBV infection (CAEBV). It has a rapid progression with multiple organ failure, sepsis and death, usually from days to weeks. This entity shows some overlapping clinicopathologic features with aggressive NK-cell leukaemia.

ICD-O code
The provisional code proposed for the fourth edition of ICD-O is *9724/3*.

Synonyms and historical annotation
Historically this process has been described under a variety of terms including: fulminant EBV+ T-cell LPD of childhood, sporadic fatal infectious mononucleosis (FIM); fulminant haemophagocytic syndrome in children in Taiwan {2115}; fatal EBV-associated haemophagocytic syndrome in Japan {1144}; and severe CAEBV {1149, 1636, 2127}.

The term fulminant or fatal haemophagocytic syndrome has been used to describe a systemic disease secondary to acute primary EBV infection affecting previously healthy children. It has been shown to be a monoclonal CD8+ EBV-associated lymphoproliferative disorder, and therefore is now considered equivalent to systemic EBV+ T-cell LPD of childhood {1797}.

The term CAEBV was coined to describe an infectious mononucleosis-like syndrome persisting for at least 6 months, and associated with high titers of antibodies to EBV-capsid antigen (VCA-IgG) and early antigen (EA-IgG) without association to malignancy, autoimmune diseases or immunodeficiency {2107}. These cases are mostly seen in Western populations; progression to EBV-positive T-cell LPD has been reported rarely in such patients {1069, 1094, 1797}.

A more severe form of CAEBV characterized by high fever, hepatosplenomegaly, extensive lymphadenopathy, and pancytopenia has been described in Japan {1149, 1150, 2127}. These patients have higher viral copy numbers in peripheral blood (PB), and instead of B-cells, T-cells or natural killer (NK)-cells are EBV-infected. These cases frequently manifest monoclonal T-cell populations and progression to overt malignant T-cell malignancy is the rule. CAEBV with monoclonal EBV+ T-cell proliferation represents part of the spectrum of systemic EBV+ T-cell LPD of childhood {1797}, and to avoid confusion should not be referred as to CAEBV.

Epidemiology
Systemic EBV+ T-cell LPD of childhood is most prevalent in Asia, primarily in Japan and Taiwan {1144, 1149, 2115, 2127}. It has been reported in Mexico and rarely in Western countries {1797}. It occurs most often in children and young adults. There is no sex predilection.

Etiology
Although the etiology is unknown, its association with primary EBV infection, and the racial predisposition, strongly suggests a genetic defect in the host immune response to EBV {1144, 1149, 1797, 2115, 2127}.

Sites of involvement
It is a systemic disease. The most commonly involved sites are liver and spleen followed by lymph nodes, bone marrow (BM), skin and lung {1144, 1149, 1797, 2115, 2127}.

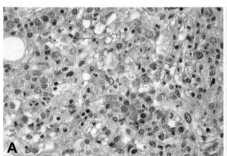 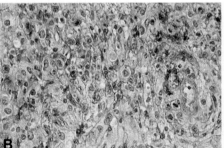 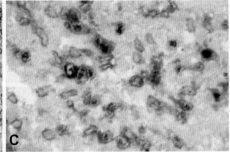

Fig.11.10 Systemic EBV+ T-cell LPD of childhood. **A** The bone marrow shows histiocytic hyperplasia with a lymphoid infiltrate composed of rather large cells with bland nuclei and inconspicuous nucleoli. **B** CD8 is positive in the large lymphoid cells. **C** Double stains demonstrate that most of the lymphocytes are EBER- and CD8-positive.

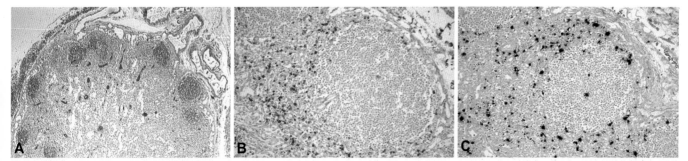

Fig. 11.11 Systemic EBV+ T-cell LPD of childhood. **A** The lymph node is unremarkable with preserved architecture and open sinuses. **B** There are numerous CD8-positive small lymphocytes surrounding the follicles. **C** Neoplastic cells are difficult to identify in H&E stained sections, but are highlighted with EBER *in situ* hybridization. The EBER-positive cells have the same distribution pattern as the CD8-positive lymphocytes.

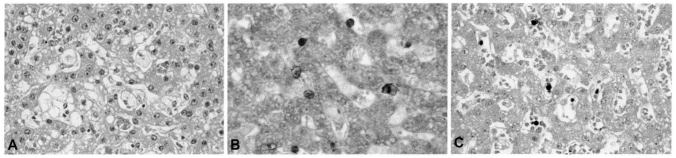

Fig. 11.12 Systemic EBV+ T-cell LPD of childhood. **A** The liver shows a subtle sinusoidal lymphoid infiltrate lacking cytologic atypia. Erythrophagocytosis is prominent. **B** The infiltrating lymphocytes are CD8-positive. **C** Nearly all lymphocytes in the sinusoids are EBER-positive.

Clinical features

Previously healthy patients present with acute onset of fever and general malaise suggestive of an acute viral respiratory illness. Within a period of weeks to months, patients develop hepatosplenomegaly and liver failure, sometimes accompanied by lymphadenopathy. Laboratory tests show pancytopenia, abnormal liver function tests and often an abnormal EBV serology with low or absent anti-VCA IgM antibodies. The disease is usually complicated by haemophagocytic syndrome, coagulopathy, multiorgan failure and sepsis {1797}. Some cases occur in patients with a well-documented history of CAEBV infection {1069, 1094}.

Morphology

The infiltrating T-cells are usually small and lack significant cytologic atypia {1797}. However, cases with pleomorphic medium-sized to large lymphoid cells, irregular nuclei and frequent mitoses have been described {2127}. The liver and spleen show mild to marked sinusoidal infiltration with striking haemophagocytosis. The splenic white pulp is depleted. The liver has prominent portal and sinusoidal infiltration, cholestasis, steatosis and necrosis. The lymph nodes usually show preserved architecture with open sinuses. A variable degree of sinus histiocytosis with erythrophagocytosis is present. Bone marrow biopsies show histiocytic hyperplasia with prominent erythrophagocytosis.

Immunophenotype

The most typical phenotype of the neoplastic cells is CD2+ CD3+ CD56- and TIA1+. Most cases secondary to acute primary EBV infection are CD8+ {1113, 1797, 2115}, whereas cases in the setting of severe CAEBV are CD4+ {1069, 1094, 1797}. Rare cases show both CD4+ and CD8+ EBV-infected T-cells {1797}. EBV-encoded RNA (EBER) is positive.

Genetics

The cells have monoclonally rearranged T-cell receptor *(TCR)* genes. All cases

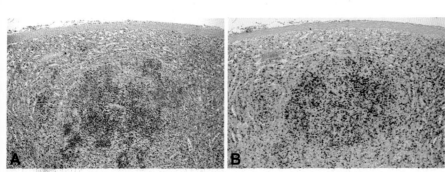

Fig. 11.13 Systemic EBV+ T-cell LPD of childhood. **A** The spleen shows depletion of the white pulp and prominent sinusoidal and nodular lymphoid infiltrates. The nodules are composed predominantly of CD4-positive cells. **B** EBER *in situ* hybridization shows that the CD4-positive cells are also positive for EBV RNA.

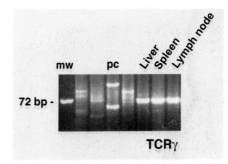

Fig.11.14 Systemic EBV+ T-cell LPD of childhood. PCR for *TRG@* gene. PCR demonstrates an identical T-cell clone in the liver, spleen and lymph nodes.

harbour EBV in a clonal episomal form {1069, 1144, 1149, 2127}. All cases analyzed carry type A EBV, either with wild-type or the 30 bp deleted product of *LMP1* gene {1113, 1797, 2127}. *In situ* hybridization for EBER shows that the majority of the infiltrating lymphoid cells are positive. No consistent chromosomal aberrations have been identified {402, 1149}.

Postulated normal counterpart
Cytotoxic CD8+ T lymphocytes or activated CD4+ T-cells.

Prognosis and predictive factors
Most cases have a fulminant clinical course resulting in death, usually from days to weeks. However, some cases show a subacute course of several months to a year.

Hydroa vacciniforme-like lymphoma

Definition
Hydroa vacciniforme-like lymphoma is an EBV-positive cutaneous T-cell lymphoma occurring in children, and associated with sun sensitivity.

ICD-O code
The provisional code proposed for the fourth edition of ICD-O is *9725/3*.

Epidemiology
This condition is seen mainly in children and adolescents from Asia, or in Native Americans from Central and South America, and Mexico. Like other EBV-positive T-cell and NK-cell lymphomas, predisposition for this condition may be related to a defective cytotoxic immune response to EBV. It is rare in adults {147, 432}.

Etiology
The neoplastic cells, usually T-cells, but sometimes NK-cells, are transformed by EBV. Patients exhibit hypersensitivity to sunlight, which precipitates clinical symptoms {1582}. A related condition is mosquito bite hypersensitivity. In the latter condition, the EBV-positive cells are of NK-cell origin.

Sites of involvement
This is a cutaneous condition that primarily affects sun-exposed skin, in particular the face {596, 1027}.

Clinical features
It is characterized by a papulovesicular eruption that generally proceeds to ulceration and scarring. In some cases, systemic symptoms including fever, wasting, lymphadenopathy and hepatosplenomegaly may be present, particularly late in the course of the disease {147, 399}.

Morphology
The neoplastic cells are generally small to medium in size without significant atypia. The infiltrates show extension from the epidermis to the subcutis, showing necrosis, angiocentricity and angioinvasion. The overlying epidermis is frequently ulcerated {147}.

Immunophenotype
The cells have a cytotoxic T-cell or, less often, NK-cell phenotype, with expression of CD56.

Genetics
Most cases have clonal rearrangements of the *TCR* genes. Some cases of NK-derivation will not show *TCR* gene rearrangement {399, 2455}.
EBER *in situ* hybridization is expressed in all of the atypical cells, but LMP1 is

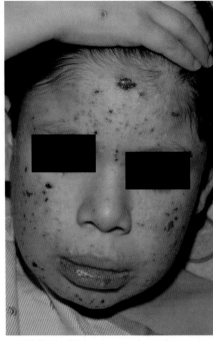

Fig. 11.15 Hydroa vacciniforme-like lymphoma. Sun-exposed areas of the skin exhibit a papulovesicular eruption. Many of the lesions are ulcerated with a haemorrhagic crust.

generally negative. EBV is monoclonal by terminal repeat analysis.

Postulated normal counterpart
Skin homing cytotoxic T-cell or NK-cell.

Prognosis and predictive factors
The clinical course is variable, and patients may have recurrent skin lesions for some time, up to 10–15 years, before progression to systemic involvement. With systemic spread, the clinical course is much more aggressive {1600}. Mosquito bite allergy is clinically more aggressive, and often associated with a haemophagocytic syndrome.

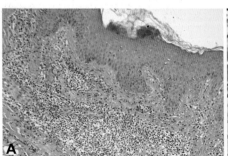
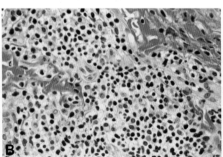
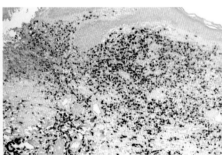

Fig. 11.16 Hydroa vacciniforme-like lymphoma. **A** The infiltrate is concentrated in the superficial dermis, but often extends to the subcutaneous tissue. **B** Neoplastic cells, which can be of T-cell or NK-cell lineage, are predominantly small, without marked atypia. **C** The lymphoid cells are positive for EBV, as demonstrated by *in situ* hybridization with the EBER probe.

Adult T-cell leukaemia/lymphoma

K. Ohshima
E.S. Jaffe
M. Kikuchi

Definition

A peripheral T-cell neoplasm most often composed of highly pleomorphic lymphoid cells. The disease is usually widely disseminated, and is caused by the human retrovirus known as human T-cell leukaemia virus type I (HTLV-I).

ICD-O code   9827/3

Epidemiology

Adult T-cell leukaemia/lymphoma (ATLL) is endemic in several regions of the world, in particular Southwestern Japan, the Caribbean basin and parts of Central Africa. The distribution of the disease is closely linked to the prevalence of HTLV-I in the population.

The disease has a long latency, and affected individuals usually are exposed to the virus very early in life. The virus may be transmitted in breast milk, and through exposure to peripheral blood (PB) and blood products. The cumulative incidence of ATLL is estimated to be 2.5% among HTLV-I carriers in Japan {2144}. Sporadic cases are described, but the affected patients often derive from an endemic region of the world. ATLL occurs only in adults and the age at onset ranges from the 20s to the 80s, with an average of 58 years. The male to female ratio is 1.5:1 {2462}.

Etiology

HTLV-I is causally linked to ATLL, but HTLV-I infection alone is not sufficient to result in neoplastic transformation of infected cells. The p40 tax viral protein leads to transcriptional activation of many genes in HTLV-I infected lymphocytes {726}. In addition, the HTLV-I basic leucine zipper factor (HBZ) is thought to be important for T-cell proliferation and oncogenesis {1940}. However, additional genetic alternations acquired over time may result in the development of a malignancy. HTLV-I also can indirectly cause other diseases, such as HTLV-I associated myelopathy/tropical spastic paraparesis {2148}.

Sites of involvement

Most ATLL patients present with widespread lymph node involvement as well as involvement of PB. The number of circulating neoplastic cells does not correlate with the degree of bone marrow (BM) involvement, suggesting that circulating cells are recruited from other organs such as the skin. In fact, the skin is the most common extralymphatic site of involvement (>50%).

The distribution of the disease is usually systemic, involving the spleen and extranodal sites including skin, lung, liver, gastrointestinal tract and central nervous system {298}. Epidemiological differences occur in patterns of presentation. For example,

Table 11.01 Clinical and morphological spectrum of HTLV-I-related diseases.

Neoplastic disorders
Peripheral blood (leukaemia)
Smoldering type
Chronic type
Acute type
Lymph node (lymphoma)
Hodgkin-like type
Pleomorphic small cell type
Pleomorphic (medium and large cells) type
Anaplastic large cell type
Skin
Erythema
Papule
Nodule
Gastrointestinal tract
Erosion
Ulceration
Tumour
Liver
Portal or sinus infiltration
Bone marrow
Infiltration with or without fibrosis
Reactive disorders
Confirmed
HTLV-I-associated myelopathy (HAM)
HTLV-I-associated uveitis
HTLV-I-associated lymphadenitis
Not-confirmed
HTLV-I-associated bronchopneumopathy (HAB)
HTLV-I-associated arthropathy (HAAP)
HTLV-I-associated nephropathy

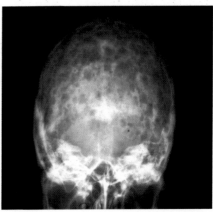

Fig. 11.17 Adult T-cell leukaemia/lymphoma. A radiograph shows extensive lytic bone lesions.

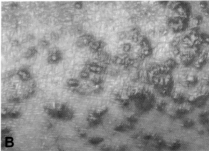

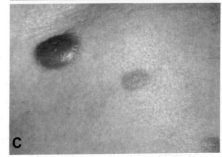

Fig.11.18 Adult T-cell leukaemia/lymphoma. Macroscopic findings of cutaneous lesions have been classified as erythema (**A**), papules (**B**) and nodules (**C**).

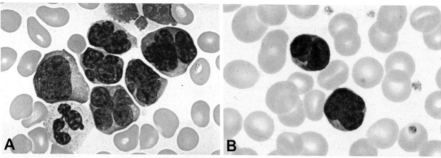

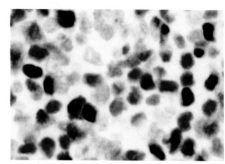

Fig. 11.19 Adult T-cell leukaemia/lymphoma. Peripheral blood films. **A** In the acute variant, the leukaemic cells are medium-sized to large lymphoid cells with irregular nuclei and basophilic cytoplasm. The characteristic Adult T-cell leukaemia/lymphoma cells have been described as "flower cells", with many nuclear convolutions and lobules. **B** Adult T-cell leukaemia/lymphoma cells in the chronic variant are generally small with slight nuclear abnormalities, such as notching, indentation, and convolution.

Fig. 11.20 Adult T-cell leukaemia/lymphoma cells frequently express FOXP3. The coexpression of FOXP3 and CD25 is characteristic of regulatory T-cells (Treg).

PB involvement is much less common in patients from the Caribbean basin than from Japan {1286}.

Clinical features

Several clinical variants have been identified: acute, lymphomatous, chronic and smoldering ATLL {2010}. The acute variant is most common and is characterized by a leukaemic phase, often with a markedly elevated white blood cell (WBC) count, skin rash and generalized lymphadenopathy. Hypercalcaemia, with or without lytic bone lesions, is a common feature. Patients with acute ATLL have a systemic disease accompanied by hepatosplenomegaly, constitutional symptoms, and elevated lactic dehydrogenase. Leukocytosis and eosinophilia are common. Many patients have an associated T-cell immunodeficiency, with frequent opportunistic infections such as *Pneumocystis jirovecii* pneumonia and Strongyloidiasis. The lymphomatous variant is characterized by prominent lymphadenopathy but without PB involvement. Most patients present with advanced stage disease similar to the acute form, although hypercalcaemia is less often seen. Cutaneous lesions are common in both the acute and lymphomatous forms of ATLL. They are clinically diverse, and include erythematous rashes, papules and nodules. Larger nodules may show ulceration.

The chronic variant is frequently associated with an exfoliative skin rash. While an absolute lymphocytosis may be present, atypical lymphocytes are not numerous in the PB. Hypercalcaemia is absent.

In the smoldering variant, the WBC count is normal with >5% circulating neoplastic cells. ATLL cells are generally small with a normal appearance. Patients frequently

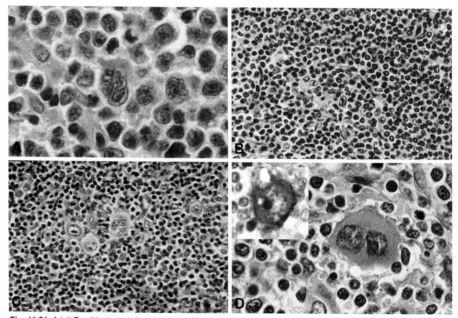

Fig. 11.21 Adult T-cell leukaemia/lymphoma. **A** The pleomorphic (medium-sized and large cell) type shows a diffuse proliferation of atypical medium-sized to large lymphoid cells with irregular nuclei, intermingled with cerebriform giant cells (centre). **B** The lymph nodes of pleomorphic small cell type show a diffuse proliferation of atypical medium-sized to small lymphoid cells. **C** The presence of pleomorphic tumour cells and background eosinophilia may simulate a classical Hodgkin lymphoma. **D** The lymph nodes of Hodgkin-like adult T-cell leukaemia/lymphoma show Reed-Sternberg-like giant cells of B-cell, not T-cell, lineage, which react with CD30 antibody (inset), and are EBV+ (not shown).

Table 11.02

Diagnostic criteria for clinical subtypes of adult T-cell leukaemia/lymphoma. Modified from Shimoyama et al. {2010}.

	Smoldering	Chronic	Acute
Lymphocytosis	No	Increased	Increased
Blood abnormal lymphocytes	> 5%	Increased	Increased
LDH	Normal	Slight increased	Increased
Calcium	Normal	Normal	Variable
Skin rash	Erythema, papules	Variable	Variable
Lymphadenopathy	No	Mild	Variable
Hepatosplenomegaly	No	Mild	Variable
Bone marrow infiltration	No	No	Variable

have skin or pulmonary lesions, but there is no hypercalcaemia. Progression from the chronic or smoldering to the acute variant occurs in 25% of the cases, but usually after a long duration {2010}.

Morphology

ATLL is characterized by a broad spectrum of cytological features {1630}. Several morphological variants have been described, reflecting this varied cytology and referred to as pleomorphic small, medium and large cell types, anaplastic, and a rare form resembling angioimmunoblastic T-cell lymphoma {1630}. Use of these variants is optional but they call attention to the spectrum of morphological appearances. Some cases exhibit a leukaemic pattern of infiltration, with preservation or dilation of lymph node sinuses that contain malignant cells. The inflammatory background is usually sparse, although eosinophilia may be present. The neoplastic lymphoid cells are typically medium-sized to large, often with pronounced nuclear pleomorphism. The nuclear chromatin is coarsely clumped with distinct, sometimes prominent, nucleoli. Blast-like cells with transformed nuclei and dispersed chromatin are present in variable proportions {2010}. Giant cells with convoluted or polylobated nuclear contours may be present. Rare cases may be composed predominantly of small lymphocytes, with irregular nuclear contours. Cell size does not correlate with the clinical course {1036}, with the exception of the chronic and smoldering forms, in which the lymphocytes have a more normal appearance.

Lymph nodes in some patients in an early phase of adult T-cell lymphoma/leukaemia may exhibit a Hodgkin-lymphoma-like histology {1632}. The lymph nodes have expanded paracortical areas containing a diffuse infiltrate of small to medium-sized lymphocytes with mild nuclear irregularities, indistinct nucleoli and scant cytoplasm. Epstein Barr virus (EBV)+ B lymphocytes with Hodgkin-like features are interspersed in this background. The expansion of EBV+ B-cells is felt to be secondary to the underlying immunodeficiency seen in patients with ATLL.

In the PB, the polylobated appearance of the neoplastic cells has led to the term flower cells. These cells have deeply basophilic cytoplasm, most readily observed with Giemsa stains of air-dried smears. Marrow infiltrates are usually patchy, ranging from sparse to moderate. Osteoclastic activity may be prominent, even in the absence of BM infiltration by neoplastic cells.

Skin lesions are seen in more than 50% of patients with ATLL. Epidermal infiltration with Pautrier-like microabscesses are common {1630}. Dermal infiltration is mainly perivascular, but larger tumour nodules with extension to subcutaneous fat may be observed.

Diffuse infiltration of many organs is indicative of the systemic nature of the disease, and presence of circulating malignant cells.

Immunophenotype

Tumour cells express T-cell-associated antigens (CD2, CD3, CD5), but usually lack CD7. While most cases are CD4+, CD8-, a few are CD4-, CD8+ or double positive for CD4 and CD8. CD25 is strongly expressed in nearly all cases. The large transformed cells may be positive for CD30, but are negative for ALK {2149} and cytotoxic molecules. In addition, tumour cells frequently express the chemokine receptor CCR4 and FOXP3, a feature of regulatory T-cells {1112}.

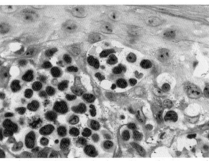

Fig. 11.22 Neoplastic cells infiltrate the epidermis, producing Pautrier-like microabscesses.

Genetics

Antigen receptor genes

T-cell receptor genes are clonally rearranged {1631}.

Oncogenes and other molecular changes

Neoplastic cells show monoclonal integration of HTLV-I. No clonal integration is present in healthy carriers {2274}. Tax, encoded by the HTLV-I pX region, is a critical nonstructural protein that plays a central role in leukaemogenesis, and activates a variety of cellular genes {1722}. Furthermore, enhancement of cyclic AMP response element binding transcription factor (CREB) phosphorylation by the

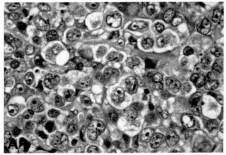 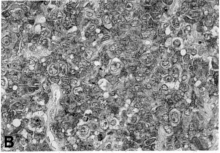

Fig. 11.23 Adult T-cell leukaemia/lymphoma. **A** In this case, the infiltrate consists of large cells with anaplastic features. **B** The cells are strongly CD30+, raising the differential diagnosis of anaplastic large cell lymphoma.

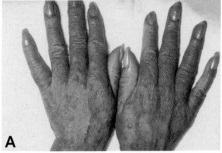 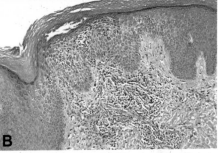

Fig. 11.24 Adult T-cell leukaemia/lymphoma, smoldering variant. **A** Clinical photo shows the diffuse exfoliative skin rash. **B** A sparse infiltrate in the skin is seen with minimal cytologic atypia.

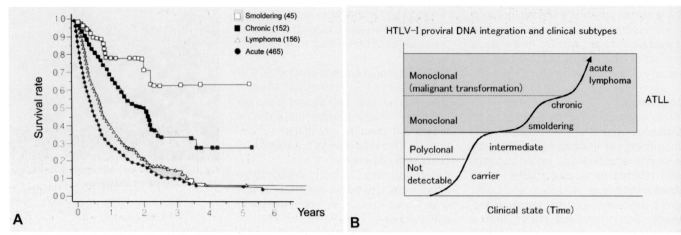

Fig. 11.25 A Survival of patients with adult T-cell leukaemia/lymphoma. Acute and lymphomatous forms have an aggressive clinical course, whereas longer survival in seen in patients with chronic or smoldering disease. **B** Adult T-cell leukaemia/lymphoma. HTLV-I proviral DNA integration and clinical subtypes.

virus appears to play a role in leukaemo-genesis {1148}.

Almost all ATLL cases have clonal chromosome numerical and structural abnormalities, but none of them is specific.

Postulated normal counterpart

Peripheral CD4+ T-cells. It has been suggested that the CD4+CD25+FOXP3+ regulatory T-cells are the closest normal counterpart {1112}. This finding correlates with the immunodeficiency characteristic of the disease.

Prognosis and predictive factors

Clinical subtypes, age, performance status, serum calcium and LDH levels are major prognostic factors {2464}. The survival time for the acute and lymphomatous variants ranges from two weeks to more than one year. Death is often caused by infectious complications including *Pneumocystis jirovecii* pneumonia, Cryptococcus meningitis, disseminated herpes zoster and hypercalcaemia {2010}. The chronic and smoldering forms have a more protracted clinical course and better survival, but can progress to an acute phase with an aggressive course {1633}.

Extranodal NK/T-cell lymphoma, nasal type

J.K.C. Chan
L. Quintanilla-Martinez
J.A. Ferry
S.-C. Peh

Definition

A predominantly extranodal lymphoma characterized by vascular damage and destruction, prominent necrosis, cytotoxic phenotype and association with Epstein-Barr virus (EBV). It is designated "NK/T" (instead of "NK"), because while most cases appear to be genuine NK-cell neoplasms, some cases show a cytotoxic T-cell phenotype.

ICD-O code   9719/3

Synonyms

Angiocentric T-cell lymphoma; malignant midline reticulosis; polymorphic reticulosis; lethal midline granuloma; angiocentric immunoproliferative lesion.

Epidemiology

Extranodal NK/T-cell lymphoma is more prevalent in Asians, and the native American population of Mexico, Central America and South America {55, 104, 381, 1795}. It occurs most often in adults, and is more common in males than females. A low frequency of HLA-A*0201 allele has been reported in patients with EBV-positive nasal NK/T lymphomas {1094A}.

Etiology

Little is known about the etiology of extranodal NK/T-cell lymphoma. However, the very strong association with EBV, irrespective of the ethnic origin of the patients, suggests a probable pathogenic role of the virus {70, 386, 389, 639, 1093, 1795, 2299}. The EBV is present in a clonal episomal form {70, 389, 639, 944, 1093, 1448, 1795, 2130, 2299} with type II latency pattern (EBNA-1+, EBNA-2-, LMP1+), and commonly shows a 30-base pair deletion in the latent membrane protein-1 gene {415, 589, 639, 1205, 2143}. Most studies show that the EBV is almost always of subtype A {148, 639, 1717, 2130, 2248}. The disease activity can also be monitored by measuring circulating EBV DNA; a high titer is furthermore correlated with extensive disease, unfavourable response to therapy and poor survival {105}.

Extranodal NK/T-cell lymphomas can occur in the setting of immunosuppression, including post-transplant {981, 1222}.

Sites of involvement

Extranodal NK/T-cell lymphoma almost always shows an extranodal presentation. The upper aerodigestive tract (nasal cavity, nasopharynx, paranasal sinuses, palate) is most commonly involved, with the nasal cavity being the prototypic site of involvement. Preferential sites of extranasal involvement include the skin, soft tissue, gastrointestinal tract and testis. Some cases may be accompanied by secondary lymph node involvement {381, 386, 1137, 1220, 1738, 2248}. Rare examples of primary lymph node disease in the absence of extranodal involvement have also been reported {421, 1082, 1905}.

Clinical features

Patients with nasal involvement present with symptoms of nasal obstruction or epistaxis due to presence of a mass lesion, or with extensive midfacial destructive

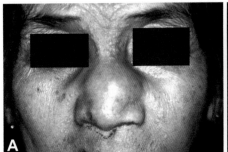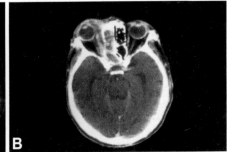

Fig. 11.26 Extranodal NK/T-cell lymphoma, nasal type. **A** Expansion of the nasal bridge. **B** Computed tomogram. The tumour in the nasal cavity extends upward into the orbit, resulting in proptosis.

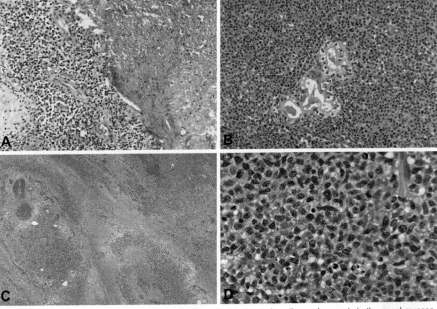

Fig. 11.27 Extranodal NK/T-cell lymphoma, nasal-type. **A** Prominent ulceration and necrosis in the nasal mucosa. **B** The nasal mucosa is diffusely infiltrated and expanded by an abnormal lymphoid infiltrate. The mucosal glands commonly show a peculiar clear cell change. **C,D** Nasal-type NK/T-cell lymphoma in the testis. **C** There is a diffuse dense lymphoid infiltrate, with prominent coagulative necrosis. **D** The neoplastic cells appear monotonous and are medium-sized.

lesions (lethal midline granuloma). The lymphoma can extend to adjacent tissues such as the nasopharynx, paranasal sinuses, orbit, oral cavity, palate and oropharynx. The disease is often localized to the upper aerodigestive tract at presentation, and bone marrow (BM) involvement is uncommon {2437}. The disease may disseminate rapidly to various sites, e.g. skin, gastrointestinal tract, testis or cervical lymph nodes during the clinical course. Some cases may be complicated by a haemophagocytic syndrome {413, 1220}.

Extranodal NK/T-cell lymphomas occurring outside the upper aerodigestive tract (often referred to as "extranasal NK/T-cell lymphomas") have variable presentations depending upon the major site of involvement. Skin lesions are commonly nodular, often with ulceration. Intestinal lesions often manifest as perforation. Other involved sites often present as mass lesions. The patients commonly have high stage disease at presentation, with involvement of multiple extranodal sites. Systemic symptoms such as fever, malaise and weight loss can be present {386, 1137, 2438}. Lymph nodes can be involved as part of disseminated disease. Marrow and peripheral blood (PB) involvement can occur, and such cases may overlap with aggressive NK-cell leukaemia.

This disease is to be distinguished from a spectrum of EBV-associated T-cell or NK-cell lymphoproliferative disorders such as chronic active EBV infection, systemic EBV+ T-cell lymphoproliferative disease of childhood and hydroa vacciniforme-like lymphoma, which occur predominantly in children {1149, 1600}.

Morphology

The histological features of extranodal NK/T-cell lymphoma are similar irrespective of the site of involvement. Mucosal sites often show extensive ulceration. The lymphomatous infiltrate is diffuse and permeative. Mucosal glands often become widely spaced or are lost. An angiocentric and angiodestructive growth pattern is frequently present, and fibrinoid changes can be seen in the blood vessels even in the absence of angioinvasion. Coagulative necrosis and admixed apoptotic bodies are very common findings. These have been attributed to vascular occlusion by lymphoma cells, but recent studies have also implicated other factors (such as chemokines, cytokines) {2185}.

The cytological spectrum of extranodal NK/T-cell lymphoma is very broad. Cells may be small, medium-sized, large or anaplastic. In most cases, the lymphoma is composed of medium-sized cells or a mixture of small and large cells. The cells often have irregularly folded nuclei which can be elongated. The chromatin is granular, except in the very large cells, which may have vesicular nuclei. Nucleoli are generally inconspicuous or small. The cytoplasm is moderate in amount and often pale to clear. Mitotic figures are easily found, even for small cell-predominant

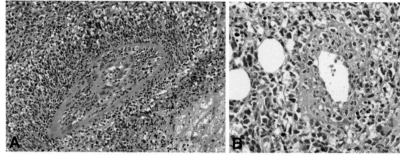

Fig. 11.28 Extranodal NK/T-cell lymphoma, nasal type. A The lymphomatous infiltrate shows infiltration and destruction of an artery. B In this case involving the skin, the lymphomatous infiltrate has an angiocentric angiodestructive quality.

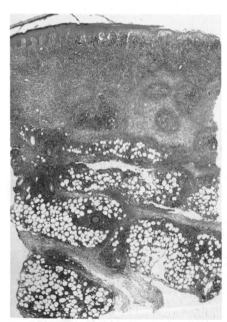

Fig. 11.29 Extranodal NK/T-cell lymphoma in the skin. The lymphomatous infiltrate involves the epidermis, dermis and subcutaneous tissue.

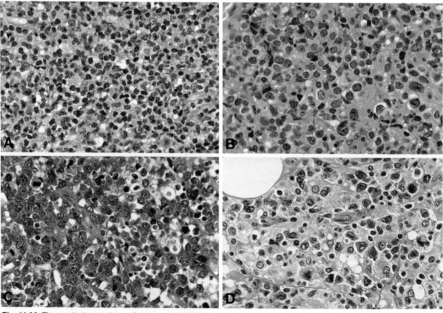

Fig. 11.30 The cytologic spectrum of extranodal NK/T-cell lymphoma, nasal type. A,B,C This nasal tumour is composed predominantly of small cells with irregular nuclei (A). Medium-sized cells with pale cytoplasm (B). Large cells (C). D Nasal type extranodal NK/T-cell lymphoma of skin, with pleomorphic large cells admixed with smaller cells.

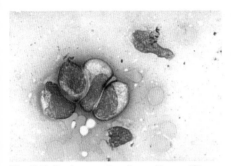

Fig. 11.31 Touch preparation of a nasal tumour (Giemsa stain). Azurophilic granules are evident in the pale cytoplasm of the lymphoma cells.

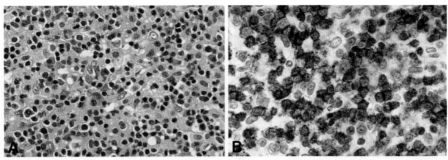

Fig. 11.32 Extranodal NK/T-cell lymphoma, nasal type. **A** This example is difficult to diagnose because the neoplastic cells are practically indistinguishable from normal small lymphocytes. There are many admixed plasma cells. **B** The presence of large numbers of cells staining for CD56 supports a diagnosis of lymphoma.

lesions. In touch preparations stained with Giemsa, azurophilic granules are commonly detected. Ultrastructurally, electron-dense membrane-bound granules are present.

Extranodal NK/T-cell lymphomas, particularly those predominated by small or mixed cell populations, or those accompanied by a heavy admixture of inflammatory cells (small lymphocytes, plasma cells, histiocytes and eosinophils) may mimic an inflammatory process {381, 911}. The lymphoma can sometimes be accompanied by florid pseudoepitheliomatous hyperplasia of the overlying epithelium.

Immunophenotype
The most typical immunophenotype of extranodal NK/T-cell lymphoma is: CD2+, CD56+, surface CD3- (as demonstrated on fresh or frozen tissue) and cytoplasmic CD3ε+ (as demonstrated on fresh, frozen or fixed tissues) {381, 388, 1032, 1037, 2273}. CD56, although a highly useful marker for NK-cells, is not specific for extranodal NK/T-cell lymphoma and can be expressed in peripheral T-cell lymphomas, particularly those that express the γδ T-cell receptor.

Cytotoxic molecules (such as granzyme B, TIA1 and perforin) are positive {639}. Other T- and NK-cell associated antigens are usually negative, including CD4, CD5, CD8, TCRδ, βF1, CD16 and CD57. CD43, CD45RO, HLA-DR, CD25, FAS (CD95) and FAS ligand are commonly expressed {1589, 1634}. Occasional cases are positive for CD7 or CD30 {1205}.

Lymphomas that demonstrate a CD3ε+, CD56- immunophenotype are also classified as extranodal NK/T-cell lymphomas if both cytotoxic molecules and EBV are positive, since these cases show a similar clinical disease as cases with CD56

expression {1590}. On the other hand, nasal or other extranodal lymphomas that are CD3+, CD56-, but negative for EBV and cytotoxic molecules should be diagnosed as peripheral T-cell lymphoma, not otherwise specified.

A diagnosis of extranodal NK/T-cell lymphoma should be accepted with some skepticism if EBV is negative {307, 389, 639, 1205, 1590, 2143}. *In situ* hybridization for EBV encoded RNA (EBER) is the most reliable way to demonstrate presence of EBV, with virtually all lymphoma cells being labeled. Immunostaining for EBV LMP1 yields variable and inconsistent results.

Genetics
Antigen receptor genes
T-cell receptor and immunoglobulin genes are in germline configuration in most cases. In a small proportion of cases, the T-cell receptor genes show clonal rearrangement, presumably corresponding to the cases of cytotoxic T lymphocyte derivation {1169, 1590, 2143}.

Cytogenetic abnormalities and oncogenes
A variety of cytogenetic aberrations have been reported, but so far no specific chromosomal translocations have been identified. The commonest cytogenetic abnormality is del(6)(q21q25) or i(6)(p10), but it is currently unclear whether this is a primary or progression-associated event {2028, 2029, 2238, 2440}. Aberrant methylation of promoter CpG regions of multiple genes is common, in particular p73 {2027}. Comparative genomic hybridization studies show that the commonest aberrations are: gain of 2q; and loss of 1p36.23-p36.33, 6q16.1-q27, 4q12, 5q34-q35.3, 7q21.3-q22.1, 11q22.3-q23.3 and 15q11.2-q14 {1567}. A proportion of cases exhibit partial deletion of *FAS* gene or mutation in *TP53*, ß-catenin, *KRAS* or *KIT* gene, but the significance is still unclear {959, 1796, 2002}.

Postulated normal counterpart
Activated NK cells and, less commonly, cytotoxic T lymphocytes.

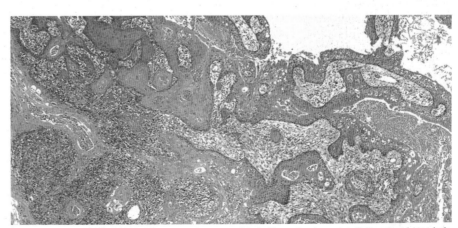

Fig. 11.33 Extranodal NK/T-cell lymphoma, nasal type associated with prominent pseudoepitheliomatous hyperplasia of the mucosal epithelium. This can potentially be misinterpreted as squamous cell carcinoma.

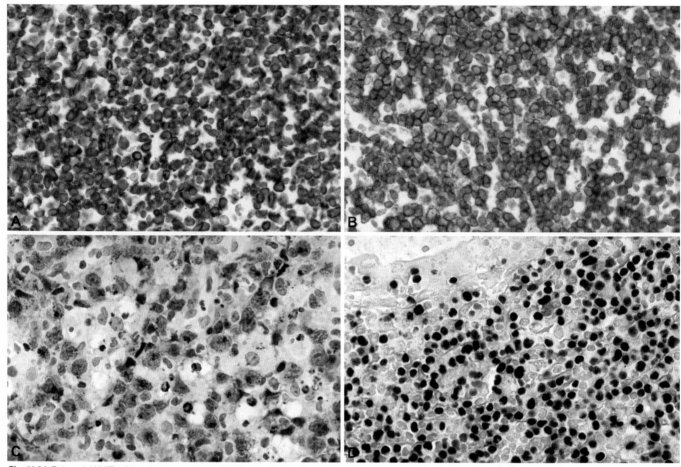

Fig. 11.34 Extranodal NK/T-cell lymphoma, nasal type. **A,B** The neoplastic cells show strong staining for cytoplasmic CD3ε (**A**) and CD56 (**B**). **C** The neoplastic cells show strong granular staining for granzyme B. **D** *In situ* hybridization for EBV-encoded RNA (EBER). In this nasal tumour, practically all the neoplastic cells show nuclear labeling.

Prognosis and predictive factors

The prognosis of nasal NK/T-cell lymphoma is variable, with some patients responding well to therapy and others dying of disseminated disease despite aggressive therapy. Historically, the survival rate has been poor (30–40%), but the survival has improved in recent years with more intensive therapy including upfront radiotherapy {148, 413, 414, 422, 493, 1169, 1220, 1293}. Significant unfavourable prognostic factors include: advanced stage disease (stage III or IV), unfavourable International Prognostic Index (2), invasion of bone or skin, high circulating EBV DNA levels and presence of EBV+ cells in BM {414, 422, 991, 1266, 1590}. The prognostic importance of cytological grade is unclear; some studies suggest that tumours composed predominantly of small cells are less aggressive, but most studies have not shown this feature to be of significance on multivariate analysis {148, 413, 943, 1205}.

Extranodal NK/T-cell lymphoma occurring outside the nasal cavity is highly aggressive, with short survival times and poor response to therapy {381, 386}. Expression of multi-drug resistance genes may contribute to chemotherapy resistance {612}.

Enteropathy-associated T-cell lymphoma

P.G. Isaacson
A. Chott
G. Ott
H. Stein

Definition

Enteropathy-associated T-cell lymphoma (EATL) is an intestinal tumour of intra-epithelial T lymphocytes, showing varying degrees of transformation but usually presenting as a tumour composed of large lymphoid cells, often with an inflammatory background. The adjacent small intestinal mucosa shows villous atrophy with crypt hyperplasia. In 10–20% of cases, the lymphoma is composed of monomorphic medium-sized cells. This monomorphic variant (type II EATL) may occur sporadically, without risk factors for coeliac disease.

ICD-O code   9717/3

Synonyms

Intestinal T-cell lymphoma (with and without enteropathy). As a variety of T-cell lymphoma subtypes can present with intestinal disease (extranodal NK/T-cell lymphoma, γδ T-cell lymphoma, anaplastic large cell lymphoma), the term intestinal T-cell lymphoma should be used only in the setting of incomplete information regarding the precise diagnosis.

Epidemiology

The disease is uncommon in most parts of the world, but is seen with greater frequency in those areas with a high prevalence of coeliac disease, in particular Northern Europe. However, the monomorphic variant appears to have a broader geographic distribution, and is encountered in Asia and other regions where coeliac disease is rare.

Etiology

In EATL, the association with coeliac disease is borne out by positive serological tests, HLA DQ2 or DQ8 expression and associated clinical findings such as dermatitis herpetiformis and hyposplenism {569, 1921, 2305}. In the monomorphic form of EATL, an association with coeliac disease and other risk factors is not proven {548}, suggesting that the monomorphic variant may represent a distinct disease entity.

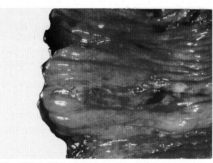

Fig. 11.35 Enteropathy-associated T-cell lymphoma. Jejunum showing circumferentially-oriented ulcers.

Sites of involvement

The lymphoma occurs most commonly in the jejunum or ileum. Presentation in the duodenum, stomach, colon or outside the gastrointestinal tract may occur but is rare.

Clinical features

In EATL, a small proportion of the patients have a history of childhood onset coeliac disease. Most show adult onset disease or are diagnosed as having coeliac disease in the same clinical episode in which the lymphoma is diagnosed. Patients present with abdominal pain, often associated with intestinal perforation. In a proportion of patients, there is a prodromal period of refractory coeliac disease that is sometimes accompanied by intestinal ulceration (ulcerative jejunitis). The clinical

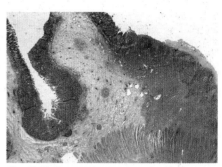

Fig. 11.36 Enteropathy-associated T-cell lymphoma, deeply infiltrating into adjacent enteropathic mucosa.

presentation of the monomorphic variant is similar, with the exception that most patients do not demonstrate evidence of coeliac disease.

Macroscopy

The tumour usually presents as multiple ulcerating raised mucosal masses, but may present as one or more ulcers or as a large exophytic mass.

Morphology

The tumour forms an ulcerating mucosal mass that invades the wall of the intestine. The tumour cells exhibit a wide range of cytological appearances {1015, 2448}. Most commonly, the tumour cells are relatively monotonous medium-sized to large cells with round or angulated vesicular nuclei, prominent nucleoli and moderate

Table 11.03 Features of enteropathy-associated intestinal T-cell lymphoma (EATL) and monomorphic intestinal T-cell lymphoma (Type II EATL).

	EATL	Type II EATL
Frequency	80–90%	10-20%
Morphology	Variable	Monomorphic small to medium
Immunophenotype {437}		
CD8	Mostly negative (20%+)	Mostly positive (80%+)
CD56	Negative (>90%)	Positive (>90%)
HLA-DQ2/-DQ8	Positive (>90%)	Positive (30-40%)*
Genetics {548}		
+ 9q31.3 or - 16q12.1	86%	83%
+ 1q32.2-q41	73%	27%
+ 5q34-q35.2	80%	20%
+ 8q24 (MYC)	27%	73%

* Corresponding to the normal frequency of HLA-DQ2/-DQ8 among the Caucasian population.

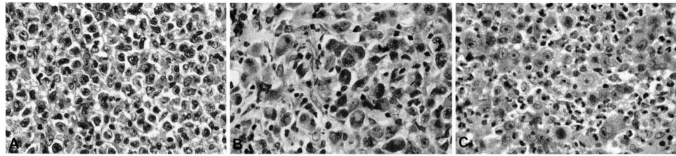

Fig. 11.37 Enteropathy-associated T-cell lymphoma. **A** Tumour cells are characterized by moderate amounts of eosinophilic cytoplasm and round or angulated nuclei with prominent nucleoli. **B** Anaplastic variant of enteropathy-associated T-cell lymphoma. **C** There is a heavy infiltrate of eosinophils between the tumour cells.

to abundant, pale-staining cytoplasm. Less commonly, the tumour exhibits marked pleomorphism with multinucleated cells bearing a resemblance to anaplastic large cell lymphoma. Most tumours show infiltration by inflammatory cells, including large numbers of histiocytes and eosinophils and in some cases these may be so abundant as to obscure the relatively small number of tumour cells present. Infiltration of the epithelium of individual crypts is present in many cases. The intestinal mucosa adjacent to the tumours, especially those in the jejunum, usually shows enteropathy comprising villous atrophy, crypt hyperplasia, increased lamina propria lymphocytes and plasma cells and intraepithelial lymphocytosis {437, 438}. The degree of enteropathy is highly variable, however, and may consist only of an increase in intraepithelial lymphocytes {124}.

In the monomorphic form of EATL (type II EATL), the neoplastic cells have medium-sized round, darkly staining nuclei with a rim of pale cytoplasm. There is usually florid infiltration of intestinal crypt epithelium. The adjacent intestinal mucosa shows villous atrophy and crypt hyperplasia with striking intraepithelial lymphocytosis involving both crypt and surface epithelium. An inflammatory background is absent, and necrosis is usually less evident than in classical EATL.

Immunophenotype

In EATL, the tumour cells are CD3+, CD5-, CD7+, CD8-/+, CD4-, CD103+, TCRß+/-, and contain cytotoxic granule associated proteins. In almost all cases, a varying proportion of the tumour cells express CD30 {2064, 2448}. The intraepithelial lymphocytes in the adjacent enteropathic mucosa may show an abnormal immunophenotype, usually CD3+, CD5-, CD8-,

CD4-, identical to that of the lymphoma. The monomorphic form of EATL has a distinctive immunophenotype. The tumour cells are CD3+, CD4-, CD8+, CD56+ and TCRß+ {437} and the intraepithelial lymphocytes in the adjacent mucosa share the identical immunophenotype {124}.

Genetics

TRB@ and *TRG@* genes are clonally rearranged {1017, 1552} in all morphological variants. More than 90% of patients with coeliac disease have the *HLADQA1*0501, DQB1*0201* genotype, also seen in patients with EATL {984}.

In contrast to primary nodal PTCL, most EATL cases (58–70%) harbour complex segmental amplifications of the 9q31.3-qter chromosome region or, alternatively, show deletions in 16q12.1. These features

are prevalent in both forms of EATL and form a common genetic link between the 2 types. However, the classical form of EATL frequently displays chromosomal gains in 1q and 5q, while the monomorphic variant is more often characterized by 8q24 *(MYC)* amplifications {548, 2491, 2494}

Precursor lesions

As indicated above, EATL may be preceded by refractory coeliac diseases (RCD) with or without ulceration. In some cases of RCD, the intraepithelial lymphocytes (IEL) are phenotypically aberrant showing down-regulation of CD8 similar to the IEL in mucosa adjacent to EATL. These cases of RCD also show monoclonal T-cell rearrangement of the IEL similar to the clonal rearrangements that may

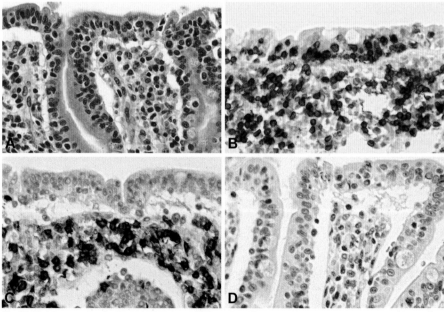

Fig. 11.38 Adjacent uninvolved mucosa in enteropathy-associated T-cell lymphoma. Increased numbers of intraepithelial lymphocytes (**A**) are CD3-positive (**B**), CD8-negative (**C**) and CD56-negative (**D**).

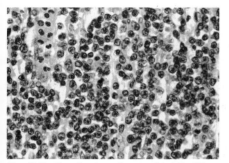

Fig. 11.39 Type II enteropathy-associated T-cell lymphoma composed of small round monomorphic cells.

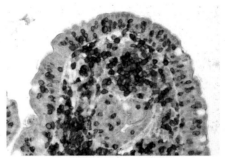

Fig. 11.40 A Small intestinal mucosa from a case of refractory coeliac disease immunostained sequentially for CD3 (alkaline phosphatase-blue) and CD8 (peroxidase-brown). Most intraepithelial lymphocytes are CD3+, CD8-.

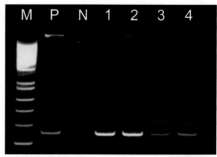

Fig. 11.41 PCR of DNA extracted from enteropathy-associated T-cell lymphoma. M, molecular weight marker; P, positive control; N, negative control; lanes 1 and 2, lymphoma; lanes 3 and 4, adjacent non-lymphomatous mucosa.

be found in the enteropathic mucosa adjacent to EATL {124}, suggesting that the immunophenotypically aberrant IEL constitute a neoplastic population. In those patients with RCD who subsequently develop EATL, the IEL share the same monoclonal *TRG@* gene rearrangement as the subsequent T-cell lymphoma {89, 358, 359, 508}. Furthermore, the IEL in these cases of RCD carry gains of chromosome 1q in common with EATL {2332}. Thus, RCD in which the IEL show these immunophenotypic and genetic features can be considered as examples of intraepithelial T-cell lymphoma or, alternatively, EATL *in situ*. In a second group of RCD patients {2332}, the IEL express a normal immunophenotype and are polyclonal. These cases probably do not progress to EATL.

The monomorphic form of EATL may also be preceded by RCD in which the immunophenotype of the IEL is similar to that of the neoplastic cells in the subsequent lymphoma, namely CD8+ and CD56+. This type of RCD has not been well characterized.

Postulated normal counterpart
Intraepithelial T-cells of the intestine.

Prognosis and predictive factors
The prognosis is usually poor with death frequently resulting from abdominal complications in patients already weakened by uncontrolled malabsorption. Recurrences are most frequent in the small intestine. Both classical EATL and the monomorphic form have a similar clinical course.

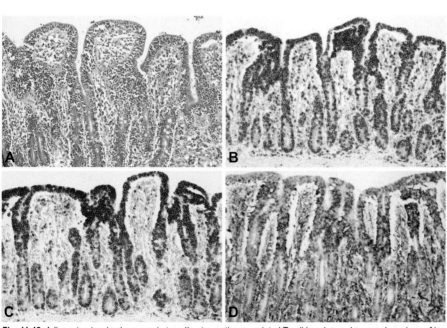

Fig. 11.42 Adjacent uninvolved mucosa in type II enteropathy-associated T-cell lymphoma. Increased numbers of intraepithelial lymphocytes (**A**) are CD3-positive (**B**), CD8-positive (**C**) and CD56-positive (**D**).

Hepatosplenic T-cell lymphoma

P. Gaulard
E.S. Jaffe
L. Krenacs
W.R. Macon

Definition
Hepatosplenic T-cell lymphoma (HSTL) is an extranodal and systemic neoplasm derived from cytotoxic T-cells usually of γδ T-cell receptor type. It is usually composed of medium-sized lymphoid cells, demonstrating marked sinusoidal infiltration of spleen, liver and bone marrow (BM).

ICD-O code   9716/3

Epidemiology
HSTL is a rare form of lymphoma, representing <1% of all non-Hodgkin lymphomas. Peak incidence occurs in adolescents and young adults, with a male predominance (median, ~35 years) {176, 465}.

Etiology
Up to 20% of HSTL arise in the setting of chronic immune suppression, most commonly long term immunosuppressive therapy for solid organ transplantation or prolonged antigenic stimulation {176, 764, 2322, 2451}. In this context, HSTL is regarded as a late-onset post-transplantation lymphoproliferative disorder of host origin. HSTL may also occur in patients, especially children, treated by azathioprine and infliximab for Crohn's disease {1355, 1872}.

Sites of involvement
Patients present with marked splenomegaly, usually with hepatomegaly, but with no lymphadenopathy {672}. Bone marrow is almost constantly involved {176, 465, 2321}.

Clinical features
HSTL typically presents with hepatosplenomegaly and systemic symptoms. Patients usually manifest marked thrombocytopenia, often with anaemia and leukopenia. Peripheral blood involvement, uncommon at presentation, may occur late in the clinical course {176, 465, 2321}. HSTL is easily distinguishable from other γδ T-cell lymphomas which involve extranodal localizations (skin and subcutaneous tissue, intestine or the nasal region) {81, 2254}.

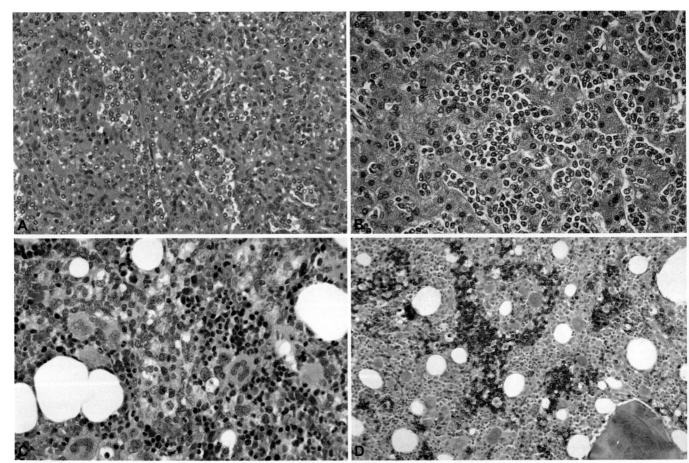

Fig. 11.43 Hepatosplenic T-cell lymphoma. **A** Cords and sinusoids of the spleen are infiltrated by a monotonous population of neoplastic lymphoid cells with medium-sized nuclei and a moderate rim of pale cytoplasm. **B** The neoplastic cells diffusely infiltrate the hepatic sinusoids. **C** The bone marrow is usually hypercellular with neoplastic cells infiltrating sinusoids. **D** Neoplastic cells highlighted with immunohistochemistry for CD3.

Morphology

The spleen is enlarged with diffuse involvement of the red pulp, without any gross lesions. Diffuse hepatic enlargement is present as well.

Histopathologically, the cells of HSTL are monotonous, with medium-sized nuclei and a rim of pale cytoplasm {465}. The nuclear chromatin is loosely condensed with small inconspicuous nucleoli. They involve the cords and sinuses of the splenic red pulp with atrophy of the white pulp. The liver shows a predominant sinusoidal infiltration. Neoplastic cells are almost constantly present in the the BM with a predominantly intrasinusoidal distribution. This may be difficult to identify without the aid of immunohistochemistry or flow cytometry. Cytologic atypia with large cell or blastic changes may be seen, especially with disease progression {176, 1414, 2321}

Immunophenotype

The neoplastic cells are CD3+ and usually TCRδ1 +, TCRαβ-, CD56+/-, CD4-, CD8-/+ and CD5-. Most γδ cases express the Vδ1 epitope {176, 1783}. A minority of cases appear to be of αβ type, which is considered a variant of the more common γδ form of the disease {1357, 2117}. The cells express the cytotoxic granule-associated proteins, TIA1 and granzyme M, but are usually negative for granzyme B and perforin {465, 678, 1191}. They often show aberrant coincident expression of multiple killer immunoglobulin-like receptors (KIR) isoforms along with dim or absent CD94 {1522}. Therefore, the cells appear to be mature, non-activated cytotoxic T-cells with phenotypic aberrancy.

Genetics

The cells have rearranged TRG@ genes. Cases of γδ origin show a biallelic rearrangement of TRG@ genes. TRB@ genes are rearranged in αβ cases; however, non-productive rearrangement of TRB@ genes have been reported in some γδ cases {764}. Isochromosome 7q is present in most cases, and with disease progression a variety of FISH patterns equivalent to two to five copies of i(7)(q10) or numerical and structural aberrations of the second chromosome 7 have been detected {27, 2425}. Ring chromosome leading to 7q amplification has also been reported {2154}. Trisomy 8 and loss of a sex chromosome may also be present. EBV is generally negative.

Postulated normal counterpart

Peripheral γδ (or less commonly αβ) cytotoxic memory T-cells of the innate immune system {1035, 1191}.

Prognosis and predictive factors

The course is aggressive. Patients may respond initially to chemotherapy, but relapses are seen in the vast majority of cases. The median survival is <2 years {176}. Platinum-cytarabine {176} and pentostatin have been shown to be active agents {473A}.

Subcutaneous panniculitis-like T-cell lymphoma

E.S. Jaffe
P. Gaulard
E. Ralfkiaer
L. Cerroni
C.J.L.M. Meijer

Definition

Subcutaneous panniculitis-like T-cell lymphoma (SPTCL) is a cytotoxic T-cell lymphoma, which preferentially infiltrates subcutaneous tissue. It is composed of atypical lymphoid cells of varying size, typically with karyorrhexis of tumour cells and associated fat necrosis. In contrast to the third edition of the WHO classification, cases expressing the γδ T-cell receptor are excluded, and now reclassified as primary cutaneous γδ T-cell lymphoma.

ICD-O code   9708/3

Epidemiology

SPTCL is a rare form of lymphoma, representing <1% of all non-Hodgkin lymphomas. It is slightly more common in females than males and has a broad age range {1202}. Approximately 20% of patients are under the age of 20 (median, 35 years) {2408}. Up to 20% of patients may have associated autoimmune disease, most commonly systemic lupus erythematosus (SLE) {2408}.

Etiology

Autoimmune disease may play a role in some patients. The lesions may show overlapping features with lupus profundus panniculitis and in some patients a diagnosis of SLE has been documented {1365, 1412}. In some patients, the early lesions may closely mimic lobular panniculitis. Whether a benign lobular panniculitis precedes the development of SPTCL in patients without SLE is not clear. Epstein-Barr virus is absent {1202}.

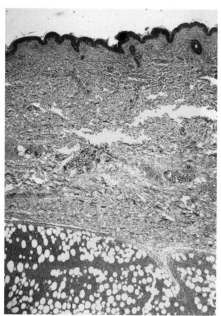

Fig. 11.44 Subcutaneous panniculitis-like lymphoma. Infiltrate is confined to the subcutaneous tissue without involvement of the overlying dermis or epidermis.

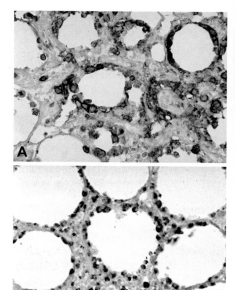

Fig. 11.45 Immunohistochemical stains highlight the rimming of individual fat spaces by tumour cells with staining for CD8 (**A**) and TIA1 (**B**).

Sites of involvement

Patients present with multiple subcutaneous nodules, usually in the absence of other sites of disease. The most common sites of localization are the extremities and trunk. The nodules range in size from 0.5 cm to several centimetres in diameter.

Table 11.04 Differential diagnosis of neoplasms expressing T-cell and NK-cell markers with frequent cutaneous involvement.

Disease	Clinical features	CD3, CD4, CD8	Cytotoxic molecules°	CD56	EBV	T-cell receptor	Lineage
SPTCL	Tumours, extremities and trunk	+, -, +	+	-	-	R	T-cell
Primary cutaneous γδ TCL	Tumours, plaques, ulcerated nodules	+, -, -/+	+	+	-	R	T-cell
Extranodal NK/T-cell lymphoma	Nodules, tumours	+, -, -	+	+	+	G	NK-cell, sometimes T-cell
Primary cutaneous ALCL	Superficial nodules with epidermal involvement	+, +, -	+	-	-	R	T-cell
Mycosis fungoides	Patches, plaques, tumours late in course	+, +, -	-	-	-	R	T-cell
Blastic plasmacytoid dendritic cell neoplasm	Nodules, tumours	-, +, -	-	+	-	G	Precursor of plasmacytoid dendritic cell

° Cytotoxic granule-associated protein, TIA1 and/or Granzyme B and/or perforin; SPTCL, subcutaneous panniculitis-like T-cell lymphoma; TCL, T-cell lymphoma; ALCL, anaplastic large cell lymphoma.

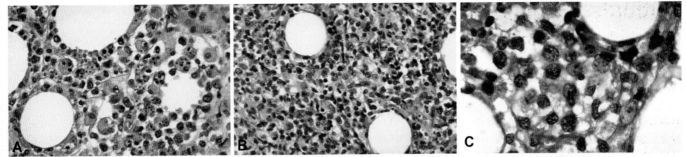

Fig. 11.46 A Subcutaneous panniculitis-like T-cell lymphoma. Tumour cells are associated with abundant histiocytes containing apoptotic debris. **B** Neoplastic cells surround fat cells, often with some admixed histiocytes. **C** Neoplastic cells have round to oval hyperchromatic nuclei with inconspicuous nucleoli and abundant pale cytoplasm.

Larger nodules may become necrotic; however, ulceration is rare {1202, 2408}.

Clinical features

Clinical symptoms are primarily related to the subcutaneous nodules. Systemic symptoms may be seen in up to 50% of patients. Laboratory abnormalities, including cytopenias and elevated liver function tests are common, and a frank haemophagocytic syndrome is seen in 15–20% {814}. Lymphadenopathy is usually absent. Hepatosplenomegaly may be seen, but almost always not due to lymphomatous involvement {1202}.

Morphology

The infiltrate involves the fat lobules, usually with sparing of septa. The overlying dermis and epidermis are typically uninvolved. The neoplastic cells range in size, but in any given case, cell size is relatively constant. The neoplastic cells have irregular and hyperchromatic nuclei. The lymphoid cells have a rim of pale-staining cytoplasm. A helpful diagnostic feature is the rimming of the neoplastic cells surrounding individual fat cells. Admixed

reactive histiocytes are frequently present, particularly in areas of fat infiltration and destruction. The histiocytes are frequently vacuolated, due to ingested lipid material. Other inflammatory cells are typically absent, notably plasma cells, which are common in lupus panniculitis. Vascular invasion may be seen in some cases, and necrosis and karyorrhexis are common {1413}. The latter feature is helpful in the differential diagnosis from other lymphomas involving skin and subcutaneous tissue{1202}. Cutaneous γδ T-cell lymphomas may show panniculitis-like features, but commonly involve the dermis and epidermis, and may show epidermal ulceration.

Immunophenotype

The cells have a mature αβ T-cell phenotype, usually CD8-positive, with expression of cytotoxic molecules including granzyme B, perforin, and T-cell intracellular antigen (TIA1) {1202, 1919}. The cells express βF1 and are negative for CD56, helping in the distinction from cutaneous γδ T-cell lymphoma {81, 2253}.

Postulated normal counterpart

Mature cytotoxic αβ T-cell.

Genetics

The neoplastic cells show rearrangement of T-cell receptor genes, and are negative for Epstein-Barr viral sequences. No specific cytogenetic features have been reported.

Prognosis and predictive factors

Dissemination to lymph nodes and other organs is rare {814, 1175, 1919}. The 5-year median survival overall is 80%; however, if a haemophagocytic syndrome is present, the prognosis is poor {1413, 2408}. Combination chemotherapy has traditionally been used, but one study suggests that more conservative immunosuppressive regimens (cyclosporine, prednisone, chlorambucil) may be effective {2273B}. A distinction from cutaneous γδ T-cell lymphomas is important, since SPTCL has a much better prognosis {2254, 2408}.

Mycosis fungoides

E. Ralfkiaer
L. Cerroni
C.A. Sander
B.R. Smoller
R. Willemze

Definition

Mycosis fungoides (MF) is an epidermotropic, primary cutaneous T-cell lymphoma (CTCL) characterized by infiltrates of small to medium-sized T lymphocytes with cerebriform nuclei. The term MF should be used only for the classical cases characterized by the evolution of patches, plaques and tumours, or for variants showing a similar clinical course.

ICD-O code   9700/3

Epidemiology

MF is the most common type of CTCL and accounts for almost 50% of all primary cutaneous lymphomas {2407}. Most patients are adults/elderly, but the disease can be observed in children and adolescents. The male:female ratio is 2:1 {2407}.

Sites of involvement

The disease is, as a rule, limited to the skin, with widespread distribution, for a protracted period. Extracutaneous dissemination may occur in advanced stages, mainly to lymph nodes, liver, spleen, lungs and blood {2407}. Involvement of the bone marrow (BM) is rare {2407}.

Clinical features

MF has an indolent clinical course with slow progression over years or sometimes decades, from patches to more infiltrated plaques and eventually tumours. Patients with tumour stage MF characteristically show a combination of patches, plaques and tumours, which often show ulceration

Table 11.05
Clinical staging system for mycosis fungoides and Sézary syndrome, as recently proposed by the ISCL-EORTC {1642}.

Stage I	Disease confined to the skin with patches/papules/plaques <10% (stage IA) or >10% (stage IB) of the skin surface; no clinically abnormal lymph nodes.
Stage II	Skin involvement with patches/papules/plaques associated with early (N1-N2) lymph node involvement (stage II A) or skin involvement with one or more tumours (>1cm) (stage IIB).
Stage III	Skin involvement with erythroderma, no or early (N1-N2) lymph node involvement and absent or low blood tumour burden (<1000/µl circulating Sézary cells).
Stage IV	High blood tumour burden (>1000/µl circulating Sézary cells) and/or extensive lymph node involvement (N3) or visceral involvement (M1).

Table 11.06
Histopathological staging for clinically abnormal lymph nodes (>1.5 cm) in mycosis fungoides and Sézary syndrome.

ISCL/EORTC {1642}	Dutch system {1958A}	NCI classification {1940A}
N1	Category 1: DL, no atypical CMC	LN0: no atypical lymphocytes LN1: occasional, isolated atypical lymphocytes LN2: clusters (3-6 cells) of atypical lymphocytes
N2*	Category 2: DL with early involvement with scattered atypical CMC	LN3: aggregates of atypical lymphocytes, but architecture preserved
N3	Category 3: partial effacement of architecture with many CMC Category 4: complete effacement of architecture	LN4: partial or complete effacement of architecture with many atypical lymphocytes

DL, dermatopathic lymphadenopathy; CMC, cerebriform mononuclear cells with nuclei >7.5µm.
*N2 is divided into 2 categories, N2a without clonally rearranged T-cells and N2b with clonally rearranged T-cells.

{2407}. Uncommonly, patients present with or develop an erythrodermic stage of disease that lack the haematologic criteria of Sézary syndrome {2342}. In some patients, lymph node and visceral organs may become involved in the later stages of the disease.

Morphology

The histology of the skin lesions varies with the stage of the disease. Early patch lesions show superficial band-like or lichenoid infiltrates, mainly consisting of lymphocytes and histiocytes. Atypical

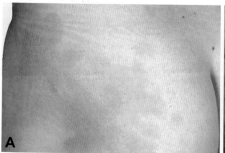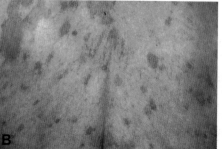

Fig.11.47 Mycosis fungoides. **A** Early stage with patches. **B** Disseminated plaque stage.

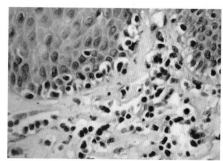

Fig.11.48 Early MF with infiltrates of atypical, haloed lymphocytes in the basal layer of epidermis.

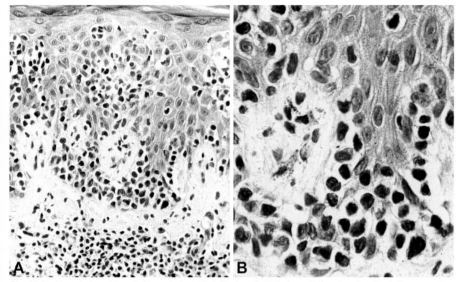

Fig. 11.49 Mycosis fungoides. **A** Plaque lesion with infiltrates of atypical, cerebriform lymphocytes in the upper dermis. **B** The epidermis is involved, mainly with single cells.

Immunophenotype

The typical phenotype is CD2+, CD3+, TCRß+, CD5+, CD4+, CD8- {1809}. Rare cases may be positive for CD8 {1809}. Such cases have the same clinical behaviour and prognosis as CD4+ cases, and should not be considered a separate entity {2407}. A CD8+ phenotype has been reported more commonly in paediatric MF. A lack of CD7 is frequent in all stages of the disease {1809}. Other alterations in the expression of T-cell antigens may be seen, but mainly occur in the advanced (tumour) stages {1809}. Cutaneous lymphocyte antigen (CLA) associated with lymphocyte homing to the skin is expressed in most cases. Cytotoxic granule-associated proteins are only rarely expressed in the early patch/plaque lesions, but may be positive in a fraction of the neoplastic cells in the more advanced lesions {2333}.

Genetics

T-cell receptor genes are clonally rearranged in a variable proportion of cases, possibly depending upon the number of tumour cells and the detection technique employed {1765, 2398}.
Complex karyotypes are present in many patients, in particular in the advanced stages {1381, 2190}. A vast number of

cells with small to medium-sized, highly indented (cerebriform) nuclei are few, and mostly confined to the epidermis where they characteristically colonize the basal layer of the epidermis often as haloed cells, either singly or in a linear distribution {1411}. In typical plaques, epidermotropism is more pronounced. The presence of intraepidermal collections of atypical cells (Pautrier microabscesses) is a highly characteristic feature, but is observed in only a minority of cases {1411}. With progression to tumour stage, the dermal infiltrates become more diffuse and epidermotropism may be lost. The tumour cells increase in number and size, showing variable proportions of small, medium-sized to large cerebriform cells, blast cells with prominent nuclei and intermediate forms {2407}. Histologic transformation, defined by presence of >25% large lymphoid cells in the dermal infiltrates may occur, mainly in the tumour stages {361, 567, 2330}. These large cells may be CD30-negative or CD30-positive. Enlarged lymph nodes from patients with MF frequently show dermatopathic lymphadenopathy with paracortical expansion due to the presence of large number of histiocytes and interdigitating cells with abundant, pale cytoplasm.
The ISCL-EORTC staging system for clinically abnormal lymph nodes (>1.5 cm) in MF and Sézary syndrome {1642} integrates the previous NCI and Dutch lymph node staging systems {1940A, 1958A}. There are 3 categories, essentially reflecting no

involvement, early involvement (with no architectural effacement), and overt involvement (with partial or complete architectural effacement). Recognition of the early infiltrates can be difficult and can be aided by T-cell receptor analysis {1642}. N3 lymph nodes may simulate peripheral T-cell lymphoma, NOS or Hodgkin lymphoma.

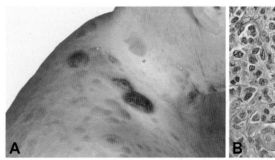

Fig. 11.50 MF tumour stage (**A**) with histological transformation to a large cell lymphoma (**B**).

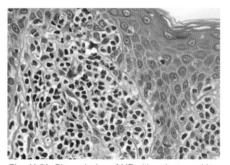

Fig. 11.51 Plaque lesion of MF with a dense, epidermotropic infiltrate of atypical, cerebriform lymphocytes and characteristic Pautrier microabscesses.

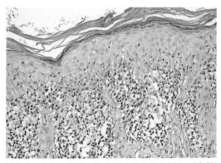

Fig. 11.52 Pagetoid reticulosis with intraepidermal infiltrates of atypical lymphocytes.

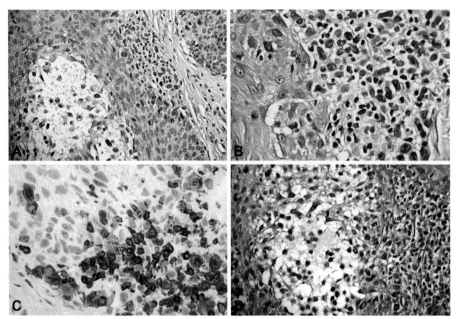

Fig. 11.53 Mycosis fungoides. **A** Folliculotropic mycosis fungoides with atypical lymphocytes infiltrating a hair follicle. **B** Note cerebriform nuclei. **C** The atypical cells are CD3-positive. **D** The involved follicle shows mucinous degeneration with accumulation of Alcian blue-positive material.

different structural and numerical alterations have been described. Constitutive activation of *STAT3* and inactivation of *CDKN2A/p16^INK4a* and *PTEN* have been identified and may be associated with disease progression {1583, 1951, 1952, 2051, 2424}. Gene expression profiling studies have shown tumour necrosis factor (TNF) anti-apoptotic pathway activation in the tumourigenesis of MF {2261}.

Postulated normal counterpart
Mature skin-homing CD4+ T-cell.

Prognosis and predictive factors
The single most important prognostic factor in MF is the extent of cutaneous and extracutaneous disease as reflected in the clinical stage. Patients with limited disease generally have an excellent prognosis with a similar survival as the general population {2298}. In the more advanced stages, the prognosis is poor, in particular

in patients with skin tumours and/or extracutaneous dissemination {2298}. Age above 60 years and elevated lactic dehydrogenase are other adverse prognostic parameters {568}. Histologic transformation with increase in blast cells (>25%) is also an adverse parameter {361}.

Variants

Folliculotropic MF
Folliculotropic MF is characterized by the presence of follicular infiltrates of atypical (cerebriform) CD4+ T lymphocytes often with sparing of the epidermis {797}. Most cases show mucinous degeneration of the hair follicles (follicular mucinosis) but similar cases without follicular mucinosis have been reported {2297}. The lesions preferentially involve the head and neck area and often present with grouped follicular papules associated with alopecia

{2297}. Due to the deep localization of the neoplastic infiltrate, the disease is less accessible to skin-targeted therapies. The disease-specific 5-year-survival is approximately 70–80%, which is significantly worse than that of patients with classical plaque stage MF {797, 2297}.

Pagetoid reticulosis
Pagetoid reticulosis is characterized by the presence of patches or plaques with an intraepidermal proliferation of neoplastic T-cells {870}. The term should only be used for the localized type (Woringer-Kolopp type) and not for the disseminated type (Ketron-Goodman type) as cases corresponding to the latter category would currently most likely be classified as aggressive epidermotropic CD8-positive CTCL or cutaneous γδ-positive T-cell lymphoma {2407}. The atypical cells have medium-sized or large, sometimes hyperchromatic and cerebriform nuclei, and either have a CD4+, CD8- or a CD4-, CD8+ phenotype. CD30 is often expressed. In contrast to classical MF, extracutaneous dissemination or disease-related deaths have never been reported {2407}.

Granulomatous slack skin
Granulomatous slack skin (GSS) is an extremely rare subtype of CTCL characterized by the slow development of folds of lax skin in the major skin folds (axillae, groin) and histologically by a granulomatous infiltrate with clonal CD4+ T cells, abundant macrophages and multinucleated giant cells {2300}. In approximately one third of the reported patients, an association with CHL has been observed. An association with classical MF has also been reported {2300}. Most patients have an indolent clinical course {1261}.

Sézary syndrome

E. Ralfkiaer
R. Willemze
S.J. Whittaker

Definition
Sézary syndrome (SS) is defined by the triad of erythroderma, generalized lymphadenopathy and the presence of clonally related neoplastic T-cells with cerebriform nuclei (Sézary cells) in skin, lymph nodes and peripheral blood (PB). In addition, one or more of the following criteria are required: an absolute Sézary cell count of at least 1000 cells per mm³, an expanded CD4+ T-cell population resulting in a CD4/CD8 ratio of more than 10 and/or loss of one or more T-cell antigens.

ICD-O code   9701/3

Epidemiology
This is a rare disease, which accounts for less than 5% of all cutaneous T-cell lymphomas {2407}. It occurs in adults, characteristically presents over the age of 60, and has a male predominance.

Sites of involvement
SS is a leukaemia and thus by definition a generalized disease. All visceral organs may be involved in the terminal stages. However, there is often a remarkable sparing of the bone marrow (BM).

Clinical features
Patients present with erythroderma and generalized lymphadenopathy. Other features are pruritus, alopecia, ectropion, palmar or plantar hyperkeratoses and onychodystrophy. An increased prevalence of secondary malignancies, both cutaneous and systemic, has been reported in SS and attributed to the immunoparesis associated with loss of normal circulating CD4 cells {989}.

Morphology
The histological features in SS may be similar to those in mycosis fungoides (MF). However, the cellular infiltrates in SS are more often monotonous, and epidermotropism may sometimes be absent. In up to one third of biopsies from patients with otherwise classical SS the histologic picture may be non-specific {2270}. Involved lymph nodes characteristically show a dense, monotonous infiltrate of Sézary cells with effacement of the normal lymph node architecture {1959}. Bone marrow may be involved, but the infiltrates are often sparse and mainly interstitial {2018}.

Immunophenotype
Tumour cells are CD2+, CD3+, TCRß+ and CD5+. Most cases are CD4+. Expression of CD8 is rare. Sézary cells express cutaneous lymphocyte antigen (CLA) and the skin-homing receptor CCR4 {703} and characteristically lack CD7 and CD26 {204, 1571, 2046}. T plastin mRNA and protein have been shown to be enhanced in Sézary cells relatively to normal helper T-cells {1110, 2116}.

Genetics
T-cell receptor genes are clonally rearranged {1765, 2397, 2398}. Recurrent chromosomal abnormalities have not been detected in SS, but complex karyotypes with numerical and structural alterations are common and similar to MF {161, 1381, 1382}.

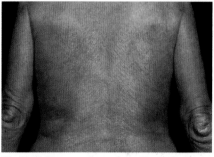

Fig. 11.54 Sézary syndrome. Generalized skin disease with erythroderma.

M-Fluorescence *in situ* hybridization (FISH) and comparative genomic hybridization (CGH) techniques have shown a high rate of unbalanced translocations and associated deletions often involving chromosomes 1p, 6q, 10q, 17p and 19, suggesting a high rate of genomic instability {1382}. Inactivation of *TP53* and *p16*^{INK4a} are frequent {1440, 1583, 1951}. Amplification of *JUNB*, has been identified in Sézary syndrome {1384}. Gene expression profiling studies have not yielded consistent findings {239, 871, 1110, 2296}.

Postulated normal counterpart
Mature epidermotropic skin homing CD4+ T-cells.

Prognosis and predictive factors
This is an aggressive disease with an overall survival rate at 5 years of 10–20% {2407}. Most patients die of opportunistic infections. Prognostic factors include the degree of lymph node and PB involvement {1161, 2342}.

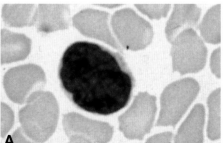
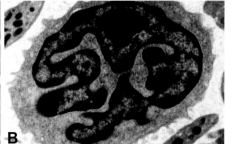

Fig. 11.55 Morphology of Sézary cells in Giemsa stained blood films (**A**) and by ultrastructural examination (**B**).

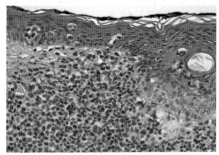

Fig. 11.56 Skin infiltrates in SS with epidermotropic infiltrates of atypical, cerebriform lymphocytes.

Primary cutaneous CD30-positive T-cell lymphoproliferative disorders

E. Ralfkiaer
R. Willemze
M. Paulli
M.E. Kadin

Primary cutaneous CD30-positive lymphoproliferative disorders (LPD) are the second most common group of the cutaneous T-cell lymphomas (CTCL), accounting for approximately 30% of the cases. This group includes primary cutaneous anaplastic large lymphoma (C-ALCL), lymphomatoid papulosis (LyP) and borderline cases.

These diseases form a spectrum that may show overlapping histopathologic and phenotypic features {2407}. The clinical appearance and course are therefore critical for the definite diagnosis. The term "borderline" refers to cases in which, despite careful clinicopathologic correlation, a definite distinction between C-ALCL and LyP cannot be made. However, clinical examination during follow-up will generally disclose whether such patients have C-ALCL or LyP {172}. From a clinical perspective LyP is not considered a malignant disorder, despite demonstration of monoclonality in many cases.

Primary cutaneous anaplastic large cell lymphoma (C-ALCL)

Definition
C-ALCL is composed of large cells with an anaplastic, pleomorphic or immunoblastic cytomorphology that express the CD30 antigen by the majority (>75%) of the tumour cells {2407}. Patients with C-ALCL should not have clinical evidence or history of mycosis fungoides (MF); in this setting the diagnosis should be considered transformation of MF to tumour stage, which may be CD30-positive or negative {2407}. The disease must also be distinguished from systemic ALCL with cutaneous involvement, which is a separate disease with different cytogenetics, clinical features and outcome {613}.

ICD-O code   9718/3

Epidemiology
C-ALCL is the second most common type of CTCL {172}. The median age is 60 years. Children are sporadically affected {172, 2407}. The M:F ratio is 2–3:1 {172}.

Sites of involvement
The most frequently affected sites include trunk, face, extremities and buttocks.

Clinical features
Most patients present with solitary or localized nodules or tumours, and sometimes papules, and often show ulceration {172, 2407}. Multifocal lesions are seen in about 20% of the patients. The skin lesions may show partial or complete spontaneous regression as in LyP. These lymphomas frequently relapse in the skin. Extracutaneous dissemination occurs in ~10% of the patients, and mainly involves the regional lymph nodes {172, 2407}.

Morphology
Histology shows diffuse, usually non-epidermotropic infiltrates with cohesive sheets of large CD30-positive tumour cells. In most cases the tumour cells have the characteristic morphology of anaplastic cells, showing round, oval or irregularly-shaped nuclei, prominent eosinophilic nucleoli and abundant cytoplasm {2407}. Less commonly (20–25%), they have a non-anaplastic (pleomorphic or immunoblastic) appearance {172, 1711}. Reactive lymphocytes are often present at the periphery of the lesions. Ulcerating lesions may show a LyP-like histology with an abundant inflammatory infiltrate of reactive T-cells, histiocytes, eosinophils, neutrophils and relatively few CD30-positive cells. In such cases epidermal hyperplasia may be prominent. The inflammatory background is especially prominent in the rare neutrophil-rich (pyogenic) variant {299}.

Immunophenotype
The neoplastic cells show an activated CD4+ T-cell phenotype with variable loss of CD2, CD5 and/or CD3 and frequent expression of cytotoxic proteins (granzyme B, TIA1, perforin) {255, 1204, 2407}. Some cases (<5%) have a CD8+ T-cell phenotype. CD30 is by definition expressed

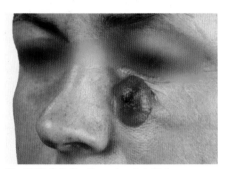

Fig. 11.57 C-ALCL with an ulcerated skin tumour.

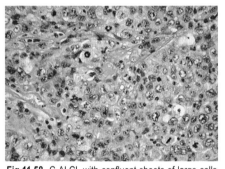

Fig.11.58 C-ALCL with confluent sheets of large cells with anaplastic morphology.

by a majority (>75%) of the neoplastic cells {2407}. Unlike systemic ALCL, most C-ALCL express the cutaneous lymphocyte antigen (CLA), but do not express EMA or ALK (anaplastic lymphoma kinase) {516, 537, 2182}. Unlike Hodgkin and Reed-Sternberg cells, staining for CD15 is generally negative. Coexpression of CD56 is observed in rare cases, but does not appear to be associated with an unfavourable prognosis {1581}.

Genetics
Most cases show clonal rearrangement of the T-cell receptor *(TCR)* genes {2407}. However, TCR proteins are often not expressed {238}.
Studies using comparative genomic hybridization have revealed chromosomal imbalances with gains of several putative oncogenes {1383}. However, specific and consistent cytogenetic abnormalities have as yet not been identified. Unlike systemic ALCL, C-ALCL does not carry translocations involving the *ALK* gene at chromosome 2 {537, 613, 2182}.

Postulated normal couterpart

Transformed/activated skin-homing T lymphocyte.

Prognosis and predictive factors

The prognosis is usually favourable, with a 10-year disease-related survival of approximately 90% {172, 1322}. Patients presenting with multifocal skin lesions and patients with involvement of regional lymph nodes have a similar prognosis to patients with only skin lesions {172}. No difference in clinical presentation, clinical behaviour or prognosis is found between cases with an anaplastic morphology and cases with a non-anaplastic (pleomorphic or immunoblastic) morphology {172, 1322, 1711}.

Lymphomatoid papulosis

Definition

Lymphomatoid papulosis (LyP) is a chronic, recurrent, self-healing skin disease composed of large atypical anaplastic, immunoblastic or Hodgkin-like cells in a marked inflammatory background. In some cases the pattern of cutaneous involvement may resemble MF (type B).

ICD-O code   9718/1

Epidemiology

LyP most often occurs in adults (median age, 45 years), but children may also be affected. The male to female ratio is 2–3:1 {172, 1322, 1996, 2303}.

Sites of involvement

LyP is a skin-limited disease that most frequently affects trunk and extremities {172}. Rarely, oral mucosal lesions may be present.

Clinical features

LyP is characterized by the presence of papular, papulonecrotic and/or nodular skin lesions at different stages of development {172}. Individual skin lesions disappear within 3–12 weeks, and may leave behind superficial scars. The duration of the disease may vary from several months to more than 40 years. In up to 20% of patients, LyP may be preceded by, associated with, or followed by another type of malignant lymphoma, generally MF, cutaneous anaplastic large cell lymphoma or Hodgkin lymphoma {172, 1079}.

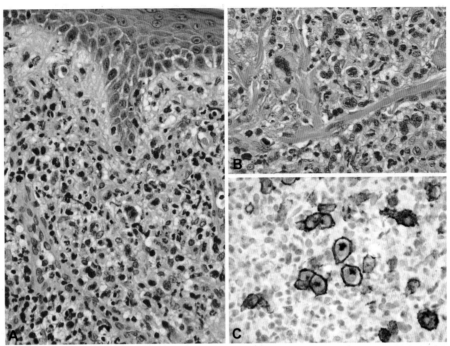

Fig. 11.59 Lymphomatoid papulosis, type A, consisting of atypical lymphoid cells admixed with many inflammatory cells (**A**). The atypical cells have a cerebriform or Hodgkin-like morphology (**B**) and are strongly positive for CD30 (**C**).

Morphology

The histologic picture of LyP is extremely variable, and in part correlates with the age of the biopsied skin lesion. Three histologic subtypes of LyP (types A, B and C) have been described, which represent a spectrum with overlapping features {172, 2407}. In LyP type A lesions, scattered or small clusters of large, sometimes multinucleated or Reed-Sternberg-like, CD30-positive cells are intermingled with numerous inflammatory cells, such as histiocytes, small lymphocytes, neutrophils and/or eosinophils. LyP, type C lesions demonstrate a monotonous population or large clusters of large CD30-positive T-cells with relatively few admixed inflammatory cells. LyP, type B is uncommon (<10%) and is characterized by an epidermotropic infiltrate of small atypical cells with cerebriform nuclei similar to that observed in MF.

Immunophenotype

The large atypical cells in the LyP type A and type C lesions have the same phenotype as the tumour cells in C-ALCL. The atypical cells with cerebriform nuclei in the LyP, type B lesions have a CD3+, CD4+, CD8- phenotype and do not express CD30 {2407}. Rare cases of LyP with CD8 and NK-cell phenotype have been reported {709, 1366}.

Genetics

Clonally rearranged T-cell receptor genes have been detected in approximately 60% of LyP lesions {1079}. Identical rearrangements have been demonstrated in LyP lesions and associated lymphomas {1079}. No consistent abnormalities have been described. The (2;5)(p23;q35) translocation is not detected in LyP {613, 614}.

Postulated normal couterpart

Activated skin-homing T lymphocyte.

Prognosis and predictive factors

LyP has an excellent prognosis. In a study of 118 LyP patients, only 2 patients (2%) died of systemic disease after a median follow-up duration of 77 months {172}. However, since risk factors for the development of a systemic lymphoma are unknown, long-term follow-up is advised.

Primary cutaneous peripheral T-cell lymphomas, rare subtypes

P. Gaulard
E. Berti
R. Willemze
E.S. Jaffe

Peripheral T-cell lymphomas (PTCL) not uncommonly involve the skin, either as primary or secondary manifestation of the disease. Within this group, three rare provisional entities were delineated in the WHO-EORTC classification for cutaneous lymphomas, including primary cutaneous γδ T-cell lymphoma, primary cutaneous aggressive epidermotropic CD8-positive cytotoxic T-cell lymphoma and primary cutaneous CD4-positive small/medium-sized pleomorphic T-cell lymphoma. The latter two entities are still considered provisional. It should be emphasized that a diagnosis of mycosis fungoides (MF) must be ruled out by complete clinical examination and an accurate clinical history.

Primary cutaneous gamma-delta T-cell lymphoma

Definition
Primary cutaneous γδ T-cell lymphoma (PCGD-TCL) is a lymphoma composed of a clonal proliferation of mature, activated γδ T-cells with a cytotoxic phenotype. This group includes cases previously known as subcutaneous panniculitis-like T-cell lymphoma (SPTCL) with a γδ phenotype. A possibly related condition may present primarily in mucosal sites. Whether cutaneous and mucosal γδ TCL are all part of a single disease, i.e. muco-cutaneous γδ TCL, is not yet clear {1040, 2432}.

ICD-O code
The provisional code proposed for the fourth edition of ICD-O is *9726/3*.

Epidemiology
PCGD-TCL are rare, representing approximately 1% of all cutaneous T-cell lymphomas {2254, 2407, 2408}. Most cases occur in adults. There is no sex predilection.

Etiology
The distribution of disease reflects the localization of normal γδ T-cells, which are believed to play a role in host mucosal and epithelial immune responses {229}.

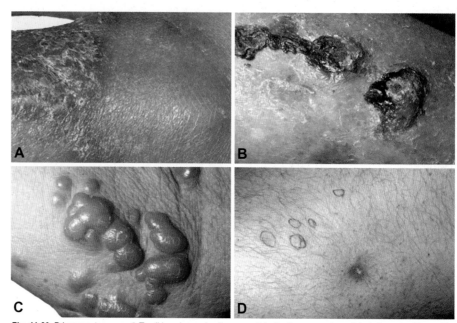

Fig. 11.60 Primary cutaneous γδ T-cell lymphoma. Lesions are clinically diverse, and consist of plaques, with or without ulceration (**A,B**), or tumours (**C**). The lesion may consist of an indurated plaque, with subcutaneous infiltration (**D**).

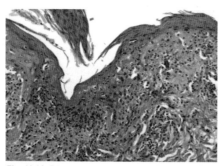

Fig. 11.61 Primary cutaneous γδ T-cell lymphoma. The epidermis is necrotic.

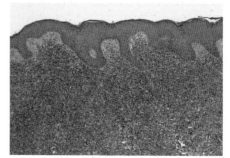

Fig. 11.62 Primary cutaneous γδ T-cell lymphoma. In this case the infiltrate is primarily dermal.

Impaired immune function associated with chronic antigen stimulation may predispose to the development of PCGD-TCL {81, 2432}.

Sites of involvement
PCGD-TCL often present with generalized skin lesions, preferentially affecting the extremities {2254, 2408}.

Clinical features
The clinical presentation of patients with PCGD-TCL is variable. The disease may be predominantly epidermotropic and present with patches/plaques. Some patients may present with deep dermal or subcutaneous tumours, with or without epidermal necrosis and ulceration {81, 207, 1068, 2254, 2408, 2432}. The lesions are most often present on the extremities, but other sites may be affected as well {1410, 2254, 2408}. Dissemination to mucosal and other extranodal sites is frequently observed, but involvement of lymph nodes, spleen or BM is uncommon. A haemophagocytic syndrome may occur

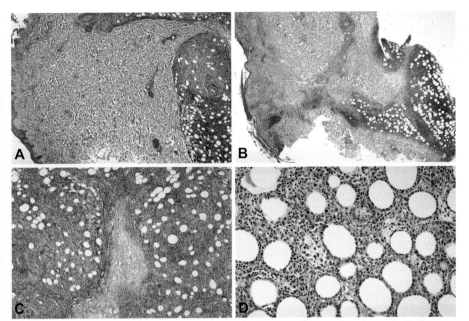

Fig. 11.63 Primary cutaneous γδ T-cell lymphoma. Histological patterns are diverse, and may be panniculitis-like in the subcutaneous fat. Dermal infiltration is usually present and the overlying epidermis may be ulcerated.

in patients with panniculitis-like tumours {2254, 2408}. B symptoms, including fever, night sweats and weight loss are seen in the majority of patients.

Morphology

Three major histologic patterns of involvement can be present in the skin: epidermotropic, dermal and subcutaneous. Often more than one histologic pattern is present in the same patient in different biopsy specimens or within a single biopsy specimen {207, 1410, 2254, 2408}. Epidermal infiltration may occur as mild epidermotropism to marked pagetoid reticulosis-like infiltrates {207, 1540, 1811}. The subcutaneous cases may show rimming of fat cells, similar to SPTCL of αβ origin, but in addition usually show dermal

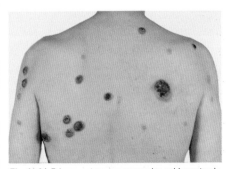

Fig. 11.64 Primary cutaneous aggressive epidermotropic CD8-positive cytotoxic T-cell lymphoma. Lesions are often haemorrhagic, and are associated with ulceration and epidermal necrosis.

and/or epidermal involvement {2254, 2408}. The neoplastic cells are generally medium to large in size with coarsely clumped chromatin {2254}. Large blastic cells with vesicular nuclei and prominent nucleoli are infrequent. Apoptosis and necrosis are common, often with angio-invasion {2254, 2408}.

Immunophenotype

The tumour cells characteristically have a βF1-, CD3+, CD2+, CD5-, CD7+/-, CD56+ phenotype with strong expression of cytotoxic proteins {1040, 1410, 1919, 2254, 2408, 2432}. Most cases lack both CD4 and CD8, although CD8 may be expressed in some cases {2254, 2408}. The cells are strongly positive for TCRδ with appropriate detection methods. If staining for TCRδ cannot be performed, the absence of βF1 may be used to infer a γδ origin under appropriate circumstances {1068, 1919, 2254, 2408}.

Genetics

The cells show clonal rearrangement of the *TRG@* and *TRD@* genes. *TRB@* may be rearranged or deleted, but is not expressed. Cases with predominant subcutaneous involvement express Vδ2, but this has not been studied in other PCGD-TCL {1783}. Epstein-Barr virus (EBV) is negative {81, 1091, 2254, 2432}.

Postulated normal counterpart

Functionally mature and activated cytotoxic γδ T-cells of the innate immune system.

Prognosis and predictive factors

PCGD-TCL are resistant to multiagent chemotherapy and/or radiation and have a poor prognosis with a median survival of approximately 15 months {2254, 2408}. Patients with subcutaneous fat involvement tend to have a more unfavourable prognosis as compared with patients with epidermal or dermal disease only {2254}.

Primary cutaneous CD8-positive aggressive epidermotropic cytotoxic T-cell lymphoma

Definition

This provisional entity is a cutaneous T-cell lymphoma (CTCL) characterized by proliferation of epidermotropic CD8-positive cytotoxic T-cells and aggressive clinical behaviour. Differentiation from other types of CTCL expressing a CD8-positive cytotoxic T-cell phenotype is based on the clinical presentation, clinical behaviour and certain histological features, such as marked epidermotropism with epidermal necrosis.

ICD-O code   9709/3

Epidemiology

This disease is rare accounting for less than 1% of all CTCL {12, 209, 2407}. It occurs mainly in adults. There are no known predisposing factors.

Sites of involvement

Most patients present with generalized skin lesions.

Clinical features

Clinically, these lymphomas are characterized by localized or disseminated eruptive papules, nodules and tumours showing central ulceration and necrosis or by superficial, hyperkeratotic patches and plaques {209, 1934}. These lymphomas may disseminate to other visceral sites (lung, testis, central nervous system, oral mucosa), but lymph nodes are often spared {209, 1404, 1790}.

Morphology

The histological appearance is very variable ranging from a lichenoid pattern with marked, pagetoid epidermotropism

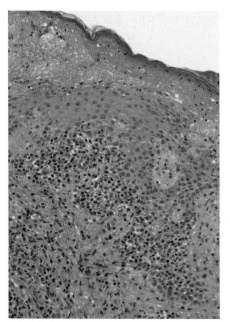

Fig. 11.65 Primary cutaneous aggressive epidermotropic CD8-positive cytotoxic T-cell lymphoma. The atypical lymphoid cells infiltrate in the superficial dermis and extend into the epidermis in a pagetoid fashion.

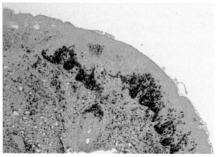

Fig. 11.66 Primary cutaneous aggressive epidermotropic CD8-positive cytotoxic T-cell lymphoma. Skin section stained for CD8, highlighting the marked epidermotropism, with the majority of the neoplastic cells localized to the epidermis.

and subepidermal edema to deeper, more nodular infiltrates. The epidermis may be acanthotic or atrophic, often with necrosis, ulceration and blister formation {12, 209}. Invasion and destruction of adnexal skin structures are commonly seen. Angiocentricity and angioinvasion may be present {1410}. Tumour cells are small-medium or medium-large with pleomorphic or blastic nuclei {209}.

Immunophenotype

The tumour cell have a ßF1+, CD3+, CD8+, granzyme B+, perforin+, TIA1+, CD45RA+/-, CD45RO-, CD2-/+, CD4-, CD5-, CD7+/- phenotype {12, 174, 209, 1410, 1934}.

Genetics

The neoplastic T-cells show clonal *TCR* gene rearrangements. Specific genetic abnormalities have not been described. EBV is negative {174, 1410}.

Postulated normal counterpart

Skin-homing, CD8-positive, cytotoxic T-cells of αβ type.

Prognosis and predictive factors

These lymphomas often have an aggressive clinical course with a median survival of 32 months {209}. There is no difference in survival between cases with a small or large cell morphology {174}.

Primary cutaneous CD4-positive small/medium T-cell lymphoma

Definition

This provisional entity is a cutaneous T-cell lymphoma characterized by a predominance of small to medium-sized CD4-positive pleomorphic T-cells without evidence of patches and plaques typical of mycosis fungoides. A majority of cases present with a solitary skin lesion.

ICD-O code   9709/3

Epidemiology

This is a rare disease, accounting for 2% of all cutaneous T-cell lymphomas {2407}.

Sites of involvement

These lesions usually present with a solitary plaque or nodule, most commonly on the face, neck or upper trunk {174, 754A}. Involvement of lower extremities is rare. By definition, there should be an absence of patches typical of mycosis fungoides {174, 734, 2098, 2341}.

Clinical features

Patients are generally asymptomatic, with the detection of a single skin lesion being the sole manifestation of disease {174, 754A}. A minority of patients may present with large tumours, or multiple skin lesions {754A}.

Morphology

These lymphomas show dense, diffuse or nodular infiltrates within the dermis with tendency to infiltrate the subcutis. Epidermotropism may be present focally, but if conspicuous, consideration should be given to the diagnosis of mycosis fungoides.

There is a predominance of small/medium-sized pleomorphic T-cells {174, 177, 734, 2098}. A small proportion (<30%) of large pleomorphic cells may be present {177}. In some cases a considerable admixture with small reactive lymphocytes and histiocytes may be observed {1950}. Eosinophils may be numerous in some cases {754A}. The principle differential diagnosis is with a reactive lymphoid infiltrate in the skin, so-called pseudolymphoma or cutaneous lymphoid hyperplasia.

Immunophenotype

By definition these lymphomas have a CD3+, CD4+, CD8-, CD30- phenotype, sometimes with loss of pan T-cell markers {174, 2098}. Cytotoxic proteins are not expressed {174}. Admixed polyclonal plasma cells and B-cells may be present, making distinction from a reactive process difficult in some cases.

Genetics

The *TCR* genes are clonally rearranged {2098, 2341}. Demonstration of an aberrant T-cell phenotype and clonality are useful criteria to differentiate these small/medium-sized pleomorphic CTCL from pseudo T-cell lymphomas, which also may present with a solitary plaque or nodule {132}. Specific genetic abnormalities have not been described. EBV is negative.

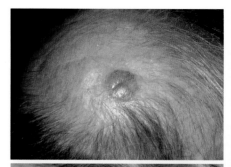

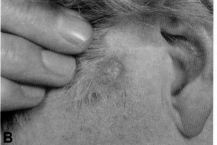

Fig. 11.67 Typical presentations of primary cutaneous small/medium CD4-positive T-cell lymphoma.

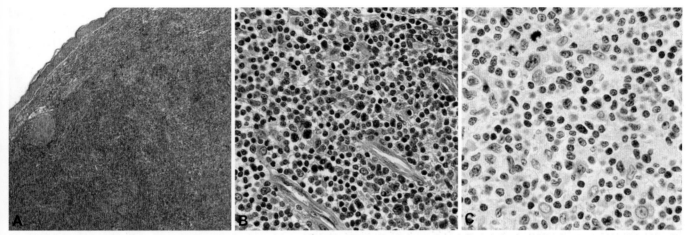

Fig. 11.68 Primary cutaneous CD4 positive small/medium T-cell lymphoma. **A,B** Atypical lymphoid cells form a dense infiltrate in the dermis, but do not extend into the epidermis. **C** The lymphoid cells are small to medium in size, with mild pleomorphism. Admixed histiocytes or plasma cells may be present, and histiocytes can be abundant in some cases.

Postulated normal counterpart
Skin homing CD4-positive T-cell.

Prognosis and predictive factors
These lymphomas have a rather favourable prognosis with an estimated 5-year survival of approximately 80% {174, 177, 706, 734, 825, 2098, 2341, 2407}. Particularly, cases presenting with a solitary or localized skin lesions seem to have an excellent prognosis {174}. In such patients surgical excision or radiotherapy is the preferred mode of treatment. Patients with multiple lesions or large tumours may have a more aggressive clinical course {754A}.

Peripheral T-cell lymphoma, not otherwise specified

S.A. Pileri   E. Ralfkiaer
D.D. Weisenburger   S. Nakamura
I. Sng   H.K. Müller-Hermelink
E.S. Jaffe

Definition

A heterogeneous category of nodal and extranodal mature T-cell lymphomas, which do not correspond to any of the specifically defined entities of mature T-cell lymphoma in the current classification.

ICD-O code

9702/3

Epidemiology

These tumours account for approximately 30% of peripheral T-cell lymphomas (PTCL) in Western countries {1849}. Most patients are adults. These lymphomas are very rare in children. The male:female ratio is 2:1.

Sites of involvement

Most patients present with peripheral lymph node involvement, but any site may be affected. Generalized disease is often encountered with infiltrates in the bone marrow (BM), liver, spleen and extranodal tissues {1849}. Peripheral blood (PB) is sometimes involved, but leukaemic presentation is uncommon. Extranodal presentations may occur, with the skin and gastrointestinal tract representing the most commonly affected sites. Under these circumstances, the diagnosis of peripheral T-cell lymphoma, not otherwise specified (PTCL, NOS) should be made only when other specific entities have been excluded. Other less frequently involved sites include the lung, salivary gland and central nervous system.

Clinical features

Patients most often present with lymph node enlargement and a majority have advanced disease with B symptoms {1849}. Paraneoplastic features such as eosinophilia, pruritus or rarely haemophagocytic syndrome may be seen {1849}.

Morphology

In the lymph node, these lymphomas show paracortical or diffuse infiltrates with effacement of the normal architecture. The cytological spectrum is extremely broad, from highly polymorphous to monomorphous. Most cases consist of numerous medium-sized and/or large cells with

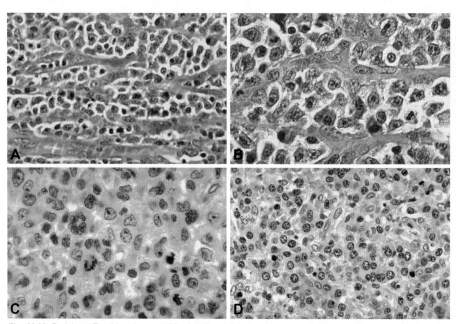

Fig. 11.69 Peripheral T-cell lymphoma, NOS. **A** Diffuse infiltrates of large lymphoid cells with pleomorphic, irregular nuclei and prominent nucleoli. **B** In between the neoplastic cells, there are scattered eosinophils and numerous vessels. **C** Nuclei are markedly pleomorphic with polylobated nuclear features. **D** In some cases, nuclei are round and monomorphic in appearance.

irregular, pleomorphic, hyperchromatic or vesicular nuclei, prominent nucleoli and many mitotic figures {898, 1035}. Clear cells and Reed-Sternberg (RS)-like cells can also be seen. Rare cases have a predominance of small lymphoid cells with atypical, irregular nuclei. High endothelial venules may be increased {898, 1035}. A T zone pattern may be observed, but is not specific for a distinct entity. An inflam-

Table 11.07 Differential diagnosis of nodal peripheral T-cell lymphoma, not otherwise specified.

Disease	Immunophenotypic features
Peripheral T-cell lymphoma, not otherwise specified	CD4>CD8, antigen loss frequent (CD7, CD5, CD4/CD8, CD52), CD30-/+, CD56 -/+, CD10-, BCL6-, CLCX13-, PD1-
Angioimmunoblastic lymphoma	CD4+ or mixed CD4/8, CD10+/-, BCL6+/-, CXCL13+, PD1+, hyperplasia of FDC, EBV+ CD20+ B blasts
Adult T-cell leukaemia/lymphoma	CD4+, CD25+, CD7-, CD30-/+, CD15-/+, FoxP3+/-
Anaplastic large cell lymphoma	CD30+, ALK+/-, EMA+, CD25+, cytotoxic granules+, CD4+/-, CD3-/+, CD43+
T-cell-rich large B-cell lymphoma	Large CD20+ blasts in background of CD3+ reactive T-cells
T zone hyperplasia	Mixed CD4/CD8, intact architecture, variable CD25 and CD30; scattered CD20+ B-cells

+, nearly always positive; +/-, majority positive; -/+, minority positive; FDC, follicular dendritic cells, EBV, Epstein-Barr virus.

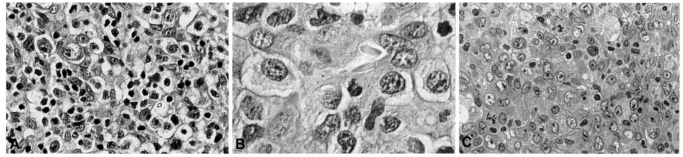

Fig. 11.70 Peripheral T-cell lymphoma, NOS, with prominent clear cell features (**A,B**) or large lymphoid cells with vesicular, immunoblast-like nuclei (**C**).

matory background is often present, including small lymphocytes, eosinophils, plasma cells, large B-cells (that may be clonal irrespective of EBV infection) {2359} and clusters of epithelioid histiocytes. Epithelioid histiocytes are particularly numerous in the lymphoepithelioid cell variant. The differential diagnosis with angioimmunoblastic T-cell lymphoma (AITL) may require extensive immunophenotyping. In one uncommon variant, the neoplastic cells selectively infiltrate the lymphoid follicles, and the resultant follicular growth pattern may suggest a B-cell lymphoma of follicular origin {524}

Extranodal involvement takes the form of diffuse infiltrates composed of similar cells. In the skin, the lymphomatous population tends to infiltrate the dermis and subcutis, often producing nodules that may undergo central ulceration {1710}. Epidermotropism, angiocentricity and adnexal involvement are at times seen {1710}. In the spleen, the pattern is very variable from solitary or multiple fleshy nodules to diffuse white pulp involvement with colonization of the periarteriolar sheath or in some cases predominant infiltration of the red pulp {382}.

Immunophenotype

PTCL, NOS is usually characterized by an aberrant T-cell phenotype with frequent downregulation of CD5 and CD7 {2390}. A CD4+/CD8- phenotype predominates in nodal cases. CD4/CD8 double-positivity or double-negativity is at times seen, as is CD8, CD56 and cytotoxic granule expression {2390}. T-cell receptor (TCR) beta-chain (βF1) is usually expressed, allowing the differentiation from γδ T-cell lymphomas and NK-cell lymphomas. CD52 is absent in 60% of cases {393, 1740, 1856}. CD30 can be expressed, exceptionally with CD15, but the global phenotypic profile and morphology allow

the distinction from anaplastic large-cell lymphoma (ALCL) and Hodgkin lymphoma {149, 2390}. Aberrant expression of CD20 and/or CD79a is occasionally encountered {2359, 2390}. Unlike AITL, PTCL, NOS usually lacks a follicular T helper (TFH) phenotype (CD10+, BCL6+, PD1+ and CXCL13+) with the exception of the follicular/perifollicular variant {99, 605, 852, 2390}. Proliferation is usually high and Ki67 rates exceeding 70% are associated with a worse prognosis {2390}.

Genetics

Antigen receptor genes

TCR genes are clonally rearranged in most cases {1849}.

Cytogenetic abnormalities and oncogenes

These are usually highly aberrant neoplasms with complex karyotypes {1849}. In both conventional and array comparative genomic hybridization (CGH) studies, recurrent chromosomal gains have been observed in chromosomes 7q, 8q, 17q and 22q, and recurrent losses in chromosomes 4q, 5q, 6q, 9p, 10q, 12q and 13q. Deletions in chromosomes 5q, 10q and 12q are associated with a better prognosis {2233, 2492}. The genetic imbalances observed in PTCL, NOS differ from those of other T-cell lymphomas, such as AITL and ALCL {2233, 2492}.

Gene expression profiling studies have provided some hints for better understanding PTCL, NOS {137, 494, 1451, 1739A}. In particular, its gene signature differs from those of AITL and ALCL {523, 1739A}.

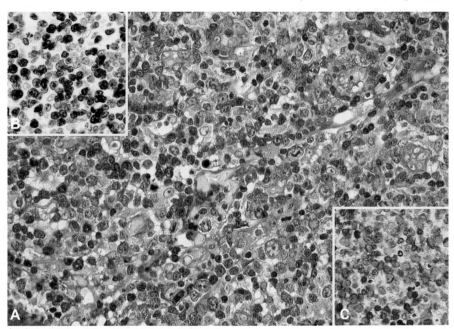

Fig. 11.71 Peripheral T-cell lymphoma, NOS. **A** Note the marked pleomorphism of the neoplastic population, **B** high Ki67 labeling. **C** βF1 staining.

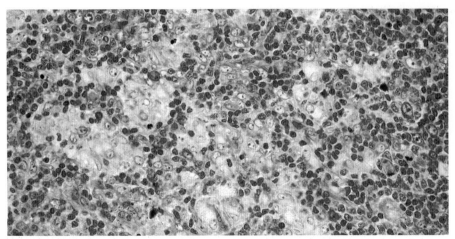

Fig. 11.72 Peripheral T-cell lymphoma, NOS, lymphoepithelioid variant. Neoplastic cells are admixed with prominent epithelioid histiocytic clusters that tend to obscure the lymphomatous growth (Giemsa).

In comparison to normal T lymphocytes, it is characterized by the recurrent deregulation of genes involved in relevant cell functions, e.g. matrix deposition, cytoskeleton organization, cell adhesion, apoptosis, proliferation, transcription and signal transduction {1739A}. The products of these genes might have therapeutic relevance {494, 1739A}.

EBV integration has been reported in some cases {632, 2390}.

Postulated normal counterpart

Activated mature T lymphocytes, mostly CD4+ central memory type of the adaptive immune sytem {523, 769, 1739A}.

Prognosis and predictive factors

These are highly aggressive lymphomas, with a poor response to therapy, frequent relapses and low 5-year overall survival and failure-free survival (20–30%) {1849}. The only factors consistently associated with prognosis are stage and IPI score {1849}. New scoring systems have recently been developed {749, 2390}. Involvement of the bone marrow (BM) has been proposed as a negative prognostic factor, but this needs further confirmation. EBV-positivity, NFκB pathway deregulation, a high proliferation signature by gene expression, and cytotoxic granule expression have been found to correlate with a poor prognosis {87, 494, 632, 2390}.

Variants

Lymphoepithelioid (Lennert lymphoma)

This variant shows diffuse or, more rarely, interfollicular growth. Cytologically, it consists predominantly of small cells with slight nuclear irregularities, confluent clusters of epithelioid histiocytes and some larger, more atypical, proliferating blasts. There can be admixed inflammatory cells and scattered Reed-Sternberg-like cells (usually EBV+). High-endothelial venules are not prominent. In the majority of cases, the neoplastic cells are CD8-positive {770}.

Follicular

This variant usually consists of atypical clear cells forming intrafollicular aggregates (mimicking follicular lymphoma), small nodular aggregates in a background of progressively-transformed germinal centres (mimicking nodular lymphocyte-predominant Hodgkin lymphoma) or enlarged perifollicular zones/nodular aggregates surrounding hyperplastic follicles (mimicking nodal marginal zone lymphoma) {524, 1894}. Despite a FTH phenotype, early stage disease, partial lymph node involvement, lack of enlarged follicular dendritic cell meshworks and lack of prominent high endothelial venules distinguish it from typical angioimmunoblastic T-cell lymphoma. Recently, a t(5;9) translocation has been reported in a subset of cases with these features {2112}. Other terms have been used for this variant, including perifollicular, intrafollicular, paracortical nodular and expanded mantle zone {1002, 1358}.

T-zone

The T-zone variant is characterized by a perifollicular growth pattern throughout the lymph node {1894, 2359}. The neoplastic cells are predominantly small with minimal cytological atypia, and the process may be mistaken for benign paracortical hyperplasia. The cells express CD3, CD4, and may show loss of CD5 or CD7. Some studies have suggested that this variant may be associated with a more indolent course than other PTCL, NOS {1894, 2359}, but data are limited. Many PTCL can show focal residual follicules; this histological feature alone does not constitute evidence for the T-zone variant.

Angioimmunoblastic T-cell lymphoma

A. Dogan
P. Gaulard
E.S. Jaffe
E. Ralfkiaer
H.K. Müller-Hermelink

Definition

Angioimmunoblastic T-cell lymphoma (AITL) is a peripheral T-cell lymphoma characterized by systemic disease, a polymorphous infiltrate involving lymph nodes, with a prominent proliferation of high endothelial venules and follicular dendritic cells.

ICD-O code 9705/3

Synonyms and historical annotation

AITL was previously felt to be an atypical reactive process, angioimmunoblastic lymphadenopathy, with an increased risk of progression to lymphoma. Currently, overwhelming evidence suggests that AITL rises de novo as a peripheral T-cell lymphoma {597}.

Epidemiology

AITL occurs in the middle-aged and elderly, with an equal incidence in males and females {597}. It is one of the more common specific subtypes of peripheral T-cell lymphoma, accounting for approximately 15–20% of cases, or 1–2% of all non-Hodgkin lymphomas {1896}.

Etiology

The nearly constant association with Epstein Barr virus (EBV) has suggested a possible role for the virus in the etiology, possibly through antigen-drive {623}. However, the neoplastic T cells are EBV negative.

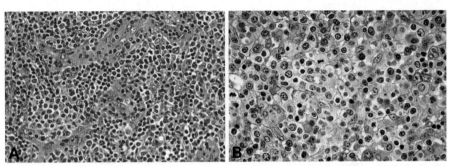

Fig. 11.73 Angioimmunoblastic T-cell lymphoma. **A** Typical cytology of neoplastic T-cells with intermediate-sized nuclei and copious pale/clear cytoplasm. **B** The infiltrate is composed of medium to large lymphoid cells with abundant clear cytoplasm.

Sites of involvement

The primary site of disease is the lymph node and virtually all patients present with generalized lymphadenopathy. In addition, spleen, liver, skin and bone marrow (BM) are frequently involved {597}.

Clinical features

AITL typically presents with advanced stage disease, generalized lymphadenopathy, hepatosplenomegaly, systemic symptoms, and polyclonal hypergammaglobulinemia {597, 1234A, 1529A, 2021}. Skin rash, often with pruritus, is frequently present. Other common findings are pleural effusion, arthritis and ascites. Laboratory findings include circulating immune complexes, cold agglutinins with haemolytic anaemia, positive rheumatoid factor and anti-smooth muscle antibodies.
Patients exhibit immunodeficiency secondary to the neoplastic process. In the

majority of the cases (75%), expansion of B-cells positive for EBV is seen, thought to be a consequence of underlying immune dysfunction {97}.

Morphology

AITL is characterized by partial effacement of the lymph node architecture, often with perinodal infiltration but sparing of the peripheral cortical sinuses. There is marked proliferation of arborizing high endothelial venules (HEV). There is predominantly paracortical polymorphic infiltrate composed of small to medium-sized lymphocytes, with clear to pale cytoplasm and distinct cell membranes and minimal cytological atypia. The neoplastic cells often form small clusters around the follicles and HEV and are admixed with variable numbers of small reactive lymphocytes, eosinophils, plasma cells and histiocytes. The polymorphic infiltrate is frequently

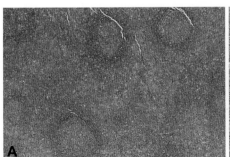
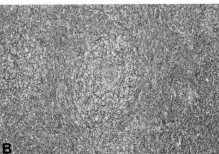
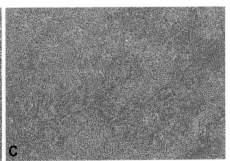

Fig. 11.74 Histological patterns of angioimmunoblastic T-cell lymphoma. **A** An early case with hyperplastic follicles and paracortical expansion (Pattern 1). **B** A case with depleted/atrophic follicles reminiscent of Castleman's disease and marked paracortical expansion (Pattern 2). **C** Classical morphology with effacement of normal architecture and marked vascular proliferation associated with aggregates of atypical lymphoid cells (Pattern 3).

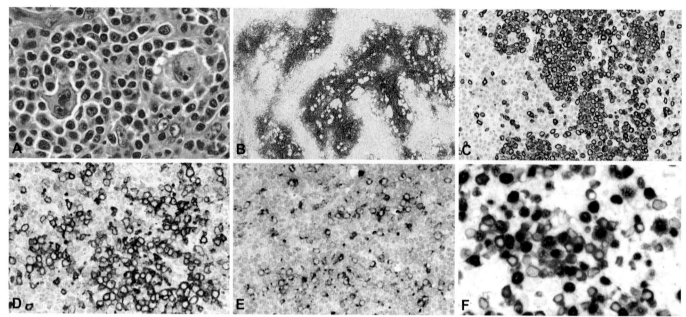

Fig. 11.75 Angioimmunoblastic T-cell lymphoma. **A** Multinucleated cells resembling Reed-Sternberg cells. **B** Low power view of CD21 immunostain highlighting marked follicular dendritic cell proliferation entrapping high endothelial venules. **C** The characteristic phenotype of tumour cells expressing CD3 (**C**), CD10 (**D**) and CXCL13 (**E**). **F** EBV-positive B-cell proliferation in angioimmunoblastic T-cell lymphoma double stained for CD79a (in brown-cytoplasmic) and EBV-EBER (in blue-nuclear).

associated with increased follicular dendritic cell meshworks. Early cases may contain hyperplastic follicles with ill-defined borders and the characteristic histology may be limited to the perifollicular areas with predominance of clear cells {1828}. The relationship between AITL showing limited paracortical involvement and the follicular variant of peripheral T-cell lymphoma, NOS remains to be clarified. An expansion of B immunoblasts is usually present in the paracortex. The expansion of normal B-cells and follicular dendritic cells in the lesions has been linked to the functional properties of the neoplastic cells as follicular helper T-cells (TFH) of the normal follicle. The expression of CXCL13 mediates expansion of follicular dendritic cells, and, adhesion of B-cells to HEV with subsequent entry to the lymph nodes. EBV-positive B-cells are nearly always present. They range in cell size and expansion of B immunoblasts may be prominent {2377, 2490}. The EBV-positive B immunoblastic proliferation may progress, either composite with AITL, or at relapse to EBV-positive diffuse large B-cell lymphoma {5, 99, 2490}. EBV-positive Reed-Sternberg-like cells of B-cell lineage may be present and may simulate classical Hodgkin lymphoma {1794}. In advanced cases, the inflammatory component is diminished, and the proportion of clear cells and large cells is increased.

Immunophenotype

The neoplastic T-cells express most pan T-cell antigens such as CD3, CD2 and CD5 and, in vast majority of the cases, CD4 although numerous reactive CD8+ T-cells are often present. Characteristically, the tumour cells show the phenotype of normal TFH expressing CD10, CXCL13 and PD-1 in 60–100% of the cases {96, 523, 605, 851}. This phenotype is helpful

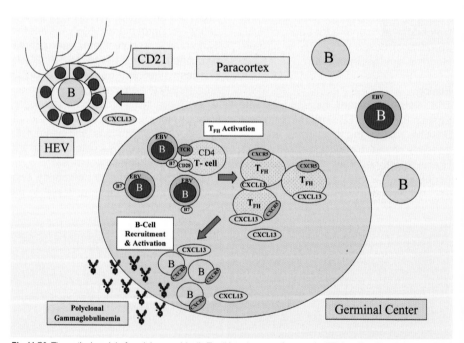

Fig.11.76 Theoretical model of angioimmunoblastic T cell lymphoma pathogenesis. EBV-positive B-cells present EBV viral proteins (e.g. EBNA-1) in association with MHC class II molecules, upregulate CD28 ligand (B7), and provide co-stimulatory signals for TFH cell activation. TFH cells upregulate CXCR5 and CXCL13. CXCL13 promotes B-cell recruitment to the lymph node through adherence of B-cells on high endothelial venules (HEV) and capillaries within germinal centres. Increased B-cells expand in the paracortex and are activated. Some paracortical B-cells become EBV transformed. CD21-positive dendritic cells expand from the HEV. Figure reproduced with permission from {623}.

in distinguishing AITL from atypical para-cortical hyperplasia and other peripheral T-cell lymphomas {631, 852} as well as diagnosing extranodal dissemination {98, 156, 1656A}. B immunoblasts and plasma cells are polytypic; however, secondary EBV-positive B-cell proliferations including diffuse large B-cell lymphoma, classical Hodgkin lymphoma or plasmacytoma may be seen. Follicular dendritic cell meshworks expressing CD21, CD23, CD35 and CNA42 are expanded, usually surrounding the high HEV.

Postulated normal counterpart
CD4+ follicular helper T-cell.

Genetics
T-cell receptor genes show clonal rearrangements in 75–90% of cases {97, 2155, 2378}. Clonal immunoglobulin gene rearrangements may be found in around 25–30% of cases {97, 2155}, and correlate with expanded EBV+ B-cells. The most frequent cytogenetic abnormalities are trisomy 3, trisomy 5 and an additional X chromosome {597, 1961} and comparative genetic hybridization has shown gains of 22q, 19 and 11q13 and losses of 13q in subset of cases {2233}. Gene expression profiling studies have shown that the neoplastic cells show features of CD4+ TFH {523}.

Prognosis and predictive factors
The clinical course is aggressive with a median survival of less than three years. Patients often succumb to infectious complications, which makes delivery of aggressive chemotherapy difficult {1336, 2021}. Supervening large B-cell lymphoma (often but not invariably EBV-positive) can occur {5, 99, 135, 2490}.

Anaplastic large cell lymphoma (ALCL), ALK-positive

G. Delsol
B. Falini
H.K. Müller-Hermelink
E. Campo

E.S. Jaffe
R.D. Gascoyne
H. Stein
M.C. Kinney

Definition

Anaplastic large cell lymphoma (ALCL), anaplastic lymphoma kinase (ALK)-positive is a T-cell lymphoma consisting of lymphoid cells that are usually large with abundant cytoplasm and pleomorphic, often horseshoe-shaped nuclei, with a translocation involving the *ALK* gene and expression of ALK protein, and expression of CD30. ALCL with comparable morphologic and phenotypic features, but lacking *ALK* rearrangement and the ALK protein, are considered as a separate category (ALCL, ALK-). ALCL, ALK+ must also be distinguished from primary cutaneous ALCL and from other subtypes of T- or B-cell lymphoma with anaplastic features and/or CD30 expression.

ICD-O code   9714/3

Epidemiology

ALCL, ALK+ accounts for approximately 3% of adult non-Hodgkin lymphomas and 10–20% of childhood lymphomas {2087}. ALCL, ALK+ is most frequent in the first three decades of life {188, 668} and shows a male predominance (M:F ratio 1.5:1).

Sites of involvement

ALCL, ALK+ frequently involves both lymph nodes and extranodal sites. The most commonly involved extranodal sites include skin, bone, soft tissues, lung and liver {285, 668, 2087}. Involvement of the gut and central nervous system (CNS) is rare. Mediastinal disease is less frequent than in classical Hodgkin lymphoma. The incidence of bone marrow (BM) involvement is approximately 10% when analyzed with H&E, but is increased significantly (30%) when immunohistochemical stains are used {724}, since BM involvement is often subtle. The small cell variant of ALCL, ALK+ may have a leukaemic presentation with peripheral blood (PB) involvement {164, 1152}.

Clinical features

The majority of patients (70%) present with advanced stage III-IV disease with peripheral and/or abdominal lymphadenopathy,

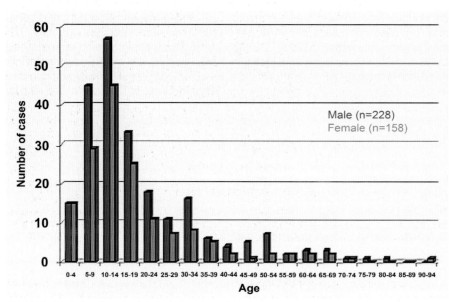

Fig. 11.77 Distribution of anaplastic large cell lymphoma (ALCL), ALK+ by age (n=386).

often associated with extranodal infiltrates and involvement of the BM {285, 668, 2091}. Patients often have B symptoms (75%), especially high fever {285, 668, 2091}.

Morphology

ALCL, ALK+ show a broad morphologic spectrum {188, 383, 551, 660, 898, 1033, 1152, 1746}. However, all cases contain a variable proportion of cells with eccentric, horseshoe- or kidney-shaped nuclei often with an eosinophilic region near the nucleus. These cells have been referred to as hallmark cells because they are present in all morphologic variants {188}. Although the hallmark cells are typically large, smaller cells with similar cytological features may be seen and can greatly aid in accurate diagnosis {188}. Depending upon the plane of section, some cells may appear to contain nuclear inclusions, but these are not true inclusions but invaginations of the nuclear membrane. Cells with these features have been referred to as doughnut cells {1033}. Morphologic features of ALCL, ALK+ range from small cell neoplasms to an opposite extreme in which very large cells

predominate. Five morphologic patterns can be recognized.
The "common pattern" accounts for 60% of cases {188, 660}. The tumour cells

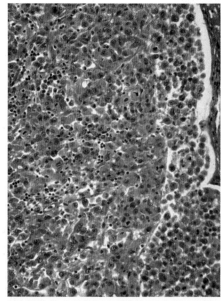

Fig. 11.78 General features of ALCL, common type. The lymph node architecture is obliterated by malignant cells and intrasinusoidal cells are observed.

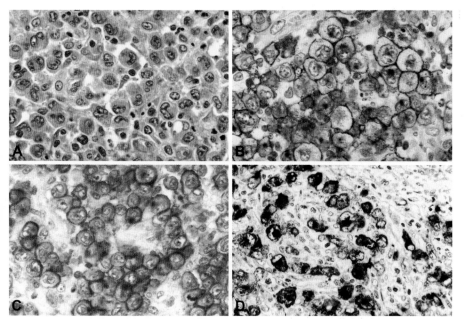

Fig. 11.79 General features of ALCL, common pattern. **A** Predominant population of large cells with irregular nuclei. Note large hallmark cells showing eccentric kidney-shaped nuclei. All malignant cells are strongly positive for CD30 (**B**), for the epithelial membrane antigen (**C**) and for granzyme B (**D**).

have abundant cytoplasm that may appear clear, basophilic or eosinophilic. Multiple nuclei may occur in a wreath-like pattern and may give rise to cells resembling Reed-Sternberg cells. The nuclear chromatin is usually finely clumped or dispersed with multiple small, basophilic nucleoli. In cases composed of larger cells, the nucleoli are more prominent, but eosinophilic, inclusion-like nucleoli are rarely seen. When the lymph node architecture is only partially effaced, the tumour characteristically grows within the sinuses and thus, may resemble a metastatic tumour.

The "lymphohistiocytic pattern" (10%) is characterized by tumour cells admixed with a large number of reactive histiocytes {188, 660, 1746}. The histiocytes may mask the malignant cells which are often smaller than in the common pattern. The neoplastic cells often cluster around blood vessels and can be highlighted by immunostaining using antibodies to CD30 and/or ALK. Occasionally, the histiocytes show signs of erythrophagocytosis.

The "small cell pattern" (5–10%) shows a predominant population of small to medium-sized neoplastic cells with irregular nuclei {188, 660, 1033, 1152}. In some cases, the majority of the cells have pale cytoplasm and centrally located nucleus, referred to as "fried egg cells". Signet ring-like cells may also be seen

rarely {188}. Hallmark cells are always present and are often concentrated around blood vessels {188, 1152}. This morphologic variant of ALCL is often misdiagnosed as peripheral T-cell lymphoma, NOS by

conventional examination. When the PB is involved, atypical cells reminiscent of flower-like cells can be noted in smear preparations.

The "Hodgkin-like pattern" (3%) is characterized by morphological features mimicking nodular sclerosis classical Hodgkin lymphoma (NSCHL) {2316}.

More than one pattern may be seen in a single lymph node biopsy ("composite pattern") (15%) {188}. Relapses may reveal morphologic features different from those seen initially {188, 946}. Other histological patterns include tumours showing cells with monomorphic, rounded nuclei, either as the predominant population or mixed with more pleomorphic cells, cases rich in multinucleated neoplastic giant cells or displaying sarcomatoid features {383}. Occasional cases may have a hypocellular appearance, with a myxoid or edematous background {410}. Spindle cells may be prominent in such cases and may simulate sarcoma in cases presenting in soft tissue {1034}. In rare cases, malignant cells are exceedingly scarce, scattered in an otherwise reactive lymph node. Capsular fibrosis and fibrosis associated with tumour nodules may be seen, mimicking metastatic nonlymphoid malignancy.

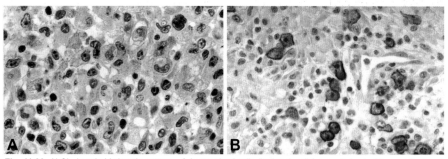

Fig. 11.80 ALCL, lymphohistiocytic pattern. **A** Large-sized cells (hallmark cells) are admixed with a predominant population of non-neoplastic cells, including histiocytes and plasma cells. **B** Malignant cells are highlighted by CD30 staining.

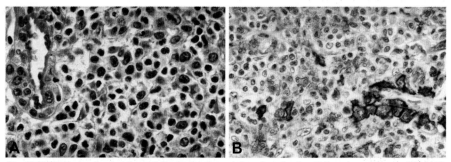

Fig. 11.81 ALCL, small cell pattern. **A** Predominant population of small cells with irregular nuclei associated with scattered hallmark cells. Note that large-sized cells predominate around the vessel. **B** CD30 staining highlights the perivascular pattern. Large cells are strongly positive for CD30 whereas small and medium-sized malignant cells are weakly stained.

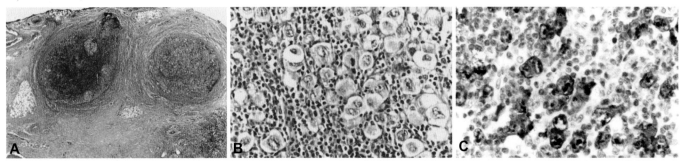

Fig. 11.82 ALCL showing "Hodgkin-like pattern". **A** Tumour nodules are surrounded by broad fibrous bands. **B** Numerous tumour cells are present, and some resemble lacunar Reed-Sternberg cells. **C** Tumour cells have cytoplasmic, nuclear and nucleolar ALK staining indicating the presence of the t(2;5)(p23;q35) and the NPM-ALK fusion protein.

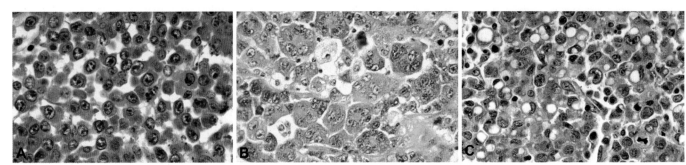

Fig. 11.83 Other histological patterns of ALCL (all these cases were positive for ALK protein). **A** ALCL showing monomorphic large cells with round nuclei. **B** ALCL consisting of pleomorphic giant cells. **C** ALCL rich in signet ring cells.

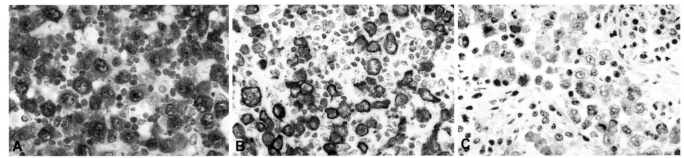

Fig. 11.84 Different ALK staining patterns. **A** Nuclear, nucleolar and cytoplasmic staining associated with the t(2;5) translocation (expression of the NPM-ALK hybrid protein). **B** Strong membranous and cytoplasmic staining sparing the nucleus in a case associated with the t(1;2) translocation (expression of the TPM3-ALK hybrid protein). **C** Finely granular cytoplasmic staining associated with the t(2;17) translocation (expression of CLTC-ALK hybrid protein).

Immunophenotype

The tumour cells are positive for CD30 on the cell membrane and in the Golgi region {2091}. The strongest immunostaining is seen in the large cells. Smaller tumour cells may be only weakly positive or even negative for CD30 {188}. In the lymphohistiocytic and small cell patterns, the strongest CD30 expression is also present in the larger tumour cells, which often cluster around blood vessels {188}. ALK expression is absent from all postnatal normal human tissues except rare cells in the brain {1786}. For this reason, immunohistochemistry has largely supplanted molecular tests for the diagnosis of ALCL, ALK+. Note that for ALK staining it is advisable to use monoclonal antibodies

(mouse or rabbit) instead of polyclonal antibodies which may give false positive staining. In the majority of the cases that have the t(2;5)/*NPM-ALK* translocation, ALK staining of large cells is both cytoplasmic and nuclear {188, 660, 2087}. In the small cell variant, ALK-positivity is usually restricted to the nucleus of tumour cells {188, 660, 1785, 2087}. In cases with variant translocations, the ALK staining may be membranous or cytoplasmic {188, 660, 1785, 2087}. Cases with t(2;5)/*NPM-ALK* translocation show aberrant cytoplasmic expression of nucleophosmin (NPM), while ALCL, ALK+ carrying variant translocations show the expected nuclear-restricted expression of NPM {669}.

The majority of ALCL, ALK+ are positive for EMA but, in some cases, only a proportion of malignant cells are positive {188, 551}. The great majority of ALCL, ALK+ express one or more T-cell antigens {188}. However, due to loss of several pan T-cell antigens, some cases may have an apparent "null cell" phenotype, but show evidence for a T-cell lineage at the genetic level {722}. Since no other distinctions can be found in cases with a T-cell versus a null-cell phenotype, T/null ALCL, ALK+ is considered a single entity {188, 898}. CD3, the most widely used pan T-cell marker, is negative in more than 75% of cases {188, 238}. CD2, CD5 and CD4 are more useful and are positive in a significant proportion of cases (70%). Furthermore, most cases

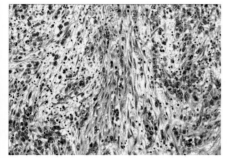

Fig. 11.85 ALCL showing sarcomatous features.

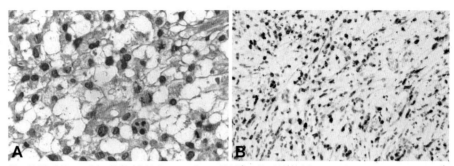

Fig. 11.86 A Hypocellular ALCL. **B** Malignant cells are highlighted by ALK staining.

exhibit positivity for the cytotoxic associated antigens TIA1, granzyme B, and/or perforin {722, 1192}. CD8 is usually negative, but rare CD8-positive cases exist. CD43 is expressed in two thirds of the cases, but this antigen lacks lineage specificity. Tumour cells are variably positive for CD45 and CD45RO and strongly positive for CD25 {551}. CD15 expression is rarely observed and when present only a small proportion of the neoplastic cells is stained {188}. Granular staining for some antibodies reactive with CD68, such as KP1, may be seen, but other antibodies directed against the macrophage-restricted form of CD68, such as PGM1, are negative. ALCL, ALK+ are BCL2 negative {484}. ALCL are also consistently negative for EBV (i.e. EBER and LMP1) {279}. A number of other antigens are expressed in ALCL but are not of diagnostic value. They include clusterin {2383}, SHP1 phosphatase {962}, BCL6, C/EBP {1798}, serpinA1 {1242} and fascin.

Differential diagnosis

A rare distinct diffuse large B-cell lymphoma with immunoblastic/plasmablastic features expressing the ALK protein may superficially resemble ALCL, ALK+ due to frequent sinusoidal growth pattern. These lymphomas express EMA (as do ALCL) but lack CD30 and show a characteristic cytoplasmic-restricted granular staining for the ALK protein {553}.

Some non-haematopoietic neoplasms such as rhabdomyosarcoma {660, 898} and inflammatory myofibroblastic tumours {843} may be positive for ALK but are morphologically distinguishable from ALCL and are negative for both CD30 and EMA.

Genetics

Antigen receptor genes

Approximately 90% of ALCL, ALK+ show clonal rearrangement of the T-cell receptor *(TCR)* genes irrespective of whether they express T-cell antigens or not. The remainder show no rearrangement of *TCR* or *IG* genes {722}.

Genetic abnormalities and oncogenes

The genes fused with *ALK* in various chromosomal translocations and the subcellular distribution of NPM-ALK and X-ALK chimeric proteins are shown in Table 11.08. The most frequent genetic alteration is a translocation, t(2;5)(p23;q35), between the *ALK* gene on chromosome 2 and the nucleophosmin *(NPM)* gene on chromosome 5 {1244, 1407, 1525}. Variant translocations involving *ALK* and other partner genes on chromosomes 1, 2, 3, 17, 19, 22 and X also occur {469, 669, 931, 1241, 1243, 1408, 1449, 1868, 2087, 2256, 2258, 2268, 2427}. The t(2;5) can be detected by RT-PCR, but cases with variant translocations will be negative by standard RT-PCR using primers that are specific for the *ALK* and *NPM* genes {660, 1762}. All these translocations result in upregulation of ALK, but the subcellular distribution of the staining varies depending on the translocation.

The *ALK* gene encodes a tyrosine kinase receptor belonging to the insulin receptor superfamily, which is normally silent in lymphoid cells {1525}. In the t(2;5)(p23;q35), the nucleophosmin *(NPM)* gene, a housekeeping gene, fuses the *ALK* gene to produce a chimeric protein in which the N-terminal portion of *NPM* is linked to the intracytoplasmic portion of *ALK* {1525}. The particular cytoplasmic, nuclear and nucleolar staining seen in cases associated with the t(2;5) can be explained by the formation of heterodimers between

Table 11.08 Translocations and fusion proteins involving *ALK* at 2p23.

Chromosomal anomaly	ALK partner	M Wt of ALK hybrid protein	ALK staining pattern	% of cases
t(2;5)(p23;q35)	NPM	80	Nuclear, diffuse cytoplasmic	84%
t(1;2)(q25;p23)	TPM3	104	Diffuse cytoplasmic with peripheral intensification	13%
Inv(2)(p23q35)	ATIC	96	Diffuse cytoplasmic	1%
t(2;3)(p23;q12)	TFG Xlong TFG long TFG short	113 97 85	Diffuse cytoplasmic Diffuse cytoplasmic Diffuse cytoplasmic	<1%
t(2;17)(p23;q23)	CLTC	250	Granular cytoplasmic	<1%
t(X;2)(q11-12;p23)	MSN	125	Membrane staining	<1%
t(2;19)(p23;p13.1)	TPM4	95	Diffuse cytoplasmic	<1%
t(2;22)(p23;q11.2)	MYH9	220	Diffuse cytoplasmic	<1%
t(2;17)(p23;q25)	ALO17	ND	Diffuse cytoplasmic	<1%
Others*	?	?	Nuclear or cytoplasmic	<1%

NPM, nucleophosmin gene; *TPM3* and *TPM4*, non-muscular tropomyosin gene; *TFG*, TRK-fused gene, three different fusion proteins of 85, 97 and 113kD (TFG-ALK$_S$, TFG-ALK$_L$, TFG-ALK$_{XL}$) are associated with the t(2;3)(p23;q35) which involves the TFG; *ATIC*, amino-terminus of 5-aminoimidazole-4-carboxamide ribonucleotide formyltransferase/IMP cyclohydrolase gene; *CLTC*, clathrin heavy polypeptide gene; *MSN*, moesin gene; *MYH9*, myosin heavy chain 9 gene; *ALO17*, ALK lymphoma oligomerization partner on chromosome 17.
*, unpublished series of 270 cases of ALCL, ALK+

wild-type NPM and the fusion NPM-ALK protein. On the other hand, the formation of NPM-ALK homodimers using dimerisation sites at the N-terminus of NPM mimicks ligand binding and is responsible for the activation of the ALK catalytic domain and for the oncogenic properties of the ALK protein {1785}.

Comparative genomic hybridization (CGH) analysis shows that ALCL, ALK+ carry frequent secondary chromosomal imbalance including losses of chromosome 4, 11q and 13q and gains of 7, 17p and 17q {1923}. In addition, this study demonstrates that ALK-positive and negative ALCL have a different representation of secondary genetic alterations, supporting the concept that they are different biological entities.

Gene expression profiling

Supervised analysis by class comparison between ALCL, ALK+ and ALCL, ALK- tumours provided distinct molecular signatures {1242}. Among the 117 genes overexpressed in ALCL, ALK+, *BCL6, PTPN12* (tyrosine phosphatase), *serpinA1* and *C/EBP* were the four top genes, being overexpressed with the most significant p-value. This overexpression was also confirmed at the protein level for C/EBP, BCL6 and serpin A1.

Postulated normal counterpart

Activated mature cytotoxic T-cell.

Prognosis and predictive factors

The international prognostic index (IPI) appears to be of some value in predicting outcome in ALCL, ALK+, although less

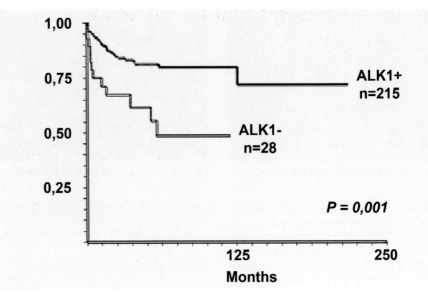

Fig. 11.87 Overall survival of ALK-positive and negative patients.

significantly than in other variants of lymphoma {668, 760}. No differences have been found between NPM-ALK-positive tumours and tumours showing variant translocations {668, 669, 760, 2013}. It might be that cases with small cell variant histology do not have the same favourable prognosis as the other ALK positive tumours since these patients often present with disseminated disease at diagnosis. ALCL, ALK+ patients have a favourable prognosis compared with ALCL, ALK- {668, 760, 2013}. The overall 5-year survival rate in ALCL, ALK+ approaches 80%, in contrast to only 48% in ALCL, ALK-. In the recent study by Savage and co-workers {1943A}, the overall 5-year survival of ALCL, ALK+ patients is slightly

lower (70%) due to the exclusion of paediatric patients. In the latter study, the 5-year failure free survival (FFS) of patients with ALCL, ALK+ was 60% *versus* 36% for ALCL, ALK-. Relapses are not uncommon (30% of cases), but often remain sensitive to chemotherapy; allogeneic BM transplant may be effective in refractory cases {1319}. Since it is now clearly demonstrated that ALK is essential for the proliferation and survival of the cells of ALCL, ALK+, it can be expected that specific ALK inhibitors, currently tested in preclinical models, may be available in the near future for clinical trials {1763}.

Anaplastic large cell lymphoma, ALK-negative

D.Y. Mason
N.L. Harris
G. Delsol
H. Stein
E. Campo
M.C. Kinney
E.S. Jaffe
B. Falini

Definition

ALK-negative anaplastic large cell lymphoma (ALCL, ALK-) is included as a provisional entity, and is defined as a CD30+ T-cell neoplasm that is not reproducibly distinguishable on morphological grounds from ALK-positive ALCL (ALCL, ALK+), but lacks anaplastic large cell lymphoma kinase (ALK) protein. Most cases express T-cell-associated markers and cytotoxic granule-associated proteins. ALCL, ALK- must be distinguished from primary cutaneous ALCL, other subtypes of CD30+ T- or B-cell lymphoma with anaplastic features, and classical Hodgkin lymphoma (CHL).

ICD-O code   9702/3

Synonyms and historical annotation

ALCL, ALK- was included in the third edition of the WHO classification, together with ALCL, ALK + in the broader entity of "anaplastic large cell lymphoma" {554}. However, it was also recognized that ALCL, ALK- (mainly because of their older median age and more aggressive clinical course) are felt to be distinct from ALCL, ALK+ {554}. However, there are also valid arguments for excluding ALCL, ALK- from the category of peripheral T-cell lymphoma (PTCL), not otherwise specified (NOS) {659, 1034, 2030, 2431}. Unfortunately, there are few detailed clinicopathological studies of ALCL, ALK- {2181} and no specific oncogenic abnormalities (e.g. comparable to ALK gene rearrangement) have been identified. Thus, the distinction between PTCL, NOS, and ALCL, ALK- is not always straightforward. The current WHO Classification considers ALCL, ALK- to be a provisional entity within the spectrum of mature T-cell lymphomas, distinct from both ALCL, ALK+ and PTCL, NOS.

Epidemiology

The peak incidence of ALCL, ALK- is in adults (40–65 years), unlike ALCL, ALK+, which occurs most commonly in children and young adults, although cases can occur at any age {659, 2087}. There is a modest male preponderance (1.5:1).

Sites of involvement

ALCL, ALK- involves both lymph nodes and extranodal tissue, although the latter sites are less commonly involved than in ALCL, ALK+. Extranodal sites include bone, soft tissues and skin. Cutaneous cases must be distinguished from primary cutaneous ALCL and cases that involve the gastrointestinal tract must be distinguished from CD30-positive enteropathy-associated T-cell lymphomas.

Clinical features

Most patients present with advanced stage III to IV disease, with peripheral and/or abdominal lymphadenopathy, and B symptoms {2180}.

Morphology

In most cases the nodal or other tissue architecture is effaced by solid, cohesive sheets of neoplastic cells. When lymph node architecture is preserved, the neoplastic cells typically grow within sinuses or within T-cell areas, commonly showing a "cohesive" pattern that may mimic carcinoma. Features such as sclerosis or eosinophils may occur, but when present should raise the suspicion of CHL. The neoplastic cells show a similar morphological spectrum to ALCL, ALK+, although a "small cell variant" is not recognized. Biopsies typically show large pleomorphic cells, sometimes containing prominent nucleoli. Multinucleated, including wreath-like, cells may also be present and mitotic figures are not infrequent. In addition, to a variable degree, "hallmark" cells with eccentric, horseshoe- or kidney-shaped nuclei are seen. The neoplastic cells in ALCL, ALK- tend to be larger and more pleomorphic than those seen in classical ALCL, ALK+ and/or have a higher nuclear:cytoplasmic ratio {668, 1565, 1762, 2013}. The latter feature may suggest a diagnosis of PTCL, NOS, but in the latter disorder abnormal small to medium-sized lymphocytes are often admixed with a morphologically homogeneous neoplastic cell population, and the sheet-like or sinus pattern of infiltration typical of ALCL is absent.

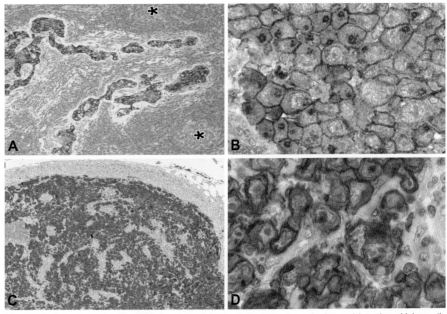

Fig. 11.88 Immunostaining for CD30 in cases of ALCL, ALK- shows the cohesive and intrasinusoidal growth pattern of the tumour and the homogeneous expression of this marker on tumour cells. Note the Golgi- and membrane-associated pattern of staining. Asterisks indicate preserved lymphoid follicles.

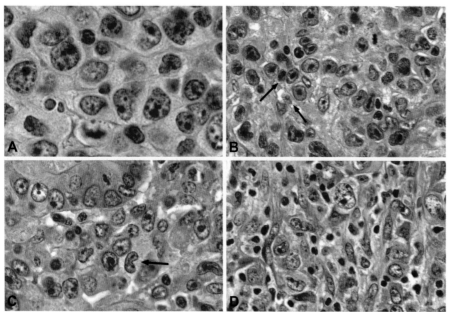

Fig. 11.89 Morphological features of four cases of ALCL, ALK-. **A** Note the high nuclear to cytoplasmic ratio. **B** Eosinophils (arrows) are present (often in clusters) but other features of Hodgkin lymphoma are absent. **C** Typical morphological and phenotypic features of ALCL (a hallmark cell is arrowed) but arose in the gastrointestinal tract (glandular epithelium is seen in the upper left). **D** Case with more cellular pleomorphism.

Emphasis should be placed on CD30 expression; if a large cell lymphoma of non-B-cell phenotype shows strong, homogeneous CD30 expression, especially if this is strongest in the Golgi and membrane regions, and the morphological features are consistent with ALCL, it should be classified as ALCL, ALK-. Fortunately the distinction between ALCL, ALK- and PTCL, NOS currently carries no major clinical implications.

Immunophenotype

All tumour cells are strongly positive for CD30, usually most strongly at the cell membrane and in the Golgi region, although diffuse cytoplasmic positivity is also common. Staining should be strong and of equal intensity in all cells, a feature that is important in distinguishing ALCL, ALK- from other PTCL, which can express CD30 in at least a proportion of the cells, and usually with variable intensity. ALK protein is by definition undetectable.

Loss of T-cell markers can occur, with greater frequency than typically seen in PTCL, NOS. In this respect, ALCL, ALK- is similar to ALCL, ALK+. However, overall more than half of all cases express one or more T-cell markers. CD2 and CD3 are found more often than CD5, and CD43 is almost always expressed. CD4 is positive in a significant proportion of cases, whereas CD8-positive cases are rare. Many cases express the cytotoxic-associated markers TIA1, granzyme B and/or perforin. A substantial minority of cases is positive for EMA (on at least a proportion of malignant cells), a marker that is almost always seen in ALCL, ALK+ but only occasionally in PTCL, NOS.

In cases that lack all T-cell/cytotoxic markers, CHL rich in neoplastic cells or another large cell malignancy (e.g. embryonal carcinoma) should be ruled out. In this regard, staining for PAX5 is useful; CHL will show weak expression of PAX5 in the majority of cases, whereas it should be negative in all cases of ALCL, ALK- or ALK+. The demonstration of CD15 should raise a suspicion for CHL. However, CD15 may be expressed in some cases of PTCL NOS, and such cases are generally strongly CD30-positive {149}. Whether peripheral T-cell neoplasms expressing both CD30 and CD15 should be classified as ALCL, ALK- or PTCL, NOS, remains to be determined. Notably, these cases have a very poor prognosis, thus clinically more closely resembling PTCL, NOS. ALCL, ALK- are consistently negative for Epstein-Barr virus (EBV) (i.e. EBER and LMP1), and the expression of these markers should strongly suggest the possibility of CHL.

A single study has reported that ALCL, ALK- and ALCL, ALK+ lack T-cell receptor proteins, and in this respect tend to differ from PTCL, NOS {238}. Clusterin is also commonly expressed in ALCL, ALK- and ALK+, but rarely in PTCL, NOS {1235, 1574, 1905}; this marker has not been examined extensively in CHL, but was negative in the cases studied {2383}.

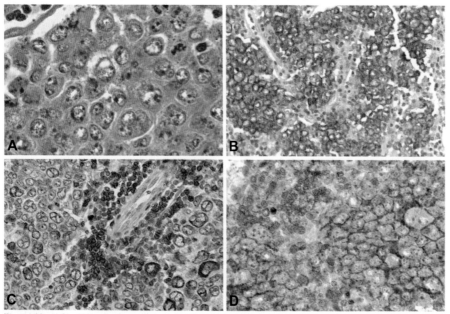

Fig. 11.90 ALCL, ALK- showing a high nuclear to cytoplasmic ratio. **A** Some features suggest peripheral T-cell lymphoma, NOS. However, extensive CD30 expression in every cell is characteristic of ALCL, ALK- (**B**). **C** Lymphoma cells express CD3 (**C**) and CD4 (**D**). Note a vessel surrounded by normal, small CD3+ T-cells.

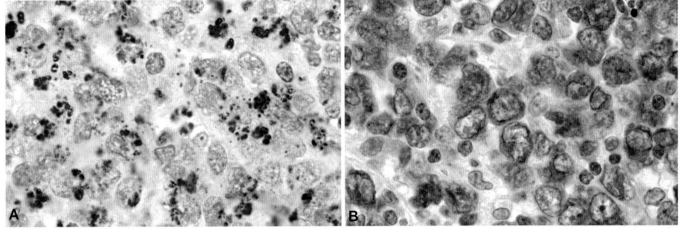

Fig. 11.91 Expression of the cytotoxic T-cell markers TIA1 (**A**) and perforin (**B**) in ALCL, ALK-.

Differential diagnosis

The principle differential diagnosis of ALCL, ALK- is with PTCL, NOS, and CHL. Historically, many cases referred to as Hodgkin-like ALCL have now been reclassified as tumour cells rich forms of CHL. With complete immunophenotypic and genetic studies, ALCL, ALK- can be distinguished from CHL in virtually all cases. By contrast, the distinction between PTCL, NOS and ALCL, ALK- is not always clear-cut, and even experts may disagree on this subject. In general, the WHO Classification advocates a conservative approach, recommending the diagnosis of ALCL, ALK-, only if both the morphology and phenotype are very close to those of ALK-positive cases, with the only distinction being the presence or absence of ALK. ALCL, ALK- must also be distinguished from primary cutaneous ALCL, which can have a similar phenotype and morphology. Clinical correlation with staging is of paramount importance in this differential. Primary cutaneous ALCL has a much better prognosis than ALCL, ALK-.

Genetics

The majority of cases show clonal rearrangement of the T-cell receptor *(TCR)* genes, whether or not they express T-cell antigens.

No recurrent primary cytogenetic abnormalities occur with any frequency. Two studies indicate a tendency of ALCL, ALK- to differ (e.g. in terms of chromosome losses or gains) both from PTCL, NOS and from ALCL, ALK+, although overlapping features can also be found {1923, 2492}. Similarly, published gene expression studies suggest that ALCL, ALK- has a distinct profile but these results do not provide definitive evidence as to whether the disease is more closely related to ALCL, ALK- or to PTCL, NOS {137, 1242, 2231}.

Postulated normal counterpart

Activated mature cytotoxic T-cell.

Prognosis and predictive factors

The clinical outcome of ALCL, ALK- with conventional therapy is clearly poorer than that of ALCL, ALK+ {668, 760, 2180}. There is some suggestion that there is a plateau of long-term survivors (not seen in PTCL, NOS), but this remains to be confirmed. In a recent report by the International Peripheral T-cell Lymphoma Project {1943A}, the clinical features of the ALCL, ALK+ and ALCL, ALK- have been compared with each other and with PTCL, NOS. The results of this study further highlight the outcome differences between PTCL, NOS and ALCL, ALK-. The 5-year FFS (36% vs 20%) and OS (49% vs 32%) were superior in ALCL, ALK- compared to PTCL, NOS. Furthermore, confining the analysis of cases of PTCL, NOS with high CD30 expression (>80% of cells), a group that can be difficult to differentiate histologically from ALCL, ALK-, magnified the difference in 5-year FFS and 5-year OS (19%) compared to ALCL, ALK-.

CHAPTER 12

Hodgkin Lymphoma

Introduction

H. Stein

Definition

Hodgkin lymphomas (HL) share the following characteristics: (1) they usually arise in lymph nodes, preferentially in the cervical region; (2) the majority of them manifest clinically in young adults; (3) neoplastic tissues usually contain a small number of scattered large mononucleated and multinucleated tumour cells (designated Hodgkin and Reed-Sternberg cells or HRS cells) residing in an abundant heterogeneous admixture of non-neoplastic inflammatory and accessory cells; (4) the tumour cells are often ringed by T lymphocytes in a rosette-like manner. Hodgkin lymphomas account for ~30% of all lymphomas. Their absolute incidence has not apparently changed, in contrast with non-Hodgkin lymphomas where there has been a steady increase in incidence.

Synonyms and historical annotation

This neoplasm was recognized in the first half of the 19th century by Thomas Hodgkin {947} and Samuel Wilks {2404, 2405}. The latter named it Hodgkin disease. The disease was also called lymphogranulomatosis, a term that is no longer in use. Since the origin of the Reed-Sternberg cell is known to be a lymphoid cell —most often of B-cell type— the term Hodgkin lymphoma is preferred over Hodgkin's disease. The modern classification of Hodgkin lymphoma is based on the Lukes-Butler scheme {1344, 1345}.

Subclassification

Biological and clinical studies in the last 30 years have shown that Hodgkin lymphomas are comprised of two disease entities {33, 573, 1406A, 1603}: nodular lymphocyte predominant Hodgkin lymphoma (NLPHL) and classical Hodgkin lymphoma (CHL). These two entities differ in their clinical features and behaviour as well as in the composition of their cellular background and —diagnostically most important— in the morphology, immunophenotype and the preservation or extinction of B-cell gene expression program. Within classical HL, four subtypes have been distinguished: nodular sclerosis, mixed cellularity, lymphocyte-rich and lymphocyte-depleted. These subtypes differ in their sites of involvement, clinical features, growth pattern, presence of fibrosis, composition of cellular background, number and/or degree of atypia of the tumour cells and frequency of Epstein-Barr virus (EBV) infection, but not in the immunophenotype of the tumour cells, which is the same in all four variants. A detailed account of the historical evolution of the subclassification of Hodgkin lymphoma is provided by Mauch *et al.* {1432} and by Anagnostopoulos *et al.* {33}.

Staging

Treatment of HL is based on clinical, and occasionally on pathological staging of the disease. The modified Ann Arbor staging system {1320B} is used (Table 12.01).

Table 12.01 Cotswold revision {1320B} of the Ann Arbor staging classification {337A}.

Stage	Definition
I	Involvement of a single lymph node region or lymphoid structure (e.g. spleen, thymus, Waldeyer ring).
II	Involvement of two or more lymph node regions on the same side of the diaphragm (the mediastinum is a single site; hilar lymph nodes are lateralized); the number of anatomic sites should be indicated by suffix (e.g. II$_3$).
III	Involvement of lymph node regions or structures on both sides of the diaphragm.
III$_1$	With or without splenic, hilar, celiac or portal nodes.
III$_2$	With paraaortic, iliac or mesenteric nodes.
IV	Involvement of extranodal site(s) beyond those designated E.

E, involvement of a single extranodal site, or contiguous or proximal to known nodal site of disease.

Nodular lymphocyte predominant Hodgkin lymphoma

S. Poppema
G. Delsol
S.A. Pileri
H. Stein

S.H. Swerdlow
R.A. Warnke
E.S. Jaffe

Definition

Nodular lymphocyte predominant Hodgkin lymphoma (NLPHL) is a monoclonal B-cell neoplasm characterized by a nodular, or a nodular and diffuse proliferation of scattered large neoplastic cells known as popcorn or lymphocyte predominant cells (LP cells) —formerly called L&H cells for lymphocytic and/or histiocytic Reed-Sternberg cell variants. These cells reside in large spherical meshworks of follicular dendritic cell processes that are filled with non-neoplastic lymphocytes and histiocytes. One third of the cases diagnosed in the past has an NLPHL were lymphocyte-rich classical HL. It is currently not clear whether a purely diffuse form of NLPHL exists. Most lesions diagnosed in the past as diffuse LPHL were probably T-cell-rich large B-cell lymphoma (TCRBCL). At present an overlap between NLPHL and TCRBCL cannot be excluded.

ICD-O code   9659/3

Epidemiology

NLPHL represents approximately 5% of all Hodgkin lymphomas. Patients are predominantly male and most frequently in the 30–50 year age group.

Sites of involvement

NLPHL usually involves cervical, axillary or inguinal lymph nodes. Mediastinal, splenic and bone marrow (BM) involvement are rare.

Clinical features

Most patients present with localized peripheral lymphadenopathy (stage I or II). 5–25% of patients present with advanced stage disease {33, 2009}.

Morphology

The lymph node architecture is totally or partially replaced by a nodular or a nodular and diffuse infiltrate, predominantly consisting of small lymphocytes, histiocytes, epithelioid histiocytes and intermingled LP cells. The latter cells are large and usually have one large nucleus and

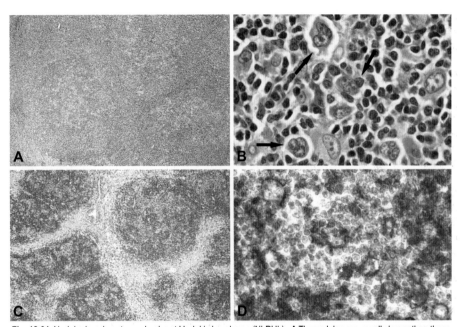

Fig. 12.01 Nodular lymphocyte predominant Hodgkin lymphoma (NLPHL). **A** The nodules are usually larger than those present in follicular lymphoma and follicular hyperplasia, and are closely packed and lack mantle zones. **B** Three popcorn cells (arrows) with the typically lobated nuclei are visible in a background of small lymphoid cells and a few histiocytes. **C** The CD20 staining reveals that the nodules of this lymphoma predominantly consist of B-cells. **D** At higher magnification, the strong membrane staining of the popcorn cells for CD20 is visible.

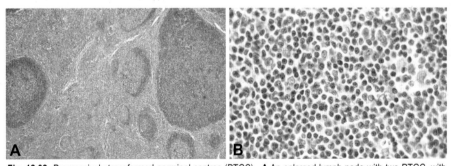

Fig. 12.02 Progressively transformed germinal centres (PTGC). **A** An enlarged lymph node with two PTGC, with several normal germinal centres in between. **B** Higher magnification shows a predominance of small lymphocytes with rare centroblasts and centrocytes.

scant cytoplasm. The nuclei are often folded or multilobated, often to such an extreme that they have also been termed "popcorn" cells. The nucleoli are usually multiple, basophilic and smaller than those seen in classical Hodgkin and Reed-Sternberg (HRS) cells. However, some LP cells may contain one prominent nucleolus and/or have more than one nucleus, and thus may be indistinguishable

from classical HRS cells on purely morphological grounds. The diffuse areas are mainly composed of small lymphocytes with admixed histiocytes which are either single or in clusters. The process is rarely totally diffuse. According to current criteria the detection of one nodule showing the typical features of NLPHL in an otherwise diffuse growth pattern is sufficient to exclude the diagnosis of a primary

T-cell/histiocyte-rich large B-cell lymphoma (THRLBCL). Histiocytes and some polyclonal plasma cells can be found at the margin of the nodules. Neutrophils and eosinophils are seldom seen in either the nodular and diffuse regions. Occasionally, there is reactive follicular hyperplasia with progressive transformation of germinal centres (PTGC) adjacent to the lesion or it may proceed or follow a diagnosis of NLPHL {33, 898}. It is uncertain whether these lesions are preneoplastic. The vast majority of patients with reactive hyperplasia and PTGC do not develop Hodgkin lymphoma {700,1657}.

Sclerosis is infrequently present in primary biopsies (7%), but can be found more frequently in recurrences (44%). Remnants of small germinal centres are infrequently present in the nodules of NLPHL, a finding more typical of lymphocyte-rich classical Hodgkin lymphoma (LRCHL) {33, 671}.

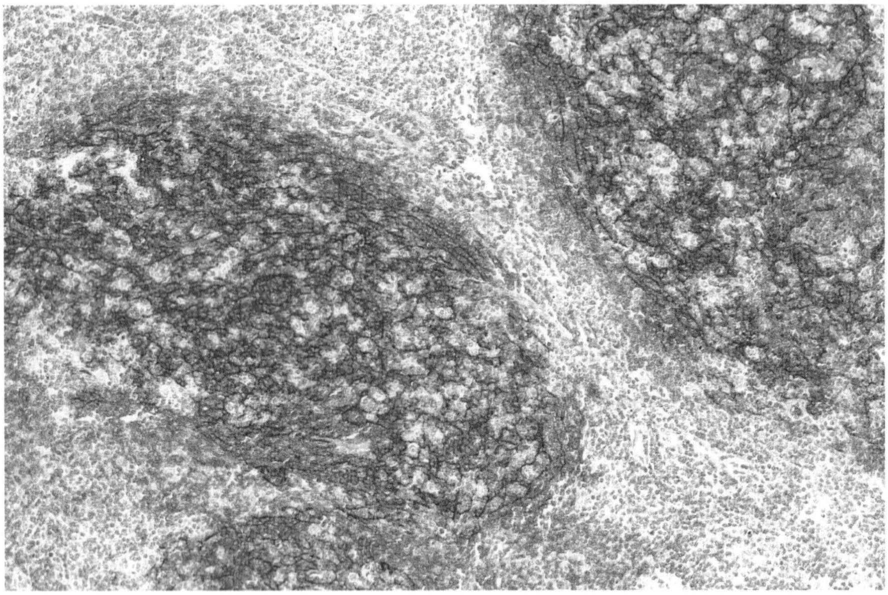

Immunophenotype

LP cells are positive for CD20 {457, 1752, 1753}, CD79a, CD75, BCL6 and CD45 in nearly all cases, J chain {1771, 2089} is present in the majority of cases, and epithelial membrane antigen (EMA) in more than 50% of cases {33, 427} (Table 12.02). In contrast to HRS cells from classical HL, OCT-2, BOB.1 and activation-induced diaminase (AID) are consistently coexpressed in NLPHL. Labeling for immunoglobulin light and/or heavy chains is frequently strong {1964, 1965, 2090}. In 9–27% of cases the LP cells are IgD-positive {837A, 1777, 2090}. The expression of IgD is more common in young males {1777}. LP cells lack CD15 and CD30 in nearly all instances. However, CD30-positive large cells may be seen: these are in most instances reactive immunoblasts unrelated to the LP cells {33}. Infrequently, the LP cells show weak expression of CD30. As revealed by their nuclear positivity for Ki67, most LP cells are in cycle. Most of the LP cells are ringed by CD3+ T cells, and to a lesser extent by CD57+ T cells.

The architectural background in NLPHL is composed of large spherical meshworks of follicular dendritic cells, which are predominantly filled with small B cells, and numerous CD4+/CD57+ T cells {1772}. These T-cells express markers like c-MAF, PD-1, BCL6, IRF4/MUM1 and CD134, all consistent with a subset of germinal centre T cells, but they do not produce IL-2 and IL-4 {95}. CD8, TIA1, and CD40L positive cells are absent, whereas CD4+/CD8+ cells are relatively frequent {1804}. Immunostaining for CD20 is helpful in detecting nodules in lesions that appear to be totally diffuse in H&E stains. T cells are numerous in the diffuse areas and tend to increase over time {33}.

A number of immunoarchitectural patterns have been described, including classic (B-cell-rich) nodular, serpiginious nodular, nodular with prominent extranodular LP cells, T-cell-rich nodular, TCRBCL-like and diffuse B-cell-rich {671}.

Fig. 12.03 Nodular lymphocyte predominant Hodgkin lymphoma (NLPHL). Immunostaining for CD21 makes visible the expanded meshwork of the follicular dendritic cells in the nodules of this lymphoma type.

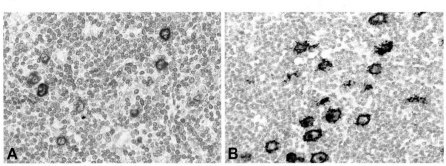

Fig. 12.04 Nodular lymphocyte predominant Hodgkin lymphoma (NLPHL). **A** Cytoplasmic positivity of the popcorn cells for J-chain is seen. **B** Membrane and dot-like staining in the Golgi region for epithelial membrane antigen (EMA) is visible in the popcorn cells.

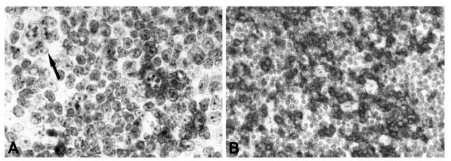

Fig. 12.05 Nodular lymphocyte predominant Hodgkin lymphoma (NLPHL). **A** Non-neoplastic bystander lymphoid blasts stain for CD30 whereas the neoplastic popcorn cell (arrow) remains unlabeled. **B** Many non-neoplastic bystander T-cells are labeled for CD57. These CD57+ cells may be involved in the rosette-like binding to the popcorn cells which is particularly pronounced in the case illustrated here.

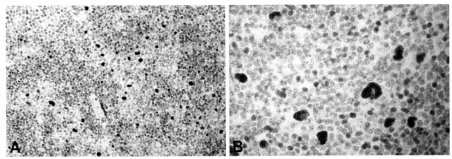

Fig. 12.06 Nodular lymphocyte predominant Hodgkin lymphoma (NLPHL). **A** Immunostaining for the transcription factor OCT-2 which is involved in the regulation of immunoglobulin expression produces a strong nuclear staining of the popcorn cells and a weaker labeling of the bystander B-cells and thus OCT-2 often highlights the presence and the nuclear atypia of popcorn cells. **B** Higher magnification of A.

A follicular dendritic cell marker, such as CD21, is essential for recognizing these different patterns. A prominence of extra-nodular LP cells is associated with a propensity to develop a diffuse pattern resembling T-cell/histiocyte-rich large B-cell lymphoma (THRLBCL-like). This is seen more frequently in patients with recurrence {671}. It is probably good practice to label cases of NLPHL that progress to a diffuse T-cell-rich pattern as NLPHL, THRLBCL-like, and distinguish these from primary THRLBCL.

In the differential diagnosis, presence of small B-cells and CD4+/CD57+ T cells favours NLPHL, whereas absence of small B-cells, and presence of CD8+ cells and TIA1+ cells favours primary THRLBCL.

Genetics

LP cells have clonally rearranged immuno-globulin *(IG)* genes {262, 1387, 1627}. The clonal rearrangements are usually not detectable in whole tissue DNA but only in the DNA of isolated single LP cells. The variable region of the *IG* heavy chain genes *(VH)* carry a high load of somatic mutations, and also show signs of ongoing mutations. The rearrangements are usually functional and *IG* mRNA transcripts are detectable in the LP cells of most cases {1387}. Latent Epstein-Barr virus (EBV) infection is consistently absent from LP cells, but may be present in bystander lymphocytes {33}. *IGH@-BCL6* translocations have been found in 5/24 NLPHL cases as well as in the NLPHL cell line DEV {94, 1838} and *BCL6* rearrangements (involving *IG, IKAROS, ABR* etc) (48%) {2426} are frequent in NLPHL. Aberrant somatic hypermutations were found in 80% of NLPHL cases, most frequently in *PAX5*, but also in *PIM1, RhoH/TTF* and *MYC* {1318}.

Postulated normal counterpart

Germinal centre B cell at the centroblastic stage of differentiation.

Prognosis and predictive factors

This disease develops slowly, with fairly frequent relapses. It usually remains responsive to therapy and thus is rarely fatal. The prognosis of patients with stage I and stage II disease is very good; with 10 year overall survival in more than 80% of cases {572, 573, 1603}. It is not clear yet whether immediate therapy is necessary to achieve this favourable prognosis. Therefore in some countries (e.g. France) stage I disease is not treated, especially in children, after the resection of the affected lymph node {1720}. Advanced stages have an unfavourable prognosis {573}. Progression to large B-cell lymphoma-like lesions has been reported in approximately 3–5% of cases {425, 884, 1476}. In some cases DLBCL was found to precede NLPHL {671}. The large B-cell lymphomas associated with NLPHL, if localized, generally have a good prognosis {884}. A clonal relationship between NLPHL and the associated DLBCL has been demonstrated {838, 2399}. Bone marrow involvement is rare in NLPHL and raises the possibility of THRLBCL in particular if there are only CD57-negative T cells and no small B cells in the background. Cases of NLPHL with BM involvement were found to show aggressive clinical behaviour {1141}.

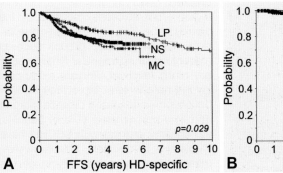

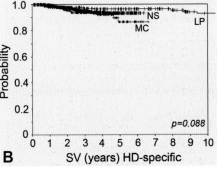

Fig. 12.07 Nodular lymphocyte predominant Hodgkin lymphoma (LP). **A** Failure free survival (FFS) (Hodgkin lymphoma specific) compared to nodular sclerosis (NS) and mixed cellularity (MC) subtypes of classical HL. **B** Overall survival (Hodgkin lymphoma specific) compared to nodular sclerosis (NS) and mixed cellularity (MC) subtypes of classical HL.

Classical Hodgkin lymphoma, introduction

H. Stein
G. Delsol
S.A. Pileri
L.M. Weiss
S. Poppema
E.S. Jaffe

Definition

Classical Hodgkin lymphoma (CHL) is a monoclonal lymphoid neoplasm (in most instances derived from B cells) composed of mononuclear Hodgkin cells and multi-nucleated Reed-Sternberg (HRS) cells residing in an infiltrate containing a variable mixture of non-neoplastic small lymphocytes, eosinophils, neutrophils, histiocytes, plasma cells, fibroblasts and collagen fibres. Based on the characteristics of the reactive infiltrate and to a certain extent on the morphology of the HRS cells (i.e. lacunar cells), four histological subtypes have been distinguished: lymphocyte-rich CHL (LRCHL), nodular sclerosis CHL (NSCHL), mixed cellularity CHL (MCCHL) and lymphocyte-depleted CHL (LDCHL). The immunophenotypic and genetic features of the mononuclear and multinucleated cells are identical in these histological subtypes, whereas their clinical features and association with Epstein-Barr virus (EBV) show differences.

ICD-O code   9650/3

Epidemiology

Classical HL accounts for 95% of all Hodgkin lymphomas, with a bimodal age curve in resource-rich countries, showing a peak at 15–35 years of age and a second peak in late life. Persons with a history of infectious mononucleosis have a higher incidence of CHL {1535}. Both familial and geographical clustering have been described {1535}.

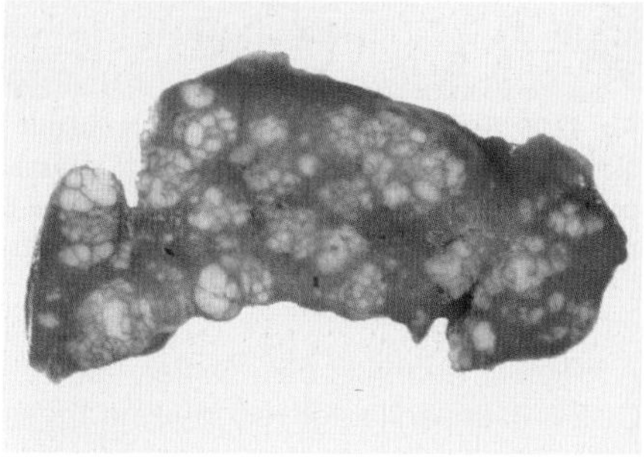

Etiology

EBV has been postulated to play a role in the pathogenesis of CHL. EBV is found in only a proportion of cases, particularly in MCCHL and LDCHL, but a search for other viruses has been unsuccessful. Loss of immune surveillance in immunodeficiency states such as HIV infection may predispose to the development of EBV-associated CHL. In tropical regions, up to 100% of CHL cases are EBV-positive {64A, 1277A, 2369, 2370}. It is possible that EBV infection of a B cell replaces one of the genetic alterations necessary for the development of CHL.

Sites of involvement

Classical Hodgkin lymphoma most often involves lymph nodes of the cervical region (75% of cases) followed by the mediastinal, axillary and paraaortic regions. Non-axial lymph node groups such as mesenteric or epitrochlear lymph nodes are rarely involved. Primary extranodal involvement is rare. More than 60% of patients have localized disease (stage I and II). Approximately 60% of patients, the majority of them with NSCHL, have mediastinal involvement. Splenic involvement is not uncommon (20%) and is associated with an increased risk of extranodal dissemination. Bone marrow (BM) involvement is much less common (5%).

Fig. 12.08 Classical Hodgkin lymphoma. Spleen.

Table 12.02 Differential diagnosis of Hodgkin lymphoma: comparative tumour cell immunophenotypes.

Marker	NLPHL	TCRBCL	CHL	DLBCL	ALCL, ALK+	ALCL, ALK-
CD30	-[1]	-[1]	+	-/+[2]	+	+
CD15	-	-	+/-	-	-[3]	-[3]
CD45	+	+	-	+	+/-	+/-
CD20	+	+	-/+[4]	+	-	-
CD79a	+	+	-/+[1]	+	-	-
PAX5	+	+	+[5]	+	-	-
J chain	+/-	+/-	-	-/+	-	-
Ig	+/-	+/-	-[6]	+/-	-	-
OCT-2	S+	S+	-/+[7]	+	n.a.	n.a.
BOB.1	+	+	-[8]	+	n.a.	n.a.
CD3	-	-	-[1]	-	-/+	-/+
CD2	-	-	-[1]	-	-/+	+/-
Perforin/Granzyme B	-	-	-[1]	-	+	+[9]
CD43	-	-	-	-/+	+/-	+/-
EMA	+/-	+/-	-[10]	-/+[11]	+/-	+/-
ALK	-	-	-	-	+	-
LMP1	-	-	+/-	-/+	-	-

NLPHL, nodular lymphocyte predominant Hodgkin lymphoma; TCRBCL, T-cell-rich large B-cell lymphoma; CHL, classical Hodgkin lymphoma; DLBCL, diffuse large B-cell lymphoma; ALCL, anaplastic large T-cell lymphoma.

+ all cases are positive, +/- majority of cases positive, -/+ minority of cases positive, - all cases are negative, S strong expression.

[1] Positive in rare cases.

[2] Prominent expression in anaplastic variant and variable expression in mediastinal large B-cell subtype.

[3] Occasional cases may show focal positivity.

[4] Present in up to 40% of the cases but usually expressed on a minority of tumour cells with variable intensity.

[5] Up to 10% might be negative.

[6] The common positivity for IgG and both Ig light chains reflects uptake of these proteins by the tumour cells rather than synthesis.

[7] Strong expression found in ~10% of the cases.

[8] Rare cases (~10%) may show scattered weak positivity.

[9] Only a minority is negative.

[10] Weak expression may be seen in tumour cells in 5% of the cases.

[11] Most frequently seen in DLBCL with anaplastic morphology.

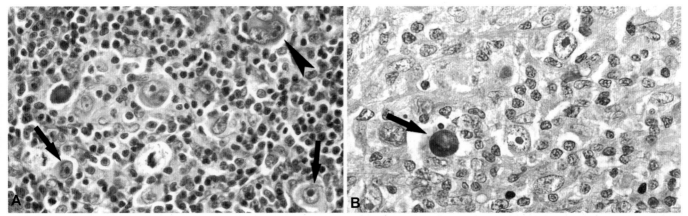

Fig. 12.09 Classical Hodgkin lymphoma. **A** Mononuclear Hodgkin cells (arrows) and a multinucleated Reed-Sternberg cell (arrowhead) are seen in a cellular background rich in lymphocytes and containing histiocytes and some eosinophils. **B** One mummified Hodgkin cell (arrow) and four vital Hodgkin cells can be seen.

As the BM lacks lymphatics, BM infiltration indicates vascular dissemination of the disease (stage IV). The anatomic distribution varies among the histological subtypes of HL {2009}.

Clinical features

Patients usually present with peripheral lymphadenopathy, localized to 1 or 2 lymph node-bearing areas. Mediastinal involvement is most frequently seen in the nodular sclerosis subtype, while abdominal and splenic involvement are more common in mixed cellularity. B symptoms consisting of fever, drenching night sweats, and significant body weight loss are present in up to 40% of patients.

Macroscopy

Lymph nodes are enlarged, encapsulated and on cut section show a fish flesh tumour. In NSCHL there is prominent nodularity, dense fibrotic bands and a thickened capsule. Splenic involvement usually shows scattered nodules within the white pulp. Sometimes very large masses are seen, these can demonstrate

fibrous bands in the nodular sclerosis subtype. Classical HL in the thymus can be associated with cystic degeneration and epithelial hyperplasia {1313}. Rare cases can be confined to the thymus.

Morphology

The lymph node architecture is effaced by variable numbers of HRS cells admixed with a rich inflammatory background. Classical diagnostic Reed-Sternberg (RS) cells are large, have abundant slightly basophilic cytoplasm and have at least two nuclear lobes or nuclei. The nuclei are large and often rounded in contour with a prominent, often irregular nuclear membrane, pale chromatin and usually one prominent eosinophilic nucleolus, with perinuclear clearing (halo), resembling a viral inclusion. Diagnostic RS cells must have at least two nucleoli in two separate nuclear lobes. Mononuclear variants are termed Hodgkin cells. Some HRS cells may have condensed cytoplasm and pyknotic reddish nuclei. These variants are known as mummified cells. Many of the neoplastic cells are not prototypic HRS cells. The lacunar

RS variant is characteristic of nodular sclerosis HL.

The neoplastic cells typically represent only a minority of the cellular infiltrate with a frequency ranging from 0.1–10%. The composition of the reactive cellular infiltrate varies according to the histological subtype. Involvement of secondary sites (BM and liver) is based on the identification of atypical mononuclear (CD30-positive Hodgkin cells with or without CD15 expression in the appropriate inflammatory background); thus diagnostic multinuclear RS cells are not required in a patient with classical HL diagnosed at another site {1819A}.

Immunophenotype

HRS cells are positive for CD30 in nearly all cases {1976A, 2088, 2091}, and for CD15 {987, 2091, 2092} in the majority (75–85%) of cases and are usually negative for CD45 and consistently negative for J chain, CD75 and macrophage specific markers such as the PG-M1-epitope of the CD68 molecule {427, 662A} (Table 12.02). Both CD30 and CD15 are typically present in a membrane pattern with

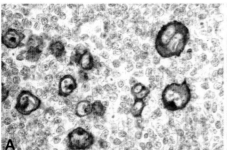
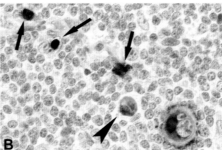
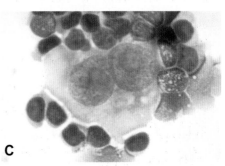

Fig. 12.10 Classical Hodgkin lymphoma. **A** The cytokine receptor CD30 is selectively expressed by the HRS cells. **B** The typical membrane and paranuclear dot-like staining of a large Reed-Sternberg cell for CD15 is seen; the small binucleated Reed-Sternberg cell (arrowhead) shows only a very faint labeling. In addition, three neutrophil granulocytes (arrows) are strongly labeled. **C** Touch imprint of a binucleated Reed-Sternberg cell ringed by lymphocytes.

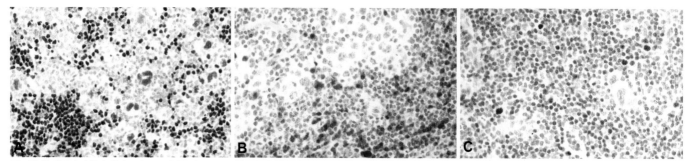

Fig. 12.11 Classical Hodgkin lymphoma. **A** The immunostaining for PAX5 labeled the nuclei of the HRS cells weakly and those of the non-neoplastic bystander B-cells strongly. **B** Immunostaining for BOB.1 (being the coactivator of the octamer-binding transcription factors OCT-1 and OCT-2) fails to stain the HRS cells in most instances. This is in difference to the non-neoplastic bystander B cells and plasma cells which show a moderately strong to strong labeling of their nuclei and in part of their cytoplasm. **C** Immunostaining for the octamer-binding transcription factor OCT-2 is negative in the HRS cells whereas the non-neoplastic bystander B cells show a nuclear positivity.

accentuation in the Golgi area of the cytoplasm; CD15 may be expressed by only a minority of the neoplastic cells and may be restricted only to the Golgi area. In 30–40% of cases, CD20 may be detectable but is usually of varied intensity and usually present only on a minority of the neoplastic cells {1964, 2507}. The B-cell-associated antigen CD79a is less often expressed. The B-cell nature of HRS cells is further demonstrable in approximately 95% of cases by their expression of the B-cell specific activator protein PAX5/BSAP {723}. The immunostaining of HRS cells for PAX5 is usually weaker than that of reactive B cells, a feature that makes the PAX5-positive HRS cells easily identifiable. The plasma cell specific transcription factor IRF4/MUM1 is consistently positive in HRS cells, usually at high intensity. In one study, BLIMP1, the key regulator of plasma cell differentiation, was expressed in only a small proportion of HRS cells in 25% of CHL {294}. The plasma-cell-associated adhesion molecule CD138 is consistently absent {294}. EBV-infected HRS cells express LMP1 and EBNA-1 without EBNA-2, a pattern characteristic of latency type II EBV

infection {552}. EBV-encoded LMP1 possesses strong transforming and anti-apoptotic potential.

Expression (usually weak membranous or sometimes globular cytoplasmic) of one or more T-cell antigens by a minority of HRS cells may be encountered in some cases {504}. This is, however, often difficult to assess because of the T cells that usually surround the HRS cells. Most of the T-cell antigen-positive classical HL cases have *IG* gene rearrangement in the HRS cells instead of T-cell receptor gene rearrangement, so that the expression of T-cell antigens is either aberrant or artifactual {1987}. Expression of epithelial membrane antigen (EMA) is rare and usually weak if present. A further characteristic finding is the absence of the transcription factor OCT-2 in ~90% of cases and absence of its coactivator BOB.1 in the same frequency. Cases in which both OCT-2 and BOB.1 are coexpressed are rare {1328}. The transcription factor PU.1 is consistently absent from HRS cells {1328, 2250A}. Most HRS cells express the proliferation-associated nuclear antigen Ki67 {775C}.

CHL cases rich in neoplastic cells may

resemble anaplastic large cell lymphoma (ALCL), a T-cell neoplasm. Their identification as classical HL is facilitated by demonstrating positivity for PAX5 and absence of EMA and ALK protein {723, 2087}. The detection of EBV-encoded RNA (EBER) or LMP1 is indicative of classical HL {992A}. The most difficult differential diagnosis is with large B-cell lymphoma displaying anaplastic morphology and expressing CD30. There may be a true biologic overlap between such cases and CHL (See Chapter 10).

Cytokines and chemokines

CHL is associated with overexpression and an abnormal pattern of cytokines and chemokines and/or their receptors in HRS cells {919, 962A, 1080, 1081, 1108, 2293}, which likely explain the abundant admixture of inflammatory cells {1067, 2186}, fibrosis {1080}, and the predominance of Th2 cells in the infiltrating T-cell population {2293}.

Genetics
Antigen receptor genes
HRS cells contain clonal immunoglobulin *(IG)* gene rearrangements in more than

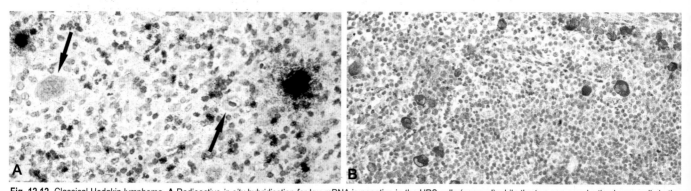

Fig. 12.12 Classical Hodgkin lymphoma. **A** Radioactive *in situ* hybridisation for Igμ mRNA is negative in the HRS cells (arrowed) while the two non-neoplastic plasma cells in the upper edges are strongly positive and the non-neoplastic bystander small B cells are moderately strongly positive. **B** Immunostaining for the antiapoptotic TRAF1 protein. The HRS cells strongly overexpress TRAF1.

98% of cases, and clonal T-cell receptor gene rearrangements in rare cases {1105, 1388, 1553, 1987, 2086}. The clonal rearrangements are usually detectable only in the DNA of isolated single HRS cells, and not in whole tissue DNA. The rearranged *IG* genes of the tumour cells harbour a high load of somatic hypermutations in the variable region of the *IG* heavy chain genes (*IGHV@*), usually without signs of ongoing mutations. These findings, in conjunction with the study of composite lymphomas consisting of classical HL and follicular non-Hodgkin lymphoma, support the view that HRS cells of B-cell lineage are derived from a germinal centre B cell {261A, 1387A}.

Abnormal gene expression
Despite their derivation from germinal centre B cells, HRS cells have lost much of the B-cell specific expression program and have acquired B-cell inappropriate gene products {636A, 1205A, 1388A, 1416A, 1977A, 2090, 1047A}. In addition, deregulated transcription factors in CHL promote proliferation and abrogate apoptosis in the neoplastic cells. The transcription factor NFκB is constitutively activated in HRS cells, and there is altered activity of the NFκB target genes, which regulate proliferation and survival {938A, 938B, 962A}, the AP-1 complex {1416A, 1416B} and the Janus kinase/-signal transducers and activators of transcription (*JAK/STAT*) signaling pathway {2030A}. Mutations of the *JAK* regulator *SOC-1* are associated with nuclear STAT5 accumulation in HRS cells, indicating a blockage of the negative feedback loop of the JAK/STAT5 pathway {1070A, 1459A, 2388}.

Epstein-Barr virus infection
The prevalence of EBV in HRS cells varies according to the histological subtype and epidemiologic factors. The highest frequency (~75%) is found in MCCHL, and the lowest (10–40%) in NSCHL {992A}. In resource-poor regions and in patients infected with the human immune deficiency virus, EBV infection is more prevalent, approaching 100% {64A, 1277A, 2369, 2370}. The type of EBV strain also varies among geographical areas. In resource-rich countries strain 1 prevails, and in resource-poor countries strain 2. A dual infection by both strains is more common in resource-poor countries {280, 2369, 2370}.

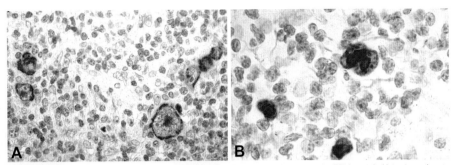

Fig. 12.13 Classical Hodgkin lymphoma. **A** EBV infected HRS cells strongly express the EBV-encoded latent membrane protein 1 (LMP1). **B** EBV-infected HRS cells consistently show a strong expression of EBER in their nuclei as revealed by non-radioactive *in situ* hybridization.

Genetic abnormalities and oncogenes
Despite the frequent overexpression of p53, mutations of *TP53* are rare or absent in primary CHL tissue, although they have been observed in Hodgkin cell lines {700A, 1504}. Conventional cytogenetic and Fluorescence *in situ* hybridization (FISH) studies show aneuploidy and hypertetraploidy, consistent with the multinucleation of the neoplastic cells; however, these techniques fail to demonstrate recurrent and specific chromosomal changes in classical HL {1935, 1960}. Comparative genomic hybridisation, however, reveals recurrent gains of the chromosomal sub-regions on chromosomal arms 2p, 9p, and 12q and distinct high-level amplifications on chromosomal bands 4p16, 4q23-q24 and 9p23-p24 {1071}. The translocations t(14;18) and t(2;5) are absent from HRS cells {831, 1244} but t(14;18) may occur in CHL arising in follicular lymphoma {1561A}. In a recent study using interphase cytogenetics breakpoints in the *IGH@* locus were

observed in HRS cells in 17% of CHL cases {1401A}.

Postulated normal counterpart
In more than 98% of CHL, the neoplastic cells are derived from mature B cells at the germinal centre stage of differentiation {1105, 1388}. In rare cases, they are derived from peripheral (post-thymic) T cells {514, 1553, 1987}.

Prognosis and predictive factors
Modern radiation and chemotherapy have made CHL curable in more than 85% of cases {462A, 571A}. Staging determines the mode of therapy, and both clinical and laboratory parameters are relevant to prognosis {904}. The response after two courses of ABVD as seen on FDG-PET imaging is an important prognostic indicator {748A}. Histologic subtype is less important as a predictive factor {25, 1076}.

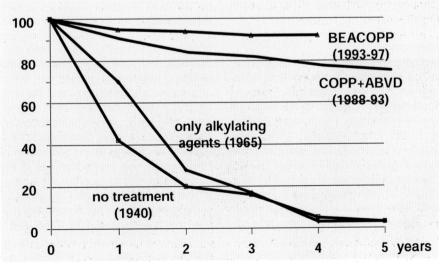

Fig. 12.14 Hodgkin lymphoma. Progress of the treatment of advanced stages since 1940.

Nodular sclerosis classical Hodgkin lymphoma

H. Stein
R. von Wasielewski
S. Poppema
K.A. MacLennan
M. Guenova

Definition

Nodular sclerosis classical Hodgkin lymphoma (NSCHL) is a subtype of CHL characterized by collagen bands that surround at least one nodule, and Hodgkin and Reed-Sternberg (HRS) cells with lacunar type morphology.

ICD-O code   9663/3

Epidemiology

NSCHL accounts for approximately 70% of CHL in Europe and USA; however, the rate varies greatly among other geographical regions; it is more common in resource-rich than in resource-poor areas, and the risk is highest among those with high socioeconomic status {445}. The incidence of NSCHL is similar in males and females and peaks at ages 15–34 years {101, 1525A}.

Sites of involvement

Mediastinal involvement occurs in 80% of cases, bulky disease in 54%, splenic and/or lung involvement in 8–10%, bone involvement in 5%, bone marrow (BM) involvement in 3% and liver involvement in 2% {456, 2009}.

Clinical features

Most patients present with Ann Arbor stage II disease. B symptoms are encountered in approximately 40% of cases {2009}.

Morphology

Lymph nodes have a nodular growth pattern, with nodules surrounded by collagen bands (nodular sclerosis). The broad fibroblast-poor collagen bands surround at least one nodule. This fibrosing process is usually associated with a thickened lymph node capsule. The lymphoma contains a highly variable number of HRS cells, small lymphocytes and other non-neoplastic inflammatory cells. The HRS cells tend to have more lobated nuclei with smaller lobes, less prominent nucleoli, and a larger amount of cytoplasm than in other types of CHL. In formalin-fixed tissues the cytoplasm of the HRS cells fre-

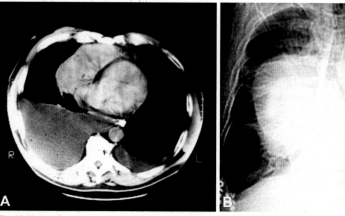

Fig. 12.15 Nodular sclerosis classical Hodgkin lymphoma. **A** CT scan shows a large anterior mediastinal mass. **B** Chest X-ray of the same patient shows mediastinal mass exceeding one-third of the chest diameter.

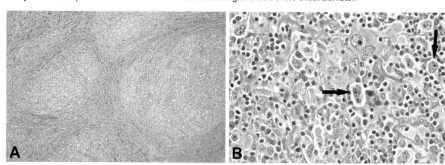

Fig. 12.16 Nodular sclerosis classical Hodgkin lymphoma. **A** Fibrous collagen bands divide the lymph node into nodules. **B** Several lacunar cells (arrowed) are present.

quently shows retraction of the cytoplasmic membrane so that the cells seem to be sitting in lacunae. These cells have therefore been designated lacunar cells. Lacunar cells may form cellular aggregates, which may be associated with necrosis and a histiocytic reaction, resembling necrotizing granulomas. When aggregates are very prominent, the term "syncytial variant" has been used. Eosinophils, histiocytes, and to a lesser extent neutrophils, are often numerous {1743}. Grading according to the proportion of HRS cells or the characteristics of the background infiltrate (such as the number of eosinophils) may predict prognosis in some settings, but is not required for routine clinical purposes {936, 1356, 2307, 2341A}; it may serve a research purpose in protocol studies.

Immunophenotype

The malignant cells exhibit the CHL phenotype (see Introduction); however, association with Epstein-Barr virus (EBV) as demonstrated by EBER or the EBV encoded LMP1 is less frequent (10–40%) than in mixed cellularity CHL {918A, 919A, 2374A, 2377A}.

Prognosis and predictive factors

NSCHL has a better prognosis overall than that of other types of CHL {25}. Massive mediastinal disease is an adverse prognostic factor {2062}.

Mixed cellularity classical Hodgkin lymphoma

L.M. Weiss
R. von Wasielewski
G. Delsol
S. Poppema
H. Stein

Definition
Mixed cellularity classical Hodgkin lymphoma (MCCHL) is a subtype of classical Hodgkin lymphoma (CHL) with scattered classical Hodgkin-Reed-Sternberg (HRS) cells in a diffuse or vaguely nodular mixed inflammatory background without nodular sclerosing fibrosis. Cases which do not fit into the other subtypes are put in this category.

ICD-O code   9652/3

Epidemiology
The mixed cellularity subtype comprises approximately 20–25% of CHL. MCCHL is more frequent in patients with HIV infection and in developing countries. A bimodal age distribution is not seen. The median age is 38 years and approximately 70% are male {2009}.

Sites of involvement
Peripheral lymph nodes are frequently involved and mediastinal involvement is uncommon. The spleen is involved in 30%, BM in 10%, liver in 3% and other organs in 1–3% {456}.

Clinical features
B symptoms are frequent.

Morphology
The lymph node architecture is usually obliterated although an interfollicular growth pattern may be seen. Interstitial

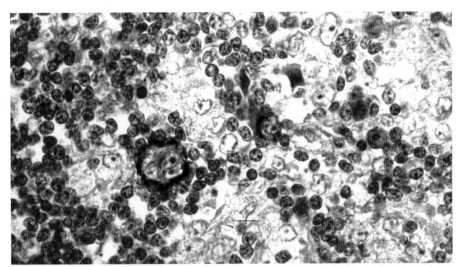

Fig. 12.17 Mixed cellularity subtype of classical Hodgkin lymphoma. CD30-negative histiocytes, with a pronounced epithelioid differentiation forming clusters, predominate. The CD30 immunostaining highlights the presence of a large Reed-Sternberg cell and a small Hodgkin cell.

fibrosis may be present, but the lymph node capsule is usually not thickened and there are no broad bands of fibrosis as seen in nodular sclerosis Hodgkin Lymphoma. The HRS cells are typical in appearance. The background cells consist of a mixture of cell types, the composition of which varies greatly. Eosinophils, neutrophils, histiocytes and plasma cells are usually present. One of these cell types may predominate. The histiocytes may show pronounced epithelioid features particularly in Epstein-Barr virus (EBV)-associated cases {552} and may form granuloma-like clusters or granulomas.

Immunophenotype
The malignant cells exhibit the CHL immunophenotype; however, the EBV-encoded LMP1 and EBER are expressed much more frequently (approximately 75% of cases) than in nodular sclerosis and lymphocyte-rich CHL {33}.

Prognosis and predictive factors
Before the introduction of modern therapy, MCCHL had a worse prognosis than nodular sclerosis and a better prognosis than lymphocyte-depleted CHL. With current regimens, these differences have largely vanished although not entirely {25}.

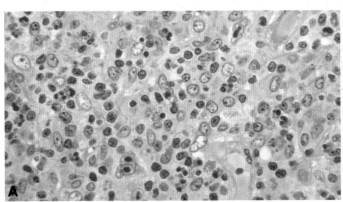
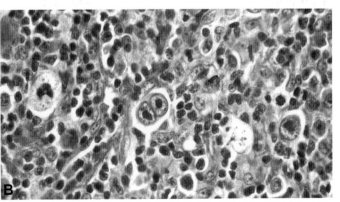

Fig. 12.18 Mixed cellularity subtype of classical Hodgkin lymphoma. **A** The mixed cellular infiltrate does not contain fibrotic bands. **B** A typical binucleated Reed-Sternberg cell in a mixed cellular infiltrate with lymphocytes, macrophages and eosinophils is visible.

Lymphocyte-rich classical Hodgkin lymphoma

I. Anagnostopoulos
P.G. Isaacson
H. Stein

Definition

Lymphocyte-rich classical Hodgkin lymphoma (LRCHL) is a subtype of classical Hodgkin lymphoma (CHL) with scattered Hodgkin and Reed-Sternberg (HRS) cells and a nodular or less often diffuse cellular background consisting of small lymphocytes and with an absence of neutrophils and eosinophils.

ICD-O code   9651/3

Epidemiology

LRCHL comprises approximately 5% of all CHL, in similar frequency to nodular lymphocyte predominant Hodgkin lymphoma (NLPHL). The median age is similar to NLPHL and significantly higher than in other subtypes of CHL {573}. There is a male predominance (70%) {2009}.

Sites of involvement

Peripheral lymph nodes are typically involved. Mediastinal involvement and bulky disease are uncommon {573, 2009}.

Clinical features

Most patients present with stage I or II disease. B symptoms are rare. The clinical features are similar to those of NLPHL with the exception that multiple relapses seem to occur less frequently {573}.

Morphology

There are two growth patterns: a common nodular one {33, 90} and a rare diffuse one {33}. The nodules of the nodular variant encompass most of the involved tissue so that the T-zone is attenuated.

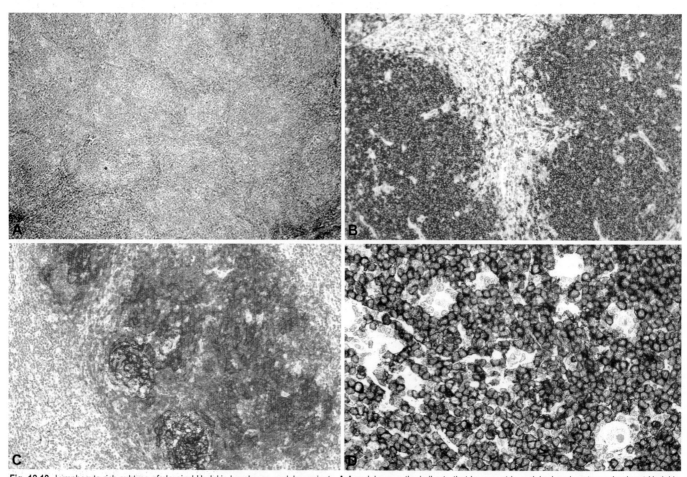

Fig. 12.19 Lymphocyte-rich subtype of classical Hodgkin lymphoma, nodular variant. **A** A nodular growth similar to that is present in nodular lymphocyte-predominant Hodgkin lymphoma. **B** Immunostaining for CD20 shows that the nodules predominantly consist of small B cells. The "holes" contain HRS cells. **C** Immunostaining for CD21 reveals that the nodules contain a meshwork of follicular dendritic cells and demonstrates that they predominantly represent follicular mantles with occasional, usually regressed germinal centres; the follicular dendritic cell meshwork is denser and more sharply defined in the germinal centres. **D** A higher magnification of one of the nodules stained for CD20 reveals a background of CD20+ B cells and CD20- HRS cells ringed by CD20-negative T cells.

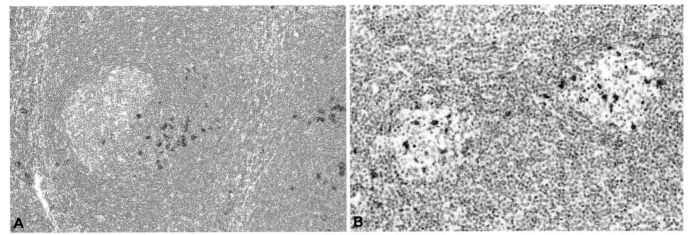

Fig. 12.20 Lymphocyte-rich subtype of classical Hodgkin lymphoma, nodular variant. **A** The CD30 staining highlights the presence of HRS cells. They are located within or at the peripheral margin of the follicular mantles but not within the germinal centres. **B** CD57+ T cells are seen in the germinal centres but not in the broadened mantle zones and not around the neoplastic cells.

The nodules are composed of small lymphocytes and may harbour germinal centres that are usually eccentrically located and relatively small or regressed. The HRS cells are predominantly found within the nodules but consistently outside of the germinal centres. A proportion of the HRS cells may resemble LP cells or mononuclear lacunar cells. This subtype can easily be confused with the NLPHL. In the past, approximately 30% of cases initially diagnosed as NLPHL were found to be LRCHL {33}. The demonstration of an immunophenotype typical for classical HRS cells is essential in making this distinction. Eosinophils and/or neutrophils are absent from the nodules and if present they are located in the interfollicular zones and are low in number. In rare instances, the LRCHL-typical nodules may be surrounded by fibrous bands associated with randomly distributed HRS cells in T-cell-rich zones. Typing of these cases as nodular sclerosis classical Hodgkin lymphoma (NSCHL) might be more appropriate. In some cases, sequential biopsies have shown NSCHL implying a possible relationship between the two subtypes of CHL and this is further inferred by the finding of HRS cells within expanded follicular mantle zones in some cases of NSCHL {1011A}. A coexistence of LRCHL and mixed cellularity classical Hodgkin lymphoma (MCCHL) occurs but is rare. In diffuse LRCHL cases the small lymphocytes of the cellular background may be admixed with histiocytes with or without epithelioid features.

Immunophenotype

The distinction of LRCHL from NLPHL is possible by immunophenotyping in all instances {33}. The atypical cells in LRCHL show the same immunophenotype (CD30+, CD15+/-, CD20-/+, CD75-, J chain-) as the HRS cells in the other subtypes of CHL. The small lymphocytes present in the nodules display the features of mantle cells (IgM+D+). Thus the nodules predominantly represent expanded mantle zones. At least some of them contain eccentrically located, usually small, germinal centres which are highlighted by a dense meshwork of CD21+ follicular dendritic cells. As intact germinal centres are infrequent in NLPHL, this feature is helpful in differential diagnosis. CD15+ granulocytes are absent from the expanded mantle zones but may be present in low numbers within the interfollicular zones. In the rare diffuse subtype the lymphocytes are nearly all of T-cell type with CD15+ granulocytes and eosinophils being absent. These features facilitate the differentiation of LRCHL from MCCHL. EBV LMP1 expression is seen more frequently than in NSCHL but less frequently than in MCCHL {33}.

Prognosis and predictive factors

With modern risk-adjusted treatment, survival and progression free survival are slightly better than in the other subtypes of CHL and similar to that of NLPHL except that relapses are more common in NLPHL than in LRCHL {33, 573, 2009}.

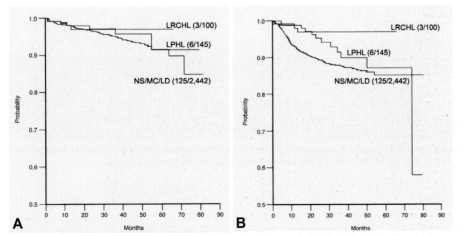

Fig. 12.21 **A** Overall survival by histologic subtype. **B** Overall event-free survival by histologic subtype {2009}. LRCHL, lymphocyte-rich classical Hodgkin lymphoma; LPHL, lymphocyte-predominant Hodgkin lymphoma; MC, mixed cellularity; NS, nodular sclerosis; LD, lymphocyte depletion.

Lymphocyte-depleted classical Hodgkin lymphoma

D. Benharroch
H. Stein
S.-C. Peh

Definition
Lymphocyte-depleted classical Hodgkin lymphoma (LDCHL) is a diffuse subtype of classical Hodgkin lymphoma (CHL) rich in Hodgkin and Reed-Stenberg (HRS) cells and/or depleted in non-neoplastic lymphocytes. The definition of LDCHL has undergone several changes in the past few decades with the result that the body of reliable clinical data on this subtype is limited. Since a proportion of these cases have been reclassified into different lymphoma entities, the previously described clinicopathological correlations are not necessarily tenable.

ICD-O code   9653/3

Epidemiology
This is the rarest CHL subtype (<1% of cases in Western countries). 60–75% of patients are male and the median age ranges from 30–37 years {25, 2009}. This subtype is often associated with HIV infection and is seen more often in developing countries {805, 2317}.

Sites of involvement
LDCHL has a predilection for retroperitoneal lymph nodes, abdominal organs, and bone marrow.

Clinical features
LDCHL presents at a more advanced stage (III-IV) and with B symptoms than the other subtypes {1585, 2009}.

Morphology
Although the appearance of LDCHL is highly variable, a unifying feature is the relative predominance of HRS cells in relation to the background lymphocytes. One pattern may resemble mixed cellularity but compared with increased numbers of prototypic HRS cells. In some cases, pleomorphic HRS cells may predominate, producing a sarcomatous appearance. These cases may be difficult to differentiate from anaplastic forms of large cell non-Hodgkin lymphoma. Another pattern is characterized by diffuse fibrosis with or without a proliferation of fibroblasts and only a few HRS cells.

If a nodular sclerosing fibrosis is present, the disease should be assigned to nodular sclerosis Hodgkin lymphoma.

Immunophenotype
The HRS cells show the same immunophenotype as in the other subtypes of classical HL. Most HIV+ cases are EBV infected and stain positively for LMP1 {932, 2020, 2276}. Coexpression of CD30 and PAX5 is very helpful in differentiating LDCHL from ALCL, ALK-.

Prognosis and predictive factors
Prior to modern therapy, the course of LDCHL was aggressive and it has remained so in some parts of Europe {25, 1782} and in developing countries. In the US and UK, the course is comparable to other CHL subtypes of similar stage. Poor prognosis is seen in HIV-related LDCHL patients.

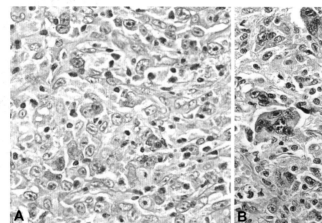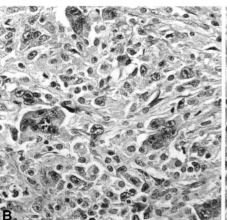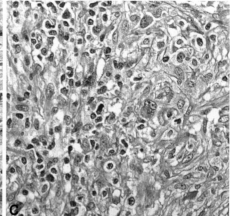

Fig. 12.22 Lymphocyte-depleted subtype of classical Hodgkin lymphoma. **A** Many Hodgkin cells with relatively few admixed lymphocytes are visible. **B** Many bizarre large and small HRS cells are present in a cellular background rich in fibrillary matrix. **C** Scattered HRS cells in a predominant fibrillary matrix with fibroblastic proliferation.

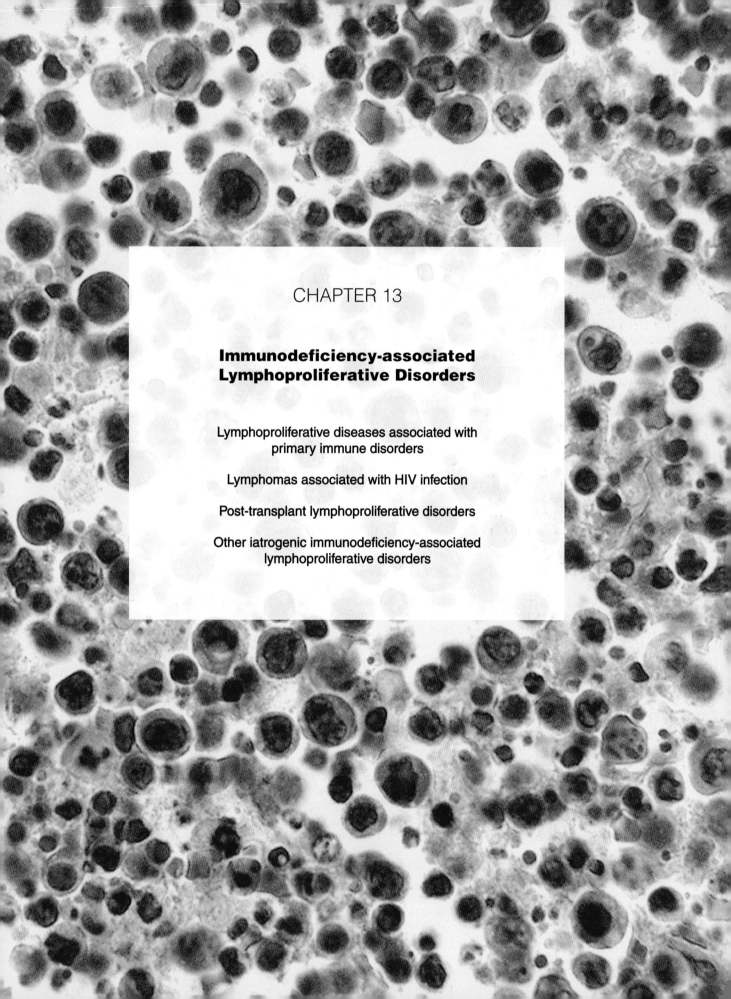

CHAPTER 13

Immunodeficiency-associated Lymphoproliferative Disorders

Lymphoproliferative diseases associated with
primary immune disorders

Lymphomas associated with HIV infection

Post-transplant lymphoproliferative disorders

Other iatrogenic immunodeficiency-associated
lymphoproliferative disorders

Lymphoproliferative diseases associated with primary immune disorders

J.H. Van Krieken
M. Onciu
K.S.J. Elenitoba-Johnson
E.S. Jaffe

Definition

Lymphoproliferative diseases (LPD) associated with primary immune disorders (PID) are lymphoid proliferations that arise as a result of immune deficiency due to a primary immunodeficiency or immuno-regulatory disorder. Because the pathology and pathogenesis of the more than 60 PID are heterogeneous, the manifestations of the lymphoproliferative diseases are highly variable. The PID most frequently associated with LPD are ataxia telangiectasia (AT), Wiskott-Aldrich syndrome (WAS), common variable immunodeficiency (CVID), severe combined immunodeficiency (SCID), X-linked lymphoproliferative disorder (XLP), Nijmegen breakage syndrome (NBS), hyper-IgM syndrome and autoimmune lymphoproliferative syndrome (ALPS).

Epidemiology

Age-specific mortality rates for all neoplasms in patients with PID are 10–200 times the expected rates for the general population. However, given that PID are rare disorders, the overall occurrence of PID-associated LPD is low. With the exception of CVID, these diseases present primarily in the paediatric age group. They are more common in males than females, primarily because several of the primary genetic abnormalities are X-linked, e.g. XLP, SCID and hyper-IgM syndrome {1063}.

Etiology

The cause of the LPD is related to the underlying primary immune defect {1606}. Epstein-Barr virus (EBV) is involved in the majority of PID-associated lymphoid proliferations {2302}. In these cases, defective T-cell immune surveillance to EBV is believed to be the primary mechanism {935, 1788}. The absence of T-cell control may be complete, resulting in fatal infectious mononucleosis, or partial, resulting in other LPD {1042}.

WAS is a complex immune disorder, with defects in function of T-cells, B-cells, neutrophils and macrophages. T-cell dysfunction is significant, and tends to increase in severity during the course of the disease. Hyper-IgM syndrome results from mutations

in the gene for CD40 or CD40 ligand, which affect interactions between T-cells and B-cells, and impair effective differentiation of B-cells into class-switched plasma cells {1008}.

In autoimmune lymphoproliferative syndrome (ALPS), mutations in the *FAS* or *FASL* gene (and rarely other abnormalities) may contribute directly to lymphoid proliferations through the accumulation of lymphoid cells that fail to undergo apoptosis, resulting in the accumulation of CD4 and CD8 double negative cells in the peripheral blood (PB) and lymphoid tissues {1300, 2042}. In ALPS, the severity of the apoptotic defect correlates directly with the risk of development of LPD {1041}. The importance of *FAS* mutations in causing LPD is supported by the fact that sporadic *FAS* mutations are associated with lymphomas in the absence of immune abnormalities {855}.

In AT, an abnormal DNA repair mechanism due to mutations of the *ATM* gene can contribute to the development of lymphoma, leukaemia and other neoplasms {638}. In these patients, non-leukaemic T-cell clones can be detected in the PB that have translocations involving the *TCR* genes similar to those seen in overt leukaemias.

NBS also results from defects in DNA repair due to mutations in the *NBS1* gene, resulting in many chromosomal breaks and translocations, including those in antigen receptor genes. In patients with NBS, LPD is the most common neoplasm {54, 339, 2314}. In patients with CVID, marked lymphoid

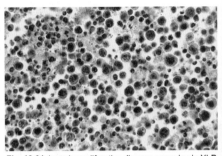

Fig. 13.01 Lymphoproliferative disease occurring in XLP with features of fatal infectious mononucleosis. There is a proliferation of B cells with plasmacytoid and immunoblastic features. Note prominent apoptosis.

hyperplasia may occur in the lung and gastrointestinal tract {1929}, a setting in which more aggressive LPD or overt lymphoma may develop {559}.

Sites of involvement

Presentation is dependent on the underlying disease. More often, LPD present in extranodal sites, most commonly the gastrointestinal tract, lung and central nervous system (CNS).

Clinical features

Patients often present with symptoms resembling those of infection or neoplasia (i.e. fever, fatigue, infectious mononucleosis-like syndromes). In some diseases, such as ALPS and XLP, the lymphoid proliferation is the first sign of the underlying immune defect, but in most patients, the diagnosis of PID has already been established because of other manifestations.

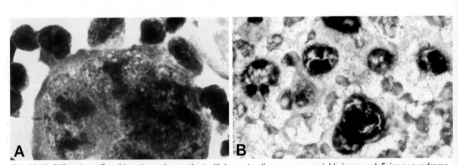

Fig. 13.02 Diffuse large B-cell lymphoma in a patient with long-standing common variable immunodeficiency syndrome. **A** Lymphoma cells are seen in ascites fluid and show marked pleomorphism. **B** Lymphoma cells are EBV-positive by EBER *in situ* hybridization.

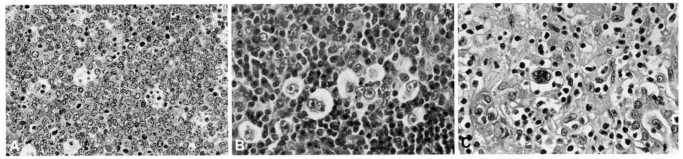

Fig. 13.03 Lymphomas in ALPS. **A** Burkitt lymphoma. **B** Classical Hodgkin lymphoma, mixed cellularity subtype. **C** T-cell-rich/histiocyte-rich large B-cell lymphoma. Histological features of these lymphoma subtypes resemble those occurring sporadically, without predisposing immune abnormalities.

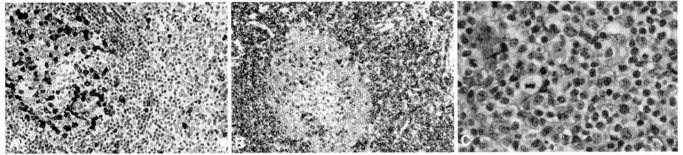

Fig. 13.04 ALPS lymph node. Paracortical T cells are CD45RO negative **(A)** and positive for CD3 **(B)**. This phenotype is characteristic of naïve T cells. **C** Paracortical T cells show varying degrees of atypia and mitotic figures may be frequent.

Morphology

As in other immune deficiency states, lymphoid proliferations in patients with primary immunodeficiency include reactive hyperplasias, polymorphous lymphoid infiltrates similar to those seen in the post-transplant setting, and frank lymphomas that do not differ from those in immuno-competent hosts. The type and frequency of each lesion differ among the PID (Table 13.01).

Non-neoplastic lesions

Primary EBV infection in PID may result in fatal infectious mononucleosis (FIM), characterized by a highly polymorphous proliferation of lymphoid cells showing evidence of plasmacytoid and immuno-blastic differentiation. Reed-Sternberg-like cells may be seen. This condition is primarily seen in patients with XLP (Duncan syndrome) {800} and SCID {1788}. The abnormal B-cell proliferation is systemic, involving both lymphoid and non-lymphoid organs, most commonly the terminal ileum. Haemophagocytic syndrome is frequent, and is most readily identified in bone marrow (BM) aspirates. In CVID, waxing and waning lymphoproliferations may occur in lymph nodes and extranodal sites, with variable morphology including follicular hyperplasia, and paracortical expansion

with many EBV-positive cells, often including large atypical cells, that may resemble Reed-Sternberg cells. CVID is characterized by nodular lymphoid hyperplasia in the gastrointestinal tract; VJ-PCR may detect clonal B-cell populations that are self-limited {1256, 1929}.

In ALPS, expansions of double-negative (CD4-/CD8-) alpha beta CD45RA+, CD45RO- T cells in PB, lymph nodes, spleen and other tissues are the hallmark of the disease. T-cell expansion can be very marked, and the T-cells may have slightly immature chromatin, which can lead to a mistaken diagnosis of T-cell lymphoma especially when, as is usual, the patient does not carry a preexisting diagnosis of ALPS {1300}. Follicular hyperplasia is often prominent, and progressively transformed germinal centres may be seen {1300}.

Hyper-IgM syndrome is characterized by circulating PB B-cells that bear only IgM and IgD. Germinal centres are absent in lymph nodes. IgM-producing plasma cells often accumulate, most commonly in extranodal sites, such as the gastrointestinal tract, liver and gallbladder. These lesions may be so extensive as to be fatal, without progression to clonal LPD.

Lymphomas

Lymphomas occurring in patients with PID do not generally differ in their morphology from those occurring in immuno-competent hosts.

Lymphomatoid granulomatosis (LYG), an EBV-driven proliferation of B-cells associated with a marked T-cell infiltration, is increased in frequency in patients with WAS {1003} (See Chapter 10). The most common sites of involvement are lung, skin, brain and kidney.

Diffuse large B-cell lymphoma (DLBCL) is the most common type of lymphoma seen in PID in general; Hodgkin and Burkitt lymphomas {2241} and peripheral T-cell lymphomas also occur {1729}. In AT, and to a lesser extent in NBS, T-cell lymphomas and leukaemias are more common than B-cell neoplasms {2164}. Rare cases of true peripheral T-cell lymphoma have been seen in patients with ALPS {1729, 2108}. Both T lymphoblastic lymphoma/leukaemia (T ALL/LBL) and T-cell prolymphocytic leukaemia (T-PLL) have been reported in PID.

Hodgkin lymphoma

Hodgkin lymphoma-like lymphoproliferations resembling those seen in the setting of methotrexate therapy as well as LPD with all morphological and phenotypic

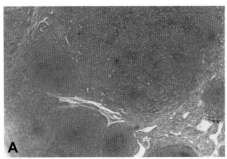 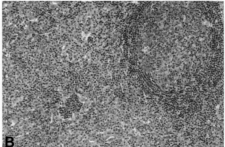 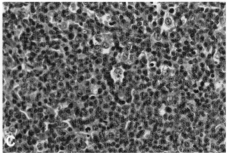

Fig. 13.05 Reactive lymph node from a patient with ALPS. **A** There is prominent paracortical expansion. **B** ALPS lymph node. Reactive germinal centres are present and the paracortex is expanded. **C** The cells are slightly larger than normal small lymphocytes, with dispersed chromatin.

features of classical Hodgkin lymphoma has been reported in patients with WAS, and AT {638, 1909}. In ALPS, nodular lymphocyte predominant Hodgkin lymphoma, classical Hodgkin lymphoma and T-cell-rich large B-cell lymphomas have been described {1300}.

Precursor lesions
The underlying primary immune disorder is the principal precursor lesion leading to the development of LPD. This morphological spectrum is accompanied by an increasing dominant clonal population: from clearly polyclonal, to oligoclonal to monoclonal. However, monoclonal expansions, particularly if they are minor clones, do not necessarily progress to major persistent clonal lesions {1256}.

Immunophenotype
Non-neoplastic proliferations
In ALPS, there is expansion of a distinctive CD3+ CD4- CD8- CD45RA+ CD45RO- naïve T-cell population in the PB and BM. The T cells may express CD57 but not CD25. Increased numbers of CD5+ polyclonal B cells may also be seen {1300}. Hyper-IgM syndrome is characterized by PB B cells that bear only IgM and IgD.

Neoplasms
Most of the lymphomas in patients with PID are of B-cell lineage, and thus express B-cell antigens corresponding to their differentiation stage. EBV infection of B cells often leads to down-regulation of B-cell antigens. Thus, CD20, CD19 and CD79a may be negative or expressed on only some of the neoplastic cells in EBV-positive LPD. Similarly, EBV leads to the expression of CD30 in most cases. In patients with EBV-positive LPD resulting from defective immune surveillance, the latency genes including LMP1 may be expressed.

In cases showing evidence of plasmacytoid differentiation, monotypic cytoplasmic immunoglobulin (Ig) may be identified. The immunophenotypes of the specific B-and T-cell lymphomas in PID do not differ from those of the same lymphomas in immunocompetent patients.

Genetics
Antigen receptor genes
Since LPD in PID is a spectrum from reactive to aggressive lymphoproliferations they can be polyclonal, oligoclonal or monoclonal. FIM is generally polyclonal; overt lymphomas such as DLBCL or Burkitt lymphoma have clonal immunoglobulin heavy and light-chain gene rearrangement {638, 1256, 1929}. Presently there is only limited experience with T-cell clonality tests in the setting of PID.

Genetic abnormalities and oncogenes
Genetic alterations may be directly related to the primary immune defect, such as *FAS* gene mutation in patients with ALPS, mutations of the gene encoding for SAP/SLAM in XLP, and many chromosomal breaks in NBS {799, 2158}. Other abnormalities may occur in the course of LPD. In AT, in addition to mutations of the

ATM gene, inversions and tranlocations of the T-cell receptor genes on chromosomes 7 and 14 are common. These often show breakpoints at 14q11-12, 7q32-35 and 7p15. These translocations may involve the *TCL1* gene, leading to T-cell lymphoproliferative diseases, including both pre T-ALL/LBL as well as T-cell PLL. Other chromosomal rearrangements/ translocations include inv(7)(p13q35), t(7;7)(p13q35), t(7;14)(p13;q11), and t(14;14)(q11;q32). The immunoglobulin gene loci also may be involved {2164}.

Prognosis and predictive factors
The prognosis is related to both the underlying primary immune disorder and the type of LPD. The immunological status of the host is an important risk factor {331}. The lymphoid proliferations in ALPS are often self-limiting. Lymphoid hyperplasias in CVID may be indolent. Most of the other LPD in patients with PID are aggressive. However, given the wide variety of underlying conditions and ensuing lymphoproliferative disorders, the prognosis must be evaluated in each case individually. In patients with EBV-driven infectious mononucleosis, a haemophagocytic syndrome may be the primary cause of death, usually

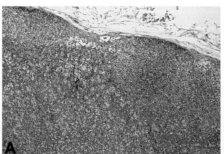 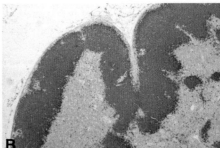

Fig. 13.06 Hyper-IgM syndrome. **A** Lymph node contains cortex with primary follicles, but lacks germinal centres. **B** CD20 stain highlights cortical areas.

associated with marked pancytopenia, liver dysfunction, coagulopathy and further infectious complications.

Treatment is based both on the nature of the neoplastic process and the underlying genetic defect. In general, less aggressive therapy than in patients without PID is needed. Allogeneic BM transplantation has been used in patients with WAS, SCID and hyper-IgM syndrome {629, 868}. Since the EBV-driven B-cell expansion in LYG is often not autonomous, it may respond to immunoregulatory therapy using interferon α-2b {2420}.

Table 13.01 Clinical features of the primary immunodeficiencies (PID).

Type of primary immunodeficiency	Frequency (among all PID*)	Gene(s) or protein(s) implicated	Most common abnormalities	Most common associated lymphoproliferative disorders (%)#
Combined T- and B-cell immunodeficiencies	9–18%			
Severe combined immunodeficiency (SCID)	1–5%	γ chain of IL-2R, IL-4R, IL-7R, IL-9R, IL15R, IL-21R; JAK3 kinase; IL-7R, CD45, CD3δ or CD3ε ; RAG1/2, Artemis, ADA	Recurrent severe bacterial, fungal and viral infections, including opportunistic infections; skin rash.	EBV-associated lesions, fatal infectious mononucleosis (nearly 100%)
CD40 ligand and CD40 deficiencies (hyper-IgM syndrome)	1–2%	CD40 ligand (CD40L, CD154) or CD40	Neutropenia, thrombocytopenia, haemolytic anaemia, biliary tract and liver disease, opportunistic infections	EBV-associated lesions, (DLBCL, Hodgkin lymphoma) Large granular lymphocyte leukaemia
Predominantly antibody PIDs	53–72%			
Common variable immunodeficiency (CVID)	21–31%	Unknown	Bacterial infections (lung, GI), autoimmune cytopenias, granulomatous disease (lung, liver)	EBV-associated lesions (DLBCL, Hodgkin lymphoma), extranodal marginal zone lymphoma, small lymphocytic lymphoma, lymphoplasmacytic lymphoma, peripheral T-cell lymphoma (rare)(2–7%)
Other well-defined immunodeficiency syndromes	5–22%			
Wiskott-Aldrich syndrome (WAS)	1–3%	WASP	Thrombocytopenia, small platelets, eczema, autoimmune disease, bacterial infections	EBV-associated lesions (DLBCL, Hodgkin lymphoma, lymphomatoid granulomatosis) (3–9%)
Ataxia-telangiectasia (AT)	2–8%	ATM	Ataxia, telangiectasias, increased AFP, increased sensitivity to ionizing radiation	Non-leukaemic clonal T-cell proliferations, DLBCL, Burkitt lymphoma, T-PLL, T-ALL, Hodgkin lymphoma (10–30%)
Nijmegen breakage syndrome (NBS)	1–2%	NBS1 (Nibrin)	Microcephaly, progressive mental retardation, sensitivity to ionizing radiation, predisposition to cancer.	DLBCL, peripheral T-cell lymphoma, T-LBL/ALL, Hodgkin lymphoma (28–36%)
Diseases of immune dysregulation	1–3%			
X-linked lymphoproliferative syndrome (XLP)	<1%	SH2D1A	EBV-triggered abnormalities (fatal IM, hepatitis, aplastic anaemia), lymphoma	EBV-associated lesions (Burkitt lymphoma, DLBCL) (nearly 100%)
Autoimmune lymphoproliferative syndrome (ALPS, Canale-Smith syndrome)	<1%	FAS (type 1a), FASL (type 1b), CASP10 (caspase 10) (type 2a) or CASP8 (caspase 8) (type 2b)	Defective lymphocyte apoptosis, splenomegaly, adenopathy, autoimmune cytopenias, recurrent infections	Nodular LP Hodgkin lymphoma, Classical Hodgkin lymphoma , DLBCL, Burkitt lymphoma, peripheral T-cell lymphoma (rare);(CHL, DLBCL and BL may be EBV+ or -) (3–10%)

* Data compiled from reports of several national and international registries. TCR, T-cell antigen receptor; NI, normal; ADA, adenosine deaminase; B, B lymphocyte; T, T lymphocytes; Ig, serum immunoglobulin; AFP, α fetoprotein. #, % where provided indicates approximate % of patients in whom LPD develops.

Lymphomas associated with HIV infection

M. Raphaël
J. Said
B. Borisch
E. Cesarman
N.L. Harris

Definition

Lymphomas that develop in HIV-positive patients are predominantly aggressive B-cell lymphomas. In a proportion of cases they are considered acquired immunodeficiency syndrome (AIDS)-defining conditions and are the initial manifestation of AIDS. These disorders are heterogeneous and include lymphomas usually diagnosed in immunocompetent patients, as well as those seen much more often in the setting of HIV infection. The most common HIV-associated lymphomas include: Burkitt lymphoma (BL), diffuse large B-cell lymphoma (DLBCL) (often involving the central nervous system), primary effusion lymphoma (PEL), and plasmablastic lymphoma. Hodgkin lymphoma (HL) is also increased in the setting of HIV.

Epidemiology

The incidence of all subtypes of non-Hodgkin lymphoma (NHL) is increased 60–200 times in HIV-positive patients. In particular, before highly active antiretroviral therapy (HAART) was available, primary central nervous system (CNS) lymphoma and BL were increased approximately 1000 times in comparison with the general population {193, 1283}. Since the introduction of HAART, the risk of NHL declined dramatically (from 53 to 23 standardized incidence ratio): the risk decreased considerably in 1996 and has remained stable thereafter {646}. Moreover, the decreased incidence of most

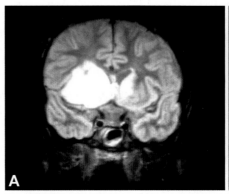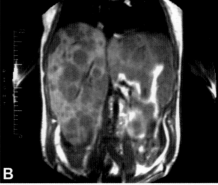

Fig. 13.07 Radiological findings in HIV-associated lymphoma. **A** Nuclear magnetic resonance (NMR) imaging scan of the brain shows a large tumour mass in the basal ganglia. **B** Multiple filling defects are seen in liver.

AIDS-associated NHL after HAART introduction is consistent with improved CD4 counts {211, 217}. HAART is also associated with enhanced survival with a 75% decrease in mortality, although lymphomas now contribute to a greater percentage of first AIDS-defining illness {570, 646}. There has been an unexpected increase in the incidence of HL since the advent of HAART therapy {451}. Since HL incidence is lower among patients with severe immunosuppression than among those with moderate immune defect, the recent increase of HL incidence could be possibly related to improvements in CD4 counts {218}.

Etiology and pathogenesis

Lymphomas in HIV-patients are heterogeneous, reflecting several pathogenetic mechanisms: chronic antigen stimulation,

genetic abnormalities, cytokine deregulation, and the role of Epstein-Barr virus (EBV) and Human Herpes Virus 8 (HHV8) {336, 337}. However, EBV-positive lymphomas decreased in the HAART era {941}. HIV-related lymphomas are consistently monoclonal and are characterized by a number of common genetic abnormalities of *MYC* and *BCL6* genes, as well as tumour suppressor genes {743, 2282}. The recognition of a polyclonal or oligoclonal nature of some HIV-related lymphoid proliferations suggests a multistep lymphomagenesis. B-cell stimulation, hypergammaglobulinemia and persistent generalized lymphadenopathy preceding the development of these lymphomas probably reflect the role of chronic antigenic stimulation. Disruption of the cytokine network leading to high serum levels of IL6 and IL10 is a feature of HIV-related lymphomas associated with EBV or HHV8. EBV is identified in the neoplastic cells of approximately 40% of HIV-related lymphomas, but the detection of EBV varies considerably with the site of presentation and histological subtype. EBV infection occurs in 80–100% of primary CNS lymphomas {325} and PEL, 80% of DLBCL with immunoblastic features and 30–50% of BL {877}. Nearly all HL cases in the setting of HIV infection are associated with EBV {107, 2068}. HHV8 is specifically associated with PEL, which usually occurs in the late stages of the disease, in the setting of profound immunosuppression {372}.

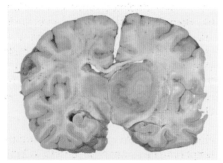

Fig. 13.08 Diffuse large B-cell lymphoma, HIV-associated. A large tumour involves the basal ganglia.

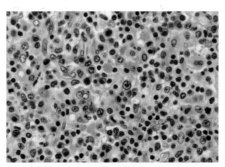

Fig. 13.09 Polymorphous lymphoid proliferation resembling PTLD with a mixture of lymphoplasmacytoid cells including large immunoblasts.

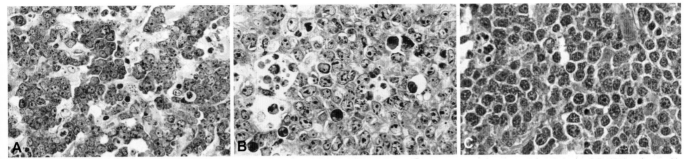

Fig. 13.10 A Burkitt lymphoma. Cell population is uniform. **B** In another case of Burkitt lymphoma, cells show much greater variation in size and shape. **C** Burkitt lymphoma with plasmacytoid differentiation. Cells have an eccentric rim of deeply stained cytoplasm.

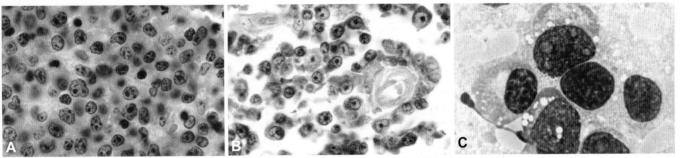

Fig. 13.11 A Primary CNS lymphoma, classified as diffuse large B-cell lymphoma in an HIV-positive patient. **B** Diffuse large B-cell lymphoma, immunoblastic variant, presenting in the central nervous system. The cells have prominent central nucleoli. **C** Cells exhibit marked plasmacytoid differentiation.

Sites of involvement

These lymphomas display a marked propensity to involve extranodal sites, in particular the gastrointestinal tract, CNS (less frequent since HAART), liver and bone marrow. The peripheral blood is rarely involved except in occasional cases of BL presenting as acute leukaemia. Unusual sites such as the oral cavity, jaw and body cavities are often involved. Many other extranodal sites, e.g. lung, skin, testis, heart and breast, can be involved. Lymph nodes are involved in about one third of patients at presentation {213}, but since the HAART era, nodal involvement accounts for half of the cases {941}.

Clinical features

Most patients present with advanced clinical stage; bulky disease with a high tumour burden is frequent. LDH is usually markedly elevated. There is a significant relationship between the subtype of lymphoma and the HIV disease status. DLBCL more often occurs in the setting of long-standing AIDS and is associated with a trend towards a higher rate of opportunistic infections and lower CD4+ T-cell counts with a mean below 100×10^6/L. In contrast, BL occurs in less immunodeficient patients, with a shorter mean interval between the diagnosis of HIV seropositivity and lymphoma and significantly higher CD4+ T-cell counts (more than 200×10^6/L) {211, 335}.

Morphology

In HIV-positive patients, different types of lymphoma can occur. Some are the same aggressive B-cell lymphomas that develop sporadically in the absence of HIV infection, while others corresponding to polymorphic lymphoid proliferations and unusual lymphoma histotypes occur more specifically in AIDS patients.

Lymphomas also occurring in immunocompetent patients

Burkitt lymphoma: Burkitt lymphoma accounts for 30% of all HIV-associated lymphomas. One third of cases display the spectrum of morphologic features described in the BL chapter, with EBV being positive in 30% of cases {1819}. Two thirds of cases show plasmacytoid differentiation, which is relatively unique to AIDS patients. They are characterized by medium-sized cells with abundant basophilic cytoplasm, and an eccentric nucleus, often with one centrally located prominent nucleolus. The cells often contain cytoplasmic immunoglobulin. EBV is positive in 50–70% of cases {511}.

Diffuse large B-cell lymphoma: The majority of these lymphomas contain numerous centroblasts, variably admixed with immunoblasts. This type accounts for 25–30% of HIV-associated lymphomas; EBV is present in 30% of cases. DLBCL containing more than 90% immunoblasts and usually exhibiting plasmacytoid features are classified as the immunoblastic variant. They account for about 10% of HIV-associated lymphomas, contain EBV in 90% of cases, and often occur late in the course of HIV disease. Primary central nervous system lymphomas are usually of the immunoblastic type {325}.

Hodgkin lymphoma: Most cases correspond to either the mixed cellularity or lymphocyte depleted forms of classical HL. Some cases of nodular sclerosis HL are also seen. HIV-related HL is associated with EBV in nearly all cases: the cells express the latent membrane protein 1 (LMP1) and are EBER-positive. Atypical forms with Hodgkin-like features may be observed in such context {1909}.

Other lymphomas: Rare cases of MALT lymphoma have been described in both paediatric and adult patients with HIV infection {1436, 2187}. Rare cases of peripheral T-cell and natural killer cell lymphoma can also occur {86, 213, 300, 330, 801, 863, 956, 1057}.

Lymphomas occurring more specifically in HIV-positive patients

Primary effusion lymphoma (PEL), Plasmablastic lymphoma, Lymphoma arising in HHV8-associated multicentric Castleman Disease (See Chapter 10).

Lymphomas occurring in other immunodeficient states

Polymorphic lymphoid proliferations resembling post-transplant associated lymphoproliferative disease (PTLD) may be seen in adults and also in children, but are much less common than in the post-transplant setting, representing less than 5% of HIV-associated lymphomas. These conform to the criteria of polymorphic B-cell PTLD. The infiltrates contain a range of lymphoid cells from small cells, often with plasmacytoid features, to immunoblasts, with scattered large bizarre cells expressing CD30. EBV is often present, but some cases are EBV-negative {1151, 1399, 1556, 2160}.

Prognosis and predictive factors

Before the HAART era, the rate of complete remissions was about 50% for most of histological subtypes. The 2-year survival was significantly lower for DLBCL than BL in univariate analysis. The International Prognostic Index (IPI) appeared to be a reliable indicator. The degree of immunodeficiency also correlated positively with the IPI score {1874}. Some other adverse prognostic factors were identified, such as age >35 years, intravenous drug use, stage III/IV and CD4 counts less than 100×10^6/L. Despite dose adjustment, the outcome of patients with lymphoma and HIV infection was closely related to the severity of immunodeficiency {253}.

Since the introduction of HAART, the overall survival of patients with DLBCL has improved, and outcomes are approaching those of patients with *de novo* lymphoma {1301}. The achievement of complete remission is the most important prognostic factor with respect to the time of survival {2434}. Long-term survival can be achieved in approximately one third of patients with favourable prognostic characteristics. PEL usually has a very poor prognosis with a low complete remission rate.

Post-transplant lymphoproliferative disorders

S.H. Swerdlow
S.A. Webber
A. Chadburn
J.A. Ferry

Definition
Post-transplant lymphoproliferative disorders (PTLD) are lymphoid or plasmacytic proliferations that develop as a consequence of immunosuppression in a recipient of a solid organ, bone marrow (BM) or stem cell allograft. PTLD comprise a spectrum ranging from usually Epstein-Barr virus (EBV)-driven infectious mononucleosis-type polyclonal proliferations to EBV-positive or EBV-negative proliferations indistinguishable from a subset of B-cell or less often T-cell lymphomas that occur in immunocompetent individuals. The monomorphic and Hodgkin-type PTLD are further categorized as in non-immunosuppressed patients, according the lymphoma they resemble. Indolent B-cell lymphomas such as follicular lymphomas and MALT

Table 13.02 Categories of post-transplant lymphoproliferative disease (PTLD).

Early lesions[1]	9971/1
Plasmacytic hyperplasia	
Infectious mononucleosis-like lesion	
Polymorphic PTLD	9971/3
Monomorphic PTLD[2]	
(classify according to lymphoma they resemble)	
B-cell neoplasms	
Diffuse large B-cell lymphoma	
Burkitt lymphoma	
Plasma cell myeloma	
Plasmacytoma-like lesion	
Other[3]	
T-cell neoplasms	
Peripheral T-cell lymphoma, NOS	
Hepatosplenic T-cell lymphoma	
Other[3]	
Classical Hodgkin lymphoma-type PTLD[2]	

[1]Some mass-like lesions in the post-transplant setting may have the morphologic appearance of florid follicular hyperplasia or other marked but non-IM-like lymphoid hyperplasias.
[2]ICD-O codes for these lesions are the same as those for the respective lymphoid or plasmacytic neoplasm.
[3]Indolent small B-cell lymphomas arising in transplant recipients are not included among the PTLD.

lymphomas in allograft recipients are designated as they are in the normal host and not considered a type of PTLD. Detection of rare EBV-positive cells in the absence of an appropriate lymphoid/plasmacytic proliferation is also not considered diagnostic of a PTLD.

Epidemiology
The characteristics of PTLD appear to differ somewhat from one institution to another, probably as a result of different patient populations, allograft types and immunosuppressive regimens. A variety of risk factors have been identified {308, 309, 1646}, but the most important risk factor for EBV-driven PTLD is EBV seronegativity at the time of transplantation {309, 2366}. Among adult solid organ recipients, the frequency of PTLD correlates, in part, with the intensity of the immunosuppressive regimen: patients receiving renal allografts have the lowest frequency of PTLD (<1%), those with hepatic and cardiac allografts have an intermediate risk (1–2%), and those receiving heart-lung/lung or intestinal allografts have the highest frequency (5% or greater) {133, 308, 309, 1646}. In children, the incidences are very much higher {562, 2367}, with the majority of cases being associated with post-transplantation primary EBV infection {2367}.
Peripheral blood (PB), stem cell and BM allograft recipients in general have a low risk of PTLD (~1%) with the risk of early-onset PTLD (<1 year) highest with unrelated or HLA mismatched related donors, selective T-cell depletion of donor BM, and use of antithymocyte globulin (ATG) or anti-CD3 monoclonal antibodies. The risk of PTLD in these patients increases up to 22% for those with two or more of these risk factors {499}. An unexpectedly high incidence of EBV-associated PTLD (17%) has been recently observed in patients undergoing unrelated umbilical cord blood transplants with a non-myeloablative preparative regimen containing ATG {291}. PTLD-like lesions are rare after autologous BMT; they may be associated with additional high-dose immunosuppressive

regimens and are best considered iatrogenic, rather than post-transplant, immunodeficiency-associated LPD {1576}.

Etiology
The majority of PTLD are associated with EBV infection (usually type A), and appear to represent EBV-induced monoclonal or, less often, polyclonal B-cell or monoclonal T-cell proliferations that occur in a setting of decreased T-cell immune surveillance {376, 450, 699, 730, 1166, 1569, 2133}. Up to 30% of PTLD are EBV-negative with some series reporting an even higher proportion of cases and with about 2/3 of T-PTLD EBV-negative {224, 699, 1260, 1586, 2133}. Furthermore, the proportion of EBV-negative PTLD appears to be increasing {1586}. EBV-negative PTLD are more common in adults, tend to occur later than EBV-positive cases and are more likely to be of monomorphic type {791, 1586}. Human herpesvirus 8 (HHV8)-associated PTLD are reported including post-transplant primary effusion lymphoma {606, 1106, 1421}; however, the etiology of the vast majority of EBV-negative PTLD is unknown. Some may be due to EBV that is no longer detectable {2073}, some due to other unknown viruses and some due to chronic antigenic stimulation, including by the transplant itself {224}. The EBV-negative cases are still considered to represent PTLD and some may respond to decreased immunosuppression {1586}.
The majority (>90%) of PTLD in solid organ recipients are of host origin and only a minority of donor origin. Donor origin PTLD appear to be most common in liver and lung allograft recipients, and frequently involve the allograft {78, 378, 1255, 2069, 2380}. In contrast, the majority of PTLD in BM allograft recipients are of donor origin, as would be expected, since successful engraftment results in an immune system that is nearly exclusively of donor origin {2510}.

Sites of involvement
Involvement of lymph node, gastrointestinal tract, lungs and liver are common in all

allograft types, whereas central nervous system (CNS) involvement is rare {699, 1569, 1723, 2367}. The CNS may be the only site of disease or may be associated with multiorgan involvement {343}. In solid organ recipients, PTLD frequently involves the allograft and this may cause diagnostic confusion since rejection and infection may result in a similar clinical picture. Allograft involvement appears more common in early-onset, EBV-positive disease {133, 791}. The heart is the only organ in which allograft involvement is very rare. "Early lesions" often present with tonsil and/or adenoid involvement but may also occur at other sites. Overt BM involvement by polymorphic and monomorphic PTLD is not common, and PB is rarely involved. Bone marrow allograft recipients tend to present with widespread disease involving nodal and extranodal sites, including liver, spleen, gastrointestinal tract and lungs {1723, 1998, 2510}.

Clinical features

The clinical features of PTLD are highly variable and correlate with the type of allograft, and to some extent, with the morphologically defined categories. Almost all solid organ transplant recipients are currently managed with a calcineurin inhibitor (cyclosporine or tacrolimus). With these agents, PTLD frequently presents in the first year after transplantation, earlier than tended to be observed in the pre-cyclosporine era {1569, 1723}. EBV-negative PTLD and T/NK-cell PTLD tend to present later (median time to occurrence 4–5 years and 6.5 years, respectively) {1260, 1586, 2133}. The majority of PTLD in BM allograft recipients develop within the first six months {499}. PTLD presentation may be non-specific with features such as malaise, lethargy, weight loss and

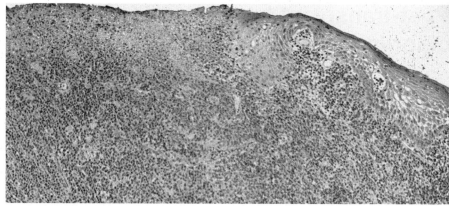

Fig. 13.12 Infectious mononucleosis-like (IM) lesion in a tonsil of an 11-year-old renal allograft recipient. There is preservation of overlying epithelium and crypts, but normal follicles are absent, and there is a diffuse lymphoid proliferation.

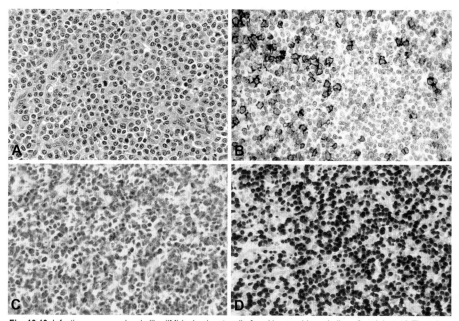

Fig. 13.13 Infectious mononucleosis-like (IM) lesion in a tonsil of an 11-year-old renal allograft recipient. **A** There is a polymorphic proliferation of immunoblasts, small lymphoid cells and plasma cells. **B** CD20 staining shows scattered B cells. **C** In contrast, a stain for CD79a shows more numerous positive cells, indicating plasmacytoid differentiation. **D** In situ hybridization identifies Epstein-Barr virus latency-associated RNA (EBER) expression in the majority of the cells.

Table 13.03 Pathologic evaluation of specimens for the diagnosis of PTLD.

Method of evaluation	Necessity	Purpose
Histopathology	Essential	Evaluate architecture and cytologic features, required for classification
Immunophenotype	Essential	Assess possible light chain class restriction* and basic lymphoid subsets, required for classification
EBER in situ hybridization	Essential**	Most sensitive method for assessing if PTLD is EBV-positive, aids in diagnosis and possibly prognostication, useful in differential diagnosis with rejection in allograft (if positive)
Genetic/cytogenetic studies	Variable	Determine clonality, lineage of clonal population(s), chromosomal and oncogene abnormalities, may be needed for classification
EBV clonality	Not required	Identification of minor clones

*Paraffin section immunohistochemistry will often fail to demonstrate monotypic B-cell populations, even if present, unless there is plasmacytic differentiation.
**If the less sensitive EBV-LMP1 stain is positive, EBER in situ hybridization is not required.

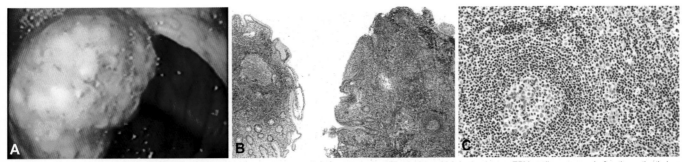

Fig. 13.14 Early lesion (follicular hyperplasia) in a 20-year-old male, 10 years after heart transplant. The lesion, which had only rare EBV+ cells, regressed after the patient's immunosuppression was reduced and did not recur. **A** Endoscopic image of ileocecal mass. **B,C** Biopsies showed a variably dense infiltrate composed of organized lymphoid tissue with scattered germinal centres, many small lymphocytes, some plasma cells and infrequent transformed cells.

fever. Lymphadenopathy and organ-specific dysfunction are also common presentations. Obstructive symptoms such as enlarged tonsils are another type of presentation. Presentation with disseminated disease seems to be less common in the current era, perhaps due to increasing awareness of the diagnosis and due to routine EBV viral load monitoring of seronegative recipients in many transplant centres.

Prognosis and predictive factors
The "early" lesions tend to regress with reduction in immune suppression, and if this can be accomplished without graft rejection, the prognosis is excellent, particularly in children {1330, 2486}. Polymorphic and less often monomorphic PTLD may also regress with reduction in immune suppression {2080, 2367}. However, rebound acute and chronic rejection may be observed and can lead to graft loss and death {2367}. A proportion of polymorphic and even more numerous monomorphic PTLD fail to regress, and require additional therapies such as monoclonal antibodies directed against B-cell antigens (most commonly anti-CD20) {435, 643}, chemotherapy {436, 643, 856} or combinations of both. Several centres are also performing phase I clinical trials of cellular immunotherapy to restore EBV-specific cytotoxic T-cell immunity in EBV-driven refractory disease {461, 889, 1946}. The myelomatous lesions usually do not regress with decreased immunosuppression, and T/NK-cell PTLD are also considered to be aggressive with the exception of those of large granular lymphocyte type {2133}. Nevertheless, some T-PTLD do respond to reconstitution of the patients' immune system. The plasmacytoma-like lesions have a variable outcome {1074}. EBV negativity in PTLD and even among the T/NK-cell PTLD, is also considered an

adverse prognostic indicator, although not all studies document a survival difference {435, 2133}.

A number of additional prognostic factors associated with an adverse outcome include multiple sites of disease and advanced stage, older age at diagnosis, late onset disease, high International Prognostic Index and elevated lactate dehydrogenase {309, 435, 643, 792, 2269}. However, risk factors for adverse outcome vary greatly between studies. Multi-site disease may not be a risk factor for adverse outcome in paediatric patients {2367}. Overall, the mortality of PTLD is greater in BM allograft recipients than solid organ allograft recipients and may be lower in children than adults.

Early lesions: plasmacytic hyperplasia (PH) and infectious mononucleosis (IM)-like PTLD

Definition
The early lesions are defined as lymphoid proliferations in an allograft recipient, characterized by architectural preservation of the involved tissue, with preservation of the nodal sinuses or tonsillar crypts, and

residual or sometimes floridly reactive follicles in some cases. In most cases, they form mass lesions. These lesions should be distinguished from lymphoid proliferations with other known explanations or other non-specific chronic inflammatory processes. Cases that have florid follicular hyperplasia but which do not fit into the PH or IM-like categories have been separately designated by some authors.

Clinical features
PH and IM-like lesions occur at a younger age than the other PTLD and are often seen in children or in adult solid organ recipients who have not had prior EBV infection {376, 1330}. Cases described as post-transplant florid follicular hyperplasia also occur most commonly in children {2284}. The early lesions involve lymph nodes or tonsils and adenoids more often than true extranodal sites {1330}. They often regress spontaneously or with reduction in immunosuppression; however, IM-like lesions can be fatal. In some cases, polymorphic or monomorphic PTLD may follow early lesions {1569, 2453}.

Morphology
Plasmacytic hyperplasia is characterized by numerous plasma cells, small

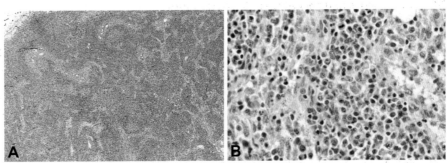

Fig. 13.15 Plasmacytic hyperplasia. **A** The normal architecture of the lymph node is intact. **B** Numerous plasma cells are present.

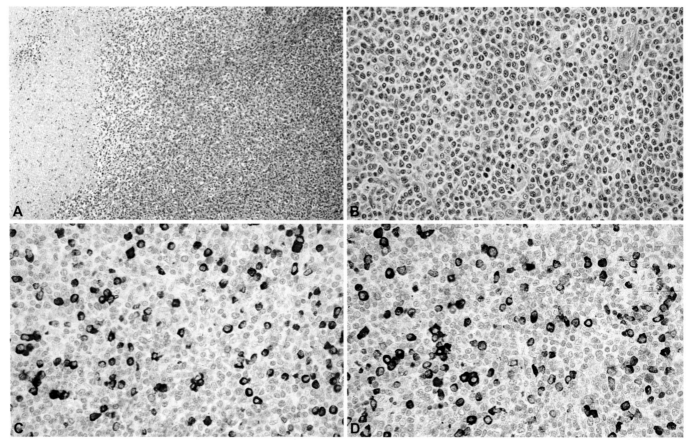

Fig. 13.16 Polymorphic PTLD. A Diffuse effacement of the nodal architecture with a large geographic area of necrosis. B Mixed proliferation of immunoblasts, plasma cells and medium-sized lymphoid cells with irregular nuclei (Giemsa stain). Immunoperoxidase stains on paraffin sections with antibodies to kappa (C) and (D) lambda immunoglobulin light chains show polyclonal staining.

lymphocytes and generally infrequent bland-appearing immunoblasts, while the IM-like lesion has the typical morphologic features of IM, with paracortical expansion and numerous immunoblasts in a background of T cells and plasma cells. Other non-destructive lymphoid hyperplasias that either show fewer immunoblasts or more prominent follicular hyperplasia than typical cases of IM may also occur in the post-transplant setting and cause mass lesions {2284}. Criteria for the distinction of these early, non-destructive PTLD from other reactive lymphoid infiltrates are not well-defined and rest on the extent of the proliferation, clinical correlations and the presence or absence of EBV.

Immunophenotype
Immunophenotypic studies show an admixture of polyclonal B cells, plasma cells and T cells without phenotypic aberrancy. EBV is present in many but not all of the cases of nodal PH and cases described as florid follicular hyperplasia {1166, 2284}. IM-like cases are typically EBV-positive with EBV-LMP1+ immunoblasts {1330}.

Genetics
Clonally rearranged immunoglobulin genes are not expected in PH, although small clonal populations may be demonstrated with Southern blot analysis using probes to the terminal repeat region of the EBV. Some IM-like PTLD may have small monoclonal or oligoclonal populations. The significance of oligoclonality or a small clonal band in these cases is unknown {1166, 2453}. Florid follicular hyperplasia (FFH) does not usually demonstrate clonal B cells but, as also reported in IM-like cases, rarely demonstrates simple clonal cytogenetic abnormalities {2284}.

Polymorphic PTLD

Definition
Polymorphic (P) PTLD are morphologically polymorphic lesions composed of immunoblasts, plasma cells and small and intermediate-sized lymphoid cells that efface the architecture of lymph nodes or form destructive extranodal masses and that

do not fulfill the criteria for any of the recognized types of lymphoma described in immunocompetent hosts. Distinction of some P-PTLD from more "monomorphic" (i.e. lymphoma-like) lesions that show plasmacytic differentiation is not well-defined.

Clinical features
The frequency of P-PTLD varies from one institution to another, ranging from 20% to over 80% of the cases {450, 699, 735, 1107, 1166, 1569, 1586}. In children this is the most common type of PTLD {2367} and frequently follows primary EBV infection. The clinical presentation of these cases is not distinguishable from PTLD in general. Reduction in immunosuppression leads to regression in a variable proportion of cases; others may progress and require treatment for lymphoma {1166, 1569, 2080, 2367}.

Morphology
In contrast to early PTLD lesions, P-PTLD show effacement of the underlying tissue architecture {735, 887}. Unlike most lymphomas, however, they show the full range

of B-cell maturation, from immunoblasts to plasma cells, with small and medium-sized lymphocytes and cells with irregular nuclear contours. There may be areas of geographic necrosis and scattered large, bizarre cells that not infrequently resemble Reed-Sternberg cells (atypical immunoblasts); numerous mitoses may be present. Some cases have areas that appear more monomorphic in the same or other tissues; thus, there may be a continuous spectrum between these lesions and the monomorphic PTLD. Other P-PTLD have features that more closely resemble Hodgkin lymphoma. Some of these cases have been referred to as "Hodgkin-like" in the past. Variably sized, but usually small, lymphoid aggregates with or without plasma cell clusters are seen in the BM in some patients with P-PTLD (and occasionally in M-PTLD) {1173}. They are more common in children than in adults. The clinical significance of these aggregates, that are not always EBV+, is uncertain.

Immunophenotype

Immunophenotypic studies demonstrate B cells with or without light chain class restriction and a variable proportion of heterogeneous T cells that sometimes predominate {625, 1569}. Light chain class restriction, when present, may be focal, and some cases may demonstrate different clonal populations in the same or different sites {1569}. Cases with clearcut light chain class restriction are recognized but this observation must be noted in the diagnostic report, as some of these cases could also be classified as a monomorphic DLBCL-like PTLD with plasmacytic differentiation, a DLBCL-like PTLD with significant polymorphism or as a plasma cell neoplasm with increased transformed cells. Reed-Sternberg-like cells when present are often CD30+, CD20+ but CD15- {406}. Most cases of P-PTLD contain numerous EBER-positive cells. Detection of EBV by EBER *in situ* hybridization is a useful tool in the differential diagnosis of PTLD versus rejection in allografts.

Genetics

P-PTLD are expected to demonstrate clonally rearranged immunoglobulin genes although the clones are less predominant than in monomorphic PTLD {449, 1107, 1166, 1327}. EBV terminal repeat analysis is the most sensitive method for demonstrating clonal populations in the EBV-positive

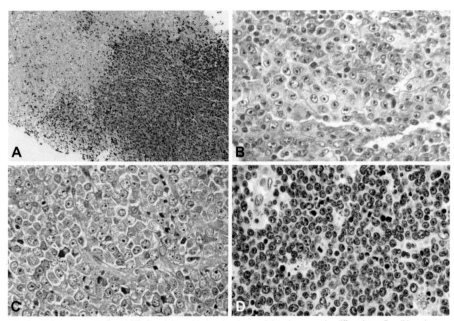

Fig. 13.17 Monomorphic B-cell PTLDs. **A** Liver biopsy showing partial replacement by diffuse large B-cell lymphoma, immunoblastic variant. **B** Diffuse large B-cell lymphoma, immunoblastic variant, EBV-positive, showing a monotonous proliferation of large immunoblast-like cells with prominent central nucleoli and basophilic cytoplasm (Giemsa stain). **C** Diffuse large B-cell lymphoma, centroblastic variant, EBV-negative, showing large transformed cells, many of which have peripheral nucleoli, consistent with centroblasts. There are also admixed immunoblasts. **D** Burkitt lymphoma showing monotonous, medium-sized cells with multiple nucleoli, basophilic cytoplasm and numerous mitoses.

cases. In some reported cases, tumours at different sites in the same patient may be clonally distinct {375}. Seventy-five percent of P-PTLD are reported to have mutated immunoglobulin gene variable regions *(IGV)* without ongoing mutations and the remainder are unmutated {334}. Significant T-cell clones are not expected. Clonal cytogenetic abnormalities may be present although less commonly detected than in monomorphic B-cell PTLD {593, 2284}. Comparative genomic hybridization studies also demonstrate abnormalities in some P-PTLD including some recurrent abnormalities also seen in monomorphic PTLD {1764}. *BCL6* somatic hypermutations may be present as well as aberrant promoter methylation, but other oncogene abnormalities are not detected {334, 371}.

Monomorphic PTLD

The group of monomorphic (M) PTLD fulfill the criteria for one of the B-cell or T/NK-cell neoplasms that are recognized in the immunocompetent host and described elsewhere in this monograph. The only exception to this is that the small B-cell lymphoid neoplasms such as follicular lymphomas or MALT lymphomas are not designated as PTLD even though

attention has been drawn to the occurrence of MALT lymphomas arising in the post-transplant setting {986}. The M-PTLD should be designated as PTLD in the diagnostic line of the pathology report, and then further categorized based on the classification of lymphomas arising in the immunocompetent host. Although the term M-PTLD reflects the fact that most cases are composed of a monotonous proliferation of transformed lymphoid cells or plasmacytic cells, there may be significant pleomorphism and variability of cell size within a given case. In addition, because polymorphic and monomorphic PTLD of B-cell origin form a spectrum, their distinction can become blurred. Currently, their distinction in problematic cases is usually based on a subjective assessment of whether there is a predominance of large transformed cells/immunoblasts. The presence of abnormalities in oncogenes and tumour suppressor genes may also favour the diagnosis of M-PTLD {1166}.

Monomorphic B-cell PTLD

Definition
The monomorphic B-cell PTLD are monoclonal transformed B lymphocytic or plasmacytic proliferations that fulfill the criteria for a diffuse large B-cell lymphoma, less

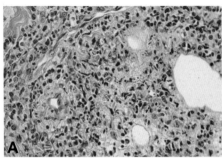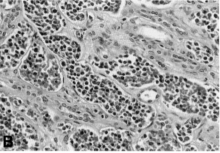

Fig. 13.18 Monomorphic T-cell PTLD. **A** Subcutaneous panniculitis-like T-cell lymphoma in an adult female renal allograft recipient, showing diffuse involvement of subcutaneous tissue. This case was EBV-negative. **B** Hepatosplenic γδ T-cell lymphoma (EBV-negative) in a 29-year-old male renal allograft recipient. There is infiltration of small blood vessels in the allograft.

often a Burkitt lymphoma or a plasma cell neoplasm. The latter may have all the features of plasma cell myeloma or of an extramedullary plasmacytoma with involvement of the gastrointestinal tract, lymph nodes or other extranodal sites.

Clinical features
The clinical presentation of patients with monomorphic B-PTLD is not distinctive and is, in general, similar to the presentation of the lymphomas or plasma cell neoplasms that they resemble.

Morphology
Monomorphic B-PTLD fulfill the conventional criteria for DLBCL, Burkitt lymphoma, plasmacytoma or myeloma {896}. This is in contrast to the full range of maturation seen in polymorphic PTLD. It is important to recognize, however, that there may be pleomorphism of the transformed cells in

monomorphic PTLD —some cells may be bizarre and multinucleated and even resemble Reed-Sternberg-like cells— and there may be plasmacytoid or plasmacytic differentiation. Thus, the term, monomorphic, does not mean complete cellular monotony, only that most of the cells appear to be transformed or more uniformly plasmacytic.

Immunophenotype
The non-plasmacytic lesions show B-cell-associated antigen expression (CD19, CD20, CD79a), with demonstrable monotypic immunoglobulin (often with expression of gamma or alpha heavy chain) in about half of the cases. Many cases are CD30+, with or without anaplastic morphology. Most M-PTLD are of non-GC type based on immunohistochemistry {332, 1061}. The EBV-positive cases usually have a late germinal centre/post germinal centre phenotype (CD10-, BCL6±, IRF4/MUM1+)

even though only a minority are CD138 positive, whereas the EBV negative cases are more likely to have a germinal centre type phenotype (CD10±, BCL6+, IRF4/MUM1-, CD138-; 60% of cases in one study) {1061}. The myelomatous or plasmacytoma-like lesions, which may be EBV-positive or negative, are phenotypically similar to those in immunocompetent patients {2165}.

Genetics
Clonal *IG* gene rearrangement is present in virtually all cases, and the majority contain EBV genomes, which, if present, are in clonal episomal form {449, 450, 1107}. Most cases have somatically mutated *IGV* with a minority showing ongoing mutations {334}. However, some cases have *IGV* loci inactivation related to crippling mutations as seen in HL {333}. As in non-PTLD DLBCL, oncogene abnormalities (*RAS* or *TP53* mutations and *MYC* rearrangements) may be found, and *BCL6* gene somatic hypermutation is common; however, *BCL6* translocations are uncommon {371, 1166}. Cytogenetic abnormalities are common, and are more frequent than in the early or polymorphic lesions {2284}. While some recurrent abnormalities are reported in PTLD such as breaks involving 1q11-q21 region, 8q24.1, 3q27, 16p13, 14q32, 11q23-24 and trisomies 9, 11, 7, X, 2 and 12, different studies find different common abnormalities {593, 2284}. Comparative genomic hybridization studies demonstrate additional gains and losses, although no individual

Table 13.04 Criteria used in the categorization of PTLD.

	Histopathology			Genetics	
Pathologic category	**Architectural effacement**	**Major findings**	**Immunophenotype/ *in situ* hybridization**	**IgH@/TCR**	**Other abnormalities**
Early lesions	Absent	Small lymphocytes, plasma cells, ± immunoblasts, ± hyperplastic follicles	Pcl B cells & admixed T cells; often EBV+	Pcl or very small mcl B-cell population(s)	None
Polymorphic PTLD	Present	Full spectrum of lymphoid maturation seen	Pcl or mcl B cells & admixed T cells; often EBV+	Mcl B cells, non-clonal T cells	Some have *BCL6* somatic hypermutations
Monomorphic PTLD	Usually present	Fulfills criteria for a NHL (other than one of the indolent B-cell neoplasms) or plasma cell neoplasm	Varies based on type of neoplasm they resemble. EBV more variable than in other categories	Clonal B cells and/or T cells (except for rare NK cases)	Usually present
Hodgkin lymphoma type PTLD	Present	Fulfills criteria for CHL	Similar to other CHL; EBV+	IgH will not be easily demonstrated.	Not known

Pcl, polyclonal; Mcl, monoclonal; NK, natural killer cell; TCR, T-cell antigen receptor.

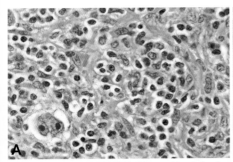 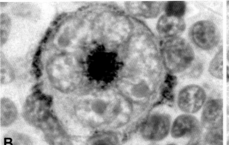 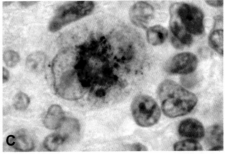

Fig. 13.19 Hodgkin-type PTLD in 52-year-old male (post renal transplant). The Reed-Sternberg cells were EBV+. **A** Reed-Sternberg cell surrounded by small lymphocytes and some eosinophils. Reed-Sternberg cells with CD30+ expression (**B**) and Golgi-type CD15 expression (**C**).

abnormality is very common; some are shared with DLBCL in immunocompetent hosts {1764, 1847}. EBV-negative monomorphic PTLD frequently lack expression of the cyclin dependent kinase inhibitor *CDKN2A* (*p16*^{INK4a}) {1397}. Aberrant promoter hypermethylation and aberrant somatic hypermutation also occur in M-PTLD {334}.

Monomorphic T/NK-cell PTLD

Definition
Monomorphic PTLD of T/NK-cell type (T/NK-PTLD) include PTLD that fulfill the criteria for any of the T- or natural killer (NK) cell lymphomas. They include almost the entire spectrum of T- or NK-cell neoplasms, with the largest group being peripheral T-cell lymphoma, not otherwise specified type, followed by hepatosplenic T-cell lymphoma. Other types of T/NK-cell PTLD include T-cell large granular lymphocyte leukaemia, adult T-cell leukaemia/lymphoma, extranodal NK/T-cell lymphoma, nasal type, mycosis fungoides/Sézary syndrome, primary cutaneous anaplastic large cell lymphoma and other anaplastic large cell lymphomas. In North America and Western Europe, they make up no more than 15% of PTLD. In some instances T-cell PTLD have occurred with, or subsequent to, other types of PTLD.

Clinical features
Clinical presentation depends on the type of T/NK-cell neoplasm. Most cases present at extranodal sites, sometimes with associated lymphadenopathy {2133}.The more common sites of involvement include the PB or BM, spleen, skin, liver, gastrointestinal tract and lung.

Morphology
The morphologic features of T/NK-PTLD do not differ from those of the same T/NK-cell lymphomas in immunocompetent hosts.

Immunophenotype
T/NK-PTLD show expression of pan-T-cell and sometimes NK-associated antigens. Depending on the specific type, they may express CD4 or CD8, CD30, ALK and either αβ or γδ T-cell receptors. About 1/3 of cases are EBV-positive.

Genetics
Cases of T-cell origin have clonal T-cell receptor gene rearrangement. Chromosomal abnormalities are common and similar to those seen in T/NK-cell neoplasms in the immunocompetent host such as i(7)(q10) and +8 in most of the hepatosplenic T-cell lymphomas {593, 2133}. *TP53* and other oncogene mutations are also reported in a high proportion of T/NK- PTLD {980}.

Classical Hodgkin lymphoma type PTLD

Classical Hodgkin lymphoma (CHL), the least common major form of PTLD, occurs in the post-transplant setting, most often in renal transplant patients, is almost always EBV-positive and should fulfill the criteria for CHL as described (See Chapter 12). Because Reed-Sternberg-like cells may be seen in early, polymorphic and some monomorphic PTLD, the diagnosis of HL must be based on both classical morphologic and immunophenotypic features, preferably including both CD15 and CD30 expression {1570, 1887}. Although CD15-negative cases occur, caution is advised in making the diagnosis of CHL-type PTLD as these cases must be distinguished from Hodgkin-like lesions, in which the EBV+ Reed-Sternberg-like cells are CD45+, CD15-, CD20+ and where one may find small and intermediate-sized EBV+ lymphoid cells as well {406, 609, 823, 1570, 1759, 1817}. Rare cases may follow other types of PTLD. Although the distinction of Hodgkin-like P-PTLD from true Hodgkin type PTLD may be difficult in some cases, the former are better characterized as either a polymorphic or monomorphic PTLD, depending on their overall morphologic features {1759, 1817}.

Other iatrogenic immunodeficiency-associated lymphoproliferative disorders

P. Gaulard
S.H. Swerdlow
N.L. Harris
E.S. Jaffe
C. Sundström

Definition

The other iatrogenic lymphoproliferative disorders (LPD) are lymphoid proliferations or lymphomas that arise in patients treated with immunosuppressive drugs for autoimmune diseases or conditions other than in the allograft/autograft transplant setting. They comprise a spectrum ranging from polymorphic proliferations resembling polymorphic post-transplant lymphoproliferative disorders (PTLD) to cases that fulfill the criteria for diffuse large B-cell lymphoma (DLBCL) or other B-cell lymphomas, peripheral T/NK-cell lymphomas or classical Hodgkin lymphoma (CHL). Iatrogenically-related lymphomas supervening on haematological malignancies are not covered here {4}.

Epidemiology

The frequency of these disorders is not well known, and it is difficult to determine how many are directly related to the iatrogenic immunosuppression rather than the underlying disorder, or to chance alone. It is likely that the risk and type of LPD that develop in this setting varies depending on the type of immunosuppressive agent and on the nature of the underlying disorder being treated (e.g. rheumatoid arthritis [RA], inflammatory bowel disease [IBD], psoriasis and psoriasic arthritis or other autoimmune disorders) {317}. Methotrexate was the first reported immunosuppressive agent associated with LPD in this

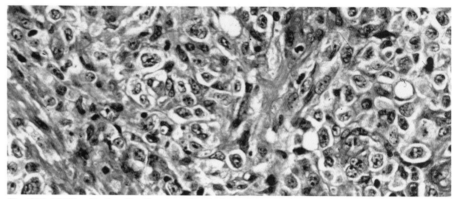

Fig. 13.20 **A** EBV-positive large B-cell lymphoproliferation in a patient with rheumatoid arthritis treated with methotrexate. This lesion regressed following cessation of therapy.

setting {1089, 1709, 1920}, predominantly in patients being treated for RA. In one survey, 479 lymphoma cases were recorded among 101,589 patients treated with methotrexate and/or anti-TNF therapy for RA {2435}. Many of these patients received a combination of several immunomodulators, complicating interpretation of the role of any specific agent. Among the TNFα antagonists (infliximab, adalimumab and etanercept), patients with Crohn's disease treated with infliximab have been reported to have a lymphoma prevalence higher than in a healthy age-matched population {1355}. A striking association between hepatosplenic T-cell lymphoma (HSTL) and young patients with Crohn's disease receiving infliximab in combination with azathioprine and/or 6-mercaptopurine has

been reported {1355, 1872}. Cases of large B-cell lymphoma and Hodgkin lymphoma have been reported in RA patients treated with TNF inhibitors, although it is not clear whether there is a significant increase in incidence {284, 2435}.

Etiology

Although some of these other iatrogenic LPD are associated with EBV, like many PTLD, the frequency of EBV infection is very variable {982, 1920}. Overall, about 40% of LPD in RA patients treated with methotrexate are EBV+, with EBV detected more frequently in Hodgkin lymphoma (~80%) than in DLBCL (~25%) or other B-cell lymphoma types. It is almost constantly found in polymorphic LPD and in LPD with Hodgkin-like features in this setting {982, 1920}. EBV is not seen in HSTL. The degree and duration of immunosuppression likely plays a role in the development of EBV-positive LPD. However, the presence of inflammation and/or chronic antigenic stimulation as well as the patient's genetic background may be important determinants of the risk and type of LPD {122}. For example, patients with RA are estimated to have a 2- to 20-fold increased risk of lymphoma even in the absence of methotrexate therapy {122, 2230}, and may have an altered Epstein-Barr virus (EBV)-host balance {316}. In addition, HSTL —a lymphoma that typically affects young men in the non-immunosuppressed population— is common in young

Table 13.05 Immunosuppressive drugs reported in the literature as associated with LPD and lymphomas.

Drug	Underlying disorder	Therapy duration	Type of LPD
Methotrexate	Autoimmune diseases, psoriasis	3 years (0.5–5 years)	DLBCL, HL Polymorphic LPD, PTCL
Antagonists of TNFα			
Infliximab (MAb)	Autoimmune diseases Crohn's disease (young patients)	6 weeks (2–44 weeks) 1–58 months	DLBCL, other types HSTL, other types
Adalimumab (MAb)	Autoimmune diseases	NA	Any type
Etanercept (fusion protein with p75)	Autoimmune diseases	8 weeks (2–52 weeks)	Any type

NA, not available; MAb, monoclonal antibody; TNF, tumour necrosis factor; DLBCL, diffuse large B-cell lymphoma, HL, Hodgkin lymphoma; LPD, lymphoproliferative disorder; PTCL, peripheral T-cell lymphoma; HSTL, hepatosplenic T-cell lymphoma (reported only in patients treated with infliximab, not with other drugs).

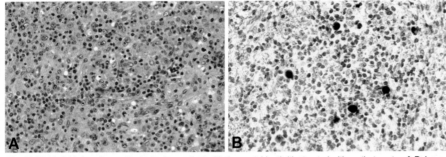

Fig. 13.21 Hodgkin lymphoma-like lesion in a patient with rheumatoid arthritis, treated with methotrexate. **A** Polymorphous infiltrate with lymphocytes, histiocytes, and Reed-Sternberg-like cells. **B** *In situ* hybridization for Epstein-Barr RNA (EBER) showing numerous positive large cells as well as many positive small lymphocytes.

men receiving infliximab for IBD, but not in older patients or in patients with RA receiving this agent.

Sites of involvement
Among the cases reported in patients receiving methotrexate, 40–50% have been extranodal, including the gastrointestinal tract, skin, liver and spleen, lung, kidney, thyroid gland, bone marrow (BM) and soft tissue {982, 1920}. As with HSTL in other settings, spleen, liver and BM are the common sites of involvement of HSTL in Crohn's disease patients receiving infliximab {1355, 1872}.

Clinical features
These do not appear to differ from those of immunocompetent patients with similar appearing lymphomas.

Histopathology
The distribution of histologic types of iatrogenic lymphoproliferations in non-transplantation settings appears to differ from that seen in other immunodeficiency settings, with a probable increase in the frequency of Hodgkin lymphoma and lymphoid proliferations with Hodgkin-like features. Among patients treated with methotrexate, the reported cases are most commonly DLBCL (35–60%) and CHL (12–25%), commonly of mixed

cellularity type, with less frequent cases of follicular lymphoma (5–10%), Burkitt lymphoma, extranodal marginal zone lymphoma of mucosa-associated lymphoid tissue and PTCL {982, 1086, 1392, 1920}. Polymorphic or lymphoplasmacytic infiltrates resembling polymorphic PTLD have been described in up to 15% of the cases in this setting. Lesions containing Reed-Sternberg-like cells but not fulfilling the criteria for Hodgkin lymphoma, that in the past were referred to as Hodgkin-like lesions, have been reported in all these settings {1090}. The HSTL in patients who have been treated with infliximab is indistinguishable from HSTL arising in immunocompetent or post-transplant patients.

Immunophenotype
The immunophenotype of the LPD does not appear to differ from those of similar histological types of lymphoma in non-immunosuppressed hosts. Immunophenotype is a useful tool in the distinction between LPD with HL-like features —that should not be considered to represent HL— and CHL, the large cells being CD20+/CD30+/CD15- and CD20-/CD30+/ CD15+ respectively. EBV is variably positive.

Genetics
The genotype of these immunodeficiency-associated LPD does not appear to differ from lymphomas of similar histological types not associated with immunosuppression.

Prognosis and predictive factors
A significant proportion of patients with methotrexate-associated LPD have shown at least partial regression in response to drug withdrawal (Table 13.06); the majority of responses have occurred in EBV-positive cases {982, 1920}. A variable proportion of DLBCL (up to 40%) and CHL (up to 30%) have regressed, while most require cytotoxic therapy; overall survival of DLBCL is approximately 50% {982, 1088, 1089, 1090}. Some patients whose LPD may initially regress after discontinuation of MTX, regrow at a later date and require chemotherapy {982}. Regression after discontinuation of drug seldom occurs in patients who develop LPD following the administration of TNFα blockers. Like in other individuals without overt immunodeficiency, cases of HSTL in patients treated with infliximab appear to be fatal {1355, 1872}.

Table 13.06 Characteristics of methotrexate–associated lymphoproliferative disorders (135 cases with details reported).

Type	Total	EBV+	Extranodal	Regress*
B-cell lymphoproliferative disorders/lymphomas				
DLBCL	64	15/58	15/27	7/41
Polymorphic/lymphoplasmacytic LPD	11	5/8	6/6	3/5
Follicular lymphoma	9	2/8	2/5	2/7
Burkitt lymphoma	3	1/3	0/1	0/3
MZL/MALT lymphoma	3	0/3	3/3	1/1
Lymphoplasmacytic lymphoma	2	0/2	-	0/2
CLL/SLL	1	0/1	0/1	0/1
T-cell lymphoproliferative disorders/lymphomas				
PTCL**	7	0/4	0/1	3/5
Extranodal NK/T lymphoma, nasal type	1	1/1	1/1	1/1
Other T-LPD	1	1/1	1/1	1/1
Hodgkin lymphomas	28	10/12	2/19	5/18
"Hodgkin-like lesions"	5	5/5	2/4	5/5
Total	135	40/106	32/69	28/90

* In about half of these cases, the duration of remission was short (1–10 months) and chemotherapy was then required.
** Includes PTCL, not otherwise specified and angioimmunoblastic T-cell lymphoma.
DLBCL, diffuse large B-cell lymphoma; MZL/MALT, marginal zone lymphoma/mucosa-associated lymphoid tissue lymphoma; CLL/SLL, chronic lymphocytic leukaemia/small lymphocytic lymphoma; PTCL, peripheral T-cell lymphoma; LPD, lymphoproliferative disorder.

CHAPTER 14

Histiocytic and Dendritic Cell Neoplasms

Histiocytic and dendritic cell neoplasms, Introduction

R. Jaffe
S.A. Pileri
F. Facchetti
D.M. Jones
E.S. Jaffe

Histiocytic neoplasms are derived from mononuclear phagocytes (macrophages and dendritic cells) or histiocytes. Dendritic cell tumours are related to several different lineages of accessory antigen-presenting cells (dendritic cells) that have a role in phagocytosis, processing and presentation of antigen to lymphoid cells. Reticulohistiocytosis and Rosai-Dorfman disease, which are covered in the WHO Classification of Tumours of the Skin, will not be included in this chapter.

Epidemiology

Tumours of histiocytes are among the rarest of tumours affecting lymphoid tissues, probably representing less than 1% of tumours presenting in lymph nodes or soft tissues {673, 1745}. As several of these tumour types were poorly recognized until recently, their true incidence remains to be determined. Historically, some large cell lymphomas of B-cell or T-cell type were thought to be histiocytic or reticulum cell sarcomas on purely morphological grounds, but only a small number

prove to be of true macrophage or dendritic cell origin. Some of the regulatory disorders such as macrophage activation or haemophagocytic syndromes may have large numbers of histiocytes but these are non-neoplastic. No sex, race or geographic predilection has yet been described.

Histogenesis

The cellular counterparts of this group of neoplasms consist of myeloid-derived macrophages, myeloid-derived dendritic cells and stromal-derived dendritic cells. The myeloid-derived macrophages and dendritic cells constitute divergent lines of differentiation from bone marrow (BM) precursors, although transdifferentiation or hybrid differentiation states likely occur.

Monocytes, macrophages, histiocytes

Metchnikoff is considered the father of the macrophage and in 1883 coined the term "phagocytosis", postulating a central role for the process in the body's innate defense against infection {821A, 1467A}. The histiocytes/macrophages are derived from

BM-derived monocytes and following migration/maturation in tissues participate in the innate response with pro- and anti-inflammatory cytokine effects as well as particulate removal and tissue reconstitution {821A, 821B}. They are derived largely from the circulating peripheral blood (PB) monocyte pool that migrates through blood vessel walls to reach their site of action, but local proliferation also contributes {1816}. Histiocytic tumours are closely related to the monocytic tumours from which their precursors are derived. The distinction between a leukaemic infiltrate of monocytic origin and histiocytic sarcoma can sometimes be difficult on morphologic grounds alone.

Macrophages display phagocytosis under some conditions of activation and, at this stage, there is heightened expression of lysosomal enzymes that can be demonstrated by histochemistry including non-specific esterases and acid phosphatase. Phagocytic activity is not a prominent feature of histiocytic malignancy but is a cardinal feature of the haemophagocytic syndromes. The haemophagocytic macrophage activation syndromes are an important group of non-neoplastic proliferative disorders that need to be differentiated from true histiocytic neoplasms, and are far more common. The haemophagocytic syndromes are the result of genetic or acquired disorders in the regulation of macrophage activation. The primary familial lymphohistiocytic disorders are due to genetically determined inability to regulate macrophage killing by NK and/or T cells because of mutations in perforin, its packaging, export or release. Acquired or secondary causes of the haemophagocytic macrophage activation syndromes follow certain infections, most notably Epstein-Barr virus (EBV) and a wide variety of other infectious agents, as well as some malignancies, rheumatic disorders and multiple organ failure {1045}. The characteristic cytopenias of the haemophagocytic syndromes are most likely due to BM suppression by the cytokine storm since the BM is often hypercellular at the outset.

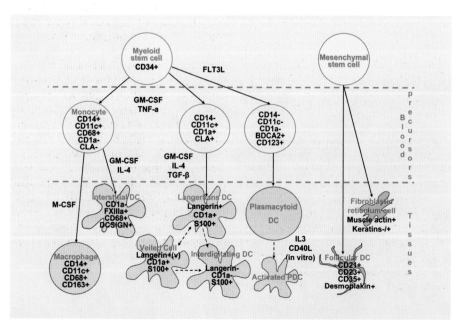

Fig.14.01 Schematic diagram of the origin. Both macrophages and dendritic cells (antigen presenting cells) are derived from a common bone marrow precursor. In contrast, follicular dendritic cells are thought to be of non-haematopoietic origin. +, most if not all cells positive; -, all cells negative; -/+, a minority of cells positive; v, variable intensity.

Table 14.01 True histiocytic malignancy, a vanishing diagnosis.

Original diagnosis	Currently considered
Histiocytic lymphoma, nodular and diffuse	Diffuse large B-cell lymphoma Follicular lymphoma, grade 3 Peripheral T-cell lymphoma Histiocyte-rich variants of B-cell, T-cell and Hodgkin lymphoma Anaplastic large cell lymphoma (ALCL)
Histiocytic medullary reticulosis	Haemophagocytic syndromes
Malignant histiocytosis	ALCL Haemophagocytic syndromes
Regressing atypical histiocytosis	Primary cutaneous CD30-positive T-cell lymphoma
Intestinal malignant histiocytosis	Enteropathy-type T-cell lymphoma
Histiocytic cytopathic panniculitis	Subcutaneous panniculitis-like T-cell lymphoma with haemophagocytosis

Table 14.02 Immunophenotypic markers of non-neoplastic macrophages and dendritic cells.

Marker	LC	IDC	FDC	PDC	Mø	DIDC
MHC-Class II	+c	++s	-	+	+	+/-
Fc-receptors	-	-	+	-	+	-
CD1a	++	-	-	-	-	-
CD4	+	+	+	+	+	+/-
CD21	-	-	++	-	-	-
CD35	-	-	++	-	-	-
CD68	+/-	+/-	-	++	++	+
CD123	-	-	-	++	-	-
CD163	-	-	-	-	++	-
Factor XIIIa	-	-	+/-	-	-	++
Fascin	-	++	+/++	-	-/+	+
Langerin	++	-	-	-	-	-
Lysozyme	+/-	-	-	-	+	-
S100	++	++	+/-	-	+/-	+/-
TCL1	-	-	-	+	-	-

FCR, Fc IgG receptors (include CD16, CD32, CD64 on some cells); LC, Langerhans cell; IDC, interdigitating dendritic cell; FDC, follicular dendritic cell; PDC, plasmacytoid dendritic cell; Mø, macrophage; DIDC, dermal/interstitial dendritic cell; c, cytoplasmic; s, surface.
Expression is semiquantitatively graded 0 through ++, + present, ++ high, +/- low or varies with cell activity.

Myeloid-derived dendritic cells

Dendritic cells or antigen presenting cells are found in various sites and at different states of activation, and no single marker will identify all dendritic cell subsets {138, 1816, 2094}. Langerhans cells (LC) are specialized dendritic cells in mucosal sites/skin that upon activation become specialized for antigen presentation to T cells, and then migrate to the lymph node through lymphatics. Lymph nodes also contain a paracortical dendritic cell type, the interdigitating cell (IDC) which may be derived in part from LC {771}. This classical dendritic cell lineage is believed to give rise to Langerhans cell histiocytosis/sarcoma and to IDC sarcoma. A third, poorly-defined DC subset, dermal/interstitial dendritic cells, are found in the soft tissue, dermis and in most organs, and can be increased in some inflammatory states {138}.
Plasmacytoid dendritic cells (PDC) (also known as plasmacytoid monocytes) are a distinct lineage of dendritic cells, which are believed to give rise to the blastic-plasmacytoid dendritic cell neoplasm (See Chapter 6) {920}. The histogenetic origins of PDC are controversial but are likely of myelomonocytic lineage. Interferon-α-producing PDC precursors, which are not strikingly dendritic in appearance, circulate in the PB and have the capacity to enter lymph nodes and tissue through high endothelial venules {1325}.

Stromal-derived dendritic cell types

Follicular dendritic cells (FDC), which are resident within primary and secondary B-cell follicles, trap and present antigen to B cells. FDC can store antigen on the cell surface as immune complexes for long periods of time {2304}. FDC appear to be closely related to BM stromal progenitors with features of myofibroblasts {1360}. They are a non-migrating population that forms a stable meshwork within the follicle via cell-to-cell attachments and desmosomes.
Fibroblastic reticular cells (FRC) are involved in maintenance of lymphoid integrity, production and transport of cytokines and other mediators. In lymph nodes, they ensheath the post-capillary venules {1115, 2320}. They are of mesenchymal origin and express smooth muscle actin. Hyperplasia of FRC (i.e. stromal overgrowth) may be seen in Castleman's disease {1028, 1309}, and tumours of FRC arise in lymph nodes and have features of myofibroblastic tumours and closely related neoplasms {44}.

Prognosis and predictive factors

Because there are few phenotypic markers unique for the dendritic or macrophage histiocytes, the investigator should use a panel appropriate to the cell in question and rigorously exclude other cell lineages (T cell, B cell, NK cell but also stromal, melanocytic and epithelial) by immunophenotypic and molecular means. It is also worth mentioning that some leukaemias and anaplastic large cell lymphoma can be accompanied in lymph nodes by an exuberant histiocytic response that may obscure the neoplastic cells.

Histiocytic sarcoma

T.M. Grogan
S.A. Pileri
J.K.C. Chan
L.M. Weiss
C.D.M. Fletcher

Definition

Histiocytic sarcoma is a malignant proliferation of cells showing morphologic and immunophenotypic features of mature tissue histiocytes. Neoplastic proliferations associated with acute monocytic leukaemia are excluded.

ICD-O code   9755/3

Epidemiology

Histiocytic sarcoma is a rare neoplasm with only limited numbers of reported series of bona fide cases {473, 886, 964, 1087, 1745, 2345}. There is a wide age range, from infancy to elderly; however, most cases occur in adults (median age, 52 years) {964, 1745, 2345}. Male predilection is found in some studies {1745, 2345} but not in others {964}.

Etiology

The etiology is unknown. A subset of cases occurs in patients with mediastinal germ cell tumour, most commonly malignant teratoma, with or without yolk sac tumour component {555}. Since teratocarcinoma cells may differentiate along haematopoietic lines in vitro {495}, histiocytic neoplasms may arise from pluripotential germ cells. Other cases may be associated with malignant lymphoma, either preceding or subsequent, or with myelodysplasia and leukaemia {677, 964, 1745, 2345}.

Sites of involvement

The majority of cases present in extranodal sites {964, 1745, 2345}, most commonly

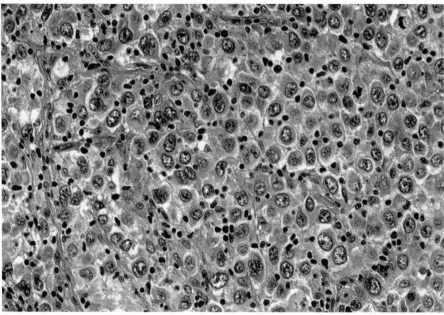

Fig. 14.02 Histiocytic sarcoma. Diffuse effacement of architecture is seen by a large cell proliferation that is indistinguishable from a diffuse large B-cell lymphoma by conventional histopathology.

intestinal tract, skin and soft tissues. Others present with lymphadenopathy. Rare patients have a systemic presentation, with multiple sites of involvement, sometimes referred to as "malignant histiocytosis" {347, 1745, 2419}.

Clinical features

Patients may present with a solitary mass, but systemic symptoms are relatively common, e.g. fever and weight loss {964, 1745, 2345}. Skin manifestations may range from a benign-appearing rash to solitary

lesions to innumerable tumours on the trunk and extremities. Patients with intestinal lesions often present with intestinal obstruction. Hepatosplenomegaly and associated pancytopenia may occur. The bone may show lytic lesions {964, 1745, 2345}.

Morphology

The tumour comprises a diffuse non-cohesive proliferation of large cells (>20 µm), but a sinusoidal distribution may be seen in lymph node, liver and spleen. The proliferating cells may be monomorphic

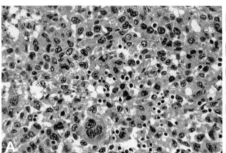
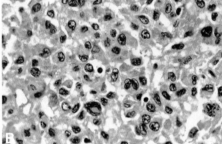
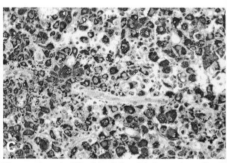

Fig. 14.03 Histiocytic sarcoma. A Note the multinucleated tumour cell. B The cytoplasm is relatively abundant, but the neoplasm is difficult to distinguish from a large B-cell lymphoma without a battery of immunohistochemical studies. C Diffuse staining for the lysosomal marker CD68.

or, more commonly, pleomorphic. The individual neoplastic cells are usually large and round to oval in shape; however, focal areas of spindling (sarcomatoid areas) may be observed. The cytoplasm is usually abundant and eosinophilic, often with some fine vacuoles. Haemophagocytosis occurs occasionally in the neoplastic cells. The nuclei are generally large, round to oval or irregularly folded, and often eccentrically placed; large multinucleated forms are commonly seen. The chromatin pattern is usually vesicular, and atypia varies from mild to marked. Immunostaining is essential for distinction from other large cell neoplasms, such as large cell lymphoma, melanoma and carcinoma.

A variable number of reactive cells may be seen, including small lymphocytes, plasma cells, benign histiocytes and eosinophils. Sometimes the neoplastic cells are obscured by a heavy inflammatory infiltrate including many neutrophils, mimicking an inflammatory lesion; this feature is particularly common in histiocytic sarcoma involving the central nervous system {411}.

Ultrastructure
The neoplastic cells show abundant cytoplasm with numerous lysosomes. Birbeck granules and cellular junctions are not seen.

Immunophenotype
By definition, there is expression of one or more histiocytic markers, including CD163, CD68 (KP1 and PGM1) and lysozyme with typical absence of Langerhans cell (CD1a, langerin), follicular dendritic cell (CD21, CD35) and myeloid cell (CD33, CD13, myeloperoxidase) markers {964, 1745, 2345}. Both CD68 and lysozyme show granular cytoplasmic staining. The lysozyme staining is accentuated in the Golgi region. CD163 staining is in the cell membrane and/or cytoplasm. Rarely, weak

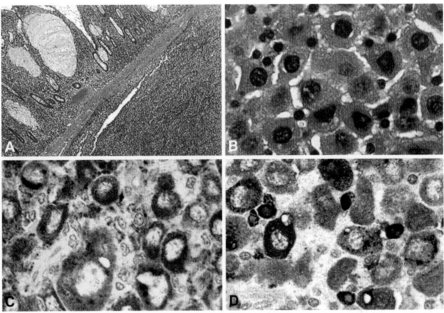

Fig. 14.04 Histiocytic sarcoma. **A** Histiocytic sarcoma involving the bowel. **B** Note the abundant cytoplasm, which stains strongly for CD68 (**C**) and lysozyme (**D**).

expression of CD15 occurs {1745}. In addition, CD45, CD45RO and HLA-DR are usually positive. There may be expression of S-100 protein, but this is usually weak or focal {1745}. There is no positivity for specific B-cell and T-cell markers. CD4 is often positive. These tumours are devoid of HMB45, epithelial membrane antigen or keratin. The Ki67 index is variable {1745}.

Genetics
Histiocytic sarcomas usually lack clonal *IgH* or *TCR* rearrangements {473}, but rare cases have been reported to show antigen receptor gene rearrangements, most likely representing examples of transdifferentiation {886, 1810, 2345}. The rare cases arising in mediastinal germ cell tumour show isochromosome 12p, identical to the genetic change in the germ cell tumour {1594}.

Postulated mormal counterpart
Mature tissue histiocyte.

Prognosis and predictive factors
Histiocytic sarcoma is usually an aggressive neoplasm, with a poor response to therapy, although some exceptions have been reported {964}. Most patients (60–80%) die of progressive disease reflecting the high clinical stage at presentation (stage III/IV) in the majority (70%) of patients {1745, 2345}. Patients with clinically localized disease and small primary tumours have a more favourable long-term outcome {964, 1745}.

Tumours derived from Langerhans cells

R. Jaffe
L.M. Weiss
F. Facchetti

The tumours discussed in this section originate from Langerhans cells of which they maintain the phenotypic profile and ultrastructural features. According to the degree of cytologic atypia and clinical aggressiveness, they are divided into two main subgroups: Langerhans cell histiocytosis and Langerhans cell sarcoma. There may be rare cases that can be difficult to assign to one or the other category; these cases need further clinicopathologic studies to clarify their nature.

Langerhans cell histiocytosis

Definition
Langerhans cell histiocytosis (LCH) is a clonal neoplastic proliferation of Langerhans-type cells that express CD1a, langerin and S100 protein, and shows Birbeck granules by ultrastructural examination.

ICD-O code
9751/3

Synonyms
Histiocytosis X, eosinophilic granuloma (if solitary lesion), Hand-Schüller-Christian disease (if multiple lesions), Letterer-Siwe disease (if disseminated or visceral involvement).

Epidemiology
The incidence is about 5 per million population per year, with most cases occurring in childhood. There is a predilection for males (M:F ratio 3.7:1) {1745}. The disease is more common in whites of northern European descent and rare in blacks. Familial clustering has shown a high concordance rate for identical twins but not dizygous pairs and no vertical inheritance {76}. Primary Langerhans cell histiocytosis of the lung is almost always a disease of smokers, usually non-clonal and thought to represent a reactive process {502, 2479}.

Sites of involvement
The disease can be localized to a single site, multiple sites within a single system, usually bone, or more disseminated and multisystem {1480, 2242}. The dominant sites of involvement in the solitary form are bone and adjacent soft tissue (skull, femur, vertebra, pelvic bones and ribs) and, less commonly, lymph node, skin and lung. The multifocal lesions are largely confined to bone and adjacent soft tissue. In multisystem disease, the skin, bone, liver, spleen and bone marrow (BM) are the preferential sites of involvement. The gonads and kidney appear to be spared even in disseminated forms.

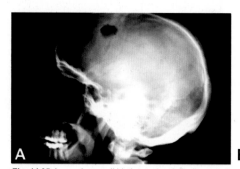
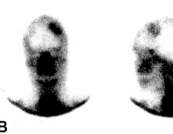

Fig. 14.05 Langerhans cell histiocytosis. **A** Radiograph from a patient with eosinophilic granuloma of bone illustrates a discrete punched-out lesion. **B** A gallium scan shows high uptake in lytic bone lesion.

Clinical features
Patients with unifocal disease are usually older children or adults who most commonly present with a lytic bone lesion, eroding the cortex. Solitary lesions at other sites present as mass lesions or enlarged lymph nodes. Patients with unisystem multifocal disease are usually young children who present with multiple or sequential destructive bone lesions often associated with adjacent soft tissue masses. Skull and mandibular involvement is common. Diabetes insipidus follows cranial involvement. Patients with multisystem involvement are infants who present with fever, cytopenias, skin and bone lesions and hepatosplenomegaly {75, 1482}. Pulmonary disease in childhood is clinically variable {1619}.

There is an association between LCH and T lymphoblastic leukaemia, with the leukaemia-associated T-cell receptor gene rearrangement present in the LCH cells; this has been considered a transdifferentiation phenomenon {676}.

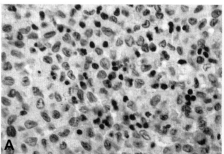
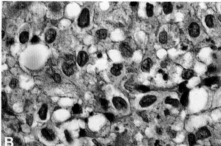
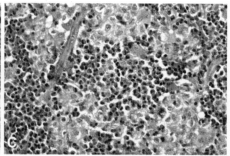

Fig. 14.06 Langerhans cell histiocytosis. **A** Numerous Langerhans cells are seen, with scattered eosinophils and small lymphocytes. **B** Note the typical cytologic features of Langerhans cells, with many nuclei containing linear grooves. **C** Eosinophilic microabscess.

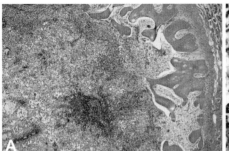
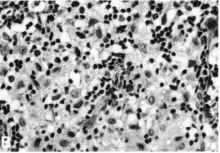
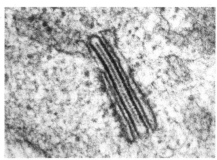

Fig. 14.07 Langerhans cell histiocytosis, at a later stage of evolution than the case illustrated in Fig. 14.06. **A** This bony lesion shows a greater number of foamy macrophages and lymphocytes. **B** A greater number of foamy macrophages and lymphocytes are present, although nuclei with typical grooves are still discernible.

Fig. 14.08 Langerhans cell histiocytosis, ultrastructure. A typical Birbeck granule is seen.

Morphology

The key feature is the identification of the LCH cells. These are oval, about 10–15 µm, recognized by their grooved, folded, indented or lobulated nuclei with fine chromatin, inconspicuous nucleoli and thin nuclear membranes. Nuclear atypia is minimal, but mitotic activity is variable and can be high without atypical forms. The cytoplasm is moderately abundant and slightly eosinophilic. Unlike epidermal Langerhans cells or dermal perivascular cells, LCH cells are oval in shape and devoid of dendritic cell processes. The characteristic milieu includes a variable number of eosinophils, histiocytes (both multinucleated LCH forms and osteoclast-type cells especially in bone), neutrophils and small lymphocytes. Plasma cells are usually sparse. Occasionally, eosinophilic abscesses with central necrosis, rich in Charcot-Leyden crystals, may be found. In early lesions, the LCH cell predominates along with eosinophils and neutrophils. In late lesions, the LCH cells are decreased in number, with increased foamy macrophages and fibrosis.

Involved lymph nodes have a sinus pattern with secondary infiltration of the paracortex. Spleen shows nodular red pulp involvement. Liver involvement has strong preference for intrahepatic biliary involvement with progressive sclerosing cholangitis. Bone marrow biopsy is preferred to aspirate for documentation of BM involvement {1481}. Large clusters or sheets of LCH cells accompanied by eosinophils can be found within other lesions, lymphomas and sarcomas. It remains to be clarified whether these represent a local reactive phenomenon or a transdifferentiation process {440}.

Ultrastructure

The ultrastructural hallmark is the cytoplasmic Birbeck granules whose presence can be confirmed by langerin expression. The Birbeck granule has a tennis racquet shape, and is 200–400 nanometers long and 33 wide, with a zipper-like appearance.

Immunophenotype

LCH consistently expresses CD1a, langerin and S100 protein {418, 1191A}. In addition, the cells are positive for vimentin, CD68 and HLA-DR. CD45 expression and lysozyme content is low. B- and T-cell

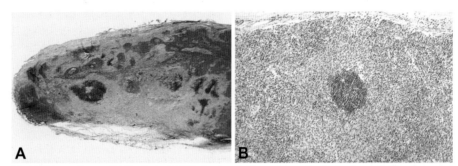

Fig.14.09 Langerhans cell histiocytosis. **A,B** This lymph node biopsy shows extensive involvement of the sinuses and paracortical regions.

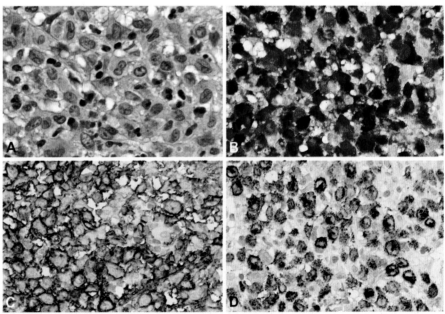

Fig. 14.10 Langerhans cell histiocytosis. **A** Contrast the bland nuclear morphology with that of the sarcoma (See Fig. 14.11 and 14.12). **B** Staining is both nuclear and cytoplasmic with S100. **C** CD1a staining is uniformly surface with a paranuclear dot. **D** Langerin staining is more granular and cytoplasmic.

lineage markers (except for CD4), CD30 and follicular dendritic cell markers are absent. Ki67 is highly variable {1745}.

Genetics
LCH has been shown to be clonal by X-linked androgen receptor gene assay (HUMARA), except in some adult pulmonary lesions {2418, 2479, 2480}. No consistent molecular genetic defect has been identified {1542}.

Postulated normal counterpart
Mature Langerhans cells.

Prognosis and predictive factors
The clinical course is related to staging of the disease at presentation, with 99% or greater survival for unifocal disease and 66% mortality for young children with multisystem involvement who do not respond promptly to therapy {740, 1480, 2242}. Involvement of BM, liver and lung are regarded as high risk factors {1480, 2242}. Progression from initial focal disease to multisystem involvement can occur, most usually in infants. Age, *per se*, is less important an indicator than extent of disease {1480, 2242}. Systemic and (rarely) multifocal disease can be complicated by haemophagocytic syndrome {674}.

Langerhans cell sarcoma

Definition
Langerhans cell sarcoma (LCS) is a high-grade neoplasm with overtly malignant cytologic features and the Langerhans cell phenotype.

ICD-O code   9756/3

Synonyms
Dendritic/histiocytic sarcoma, Langerhans cell type, malignant histiocytosis X.

Epidemiology
Langerhans cell sarcoma is rare {183, 232, 1745}, and almost all reported cases are in adults. The median age is 39 years (range, 10–72 years). A female predominance is described (M:F ratio 2:1) {1745}.

Sites of involvement
Skin and underlying soft tissue are the most common, with multiorgan involvement that includes lymph nodes, lung, liver, spleen and bone {232, 696, 1745}.

Clinical features
Most instances are extranodal involving skin and bone and multifocal, high-stage disease (III-IV) is seen in 44%. Only 22% are primarily nodal. Hepatosplenomegaly is noted in 22% and pancytopenia in 11%.

Morphology
The most prominent feature is the overtly malignant cytology of a pleomorphic tumour, and only the phenotype and/or ultrastructure will reveal the Langerhans cell derivation. Chromatin is clumped and nucleoli are conspicuous. Some cells may have the complex grooves of the LCH cell, a key clue to the diagnosis. The mitotic rate is high, usually more than 50 per 10 high power fields. Rare eosinophils may be admixed.

Ultrastructure
Birbeck granules are present, while desmosomes/junctional specializations are absent {1745}.

Immunophenotype
The immunophenotype is identical to that of Langerhans cell histiocytosis, although the staining for the individual markers can be focal and patchy.

Postulated normal counterpart
Mature Langerhans cell.

Prognosis and predictive factors
Langerhans cell sarcoma is an aggressive, high-grade malignancy with > 50% mortality from progressive disease.

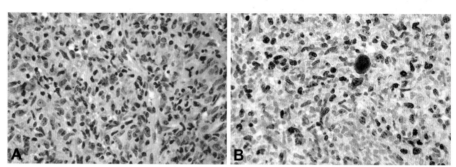

Fig.14.11 Langerhans cell sarcoma. **A** A tonsillar lesion in a 31-year-old male. The nuclear profiles and abundant cytoplasm are pointers to a histiocytic lesion. Nuclear pleomorphism and atypical mitosis indicate high-grade disease. **B** Ki67 immunostain showing the high proliferative index.

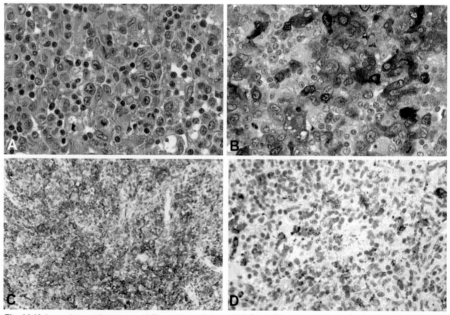

Fig.14.12 Langerhans cell sarcoma. **A** The nuclear pleomorphism is not a feature of LCH but should raise the possibility of malignancy. **B** S100 is widely represented, nuclear and cytoplasmic, but variable in intensity. **C** Lesional cells have surface CD1a, more variable than LCH. **D** Langerin is demonstrable, not as much as in LCH in this example.

Interdigitating dendritic cell sarcoma

L.M. Weiss
T.M. Grogan
J.K.C. Chan

Definition

Interdigitating dendritic cell (IDC) sarcoma is a neoplastic proliferation of spindle to ovoid cells with phenotypic features similar to those of interdigitating dendritic cells.

ICD-O code

Interdigitating dendritic
cell sarcoma   9757/3

Epidemiology

Interdigitating dendritic cell sarcoma is an extremely rare neoplasm, with most studies representing single case reports or very small series {44, 681, 1343, 1475, 1563, 1564, 1745, 1881, 2375}. The largest series to date have consisted of four cases {741, 1745, 1748}. The reported cases have occurred predominantly in adults, although one paediatric series has been reported {1748}. There is a slight male predominance. Occasional cases have been associated with low-grade B-cell lymphoma and rare cases have been associated with T-cell lymphoma {741}.

Sites of involvement

The presentation has shown wide variation. Solitary lymph node involvement is most common, but extranodal presentations, particularly the skin and soft tissue, have been reported.

Clinical features

Patients usually present with an asymptomatic mass, although systemic symptoms, such as fatigue, fever and night sweats, have been reported. Rarely, there may be generalized lymphadenopathy, splenomegaly or hepatomegaly.

Morphology

The lesional tissue in lymph nodes is present in a paracortical distribution with residual follicles. The neoplastic proliferation usually forms fascicles, a storiform pattern, and whorls of spindled to ovoid cells. Sheets of round cells are occasionally found. The cytoplasm of the neoplastic cells is usually abundant, slightly eosinophilic, and often has an indistinct border.

The nuclei also appear spindled to ovoid, and may show indentations; occasional multinucleate cells may be seen. The chromatin is often vesicular, with small to large, distinct nucleoli. Cytologic atypia varies from case to case, although the mitotic rate is usually low (<5 per 10 high power fields). Necrosis is usually not present. There are often numerous admixed lymphocytes, and less commonly, plasma cells. The histological appearance is sometimes indistinguishable from a follicular dendritic cell sarcoma and phenotyping is necessary for precise diagnosis.

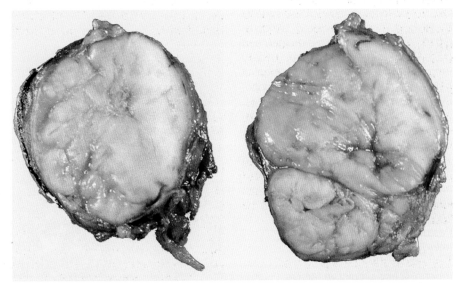

Fig. 14.13 Interdigitating dendritic cell sarcoma. Tumour is vaguely lobulated in lymph node, and firm in consistency.

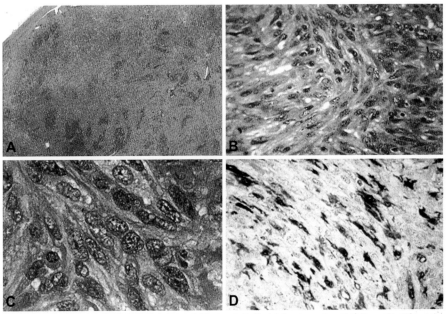

Fig. 14.14 Interdigitating dendritic cell sarcoma. **A** The tumour infiltrates the paracortex. Note the residual lymphoid tissue in one corner. **B** Sheets of spindled cells with a whorled pattern are seen. **C** The cells show marked cytologic atypia. **D** The stain for S100 protein is focally positive.

Ultrastructure

The neoplastic cells show complex inter-digitating cell processes, but well-formed desmosomes are not present. Scattered lysosomes may be present, but Birbeck granules are not seen.

Immunophenotype

The neoplastic cells consistently express S100 protein and vimentin with CD1a and langerin being negative. They are usually positive for fascin and variably, weakly positive for CD68, lysozyme and CD45. Strong nuclear staining for p53 may be present. They are negative for markers of follicular dendritic cells (CD21, CD23 and CD35), myeloperoxidase, CD34, specific B-cell and T-cell associated antigens, CD30, epithelial membrane antigen and cytokeratins. The Ki67 index usually ranges between 10 and 20% (median 11%) {681}. The admixed small lymphocytes are almost always of T-cell lineage, with near absence of B cells.

Genetics

The immunoglobulin heavy chain gene and the beta, delta and gamma chain genes of the T-cell receptor are in a germline configuration {2375}.

Postulated normal counterpart

Interdigitating dendritic cell.

Prognosis and predictive factors

The clinical course is generally aggressive, with about one half of patients dying of their disease. Visceral organs that are commonly affected include the liver, spleen, kidney and lung. Stage may be an important prognostic factor, however histologic features have not been correlated with clinical outcome.

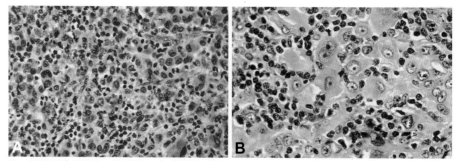

Fig. 14.15 Interdigitating dendritic cell sarcoma. **A** The cells are rounded, and the nuclei are relatively bland. **B** The nuclei are relatively bland, but have a vesicular chromatin pattern and a single medium-sized nucleolus.

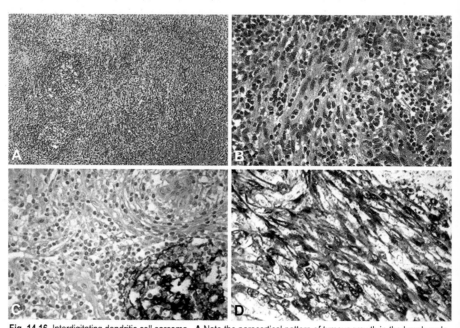

Fig. 14.16 Interdigitating dendritic cell sarcoma. **A** Note the paracortical pattern of tumour growth in the lymph node. **B** There are scattered small lymphocytes throughout the lesion. **C** The CD21 stain is negative on the tumour cells, but labels follicular dendritic cells in residual follicles. **D** In contrast, the stain for S100 protein is strongly positive in the tumour cells.

Follicular dendritic cell sarcoma

J.K.C. Chan
S.A. Pileri
G. Delsol
C.D.M. Fletcher
L.M. Weiss
K.L. Grogg

Definition
Follicular dendritic cell (FDC) sarcoma is a neoplastic proliferation of spindled to ovoid cells showing morphologic and immunophenotypic features of follicular dendritic cells.

ICD-O code   9758/3

Epidemiology
Follicular dendritic cell sarcoma is a rare neoplasm {44, 385, 1501, 1591, 1724, 1745, 2375}. There is a wide age range, with an adult predominance (mean age, 44 years) {1591, 1745}. The sex distribution is about even, but there is marked female predilection for the inflammatory pseudotumour-like variant {409, 1745, 2313}. Follicular dendritic cell sarcoma occurs in association with Castleman disease in a small proportion of cases, usually the hyaline-vascular type {387}. In these cases, either the Castleman disease precedes the follicular dendritic cell sarcoma or the two lesions occur simultaneously.

Etiology
There is no known etiology for most cases. The inflammatory pseudo-tumour-like variant of follicular dendritic cell sarcoma is consistently associated with Epstein-Barr virus (EBV) {71}, with EBV-encoded RNA (EBER) being demonstrable in virtually all the neoplastic spindle cells, and Southern blot studies have demonstrated the virus to be present in a monoclonal episomal form {1991}.

Precursor lesions
In rare cases of Castleman disease, there is a proliferation of follicular dendritic cells outside of the follicles forming clusters and small sheets {1893}. Follicular dendritic cell sarcoma may evolve in this setting of follicular dendritic cell hyperplasia and overgrowth.

Sites of involvement
Follicular dendritic cell sarcoma presents as lymphadenopathy in one half to two thirds of cases, with one of the cervical lymph nodes being most often affected. The tumour can also present in a wide variety of extranodal sites, such as the tonsil, oral cavity, gastrointestinal tract, soft tissue, skin, mediastinum, liver and spleen {957}. Common sites for metastasis include lymph nodes, lung and liver {434}.

Clinical features
Patients most often present with a slow-growing, painless mass, although patients with abdominal disease may present with abdominal pain. The tumours are often large, with a median size of 5 cm. Systemic symptoms are uncommon in conventional follicular dendritic cell sarcoma, but are common in the inflammatory pseudo-tumour-like variant {409}. Rare patients have paraneoplastic pemphigus {1265, 1405, 2357}.

Morphology
The neoplasm comprises spindled to ovoid cells forming fascicles, storiform arrays, whorls (at times reminiscent of the 360° pattern observed in meningioma), diffuse

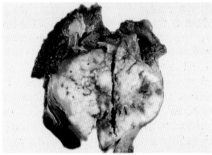

Fig. 14.17 Follicular dendritic cell sarcoma. This mass occurred in the soft tissues, and has the appearance of a sarcoma.

sheets or vague nodules. The individual neoplastic cells generally show indistinct cell borders and a moderate amount of eosinophilic cytoplasm. The nuclei are oval or elongated, with vesicular or granular finely dispersed chromatin, small but distinct nucleoli, and a delicate nuclear membrane. The nuclei tend to be unevenly spaced, with areas showing clustering. Nuclear pseudo-inclusions are common. Binucleated and multinucleated tumour cells are often seen. Although the cytologic features are usually relatively bland, significant cytologic atypia may be found in some cases. The mitotic rate is usually between 0 and 10 per 10 high-power fields, although the more pleomorphic cases can show much higher mitotic rates (>30 per 10 high-power fields), easily found atypical mitoses and coagulative necrosis.

The tumour is typically lightly infiltrated by small lymphocytes, which can sometimes be aggregated around the blood vessels

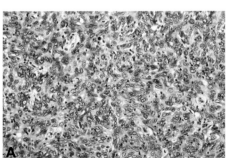 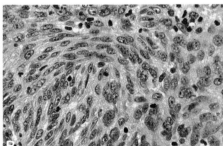 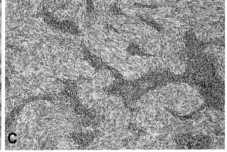

Fig. 14.18 Follicular dendritic cell sarcoma. **A** Spindle cell proliferation. **B** A 360° whorl is seen. Note the occasional multinucleated cells. **C** Residual small lymphocytes, particularly in a perivascular location.

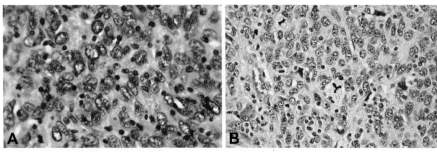

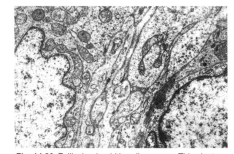

Fig. 14.19 Follicular dendritic cell sarcoma. **A** These ovoid cells have indistinct cytoplasmic outlines. **B** A greater than usual degree of cytologic atypia is present. Note the atypical mitotic figure.

Fig. 14.20 Follicular dendritic cell sarcoma. This electron micrograph shows numerous cytoplasmic processes, with one well-formed desmosome present in the centre.

as well {384}. Less common morphologic features include: epithelioid tumour cells with hyaline cytoplasm, clear cells, oncocytic cells, myxoid stroma, fluid-filled cystic spaces, prominent fibrovascular septa and admixed osteoclastic giant cells {384, 385, 1724, 1725}. In rare cases, the large neoplastic cells are scattered singly in a background of small lymphocytes, mimicking Hodgkin lymphoma. Rare cases may also show jigsaw puzzle-like lobulation and perivascular spaces, mimicking thymoma or carcinoma showing thymus-like element (CASTLE) {434}.

The inflammatory pseudo-tumour-like variant of follicular dendritic cell sarcomas occurs exclusively as primary tumours in the liver or spleen {71, 409, 1991}. The neoplastic spindled cells are dispersed within a prominent lymphoplasmacytic infiltrate. The nuclei usually show vesicular chromatin pattern and distinct nucleoli. Nuclear atypia is highly variable; usually many cells are bland-looking, but some cells with enlarged, irregularly-folded or hyperchromatic nuclei are always found. Some tumour cells may even resemble Reed-Sternberg cells {1991}. Necrosis and haemorrhage are often present. The blood vessels frequently show fibrinoid deposits in the walls.

Ultrastructure
The neoplastic cells have elongated nuclei, often with cytoplasmic invaginations. There are characteristically numerous long, slender cytoplasmic processes, often connected by scattered, mature desmosomes. Birbeck granules and numerous lysosomes are not seen.

Immunophenotype
Follicular dendritic cell sarcoma is positive for one or more of the follicular dendritic markers, such as CD21, CD35, CD23, KiM4p and CNA.42 {1591}. Clusterin is almost always strongly positive, while this marker is usually negative or only weakly positive in other dendritic cell tumours {853, 854}. In addition, the tumour is usually positive for desmoplakin, vimentin, fascin, epidermal growth factor receptor and HLA-DR {384, 2122}. It is variably positive for epithelial membrane antigen, S100 protein and CD68. Exceptionally, cytokeratin, CD45 or CD20 can be expressed. Staining for CD1a, lysozyme, myeloperoxidase, CD34, CD3, CD79a, CD30 and HMB45 are negative. Ki67 labeling ranges from 1 to 25% (mean, 13%).

The admixed small lymphocytes are predominantly B cells in some cases,

predominantly T cells in some, and mixed B and T cells in others {385,1745}.

Genetics
The immunoglobulin and T-cell receptor genes are in a germline configuration {2375}. Data on genetic changes are currently very limited {1927}.

Postulated normal counterpart
Follicular dendritic cell of the lymphoid follicle.

Prognosis and predictive factors
The behaviour is usually indolent, much like a low or intermediate-grade soft tissue sarcoma {385}. Most patients are treated by complete surgical excision, with or without adjuvant radiotherapy or chemotherapy. Local recurrences occur in more than 50% of cases, and metastases occur in about 25% of patients; such occurrences may be delayed after many years {384, 1725, 2054, 2313}. At least 10–20% of patients ultimately die of the disease, often after a long period of time. Cases showing high-grade features (significant cytologic atypia, extensive coagulative necrosis and a high proliferative index), large tumour size (greater than 6 cm) or intraabdominal location can pursue a rapidly fatal course {385, 1745}.

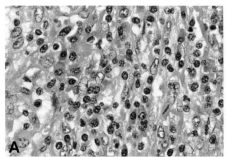

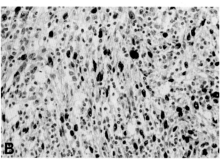

Fig. 14.21 Inflammatory pseudotumour-like follicular dendritic cell sarcoma. **A** Typically spindled cells are masked by numerous small lymphocytes and plasma cells. The spindled cells show indistinct cell borders and vesicular nuclei. Some are bland-looking, while others are enlarged or overtly atypical. **B** *In situ* hybridization for EBER selectively highlights the nuclei of the spindled cells. The nuclei show a range of size and atypia.

Other rare dendritic cell tumours

L.M. Weiss
J.K.C. Chan
C.D.M. Fletcher

There are rare types of dendritic cell tumour other than the better-delineated entities covered in the previous chapters. These may be derived either from myeloid-derived dendritic cells, such as indeterminate dendritic cell tumour; or from stroma-derived dendritic cells, such as fibroblastic reticular cell tumour. Some dendritic cell tumours may remain unclassifiable despite extensive work-up or show hybrid features, and such cases may be tentatively designated "dendritic cell tumour, not otherwise specified".

Fibroblastic reticular cell tumour

ICD-O code   9759/3

Fibroblastic reticular cell tumour is very rare, and the entity reported as "cytokeratin-positive interstitial reticulum cell tumour" probably represents the same entity {44, 380}. This tumour can occur in lymph node, spleen or soft tissue {44, 380, 822, 1065}. The clinical outcome is variable, with some patients dying of the disease.

The tumour is histologically similar to follicular dendritic cell sarcoma or interdigitating dendritic cell sarcoma, but lacks the immunophenotypic profile of these tumour types. There are often interspersed delicate collagen fibres. Ultrastructurally, the spindle cells show delicate cytoplasmic extensions and features reminiscent of myofibroblasts (filaments with occasional fusiform densities, well-developed desmosomal attachments, rough endoplasmic reticulum and basal lamina-like material). The tumour cells show variable immunoreactivity for smooth muscle actin, desmin, cytokeratin (in a dendritic pattern) and CD68.

Indeterminate dendritic cell tumour

ICD-O code   9757/3

Indeterminate dendritic cell tumour, also known as indeterminate cell histiocytosis, is a neoplastic proliferation of spindled to ovoid cells with phenotypic features similar to those of normal indeterminate cells, the alleged precursor cells of Langerhans cells. These neoplasms are extraordinarily rare {44, 208, 236, 391, 1177, 1859, 1865, 2019, 2315, 2325, 2441, 2450}. There may be an association with low-grade B-cell lymphoma {2315}.

Patients typically present with one or, more commonly, multiple generalized papules, nodules or plaques. Systemic symptoms are usually not present.

The lesions are usually based in the dermis, but may extend into the subcutaneous fat. The infiltrate is diffuse, comprising cells resembling Langerhans cells, with irregular nuclear grooves and clefts. Cytoplasm is typically abundant and usually eosinophilic. Multinucleated giant cells may be present. In some cases, there may be spindling of the cells. The mitotic rate varies widely from case to case. An accompanying eosinophilic infiltrate is usually not present. By definition, these cells lack Birbeck granules on ultrastructural examination. There can be complex interdigitating cell processes, but desmosomes are lacking.

The proliferating cells consistently express S100 protein and CD1a. Langerin has been negative in one studied case. They are negative for specific B- and T-cell markers, CD30, the histiocytic marker CD163, and the follicular dendritic cell markers CD21, CD23 and CD35. They are variably positive for CD45, CD68, lysozyme and CD4. The Ki67 index is highly variable. One case has been shown to be clonal by human androgen receptor gene assay.

The clinical course has been highly variable, ranging from spontaneous regression to rapid progression. There are no known prognostic factors. One case has been associated with the development of acute myeloid leukaemia {2325}.

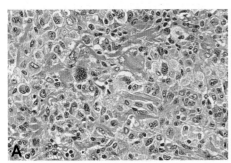
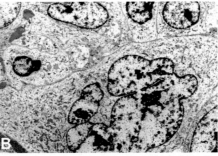

Fig. 14.22 Indeterminate dendritic cell tumour. **A** This is a histiocytic-appearing neoplasm. A multinucleated cell is seen. **B** Ultrastructural feature showing complex interdigitating process, but no Birbeck granules.

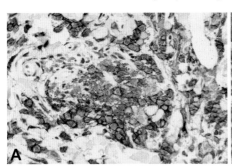
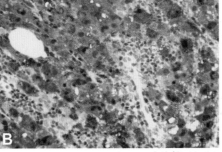

Fig. 14.23 Indeterminate dendritic cell tumour. The lesion is positive for CD1a (**A**) and S100-protein (**B**).

Disseminated juvenile xanthogranuloma

R. Jaffe
C.D.M. Fletcher
W. Burgdorf

Definition

Disseminated juvenile xanthogranuloma (JXG) is characterized by a proliferation of histiocytes similar to those of the dermal JXG, commonly having a foamy (xanthomatous) component with Touton-type giant cells. There is evidence for clonality in some instances.

Synonyms

Deep JXG (if soft tissue involvement).
Benign cephalic histiocytosis, progressive nodular histiocytosis or generalized (non-lipidemic) eruptive histiocytosis (cutaneous disorders with multiple JXG but without systemic involvement).
Xanthoma disseminatum (if skin and mucosal lesions).
Erdheim-Chester disease (possible adult form with bone and lung involvement) {2488A, 2381A}.

Epidemiology

Solitary dermal JXG is vastly more common than other forms and does not progress to more disseminated forms {538A}. The majority of deep, visceral and disseminated forms occur by age 10 years, half within the first year of life, except for the adult Erdheim-Chester form {1045B}.

Etiology

There is a known association with neurofibromatosis type 1 (NF1); patients with both are at slightly higher risk of juvenile myelomonocytic leukaemia (JMML) {2510A}. Patients with both Langerhans cell disease (LCH) and JXG are encountered.

Sites of involvement

Skin and soft tissues are most common, and, in disseminated forms, mucosal surfaces especially upper aerodigestive tract. The central nervous system, dura and pituitary stalk can be affected as well as eye, liver, lung, lymph node and bone marrow (BM). Retroperitoneal and periaortic involvement is noted in Erdheim-Chester disease {538A, 733A, 1045B}.

Clinical features

Skin lesions other than the common papular solitary form are small (1–2 mm) and multiple. Soft tissue lesions can be large, and the lesions present as mass effect. Optic lesions can cause glaucoma. CNS and pituitary lesions, like LCH, can cause diabetes insipidus, seizures, hydrocephalus and mental status changes {538A, 733A, 1045B}. In contrast to LCH, liver involvement does not target the biliary system or lead to sclerosing cholangitis {1042A}. There is some capacity for lesions to slowly regress. While JXG appears to be benign, a concomitant macrophage activation syndrome can lead to cytopenias, liver damage and death in the systemic forms.

Morphology

The JXG cell is small and oval, sometimes slightly spindled with a bland round-to-oval nucleus without grooves and pink cytoplasm. Touton cells are less common at non-dermal sites. The cells become progressively lipidized (xanthomatous). A mixed inflammatory component is invariable. Variants include epithelioid cells with glassy cytoplasm. The ultrastructural features are histiocytic without distinguishing features {2488A}.

Immunophenotype

In common with macrophages, cells express vimentin, surface CD14, CD68 (PGM1) in a coarse granular pattern, CD163 in surface and cytoplasmic pattern and Stabilin-1 (MS-1 antigen). Factor XIIIa staining is common but not universal. Fascin stains the cell cytoplasm and S100 is variably positive in less than 20% of the cases; however, none of these markers is specific for JXG. CD1a and Langerin are negative {392A, 1188A, 1931A, 2488A}.

Genetics

No consistent cytogenetic or molecular genetic change has been identified. B and T-cell receptor gene rearrangement are germline. An association with NF1 is known in some. There is evidence for clonality in some instances {1045A}.

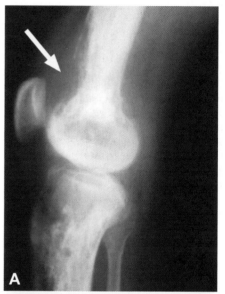

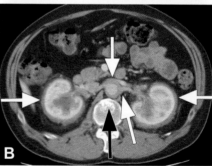

Fig. 14.24 A Radiograph of a case of Erdheim-Chester disease showing a lytic and sclerotic lesion in the distal femur and the proximal tibia. There is destruction of the anterior femoral cortex, with an impacted pathologic fracture through the lesion and an anterolateral soft-tissue mass extending from the destroyed femur (arrow). Reprinted from {1872A}. Courtesy of Dr. Susan Kattapuram. **B** Abdominal CT from a patient with Erdheim-Chester disease showing a soft tissue infiltrate surrounding the aorta and kidneys (white arrows). There is a sclerotic lesion in the vertebra (black arrow). Reprinted from {1479A}. Courtesy of Dr. R.Gilberto Gonzalez.

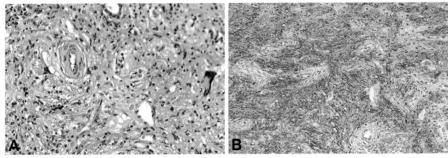

Fig. 14.25 Systemic JXG involving liver. **A** The infiltrate is portal in nature but spares the bile duct. Few Touton cells are present. **B** Factor XIIIa. There is diffuse staining of the portal histiocytes.

Postulated normal counterpart

The cell of origin is debated. In spite of macrophage phenotype, it has been said to be a dermal/interstitial dendritic cell on the basis of shared Factor XIIIa and fascin immunostaining, but these have limited specificity {1188A}.

Prognosis and predictive factors

All clinical forms are benign, though multiple lesions in brain, dura, or pituitary can cause local consequences and even death. Systemic forms that involve liver and BM have been treated with LCH-type therapy.

Contributors

Dr Cem AKIN
Department of Internal Medicine
University of Michigan
1150 West Medical Center Drive
Ann Arbor, MI 48109-5600
USA
Tel. +1 734 647 6234 / 936 5634
Fax. +1 734 763 4151
cemakin@umich.edu

Dr Ioannis ANAGNOSTOPOULOS
Charité Medical University of Berlin
Institute of Pathology
Hindenburgdamm 30
12200 Berlin
GERMANY
Tel. +49 30 8445 2296
Fax. +49 30 8445 4473
Ioannis.Anagnostopoulos@charite.de

Dr Katsuyuki AOZASA
Department of Pathology (C3)
Osaka University Graduate School of
Medicine
Yamada-oka 2-2
565-0871 Suita, Osaka
JAPAN
Tel. +81 6 6879 3710
Fax. +81 6 6879 3713
aozasa@molpath.med.osaka-u.ac.jp

Dr Daniel A. ARBER*
Stanford University Medical Center
300 Pasteur Drive H1507 M/C 5627
Stanford, CA 94305-5627
USA
Tel. +1 650 725 5604
Fax. +1 650 736 1473
darber@stanfordmed.org

Dr Michele BACCARANI
Department of Haematology and
Oncological Sciences, L. and A. Seràgnoli
University of Bologna
Via G. Massarenti 9
40138 Bologna
ITALY
Tel. +39 051 636 3680
Fax. +39 051 398 973
baccarani@med.unibo.it

Dr Barbara J. BAIN*
Department of Haematology
Imperial College Faculty of Medicine
St. Mary's Hospital
Praed Street, London W2 1NY
UK
Tel. +44 207 886 1939
Fax. +44 207 886 6809
b.bain@ic.ac.uk

Dr Giovanni BAROSI
Unit of Clinical Epidemiology
and Center for the Study of
Myelofibrosis
IRCCS Policlinico S. Matteo
27100 Pavia
ITALY
Tel. +39 038 250 3636
Fax. +39 038 250 3917
barosig@smatteo.pv.it

Dr Irith BAUMANN
Institute of Pathology
Bayreuth Clinic
Preuschwitzer Street 101
95445 Bayreuth
GERMANY
Tel. +49 921 400 5612
Fax. +49 921 400 5609
iirith.baumann@klinikum-bayreuth.de

Dr Marie-Christine BENE
Laboratory of Immunology
Nancy University UHP & Nancy CHU
9 Avenue de la Forêt de Haye
54505 Vandoeuvre-Les-Nancy
FRANCE
Tel. +33 383 68 36 60 / 15 76 15
Fax. +33 383 44 60 22
marie-christine.bene@medecine.uhp-
nancy.fr

Dr Daniel BENHARROCH
Department of Pathology
Ben Gurion University
Soroka University Medical Center
84101 Beer-Sheva
ISRAEL
Tel. +972 8 640 0920
Fax. +972 8 623 2770
benaroch@bgu.ac.il

Dr John M. BENNETT
Departments of Medicine and Pathology
University of Rochester Medical Center
and the James P. Wilmot Cancer Center
601 Elmwood Avenue
Rochester, NY 14642
USA
Tel. +1 585 275 4915
Fax. +1 585 442 0039
John_Bennett@URMC.Rochester.edu

Dr Françoise BERGER
Department of Pathological Anatomy
Lyon-Sud Hospital
69495 Pierre-Bénite
FRANCE
Tel. +33 4 78 86 11 87
Fax. +33 4 78 86 57 13
francoise.berger@chu-lyon.fr

Dr Emilio BERTI
Institute of Dermatological Sciences,
University of Milan, IRCCS Ospedale
Maggiore, Policlinico, Mangiagalli and
Regina Elena
Via Pace 9, 20122 Milano
ITALY
Tel. +39 025 503 5107 / 5200
Fax. +39 025 032 0779
emilio.berti@unimib.it

Dr Gunnar BIRGEGARD
Department of Hematology
University Hospital
SE-75185 Uppsala
SWEDEN
Tel. +46 18 61 10 000
Fax. +46 18 50 92 97
gunnar.birgegard@medsci.uu.se

Dr Clara D. BLOOMFIELD
The Ohio State University
519 James Cancer Hospital
300 West 10th Avenue
Columbus, OH 43210
USA
Tel. +1 614 293 7518
Fax. +1 614 293 3132
clara.bloomfield@osumc.edu

Dr Bettina BORISCH
Department of Pathology - CMU
University of Geneva
1, Rue Michel Servet
1211 Geneva 4
SWITZERLAND
Tel. +41 22 379 5893 / 5954
Fax. +41 22 379 5912
Bettina.Borisch@medecine.unige.ch

Dr Michael J. BOROWITZ*
Department of Pathology and Oncology
The John Hopkins Medical Institutions
401 North Broadway
Baltimore, MD 21231
USA
Tel. +1 410 614 2889
Fax. +1 410 502 1493
mborowit@jhmi.edu

Dr Richard D. BRUNNING*
Department of Laboratory Medicine
and Pathology, University of Minnesota
420 Delaware Street SE
Minneapolis, MN 55455
USA
Tel. +1 612 332 8001
Fax. +1 612 624 6662
Brunn001@umn.edu

Dr Walter BURGDORF
Traubinger Strasse 45A
82327 Tutzing
GERMANY
Tel. +49 8158 7159
wburgdorf@gmx.de

Dr Elias CAMPO*
Department of Pathology
Hospital Clinic, University of Barcelona
Villarroel 170
08036 Barcelona
SPAIN
Tel. +34 93 227 5450
Fax. +34 93 227 5717
ecampo@clinic.ub.es

Dr Daniel CATOVSKY
Section of Haemato-oncology
Institute of Cancer Research
15 Cotswold Road
Sutton, Surrey SM2 5NG
UK
Tel. +44 208 722 4114
Fax. +44 207 795 0310
Daniel.Catovsky@icr.ac.uk

Dr Lorenzo CERRONI
Department of Dermatology
Medical University of Graz
Auenbruggerplatz 8
8036 Graz
AUSTRIA
Tel. +43 3 16385 2423
Fax. +43 3 16385 2466
lorenzo.cerroni@meduni-graz.at

Dr Ethel CESARMAN
Department of Pathology and
Laboratory, Medicine
Weill Cornell Medical College
New York, NY 10065
USA
Tel. +1 212 746 8838
Fax. +1 212 746 4483
ecesarm@med.cornell.edu

*The asterisk indicates participation in the Working Group Meeting on the WHO Classification of Tumours of Haematopoietic and Lymphoid Tissues that was held in Lyon, France, October 25-27, 2007.

Dr Amy CHADBURN
Department of Pathology and
Laboratory Medicine
Weill Cornell Medical College
New York, NY 10065
USA
Tel. +1 212 746 2442
Fax. +1 212 746 8173
achadbur@med.cornell.edu

Dr John K.C. CHAN*
Department of Pathology
Queen Elizabeth Hospital
Wylie Road, Kowloon
Hong Kong
SAR CHINA
Tel. +852 2958 6830
Fax. +852 2385 2455
jkcchan@ha.org.hk

Dr Wing Chung CHAN*
Department of Pathology
University of Nebraska Medical Center
983135 Nebraska Medical Center
Omaha, NE 68198
USA
Tel. +1 402 559 7689
Fax. +1 402 559 6018
jchan@unmc.edu

Dr Andreas CHOTT
Institute of Pathology and Microbiology
Wilhelminenspital
Montleartstrasse 37
1160 Vienna
AUSTRIA
Tel. +43 1 49150 3201
Fax. +43 1 49150 3209
andreas.chott@wienkav.at

Dr Robert W. COUPLAND
Department of Pathology
Vancouver General Hospital
855 West 12th Avenue
Vancouver, BC V5Z 1M9
CANADA
Tel. +1 604 875 5273
Fax. +1 604 875 5707
Robert.Coupland@vch.ca

Dr Daphne DE JONG
Department of Pathology
The Netherlands Cancer Institute
Antoni van Leeuwenhoek Hospital
Plesmanlaan 121, 1066 CX Amsterdam
THE NETHERLANDS
Tel. +31 20 512 2752
Fax. +31 20 512 2759
d.d.jong@nki.nl

Dr Christiane DE WOLF-PEETERS*
Department of Pathology
University Hospitals K.U. Leuven
Minderbroederstraat 12
3000 Leuven
BELGIUM
Tel. +32 16 336 582
Fax. +32 16 336 548
christiane.peeters@uz.kuleuven.ac.be

Dr Martina DECKERT
Department of Neuropathology
University of Cologne
Kerpener Str. 62
50924 Cologne
GERMANY
Tel. +49 221 478 5265
Fax. +49 221 478 7237
martina.deckert@uni-koeln.de

Dr Jan DELABIE
Department of Pathology
The Norwegian Radium Hospital
University of Oslo
0310 Oslo
NORWAY
Tel. +47 22 93 4879
Fax. +47 22 73 0164
jan.delabie@labmed.uio.no

Dr Georges DELSOL*
Laboratory of Pathological Anatomy
CHU Purpan, Place du Docteur Baylac
31059 Toulouse Cedex
FRANCE
Tel. +33 5 61 77 75 25
Fax. +33 5 61 77 76 03
gdelsol@toulouse.inserm.fr

Dr Ahmet DOGAN
Mayo Clinic, Department of Laboratory
Medicine and Pathology
200 First Street SW
Rochester, MN 55905
USA
Tel. +1 507 538 4907
Fax. +1 507 284 1599
dogan.ahmet@mayo.edu

Dr Lyn M. DUNCAN
Department of Dermatopathology
Massachusetts General Hospital
55 Fruit Street, Warren 820
Boston, MA 02114
USA
Tel. +1 617 726 8890
Fax. +1 617 726 8711
duncan@helix.mgh.harvard.edu

Dr Kojo S.J. ELENITOBA-JOHNSON
University of Michigan Medical School
109 Zina Pitcher Place
Ann Arbor, MI 48109-2200
USA
Tel. +1 734 647 8153
Fax. +1 734 615 2331
kojoelen@umich.edu

Dr Luis ESCRIBANO
Centro de Estudios de Mastocitosis de
Castilla La Mancha, Hospital Virgen del Valle
Carretera de Cobisa s/n 45071 Toledo
SPAIN
Tel. +34 925 269 200 Ext. 49335
Fax. +34 925 269 355
lescribanom@sescam.jccm.es
luisescribanomora@hotmail.com

Dr Fabio FACCHETTI
Department of Pathology I
University of Brescia, Hospital of Brescia
Piazzale Spedali Civili 1
25124 Brescia
ITALY
Tel. +39 030 399 5426
Fax. +39 030 338 4418
facchett@med.unibs.it

Dr Brunangelo FALINI*
Institute of Haematology, University of
Perugia Policlinico Monteluce
Via Brunamonti
06122 Perugia
ITALY
Tel. +39 075 578 3219
Fax. +39 075 578 3834 / 3691
faliniem@unipg.it

Dr Judith A. FERRY
Pathology Department, Warren 2
Massachusetts General Hospital
55 Fruit Street
Boston, MA 02114
USA
Tel. +1 617 726 3978
Fax. +1 617 726 7474
jferry@partners.org

Dr Christopher D.M. FLETCHER
Department of Pathology
Brigham and Women's Hospital
75 Francis Street
Boston, MA 02115
USA
Tel. +1 617 732 8558
Fax. +1 617 566 3897
cfletcher@partners.org

Dr Kathryn FOUCAR
Department of Pathology, University of
New Mexico Health Sciences Center
1001 Woodward Place NE
Albuquerque, NM 87102
USA
Tel. +1 505 938 8457
Fax. +1 505 938 8414
Kfoucar@salud.unm.edu

Dr Randy D. GASCOYNE
Department of Pathology
British Columbia Cancer Agency
600 W 10th Avenue
Vancouver, BC V5Z 4E6
CANADA
Tel. +1 604 877 6098 Ext 2097
Fax. +1 604 877 6178
rgascoyn@bccancer.bc.ca

Dr Kevin C. GATTER
Nuffield Department of Clinical Laboratory
Sciences, John Radcliffe Hospital
Level 4, Academic Block
Oxford OX3 9DU
UK
Tel. +44 1865 220 556
Fax. +44 1865 228 980
kevin.gatter@ndcls.ox.ac.uk

Dr Norbert GATTERMANN
Department of Hematology/Oncology
Heinrich Heine University
Moorenstrasse 5
40225 Düsseldorf
GERMANY
Tel. +49 211 811 6500
Fax. +49 211 811 8853
gattermann@med.uni-duesseldorf.de

Dr Philippe GAULARD*
Department of Pathology,
Henri Mondor Hospital, INSERM U 841
51, Avenue Maréchal de Lattre de Tassigny
94010 Créteil
FRANCE
Tel. +33 1 49 81 27 43
Fax. +33 1 49 81 27 33
philippe.gaulard@hmn.aphp.fr

Dr Ulrich GERMING
Department of Hematology/Oncology
and Clinical Immunology
Heinrich Heine University
Moorenstrasse 5, 40225 Düsseldorf
GERMANY
Tel. +49 211 811 7780
Fax. +49 211 811 8853
germing@med.uni-duesseldorf.de

Dr D. Gary GILLILAND
Brigham and Women's Hospital
Harvard Medical School
1 Flackfan Circle
Boston, MA 02115
USA
Tel. +1 617 355 9092
Fax. +1 617 355 9093
ggilliland@rics.bwh.harvard.edu

Dr Heinz GISSLINGER
Department of Internal Medicine I
Medical University of Vienna
Waehringer Guertel 18-20
1090 Wien
AUSTRIA
Tel. +43 1 40400 5464
Fax. +43 1 40400 4030
heinz.gisslinger@meduniwien.ac.at

Dr Peter L. GREENBERG
Haematology Division
Stanford University Cancer Center
875 Blake Wilbur Drive, Room 2335
Stanford, CA 94305-5821
USA
Tel. +1 650 725 8355
Fax. +1 650 723 1269
peterg@stanford.edu

Dr Thomas M. GROGAN
Department of Pathology
University of Arizona
1501 N. Campbell Avenue
Tucson, AZ 85724
USA
Tel. +1 520 906 2989
Fax. +1 520 229 4074
tgrogan@ventanamed.com

Dr Karen L. GROGG
Department of Laboratory Medicine and
Pathology, Mayo Clinic
200 First Street, SW
Rochester, MN 55905
USA
Tel. +1 507 538 1180
Fax. +1 507 284 1599
grogg.karen@mayo.edu

Dr Margarita GUENOVA
Laboratory of Cytopathology, Histopathology
and Immunology, National Center of
Haematology and Transfusiology
6 Plovdivsko pole Str, 1756 Sofia
BULGARIA
Tel. +359 888 248 324
Fax. +359 287 073 16
margenova@mail.bg

Dr Nancy Lee HARRIS*
Pathology-Warren 2
Massachusetts General Hospital
55 Fruit Street
Boston, MA 02114
USA
Tel. +1 617 726 5155
Fax. +1 617 726 7474
nlharris@partners.org

Dr Robert Paul HASSERJIAN
Department of Pathology
Massachusetts General Hospital
55 Fruit Street
Boston, MA 02114-2698
USA
Tel. +1 617 724 1445
Fax. +1 617 726 7474
rhasserjian@partners.org

Dr Eva HELLSTROM-LINDBERG
Department of Medicine, Division of
Hematology, Karolinska Institute
Karolinska University Hospital,
Huddinge
14186 Stockholm
SWEDE
Tel. +46 8 5858 2506
Fax. +46 8 774 8725
Eva.Hellstrom-Lindberg@ki.se

Dr Hans-Peter HORNY
Clinic of Ansbach
Institute of Pathology
Escherichstr. 6
91522 Ansbach
GERMANY
Tel. +49 981 488 8344
Fax. +49 981 488 8310
horny@pathologie-ansbach.com

Dr Peter G. ISAACSON*
Department of Histopathology
Royal Free and University College Medical
School, University College London
Hospitals Trusts
London WC1E6JJ
UK
Tel. +44 207 679 6045
Fax. +44 207 387 3674
p.isaacson@ucl.ac.uk

Dr Elaine S. JAFFE*
Laboratory of Pathology
Center for Cancer Research
National Cancer Institute
10 Center Drive MSC 1500
Bethesda, MD 20892
USA
Tel. +1 301 496 0183
Fax. +1 301 402 2415
elainejaffe@nih.gov

Dr Ronald JAFFE
Department of Pathology
Children's Hospital
3705 5th Avenue
Pittsburgh, PA 15213
USA
Tel. +1 412 692 5657
Fax. +1 412 692 6550
ronald.jaffe@chp.edu

Dr Daniel M. JONES
Department of Pathology
U-T - M.D. Anderson Cancer Center
1515 Holcombe Boulevard
Houston, TX 77030
USA
Tel. +1 713 745 2598
Fax. +1 713 745 0736
dajones@mdanderson.org

Dr Marshall E. KADIN
Department of Dermatology and Skin
Surgery, Roger Williams Medical Center
50 Maude Street
Providence, RI 02908
USA
Tel. +1 401 456 2521
Fax. +1 401 456 6449
mkadin@rwmc.org

Dr Masahiro KIKUCHI
Karindoh Hospital
Ozasa 5-21-34, Chuo-ku
810-0033 Fukuoka
JAPAN
Tel. +81 92 522 3574
Fax. +81 92 522 3574
masakiku@karindoh.or.jp

Dr Hiroshi KIMURA
Department of Virology
Nagoya University,
Graduate School of Medicine
65 Tsurumai-Cho, Showa-ku
466-8550 Nagoya
JAPAN
Tel. +81 52 744 2207
Fax. +81 52 744 2452
hkimura@med.nagoya-u.ac.jp

Dr Marsha C. KINNEY
Department of Pathology
Health Science Center, University of
Texas
7703 Floyd Curl Drive
San Antonio, TX 78229-3900
USA
Tel. +1 210 567 4098
Fax. +1 210 567 0409
kinneym@uthscsa.edu

Dr Philip M. KLUIN*
Department of Pathology and Laboratory
Medicine
University Medical Center Groningen
UMCG University of Groningen
Hanzeplein 1, 9713 GZ, Groningen
THE NETHERLANDS
Tel. +31 50 361 0020 / 6161
Fax. +31 50 361 9107
p.m.kluin@path.umcg.nl

Dr Young-Hyeh KO
Department of Pathology, Samsung
Medical Center, Sungkyunkwan
University School of Medicine
Kangnam-gu, Ilwon-dong 50
135-710 Seoul
REPUBLIC OF KOREA
Tel.: +82 2 3410 2762
Fax. +82 2 3410 0025
yhko310@skku.edu

Dr Alla M. KOVRIGINA
N. N. Blokhin Cancer Research Centre
Russian Academy of Medical Sciences
24, Kashyrskoe Shosse,
115478 Moscow
RUSSIAN FEDERATION
Tel. +7 495 324 61 02
Fax. +7 495 323 57 10
kovrigina-alla@mail.ru

Dr Laszlo KRENACS
Laboratory of Tumor Pathology
Institute for Biotechnology
Bay Zoltan Foundation for Applied Research
Derkovits Fasor 2, 6726 Szeged
HUNGARY
Tel. +36 62 432 248
Fax. +36 62 432 250
krenacsl@bay.u-szeged.hu

Dr W. Michael KUEHL
Genetics Branch, National Cancer
Institute, Bethesda Naval Hospital
8901 Wisconsin Avenue
Bethesda, MD 20889-5101
USA
Tel. +1 301 435 5421
Fax. +1 301 496 0047
wmk@helix.nih.gov

Dr Jeffery L. KUTOK
Department of Pathology
Brigham and Women's Hospital
75 Francis Street
Boston, MA 02115
USA
Tel. +1 617 732 5714
Fax. +1 617 264 5169
jkutok@partners.org

Dr Hans Michael KVASNICKA
Institute for Pathology
University of Cologne
Kerpener Str. 62
50924 Cologne
GERMANY
Tel. +49 221 478 6369
Fax. +49 221 478 6360
hm.kvasnicka@uni-koeln.de

Dr ROBERT A. KYLE
Department of Laboratory Medicine and
Pathology
Mayo Clinic
200 First Street SW
Rochester, MN 55905
USA
Tel. +1 507 284 3039
Fax. +1 507 266 9277
Kyle.Robert@mayo.edu

Dr Richard A. LARSON
Department of Medicine
University of Chicago,
Cancer Research Center
5841 S. Maryland Avenue, MC2115
Chicago, IL 60637
USA
Tel. +1 773 702 6783
Fax. +1 773 702 3002
rlarson@medicine.bsd.uchicago.edu

Dr Michelle M. LE BEAU
Cancer Cytogenetics Laboratory
University of Chicago
5841 S. Maryland Avenue MC1140
Chicago, IL 60637
USA
Tel. +1 773 702 0795
Fax. +1 773 702 9311
mlebeau@medicine.bsd.uchicago.edu

Dr Lorenzo LEONCINI
Institute of Human Pathology and
Oncology, University of Siena
Via delle Scotte, 6
53100 Siena
ITALY
Tel. +39 057 723 3237
Fax. +39 057 723 3235
leoncinil@unisi.it

Dr Alan F. LIST
Dept. of Malignant Hematology,
H. Lee Moffitt Cancer Center
and Research Institute
12902 Magnolia Drive
Tampa, FL 33612-9497
USA
Tel. +1 813 745 6083
Fax. +1 813 745 3727
Alan.List@Moffitt.org

Dr Kenneth A. MACLENNAN
ICRF, Cancer Medicine Research Unit
St. James's University Hospital
Leeds LS9 7TF
UK
Tel. +44 113 392 6049
Fax. +44 113 392 6483
kenneth.maclennan@leedsth.nhs.uk

Dr William R. MACON
Department of Laboratory Medicine and
Pathology, Mayo Clinic
200 First Street SW
Rochester, MN 55905
USA
Tel. +1 507 284 1198
Fax. +1 507 284 1599
macon.william@mayo.edu

Dr David Y. MASON (deceased)
Haematology Department
John Radcliffe Hospital
Level 4
Oxford OX3 9DU
UK
Tel. +44 1865 220 356 / 7850 066 416
Fax. +44 1865 740 811
david.mason@ndcls.ox.ac.uk

Dr Estella MATUTES
Section of Haemato-Oncology
Institute of Cancer Research/Royal
Marsden Hospital, 203 Fulham Road
London SW3 6JJ
UK
Tel. +44 207 808 2609
Fax. +44 207 808 2955
Estella.Matutes@icr.ac.uk

Dr Robert W. MCKENNA
Department of Laboratory Medicine and
Pathology, University of Minnesota
420 Delaware Street SE, MMC 609
Minneapolis, MN 55455
USA
Tel. +1 612 273 3137
Fax. +1 612 624 6662
mcken138@umn.edu

Dr Chris J.L.M. MEIJER
Department of Pathology
Free University Medical Center
De Boelelaan 1117, PO Box 7057
1007 MB Amsterdam
THE NETHERLANDS
Tel. +31 20 444 4070
Fax. +31 20 444 2964
cjlm.meijer@vumc.nl

Dr Junia V. MELO
Division of Haematology, Institute of
Medical & Veterinary Sciences
Frome Road
Adelaide, SA 5000
AUSTRALIA
Tel. +61 8 8222 3441
Fax. + 61 8 8222 3139
junia.melo@imvs.sa.gov.au

Dr Dean D. METCALFE
Laboratory of Allergic Diseases, NIAID
National Institutes of Health
10 Center Drive, MSC 1881
Bethesda, MD 20892 1881
USA
Tel. +1 301 496 2165
Fax. +1 301 480 8384
dmetcalfe@niaid.nih.gov

Dr Manuela MOLLEJO
Department of Pathology
Hospital Virgen de la Salud
Avd. Barber, 30
45004 Toledo
SPAIN
Tel. +34 925 269 245
Fax. +34 925 253 613
mmollejov@sescam.jccm.es

Dr Peter MÖLLER
Department of Pathology
University of Ulm
89069 Ulm
GERMANY
Tel. +49 731 5005 6320
Fax. +49 731 5005 6384
peter.moeller@uniklinik-ulm.de

Dr Emili MONTSERRAT
Department of Hematology, Hospital
Clinic IDIBAPS, University of Barcelona
Villarroel, 170
08036 Barcelona
SPAIN
Tel. +34 93 227 5475
Fax. +34 93 227 9811
emontse@clinic.ub.es

Dr William G. MORICE
Department of Laboratory Medicine and
Pathology, Mayo Clinic
200 First Street SW
Rochester, MN 55905
USA
Tel. +1 507 284 2511
Fax. +1 507 284 5115
morice.william@mayo.edu

Dr Hans Konrad MÜLLER-HERMELINK*
Department of Pathology
University of Würzburg
Josef-Schneider-Str. 2
97080 Würzburg
GERMANY
Tel. +49 931 2014 7776
Fax. +49 931 2014 7440
path062@uni-wuerzburg.de

Dr Shigeo NAKAMURA*
Department of Pathology and Clinical
Laboratories
Nagoya University Hospital
65 Tsurumai-cho, Showa-ku
466-8560 Nagoya
JAPAN
Tel. +81 52 744 2896
Fax. +81 52 744 2897
snakamur@med.nagoya-u.ac.jp

Dr Bharat N. NATHWANI
Department of Hematopathology
University of Southern California
Keck School of Medicine
1200 North State Street
Los Angeles, CA 90033
USA
Tel. +1 323 226 7063
Fax. +1 323 226 7119
nathwani@usc.edu

Dr Charlotte M. NIEMEYER
Department of Pediatrics and Adolescent
Medicine, University of Freiburg
Mathildengasse 11
79106 Freiburg
GERMANY
Tel. +49 761 270 4506
Fax. +49 761 270 4518
charlotte.niemeyer@uniklinik-freiburg.de

Dr Hiroko OHGAKI*
International Agency for Research on
Cancer (IARC)
150, Cours Albert Thomas
69008 Lyon
FRANCE
Tel. +33 4 72 73 85 34
Fax. +33 4 72 73 86 98
ohgaki@iarc.fr

Dr Koichi OHSHIMA
Department of Pathology
Kurume University, School of Medicine
Asahimati 67
830-0011 Kurume
JAPAN
Tel. +81 942 317 547
Fax. +81 942 310 342
ohshima_kouichi@med.kurume-u.ac.jp

Dr Mihaela ONCIU
Department of Pathology
St. Jude Children's Research Hospital
332 North Lauderdale Street
Memphis, TN 38128
USA
Tel. +1 901 495 5347
Fax. +1 901 495 3100
Mihaela.Onciu@StJude.org

Dr Attilio ORAZI
Department of Pathology and Laboratory
Medicine, Weill Medical College of
Cornell University, 525 E. 68th street
New York, NY 10021
USA
Tel. +1 212 746 2442
Fax. +1 212 746 8173
ato9002@med.cornell.edu

Dr German OTT
Department of Clinical Pathology
Robert Bosch Hospital
Auerbachstrasse 110
70376 Stuttgart
GERMANY
Tel. +49 711 8101 3394
Fax. +49 711 8101 3619
German.Ott@rbk.de

Dr Marco PAULLI
Department of Pathology
University of Pavia
Policlinico San Matteo Foundation,
Via Forlanini 14, 27100 Pavia
ITALY
Tel. +39 038 250 1241 / 2953
Fax. +39 038 252 5866
m.paulli@smatteo.pv.it

Dr Suat-Cheng PEH
Department of Pathology
University of Malaya Kuala Lumpur
50603 Kuala Lumpur
MALAYSIA
Tel. +60 3 796 75797 / 794 92064
Fax. +60 3 755 6845 / 795 5021
chensuat@netscape.net
pehsc@um.edu.my

Dr LoAnn PETERSON
Department of Pathology
Northwestern University
Feinberg School of Medicine
251 E.Huron Street, Chicago, IL 60611
USA
Tel. +1 312 926 8540
Fax. +1 312 926 0560
loannc@northwestern.edu

Dr Tony PETRELLA
Center of Pathology
Laboratory of Pathological Anatomy,
CHU
33 Rue Nicolas Bornier BP 189
21000 Dijon
FRANCE
Tel. +33 3 80 66 43 30
Fax. +33 3 80 66 79 70
T.PETRELLA@centre-de-pathologie.fr

Dr Stefano A. PILERI*
Department of Haematology and
Oncological Sciences, "Seràgnoli"
St Orsola- Malpighi Hospital, University
of Bologna, School of Medicine
Via G. Massarenti 9, 40138 Bologna
ITALY
Tel. +39 051 636 3044
Fax. +39 051 636 3606
stefano.pileri@unibo.it

Dr Miguel A. PIRIS*
Molecular Pathology Programme
Spanish National Cancer Centre
(CNIO) Melchor Fernandez Almagro 3
28029 Madrid
SPAIN
Tel. +34 91 224 6965
Fax. +34 91 224 6923
mapiris@cnio.es

Dr Stefania PITTALUGA
Laboratory of Pathology
National Institutes of Health
10 Center Drive MSC-1500
Bethesda, MD 20892-1500
USA
Tel. +1 301 402 0297
Fax. +1 301 402 2415
stefpitt@mail.nih.gov

Dr Maurilio PONZONI
Unit of Lymphoid Malignancies
San Raffaele Scientific Institute
Via Olgettina 60
20132 Milano
ITALY
Tel. +39 02 2643 2544
Fax. +39 02 2643 2409
ponzoni.maurilio@hsr.it

Dr Sibrand POPPEMA
Dept. of Pathology and Laboratory
Medicine, University Medical Centre
Groningen, Hanzeplein 1
P.O. Box 30.001
9700 RB Groningen
THE NETHERLANDS
Tel. +31 50 361 0281
Fax. +31 50 361 4351
s.poppema@rvb.umcg.nl

Dr Anna PORWIT*
Department of Pathology
Karolinska University Hospital
171 76 Stockholm
SWEDEN
Tel. +46 8 51 77 55 14
Fax. +46 8 51 77 58 43
Anna.porwit@karolinska.se

Dr Kevin SHANNON
University of California
at San Francisco
513 Parnassus Avenue
San Francisco, CA 94143-0519
USA
Tel. +1 415 476 7932
Fax. +1 415 502 5127
shannonk@peds.ucsf.edu

Dr Ayalew TEFFERI
Division of Hematology
Mayo Clinic
200 First Street, S.W.
Rochester, MN 55905
USA
Tel. +1 507 284 3159
Fax. +1 507 266 4972
tefferi.ayalew@mayo.edu

Dr Neus VILLAMOR
Hematopathology Unit, IDIBAPS
Hospital Clinic
Villarroel 170
08036 Barcelona
SPAIN
Tel. +34 93 227 5572
Fax. +34 93 227 5572
villamor@clinic.ub.es

Dr Leticia QUINTANILLA-MARTINEZ
Institute of Pathology, University Hospital
Tuebingen, Eberhard Karls University
Liebermeisterstrasse 8
72076 Tuebingen
GERMANY
Tel. +49 707 1298 2266
Fax. +49 707 1292 258
leticia.quintanilla-fend@med.uni-tuebingen.de

Dr Bruce R. SMOLLER
Dept. of Pathology, College of Medicine,
University of Arkansas for Medical Sciences
4301 West Markham Street
Little Rock, AR 72205
USA
Tel. +1 501 686 5170
Fax. +1 501 296 1184
smollerbrucer@uams.edu

Dr Catherine THIEBLEMONT
Unit of Onco-Haematology
Saint-Louis Hospital
1, Avenue Calude Vellefaux
75010 Paris
FRANCE
Tel. +33 1 42 49 98 37
Fax. +33 1 42 49 96 41
catherine.thieblemont@sls.aphp.fr

Dr Reinhard VON WASIELEWSKI
Institute of Pathology
Hannover School of Medicine
Carl-Neubergstrasse 1
30625 Hannover
GERMANY
Tel. +49 511 532 4470
Fax. +49 511 532 5799
Wasielewski.reinhard.von@mh-hannover.de

Dr Elisabeth RALFKIAER
Department of Pathology
Copenhagen University Hospital
Blegdamsvej 9
2100 Copenhagen
DENMARK
Tel. +45 3545 5346
Fax. +45 3545 6380
e.ralfkiaer@rh.regionh.dk

Dr Ivy SNG
Department of Pathology
Singapore General Hospital
Outram Road
Singapore 169608
SINGAPORE
Tel. +65 6321 4926
Fax. +65 6222 6826
ivy.sng.t.y@sgh.com.sg

Dr Jürgen THIELE*
Institute of Pathology
University of Cologne
Kerpener Str. 62
50924 Cologne
GERMANY
Tel. +49 221 478 5008
Fax. +49 221 478 6360
j.thiele@uni-koeln.de

Dr Roger A. WARNKE*
Department of Pathology
Stanford University School of Medicine
300 Pasteur Drive
Stanford, CA 94305-5324
USA
Tel. +1 650 725 5167
Fax. +1 650 725 6902
rwarnke@stanford.edu

Dr Martine RAPHAËL
Unit of Haematology and Biological
Immunology, Cytogenetics
INSERM U802, CHU Bicêtre
78 rue du Général Leclerc,
94270 Le Kremlin Bicêtre, FRANCE
Tel. +33 1 45 21 20 06
Fax. +33 1 45 21 28 47
martine.raphael@bct.aphp.fr

Dr Dominic SPAGNOLO
Path West Laboratory Medicine WA
Locked Bag 2009
Western Australia 6909 Nedlands
AUSTRALIA
Tel. +61 8 9346 2953
Fax. +61 8 9346 4122
Dominic.spagnolo@health.wa.gov.au

Dr Peter VALENT
Medical University of Vienna
Wahringer Gurtel 18-20
1090 Vienna
AUSTRIA
Tel. +43 1 40400 6085
Fax. +43 1 40400 4030
peter.valent@meduniwien.ac.at

Dr Steven A. WEBBER
Cardiology Department
Children's Hospital of Pittsburgh
3705 Fifth Avenue
Pittsburgh, PA 15213
USA
Tel. +1 412 692 6995
Fax. +1 412 692 6870
steve.webber@chp.edu

Dr Jonathan SAID
Department of Pathology and Laboratory
Medicine, Center for the Health
Sciences 13-226 UCLA
10833 Le Conte Avenue
Los Angeles, CA 90095-1732
USA
Tel. +1 310 825 1149
Fax. +1 310 794 4161
jsaid@mednet.ucla.edu

Dr Harald STEIN*
Institute for Pathology
Campus Benjamin Franklin
Charité University Medicine Berlin
12200 Berlin
GERMANY
Tel. +49 30 8445 2295
Fax. +49 30 8445 4473
harald.stein@charite.de

Dr J. H. VAN KRIEKEN
Department of Pathology, Radboud
University Nijmegen Medical Centre
P.O. Box 9101
6500 HB Nijmegen
The NETHERLANDS
Tel. +31 24 361 4352
Fax. +31 24 354 0520
J.vanKrieken@pathol.umcn.nl

Dr Dennis D. WEISENBURGER
Department of Pathology and
Microbiology
University of Nebraska Medical Center
Omaha, NE 68198-3135
USA
Tel. +1 402 559 7688
Fax. +1 402 559 6018
dweisenb@unmc.edu

Dr Christian A. SANDER
Department of Dermatology
Asklepios Klinik St. Georg
Lohmuehlenstr. 5
20099 Hamburg
GERMANY
Tel. +49 40 181 885 2220
Fax. +49 40 181 885 2462
c.sander@asklepios.com

Dr Christer SUNDSTRÖM
Department of Pathology
Uppsala University Hospital
75185 Uppsala
SWEDEN
Tel. +46 18 61 13 806
Fax. +46 18 61 12 665
christer.sundstrom@akademiska.se

Dr James W. VARDIMAN*
Department of Pathology
University of Chicago Medical Center
5841 S. Maryland Avenue
Chicago, IL 60637-1470
USA
Tel. +1 773 702 6196
Fax. +1 773 702 1200
James.Vardiman@uchospitals.edu

Dr Lawrence M. WEISS
Division of Pathology
City of Hope National Medical Center
1500 East Duarte Road
Duarte, CA 91010-0269
USA
Tel. +1 626 256 4673
Fax. +1 626 301 8145
lweiss@coh.org

Dr Masao SETO
Division of Molecular Medicine
Aichi Cancer Center Research Institute
Kanokoden Chikusa-ku
464-8681 Nagoya
JAPAN
Tel. +81 52 762 6111 Ext. 7080 / 7082
Fax. +81 52 764 2982
mseto@aichi-cc.jp

Dr Steven H. SWERDLOW*
Department of Pathology
Division of Hematopathology
UPMC Presbyterian
200 Lothrop Street, Pittsburgh, PA 15213
USA
Tel. +1 412 647 5191
Fax. +1 412 647 4008
swerdlowsh@upmc.edu

Dr Beatrice VERGIER
Department of Pathology, EA 2406
CHU Bordeaux - Victor Segalen
University, Haut-Lévêque Hospital
Avenue de Magellan
33604 Pessac - Bordeaux
FRANCE
Tel. +33 5 57 65 60 26
Fax. +33 5 57 65 63 72
beatrice.vergier@chu-bordeaux.fr

Dr Sean J. WHITTAKER
Skin Cancer Unit
St. John's Institute of Dermatology
St. Thomas's Hospital
Lambeth Palace Road, London SE1 7EM
UK
Tel. +44 207 188 6396
Fax. +44 207 188 6257
Sean.whittaker@kcl.ac.uk

Dr Rein WILLEMZE*
Department of Dermatology
Leiden University Medical Center
PO Box 9600
2300 RC Leiden
THE NETHERLANDS
Tel. +31 71 526 2421
Fax. +31 71 524 8106
willemze.dermatology@lumc.nl

Dr Wyndham H. WILSON
Lymphoma Therapeutics Section,
Metabolism Branch, National Cancer
Institute
10 Center Drive 10/12C42
Bethesda, MD 20892
USA
Tel. +1 301 435 2415
Fax. +1 301 402 0172
wilsonw@mail.nih.gov

Dr Tadashi YOSHINO
Department of Pathology, Okayama
University Graduate School of Medicine
Dentistry and Pharmaceutical Sciences
2-5-1, Shikata-cho, 700-8558 Okayama
JAPAN
Tel. +81 86 235 7149
Fax. +81 86 235 7156
yoshino@md.okayama-u.ac.jp

Clinical Advisory Committee

Dr Kenneth C. ANDERSON
Dana Farber Cancer Institute
Boston, MA, USA

Dr Robert ARCECI
Kimmel Comprehensive Cancer Center
Johns Hopkins Oncology Center
Baltimore, MD, USA

Dr James O. ARMITAGE
University of Nebraska Medical Center
Omaha, NE, USA

Dr Tiziano BARBUI
Hospitals of Bergamo
Bergamo, ITALY

Dr John BENNETT**
University of Rochester Medical Center
Rochester, NY, USA

Dr Peter Leif BERGSAGEL
Mayo Clinic
Scottsdale, AZ, USA

Dr Clara D. BLOOMFIELD**
(Myeloid chair)
Ohio State University
Columbus, OH, USA

Dr William CARROLL
NYU School of Medicine
New York, NY, USA

Dr Daniel CATOVSKY**
Institute of Cancer Research
Sutton, U.K.

Dr Franco CAVALLI
San Giovannni Hospital
Bellinzona, SWITZERLAND

Dr Bruce CHESON
Georgetown University Hospital
Washington, DC, USA

Dr Bertrand COIFFIER
Lyon-Sud Hospital
Pierre Bénite, FRANCE

Dr Joseph CONNORS
B.C. Cancer Agency
Vancouver Clinic
Vancouver, CANADA

Dr Theo M. DE WITTE
University Hospital Nijmegen
Nijmegen, THE NETHERLANDS

Dr Volker DIEHL
University Hospital of Köln
Köln, GERMANY

Dr Meletios A. DIMOPOULOS
University of Athens
Athens, GREECE

Dr Hartmut DOHNER
University of Ulm
Ulm, GERMANY

Dr Andreas ENGERT
University Hospital of Köln
Köln, GERMANY

Dr Elihu H. ESTEY
Fred Hutchinson Cancer Research
Center, University of Washington,
Seattle, WA, USA

Dr Brunangelo FALINI**
Institute of Haematology, Policlinico
Monteluce
Perugia, ITALY

Dr Pierre FENAUX
Avicenne Hospital
University Paris XIII
Bobigny, FRANCE

Dr Richard I. FISHER
University of Rochester Medical Center
Rochester, NY, USA

Dr Robin FOA
University "La Sapienza"
Rome, ITALY

Dr Ulrich GERMING**
Heinrich Heine University
Duesseldorf, GERMANY

Dr D. Gary GILLILAND**
Brigham and Women's Hospital
Harvard Medical School
Boston, MA, USA

Dr Peter L. GREENBERG**
Stanford University Cancer Center
Stanford, CA, USA

Dr Anton HAGENBEEK
Academic Medical Center
Amsterdam, THE NETHERLANDS

Dr Eva HELLSTROM-LINDBERG**
Karolinska Institute
Karolinska University, Hospital
Huddinge, Stockholm, SWEDEN

Dr Wolfgang HIDDEMANN
University of Munich
Munich, GERMANY

Dr Richard HOPPE
Stanford University Medical Center
Palo Alto, CA, USA

Dr Sandra J. HORNING
(Lymphoid co-chair)
Stanford University Medical Center
Palo Alto, CA, USA

Dr Melissa M. HUDSON
St. Jude Children's Hospital
Memphis, TN, USA

Source of charts and photographs

1.01	Vardiman J.W.	2.36	Horny H.-P.	5.08	Brunning R.D.
1.02	Vardiman J.W.	2.37	Horny H.-P.	5.09	Brunning R.D.
1.03	Vardiman J.W.	2.38 A,B	Horny H.-P.	5.10	Brunning R.D.
1.04	Goasguen J.	2.39	Brunning R.D.	5.11	Brunning R.D.
	Université de Rennes 1	2.40	Longley J.B.	5.12 A	Orazi A.
	France	2.41	Vardiman J.W.	5.12 B	Thiele J.
1.05	Porwit A.	2.42	Vardiman J.W.	5.13	Brunning R.D.
1.06	Vardiman J.W.	2.43 A	Valent P.	5.14 A,B	Brunning R.D.
1.07	Gilliland D.G.	2.43 B	Vardiman J.W.	5.15 A	Brunning R.D.
1.08	Doehner H.	2.44 A,B	Longley J.B.	5.15 B,C	Hasserjian R.P.
		2.45 A,B	Vardiman J.W.	5.16	Hasserjian R.P.
		2.46 A	Jaffe E.S.	5.17 A,B	Brunning R.D.
2.01 A	Vardiman J.W.	2.46 B	Vardiman J.W.	5.18	Brunning R.D.
2.01 B	Vardiman J.W.	2.47 A,B	Vardiman J.W.	5.19	Brunning R.D.
2.01 C	Vardiman J.W.	2.48 A,B	Vardiman J.W.	5.20 A	Brunning R.D.
2.02 A,B	Thiele J.	2.49 A-D	Vardiman J.W.	5.20 B	Hasserjian R.P.
2.03 A,B	Thiele J.	2.50 A,B	Brunning R.D.	5.21	Baumann I.
2.04 A	Vardiman J.W.	2.51 A-C	Vardiman J.W.	5.22 A	Baumann I.
2.04 B	Thiele J.	2.52 A-C	Vardiman J.W.	5.22 B	Baumann I.
2.05 A-C	Vardiman J.W.	2.53 A-D	Vardiman J.W.	5.22 C	Brunning R.D.
2.06 A-F	Thiele J.	2.54 A,B	Horny H.-P.	5.22 D	Baumann I.
2.07 A,B	Vardiman J.W.	2.55 A,B	Kvasnicka H.M.		
2.07 C	Thiele J.	2.56	Kvasnicka H.M.		
2.08 A-D	Vardiman J.W.			6.01	Arber D.A.
2.09 A-C	Vardiman J.W.			6.02	Brunning R.D.
2.10 A-C	Vardiman J.W.			6.03 A,B	Hirsch B.
2.11 A,B	Le Beau M.M.	3.01 A-D	Bain B.J.		University of Minnesota
2.12 A,B	Melo J.V.	3.02	Bain B.J.		School of Medicine,
2.13 A-D	Vardiman J.W.	3.03 A,B	Vardiman J.W.		Minneapolis, MN, USA
2.14	Thiele J.	3.04	Vardiman J.W.	6.04	Flandrin G.
2.15 A,B	Thiele J.				Lab. Central d'Hématologie
2.16 A-D	Thiele J.				Hopital Necker, Paris, France
2.17	Vardiman J.W.	4.01 A,B	Vardiman J.W.	6.05 A	Flandrin G.
2.18 A	Vardiman J.W.	4.01 C	Orazi A.	6.05 B	Brunning R.D.
2.18 B-D	Thiele J.	4.02 A-D	Vardiman J.W.	6.06 A,B	Hirsch B.
2.19	Vardiman J.W.	4.03 A-C	Vardiman J.W.	6.07	Brunning R.D.
2.20 A-C	Thiele J.	4.04 A,B	Vardiman J.W.	6.08	Falini B.
2.21	Thiele J.	4.05 A,B	Orazi A.	6.09 A,B	Brunning R.D.
2.22 A-D	Thiele J.	4.06 A,B	Vardiman J.W.	6.10 A,B	Brunning R.D.
2.23 A,B	Vardiman J.W.	4.07 A-C	Vardiman J.W.	6.11	Vardiman J.W.
2.24 A	Vardiman J.W.	4.08	Baumann I.	6.12	Arber D.A.
2.24 B-D	Thiele J.	4.09 A,B	Vardiman J.W.	6.13 A-C	Brunning R.D.
2.25 A,B	Thiele J.	4.10 A,B	Vardiman J.W.	6.14 A-D	Falini B.
2.26	Vardiman J.W.	4.11 A,B	Vardiman J.W.	6.15	Mrózek K
2.27 A,B	Vardiman J.W.	4.11 C,D	Hussain A.		The Ohio State University, USA
2.28 A-D	Thiele J.		Lyola University Med. Center	6.16 A-D	Falini B.
2.29 A,B	Thiele J.		Maywood, IL, USA	6.17	Falini B.
2.30 A,B	Vardiman J.W.	4.12	Shannon K.	6.18	Döhner H.
2.31	Vardiman J.W.	4.13 A-D	Vardiman J.W.		University of Ulm, Germany
2.32	Vardiman J.W.			6.19 A,B	Arber D.A.
2.33	Medenica M.			6.20	Grimwade D.
	Dept of Medicine,	5.01	Brunning R.D.		King's College, London, UK
	University of Chicago, IL, USA	5.02	Brunning R.D.	6.21	Vardiman J.W.
2.34	Medenica M.	5.03	Brunning R.D.	6.22 A-C	Vardiman J.W.
2.35	Longley J.B.	5.04	Brunning R.D.	6.23 A	Flandrin G.
	Dept. of Dermatology,	5.05 A,B	Brunning R.D.	6.23 B	Brunning R.D.
	Columbia University, NY, USA	5.06 A,B	Brunning R.D.	6.24 A	Arber D.A.
		5.07 A,B	Orazi A.		

6.24 B — Flandrin G.
6.25 — Brunning R.D.
6.26 A-C — Brunning R.D.
6.27 A-C — Flandrin G.
6.28 A,B — Brunning R.D.
6.29 A,B — Brunning R.D.
6.30 A — Arber D.A.
6.30 B — Brunning R.D.
6.31 — Brunning R.D.
6.32 — Brunning R.D.
6.33 A,B — Falini B.
6.34 A,B — Flandrin G.
6.35 A,B — Brunning R.D.
6.36 A,B — Flandrin G.
6.37 — Brunning R.D.
6.38 A — Flandrin G.
6.38 B — Brunning R.D.
6.39 A — Brunning R.D.
6.39 B-D — Orazi A.
6.40 A,B — Pileri S.A.
6.41 — Baumann I.
6.42 A,B — Baumann I.
6.42 C — Brunning R.D.
6.43 — Baumann I.
6.44 A-C — Facchetti F.
6.45 A-F — Facchetti F
6.46 A,B — Facchetti F

7.01 — Matutes E.
7.02 — Borowitz M.J.
7.03 A-D — Borowitz M.J.
7.04 — Borowitz M.J.
7.05 — Borowitz M.J.

8.01 — Jaffe E.S.
8.02 — Stein H.
8.03 — Jaffe E.S. & Stein H.
8.04 — Stein H.
8.05 — Jaffe E.S.
8.06 — Jaffe E.S.
8.07 — Vose J.M.
University of Nebraska Medical Center, Omaha, USA

9.01 A,B — Brunning R.D.
9.02 — Brunning R.D.
9.03 A,B — Jaffe E.S.
9.04 A,B — Brunning R.D.
9.05 — Brunning R.D.
9.06 — Brunning R.D.
9.07 — Carroll A.J.
University of Alabama Birmingham, AL, USA
9.08 — Carroll A.J.
9.09 — Carroll A.J.
9.10 — Hasserjian R.P.
9.11 A,B — Brunning R.D.
9.12 A,B — Nathwani B.
9.13 — Jaffe E.S.
9.14 — Chan J.K.C.

10.01 A,B — Muller-Hermelink H.-K.

10.02 A,B — Muller-Hermelink H.-K.
10.03 A,B — Catovski D.
10.03 C — Rozman M. Hospital Clinic, Barcelona, Spain
10.04 A-C — Harris N.L.
10.05 — Villamor N. Hospital Clinic, Barcelona, Spain
10.06 A — Catovski D.
10.06 B — Jaffe E.S.
10.07 A,B — Isaacson P.G.
10.08 — Jaffe E.S.
10.09 — Isaacson P.G.
10.10 A,B — Isaacson P.G.
10.11 A-C — Isaacson P.G.
10.12 A-C — Isaacson P.G.
10.13 A-C — Foucar K.
10.14 — Harris N.L.
10.15 A-D — Foucar K.
10.16 A-D — Foucar K.
10.17 A,B — Foucar K.
10.17 C,D — Falini B.
10.18 A-C — Piris M.
10.19 A-D — Piris M.
10.20 A,B — Catovski D
10.21 A-C — Swerdlow S.H.
10.22 A,B — Swerdlow S.H.
10.23 A,B — Swerdlow S.H.
10.23 C — Pileri S.A.
10.24 A,B — Grogan T.
10.25 A-C — Rahemtullah A. Massachusetts General Hospital, Boston, MA, USA
10.26 — Grogan T.
10.27 — Murali M. Massachusetts General Hospital, Boston, MA, USA
10.28 — Munshi N. Dana Farber Cancer Institute, Boston, MA, USA
10.29 A — Jaffe E.S.
10.29 B — Grogan T.
10.30 A — Grogan T.
10.30 B — Jaffe E.S.
10.31 A,B — McKenna R.W.
10.32 A,B — Grogan T.
10.33 — Wians F.H. Jr & Wooten D.C. Dept of Pathology, UT Southwestern Med. Center, Dallas, TX, USA
10.34 — Grogan T.
10.35 A — McKenna R.W.
10.35 B — Grogan T.
10.36 A-D — Grogan T.
10.37 A,B — Grogan T.
10.38 — McKenna R.W.
10.39 A-D — Van Wier S.& Fonseca R. Mayo Clinic, USA
10.40 — Roschke A & Gabrea A. National Cancer Institute, Bethesda, MD, USA
10.41 A,B — Grogan T.
10.42 A-F — Grogan T.
10.43 A-C — Grogan T.
10.44 A-D — Grogan T.

10.45 A-C — Grogan T.
10.46 A,B — Grogan T.
10.47 A-C — Grogan T.
10.48 A,B — Grogan T.
10.49 A,B — Isaacson P.G.
10.50 A,B — Isaacson P.G.
10.51 A,B — Isaacson P.G.
10.52 A-D — Isaacson P.G.
10.53 A,B — Isaacson P.G.
10.54 — Isaacson P.G.
10.55 — Isaacson P.G.
10.56 — Isaacson P.G.
10.57 A,B — Isaacson P.G.
10.58 A,B — Isaacson P.G.
10.59 A — Campo E & Swerdlow S.H.
10.59 B-E — Campo E. & Jaffe E.S.
10.60 A,B — Jaffe E.S.
10.61 — Nathwani B.N.
10.62 — Nathwani B.N.
10.63 A-D — de Leval L. Dept of pathology CHU Sart Tilman, Liege, Belgium
10.64 A-C — Nathwani B.N.
10.65 A,B — de Leval L.
10.66 A,B — de Leval L.
10.67 A-D — de Leval L.
10.68 A-C — Weisenburger D.D.. et al. {2374}
10.69 A-C — de Leval L.
10.70 A-C — Yoshino T.
10.71 A-D — de Leval L.
10.72 — Willemze R.
10.73 — Willemze R.
10.74 A-C — Willemze R.
10.75 A-C — Willemze R.
10.76 A-C — Willemze R.
10.77 A,B — Harris N.L.
10.78 A-C — Swerdlow S.H.
10.79 A-D — Swerdlow S.H.
10.80 — Swerdlow S.H.
10.81 — Jares P. et al. {1048A}
10.82 — Jaffe E.S.
10.83 A,B — Jaffe E.S.
10.84 A — Harris N.L.
10.84 B,C — Warnke R.A.
10.85 — Coiffier B. Lyon-Sud Hospital, Lyon, France
10.86 A-D — De Wolf-Peeters C.
10.87 A,B — Graus F. Hospital Clinic, Barcelona, Spain
10.88 A-C — Kluin P.M.
10.89 — Kluin P.M.
10.90 A-D — Willemze R.
10.91 — Willemze R.
10.92 A-C — Nakamura S. & Murase T.
10.93 A-C — Nakamura S. & Murase T.
10.94 A,B — Aozasa K.
10.95 — Aozasa K.
10.96 A-C — Aozasa K.
10.97 — Aozasa K.
10.98 A,B — Jaffe E.S.
10.99 — Jaffe E.S.
10.100 — Jaffe E.S.

10.101 A-D	Jaffe E.S.	11.21 A	Ohshima K.	11.76	Jaffe E.S.
10.102 A,B	Diebold J.	11.21 B,C	Kikuchi M.	11.77	Delsol G.
	Hotel Dieu, Paris, France	11.21 D	Ohshima K.	11.78	Delsol G.
10.102 C	Harris N.L.	11.22	Jaffe E.S.	11.79 A,B	Delsol G.
10.103	Harris N.L.	11.23 A,B	Kikuchi M.	11.80 A	Ralfkiaer E.
10.104	Banks P.M.	11.24 A,B	Jaffe E.S.	11.80 B	Delsol G.
	Carolinas Med. Center	11.25 A,B	Ohshima K.	11.81 A,B	Delsol G.
	Charlotte, NC, USA	11.26 A,B	Chan J.K.C.	11.82 A-C	Delsol G.
10.105 A,B	Diebold J.	11.27 A-D	Chan J.K.C.	11.83 A-C	Delsol G.
10.106 A,B	Diebold J.	11.28 A,B	Chan J.K.C.	11.84 A-C	Delsol G.
10.107 A,B	Gaulard P.	11.29	Chan J.K.C.	11.85	Delsol G.
10.108 A-C	Nakamura S & Murase T.	11.30 A-D	Chan J.K.C.	11.86 A,B	Chan J.K.C.
10.108 D	Diebold J.	11.31	Chan J.K.C.	11.87	Delsol G.
10.109	Nakamura S & Murase T	11.32 A,B	Chan J.K.C.	11.88 A-D	Mason D.Y.
10.110	Diebold J.	11.33	Chan J.K.C.	11.89 A-D	Mason D.Y.
10.111 A-C	Diebold J.	11.34 A-D	Chan J.K.C.	11.90 A-D	Mason D.Y.
10.112 A,B	Delsol G.	11.35	Harris N.L.	11.91 A,B	Mason D.Y.
10.113 A,B	Stein H.	11.36	Wright D.H.		
10.114 A,B	Stein H.		Winchester, UK		
10.114 C	Harris N.L.	11.37 A,B	Isaacson P.G.	12.01 A-D	Stein H.
10.115	Issacson P.G.	11.37 C	Wright D.H.	12.02 A,B	Stein H.
10.116 A-D	Issacson P.G.	11.38 A-D	Isaacson P.G.	12.03	Stein H.
10.117 A-D	Issacson P.G.	11.39	Isaacson P.G.	12.04 A,B	Stein H.
10.118 A-D	Issacson P.G.	11.40	Isaacson P.G.	12.05 A,B	Stein H.
10.119 A,B	Said J.	11.41	Isaacson P.G.	12.06 A,B	Stein H.
10.120	Said J.	11.42 A-D	Isaacson P.G.	12.07 A,B	Stein H.
10.121	Jaffe E.S.	11.43 A	Gaulard P.	12.08	Stein H.
10.122	Jaffe E.S.	11.43 B-D	Jaffe E.S.	12.09 A,B	Stein H.
10.123	Jaffe E.S.	11.44	Jaffe E.S.	12.10 A-C	Stein H.
10.124 A,B	Jaffe E.S.	11.45 A,B	Jaffe E.S.	12.11 A-C	Stein H.
10.125 A	Pileri S.A.	11.46 A-C	Jaffe E.S.	12.12 A,B	Stein H.
10.125 B	Leoncini L.	11.47 A	Willemze R.	12.13 A,B	Stein H.
10.125 C,D	Kluin P.M.	11.47 B	Ralfkiaer E.	12.14	Stein H.
10.126	Kluin P.M.	11.48	Ralfkiaer E.	12.15 A,B	Jaffe E.S.
10.127 A-C	Harris N.L. and	11.49 A,B	Ralfkiaer E.	12.16 A,B	Stein H.
	Horning S.J.	11.50 A	Willemze R.	12.17	Stein H.
	Stanford University	11.50 B	Ralfkiaer E.	12.18 A,B	Stein H.
	Palo Alta, CA, USA	11.51	Ralfkiaer E.	12.19 A-D	Stein H.
10.128	Kluin P.M.	11.52	Ralfkiaer E.	12.20 A,B	Stein H.
10.129 A,B	Jaffe E.S.	11.53 A-D	Ralfkiaer E.	12.21 A,B	Josting A.
10.130	Jaffe E.S.	11.54	Ralfkiaer E.		University Hospital Cologne
10.131 A-C	Jaffe E.S.	11.55 A,B	Ralfkiaer E.		Germany
		11.56	Ralfkiaer E.	12.22 A-C	Stein H.
		11.57	Willemze R.		
11.01 A,B	Muller-Hermelink H.-K.	11.58	Ralfkiaer E.		
11.02	Muller-Hermelink H.-K.	11.59 A-C	Ralfkiaer E.	13.01	Pittaluga S.
11.03 A,B	Muller-Hermelink H.-K.	11.60 A-D	Toro J.	13.02 A,B	Jaffe E.S.
11.04	Chan W.C.		National Cancer Institute	13.03 A-C	Jaffe E.S.
11.05 A	Morice W.		Bethesda, USA	13.04 A-C	Jaffe E.S.
11.05 B,C	Osuji N.	11.61	Jaffe E.S.	13.05 A	Harris N.L.
11.06 A-C	Villamor N.	11.62	Jaffe E.S.	13.05 B	Jaffe E.S.
11.06 D	Morice W.	11.63 A-D	Jaffe E.S.	13.05 C	Harris N.L.
11.07 A-D	Chan J.K.C.	11.64	Willemze R.	13.06 A,B	Jaffe E.S.
11.08 A,B	Ko Y.H.	11.65	Jaffe E.S.	13.07 A,B	Jaffe E.S.
11.09 A-D	Ko Y.H.	11.66	Jaffe E.S.	13.08	Jaffe E.S.
11.10 A-C	Quintanilla-Martinez L.	11.67 A-B	Willemze R.	13.09	Jaffe E.S.
11.11 A-C	Quintanilla-Martinez L.	11.68 A-C	Willemze R.	13.10 A,B	Raphael M.
11.12 A-C	Quintanilla-Martinez L.	11.69 A,B	Ralfkiaer E.	13.10 C	Jaffe E.S.
11.13 A,B	Quintanilla-Martinez L.	11.69 C,D	Jaffe E.S.	13.11 A	Jaffe E.S.
11.14	Quintanilla-Martinez L.	11.70 A-C	Ralfkiaer E.	13.11 B,C	Raphael M.
11.15	Jaffe E.S.	11.71	Pileri S.A.	13.12	Harris N.L.
11.16 A-C	Jaffe E.S.	11.72	Pileri S.A.	13.13 A-D	Harris N.L.
11.17	Jaffe E.S.	11.73 A	Dogan A.	13.14 A	Webber S.A.
11.18 A-C	Ohshima K.	11.73 B	Jaffe E.S.	13.14 B,C	Swerdlow S.H.
11.19 A,B	Kikuchi M.	11.74 A-D	Dogan A.	13.15 A,B	Swerdlow S.H. & Nelson BP
11.20	Ohshima K.	11.75 A-F	Dogan A.	13.16 A	Swerdlow S.H. & Nelson BP

13.16 B-D	Harris N.L.
13.17 A	Harris N.L.
13.17 B	Swerdlow S.H.
13.17 C,D	Harris N.L.
13.18 A,B	Harris N.L.
13.19 A-C	Swerdlow S.H.
13.20	Harris N.L.
13.21 A,B	Harris N.L.
14.01	Pileri S.A.
14.02	Grogan T.
14.03 A,B	Weiss L.M.
14.03 C	Grogan T.
14.04 A-D	Grogan T.
14.05 A,B	Jaffe E.S.
14.06 A-C	Weiss L.M.
14.07 A,B	Weiss L.M.
14.08	Weiss L.M.
14.09 A	Grogan T.
14.09 B	Weiss L.M.
14.10 A-D	Falini B.
14.11 A,B	Jaffe R.
14.12 A-D	Jaffe R.
14.13 A,B	Jaffe E.S.
14.14 A-D	Grogan T.
14.15 A,B	Weiss L.M.
14.16 A-D	Grogan T.
14.17	Weiss L.M.
14.18 A-C	Weiss L.M.
14.19 A,B	Weiss L.M.
14.20	Weiss L.M.
14.21 A,B	Chan J.K.C.
14.22 A	Weiss L.M.
14.22 B	Spagnolo D.V.
14.23 A,B	Weiss L.M.
14.24 A	Kattapuram S. Massachusetts General Hospital, Boston, USA
14.24 B	Gonzalez R.G. Massachusetts General Hospital, Boston, USA
14.25 A,B	Jaffe R.

References

1. Aarts WM, Willemze R, Bende RJ, Meijer CJ, Pals ST, van Noesel CJ (1998). VH gene analysis of primary cutaneous B-cell lymphomas: evidence for ongoing somatic hypermutation and isotype switching. Blood 92: 3857-3864.
2. Abramson JS (2006). T-cell/histiocyte-rich B-cell lymphoma: biology, diagnosis, and management. Oncologist 11: 384-392.
3. Abruzzo LV, Jaffe ES, Cotelingam JD, Whang-Peng J, Del DV, Jr., Medeiros LJ (1992). T-cell lymphoblastic lymphoma with eosinophilia associated with subsequent myeloid malignancy. Am J Surg Pathol 16: 236-245.
4. Abruzzo LV, Rosales CM, Medeiros LJ, Vega F, Luthra R, Manning JT, Keating MJ, Jones D (2002). Epstein-Barr virus-positive B-cell lymphoproliferative disorders arising in immunodeficient patients previously treated with fludarabine for low-grade B-cell neoplasms. Am J Surg Pathol 26: 630-636.
5. Abruzzo LV, Schmidt K, Weiss LM, Jaffe ES, Medeiros LJ, Sander CA, Raffeld M (1993). B-cell lymphoma after angioimmunoblastic lymphadenopathy: a case with oligoclonal gene rearrangements associated with Epstein-Barr virus. Blood 82: 241-246.
6. Achten R, Verhoef G, Vanuytsel L, Wolf-Peeters C (2002). Histiocyte-rich, T-cell-rich B-cell lymphoma: a distinct diffuse large B-cell lymphoma subtype showing characteristic morphologic and immunophenotypic features. Histopathology 40: 31-45.
7. Achten R, Verhoef G, Vanuytsel L, Wolf-Peeters C (2002). T-cell/histiocyte-rich large B-cell lymphoma: a distinct clinicopathologic entity. J Clin Oncol 20: 1269-1277.
8. Adam P, Katzenberger T, Eifert M, Ott MM, Rosenwald A, Muller-Hermelink HK, Ott G (2005). Presence of preserved reactive germinal centers in follicular lymphoma is a strong histopathologic indicator of limited disease stage. Am J Surg Pathol 29: 1661-1664.
9. Adam P, Katzenberger T, Seeberger H, Gattenlohner S, Wolf J, Steinlein C, Schmid M, Muller-Hermelink HK, Ott G (2003). A case of a diffuse large B-cell lymphoma of plasmablastic type associated with the t(2;5)(p23;q35) chromosome translocation. Am J Surg Pathol 27: 1473-1476.
10. Adida C, Haioun C, Gaulard P, Lepage E, Morel P, Briere J, Dombret H, Reyes F, Diebold J, Gisselbrecht C, Salles G, Altieri DC, Molina TJ (2000). Prognostic significance of survivin expression in diffuse large B-cell lymphomas. Blood 96: 1921-1925.
11. Adolfsson J, Mansson R, Buza-Vidas N, Hultquist A, Liuba K, Jensen CT, Bryder D, Yang L, Borge OJ, Thoren LA, Anderson K, Sitnicka E, Sasaki Y, Sigvardsson M, Jacobsen SE (2005). Identification of Flt3+ lympho-myeloid stem cells lacking erythro-megakaryocytic potential a revised road map for adult blood lineage commitment. Cell 121: 295-306.
12. Agnarsson BA, Vonderheid EC, Kadin ME (1990). Cutaneous T cell lymphoma with suppressor/cytotoxic (CD8) phenotype: identification of rapidly progressive and chronic subtypes. J Am Acad Dermatol 22: 569-577.
12A. Agnello V, Chung RT, Kaplan LM (1992). A role for hepatitis C virus infection in type II cryoglobulinemia. N Engl J Med 327: 1490-1495.
13. Aguilera NS, Tomaszewski MM, Moad JC, Bauer FA, Taubenberger JK, Abbondanzo SL (2001). Cutaneous follicle center lymphoma: a clinicopathologic study of 19 cases. Mod Pathol 14: 828-835.
13A. Aki H, Tuzuner N, Ongoren S, Baslar Z, Soysal T, Ferhanoglu B, Sahinler I, Aydin Y, Ulku B, Aktuglu G (2004). T-cell-rich B-cell lymphoma: a clinicopathologic study of 21 cases and comparison with 43 cases of diffuse large B-cell lymphoma. Leuk. Res 28: 229-236.
14. Akin C, Fumo G, Yavuz AS, Lipsky PE, Neckers L, Metcalfe DD (2004). A novel form of mastocytosis associated with a transmembrane c-kit mutation and response to imatinib. Blood 103: 3222-3225.
15. Akin C, Kirshenbaum AS, Semere T, Worobec AS, Scott LM, Metcalfe DD (2000). Analysis of the surface expression of c-kit and occurrence of the c-kit Asp816Val activating mutation in T cells, B cells, and myelomonocytic cells in patients with mastocytosis. Exp Hematol 28: 140-147.
16. Al Saleem T, Al Mondhiry H (2005). Immunoproliferative small intestinal disease (IPSID): a model for mature B-cell neoplasms. Blood 105: 2274-2280.
16A. Al-Dayel F, Al-Rasheed M, Ibrahim M, Bu R, Bavi P, Abubaker J, Al-Jomah N, Mohamed GH, Moorji A, Uddin S, Siraj AK, Al-Kuraya K (2008). Polymorphisms of drug-metabolizing enzymes CYP1A1, GSTT and GSTP contribute to the development of diffuse large B-cell lymphoma risk in the Saudi Arabian population. Leuk Lymphoma 49: 122-129.
17. Albiero E, Madeo D, Bolli N, Giaretta I, Bona ED, Martelli MF, Nicoletti I, Rodeghiero F, Falini B (2007). Identification and functional characterization of a cytoplasmic nucleophosmin leukaemic mutant generated by a novel exon-11 NPM1 mutation. Leukemia 21: 1099-1103.
18. Albinger-Hegyi A, Hochreutener B, Abdou MT, Hegyi I, Dours-Zimmermann MT, Kurrer MO, Heitz PU, Zimmermann DR (2002). High frequency of t(14;18)-translocation breakpoints outside of major breakpoint and minor cluster regions in follicular lymphomas: improved polymerase chain reaction protocols for their detection. Am J Pathol 160: 823-832.
19. Alcalay M, Tiacci E, Bergomas R, Bigerna B, Venturini E, Minardi SP, Meani N, Diverio D, Bernard L, Tizzoni L, Volorio S, Luzi L, Colombo E, Lo Coco F, Mecucci C, Falini B, Pelicci PG (2005). Acute myeloid leukemia bearing cytoplasmic nucleophosmin (NPMc+ AML) shows a distinct gene expression profile characterized by up-regulation of genes involved in stem-cell maintenance. Blood 106: 899-902.
20. Alcindor T, Bridges KR (2002). Sideroblastic anaemias. Br J Haematol 116: 733-743.
21. Alexander A, Anicito I, Buxbaum J (1988). Gamma heavy chain disease in man. Genomic sequence reveals two noncontiguous deletions in a single gene. J Clin Invest 82: 1244-1252.
22. Alexiou C, Kau RJ, Dietzfelbinger H, Kremer M, Spiess JC, Schratzenstaller B, Arnold W (1999). Extramedullary plasmacytoma: tumor occurrence and therapeutic concepts. Cancer 85: 2305-2314.
23. Algara P, Mateo MS, Sanchez-Beato M, Mollejo M, Navas IC, Romero L, Sole F, Salido M, Florensa L, Martinez P, Campo E, Piris MA (2002). Analysis of the IgV(H) somatic mutations in splenic marginal zone lymphoma defines a group of unmutated cases with frequent 7q deletion and adverse clinical course. Blood 99: 1299-1304.
24. Alizadeh AA, Eisen MB, Davis RE, Ma C, Lossos IS, Rosenwald A, Boldrick JC, Sabet H, Tran T, Yu X, Powell JI, Yang L, Marti GE, Moore T, Hudson J, Jr., Lu L, Lewis DB, Tibshirani R, Sherlock G, Chan WC, Greiner TC, Weisenburger DD, Armitage JO, Warnke R, Staudt LM (2000). Distinct types of diffuse large B-cell lymphoma identified by gene expression profiling. Nature 403: 503-511.
25. Allemani C, Sant M, De Angelis R, Marcos-Gragera R, Coebergh JW (2006). Hodgkin disease survival in Europe and the U.S.: prognostic significance of morphologic groups. Cancer 107: 352-360.
26. Almeida J, Orfao A, Ocqueteau M, Mateo G, Corral M, Caballero MD, Blade J, Moro MJ, Hernandez J, San Miguel JF (1999). High-sensitive immunophenotyping and DNA ploidy studies for the investigation of minimal residual disease in multiple myeloma. Br J Haematol 107: 121-131.
27. Alonsozana EL, Stamberg J, Kumar D, Jaffe ES, Medeiros LJ, Frantz C, Schiffer CA, O'Connell BA, Kerman S, Stass SA, Abruzzo LV (1997). Isochromosome 7q: the primary cytogenetic abnormality in hepatosplenic gammadelta T cell lymphoma. Leukemia 11: 1367-1372.
28. Alsabeh R, Brynes RK, Slovak ML, Arber DA (1997). Acute myeloid leukemia with t(6;9) (p23;q34): association with myelodysplasia, basophilia, and initial CD34 negative immunophenotype. Am J Clin Pathol 107: 430-437.
28A. Alsabeh R, Medeiros LJ, Glackin C, Weiss LM. Transformation of follicular lymphoma into CD30-large cell lymphoma with anaplastic cytologic features. Am J Surg Pathol 1997; 21:528-536.
29. Altieri A, Bermejo JL, Hemminki K (2005). Familial aggregation of lymphoplasmacytic lymphoma with non-Hodgkin lymphoma and other neoplasms. Leukemia 19: 2342-2343.
30. Amato D, Oscier DG, Davis Z, Mould S, Zheng J, Kolomietz E, Wang C (2007). Cytogenetic aberrations and immunoglobulin VH gene mutations in clinically benign CD5-monoclonal B-cell lymphocytosis. Am J Clin Pathol 128: 333-338.
31. Amen F, Horncastle D, Elderfield K, Banham AH, Bower M, Macdonald D, Kanfer E, Naresh KN (2007). Absence of cyclin-D2 and Bcl-2 expression within the germinal centre type of diffuse large B-cell lymphoma identifies a very good prognostic subgroup of patients. Histopathology 51: 70-79.
32. Amenomori T, Tomonaga M, Yoshida Y, Kuriyama K, Matsuo T, Jinnai I, Ichimaru M, Omiya A, Tsuji Y (1986). Cytogenetic evidence for partially committed myeloid progenitor cell origin of chronic myelomonocytic leukaemia and juvenile chronic myeloid leukaemia: both granulocyte-macrophage precursors and erythroid precursors carry identical marker chromosome. Br J Haematol 64: 539-546.
33. Anagnostopoulos I, Hansmann ML, Franssila K, Harris M, Harris NL, Jaffe ES, Han J, van Krieken JM, Poppema S, Marafioti T, Franklin J, Sextro M, Diehl V, Stein H (2000). European Task Force on Lymphoma project on lymphocyte predominance Hodgkin disease: histologic and immunohistologic analysis of submitted cases reveals 2 types of Hodgkin disease with a nodular growth pattern and abundant lymphocytes. Blood 96: 1889-1899.
34. Anastasi J, Feng J, Dickstein JI, Le Beau MM, Rubin CM, Larson RA, Rowley JD, Vardiman JW (1996). Lineage involvement by BCR/ABL in Ph+ lymphoblastic leukemias: chronic myelogenous leukemia presenting in lymphoid blast vs Ph+ acute lymphoblastic leukemia. Leukemia 10: 795-802.
35. Anastasi J, Musvee T, Roulston D, Domer PH, Larson RA, Vardiman JW (1998). Pseudo-Gaucher histiocytes identified up to 1 year after transplantation for CML are BCR/ABL-positive. Leukemia 12: 233-237.
35A. Anastasi J, Vardiman JW (2001). Chronic myelogenous leukemia and the chronic myeloproliferative diseases In: Neoplastic Hematopathology. 2nd Edition.Knowles,D.M. (ed). Lippincott Williams & Wilkins.Philadelphia.
36. Andersen MK, Larson RA, Mauritzson N, Schnittger S, Jhanwar SC, Pedersen-Bjergaard J (2002). Balanced chromosome abnormalities inv(16) and t(15;17) in therapy-related myelodysplastic syndromes and acute leukemia: report from an international workshop. Genes Chromosomes Cancer 33: 395-400.
37. Anderson JR, Armitage JO, Weisenburger DD (1998). Epidemiology of the non-Hodgkin's lymphomas: distributions of the major subtypes differ by geographic locations. Non-Hodgkin's Lymphoma Classification Project. Ann Oncol 9: 717-720.
38. Anderson JR, Vose JM, Bierman PJ, Weisenberger DD, Sanger WG, Pierson J, Bast M, Armitage JO (1993). Clinical features and prognosis of follicular large-cell lymphoma: a report from the Nebraska Lymphoma Study Group. J Clin Oncol 11: 218-224.
39. Anderson K, Arvidsson I, Jacobsson B, Hast R (2002). Fluorescence in situ hybridization for the study of cell lineage involvement in myelodysplastic syndromes with chromosome 5 anomalies. Cancer Genet Cytogenet 136: 101-107.
40. Anderson T, Bender RA, Fisher RI, DeVita VT, Chabner BA, Berard CW, Norton L, Young RC (1977). Combination chemotherapy in non-Hodgkin's lymphoma: results of long-term followup. Cancer Treat Rep 61: 1057-1066.
41. Andreasson B, Swolin B, Kutti J (2002). Patients with idiopathic myelofibrosis show increased CD34+ cell concentrations in peripheral blood compared to patients with polycythaemia vera and essential thrombocythaemia. Eur J Haematol 68: 189-193.
42. Andrieux JL, Demory JL (2005).

Karyotype and molecular cytogenetic studies in polycythemia vera. Curr Hematol Rep 4: 224-229.
43. Andriko JA, Swerdlow SH, Aguilera NI, Abbondanzo SL (2001). Is lymphoplasmacytic lymphoma/immunocytoma a distinct entity? A clinicopathologic study of 20 cases. Am J Surg Pathol 25: 742-751.
44. Andriko JW, Kaldjian EP, Tsokos M, Abbondanzo SL, Jaffe ES (1998). Reticulum cell neoplasms of lymph nodes: a clinicopathologic study of 11 cases with recognition of a new subtype derived from fibroblastic reticular cells. Am J Surg Pathol 22: 1048-1058.
45. Annunziata CM, Davis RE, Demchenko Y, Bellamy W, Gabrea A, Zhan F, Lenz G, Hanamura I, Wright G, Xiao W, Dave S, Hurt EM, Tan B, Zhao H, Stephens O, Santra M, Williams DR, Dang L, Barlogie B, Shaughnessy JD, Jr., Kuehl WM, Staudt LM (2007). Frequent engagement of the classical and alternative NF-kappaB pathways by diverse genetic abnormalities in multiple myeloma. Cancer Cell 12: 115-130.
46. Anon. (1969). Histopathological definition of Burkitt's tumour. Bull World Health Organ 40: 601-607.
47. Anon. (1982). National Cancer Institute sponsored study of classifications of non-Hodgkin's lymphomas: summary and description of a working formulation for clinical usage. The Non-Hodgkin's Lymphoma Pathologic Classification Project. Cancer 49: 2112-2135.
47A. Anon. (1987). Recommendations for a morphologic, immunologic, and cytogenetic (MIC) working classification of the primary and therapy-related myelodysplastic disorders. Report of the workshop held in Scottsdale, Arizona, USA, on February 23-25, 1987. Third MIC Cooperative Study Group
47B. Anon. (1987). Histiocytosis syndromes in children. Writing Group of the Histiocyte Society. Lancet 1: 208-209.
48. Anon. (1991). Chronic myelomonocytic leukemia: single entity or heterogeneous disorder? A prospective multicenter study of 100 patients. Groupe Francais de Cytogenetique Hematologique. Cancer Genet Cytogenet 55: 57-65.
49. Anon. (1993). A predictive model for aggressive non-Hodgkin's lymphoma. The International Non-Hodgkin's Lymphoma Prognostic Factors Project. N Engl J Med 329: 987-994.
50. Anon. (1995). Polycythemia vera: the natural history of 1213 patients followed for 20 years. Gruppo Italiano Studio Policitemia. Ann Intern Med 123: 656-664.
51. Anon. (1997). A clinical evaluation of the International Lymphoma Study Group classification of non-Hodgkin's lymphoma. The Non-Hodgkin's Lymphoma Classification Project. Blood 89: 3909-3918.
52. Anon. (1997). Primary immunodeficiency diseases. Report of a WHO scientific group. Clin Exp Immunol 109 Suppl 1:1-28: 1-28.
53. Anon. (1998). The value of c-kit in the diagnosis of biphenotypic acute leukemia. EGIL (European Group for the Immunological Classification of Leukaemias). Leukemia 12: 2038.
54. Anon. (2000). Nijmegen breakage syndrome. The International Nijmegen Breakage Syndrome Study Group. Arch Dis Child 82: 400-406.
55. Anon. (2000). The world health organization classification of malignant lymphomas in Japan: incidence of recently recognized entities. Lymphoma Study Group of Japanese Pathologists. Pathol Int 50: 696-702.
56. Anon. (2003). Criteria for the classification of monoclonal gammopathies, multiple myeloma and related disorders: a report of the International Myeloma Working Group. Br J Haematol 121: 749-757.
57. Anon. (2004). Guidelines on the diagnosis and management of AL amyloidosis. Br J Haematol 125: 681-700.
57A. Armitage J, Vose J, Weisenburger D (2008). International Peripheral T-Cell and NK/T-Cell Lymphoma study: Pathology findings and clinical outcomes. J Clin Oncol 26:4124-4130.
58. Ansari MQ, Dawson DB, Nador R, Rutherford C, Schneider NR, Latimer MJ, Picker L, Knowles DM, McKenna RW (1996). Primary body cavity-based AIDS-related lymphomas. Am J Clin Pathol 105: 221-229.
59. Aoki Y, Yarchoan R, Braun J, Iwamoto A, Tosato G (2000). Viral and cellular cytokines in AIDS-related malignant lymphomatous effusions. Blood 96: 1599-1601.
60. Aozasa K (1990). Hashimoto's thyroiditis as a risk factor of thyroid lymphoma. Acta Pathol Jpn 40: 459-468.
61. Aozasa K, Ohsawa M, Iuchi K, Mori T, Komatsu H, Tajima K, Minato K, Tajima K, Shimoyama M (1991). Prognostic factors for pleural lymphoma patients. Jpn J Clin Oncol 21: 417-421.
62. Aozasa K, Ohsawa M, Iuchi K, Tajima K, Komatsu H, Shimoyama M (1993). Artificial pneumothorax as a risk factor for development of pleural lymphoma. Jpn J Cancer Res 84: 55-57.
63. Aozasa K, Takakuwa T, Nakatsuka S (2005). Pyothorax-associated lymphoma: a lymphoma developing in chronic inflammation. Adv Anat Pathol 12: 324-331.
64. Apperley JF, Gardembas M, Melo JV, Russell-Jones R, Bain BJ, Baxter EJ, Chase A, Chessells JM, Colombat M, Dearden CE, Dimitrijevic S, Mahon FX, Marin D, Nikolova Z, Olavarria E, Silberman S, Schultheis B, Cross NC, Goldman JM (2002). Response to imatinib mesylate in patients with chronic myeloproliferative diseases with rearrangements of the platelet-derived growth factor receptor beta. N Engl J Med 347: 481-487.
64A. Araujo I, Bittencourt AL, Barbosa HS, Netto EM, Mendonça N, Foss HD, Hummel M, Stein H (2006). The high frequency of EBV infection in pediatric Hodgkin lymphoma is related to the classical type in Bahia, Brazil. Virchows Arch 449:315-319
65. Arber DA, Carter NH, Ikle D, Slovak ML (2003). Value of combined morphologic, cytochemical, and immunophenotypic features in predicting recurrent cytogenetic abnormalities in acute myeloid leukemia. Hum Pathol 34: 479-483.
66. Arber DA, Chang KL, Lyda MH, Bedell V, Spielberger R, Slovak ML (2003). Detection of NPM/MLF1 fusion in t(3;5)-positive acute myeloid leukemia and myelodysplasia. Hum Pathol 34: 809-813.
67. Arber DA, George TI (2005). Bone marrow biopsy involvement by non-Hodgkin's lymphoma: frequency of lymphoma types, patterns, blood involvement, and discordance with other sites in 450 specimens. Am J Surg Pathol 29: 1549-1557.
68. Arber DA, Slovak ML, Popplewell L, Bedell V, Ikle D, Rowley JD (2002). Therapy-related acute myeloid leukemia/myelodysplasia with balanced 21q22 translocations. Am J Clin Pathol 117: 306-313.
69. Arber DA, Stein AS, Carter NH, Ikle D, Forman SJ, Slovak ML (2003). Prognostic impact of acute myeloid leukemia classification. Importance of detection of recurring cytogenetic abnormalities and multilineage dysplasia on survival. Am J Clin Pathol 119: 672-680.
70. Arber DA, Weiss LM, Albujar PF, Chen YY, Jaffe ES (1993). Nasal lymphomas in Peru. High incidence of T-cell immunophenotype and Epstein-Barr virus infection. Am J Surg Pathol 17: 392-399.
71. Arber DA, Weiss LM, Chang KL (1998). Detection of Epstein-Barr Virus in inflammatory pseudotumor. Semin Diagn Pathol 15: 155-160.
72. Arcaini L, Lazzarino M, Colombo N, Burcheri S, Boveri E, Paulli M, Morra E, Gambacorta M, Cortelazzo S, Tucci A, Ungari M, Ambrosetti A, Menestrina F, Orsucci L, Novero D, Pulsoni A, Frezzato M, Gaidano G, Vallisa D, Minardi V, Tripodo C, Callea V, Baldini L, Merli F, Federico M, Franco V, Iannitto E (2006). Splenic marginal zone lymphoma: a prognostic model for clinical use. Blood 107: 4643-4649.
73. Arcaini L, Paulli M, Burcheri S, Rossi A, Spina M, Passamonti F, Lucioni M, Motta T, Canzonieri V, Montanari M, Bonoldi E, Gallamini A, Uziel L, Crugnola M, Ramponi A, Montanari F, Pascutto C, Morra E, Lazzarino M (2007). Primary nodal marginal zone B-cell lymphoma: clinical features and prognostic assessment of a rare disease. Br J Haematol 136: 301-304.
74. Argatoff LH, Connors JM, Klasa RJ, Horsman DE, Gascoyne RD (1997). Mantle cell lymphoma: a clinicopathologic study of 80 cases. Blood 89: 2067-2078.
75. Arico M, Girschikofsky M, Genereau T, Klersy C, McClain K, Grois N, Emile JF, Lukina E, De Juli E, Danesino C (2003). Langerhans cell histiocytosis in adults. Report from the International Registry of the Histiocyte Society. Eur J Cancer 39: 2341-2348.
76. Arico M, Nichols K, Whitlock JA, Arceci R, Haupt R, Mittler U, Kuhne T, Lombardi A, Ishii E, Egeler RM, Danesino C (1999). Familial clustering of Langerhans cell histiocytosis. Br J Haematol 107: 883-888.
77. Arico M, Valsecchi MG, Camitta B, Schrappe M, Chessells J, Baruchel A, Gaynon P, Silverman L, Janka-Schaub G, Kamps W, Pui CH, Masera G (2000). Outcome of treatment in children with Philadelphia chromosome-positive acute lymphoblastic leukemia. N Engl J Med 342: 998-1006.
78. Armes JE, Angus P, Southey MC, Battaglia SE, Ross BC, Jones RM, Venter DJ (1994). Lymphoproliferative disease of donor origin arising in patients after orthotopic liver transplantation. Cancer 74: 2436-2441.
79. Armitage JO, Weisenburger DD (1998). New approach to classifying non-Hodgkin's lymphomas: clinical features of the major histologic subtypes. Non-Hodgkin's Lymphoma Classification Project. J Clin Oncol 16: 2780-2795.
80. Armstrong SA, Kung AL, Mabon ME, Silverman LB, Stam RW, Den Boer ML, Pieters R, Kersey JH, Sallan SE, Fletcher JA, Golub TR, Griffin JD, Korsmeyer SJ (2003). Inhibition of FLT3 in MLL. Validation of a therapeutic target identified by gene expression based classification. Cancer Cell 3: 173-183.
81. Arnulf B, Copie-Bergman C, Delfau-Larue MH, Lavergne-Slove A, Bosq J, Wechsler J, Wassef M, Matuchansky C, Epardeau B, Stern M, Bagot M, Reyes F, Gaulard P (1998). Nonhepatosplenic gammadelta T-cell lymphoma: a subset of cytotoxic lymphomas with mucosal or skin localization. Blood 91: 1723-1731.
82. Arons E, Sorbara L, Raffeld M, Stetler-Stevenson M, Steinberg SM, Liewehr DJ, Pastan I, Kreitman RJ (2006). Characterization of T-cell repertoire in hairy cell leukemia patients before and after recombinant immunotoxin BL22 therapy. Cancer Immunol Immunother 55: 1100-1110.
83. Arons E, Sunshine J, Suntum T, Kreitman RJ (2006). Somatic hypermutation and VH gene usage in hairy cell leukaemia. Br J Haematol 133: 504-512.
84. Arvanitakis L, Geras-Raaka E, Varma A, Gershengorn MC, Cesarman E (1997). Human herpesvirus KSHV encodes a constitutively active G-protein-coupled receptor linked to cell proliferation. Nature 385: 347-350.
85. Arvanitakis L, Mesri EA, Nador RG, Said JW, Asch AS, Knowles DM, Cesarman E (1996). Establishment and characterization of a primary effusion (body cavity-based) lymphoma cell line (BC-3) harboring kaposi's sarcoma-associated herpesvirus (KSHV/HHV-8) in the absence of Epstein-Barr virus. Blood 88: 2648-2654.
86. Arzoo KK, Bu X, Espina BM, Seneviratne L, Nathwani B, Levine AM (2004). T-cell lymphoma in HIV-infected patients. J Acquir Immune Defic Syndr 36: 1020-1027.
87. Asano N, Suzuki R, Kagami Y, Ishida F, Kitamura K, Fukutani H, Morishima Y, Takeuchi K, Nakamura S (2005). Clinicopathologic and prognostic significance of cytotoxic molecule expression in nodal peripheral T-cell lymphoma, unspecified. Am J Surg Pathol 29: 1284-1293.
88. Ascani S, Piccioli M, Poggi S, Briskomatis A, Bolis GB, Liberati F, Frongillo R, Caramatti C, Fraternali-Orcioni G, Gamberi B, Zinzani PL, Lazzi S, Leoncini L, O'Leary J, Piccaluga PP, Pileri SA (1997). Pyothorax-associated lymphoma: description of the first two cases detected in Italy. Ann Oncol 8: 1133-1138.
88A. Ascoli V, Lo CF, Artini M, Levrero M, Martelli M, Negro F (1998). Extranodal lymphomas associated with hepatitis C virus infection. Am J Clin Pathol 109: 600-609.
88B Ascani S, Zinzani PL, Gherlinzoni F, Sabattini E, Briskomatis A, de Vivo A, Piccioli M, Fraternali OG, Pieri F, Goldoni A, Piccaluga PP, Zallocco D, Burnelli R, Leoncini L, Falini B, Tura S, Pileri SA (1997). Peripheral T-cell lymphomas. Clinico-pathologic study of 168 cases diagnosed according to the R.E.A.L. Classification. Ann Oncol 8:583-592.
89. Ashton-Key M, Diss TC, Pan L, Du MQ, Isaacson PG (1997). Molecular analysis of T-cell clonality in ulcerative jejunitis and enteropathy-associated T-cell lymphoma. Am J Pathol 151: 493-498.
90. Ashton-Key M, Thorpe PA, Allen JP, Isaacson PG (1995). Follicular Hodgkin's disease. Am J Surg Pathol 19: 1294-1299.
91. Asou H, Said JW, Yang R, Munker R, Park DJ, Kamada N, Koeffler HP (1998). Mechanisms of growth control of Kaposi's sarcoma-associated herpes virus-associated primary effusion lymphoma cells. Blood 91: 2475-2481.
92. Assaf C, Gellrich S, Whittaker S, Robson A, Cerroni L, Massone C, Kerl H, Rose C, Chott A, Chimenti S, Hallermann C, Petrella T, Wechsler J, Bagot M, Hummel M, Bullani-Kerl K, Bekkenk M, Kempf W, Meijer C, Willemze R, Sterry W (2006). CD56 lymphoproliferative disorders of the skin: A multicenter study of the Cutaneous Lymphoma Project Group of the European Organization for Research and Treatment of Cancer (EORTC). J Clin Pathol 60: 981-989.
93. Aster JC, Longtine JA (2002). Detection of BCL2 rearrangements in follicular lymphoma. Am J Pathol 160: 759-763.
94. Atayar C, Kok K, Kluiver J, Bosga A, van den BE, van d, V, Blokzijl T, Harms G, Davelaar I, Sikkema-Raddatz B, Martin-Subero JI, Siebert R, Poppema S, van den BA (2006). BCL6 alternative breakpoint region break and homozygous deletion of 17q24 in the nodular lymphocyte predominance type of Hodgkin's lymphoma-derived cell line DEV. Hum Pathol 37: 675-683.
95. Atayar C, Poppema S, Visser L, van den Berg A (2006). Cytokine gene expression

profile distinguishes CD4+/CD57+ T cells of the nodular lymphocyte predominance type of Hodgkin's lymphoma from their tonsillar counterparts. J Pathol 208: 423-430.

96. Attygalle A, Al Jehani R, Diss TC, Munson P, Liu H, Du MQ, Isaacson PG, Dogan A (2002). Neoplastic T cells in angioimmunoblastic T-cell lymphoma express CD10. Blood 99: 627-633.

97. Attygalle AD, Chuang SS, Diss TC, Du MQ, Isaacson PG, Dogan A (2007). Distinguishing angioimmunoblastic T-cell lymphoma from peripheral T-cell lymphoma, unspecified, using morphology, immunophenotype and molecular genetics. Histopathology 50: 498-508.

98. Attygalle AD, Diss TC, Munson P, Isaacson PG, Du MQ, Dogan A (2004). CD10 expression in extranodal dissemination of angioimmunoblastic T-cell lymphoma. Am J Surg Pathol 28: 54-61.

99. Attygalle AD, Kyriakou C, Dupuis J, Grogg KL, Diss TC, Wotherspoon AC, Chuang SS, Cabecadas J, Isaacson PG, Du MQ, Gaulard P, Dogan A (2007). Histologic Evolution of Angioimmunoblastic T-cell Lymphoma in Consecutive Biopsies: Clinical Correlation and Insights Into Natural History and Disease Progression. Am J Surg Pathol 31: 1077-1088.

100. Attygalle AD, Liu H, Shirali S, Diss TC, Loddenkemper C, Stein H, Dogan A, Du MQ, Isaacson PG (2004). Atypical marginal zone hyperplasia of mucosa-associated lymphoid tissue: a reactive condition of childhood showing immunoglobulin lambda light-chain restriction. Blood 104: 3343-3348.

101. Au WY, Gascoyne RD, Gallagher RE, Le N, Klasa RD, Liang RH, Choy C, Foo W, Connors JM (2004). Hodgkin's lymphoma in Chinese migrants to British Columbia: a 25-year survey. Ann Oncol 15: 626-630.

102. Au WY, Horsman DE, Gascoyne RD, Viswanatha DS, Klasa RJ, Connors JM (2004). The spectrum of lymphoma with 8q24 aberrations: a clinical, pathological and cytogenetic study of 87 consecutive cases. Leuk Lymphoma 45: 519-528.

103. Au WY, Lam CC, Lie AK, Pang A, Kwong YL (2003). T-cell large granular lymphocyte leukemia of donor origin after allogeneic bone marrow transplantation. Am J Clin Pathol 120: 626-630.

104. Au WY, Ma SY, Chim CS, Choy C, Loong F, Lie AK, Lam CC, Leung AY, Tse E, Yau CC, Liang R, Kwong YL (2005). Clinicopathologic features and treatment outcome of mature T-cell and natural killer-cell lymphomas diagnosed according to the World Health Organization classification scheme: a single center experience of 10 years. Ann Oncol 16: 206-214.

105. Au WY, Pang A, Choy C, Chim CS, Kwong YL (2004). Quantification of circulating Epstein-Barr virus (EBV) DNA in the diagnosis and monitoring of natural killer cell and EBV-positive lymphomas in immunocompetent patients. Blood 104: 243-249.

106. Aucouturier P, Khamlichi AA, Touchard G, Justrabo E, Cogne M, Chauffert B, Martin F, Preud'Homme JL (1993). Brief report: heavy-chain deposition disease. N Engl J Med 329: 1389-1393.

107. Audouin J, Diebold J, Pallesen G (1992). Frequent expression of Epstein-Barr virus latent membrane protein-1 in tumour cells of Hodgkin's disease in HIV-positive patients. J Pathol 167: 381-384.

108. Aul C, Bowen DT, Yoshida Y (1998). Pathogenesis, etiology and epidemiology of myelodysplastic syndromes. Haematologica 83: 71-86.

109. Aul C, Gattermann N, Schneider W (1992). Age-related incidence and other epidemiological aspects of myelodysplastic syndromes. Br J Haematol 82: 358-367.

110. Ault P, Lynn A, Tam CS, Medeiros LJ, Keating MJ (2007). Systemic mastocytosis in association with chronic lymphocytic leukemia: A rare diagnosis. Leuk Res 31: 1755-1758.

111. Avet-Loiseau H, Attal M, Moreau P, Charbonnel C, Garban F, Hulin C, Leyvraz S, Michallet M, Yakoub-Agha I, Garderet L, Marit G, Michaux L, Voillat L, Renaud M, Grosbois B, Guillerm G, Benboubker L, Monconduit M, Thieblemont C, Casassus P, Caillot D, Stoppa AM, Sotto JJ, Wetterwald M, Dumontet C, Fuzibet JG, Azais I, Dorvaux V, Zandecki M, Bataille R, Minvielle S, Harousseau JL, Facon T, Mathiot C (2007). Genetic abnormalities and survival in multiple myeloma: the experience of the Intergroupe Francophone du Myelome. Blood 109: 3489-3495.

112. Avet-Loiseau H, Daviet A, Brigaudeau C, Callet-Bauchu E, Terre C, Lafage-Pochitaloff M, Desangles F, Ramond S, Talmant P, Bataille R (2001). Cytogenetic, interphase, and multicolor fluorescence in situ hybridization analyses in primary plasma cell leukemia: a study of 40 patients at diagnosis, on behalf of the Intergroupe Francophone du Myelome and the Groupe Francais de Cytogenetique Hematologique. Blood 97: 822-825.

113. Avet-Loiseau H, Facon T, Grosbois B, Magrangeas F, Rapp MJ, Harousseau JL, Minvielle S, Bataille R (2002). Oncogenesis of multiple myeloma: 14q32 and 13q chromosomal abnormalities are not randomly distributed, but correlate with natural history, immunological features, and clinical presentation. Blood 99: 2185-2191.

114. Ayton PM, Cleary ML (2001). Molecular mechanisms of leukemogenesis mediated by MLL fusion proteins. Oncogene 20: 5695-5707.

115. Baccarani M, Russo D, Rosti G, Martinelli G (2003). Interferon-alfa for chronic myeloid leukemia. Semin Hematol 40: 22-33.

116. Baccarani M, Saglio G, Goldman J, Hochhaus A, Simonsson B, Appelbaum F, Apperley J, Cervantes F, Cortes J, Deininger M, Gratwohl A, Guilhot F, Horowitz M, Hughes T, Kantarjian H, Larson R, Niederwieser D, Silver R, Hehlmann R (2006). Evolving concepts in the management of chronic myeloid leukemia: recommendations from an expert panel on behalf of the European Leukemia Net. Blood 108: 1809-1820.

117. Bacher U, Haferlach C, Kern W, Haferlach T, Schnittger S (2008). Prognostic relevance of FLT3-TKD mutations in AML: the combination matters - an analysis of 3082 patients. Blood 111: 2527-2537.

118. Bacher U, Kern W, Schnittger S, Hiddemann W, Schoch C, Haferlach T (2005). Blast count and cytogenetics correlate and are useful parameters for the evaluation of different phases in chronic myeloid leukemia. Leuk Lymphoma 46: 357-366.

119. Bacon CM, Ye H, Diss TC, McNamara C, Kueck B, Hasserjian RP, Rohatiner AZ, Ferry J, Du MQ, Dogan A (2007). Primary follicular lymphoma of the testis and epididymis in adults. Am J Surg Pathol 31: 1050-1058.

120. Baddoura FK, Hanson C, Chan WC (1992). Plasmacytoid monocyte proliferation associated with myeloproliferative disorders. Cancer 69: 1457-1467.

121. Bader-Meunier B, Tchernia G, Mielot F, Fontaine JL, Thomas C, Lyonnet S, Lavergne JM, Dommergues JP (1997). Occurrence of myeloproliferative disorder in patients with Noonan syndrome. J Pediatr 130: 885-889.

122. Baecklund E, Sundstrom C, Ekbom A, Catrina AI, Biberfeld P, Feltelius N, Klareskog L (2003). Lymphoma subtypes in patients with rheumatoid arthritis: increased proportion of diffuse large B cell lymphoma. Arthritis Rheum 48: 1543-1550.

123. Baer MR, Stewart CC, Lawrence D, Arthur DC, Byrd JC, Davey FR, Schiffer CA, Bloomfield CD (1997). Expression of the neural cell adhesion molecule CD56 is associated with short remission duration and survival in acute myeloid leukemia with t(8;21)(q22;q22). Blood 90: 1643-1648.

124. Bagdi E, Diss TC, Munson P, Isaacson PG (1999). Mucosal intra-epithelial lymphocytes in enteropathy-associated T-cell lymphoma, ulcerative jejunitis, and refractory celiac disease constitute a neoplastic population. Blood 94: 260-264.

125. Bahler DW, Pindzola JA, Swerdlow SH (2002). Splenic marginal zone lymphomas appear to originate from different B cell types. Am J Pathol 161: 81-88.

126. Bai M, Tsanou E, Skyrlas A, Sainis I, Agnantis N, Kanavaros P (2007). Alterations of the p53, Rb and p27 tumor suppressor pathways in diffuse large B-cell lymphomas. Anticancer Res 27: 2345-2352.

127. Bain B (2006). Ringed sideroblasts with thrombocytosis: an uncommon mixed myelodysplastic/myeloproliferative disease in older adults. Br J Haematol 134: 340-341.

128. Bain BJ (1996). Eosinophilic leukaemias and the idiopathic hypereosinophilic syndrome. Br J Haematol 95: 2-9.

129. Bain BJ (1999). The relationship between the myelodysplastic syndromes and the myeloproliferative disorders. Leuk Lymphoma 34: 443-449.

130. Bain BJ (2004). Relationship between idiopathic hypereosinophilic syndrome, eosinophilic leukemia, and systemic mastocytosis. Am J Hematol 77: 82-85.

131. Bain BJ, Fletcher SH (2007). Chronic eosinophilic leukemias and the myeloproliferative variant of the hypereosinophilic syndrome. Immunol Allergy Clin North Am 27: 377-388.

132. Bakels V, Van Oostveen JW, Van der Putte SC, Meijer CJ, Willemze R (1997). Immunophenotyping and gene rearrangement analysis provide additional criteria to differentiate between cutaneous T-cell lymphomas and pseudo-T-cell lymphomas. Am J Pathol 150: 1941-1949.

133. Bakker NA, van Imhoff GW, Verschuuren EA, van Son WJ, Homan van der Heide JJ, Veeger NJ, Kluin PM, Kluin-Nelemans HC (2005). Early onset post-transplant lymphoproliferative disease is associated with allograft localization. Clin Transplant 19: 327-334.

134. Bakkus MH, Heirman C, Van R, I, Van Camp B, Thielemans K (1992). Evidence that multiple myeloma Ig heavy chain VDJ genes contain somatic mutations but show no intraclonal variation. Blood 80: 2326-2335.

135. Balague O, Martinez A, Colomo L, Rosello E, Garcia A, Martinez-Bernal M, Palacin A, Fu K, Weisenburger D, Colomer D, Burke JS, Warnke RA, Campo E (2007). Epstein-Barr virus negative clonal plasma cell proliferations and lymphomas in peripheral T-cell lymphomas: a phenomenon with distinctive clinicopathologic features. Am J Surg Pathol 31: 1310-1322.

135A. Baldus CD, Tanner SM, Ruppert AS, Whitman SP, Archer KJ, Marcucci G, Caligiuri MA, Carroll AJ, Vardiman JW, Powell BL, Allen SL, Moore JO, Larson RA, Kolitz JE, de la Chapelle A, Bloomfield CD (2003). BAALC expression predicts clinical outcome of de novo acute myeloid leukemia patients with normal cytogenetics: a Cancer and Leukemia Group B study. Blood 102: 1613-1618.

135B. Baldus CD, Thiede C, Soucek S, Bloomfield CD, Thiel E, Ehninger G (2006). BAALC expression and FLT3 internal tandem duplication mutations in acute myeloid leukemia patients with normal cytogenetics: prognostic implications. J Clin Oncol 24: 790- 797.

136. Ballard HS, Hamilton LM, Marcus AJ, Illes CH (1970). A new variant of heavy-chain disease (mu-chain disease). N Engl J Med 282: 1060-1062.

137. Ballester B, Ramuz O, Gisselbrecht C, Doucet G, Loi L, Loriod B, Bertucci F, Bouabdallah R, Devilard E, Carbuccia N, Mozziconacci MJ, Birnbaum D, Brousset P, Berger F, Salles G, Briere J, Houlgatte R, Gaulard P, Xerri L (2006). Gene expression profiling identifies molecular subgroups among nodal peripheral T-cell lymphomas. Oncogene 25: 1560-1570.

138. Banchereau J, Briere F, Caux C, Davoust J, Lebecque S, Liu YJ, Pulendran B, Palucka K (2000). Immunobiology of dendritic cells. Annu Rev Immunol 18: 767-811.

139. Banks PM, Chan J, Cleary ML, Delsol G, Wolf-Peeters C, Gatter K, Grogan TM, Harris NL, Isaacson PG, Jaffe ES (1992). Mantle cell lymphoma. A proposal for unification of morphologic, immunologic, and molecular data. Am J Surg Pathol 16: 637-640.

139A Bardet V, Costa LD, Elie C, Malinge S, Demur C, Tamburini J, Lefebvre PC, Witz F, Lioure B, Jourdan E, Pigneux A, Ifrah N, Attal M, Dreyfus F, Mayeux P, Lacombe C, Bennaceur-Griscelli A, Bernard OA, Bouscary D, Recher C (2006). Nucleophosmin status may influence the therapeutic decision in de novo acute myeloid leukemia with normal karyotype. Leukemia 20: 1644-1646.

140. Barlogie B, Epstein J, Selvanayagam P, Alexanian R (1989). Plasma cell myeloma— new biological insights and advances in therapy. Blood 73: 865-879.

141. Baro C, Salido M, Domingo A, Granada I, Colomo L, Serrano S, Sole F (2006). Translocation t(9;14)(p13;q32) in cases of splenic marginal zone lymphoma. Haematologica 91: 1289-1291.

142. Barosi G (1999). Myelofibrosis with myeloid metaplasia: diagnostic definition and prognostic classification for clinical studies and treatment guidelines. J Clin Oncol 17: 2954-2970.

143. Barosi G, Hoffman R (2005). Idiopathic myelofibrosis. Semin Hematol 42: 248-258.

143A. Barosi G, Mesa RA, Thiele J, Cervantes F, Campbell PJ, Verstovsek S, Dupriez B, Levine RL, Passamonti F, Gotlib J, Reilly JT, Vannucchi AM, Hanson CA, Solberg LA, Orazi A, Tefferi A; International Working Group for Myelofibrosis Research and Treatment (IWG-MRT) (2008). Proposed criteria for the diagnosis of post-polycythemia vera and post-essential thrombocythemia myelofibrosis: a consensus statement from the International Working Group for Myelofibrosis Research and Treatment. Leukemia 22: 437-438.

144. Barosi G, Rosti V, Massa M, Viarengo GL, Pecci A, Necchi V, Ramaioli I, Campanelli R, Marchetti M, Bazzan M, Magrini U (2004). Spleen neoangiogenesis in patients with myelofibrosis with myeloid metaplasia. Br J Haematol 124: 618-625.

145. Barosi G, Viarengo G, Pecci A, Rosti V, Piaggio G, Marchetti M, Frassoni F (2001). Diagnostic and clinical relevance of the number of circulating CD34(+) cells in myelofibrosis with myeloid metaplasia. Blood 98: 3249-3255.

146. Barrans SL, Fenton JA, Banham A, Owen RG, Jack AS (2004). Strong expression of FOXP1 identifies a distinct subset of diffuse large B-cell lymphoma (DLBCL) patients with poor outcome. Blood 104: 2933-2935.

147. Barrionuevo C, Anderson VM, Zevallos-Giampietri E, Zaharia M, Misad O, Bravo F, Caceres H, Taxa L, Martinez MT, Wachtel A, Piris MA (2002). Hydroa-like cutaneous T-cell lymphoma: a clinicopathologic and molecular genetic study of 16 pediatric cases from Peru. Appl Immunohistochem Mol Morphol 10: 7-14.
148. Barrionuevo C, Zaharia M, Martinez MT, Taxa L, Misad O, Moscol A, Sarria G, Guerrero I, Casanova L, Flores C, Zevallos-Giampietri EA (2007). Extranodal NK/T-cell lymphoma, nasal type: study of clinicopathologic and prognosis factors in a series of 78 cases from Peru. Appl Immunohistochem Mol Morphol 15: 38-44.
149. Barry TS, Jaffe ES, Sorbara L, Raffeld M, Pittaluga S (2003). Peripheral T-cell lymphomas expressing CD30 and CD15. Am J Surg Pathol 27: 1513-1522.
150. Barth TF, Leithauser F, Joos S, Bentz M, Moller P (2002). Mediastinal (thymic) large B-cell lymphoma: where do we stand? Lancet Oncol 3: 229-234.
151. Barth TF, Muller S, Pawlita M, Siebert R, Rother JU, Mechtersheimer G, Kitinya J, Bentz M, Moller P (2004). Homogeneous immunophenotype and paucity of secondary genomic aberrations are distinctive features of endemic but not of sporadic Burkitt's lymphoma and diffuse large B-cell lymphoma with MYC rearrangement. J Pathol 203: 940-945.
152. Bartl R, Frisch B, Fateh-Moghadam A, Kettner G, Jaeger K, Sommerfeld W (1987). Histologic classification and staging of multiple myeloma. A retrospective and prospective study of 674 cases. Am J Clin Pathol 87: 342-355.
153. Bartlett NL, Rizeq M, Dorfman RF, Halpern J, Horning SJ (1994). Follicular large-cell lymphoma: intermediate or low grade? J Clin Oncol 12: 1349-1357.
154. Bartram CR, de Klein A, Hagemeijer A, van Agthoven T, Geurts vK, Bootsma D, Grosveld G, Ferguson-Smith MA, Davies T, Stone M (1983). Translocation of c-ab1 oncogene correlates with the presence of a Philadelphia chromosome in chronic myelocytic leukaemia. Nature 306: 277-280.
155. Baruchel A, Cayuela JM, Ballerini P, Landman-Parker J, Cezard V, Firat H, Haddad E, Auclerc MF, Valensi F, Cayre YE, Macintyre EA, Sigaux F (1997). The majority of myeloid-antigen-positive (My+) childhood B-cell precursor acute lymphoblastic leukaemias express TEL-AML1 fusion transcripts. Br J Haematol 99: 101-106.
156. Baseggio L, Berger F, Morel D, Delfau-Larue MH, Goedert G, Salles G, Magaud JP, Felman P (2006). Identification of circulating CD10 positive T cells in angioimmunoblastic T-cell lymphoma. Leukemia 20: 296-303.
157. Basso K, Liso A, Tiacci E, Benedetti R, Pulsoni A, Foa R, Di Raimondo F, Ambrosetti A, Califano A, Klein U, Dalla FR, Falini B (2004). Gene expression profiling of hairy cell leukemia reveals a phenotype related to memory B cells with altered expression of chemokine and adhesion receptors. J Exp Med 199: 59-68.
158. Bastard C, Deweindt C, Kerckaert JP, Lenormand B, Rossi A, Pezzella F, Fruchart C, Duval C, Monconduit M, Tilly H (1994). LAZ3 rearrangements in non-Hodgkin's lymphoma: correlation with histology, immunophenotype, karyotype, and clinical outcome in 217 patients. Blood 83: 2423-2427.
159. Bataille R, Boccadoro M, Klein B, Durie B, Pileri A (1992). C-reactive protein and beta-2 microglobulin produce a simple and powerful myeloma staging system. Blood 80: 733-737.
160. Bataille R, Durie BG, Grenier J, Sany J (1986). Prognostic factors and staging in multiple myeloma: a reappraisal. J Clin Oncol 4: 80-87.
161. Batista DA, Vonderheid EC, Hawkins A, Morsberger L, Long P, Murphy KM, Griffin CA (2006). Multicolor fluorescence in situ hybridization (SKY) in mycosis fungoides and Sezary syndrome: search for recurrent chromosome abnormalities. Genes Chromosomes Cancer 45: 383-391.
162. Baxter EJ, Hochhaus A, Bolufer P, Reiter A, Fernandez JM, Senent L, Cervera J, Moscardo F, Sanz MA, Cross NC (2002). The t(4;22)(q12;q11) in atypical chronic myeloid leukaemia fuses BCR to PDGFRA. Hum Mol Genet 11: 1391-1397.
163. Baxter EJ, Scott LM, Campbell PJ, East C, Fourouclas N, Swanton S, Vassiliou GS, Bench AJ, Boyd EM, Curtin N, Scott MA, Erber WN, Green AR (2005). Acquired mutation of the tyrosine kinase JAK2 in human myeloproliferative disorders. Lancet 365: 1054-1061.
164. Bayle C, Charpentier A, Duchayne E, Manel AM, Pages MP, Robert A, Lamant L, Dastugue N, Bertrand Y, Dijoud F, Emile JF, Machover D, Brugieres L, Delsol G (1999). Leukaemic presentation of small cell variant anaplastic large cell lymphoma: report of four cases. Br J Haematol 104: 680-688.
165. Bea S, Ribas M, Hernandez JM, Bosch F, Pinyol M, Hernandez L, Garcia JL, Flores T, Gonzalez M, Lopez-Guillermo A, Piris MA, Cardesa A, Montserrat E, Miro R, Campo E (1999). Increased number of chromosomal imbalances and high-level DNA amplifications in mantle cell lymphoma are associated with blastoid variants. Blood 93: 4365-4374.
166. Bea S, Tort F, Pinyol M, Puig X, Hernandez L, Hernandez S, Fernandez PL, van Lohuizen M, Colomer D, Campo E (2001). BMI-1 gene amplification and overexpression in hematological malignancies occur mainly in mantle cell lymphomas. Cancer Res 61: 2409-2412.
167. Bea S, Zettl A, Wright G, Salaverria I, Jehn P, Moreno V, Burek C, Ott G, Puig X, Yang L, Lopez-Guillermo A, Chan WC, Greiner TC, Weisenburger DD, Armitage JO, Gascoyne RD, Connors JM, Grogan TM, Braziel R, Fisher RI, Smeland EB, Kvaloy S, Holte H, Delabie J, Simon R, Powell J, Wilson WH, Jaffe ES, Montserrat E, Muller-Hermelink HK, Staudt LM, Campo E, Rosenwald A (2005). Diffuse large B-cell lymphoma subgroups have distinct genetic profiles that influence tumor biology and improve gene-expression-based survival prediction. Blood 106: 3183-3190.
168. Bearman RM, Pangalis GA, Rappaport H (1979). Acute ("malignant") myelosclerosis. Cancer 43: 279-293.
169. Beaty MW, Kumar S, Sorbara L, Miller K, Raffeld M, Jaffe ES (1999). A biophenotypic human herpesvirus 8—associated primary bowel lymphoma. Am J Surg Pathol 23: 992-994.
170. Beaty MW, Toro J, Sorbara L, Stern JB, Pittaluga S, Raffeld M, Wilson WH, Jaffe ES (2001). Cutaneous lymphomatoid granulomatosis: correlation of clinical and biologic features. Am J Surg Pathol 25: 1111-1120.
171. Bedeir A, Jukic DM, Wang L, Mullady DK, Regueiro M, Krasinskas AM (2006). Systemic mastocytosis mimicking inflammatory bowel disease: A case report and discussion of gastrointestinal pathology in systemic mastocytosis. Am J Surg Pathol 30: 1478-1482.
172. Bekkenk MW, Geelen FA, Voorst Vader PC, Heule F, Geerts ML, van Vloten WA, Meijer CJ, Willemze R (2000). Primary and secondary cutaneous CD30(+) lymphoproliferative disorders: a report from the Dutch Cutaneous Lymphoma Group on the long-term follow-up data of 219 patients and guidelines for diagnosis and treatment. Blood 95: 3653-3661.
173. Bekkenk MW, Jansen PM, Meijer CJ, Willemze R (2004). CD56+ hematological neoplasms presenting in the skin: a retrospective analysis of 23 new cases and 130 cases from the literature. Ann Oncol 15: 1097-1108.
174. Bekkenk MW, Vermeer MH, Jansen PM, van Marion AM, Canninga-van Dijk MR, Kluin PM, Geerts ML, Meijer CJ, Willemze R (2003). Peripheral T-cell lymphomas unspecified presenting in the skin: analysis of prognostic factors in a group of 82 patients. Blood 102: 2213-2219.
175. Belec L, Mohamed AS, Authier FJ, Hallouin MC, Soe AM, Cotigny S, Gaulard P, Gherardi RK (1999). Human herpesvirus 8 infection in patients with POEMS syndrome-associated multicentric Castleman's disease. Blood 93: 3643-3653.
176. Belhadj K, Reyes F, Farcet JP, Tilly H, Bastard C, Angonin R, Deconinck E, Charlotte F, Leblond V, Labouyrie E, Lederlin P, Emile JF, Delmas-Marsalet B, Arnulf B, Zafrani ES, Gaulard P (2003). Hepatosplenic gammadelta T-cell lymphoma is a rare clinicopathologic entity with poor outcome: report on a series of 21 patients. Blood 102: 4261-4269.
177. Beljaards RC, Meijer CJ, Van der Putte SC, Hollema H, Geerts ML, Bezemer PD, Willemze R (1994). Primary cutaneous T-cell lymphoma: clinicopathological features and prognostic parameters of 35 cases other than mycosis fungoides and CD30-positive large cell lymphoma. J Pathol 172: 53-60.
178. Bellan C, De Falco G, Lazzi S, Leoncini L (2003). Pathologic aspects of AIDS malignancies. Oncogene 22: 6639-6645.
179. Bellan C, Lazzi S, De Falco G, Nyongo A, Giordano A, Leoncini L (2003). Burkitt's lymphoma: new insights into molecular pathogenesis. J Clin Pathol 56: 188-192.
180. Bellan C, Lazzi S, Hummel M, Palummo N, de Santi M, Amato T, Nyagol J, Sabattini E, Lazure T, Pileri SA, Raphael M, Stein H, Tosi P, Leoncini L (2005). Immunoglobulin gene analysis reveals 2 distinct cells of origin for EBV-positive and EBV-negative Burkitt lymphomas. Blood 106: 1031-1036.
181. Beltrani G, Carlesimo OA (1966). [Telangiectasia macularis eruptiva perstans with mastocytosis]. Minerva Dermatol 41: 436-442.
182. Ben Ayed F, Halphen M, Najjar T, Boussene H, Jaafoura H, Bouguerra A, Ben Salah N, Mourali N, Ayed K, Ben Khalifa H (1989). Treatment of alpha chain disease. Results of a prospective study in 21 Tunisian patients by the Tunisian-French intestinal Lymphoma Study Group. Cancer 63: 1251-1256.
183. Ben Ezra J, Bailey A, Azumi N, Delsol G, Stroup R, Sheibani K, Rappaport H (1991). Malignant histiocytosis X. A distinct clinicopathologic entity. Cancer 68: 1050-1060.
184. Ben Ezra J, Burke JS, Swartz WG, Brownell MD, Brynes RK, Hill LR, Nathwani BN, Oken MM, Wolf BC, Woodruff R (1989). Small lymphocytic lymphoma: a clinicopathologic analysis of 268 cases. Blood 73: 579-587.
185. Bendriss-Vermare N, Chaperot L, Peoc'h M, Vanbervliet B, Jacob MC, Briere F, Bensa JC, Caux C, Plumas J (2004). In situ leukemic plasmacytoid dendritic cells pattern of chemokine receptors expression and in vitro migratory response. Leukemia 18: 1491-1498.
186. Bene MC, Bernier M, Casasnovas RO, Castoldi G, Doekharan D, van der HB, Knapp W, Lemez P, Ludwig WD, Matutes E, Orfao A, Schoch C, Sperling C, van't Veer MB (2001). Acute myeloid leukaemia M0: haematological, immunophenotypic and cytogenetic characteristics and their prognostic significance: an analysis in 241 patients. Br J Haematol 113: 737-745.
187. Bene MC, Castoldi G, Knapp W, Ludwig WD, Matutes E, Orfao A, van't Veer MB (1995). Proposals for the immunological classification of acute leukemias. European Group for the Immunological Characterization of Leukemias (EGIL). Leukemia 9: 1783-1786.
188. Benharroch D, Meguerian-Bedoyan Z, Lamant L, Amin C, Brugieres L, Terrier-Lacombe MJ, Haralambieva E, Pulford K, Pileri S, Morris SW, Mason DY, Delsol G (1998). ALK-positive lymphoma: a single disease with a broad spectrum of morphology. Blood 91: 2076-2084.
189. Bennett JM, Catovsky D, Daniel MT, Flandrin G, Galton DA, Gralnick H, Sultan C, Cox C (1994). The chronic myeloid leukaemias: guidelines for distinguishing chronic granulocytic, atypical chronic myeloid, and chronic myelomonocytic leukaemia. Proposals by the French-American-British Cooperative Leukaemia Group. Br J Haematol 87: 746-754
189A. Bennett JM, Catovsky D, Daniel MT, Flandrin G, Galton DA, Gralnick HR, Sultan C. (1976) Proposals for the classification of the acute leukaemias. French-American-British (FAB) co-operative group. Br J Haematol. 33: 451-458.
190. Bennett JM, Catovsky D, Daniel MT, Flandrin G, Galton DA, Gralnick HR, Sultan C (1982). Proposals for the classification of the myelodysplastic syndromes. Br J Haematol 51: 189-199.
191. Bennett JM, Catovsky D, Daniel MT, Flandrin G, Galton DA, Gralnick HR, Sultan C (1989). Proposals for the classification of chronic (mature) B and T lymphoid leukaemias. French-American-British (FAB) Cooperative Group. J Clin Pathol 42: 567-584.
192. Bentz M, Barth TF, Bruderlein S, Bock D, Schwerer MJ, Baudis M, Joos S, Viardot A, Feller AC, Muller-Hermelink HK, Lichter P, Dohner H, Moller P (2001). Gain of chromosome arm 9p is characteristic of primary mediastinal B-cell lymphoma (MBL): comprehensive molecular cytogenetic analysis and presentation of a novel MBL cell line. Genes Chromosomes Cancer 30: 393-401.
193. Beral V, Peterman T, Berkelman R, Jaffe H (1991). AIDS-associated non-Hodgkin lymphoma. Lancet 337: 805-809.
193A. Beran M, Luthra R, Kantarjian H, Estey E (2004). FLT3 mutation and response to intensive chemotherapy in young adult and elderly patients with normal karyotype. Leuk Res 28: 547-550.
194. Berger F, Felman P, Sonet A, Salles G, Bastion Y, Bryon PA, Coiffier B (1994). Nonfollicular small B-cell lymphomas: a heterogeneous group of patients with distinct clinical features and outcome. Blood 83: 2829-2835.
195. Berger F, Felman P, Thieblemont C, Pradier T, Baseggio L, Bryon PA, Salles G, Callet-Bauchu E, Coiffier B (2000). Non-MALT marginal zone B-cell lymphomas: a description of clinical presentation and outcome in 124 patients. Blood 95: 1950-1956.
196. Berglund M, Thunberg U, Amini RM, Book M, Roos G, Erlanson M, Linderoth J, Dictor M, Jerkeman M, Cavallin-Stahl E, Sundstrom C, Rehn-Eriksson S, Backlin C, Hagberg H, Rosenquist R, Enblad G (2005). Evaluation of immunophenotype in diffuse large B-cell lymphoma and its impact on prognosis. Mod Pathol 18: 1113-1120.
197. Berglund S, Zettervall O (1992). Incidence of polycythemia vera in a defined population. Eur J Haematol 48: 20-26.
198. Bergman R (1999). How useful are T-cell receptor gene rearrangement studies as an adjunct to the histopathologic diagnosis of mycosis fungoides? Am J Dermatopathol 21: 498-502.
199. Bergsagel PL, Kuehl WM (2001). Chromosome translocations in multiple myelo-

ma. Oncogene 20: 5611-5622.
200. Bergsagel PL, Kuehl WM (2005). Molecular pathogenesis and a consequent classification of multiple myeloma. J Clin Oncol 23: 6333-6338.
201. Bergsagel PL, Kuehl WM, Zhan F, Sawyer J, Barlogie B, Shaughnessy J, Jr. (2005). Cyclin D dysregulation: an early and unifying pathogenic event in multiple myeloma. Blood 106: 296-303.
202. Bernard A, Murphy SB, Melvin S, Bowman WP, Caillaud J, Lemerle J, Boumsell L (1982). Non-T, non-B lymphomas are rare in childhood and associated with cutaneous tumor. Blood 59: 549-554.
203. Bernasconi NL, Onai N, Lanzavecchia A (2003). A role for Toll-like receptors in acquired immunity: up-regulation of TLR9 by BCR triggering in naive B cells and constitutive expression in memory B cells. Blood 101: 4500-4504.
204. Bernengo MG, Novelli M, Quaglino P, Lisa F, De Matteis A, Savoia P, Cappello N, Fierro MT (2001). The relevance of the CD4+. CO26- subset in the identification of circulating Sezary cells. Br J Dermatol 144: 125-135.
205. Bernstein J, Dastugue N, Haas OA, Harbott J, Heerema NA, Huret JL, Landman-Parker J, LeBeau MM, Leonard C, Mann G, Pages MP, Perot C, Pirc-Danoewinata H, Roitzheim B, Rubin CM, Slociak M, Viguie F (2000). Nineteen cases of the t(1;22)(p13;q13) acute megakaryoblastic leukaemia of infants/children and a review of 39 cases: report from a t(1;22) study group. Leukemia 14: 216-218.
206. Berti E, Alessi E, Caputo R, Gianotti R, Delia D, Vezzoni P (1988). Reticulohistiocytoma of the dorsum. J Am Acad Dermatol 19: 259-272.
207. Berti E, Cerri A, Cavicchini S, Delia D, Soligo D, Alessi E, Caputo R (1991). Primary cutaneous gamma/delta T-cell lymphoma presenting as disseminated pagetoid reticulosis. J Invest Dermatol 96: 718-723.
208. Berti E, Gianotti R, Alessi E (1988). Unusual cutaneous histiocytosis expressing an intermediate immunophenotype between Langerhans' cells and dermal macrophages. Arch Dermatol 124: 1250-1253.
209. Berti E, Tomasini D, Vermeer MH, Meijer CJ, Alessi E, Willemze R (1999). Primary cutaneous CD8-positive epidermotropic cytotoxic T cell lymphomas. A distinct clinicopathological entity with an aggressive clinical behavior. Am J Pathol 155: 483-492.
210. Besses C, Cervantes F, Pereira A, Florensa L, Sole F, Hernandez-Boluda JC, Woessner S, Sans-Sabrafen J, Rozman C, Montserrat E (1999). Major vascular complications in essential thrombocythemia: a study of the predictive factors in a series of 148 patients. Leukemia 13: 150-154.
211. Besson C, Goubar A, Gabarre J, Rozenbaum W, Pialoux G, Chatelet FP, Katlama C, Charlotte F, Dupont B, Brousse N, Huerre M, Mikol J, Camparo P, Mokhtari K, Tulliez M, Salmon-Ceron D, Boue F, Costagliola D, Raphael M (2001). Changes in AIDS-related lymphoma since the era of highly active antiretroviral therapy. Blood 98: 2339-2344.
212. Bethel KJ, Sharpe RW (2003). Pathology of hairy-cell leukaemia. Best Pract Res Clin Haematol 16: 15-31.
213. Beylot-Barry M, Vergier B, Masquelier B, Bagot M, Joly P, Souteyrand P, Vaillant L, Avril MF, Franck N, Fraitag S, Delaunay M, Laroche L, Esteve E, Courville P, Dechelotte P, Beylot C, de Mascarel A, Wechsler J, Merlio JP (1999). The Spectrum of Cutaneous Lymphomas in HIV infection: a study of 21 cases. Am J Surg Pathol 23: 1208-1216.
214. Bhargava P, Rushin JM, Rusnock EJ, Hefter LG, Franks TJ, Sabnis SG, Travis WD (2007). Pulmonary light chain deposition disease: report of five cases and review of the literature. Am J Surg Pathol 31: 267-276.
215. Biagi JJ, Seymour JF (2002). Insights into the molecular pathogenesis of follicular lymphoma arising from analysis of geographic variation. Blood 99: 4265-4275.
216. Bienz M, Ludwig M, Leibundgut EO, Mueller BU, Ratschiller D, Solenthaler M, Fey MF, Pabst T (2005). Risk assessment in patients with acute myeloid leukemia and a normal karyotype. Clin Cancer Res 11: 1416-1424.
217. Biggar RJ, Chaturvedi AK, Goedert JJ, Engels EA (2007). AIDS-related cancer and severity of immunosuppression in persons with AIDS. J Natl Cancer Inst 99: 962-972.
218. Biggar RJ, Jaffe ES, Goedert JJ, Chaturvedi A, Pfeiffer R, Engels EA (2006). Hodgkin lymphoma and immunodeficiency in persons with HIV/AIDS. Blood 108: 3786-3791.
219. Bigoni R, Cuneo A, Milani R, Cavazzini F, Bardi A, Roberti MG, Agostini P, della PM, Specchia G, Rigolin GM, Castoldi G (2001). Multilineage involvement in the 5q- syndrome: a fluorescent in situ hybridization study on bone marrow smears. Haematologica 86: 375-381.
220. Bigouret V, Hoffmann T, Arlettaz L, Villard J, Colonna M, Ticheli A, Gratwohl A, Samii K, Chapuis B, Rufer N, Roosnek E (2003). Monoclonal T-cell expansions in asymptomatic individuals and in patients with large granular leukemia consist of cytotoxic effector T cells expressing the activating CD94:NKG2C/E and NKD2D killer cell receptors. Blood 101: 3198-3204.
221. Binet JL, Auquier A, Dighiero G, Chastang C, Piguet H, Goasguen J, Vaugier G, Potron G, Colona P, Oberling F, Thomas M, Tchernia G, Jacquillat C, Boivin P, Lesty C, Duault MT, Monconduit M, Belabbes S, Gremy F (1981). A new prognostic classification of chronic lymphocytic leukemia derived from a multivariate survival analysis. Cancer 48: 198-206.
222. Binet JL, Caligaris-Cappio F, Catovsky D, Cheson B, Davis T, Dighiero G, Dohner H, Hallek M, Hillmen P, Keating M, Montserrat E, Kipps TJ, Rai K (2006). Perspectives on the use of new diagnostic tools in the treatment of chronic lymphocytic leukemia. Blood 107: 859-861.
223. Birgegard G, Wide L (1992). Serum erythropoietin in the diagnosis of polycythaemia and after phlebotomy treatment. Br J Haematol 81: 603-606.
224. Birkeland SA, Hamilton-Dutoit S (2003). Is posttransplant lymphoproliferative disorder (PTLD) caused by any specific immunosuppressive drug or by the transplantation per se? Transplantation 76: 984-988.
225. Bitter MA, Neilly ME, Le Beau MM, Pearson MG, Rowley JD (1985). Rearrangements of chromosome 3 involving bands 3q21 and 3q26 are associated with normal or elevated platelet counts in acute nonlymphocytic leukemia. Blood 66: 1362-1370.
226. Bizzozero OJ, Jr., Johnson KG, Ciocco A (1966). Radiation-related leukemia in Hiroshima and Nagasaki, 1946-1964. I. Distribution, incidence and appearance time. N Engl J Med 274: 1095-1101.
227. Bloomfield CD, Archer KJ, Mrózek K, Lillington DM, Kaneko Y, Head DR, Dal Cin P, Raimondi SC (2002). 11q23 balanced chromosome aberrations in treatment-related myelodysplastic syndromes and acute leukemia: report from an International Workshop. Genes Chromosomes Cancer 33: 362-378.
228. Bloomfield CD, Lawrence D, Byrd JC, Carroll A, Pettenati MJ, Tantravahi R, Patil SR, Davey FR, Berg DT, Schiffer CA, Arthur DC, Mayer RJ (1998). Frequency of prolonged remission duration after high-dose cytarabine intensification in acute myeloid leukemia varies by cytogenetic subtype. Cancer Res 58: 4173-4179.
229. Bluestone JA, Khattri R, Sciammas R, Sperling AI (1995). TCR gamma delta cells: a specialized T-cell subset in the immune system. Annu Rev Cell Dev Biol 11:307-53.: 307-353.
230. Boerma EG, van Imhoff GW, Appel IM, Veeger NJ, Kluin PM, Kluin-Nelemans JC (2004). Gender and age-related differences in Burkitt lymphoma—epidemiological and clinical data from The Netherlands. Eur J Cancer 40: 2781-2787.
231. Bohm J, Schaefer HE (2002). Chronic neutrophilic leukaemia: 14 new cases of an uncommon myeloproliferative disease. J Clin Pathol 55: 862-864.
232. Bohn OL, Ruiz-Arguelles G, Navarro L, Saldivar J, Sanchez-Sosa S (2007). Cutaneous Langerhans cell sarcoma: a case report and review of the literature. Int J Hematol 85: 116-120.
233. Boissel N, Auclerc MF, Lheritier V, Perel Y, Thomas X, Leblanc T, Rousselot P, Cayuela JM, Gabert J, Fegueux N, Piguet C, Huguet-Rigal F, Berthou C, Boiron JM, Pautas C, Michel G, Fiere D, Leverger G, Dombret H, Baruchel A (2003). Should adolescents with acute lymphoblastic leukemia be treated as old children or young adults? Comparison of the French FRALLE-93 and LALA-94 trials. J Clin Oncol 21: 774-780.
233A. Boissel N, Leroy H, Brethon B, Philippe N, de Botton S, Auvrignon A, Raffoux E, Leblanc T, Thomas X, Hermine O, Quesnel B, Baruchel A, Leverger G, Dombret H, Preudhomme C (2006). Incidence and prognostic impact of c-Kit, FLT3, and Ras gene mutations in core binding factor acute myeloid leukemia (CBF-AML). Leukemia 20: 965-970.
233B. Boissel N, Renneville A, Biggio V, Philippe N, Thomas X, Cayuela JM, Terre C, Tigaud I, Castaigne S, Raffoux E, de Botton S, Fenaux P, Dombret H, Preudhomme C (2005). Prevalence, clinical profile, and prognosis of *NPM* mutations in AML with normal karyotype. Blood 106: 3618-3620.
234. Boissinot M, Garand R, Hamidou M, Hermouet S (2006). The JAK2-V617F mutation and essential thrombocythemia features in a subset of patients with refractory anemia with ring sideroblasts (RARS). Blood 108: 1781-1782.
235. Bonato M, Pittaluga S, Tierens A, Criel A, Verhoef G, Wlodarska I, Vanutysel L, Michaux L, Vandekerckhove P, Van den BH, Wolf-Peeters C (1998). Lymph node histology in typical and atypical chronic lymphocytic leukemia. Am J Surg Pathol 22: 49-56.
236. Bonetti F, Knowles DM, Chilosi M, Pisa R, Fiaccavento S, Rizzuto N, Zamboni G, Menestrina F, Fiore-Donati L (1985). A distinctive cutaneous malignant neoplasm expressing the Langerhans cell phenotype. Synchronous occurrence with B-chronic lymphocytic leukemia. Cancer 55: 2417-2425.
237. Bonifacio SL, Kitterman JA, Ursell PC (2003). Pseudomonas pneumonia in infants: an autopsy study. Hum Pathol 34: 929-938.
238. Bonzheim I, Geissinger E, Roth S, Zettl A, Marx A, Rosenwald A, Muller-Hermelink HK, Rudiger T (2004). Anaplastic large cell lymphomas lack the expression of T-cell receptor molecules or molecules of proximal T-cell receptor signaling. Blood 104: 3358-3360.
239. Booken N, Gratchev A, Utikal J, Weiss C, Yu X, Qadoumi M, Schmuth M, Sepp N, Nashan D, Rass K, Tuting T, Assaf C, Dippel E, Stadler R, Klemke CD, Goerdt S (2008). Sezary syndrome is a unique cutaneous T-cell lymphoma as identified by an expanded gene signature including diagnostic marker molecules CDO1 and DNM3. Leukemia 22: 393-399.
240. Booman M, Douwes J, Glas AM, Riemersma SA, Jordanova ES, Kok K, Rosenwald A, De Jong D, Schuuring E, Kluin PM (2006). Mechanisms and effects of loss of human leukocyte antigen class II expression in immune-privileged site-associated B-cell lymphoma. Clin Cancer Res 12: 2698-2705.
241. Borenstein J, Pezzella F, Gatter KC (2007). Plasmablastic lymphomas may occur as post-transplant lymphoproliferative disorders. Histopathology 51: 774-777.
242. Borowitz MJ, Croker BP, Metzgar RS (1983). Lymphoblastic lymphoma with the phenotype of common acute lymphoblastic leukemia. Am J Clin Pathol 79: 387-391.
243. Borowitz MJ, Guenther KL, Shults KE, Stelzer GT (1993). Immunophenotyping of acute leukemia by flow cytometric analysis. Use of CD45 and right-angle light scatter to gate on leukemic blasts in three-color analysis. Am J Clin Pathol 100: 534-540.
244. Borowitz MJ, Hunger SP, Carroll AJ, Shuster JJ, Pullen DJ, Steuber CP, Cleary ML (1993). Predictability of the t(1;19)(q23;p13) from surface antigen phenotype: implications for screening cases of childhood acute lymphoblastic leukemia for molecular analysis: a Pediatric Oncology Group study. Blood 82: 1086-1091.
245. Borowitz MJ, Rubnitz J, Nash M, Pullen DJ, Camitta B (1998). Surface antigen phenotype can predict TEL-AML1 rearrangement in childhood B-precursor ALL: a Pediatric Oncology Group study. Leukemia 12: 1764-1770.
246. Bosch F, Campo E, Jares P, Pittaluga S, Munoz J, Nayach I, Piris MA, Dewolf-Peeters C, Jaffe ES, Rozman C (1995). Increased expression of the PRAD-1/CCND1 gene in hairy cell leukaemia. Br J Haematol 91: 1025-1030.
247. Bosch F, Lopez-Guillermo A, Campo E, Ribera JM, Conde E, Piris MA, Vallespi T, Woessner S, Montserrat E (1998). Mantle cell lymphoma: presenting features, response to therapy, and prognostic factors. Cancer 82: 567-575.
248. Bosga-Bouwer AG, van den Berg A, Haralambieva E, De Jong D, Boonstra R, Kluin P, van den Berg E, Poppema S (2006). Molecular, cytogenetic, and immunophenotypic characterization of follicular lymphoma grade 3B; a separate entity or part of the spectrum of diffuse large B-cell lymphoma or follicular lymphoma? Hum Pathol 37: 528-533.
249. Bosga-Bouwer AG, van Imhoff GW, Boonstra R, van der Veen A, Haralambieva E, van den Berg A, de Jong B, Krause V, Palmer MC, Coupland R, Kluin PM, van den Berg E, Poppema S (2003). Follicular lymphoma grade 3B includes 3 cytogenetically defined subgroups with primary t(14;18), 3q27, or other translocations: t(14;18) and 3q27 are mutually exclusive. Blood 101: 1149-1154.
250. Boshoff C, Weiss RA (2001). Epidemiology and pathogenesis of Kaposi's sarcoma-associated herpesvirus. Philos Trans R Soc Lond B Biol Sci 356: 517-534.
251. Bouabdallah R, Mounier N, Guettier C, Molina T, Ribrag V, Thieblemont C, Sonet A, Delmer A, Belhadj K, Gaulard P, Gisselbrecht C, Xerri L (2003). T-cell/histiocyte-rich large B-cell lymphomas and classical diffuse large B-cell lymphomas have similar outcome after chemotherapy: a matched-control analysis. J Clin Oncol 21: 1271-1277.
252. Boudova L, Torlakovic E, Delabie J, Reimer P, Pfistner B, Wiedenmann S, Diehl V, Muller-Hermelink HK, Rudiger T (2003). Nodular lymphocyte-predominant Hodgkin lym-

phoma with nodules resembling T-cell/histiocyte-rich B-cell lymphoma: differential diagnosis between nodular lymphocyte-predominant Hodgkin lymphoma and T-cell/histiocyte-rich B-cell lymphoma. Blood 102: 3753-3758.
253. Boue F, Gabarre J, Gisselbrecht C, Reynes J, Cheret A, Bonnet F, Billaud E, Raphael M, Lancar R, Costagliola D (2006). Phase II trial of CHOP plus rituximab in patients with HIV-associated non-Hodgkin's lymphoma. J Clin Oncol 24: 4123-4128.
254. Boulanger E, Hermine O, Fermand JP, Radford-Weiss I, Brousse N, Meignin V, Gessain A (2004). Human herpesvirus 8 (HHV-8)-associated peritoneal primary effusion lymphoma (PEL) in two HIV-negative elderly patients. Am J Hematol 76: 88-91.
255. Boulland ML, Wechsler J, Bagot M, Pulford K, Kanavaros P, Gaulard P (2000). Primary CD30-positive cutaneous T-cell lymphomas and lymphomatoid papulosis frequently express cytotoxic proteins. Histopathology 36: 136-144.
256. Boultwood J, Fidler C, Strickson AJ, Watkins F, Gama S, Kearney L, Tosi S, Kasprzyk A, Cheng JF, Jaju RJ, Wainscoat JS (2002). Narrowing and genomic annotation of the commonly deleted region of the 5q- syndrome. Blood 99: 4638-4641.
257. Boultwood J, Lewis S, Wainscoat JS (1994). The 5q-syndrome. Blood 84: 3253-3260.
258. Bourquin JP, Subramanian A, Langebrake C, Reinhardt D, Bernard O, Ballerini P, Baruchel A, Cave H, Dastugue N, Hasle H, Kaspers GL, Lessard M, Michaux L, Vyas P, van Wering E, Zwaan CM, Golub TR, Orkin SH (2006). Identification of distinct molecular phenotypes in acute megakaryoblastic leukemia by gene expression profiling. Proc Natl Acad Sci U S A 103: 3339-3344.
259. Bousquet M, Quelen C, De M, V, Duchayne E, Roquefeuil B, Delsol G, Laurent G, Dastugue N, Brousset P (2005). The t(8;9)(p22;p24) translocation in atypical chronic myeloid leukaemia yields a new PCM1-JAK2 fusion gene. Oncogene 24: 7248-7252.
260. Bowen D, Culligan D, Jowitt S, Kelsey S, Mufti G, Oscier D, Parker J (2003). Guidelines for the diagnosis and therapy of adult myelodysplastic syndromes. Br J Haematol 120: 187-200.
261. Braaten KM, Betensky RA, de Leval L, Okada Y, Hochberg FH, Louis DN, Harris NL, Batchelor TT (2003). BCL-6 expression predicts improved survival in patients with primary central nervous system lymphoma. Clin Cancer Res 9: 1063-1069.
261A. Bräuninger A, Hansmann ML, Strickler JG, Dummer R, Burg G, Rajewsky K, Küppers R (1999). Identification of common germinal-center B-cell precursors in two patients with both Hodgkin's disease and non-Hodgkin's lymphoma. NEJM 340:1239-1247.
262. Braeuninger A, Kuppers R, Strickler JG, Wacker HH, Rajewsky K, Hansmann ML (1997). Hodgkin and Reed-Sternberg cells in lymphocyte predominant Hodgkin disease represent clonal populations of germinal center-derived tumor B cells. Proc Natl Acad Sci U S A 94: 9337-9342.
263. Brauninger A, Kuppers R, Spieker T, Siebert R, Strickler JG, Schlegelberger B, Rajewsky K, Hansmann ML (1999). Molecular analysis of single B cells from T-cell-rich B-cell lymphoma shows the derivation of the tumor cells from mutating germinal center B cells and exemplifies means by which immunoglobulin genes are modified in germinal center B cells. Blood 93: 2679-2687.
264. Braziel RM, Arber DA, Slovak ML, Gulley ML, Spier C, Kjeldsberg C, Unger J, Miller TP, Tubbs R, Leith C, Fisher RI, Grogan TM (2001). The Burkitt-like lymphomas: a Southwest Oncology Group study delineating phenotypic, genotypic, and clinical features. Blood 97: 3713-3720.
265. Brcic L, Vuletic LB, Stepan J, Bonevski A, Jakovljevic G, Gasparov S, Marjanovic K, Seiwerth S (2007). Mast-cell sarcoma of the tibia. J Clin Pathol 60: 424-425.
266. Breccia M, Biondo F, Latagliata R, Carmosino I, Mandelli F, Alimena G (2006). Identification of risk factors in atypical chronic myeloid leukemia. Haematologica 91: 1566-1568.
267. Breccia M, Carmosino I, Biondo F, Mancini M, Russo E, Latagliata R, Alimena G (2006). Usefulness and prognostic impact on survival of WHO reclassification in FAB low risk myelodyplastic syndromes. Leuk Res 30: 178-182.
268. Breccia M, Mandelli F, Petti MC, D'Andrea M, Pescarmona E, Pileri SA, Carmosino I, Russo E, De Fabritiis P, Alimena G (2004). Clinico-pathological characteristics of myeloid sarcoma at diagnosis and during follow-up: report of 12 cases from a single institution. Leuk Res 28: 1165-1169.
269. Brecher M, Banks PM (1990). Hodgkin's disease variant of Richter's syndrome. Report of eight cases. Am J Clin Pathol 93: 333-339.
270. Briere JB (2006). Budd-Chiari syndrome and portal vein thrombosis associated with myeloproliferative disorders: diagnosis and management. Semin Thromb Hemost 32: 208-218.
271. Brink DS (2006). Transient leukemia (transient myeloproliferative disorder, transient abnormal myelopoiesis) of Down syndrome. Adv Anat Pathol 13: 256-262.
272. Brito-Babapulle V, Catovsky D (1991). Inversions and tandem translocations involving chromosome 14q11 and 14q32 in T-prolymphocytic leukemia and T-cell leukemias in patients with ataxia telangiectasia. Cancer Genet Cytogenet 55: 1-9.
273. Brito-Babapulle V, Hamoudi R, Matutes E, Watson S, Kaczmarek P, Maljaie H, Catovsky D (2000). p53 allele deletion and protein accumulation occurs in the absence of p53 gene mutation in T-prolymphocytic leukaemia and Sezary syndrome. Br J Haematol 110: 180-187.
274. Brito-Babapulle V, Pittman S, Melo JV, Pomfret M, Catovsky D (1987). Cytogenetic studies on prolymphocytic leukemia. 1. B-cell prolymphocytic leukemia. Hematol Pathol 1: 27-33.
275. Brittinger G, Bartels H, Common H, Duhmke E, Fulle HH, Gunzer U, Gyenes T, Heinz R, Konig E, Meusers P (1984). Clinical and prognostic relevance of the Kiel classification of non-Hodgkin lymphomas results of a prospective multicenter study by the Kiel Lymphoma Study Group. Hematol Oncol 2: 269-306.
276. Brizard A, Huret JL, Lamotte F, Guilhot F, Benz-Lemoine E, Giraud C, Desmarest MC, Tanzer J (1989). Three cases of myelodysplastic-myeloproliferative disorder with abnormal chromatin clumping in granulocytes. Br J Haematol 72: 294-295.
277. Brody JP, Allen S, Schulman P, Sun T, Chan WC, Friedman HD, Teichberg S, Koduru P, Cone RW, Loughran TP, Jr. (1995). Acute agranular CD4-positive natural killer cell leukemia. Comprehensive clinicopathologic studies including virologic and in vitro culture with inducing agents. Cancer 75: 2474-2483.
278. Brouet JC, Sasportes M, Flandrin G, Preud'Homme JL, Seligmann M (1975). Chronic lymphocytic leukaemia of T-cell origin. Immunological and clinical evaluation in eleven patients. Lancet 2: 890-893.
279. Brousset P, Rochaix P, Chittal S, Rubie H, Robert A, Delsol G (1993). High incidence of Epstein-Barr virus detection in Hodgkin's disease and absence of detection in anaplastic large-cell lymphoma in children. Histopathology 23: 189-191.
280. Brousset P, Schlaifer D, Meggetto F, Bachmann E, Rothenberger S, Pris J, Delsol G, Knecht H (1994). Persistence of the same viral strain in early and late relapses of Epstein-Barr virus-associated Hodgkin's disease. Blood 84: 2447-2451.
281. Brown L, Cheng JT, Chen Q, Siciliano MJ, Crist W, Buchanan G, Baer R (1990). Site-specific recombination of the tal-1 gene is a common occurrence in human T cell leukemia. EMBO J 9: 3343-3351.
282. Brown LM, Linet MS, Greenberg RS, Silverman DT, Hayes RB, Swanson GM, Schwartz AG, Schoenberg JB, Pottern LM, Fraumeni JF, Jr. (1999). Multiple myeloma and family history of cancer among blacks and whites in the U.S. Cancer 85: 2385-2390.
283. Brown P, McIntyre E, Rau R, Meshinchi S, Lacayo N, Dahl G, Alonzo TA, Chang M, Arceci RJ, Small D (2007). The incidence and clinical significance of nucleophosmin mutations in childhood AML. Blood 110: 979-985.
284. Brown SL, Greene MH, Gershon SK, Edwards ET, Braun MM (2002). Tumor necrosis factor antagonist therapy and lymphoma development: twenty-six cases reported to the Food and Drug Administration. Arthritis Rheum 46: 3151-3158.
285. Brugieres L, Deley MC, Pacquement H, Meguerian-Bedoyan Z, Terrier-Lacombe MJ, Robert A, Pondarre C, Leverger G, Devalck C, Rodary C, Delsol G, Hartmann O (1998). CD30(+) anaplastic large-cell lymphoma in children: analysis of 82 patients enrolled in two consecutive studies of the French Society of Pediatric Oncology. Blood 92: 3591-3598.
286. Brugnoni D, Airo P, Rossi G, Bettinardi A, Simon HU, Garza L, Tosoni C, Cattaneo R, Blaser K, Tucci A (1996). A case of hypereosinophilic syndrome is associated with the expansion of a CD3-CD4+ T-cell population able to secrete large amounts of interleukin-5. Blood 87: 1416-1422.
287. Brunning RD, McKenna RW (1994). Mast cell disease. In: Atlas of tumor pathology. Tumors of the bone marrow. Atlas of tumor pathology. Tumors of the bone marrow. Armed Forces Institute of Pathology: Washington, D.C., pp. 419-434.
288. Brunning RD, McKenna RW (1994). Plasma cell dyscrasias and related disorders. In: Atlas of Tumor Pathology. Armed Forces Institute of Pathology, ed. Washington, D.C., pp. 323-367.
289. Brunning RD, McKenna RW (1994). Tumors of the bone marrow. Armed Forces Institute of Pathology: Washington, D.C.
290. Brunning RD, McKenna RW, Rosai J, Parkin JL, Risdall R (1983). Systemic mastocytosis. Extracutaneous manifestations. Am J Surg Pathol 7: 425-438.
291. Brunstein CG, Weisdorf DJ, DeFor T, Barker JN, Tolar J, van Burik JA, Wagner JE (2006). Marked increased risk of Epstein-Barr virus-related complications with the addition of antithymocyte globulin to a nonmyeloablative conditioning prior to unrelated umbilical cord blood transplantation. Blood 108: 2874-2880.
292. Buesche G, Ganser A, Schlegelberger B, von Neuhoff N, Gadzicki D, Hecker H, Bock O, Frye B, Kreipe H (2007). Marrow fibrosis and its relevance during imatinib treatment of chronic myeloid leukemia. Leukemia 21: 2420-2427.
293. Buesche G, Hehlmann R, Hecker H, Heimpel H, Heinze B, Schmeil A, Pfirrmann M, Gomez G, Tobler A, Herrmann H, Kappler M, Hasford J, Buhr T, Kreipe HH, Georgii A (2003). Marrow fibrosis, indicator of therapy failure in chronic myeloid leukemia - prospective long-term results from a randomized-controlled trial. Leukemia 17: 2444-2453.
294. Buettner M, Greiner A, Avramidou A, Jack HM, Niedobitek G (2005). Evidence of abortive plasma cell differentiation in Hodgkin and Reed-Sternberg cells of classical Hodgkin lymphoma. Hematol Oncol 23: 127-132.
295. Buhr T, Busche G, Choritz H, Langer F, Kreipe H (2003). Evolution of myelofibrosis in chronic idiopathic myelofibrosis as evidenced in sequential bone marrow biopsy specimens. Am J Clin Pathol 119: 152-158.
296. Buhr T, Choritz H, Georgii A (1992). The impact of megakaryocyte proliferation of the evolution of myelofibrosis. Histological follow-up study in 186 patients with chronic myeloid leukaemia. Virchows Arch A Pathol Anat Histopathol 420: 473-478.
297. Buhr T, Georgii A, Choritz H (1993). Myelofibrosis in chronic myeloproliferative disorders. Incidence among subtypes according to the Hannover Classification. Pathol Res Pract 189: 121-132.
298. Bunn PA, Jr., Schechter GP, Jaffe E, Blayney D, Young RC, Matthews MJ, Blattner W, Broder S, Robert-Guroff M, Gallo RC (1983). Clinical course of retrovirus-associated adult T-cell lymphoma in the United States. N Engl J Med 309: 257-264.
299. Burg G, Kempf W, Kazakov DV, Dummer R, Frosch PJ, Lange-Ionescu S, Nishikawa T, Kadin ME (2003). Pyogenic lymphoma of the skin: a peculiar variant of primary cutaneous neutrophil-rich CD30+ anaplastic large-cell lymphoma. Clinicopathological study of four cases and review of the literature. Br J Dermatol 148: 580-586.
300. Burke AP, Andriko JA, Virmani R (2000). Anaplastic large cell lymphoma (CD 30+), T-phenotype, in the heart of an HIV-positive man. Cardiovasc Pathol 9: 49-52.
301. Burkitt DP (1958). A sarcoma involving the jaws in African children. Br J Surg 1958; 46: 218. Br J Surg 46: 218-223.
302. Burkitt DP (1970). General features and facial tumours. In: Burkitt's lymphoma. Burkitt DP, Wright DH, eds. Livingstone: Edinburgh and London.
303. Busque L, Gilliland DG, Prchal JT, Sieff CA, Weinstein HJ, Sokol JM, Belickova M, Wayne AS, Zuckerman KS, Sokol L (1995). Clonality in juvenile chronic myelogenous leukemia. Blood 85: 21-30.
303A. Butcher EC (1990). Cellular and molecular mechanisms that direct leukocyte traffic. Am J Pathol 136:3-11.
304. Buxbaum J (1992). Mechanisms of disease: monoclonal immunoglobulin deposition. Amyloidosis, light chain deposition disease, and light and heavy chain deposition disease. Hematol Oncol Clin North Am 6: 323-346.
305. Buxbaum J, Gallo G (1999). Nonamyloidotic monoclonal immunoglobulin deposition disease. Light-chain, heavy-chain, and light- and heavy-chain deposition diseases. Hematol Oncol Clin North Am 13: 1235-1248.
306. Byrd JC, Mrózek K, Dodge RK, Carroll AJ, Edwards CG, Arthur DC, Pettenati MJ, Patil SR, Rao KW, Watson MS, Koduru PR, Moore JO, Stone RM, Mayer RJ, Feldman EJ, Davey FR, Schiffer CA, Larson RA, Bloomfield CD (2002). Pretreatment cytogenetic abnormalities are predictive of induction success, cumulative incidence of relapse, and overall survival in adult patients with de novo acute myeloid leukemia: results from Cancer and Leukemia Group B (CALGB 8461). Blood 100: 4325-4336.

307. Cabrera ME, Eizuru Y, Itoh T, Koriyama C, Tashiro Y, Ding S, Rey S, Akiba S, Corvalan A (2007). Nasal natural killer/T-cell lymphoma and its association with type "i"/XhoI loss strain Epstein-Barr virus in Chile. J Clin Pathol 60: 656-660.

308. Caillard S, Dharnidharka V, Agodoa L, Bohen E, Abbott K (2005). Posttransplant lymphoproliferative disorders after renal transplantation in the United States in era of modern immunosuppression. Transplantation 80: 1233-1243.

309. Caillard S, Lelong C, Pessione F, Moulin B (2006). Post-transplant lymphoproliferative disorders occurring after renal transplantation in adults: report of 230 cases from the French Registry. Am J Transplant 6: 2735-2742.

310. Cairo MS, Gerrard M, Sposto R, Auperin A, Pinkerton CR, Michon J, Weston C, Perkins SL, Raphael M, McCarthy K, Patte C (2007). Results of a randomized international study of high-risk central nervous system B non-Hodgkin lymphoma and B acute lymphoblastic leukemia in children and adolescents. Blood 109: 2736-2743.

310A. Cairoli R, Beghini A, Grillo G, Nadali G, Elice F, Ripamonti CB, Colapietro P, Nichelatti M, Pezzetti L, Lunghi M, Cuneo A, Viola A, Ferrara F, Lazzarino M, Rodeghiero F, Pizzolo G, Larizza L, and Morra E (2006). Prognostic impact of c-KIT mutations in core binding factor leukemias: an Italian retrospective study. Blood 107: 3463-3468.

311. Calaminici M, Piper K, Lee AM, Norton AJ (2004). CD23 expression in mediastinal large B-cell lymphomas. Histopathology 45: 619-624.

312. Caldwell GG, Kelley DB, Heath CW, Jr., Zack M (1984). Polycythemia vera among participants of a nuclear weapons test. JAMA 252: 662-664.

313. Caligiuri MA, Strout MP, Lawrence D, Arthur DC, Baer MR, Yu F, Knuutila S, Mrózek K, Oberkircher AR, Marcucci G, de la Chapelle A, Elonen E, Block AW, Rao PN, Herzig GP, Powell BL, Ruutu T, Schiffer CA, Bloomfield CD (1998). Rearrangement of ALL1 (MLL) in acute myeloid leukemia with normal cytogenetics. Cancer Res 58: 55-59.

314. Caligiuri MA, Strout MP, Schichman SA, Mrózek K, Arthur DC, Herzig GP, Baer MR, Schiffer CA, Heinonen K, Knuutila S, Nousiainen T, Ruutu T, Block AW, Schulman P, Pedersen-Bjergaard J, Croce CM, Bloomfield CD (1996). Partial tandem duplication of ALL1 as a recurrent molecular defect in acute myeloid leukemia with trisomy 11. Cancer Res 56: 1418-1425.

315. Calin GA, Ferracin M, Cimmino A, Di Leva G, Shimizu M, Wojcik SE, Iorio MV, Visone R, Sever NI, Fabbri M, Iuliano R, Palumbo T, Pichiorri F, Roldo C, Garzon R, Sevignani C, Rassenti L, Alder H, Volinia S, Liu CG, Kipps TJ, Negrini M, Croce CM (2005). A MicroRNA signature associated with prognosis and progression in chronic lymphocytic leukemia. N Engl J Med 353: 1793-1801.

316. Callan MF (2004). Epstein-Barr virus, arthritis, and the development of lymphoma in arthritis patients. Curr Opin Rheumatol 16: 399-405.

317. Callen JP (2007). Complications and adverse reactions in the use of newer biologic agents. Semin Cutan Med Surg 26: 6-14.

318. Callens C, Chevret S, Cayuela JM, Cassinat B, Raffoux E, de Botton S, Thomas X, Guerci A, Fegueux N, Pigneux A, Stoppa AM, Lamy T, Rigal-Huguet F, Vekhoff A, Meyer-Monard S, Ferrand A, Sanz M, Chomienne C, Fenaux P, Dombret H (2005). Prognostic implication of FLT3 and Ras gene mutations in patients with acute promyelocytic leukemia (APL): a retrospective study from the European APL Group. Leukemia 19: 1153-1160.

319. Callet-Bauchu E, Baseggio L, Felman P, Traverse-Glehen A, Berger F, Morel D, Gazzo S, Poncet C, Thieblemont C, Coiffier B, Magaud JP, Salles G (2005). Cytogenetic analysis delineates a spectrum of chromosomal changes that can distinguish non-MALT marginal zone B-cell lymphomas among mature B-cell entities: a description of 103 cases. Leukemia 19: 1818-1823.

320. Camacho E, Hernandez L, Hernandez S, Tort F, Bellosillo B, Bea S, Bosch F, Montserrat E, Cardesa A, Fernandez PL, Campo E (2002). ATM gene inactivation in mantle cell lymphoma mainly occurs by truncating mutations and missense mutations involving the phosphatidylinositol-3 kinase domain and is associated with increasing numbers of chromosomal imbalances. Blood 99: 238-244.

321. Camacho FI, Algara P, Mollejo M, Garcia JF, Montalban C, Martinez N, Sanchez-Beato M, Piris MA (2003). Nodal marginal zone lymphoma: a heterogeneous tumor: a comprehensive analysis of a series of 27 cases. Am J Surg Pathol 27: 762-771.

322. Camacho FI, Algara P, Rodriguez A, Ruiz-Ballesteros E, Mollejo M, Martinez N, Martinez-Climent JA, Gonzalez M, Mateo M, Caleo A, Sanchez-Beato M, Menarguez J, Garcia-Conde J, Sole F, Campo E, Piris MA (2003). Molecular heterogeneity in MCL defined by the use of specific VH genes and the frequency of somatic mutations. Blood 101: 4042-4046.

323. Camacho FI, Garcia JF, Cigudosa JC, Mollejo M, Algara P, Ruiz-Ballesteros E, Gonzalvo P, Martin P, Perez-Seoane C, Sanchez-Garcia J, Piris MA (2004). Aberrant Bcl6 protein expression in mantle cell lymphoma. Am J Surg Pathol 28: 1051-1056.

324. Camilleri-Broet S, Criniere E, Broet P, Delwail V, Mokhtari K, Moreau A, Kujas M, Raphael M, Iraqi W, Sautes-Fridman C, Colombat P, Hoang-Xuan K, Martin A (2006). A uniform activated B-cell-like immunophenotype might explain the poor prognosis of primary central nervous system lymphomas: analysis of 83 cases. Blood 107: 190-196.

325. Camilleri-Broet S, Davi F, Feuillard J, Seilhean D, Michiels JF, Brousset P, Epardeau B, Navratil E, Mokhtari K, Bourgeois C, Marelle L, Raphael M, Hauw JJ (1997). AIDS-related primary brain lymphomas: histopathologic and immunohistochemical study of 51 cases. The French Study Group for HIV-Associated Tumors. Hum Pathol 28: 367-374.

326. Campana D, Coustan-Smith E (2004). Minimal residual disease studies by flow cytometry in acute leukemia. Acta Haematol 112: 8-15.

327. Campbell J, Seymour JF, Matthews J, Wolf M, Stone J, Juneja S (2006). The prognostic impact of bone marrow involvement in patients with diffuse large cell lymphoma varies according to the degree of infiltration and presence of discordant marrow involvement. Eur J Haematol 76: 473-480.

328. Campo E, Miquel R, Krenacs L, Sorbara L, Raffeld M, Jaffe ES (1999). Primary nodal marginal zone lymphomas of splenic and MALT type. Am J Surg Pathol 23: 59-68.

329. Campo E, Raffeld M, Jaffe ES (1999). Mantle-cell lymphoma. Semin Hematol 36: 115-127.

330. Canioni D, Arnulf B, Asso-Bonnet M, Raphael M, Brousse N (2001). Nasal natural killer lymphoma associated with Epstein-Barr virus in a patient infected with human immunodeficiency virus. Arch Pathol Lab Med 125: 660-662.

331. Canioni D, Jabado N, Macintyre E, Patey N, Emile JF, Brousse N (2001). Lymphoproliferative disorders in children with primary immunodeficiencies: immunological status may be more predictive of the outcome than other criteria. Histopathology 38: 146-159.

332. Capello D, Cerri M, Muti G, Berra E, Oreste P, Deambrogi C, Rossi D, Dotti G, Conconi A, Vigano M, Magrini U, Ippoliti G, Morra E, Gloghini A, Rambaldi A, Paulli M, Carbone A, Gaidano G (2003). Molecular histogenesis of posttransplantation lymphoproliferative disorders. Blood 102: 3775-3785.

333. Capello D, Cerri M, Muti G, Lucioni M, Oreste P, Gloghini A, Berra E, Deambrogi C, Franceschetti S, Rossi D, Alabiso O, Morra E, Rambaldi A, Carbone A, Paulli M, Gaidano G (2006). Analysis of immunoglobulin heavy and light chain variable genes in post-transplant lymphoproliferative disorders. Hematol Oncol 24: 212-219.

334. Capello D, Rossi D, Gaidano G (2005). Post-transplant lymphoproliferative disorders: molecular basis of disease histogenesis and pathogenesis. Hematol Oncol 23: 61-67.

335. Carbone A (1997). The Spectrum of AIDS-Related Lymphoproliferative Disorders. Adv Clin Path 1: 13-19.

336. Carbone A (2003). Emerging pathways in the development of AIDS-related lymphomas. Lancet Oncol 4: 22-29.

337. Carbone A, Gloghini A (2005). AIDS-related lymphomas: from pathogenesis to pathology. Br J Haematol 130: 662-670.

337A. Carbone PP, Kaplan HS, Musshoff K, Smithers DW, Tubiana M (1971). Report of the committee on Hodgkin's Disease Staging Classification. Cancer Res 31: 1860-1861.

338. Carbonell F, Swansbury J, Min T, Matutes E, Farahat N, Buccheri V, Morilla R, Secker-Walker L, Catovsky D (1996). Cytogenetic findings in acute biphenotypic leukaemia. Leukemia 10: 1283-1287.

338A. Care RS, Valk PJ, Goodeve AC, Abu-Duhier FM, Geertsma-Kleinekoort WM, Wilson GA, Gari MA, Peake IR, Lowenberg B, Reilly JT (2003). Incidence and prognosis of c-KIT and FLT3 mutations in core binding factor (CBF) acute myeloid leukaemias. Br J Haematol 121: 775-777.

339. Carney JP, Maser RS, Olivares H, Davis EM, Le Beau M, Yates JR, III, Hays L, Morgan WF, Petrini JH (1998). The hMre11/hRad50 protein complex and Nijmegen breakage syndrome: linkage of double-strand break repair to the cellular DNA damage response. Cell 93: 477-486.

340. Carreras J, Villamor N, Colomo L, Moreno C, Cajal S, Crespo M, Tort F, Bosch F, Lopez-Guillermo A, Colomer D, Montserrat E, Campo E (2005). Immunohistochemical analysis of ZAP-70 expression in B-cell lymphoid neoplasms. J Pathol 205: 507-513.

341. Carroll A, Civin C, Schneider N, Dahl G, Pappo A, Bowman P, Emami A, Gross S, Alvarado C, Phillips C et al. (1991). The t(1;22) (p13;q13) is nonrandom and restricted to infants with acute megakaryoblastic leukemia: a Pediatric Oncology Group Study. Blood 78: 748-752.

342. Castaigne S, Chomienne C, Daniel MT, Ballerini P, Berger R, Fenaux P, Degos L (1990). All-trans retinoic acid as a differentiation therapy for acute promyelocytic leukemia. I. Clinical results. Blood 76: 1704-1709.

343. Castellano-Sanchez AA, Li S, Qian J, Lagoo A, Weir E, Brat DJ (2004). Primary central nervous system posttransplant lymphoproliferative disorders. Am J Clin Pathol 121: 246-253.

344. Castor A, Nilsson L, Astrand-Grundstrom I, Buitenhuis M, Ramirez C, Anderson K, Strombeck B, Garwicz S, Bekassy AN, Schmiegelow K, Lausen B, Hokland P, Lehmann S, Juliusson G, Johansson B, Jacobsen SE (2005). Distinct patterns of hematopoietic stem cell involvement in acute lymphoblastic leukemia. Nat Med 11: 630-637.

345. Castro-Malaspina H, Schaison G, Passe S, Pasquier A, Berger R, Bayle-Weisgerber C, Miller D, Seligmann M, Bernard J (1984). Subacute and chronic myelomonocytic leukemia in children (juvenile CML). Clinical and hematologic observations, and identification of prognostic factors. Cancer 54: 675-686.

346. Cattoretti G, Chang CC, Cechova K, Zhang J, Ye BH, Falini B, Louie DC, Offit K, Chaganti RS, Dalla-Favera R (1995). BCL-6 protein is expressed in germinal-center B cells. Blood 86: 45-53.

347. Cattoretti G, Villa A, Vezzoni P, Giardini R, Lombardi L, Rilke F (1990). Malignant histiocytosis. A phenotypic and genotypic investigation. Am J Pathol 136: 1009-1019.

348. Cawley JC (2006). The pathophysiology of the hairy cell. Hematol Oncol Clin North Am 20: 1011-1021.

349. Cazals-Hatem D, Andre M, Mounier N, Copin MC, Divine M, Berger F, Bosly A, Kerneis Y, Briere J, Quesnel B, Diebold J, Gaulard P (2001). Pathologic and clinical features of 77 Hodgkin's lymphoma patients treated in a lymphoma protocol (LNH87): a GELA study. Am J Surg Pathol 25: 297-306.

350. Cazals-Hatem D, Lepage E, Brice P, Ferrant A, d'Agay MF, Baumelou E, Briere J, Blanc M, Gaulard P, Biron P, Schlaifer D, Diebold J, Audouin J (1996). Primary mediastinal large B-cell lymphoma. A clinicopathologic study of 141 cases compared with 916 non-mediastinal large B-cell lymphomas, a GELA ("Groupe d'Etude des Lymphomes de l'Adulte") study. Am J Surg Pathol 20: 877-888.

351. Cazzaniga G, Dell'Oro MG, Mecucci C, Giarin E, Masetti R, Rossi V, Locatelli F, Martelli MF, Basso G, Pession A, Biondi A, Falini B (2005). Nucleophosmin mutations in childhood acute myelogenous leukemia with normal karyotype. Blood 106: 1419-1422.

352. Cazzola M, Invernizzi R, Bergamaschi G, Levi S, Corsi B, Travaglino E, Rolandi V, Biasiotto G, Drysdale J, Arosio P (2003). Mitochondrial ferritin expression in erythroid cells from patients with sideroblastic anemia. Blood 101: 1996-2000.

353. Cazzola M, Malcovati L (2005). Myelodysplastic syndromes—coping with ineffective hematopoiesis. N Engl J Med 352: 536-538.

354. Ceesay MM, Lea NC, Ingram W, Westwood NB, Gaken J, Mohamedali A, Cervera J, Germing U, Gattermann N, Giagounidis A, Garcia-Casado Z, Sanz G, Mufti GJ (2006). The JAK2 V617F mutation is rare in RARS but common in RARS-T. Leukemia 20: 2060-2061.

355. Cehreli C, Undar B, Akkoc N, Onvural B, Altungoz O (1994). Coexistence of chronic neutrophilic leukemia with light chain myeloma. Acta Haematol 91: 32-34.

356. Cella M, Facchetti F, Lanzavecchia A, Colonna M (2000). Plasmacytoid dendritic cells activated by influenza virus and CD40L drive a potent TH1 polarization. Nat Immunol 1: 305-310.

357. Cella M, Jarrossay D, Facchetti F, Alebardi O, Nakajima H, Lanzavecchia A, Colonna M (1999). Plasmacytoid monocytes migrate to inflamed lymph nodes and produce large amounts of type I interferon. Nat Med 5: 919-923.

358. Cellier C, Delabesse E, Helmer C, Patey N, Matuchansky C, Jabri B, Macintyre E, Cerf-Bensussan N, Brousse N (2000). Refractory sprue, coeliac disease, and enteropathy-associated T-cell lymphoma. French Coeliac Disease Study Group. Lancet 356: 203-208.

359. Cellier C, Patey N, Mauvieux L, Jabri B,

Delabesse E, Cervoni JP, Burtin ML, Guy-Grand D, Bouhnik Y, Modigliani R, Barbier JP, Macintyre E, Brousse N, Cerf-Bensussan N (1998). Abnormal intestinal intraepithelial lymphocytes in refractory sprue. Gastroenterology 114: 471-481.
359A. Cerhan JR, Wang S, Maurer MJ, Ansell SM, Geyer SM, Cozen W, Morton LM, Davis S, Severson RK, Rothman N, Lynch CF, Wacholder S, Chanock SJ, Habermann TM, Hartge P (2007). Prognostic significance of host immune gene polymorphisms in follicular lymphoma survival. Blood 109: 5439-5346.
360. Cerroni L, Arzberger E, Putz B, Hofler G, Metze D, Sander CA, Rose C, Wolf P, Rutten A, McNiff JM, Kerl H (2000). Primary cutaneous follicle center cell lymphoma with follicular growth pattern. Blood 95: 3922-3928.
361. Cerroni L, Rieger E, Hodl S, Kerl H (1992). Clinicopathologic and immunologic features associated with transformation of mycosis fungoides to large-cell lymphoma. Am J Surg Pathol 16: 543-552.
362. Cerroni L, Shabrawi-Caelen L, Fink-Puches R, LeBoit PE, Kerl H (2000). Cutaneous spindle-cell B-cell lymphoma: a morphologic variant of cutaneous large B-cell lymphoma. Am J Dermatopathol 22: 299-304.
363. Cerroni L, Volkenandt M, Rieger E, Soyer HP, Kerl H (1994). bcl-2 protein expression and correlation with the interchromosomal 14;18 translocation in cutaneous lymphomas and pseudolymphomas. J Invest Dermatol 102: 231-235.
364. Cerroni L, Zochling N, Putz B, Kerl H (1997). Infection by Borrelia burgdorferi and cutaneous B-cell lymphoma. J Cutan Pathol 24: 457-461.
365. Cervantes F, Alvarez-Larran A, Talarn C, Gomez M, Montserrat E (2002). Myeliofibrosis with myeloid metaplasia following essential thrombocythaemia: actuarial probability, presenting characteristics and evolution in a series of 195 patients. Br J Haematol 118: 786-790.
366. Cervantes F, Barosi G (2005). Myelofibrosis with myeloid metaplasia: diagnosis, prognostic factors, and staging. Semin Oncol 32: 395-402.
367. Cervantes F, Barosi G, Demory JL, Reilly J, Guarnone R, Dupriez B, Pereira A, Montserrat E (1998). Myelofibrosis with myeloid metaplasia in young individuals: disease characteristics, prognostic factors and identification of risk groups. Br J Haematol 102: 684-690.
368. Cervantes F, Lopez-Guillermo A, Bosch F, Terol MJ, Rozman C, Montserrat E (1996). An assessment of the clinicohematological criteria for the accelerated phase of chronic myeloid leukemia. Eur J Haematol 57: 286-291.
369. Cervantes F, Ribera JM, Sanchez-Bisono J, Brugues R, Rozman C (1984). Myeloproliferative disease in two young siblings. Cancer 54: 899-902.
370. Cesana C, Barbarano L, Miqueleiz S, Lucchesini C, Ricci F, Varettoni M, Filippini D, Lazzarino M, Morra E (2005). Clinical characteristics and outcome of immunoglobulin M-related disorders. Clin Lymphoma 5: 261-264.
371. Cesarman E, Chadburn A, Liu YF, Migliazza A, Dalla-Favera R, Knowles DM (1998). BCL-6 gene mutations in posttransplantation lymphoproliferative disorders predict response to therapy and clinical outcome. Blood 92: 2294-2302.
372. Cesarman E, Chang Y, Moore PS, Said JW, Knowles DM (1995). Kaposi's sarcoma-associated herpesvirus-like DNA sequences in AIDS-related body-cavity-based lymphomas. N Engl J Med 332: 1186-1191.
373. Cessna MH, Hartung L, Tripp S, Perkins SL, Bahler DW (2005). Hairy cell leukemia variant: fact or fiction. Am J Clin Pathol 123: 132-138.
374. Chacon JI, Mollejo M, Munoz E, Algara P, Mateo M, Lopez L, Andrade J, Carbonero IG, Martinez B, Piris MA, Cruz MA (2002). Splenic marginal zone lymphoma: clinical characteristics and prognostic factors in a series of 60 patients. Blood 100: 1648-1654.
375. Chadburn A, Cesarman E, Liu YF, Addonizio L, Hsu D, Michler RE, Knowles DM (1995). Molecular genetic analysis demonstrates that multiple posttransplantation lymphoproliferative disorders occurring in one anatomic site in a single patient represent distinct primary lymphoid neoplasms. Cancer 75: 2747-2756.
376. Chadburn A, Chen JM, Hsu DT, Frizzera G, Cesarman E, Garrett TJ, Mears JG, Zangwill SD, Addonizio LJ, Michler RE, Knowles DM (1998). The morphologic and molecular genetic categories of posttransplantation lymphoproliferative disorders are clinically relevant. Cancer 82: 1978-1987.
377. Chadburn A, Hyjek E, Mathew S, Cesarman E, Said J, Knowles DM (2004). KSHV-positive solid lymphomas represent an extra-cavitary variant of primary effusion lymphoma. Am J Surg Pathol 28: 1401-1416.
378. Chadburn A, Suciu-Foca N, Cesarman E, Reed E, Michler RE, Knowles DM (1995). Post-transplantation lymphoproliferative disorders arising in solid organ transplant recipients are usually of recipient origin. Am J Pathol 147: 1862-1870.
379. Chait Y, Condat B, Cazals-Hatem D, Rufat P, Atmani S, Chaoui D, Guilmin F, Kiladjian JJ, Plessier A, Denninger MH, Casadevall N, Valla D, Briere JB (2005). Relevance of the criteria commonly used to diagnose myeloproliferative disorder in patients with splanchnic vein thrombosis. Br J Haematol 129: 553-560.
380. Chan AC, Serrano-Olmo J, Erlandson RA, Rosai J (2000). Cytokeratin-positive malignant tumors with reticulum cell morphology: a subtype of fibroblastic reticulum cell neoplasm? Am J Surg Pathol 24: 107-116.
381. Chan JK (1998). Natural killer cell neoplasms. Anat Pathol 3:77-145: 77-145.
382. Chan JK (2003). Splenic involvement by peripheral T-cell and NK-cell neoplasms. Semin Diagn Pathol 20: 105-120.
383. Chan JK, Buchanan R, Fletcher CD (1990). Sarcomatoid variant of anaplastic large-cell Ki-1 lymphoma. Am J Surg Pathol 14: 983-988.
384. Chan JK, Chan JK (1997). Proliferative lesions of follicular dendritic cells: An overview, including a detailed account of follicular dendritic cell sarcoma, a neoplasm with many faces and uncommon etiologic associations. Adv Anat Pathol 4: 387-411.
385. Chan JK, Fletcher CD, Nayler SJ, Cooper K (1997). Follicular dendritic cell sarcoma. Clinicopathologic analysis of 17 cases suggesting a malignant potential higher than currently recognized. Cancer 79: 294-313.
386. Chan JK, Sin VC, Wong KF, Ng CS, Tsang WY, Chan CH, Cheung MM, Lau WH (1997). Nonnasal lymphoma expressing the natural killer cell marker CD56: a clinicopathologic study of 49 cases of an uncommon aggressive neoplasm. Blood 89: 4501-4513.
387. Chan JK, Tsang WY, Ng CS (1994). Follicular dendritic cell tumor and vascular neoplasm complicating hyaline-vascular Castleman's disease. Am J Surg Pathol 18: 517-525.
388. Chan JK, Tsang WY, Ng CS (1996). Clarification of CD3 immunoreactivity in nasal T/natural killer cell lymphomas: the neoplastic cells are often CD3 epsilon+. Blood 87: 839-841.
389. Chan JK, Yip TT, Tsang WY, Ng CS, Lau WH, Poon YF, Wong CC, Ma VW (1994). Detection of Epstein-Barr viral RNA in malignant lymphomas of the upper aerodigestive tract. Am J Surg Pathol 18: 938-946.
390. Chan WC, Link S, Mawle A, Check I, Brynes RK, Winton EF (1986). Heterogeneity of large granular lymphocyte proliferations: delineation of two major subtypes. Blood 68: 1142-1153.
391. Chan WC, Zaatari G (1986). Lymph node interdigitating reticulum cell sarcoma. Am J Clin Pathol 85: 739-744.
392. Chang HW, Leong KH, Koh DR, Lee SH (1999). Clonality of isolated eosinophils in the hypereosinophilic syndrome. Blood 93: 1651-1657.
392A. Chang SE, Cho S, Choi JC, Choi JH, Sung KJ, Moon KC, Koh JK (2001). Clinicohistopathologic comparison of adult type and juvenile type xanthogranulomas in Korea. J Dermatol 28: 413-418.
393. Chang ST, Lu CL, Chuang SS (2007). CD52 expression in non-mycotic T- and NK/T-cell lymphomas. Leuk Lymphoma 48: 117-121.
394. Chanudet E, Zhou Y, Bacon CM, Wotherspoon AC, Muller-Hermelink HK, Adam P, Dong HY, De Jong D, Li Y, Wei R, Gong X, Wu Q, Ranaldi R, Goteri G, Pileri SA, Ye H, Hamoudi RA, Liu H, Radford J, Du MQ (2006). Chlamydia psittaci is variably associated with ocular adnexal MALT lymphoma in different geographical regions. J Pathol 209: 344-351.
395. Chaperot L, Bendriss N, Manches O, Gressin R, Maynadie M, Trimoreau F, Orfeuvre H, Corront B, Feuillard J, Sotto JJ, Bensa JC, Briere F, Plumas J, Jacob MC (2001). Identification of a leukemic counterpart of the plasmacytoid dendritic cells. Blood 97: 3210-3217.
396. Chaperot L, Perrot I, Jacob MC, Blanchard D, Salaun V, Deneys V, Lebecque S, Briere F, Bensa JC, Plumas J (2004). Leukemic plasmacytoid dendritic cells share phenotypic and functional features with their normal counterparts. Eur J Immunol 34: 418-426.
397. Chapman AL, Rickinson AB (1998). Epstein-Barr virus in Hodgkin's disease. Ann Oncol 9 Suppl 5: S5-16.
398. Charrette EE, Mariano AV, Laforet EG (1966). Solitary mast cell "tumor" of lung. Its place in the spectrum of mast cell disease. Arch Intern Med 118: 358-362.
399. Chen HH, Hsiao CH, Chiu HC (2002). Hydroa vacciniforme-like primary cutaneous CD8-positive T-cell lymphoma. Br J Dermatol 147: 587-591.
400. Chen J, DeAngelo DJ, Kutok JL, Williams IR, Lee BH, Wadleigh M, Duclos N, Cohen S, Adelsperger J, Okabe R, Coburn A, Galinsky I, Huntly B, Cohen PS, Meyer T, Fabbro D, Roesel J, Banerji L, Griffin JD, Xiao S, Fletcher JA, Stone RM, Gilliland DG (2004). PKC412 inhibits the zinc finger 198-fibroblast growth factor receptor 1 fusion tyrosine kinase and is active in treatment of stem cell myeloproliferative disorder. Proc Natl Acad Sci U S A 101: 14479-14484.
401. Chen JS, Coustan-Smith E, Suzuki T, Neale GA, Mihara K, Pui CH, Campana D (2001). Identification of novel markers for monitoring minimal residual disease in acute lymphoblastic leukemia. Blood 97: 2115-2120.
402. Chen JS, Tzeng CC, Tsao CJ, Su WC, Chen TY, Jung YC, Su IJ (1997). Clonal karyotype abnormalities in EBV-associated hemophagocytic syndrome. Haematologica 82: 572-576.
403. Chen L, Widhopf G, Huynh L, Rassenti L, Rai KR, Weiss A, Kipps TJ (2002). Expression of ZAP-70 is associated with increased B-cell receptor signaling in chronic lymphocytic leukemia. Blood 100: 4609-4614.
404. Chen YH, Tallman MS, Goolsby C, Peterson L (2006). Immunophenotypic variations in hairy cell leukemia. Am J Clin Pathol 125: 251-259.
405. Chesi M, Bergsagel PL, Brents LA, Smith CM, Gerhard DS, Kuehl WM (1996). Dysregulation of cyclin D1 by translocation into an IgH gamma switch region in two multiple myeloma cell lines. Blood 88: 674-681.
406. Chetty R, Biddolph S, Gatter K (1997). An immunohistochemical analysis of Reed-Sternberg-like cells in posttransplantation lymphoproliferative disorders: the possible pathogenetic relationship to Reed-Sternberg cells in Hodgkin's disease and Reed-Sternberg-like cells in non-Hodgkin's lymphomas and reactive conditions. Hum Pathol 28: 493-498.
407. Chetty R, Pulford K, Jones M, Mathieu-Mahul D, Close P, Hussein S, Pallesen G, Ralfkiaer E, Stein H, Gatter K. *et al.* (1995). SCL/Tal-1 expression in T-acute lymphoblastic leukemia: an immunohistochemical and genotypic study. Hum Pathol 26: 994-998.
408. Cheuk W, Chan AC, Chan JK, Lau GT, Chan VN, Yiu HH (2005). Metallic implant-associated lymphoma: a distinct subgroup of large B-cell lymphoma related to pyothorax-associated lymphoma? Am J Surg Pathol 29: 832-836.
409. Cheuk W, Chan JK, Shek TW, Chang JH, Tsou MH, Yuen NW, Ng WF, Chan AC, Prat J (2001). Inflammatory pseudotumor-like follicular dendritic cell tumor: a distinctive low-grade malignant intra-abdominal neoplasm with consistent Epstein-Barr virus association. Am J Surg Pathol 25: 721-731.
410. Cheuk W, Hill RW, Bacchi C, Dias MA, Chan JK (2000). Hypocellular anaplastic large cell lymphoma mimicking inflammatory lesions of lymph nodes. Am J Surg Pathol 24: 1537-1543.
411. Cheuk W, Walford N, Lou J, Lee AK, Fung CF, Au KH, Mak LS, Chan JK (2001). Primary histiocytic lymphoma of the central nervous system: a neoplasm frequently overshadowed by a prominent inflammatory component. Am J Surg Pathol 25: 1372-1379.
412. Cheuk W, Wong KO, Wong CS, Chan JK (2004). Consistent immunostaining for cyclin D1 can be achieved on a routine basis using a newly available rabbit monoclonal antibody. Am J Surg Pathol 28: 801-807.
413. Cheung MM, Chan JK, Lau WH, Foo W, Chan PT, Ng CS, Ngan RK (1998). Primary non-Hodgkin's lymphoma of the nose and nasopharynx: clinical features, tumor immunophenotype, and treatment outcome in 113 patients. J Clin Oncol 16: 70-77.
414. Cheung MM, Chan JK, Lau WH, Ngan RK, Foo WW (2002). Early stage nasal NK/T-cell lymphoma: clinical outcome, prognostic factors, and the effect of treatment modality. Int J Radiat Oncol Biol Phys 54: 182-190.
415. Chiang AK, Wong KY, Liang AC, Srivastava G (1999). Comparative analysis of Epstein-Barr virus gene polymorphisms in nasal T/NK-cell lymphomas and normal nasal tissues: implications on virus strain selection in malignancy. Int J Cancer 80: 356-364.
416. Chiecchio L, Protheroe RK, Ibrahim AH, Cheung KL, Rudduck C, Dagrada GP, Cabanas ED, Parker T, Nightingale M, Wechalekar A, Orchard KH, Harrison CJ, Cross NC, Morgan GJ, Ross FM (2006). Deletion of chromosome 13 detected by conventional cytogenetics is a critical prognostic factor in myeloma. Leukemia 20: 1610-1617.
417. Chikatsu N, Kojima H, Suzukawa K, Shinagawa A, Nagasawa T, Ozawa H, Yamashita Y, Mori N (2003). ALK+, CD30-, CD20- large B-cell lymphoma containing anaplastic lymphoma kinase (ALK) fused to clathrin heavy chain gene (CLTC). Mod Pathol

16: 828-832.

418. Chikwava K, Jaffe R (2004). Langerin (CD207) staining in normal pediatric tissues, reactive lymph nodes, and childhood histiocytic disorders. Pediatr Dev Pathol 7: 607-614.

419. Child FJ, Russell-Jones R, Woolford AJ, Calonje E, Photiou A, Orchard G, Whittaker SJ (2001). Absence of the t(14;18) chromosomal translocation in primary cutaneous B-cell lymphoma. Br J Dermatol 144: 735-744.

420. Chilosi M, Doglioni C, Magalini A, Inghirami G, Krampera M, Nadali G, Rahal D, Pedron S, Benedetti A, Scardoni M, Macri E, Lestani M, Menestrina F, Pizzolo G, Scarpa A (1996). p21/WAF1 cyclin-kinase inhibitor expression in non-Hodgkin's lymphomas: a potential marker of p53 tumor-suppressor gene function. Blood 88: 4012-4020.

421. Chim CS, Ma ES, Loong F, Kwong YL (2005). Diagnostic cues for natural killer cell lymphoma: primary nodal presentation and the role of in situ hybridisation for Epstein-Barr virus encoded early small RNA in detecting occult bone marrow involvement. J Clin Pathol 58: 443-445.

422. Chim CS, Ma SY, Au WY, Choy C, Lie AK, Liang R, Yau CC, Kwong YL (2004). Primary nasal natural killer cell lymphoma: long-term treatment outcome and relationship with the International Prognostic Index. Blood 103: 216-221.

423. Chiorazzi N, Hatzi K, Albesiano E (2005). B-cell chronic lymphocytic leukemia, a clonal disease of B lymphocytes with receptors that vary in specificity for (auto)antigens. Ann N Y Acad Sci 1062: 1-12.

424. Chiorazzi N, Rai KR, Ferrarini M (2005). Chronic lymphocytic leukemia. N Engl J Med 352: 804-815.

425. Chittal SM, Alard C, Rossi JF, al Saati T, Le Tourneau A, Diebold J, Delsol G (1990). Further phenotypic evidence that nodular, lymphocyte-predominant Hodgkin's disease is a large B-cell lymphoma in evolution. Am J Surg Pathol 14: 1024-1035.

426. Chittal SM, Brousset P, Voigt JJ, Delsol G (1991). Large B-cell lymphoma rich in T-cells and simulating Hodgkin's disease. Histopathology 19: 211-220.

427. Chittal SM, Caveriviere P, Schwarting R, Gerdes J, al Saati T, Rigal-Huguet F, Stein H, Delsol G (1988). Monoclonal antibodies in the diagnosis of Hodgkin's disease. The search for a rational panel. Am J Surg Pathol 12: 9-21.

428. Chng WJ, Santana-Davila R, Van Wier SA, Ahmann GJ, Jalal SM, Bergsagel PL, Chesi M, Trendle MC, Jacobus S, Blood E, Oken MM, Henderson K, Kyle RA, Gertz MA, Lacy MQ, Dispenzieri A, Greipp PR, Fonseca R (2006). Prognostic factors for hyperdiploid-myeloma: effects of chromosome 13 deletions and IgH translocations. Leukemia 20: 807-813.

429. Chng WJ, Schop RF, Price-Troska T, Ghobrial I, Kay N, Jelinek DF, Gertz MA, Dispenzieri A, Lacy M, Kyle RA, Greipp PR, Tschumper RC, Fonseca R, Bergsagel PL (2006). Gene-expression profiling of Waldenstrom macroglobulinemia reveals a phenotype more similar to chronic lymphocytic leukemia than multiple myeloma. Blood 108: 2755-2763.

430. Chng WJ, Van Wier SA, Ahmann GJ, Winkler JM, Jalal SM, Bergsagel PL, Chesi M, Trendle MC, Oken MM, Blood E, Henderson K, Santana-Davila R, Kyle RA, Gertz MA, Lacy MQ, Dispenzieri A, Greipp PR, Fonseca R (2005). A validated FISH trisomy index demonstrates the hyperdiploid and nonhyperdiploid dichotomy in MGUS. Blood 106: 2156-2161.

431. Chng WJ, Winkler JM, Greipp PR, Jalal SM, Bergsagel PL, Chesi M, Trendle MC, Ahmann GJ, Henderson K, Blood E, Oken MM,

Hulbert A, Van Wier SA, Santana-Davila R, Kyle RA, Gertz MA, Lacy MQ, Dispenzieri A, Fonseca R (2006). Ploidy status rarely changes in myeloma patients at disease progression. Leuk Res 30: 266-271.

432. Cho KH, Kim CW, Heo DS, Lee DS, Choi WW, Rim JH, Han WS (2001). Epstein-Barr virus-associated peripheral T-cell lymphoma in adults with hydroa vacciniforme-like lesions. Clin Exp Dermatol 26: 242-247.

433. Choi IK, Kim BS, Lee KA, Ryu S, Seo HY, Sul H, Choi JG, Sung HJ, Park KH, Yoon SY, Oh SC, Seo JH, Choi CW, Shin SW, Yoon SY, Cho Y, Kim YK, Kim YH, Kim JS (2004). Efficacy of imatinib mesylate (STI571) in chronic neutrophilic leukemia with t(15;19): case report. Am J Hematol 77: 366-369.

434. Choi PC, To KF, Lai FM, Lee TW, Yim AP, Chan JK (2000). Follicular dendritic cell sarcoma of the neck: report of two cases complicated by pulmonary metastases. Cancer 89: 664-672.

435. Choquet S, Leblond V, Herbrecht R, Socie G, Stoppa AM, Vandenberghe P, Fischer A, Morschhauser F, Salles G, Feremans W, Vilmer E, Peraldi MN, Lang P, Lebranchu Y, Oksenhendler E, Garnier JL, Lamy T, Jaccard A, Ferrant A, Offner F, Hermine O, Moreau A, Fafi-Kremer S, Morand P, Chatenoud L, Berriot-Varoqueaux N, Bergougnoux L, Milpied N (2006). Efficacy and safety of rituximab in B-cell post-transplantation lymphoproliferative disorders: results of a prospective multicenter phase 2 study. Blood 107: 3053-3057.

436. Choquet S, Trappe R, Leblond V, Jager U, Davi F, Oertel S (2007). CHOP-21 for the treatment of post-transplant lymphoproliferative disorders (PTLD) following solid organ transplantation. Haematologica 92: 273-274.

437. Chott A, Haedicke W, Mosberger I, Fodinger M, Winkler K, Mannhalter C, Muller-Hermelink HK (1998). Most CD56+ intestinal lymphomas are CD8+CD5-T-cell lymphomas of monomorphic small to medium size histology. Am J Pathol 153: 1483-1490.

438. Chott A, Vesely M, Simonitsch I, Mosberger I, Hanak H (1999). Classification of intestinal T-cell neoplasms and their differential diagnosis. Am J Clin Pathol 111: S68-S74.

439. Chou WC, Tang JL, Lin LI, Yao M, Tsay W, Chen CY, Wu SJ, Huang CF, Chiou RJ, Tseng MH, Lin DT, Lin KH, Chen YC, Tien HF (2006). Nucleophosmin mutations in de novo acute myeloid leukemia: the age-dependent incidences and the stability during disease evolution. Cancer Res 66: 3310-3316.

440. Christie LJ, Evans AT, Bray SE, Smith ME, Kernohan NM, Levison DA, Goodlad JR (2006). Lesions resembling Langerhans cell histiocytosis in association with other lymphoproliferative disorders: a reactive or neoplastic phenomenon? Hum Pathol 37: 32-39.

441. Chuang SS, Ye H, Du MQ, Lu CL, Dogan A, Hsieh PP, Huang WT, Jung YC (2007). Histopathology and immunohistochemistry in distinguishing Burkitt lymphoma from diffuse large B-cell lymphoma with very high proliferation index and with or without a starry-sky pattern: a comparative study with EBER and FISH. Am J Clin Pathol 128: 558-564.

442. Chung R, Lai R, Wei P, Lee J, Hanson J, Belch AR, Turner AR, Reiman T (2007). Concordant but not discordant bone marrow involvement in diffuse large B-cell lymphoma predicts a poor clinical outcome independent of the International Prognostic Index. Blood 110: 1278-1282.

443. Chusid MJ, Dale DC, West BC, Wolff SM (1975). The hypereosinophilic syndrome: analysis of fourteen cases with review of the literature. Medicine (Baltimore) 54: 1-27.

444. Claessens YE, Bouscary D, Dupont

JM, Picard F, Melle J, Gisselbrecht S, Lacombe C, Dreyfus F, Mayeux P, Fontenay-Roupie M (2002). In vitro proliferation and differentiation of erythroid progenitors from patients with myelodysplastic syndromes: evidence for Fas-dependent apoptosis. Blood 99: 1594-1601.

445. Clarke CA, Glaser SL, Keegan TH, Stroup A (2005). Neighborhood socioeconomic status and Hodgkin's lymphoma incidence in California. Cancer Epidemiol Biomarkers Prev 14: 1441-1447.

446. Clarke M, Gaynon P, Hann I, Harrison G, Masera G, Peto R, Richards S (2003). CNS-directed therapy for childhood acute lymphoblastic leukemia: Childhood ALL Collaborative Group overview of 43 randomized trials. J Clin Oncol 21: 1798-1809.

447. Claviez A, Tiemann M, Luders H, Krams M, Parwaresch R, Schellong G, Dorffel W (2005). Impact of latent Epstein-Barr virus infection on outcome in children and adolescents with Hodgkin's lymphoma. J Clin Oncol 23: 4048-4056.

448. Cleary ML, Meeker TC, Levy S, Lee E, Trela M, Sklar J, Levy R (1986). Clustering of extensive somatic mutations in the variable region of an immunoglobulin heavy chain gene from a human B cell lymphoma. Cell 44: 97-106.

449. Cleary ML, Nalesnik MA, Shearer WT, Sklar J (1988). Clonal analysis of transplant-associated lymphoproliferations based on the structure of the genomic termini of the Epstein-Barr virus. Blood 72: 349-352.

450. Cleary ML, Warnke R, Sklar J (1984). Monoclonality of lymphoproliferative lesions in cardiac-transplant recipients. Clonal analysis based on immunoglobulin-gene rearrangements. N Engl J Med 310: 477-482.

451. Clifford GM, Polesel J, Rickenbach M, Dal Maso L, Keiser O, Kofler A, Rapiti E, Levi F, Jundt G, Fisch T, Bordoni A, De Weck D, Franceschi S (2005). Cancer risk in the Swiss HIV Cohort Study: associations with immunodeficiency, smoking, and highly active antiretroviral therapy. J Natl Cancer Inst 97: 425-432.

451A. Cobaleda C, Busslinger M (2008). Developmental plasticity of lymphocytes. Curr Opin Immunol. 20:139-148

452. Cobaleda C, Gutierrez-Cianca N, Perez-Losada J, Flores T, Garcia-Sanz R, Gonzalez M, Sanchez-Garcia I (2000). A primitive hematopoietic cell is the target for the leukemic transformation in human philadelphia-positive acute lymphoblastic leukemia. Blood 95: 1007-1013.

453. Cobbers JM, Wolter M, Reifenberger J, Ring GU, Jessen F, An HX, Niederacher D, Schmidt EE, Ichimura K, Floeth F, Kirsch L, Borchard F, Louis DN, Collins VP, Reifenberger G (1998). Frequent inactivation of CDKN2A and rare mutation of TP53 in PCNSL. Brain Pathol 8: 263-276.

454. Cobo F, Hernandez S, Hernandez L, Pinyol M, Bosch F, Esteve J, Lopez-Guillermo A, Palacin A, Raffeld M, Montserrat E, Jaffe ES, Campo E (1999). Expression of potentially oncogenic HHV-8 genes in an EBV-negative primary effusion lymphoma occurring in an HIV-seronegative patient. J Pathol 189: 288-293.

455. Coiffier B (2007). Rituximab therapy in malignant lymphoma. Oncogene 26: 3603-3613.

456. Colby TV, Hoppe RT, Warnke RA (1982). Hodgkin's disease: a clinicopathologic study of 659 cases. Cancer 49: 1848-1858.

457. Coles FB, Cartun RW, Pastuszak WT (1988). Hodgkin's disease, lymphocyte-predominant type: immunoreactivity with B-cell antibodies. Mod Pathol 1: 274-278.

458. Colombi M, Radaelli F, Zocchi L, Maiolo AT (1991). Thrombotic and hemorrhagic complications in essential thrombocythemia. A ret-

rospective study of 103 patients. Cancer 67: 2926-2930.

459. Colomo L, Loong F, Rives S, Pittaluga S, Martinez A, Lopez-Guillermo A, Ojanguren J, Romagosa V, Jaffe ES, Campo E (2004). Diffuse large B-cell lymphomas with plasmablastic differentiation represent a heterogeneous group of disease entities. Am J Surg Pathol 28: 736-747.

460. Colomo L, Lopez-Guillermo A, Perales M, Rives S, Martinez A, Bosch F, Colomer D, Falini B, Montserrat E, Campo E (2003). Clinical impact of the differentiation profile assessed by immunophenotyping in patients with diffuse large B-cell lymphoma. Blood 101: 78-84.

460A. Colt JS, Davis S, Severson RK, Lynch CF, Cozen W, Camann D, Engels EA, Blair A, Hartge P (2006). Residential insecticide use and risk of non-Hodgkin's lymphoma. Cancer Epidemiol Biomarkers Prev 15: 251-257.

461. Comoli P, Basso S, Zecca M, Pagliara D, Baldanti F, Bernardo ME, Barberi W, Moretta A, Labirio M, Paulli M, Furione M, Maccario R, Locatelli F (2007). Preemptive therapy of EBV-related lymphoproliferative disease after pediatric haploidentical stem cell transplantation. Am J Transplant 7: 1648-1655.

462. Cong P, Raffeld M, Teruya-Feldstein J, Sorbara L, Pittaluga S, Jaffe ES (2002). In situ localization of follicular lymphoma: description and analysis by laser capture microdissection. Blood 99: 3376-3382.

462A. Connors JM (2005). State-of-the-art therapeutics: Hodgkin's lymphoma. J Clin Oncol 23: 6400-6408.

463. Cook JR, Aguilera NI, Reshmi-Skarja S, Huang X, Yu Z, Gollin SM, Abbondanzo SL, Swerdlow SH (2004). Lack of PAX5 rearrangements in lymphoplasmacytic lymphomas: reassessing the reported association with t(9;14). Hum Pathol 35: 447-454.

464. Cook JR, Aguilera NI, Reshmi S, Huang X, Yu Z, Gollin SM, Abbondanzo SL, Swerdlow SH (2005). Deletion 6q is not a characteristic marker of nodal lymphoplasmacytic lymphoma. Cancer Genet Cytogenet 162: 85-88.

465. Cooke CB, Krenacs L, Stetler-Stevenson M, Greiner TC, Raffeld M, Kingma DW, Abruzzo L, Frantz C, Kaviani M, Jaffe ES (1996). Hepatosplenic T-cell lymphoma: a distinct clinicopathologic entity of cytotoxic gamma delta T-cell origin. Blood 88: 4265-4274.

466. Cools J, DeAngelo DJ, Gotlib J, Stover EH, Legare RD, Cortes J, Kutok J, Clark J, Galinsky I, Griffin JD, Cross NC, Tefferi A, Malone J, Alam R, Schrier SL, Schmid J, Rose M, Vandenberghe P, Verhoef G, Boogaerts M, Wlodarska I, Kantarjian H, Marynen P, Coutre SE, Stone R, Gilliland DG (2003). A tyrosine kinase created by fusion of the PDGFRA and FIP1L1 genes as a therapeutic target of imatinib in idiopathic hypereosinophilic syndrome. N Engl J Med 348: 1201-1214.

467. Cools J, Mentens N, Odero MD, Peeters P, Wlodarska I, Delforge M, Hagemeijer A, Marynen P (2002). Evidence for position effects as a variant ETV6-mediated leukemogenic mechanism in myeloid leukemias with a t(4;12)(q11-q12;p13) or t(5;12)(q31;p13). Blood 99: 1776-1784.

468. Cools J, Stover EH, Boulton CL, Gotlib J, Legare RD, Amaral SM, Curley DP, Duclos N, Rowan R, Kutok JL, Lee BH, Williams IR, Coutre SE, Stone RM, DeAngelo DJ, Marynen P, Manley PW, Meyer T, Fabbro D, Neuberg D, Weisberg E, Griffin JD, Gilliland DG (2003). PKC412 overcomes resistance to imatinib in a murine model of FIP1L1-PDGFRalpha-induced myeloproliferative disease. Cancer Cell 3: 459-469.

469. Cools J, Wlodarska I, Somers R, Mentens N, Pedeutour F, Maes B, Wolf-

Peeters C, Pauwels P, Hagemeijer A, Marynen P (2002). Identification of novel fusion partners of ALK, the anaplastic lymphoma kinase, in anaplastic large-cell lymphoma and inflammatory myofibroblastic tumor. Genes Chromosomes Cancer 34: 354-362.
470. Copie-Bergman C, Gaulard P, Maouche-Chretien L, Briere J, Haioun C, Alonso MA, Romeo PH, Leroy K (1999). The MAL gene is expressed in primary mediastinal large B-cell lymphoma. Blood 94: 3567-3575.
471. Copie-Bergman C, Niedobitek G, Mangham DC, Selves J, Baloch K, Diss TC, Knowles DN, Delsol G, Isaacson PG (1997). Epstein-Barr virus in B-cell lymphomas associated with chronic suppurative inflammation. J Pathol 183: 287-292.
472. Copie-Bergman C, Plonquet A, Alonso MA, Boulland ML, Marquet J, Divine M, Moller P, Leroy K, Gaulard P (2002). MAL expression in lymphoid cells: further evidence for MAL as a distinct molecular marker of primary mediastinal large B-cell lymphomas. Mod Pathol 15: 1172-1180.
473. Copie-Bergman C, Wotherspoon AC, Norton AJ, Diss TC, Isaacson PG (1998). True histiocytic lymphoma: a morphologic, immunohistochemical, and molecular genetic study of 13 cases. Am J Surg Pathol 22: 1386-1392.
473A. Corazzelli G, Capobianco G, Russo F, Frigeri F, Aldinucci D, and Pinto A (2005). Pentostatin (2'-deoxycoformycin) for the treatment of hepatosplenic gammadelta T-cell lymphomas. Haematologica 90: 39-41.
474. Corcoran MM, Mould SJ, Orchard JA, Ibbotson RE, Chapman RM, Boright AP, Platt C, Tsui LC, Scherer SW, Oscier DG (1999). Dysregulation of cyclin dependent kinase 6 expression in splenic marginal zone lymphoma through chromosome 7q translocations. Oncogene 18: 6271-6277.
475. Cordone I, Masi S, Mauro FR, Soddu S, Morsilli O, Valentini T, Vegna ML, Guglielmi C, Mancini F, Giuliacci S, Sacchi A, Mandelli F, Foa R (1998). p53 expression in B-cell chronic lymphocytic leukemia: a marker of disease progression and poor prognosis. Blood 91: 4342-4349.
476. Corey SJ, Locker J, Oliveri DR, Shekhter-Levin S, Redner RL, Penchansky L, Gollin SM (1994). A non-classical translocation involving 17q12 (retinoic acid receptor alpha) in acute promyelocytic leukemia (APML) with atypical features. Leukemia 8: 1350-1353.
477. Coriu D, Weaver K, Schell M, Eulitz M, Murphy CL, Weiss DT, Solomon A (2004). A molecular basis for nonsecretory myeloma. Blood 104: 829-831.
478. Cormier V, Rotig A, Quartino AR, Forni GL, Cerone R, Maier M, Saudubray JM, Munnich A (1990). Widespread multi-tissue deletions of the mitochondrial genome in the Pearson marrow-pancreas syndrome. J Pediatr 117: 599-602.
479. Corso A, Lazzarino M, Morra E, Merante S, Astori C, Bernasconi P, Boni M, Bernasconi C (1995). Chronic myelogenous leukemia and exposure to ionizing radiation—a retrospective study of 443 patients. Ann Hematol 70: 79-82.
480. Cortes J (2003). CMML: a biologically distinct myeloproliferative disease. Curr Hematol Rep 2: 202-208.
481. Cortes JE, Talpaz M, Giles F, O'Brien S, Rios MB, Shan J, Garcia-Manero G, Faderl S, Thomas DA, Wierda W, Ferrajoli A, Jeha S, Kantarjian HM (2003). Prognostic significance of cytogenetic clonal evolution in patients with chronic myelogenous leukemia on imatinib mesylate therapy. Blood 101: 3794-3800.
482. Cortes JE, Talpaz M, O'Brien S, Faderl S, Garcia-Manero G, Ferrajoli A, Verstovsek S, Rios MB, Shan J, Kantarjian HM (2006). Staging of chronic myeloid leukemia in the imatinib era: an evaluation of the World Health Organization proposal. Cancer 106: 1306-1315.
483. Costa D, Queralt R, Aymerich M, Carrio A, Rozman M, Vallespi T, Colomer D, Nomdedeu B, Montserrat E, Campo E (2003). High levels of chromosomal imbalances in typical and small-cell variants of T-cell prolymphocytic leukemia. Cancer Genet Cytogenet 147: 36-43.
484. Costes-Martineau V, Delfour C, Obled S, Lamant L, Pageaux GP, Baldet P, Blanc P, Delsol G (2002). Anaplastic lymphoma kinase (ALK) protein expressing lymphoma after liver transplantation: case report and literature review. J Clin Pathol 55: 868-871.
485. Cote TR, Manns A, Hardy CR, Yellin FJ, Hartge P (1996). Epidemiology of brain lymphoma among people with or without acquired immunodeficiency syndrome. AIDS/Cancer Study Group. J Natl Cancer Inst 88: 675-679.
486. Cotta CV, Bueso-Ramos CE (2007). New insights into the pathobiology and treatment of chronic myelogenous leukemia. Ann Diagn Pathol 11: 68-78.
487. Coupland SE, Charlotte F, Mansour G, Maloum K, Hummel M, Stein H (2005). HHV-8-associated T-cell lymphoma in a lymph node with concurrent peritoneal effusion in an HIV-positive man. Am J Surg Pathol 29: 647-652.
488. Coustan-Smith E, Sancho J, Hancock ML, Boyett JM, Behm FG, Raimondi SC, Sandlund JT, Rivera GK, Rubnitz JE, Ribeiro RC, Pui CH, Campana D (2000). Clinical importance of minimal residual disease in childhood acute lymphoblastic leukemia. Blood 96: 2691-2696.
489. Crescenzi B, La Starza R, Nozzoli C, Ciolli S, Matteucci C, Romoli S, Rigacci L, Gorello P, Bosi A, Martelli MF, Marynen P, Mecucci C (2007). Molecular cytogenetic findings in a four-way t(1;12;5;12)(p36;p13;q33;q24) underlying the ETV6-PDGFRB fusion gene in chronic myelomonocytic leukemia. Cancer Genet Cytogenet 176: 67-71.
490. Crespo M, Bosch F, Villamor N, Bellosillo B, Colomer D, Rozman M, Marce S, Lopez-Guillermo A, Campo E, Montserrat E (2003). ZAP-70 expression as a surrogate for immunoglobulin-variable-region mutations in chronic lymphocytic leukemia. N Engl J Med 348: 1764-1775.
491. Creutzig U, Harbott J, Sperling C, Ritter J, Zimmermann M, Loffler H, Riehm H, Schellong G, Ludwig WD (1995). Clinical significance of surface antigen expression in children with acute myeloid leukemia: results of study AML-BFM-87. Blood 86: 3097-3108.
492. Criel A, Michaux L, Wolf-Peeters C (1999). The concept of typical and atypical chronic lymphocytic leukaemia. Leuk Lymphoma 33: 33-45.
492A. Criscione VD, Weinstock MA (2007). Incidence of cutaneous T-cell lymphoma in the United States, 1973-2002. Arch Dermatol 143: 854-859.
493. Cuadra-Garcia I, Proulx GM, Wu CL, Wang CC, Pilch BZ, Harris NL, Ferry JA (1999). Sinonasal lymphoma: a clinicopathologic analysis of 58 cases from the Massachusetts General Hospital. Am J Surg Pathol 23: 1356-1369.
494. Cuadros M, Dave SS, Jaffe ES, Honrado E, Milne R, Alves J, Rodriguez J, Zajac M, Benitez J, Staudt LM, Martinez-Delgado B (2007). Identification of a Proliferation Signature Related to Survival in Nodal Peripheral T-Cell Lymphomas. J Clin Oncol 25: 3321-3329.
495. Cudennec CA, Johnson GR (1981). Presence of multipotential hemopoietic cells in teratocarcinoma cultures. J Embryol Exp Morphol 61: 51-59.
496. Cuneo A, Bigoni R, Rigolin GM, Roberti MG, Bardi A, Piva N, Milani R, Bullrich F, Veronese ML, Croce C, Birg F, Dohner H, Hagemeijer A, Castoldi G (1999). Cytogenetic profile of lymphoma of follicle mantle lineage: correlation with clinicobiologic features. Blood 93: 1372-1380.
497. Curtis CE, Grand FH, Musto P, Clark A, Murphy J, Perla G, Minervini MM, Stewart J, Reiter A, Cross NC (2007). Two novel imatinib-responsive PDGFRA fusion genes in chronic eosinophilic leukaemia. Br J Haematol 138: 77-81.
498. Curtis CE, Grand FH, Waghorn K, Sahoo TP, George J, Cross NC (2007). A novel ETV6-PDGFRB fusion transcript missed by standard screening in a patient with an imatinib responsive chronic myeloproliferative disease. Leukemia 21: 1839-1841.
499. Curtis RE, Travis LB, Rowlings PA, Socie G, Kingma DW, Banks PM, Jaffe ES, Sale GE, Horowitz MM, Witherspoon RP, Shriner DA, Weisdorf DJ, Kolb HJ, Sullivan KM, Sobocinski KA, Gale RP, Hoover RN, Fraumeni JF, Jr., Deeg HJ (1999). Risk of lymphoproliferative disorders after bone marrow transplantation: a multi-institutional study. Blood 94: 2208-2216.
500. Czuczman MS, Dodge RK, Stewart CC, Frankel SR, Davey FR, Powell BL, Szatrowski TP, Schiffer CA, Larson RA, Bloomfield CD (1999). Value of immunophenotype in intensively treated adult acute lymphoblastic leukemia: cancer and leukemia Group B study 8364. Blood 93: 3931-3939.
501. D'Achille P, Seymour JF, Campbell LJ (2006). Translocation (14;18)(q32;q21) in acute lymphoblastic leukemia: a study of 12 cases and review of the literature. Cancer Genet Cytogenet 171: 52-56.
502. Dacic S, Trusky C, Bakker A, Finkelstein SD, Yousem SA (2003). Genotypic analysis of pulmonary Langerhans cell histiocytosis. Hum Pathol 34: 1345-1349.
503. Dalal BI, Horsman DE, Bruyere H, Forrest DL (2007). Imatinib mesylate responsiveness in aggressive systemic mastocytosis: novel association with a platelet derived growth factor receptor beta mutation. Am J Hematol 82: 77-79.
504. Dallenbach FE, Stein H (1989). Expression of T-cell-receptor beta chain in Reed-Sternberg cells. Lancet 2: 828-830.
505. Damle RN, Wasil T, Fais F, Ghiotto F, Valetto A, Allen SL, Buchbinder A, Budman D, Dittmar K, Kolitz J, Lichtman SM, Schulman P, Vinciguerra VP, Rai KR, Ferrarini M, Chiorazzi N (1999). Ig V gene mutation status and CD38 expression as novel prognostic indicators in chronic lymphocytic leukemia. Blood 94: 1840-1847.
506. Dash A, Gilliland DG (2001). Molecular genetics of acute myeloid leukaemia. Best Pract Res Clin Haematol 14: 49-64.
507. Dastugue N, Lafage-Pochitaloff M, Pages MP, Radford I, Bastard C, Talmant P, Mozziconacci MJ, Leonard C, Bilhou-Nabera C, Cabrol C, Capodano AM, Cornillet-Lefebvre P, Lessard M, Mugneret F, Perot C, Taviaux S, Fenneteaux O, Duchayne E, Berger R (2002). Cytogenetic profile of childhood and adult megakaryoblastic leukemia (M7): a study of the Groupe Francais de Cytogenetique Hematologique (GFCH). Blood 100: 618-626.
508. Daum S, Cellier C, Mulder CJ (2005). Refractory coeliac disease. Best Pract Res Clin Gastroenterol 19: 413-424.
509. Dave SS, Fu K, Wright GW, Lam LT, Kluin P, Boerma EJ, Greiner TC, Weisenburger DD, Rosenwald A, Ott G, Muller-Hermelink HK, Gascoyne RD, Delabie J, Rimsza LM, Braziel RM, Grogan TM, Campo E, Jaffe ES, Dave BJ, Sanger W, Bast M, Vose JM, Armitage JO, Connors JM, Smeland EB, Kvaloy S, Holte H, Fisher RI, Miller TP, Montserrat E, Wilson WH, Bahl M, Zhao H, Yang L, Powell J, Simon R, Chan WC, Staudt LM (2006). Molecular diagnosis of Burkitt's lymphoma. N Engl J Med 354: 2431-2442.
510. Dave SS, Wright G, Tan B, Rosenwald A, Gascoyne RD, Chan WC, Fisher RI, Braziel RM, Rimsza LM, Grogan TM, Miller TP, LeBlanc M, Greiner TC, Weisenburger DD, Lynch JC, Vose J, Armitage JO, Smeland EB, Kvaloy S, Holte H, Delabie J, Connors JM, Lansdorp PM, Ouyang Q, Lister TA, Davies AJ, Norton AJ, Muller-Hermelink HK, Ott G, Campo E, Montserrat E, Wilson WH, Jaffe ES, Simon R, Yang L, Powell J, Zhao H, Goldschmidt N, Chiorazzi M, Staudt LM (2004). Prediction of survival in follicular lymphoma based on molecular features of tumor-infiltrating immune cells. N Engl J Med 351: 2159-2169.
511. Davi F, Delecluse HJ, Guiet P, Gabarre J, Fayon A, Gentilhomme O, Felman P, Bayle C, Berger F, Audouin J, Bryon PA, Diebold J, Raphael M (1998). Burkitt-like lymphomas in AIDS patients: characterization within a series of 103 human immunodeficiency virus-associated non-Hodgkin's lymphomas. Burkitt's Lymphoma Study Group. J Clin Oncol 16: 3788-3795.
512. David M, Cross NC, Burgstaller S, Chase A, Curtis C, Dang R, Gardembas M, Goldman JM, Grand F, Hughes G, Huguet F, Lavender L, McArthur GA, Mahon FX, Massimini G, Melo J, Rousselot P, Russell-Jones RJ, Seymour JF, Smith G, Stark A, Waghorn K, Nikolova Z, Apperley JF (2007). Durable responses to imatinib in patients with PDGFRB fusion gene-positive and BCR-ABL-negative chronic myeloproliferative disorders. Blood 109: 61-64.
513. Davies AJ, Rosenwald A, Wright G, Lee A, Last KW, Weisenburger DD, Chan WC, Delabie J, Braziel RM, Campo E, Gascoyne RD, Jaffe ES, Muller-Hermelink K, Ott G, Calaminici M, Norton AJ, Goff LK, Fitzgibbon J, Staudt LM, Andrew LT (2007). Transformation of follicular lymphoma to diffuse large B-cell lymphoma proceeds by distinct oncogenic mechanisms. Br J Haematol 136: 286-293.
514. Davis TH, Morton CC, Miller-Cassman R, Balk SP, Kadin ME (1992). Hodgkin's disease, lymphomatoid papulosis, and cutaneous T-cell lymphoma derived from a common T-cell clone. N Engl J Med 326: 1115-1122.
515. De Boer CJ, Van Krieken JH, Kluin-Nelemans HC, Kluin PM, Schuuring E (1995). Cyclin D1 messenger RNA overexpression as a marker for mantle cell lymphoma. Oncogene 10: 1833-1840.
516. de Bruin PC, Beljaards RC, van Heerde P, van d, V, Noorduyn LA, Van Krieken JH, Kluin-Nelemans JC, Willemze R, Meijer CJ (1993). Differences in clinical behaviour and immunophenotype between primary cutaneous and primary nodal anaplastic large cell lymphoma of T-cell or null cell phenotype. Histopathology 23: 127-135.
517. De Falco G, Leucci E, Lenze D, Piccaluga PP, Claudio PP, Onnis A, Cerino G, Nyagol J, Mwanda W, Bellan C, Hummel M, Pileri S, Tosi P, Stein H, Giordano A, Leoncini L (2007). Gene-expression analysis identifies novel RBL2/p130 target genes in endemic Burkitt lymphoma cell lines and primary tumors. Blood 110: 1301-1307.
518. De Jong D, Rosenwald A, Chhanabhai M, Gaulard P, Klapper W, Lee A, Sander B,

Thorns C, Campo E, Molina T, Norton A, Hagenbeek A, Horning S, Lister A, Raemaekers J, Gascoyne RD, Salles G, Weller E (2007). Immunohistochemical prognostic markers in diffuse large B-cell lymphoma: validation of tissue microarray as a prerequisite for broad clinical applications—a study from the Lunenburg Lymphoma Biomarker Consortium. J Clin Oncol 25: 805-812.
518A de Jong D, Voetdujk B, Baverstock G, et al. Activation of the c-myc oncogene in a precursor B-cell blast crisis of follicular lymphoma, presenting as composite lymphoma. N Engl J Med 1988; 318:1373-.
519. De Keersmaecker K, Marynen P, Cools J (2005). Genetic insights in the pathogenesis of T-cell acute lymphoblastic leukemia. Haematologica 90: 1116-1127.
520. de Leval L, Ferry JA, Falini B, Shipp M, Harris NL (2001). Expression of bcl-6 and CD10 in primary mediastinal large B-cell lymphoma: evidence for derivation from germinal center B cells? Am J Surg Pathol 25: 1277-1282.
521. de Leval L, Harris NL (2003). Variability in immunophenotype in diffuse large B-cell lymphoma and its clinical relevance. Histopathology 43: 509-528.
522. de Leval L, Harris NL, Longtine J, Ferry JA, Duncan LM (2001). Cutaneous B-cell lymphomas of follicular and marginal zone types: use of Bcl-6, CD10, Bcl-2, and CD21 in differential diagnosis and classification. Am J Surg Pathol 25: 732-741.
523. de Leval L, Rickman DS, Thielen C, Reynies A, Huang YL, Delsol G, Lamant L, Leroy K, Briere J, Molina T, Berger F, Gisselbrecht C, Xerri L, Gaulard P (2007). The gene expression profile of nodal peripheral T-cell lymphoma demonstrates a molecular link between angioimmunoblastic T-cell lymphoma (AITL) and follicular helper T (TFH) cells. Blood 109: 4952-4963.
524. de Leval L, Savilo E, Longtine J, Ferry JA, Harris NL (2001). Peripheral T-cell lymphoma with follicular involvement and a CD4+/bcl-6+ phenotype. Am J Surg Pathol 25: 395-400.
525. de Lima M, O'Brien S, Lerner S, Keating MJ (1998). Chronic lymphocytic leukemia in the young patient. Semin Oncol 25: 107-116.
526. De Paepe P, Achten R, Verhoef G, Wlodarska I, Stul M, Vanhentenrijk V, Praet M, Wolf-Peeters C (2005). Large cleaved and immunoblastic lymphoma may represent two distinct clinicopathologic entities within the group of diffuse large B-cell lymphomas. J Clin Oncol 23: 7060-7068.
527. De Paepe P, Baens M, van Krieken H, Verhasselt B, Stul M, Simons A, Poppe B, Laureys G, Brons P, Vandenberghe P, Speleman F, Praet M, Wolf-Peeters C, Marynen P, Wlodarska I (2003). ALK activation by the CLTC-ALK fusion is a recurrent event in large B-cell lymphoma. Blood 102: 2638-2641.
527A. de Sanjose S, Benavente Y, Vajdic CM, Engels EA, Morton LM, Bracci PM, Spinelli JJ, Zheng T, Zhang Y, Franceschi S, Talamini R, Holly EA, Grulich AE, Cerhan JR, Hartge P, Cozen W, Boffetta P, Brennan P, Maynadié M, Cocco P, Bosch R, Foretova L, Staines A, Becker N, Nieters A (2008). Hepatitis C and non-Hodgkin lymphoma among 4784 cases and 6269 controls from the International Lymphoma Epidemiology Consortium. Clin Gastroenterol Hepatol 6: 451-458.
528. De The G, Geser A, Day NE, Tukei PM, Williams EH, Beri DP, Smith PG, Dean AG, Bronkamm GW, Feorino P, Henle W (1978). Epidemiological evidence for causal relationship between Epstein-Barr virus and Burkitt's lymphoma from Ugandan prospective study. Nature 274: 756-761.
529. de The H, Chomienne C, Lanotte M, Degos L, Dejean A (1990). The t(15;17) translocation of acute promyelocytic leukaemia fuses the retinoic acid receptor alpha gene to a novel transcribed locus. Nature 347: 558-561.
530. de Tute R, Yuille M, Catovsky D, Houlston RS, Hillmen P, Rawstron AC (2006). Monoclonal B-cell lymphocytosis (MBL) in CLL families: substantial increase in relative risk for young adults. Leukemia 20: 728-729.
531. de Vries MJ, Veerman AJ, Zwaan CM (2004). Rituximab in three children with relapsed/refractory B-cell acute lymphoblastic leukaemia/Burkitt non-Hodgkin's lymphoma. Br J Haematol 125: 414-415.
532. de Witte T, Oosterveld M, Muus P (2007). Autologous and allogeneic stem cell transplantation for myelodysplastic syndrome. Blood Rev 21: 49-59.
533. De Zen A, Orfao A, Cazzaniga G, Masiero L, Cocito MG, Spinelli M, Rivolta A, Biondi A, Zanesco L, Basso G (2000). Quantitative multiparametric immunophenotyping in acute lymphoblasticleukemia; correlation with specific genotype. I. ETV6/AML1 ALLs identification. Leukemia 14: 1225-1231.
534. De Re, V, De Vita S, Marzotto A, Rupolo M, Gloghini A, Pivetta B, Gasparotto D, Carbone A, Boiocchi M (2000). Sequence analysis of the immunoglobulin antigen receptor of hepatitis C virus-associated non-Hodgkin lymphomas suggests that the malignant cells are derived from the rheumatoid factor-producing cells that occur mainly in type II cryoglobulinemia. Blood 96: 3578-3584.
534A. De Vita S, Sacco C, Sansonno D, Gloghini A, Dammacco F, Crovatto M, Santini G, Dolcetti R, Boiocchi M, Carbone A, Zagonel V (1997). Characterization of overt B-cell lymphomas in patients with hepatitis C virus infection. Blood 90: 776-782.
535. Dearden CE (2006). T-cell prolymphocytic leukemia. Med Oncol 23: 17-22.
536. Dearden CE, Matutes E, Cazin B, Tjonnfjord GE, Parreira A, Nomdedeu B, Leoni P, Clark FJ, Radia D, Rassam SM, Roques T, Ketterer N, Brito-Babapulle V, Dyer MJ, Catovsky D (2001). High remission rate in T-cell prolymphocytic leukemia with CAMPATH-1H. Blood 98: 1721-1726.
537. DeCoteau JF, Butmarc JR, Kinney MC, Kadin ME (1996). The t(2;5) chromosomal translocation is not a common feature of primary cutaneous CD30+ lymphoproliferative disorders: comparison with anaplastic large-cell lymphoma of nodal origin. Blood 87: 3437-3441.
538. Deglesne PA, Chevallier N, Letestu R, Baran-Marszak F, Beitar T, Salanoubat C, Sanhes L, Nataf J, Roger C, Varin-Blank N, Ajchenbaum-Cymbalista F (2006). Survival response to B-cell receptor ligation is restricted to progressive chronic lymphocytic leukemia cells irrespective of Zap70 expression. Cancer Res 66: 7158-7166.
538A. Dehner LP (2003). Juvenile xanthogranulomas in the first two decades of life: a clinicopathologic study of 174 cases with cutaneous and extracutaneous manifestations.Am J Surg Pathol 27: 579-953.
539. Deininger MW, Goldman JM, Melo JV (2000). The molecular biology of chronic myeloid leukemia. Blood 96: 3343-3356.
540. Dekmezian R, Kantarjian HM, Keating MJ, Talpaz M, McCredie KB, Freireich EJ (1987). The relevance of reticulin stain-measured fibrosis at diagnosis in chronic myelogenous leukemia. Cancer 59: 1739-1743.
541. Del Giudice I, Matutes E, Morilla R, Morilla A, Owusu-Ankomah K, Rafiq F, A'Hern R, Delgado J, Bazerbashi MB, Catovsky D (2004). The diagnostic value of CD123 in B-cell disorders with hairy or villous lymphocytes. Haematologica 89: 303-308.
542. Del G, I, Davis Z, Matutes E, Osuji N, Parry-Jones N, Morilla A, Brito-Babapulle V, Oscier D, Catovsky D (2006). IgVH genes mutation and usage, ZAP-70 and CD38 expression provide new insights on B-cell prolymphocytic leukemia (B-PLL). Leukemia 20: 1231-1237.
543. Delabesse E, Bernard M, Meyer V, Smit L, Pulford K, Cayuela JM, Ritz J, Bourquelot P, Strominger JL, Valensi F, Macintyre EA (1998). TAL1 expression does not occur in the majority of T-ALL blasts. Br J Haematol 102: 449-457.
544. Delabie J, Vandenberghe E, Kennes C, Verhoef G, Foschini MP, Stul M, Cassiman JJ, Wolf-Peeters C (1992). Histiocyte-rich B-cell lymphoma. A distinct clinicopathologic entity possibly related to lymphocyte predominant Hodgkin's disease, paragranuloma subtype. Am J Surg Pathol 16: 37-48.
545. Delauche-Cavallier MC, Laredo JD, Wybier M, Bard M, Mazabraud A, Bail Darne JL, Kuntz D, Ryckewaert A (1988). Solitary plasmacytoma of the spine. Long-term clinical course. Cancer 61: 1707-1714.
546. Delaunay J, Vey N, Leblanc T, Fenaux P, Rigal-Huguet F, Witz F, Lamy T, Auvrignon A, Blaise D, Pigneux A, Mugneret F, Bastard C, Dastugue N, Van den AJ, Fiere D, Reiffers J, Castaigne S, Leverger G, Harousseau JL, Dombret H (2003). Prognosis of inv(16)/t(16;16) acute myeloid leukemia (AML): a survey of 110 cases from the French AML Intergroup. Blood 102: 462-469.
547. Delecluse HJ, Anagnostopoulos I, Dallenbach F, Hummel M, Marafioti T, Schneider U, Huhn D, Schmidt-Westhausen A, Reichart PA, Gross U, Stein H (1997). Plasmablastic lymphomas of the oral cavity: a new entity associated with the human immunodeficiency virus infection. Blood 89: 1413-1420.
548. Deleeuw RJ, Zettl A, Klinker E, Haralambieva E, Trottier M, Chari R, Ge Y, Gascoyne RD, Chott A, Muller-Hermelink HK, Lam WL (2007). Whole-genome analysis and HLA genotyping of enteropathy-type T-cell lymphoma reveals 2 distinct lymphoma subtypes. Gastroenterology 132: 1902-1911.
549. Della Porta MG, Malcovati L, Galli A, Boggi S, Travaglino E, Marseglia C, Maffioli M, Levi S, Arosio P, Invernizzi R, Lazzarino M, Cazzola M (2005). Mitochondrial ferritin expression and clonality of hematopoiesis in patients with refractory anemia with ringed sideroblasts. Blood 106: Abstract 3444.
550. Della Porta MG, Malcovati L, Invernizzi R, Travaglino E, Pascutto C, Maffioli M, Galli A, Boggi S, Pietra D, Vanelli L, Marseglia C, Levi S, Arosio P, Lazzarino M, Cazzola M (2006). Flow cytometry evaluation of erythroid dysplasia in patients with myelodysplastic syndrome. Leukemia 20: 549-555.
551. Delsol G, al Saati T, Gatter KC, Gerdes J, Schwarting R, Caveriviere P, Rigal-Huguet F, Robert A, Stein H, Mason DY (1988). Coexpression of epithelial membrane antigen (EMA), Ki-1, and interleukin-2 receptor by anaplastic large cell lymphomas. Diagnostic value in so-called malignant histiocytosis. Am J Pathol 130: 59-70.
552. Delsol G, Brousset P, Chittal S, Rigal-Huguet F (1992). Correlation of the expression of Epstein-Barr virus latent membrane protein and in situ hybridization with biotinylated BamHI-W probes in Hodgkin's disease. Am J Pathol 140: 247-253.
553. Delsol G, Lamant L, Mariame B, Pulford K, Dastugue N, Brousset P, Rigal-Huguet F, al Saati T, Cerretti DP, Morris SW, Mason DY (1997). A new subtype of large B-cell lymphoma expressing the ALK kinase and lacking the 2;5 translocation. Blood 89: 1483-1490.
554. Delsol G, Ralfkiaer E, Stein H, Wright D, Jaffe ES (2001). Anaplastic large cell lymphoma. In: WHO Classification of Tumours of the Haematopoietic and Lymphoid Tissues. IARCPress: Lyon, pp. 230-235.
555. deMent SH (1990). Association between mediastinal germ cell tumors and hematologic malignancies: an update. Hum Pathol 21: 699-703.
556. DePond W, Said JW, Tasaka T, de Vos S, Kahn D, Cesarman E, Knowles DM, Koeffler HP (1997). Kaposi's sarcoma-associated herpesvirus and human herpesvirus 8 (KSHV/HHV8)-associated lymphoma of the bowel. Report of two cases in HIV-positive men with secondary effusion lymphomas. Am J Surg Pathol 21: 719-724.
557. Derderian PM, Kantarjian HM, Talpaz M, O'Brien S, Cork A, Estey E, Pierce S, Keating M (1993). Chronic myelogenous leukemia in the lymphoid blastic phase: characteristics, treatment response, and prognosis. Am J Med 94: 69-74.
558. Derringer GA, Thompson LD, Frommelt RA, Bijwaard KE, Heffess CS, Abbondanzo SL (2000). Malignant lymphoma of the thyroid gland: a clinicopathologic study of 108 cases. Am J Surg Pathol 24: 623-639.
559. Desar IM, Keuter M, Raemaekers JM, Jansen JB, Van Krieken JH, van der Meer JW (2006). Extranodal marginal zone (MALT) lymphoma in common variable immunodeficiency. Neth J Med 64: 136-140.
559A. Deschler B, Lübbert M (2006). Acute myeloid leukemia: epidemiology and etiology. Cancer 107: 2099-2107.
560. Despouy G, Joiner M, Le Toriellec E, Weil R, Stern MH (2007). The TCL1 oncoprotein inhibits activation-induced cell death by impairing PKC{theta} and ERK pathways. Blood 110: 4406-4416.
561. Dewald GW, Kyle RA, Hicks GA, Greipp PR (1985). The clinical significance of cytogenetic studies in 100 patients with multiple myeloma, plasma cell leukemia, or amyloidosis. Blood 66: 380-390.
562. Dharnidharka VR, Tejani AH, Ho PL, Harmon WE (2002). Post-transplant lymphoproliferative disorder in the United States: young Caucasian males are at highest risk. Am J Transplant 2: 993-998.
563. Dhodapkar MV, Li CY, Lust JA, Tefferi A, Phyliky RL (1994). Clinical spectrum of clonal proliferations of T-large granular lymphocytes: a T-cell clonopathy of undetermined significance? Blood 84: 1620-1627.
564. Dhodapkar MV, Merlini G, Solomon A (1997). Biology and therapy of immunoglobulin deposition diseases. Hematol Oncol Clin North Am 11: 89-110.
565. Di Benedetto G, Cataldi A, Verde A, Gloghini A, Nicolo G, Pistoia V (1989). Gamma heavy chain disease associated with Hodgkin's disease. Clinical, pathologic, and immunologic features of one case. Cancer 63: 1804-1809.
566. Di Donato C, Croci G, Lazzari S, Scarduelli L, Vignoli R, Buia M, Tramaloni C, Maccari S, Plancher AC (1986). Chronic neutrophilic leukemia: description of a new case with karyotypic abnormalities. Am J Clin Pathol 85: 369-371.
567. Diamandidou E, Colome-Grimmer M, Fayad L, Duvic M, Kurzrock R (1998). Transformation of mycosis fungoides/Sezary syndrome: clinical characteristics and prognosis. Blood 92: 1150-1159.
568. Diamandidou E, Colome M, Fayad L, Duvic M, Kurzrock R (1999). Prognostic factor analysis in mycosis fungoides/Sezary syn-

drome. J Am Acad Dermatol 40: 914-924.
569. Diamanti A, Colistro F, Calce A, Devito R, Ferretti F, Minozzi A, Santoni A, Castro M (2006). Clinical value of immunoglobulin A anti-transglutaminase assay in the diagnosis of celiac disease. Pediatrics 118: e1696-e1700.
570. Diamond C, Taylor TH, Im T, Anton-Culver H (2006). Presentation and outcomes of systemic non-Hodgkin's lymphoma: a comparison between patients with acquired immunodeficiency syndrome (AIDS) treated with highly active antiretroviral therapy and patients without AIDS. Leuk Lymphoma 47: 1822-1829.
571. Dib A, Peterson TR, Raducha-Grace L, Zingone A, Zhan F, Hanamura I, Barlogie B, Shaughnessy J, Jr., Kuehl WM (2006). Paradoxical expression of INK4c in proliferative multiple myeloma tumors: bi-allelic deletion vs increased expression. Cell Div 1: 23.
571A. Diehl V, Engert A, Re D (2007). New strategies for the treatment of advanced-stage Hodgkin's lymphoma. Hematol Oncol Clin North Am 21:897-914.
572. Diehl V, Franklin J, Sextro M, Mauch P (1999). Clinical presentation and treatment of Lymphocyte Predominance Hodgkin's Disease. In: Hodgkin's Disease. Mauch P, Armitage JO, Diehl V, eds. Lippincott Williams & Wilkins: Philadelphia, pp. 563.
573. Diehl V, Sextro M, Franklin J, Hansmann ML, Harris N, Jaffe E, Poppema S, Harris M, Franssila K, van Krieken J, Marafioti T, Anagnostopoulos I, Stein H (1999). Clinical presentation, course, and prognostic factors in lymphocyte-predominant Hodgkin's disease and lymphocyte-rich classical Hodgkin's disease: report from the European Task Force on Lymphoma Project on Lymphocyte-Predominant Hodgkin's Disease. J Clin Oncol 17: 776-783.
574. Dierlamm J, Baens M, Wlodarska I, Stefanova-Ouzounova M, Hernandez JM, Hossfeld DK, Wolf-Peeters C, Hagemeijer A, Van den Berghe H, Marynen P (1999). The apoptosis inhibitor gene API2 and a novel 18q gene, MLT, are recurrently rearranged in the t(11;18)(q21;q21)p6ssociated with mucosa-associated lymphoid tissue lymphomas. Blood 93: 3601-3609.
575. Dierlamm J, Wlodarska I, Michaux L, Stefanova M, Hinz K, Van den BH, Hagemeijer A, Hossfeld DK (2000). Genetic abnormalities in marginal zone B-cell lymphoma. Hematol Oncol 18: 1-13.
576. DiGiuseppe JA, Louie DC, Williams JE, Miller DT, Griffin CA, Mann RB, Borowitz MJ (1997). Blastic natural killer cell leukemia/lymphoma: a clinicopathologic study. Am J Surg Pathol 21: 1223-1230.
577. Dijkman R, Tensen CP, Jordanova ES, Knijnenburg J, Hoefnagel JJ, Mulder AA, Rosenberg C, Raap AK, Willemze R, Szuhai K, Vermeer MH (2006). Array-based comparative genomic hybridization analysis reveals recurrent chromosomal alterations and prognostic parameters in primary cutaneous large B-cell lymphoma. J Clin Oncol 24: 296-305.
578. Dijkman R, van Doorn R, Szuhai K, Willemze R, Vermeer MH, Tensen CP (2007). Gene-expression profiling and array-based CGH classify CD4+CD56+ hematodermic neoplasm and cutaneous myelomonocytic leukemia as distinct disease entities. Blood 109: 1720-1727.
579. Dimopoulos MA, Hamilos G (2002). Solitary bone plasmacytoma and extramedullary plasmacytoma. Curr Treat Options Oncol 3: 255-259.
580. Dimopoulos MA, Kiamouris C, Moulopoulos LA (1999). Solitary plasmacytoma of bone and extramedullary plasmacytoma. Hematol Oncol Clin North Am 13: 1249-1257.
581. Dimopoulos MA, Kyle RA, Anagnostopoulos A, Treon SP (2005). Diagnosis and management of Waldenstrom's macroglobulinemia. J Clin Oncol 23: 1564-1577.
582. Dimopoulos MA, Moulopoulos LA, Maniatis A, Alexanian R (2000). Solitary plasmacytoma of bone and asymptomatic multiple myeloma. Blood 96: 2037-2044.
583. Dimopoulos MA, Palumbo A, Delasalle KB, Alexanian R (1994). Primary plasma cell leukaemia. Br J Haematol 88: 754-759.
584. Dincol G, Nalcaci M, Dogan O, Aktan M, Kucukkaya R, Agan M, Dincol K (2002). Coexistence of chronic neutrophilic leukemia with multiple myeloma. Leuk Lymphoma 43: 649-651.
585. Ding J, Komatsu H, Wakita A, Kato-Uranishi M, Ito M, Satoh A, Tsuboi K, Nitta M, Miyazaki H, Iida S, Ueda R (2004). Familial essential thrombocythemia associated with a dominant-positive activating mutation of the c-MPL gene, which encodes for the receptor for thrombopoietin. Blood 103: 4198-4200.
586. Dingli D, Grand FH, Mahaffey V, Spurbeck J, Ross FM, Watmore AE, Reilly JT, Cross NC, Dewald GW, Tefferi A (2005). Der(6)t(1;6)(q21-23;p21.3): a specific cytogenetic abnormality in myelofibrosis with myeloid metaplasia. Br J Haematol 130: 229-232.
587. Dingli D, Kyle RA, Rajkumar SV, Nowakowski GS, Larson DR, Bida JP, Gertz MA, Therneau TM, Melton LJ, III, Dispenzieri A, Katzmann JA (2006). Immunoglobulin free light chains and solitary plasmacytoma of bone. Blood 108: 1979-1983.
588. Dingli D, Mesa RA, Tefferi A (2004). Myelofibrosis with myeloid metaplasia: new developments in pathogenesis and treatment. Intern Med 43: 540-547.
589. Dirnhofer S, Angeles-Angeles A, Ortiz-Hidalgo C, Reyes E, Gredler E, Krugmann J, Fend F, Quintanilla-Martinez L (1999). High prevalence of a 30-base pair deletion in the Epstein-Barr virus (EBV) latent membrane protein 1 gene and of strain type B EBV in Mexican classical Hodgkin's disease and reactive lymphoid tissue. Hum Pathol 30: 781-787.
590. Dispenzieri A, Kyle RA, Lacy MQ, Rajkumar SV, Therneau TM, Larson DR, Greipp PR, Witzig TE, Basu R, Suarez GA, Fonseca R, Lust JA, Gertz MA (2003). POEMS syndrome: definitions and long-term outcome. Blood 101: 2496-2506.
591. Divine M, Casassus P, Koscielny S, Bosq J, Sebban C, Le Maignan C, Stamattoulas A, Dupriez B, Raphael M, Pico JL, Ribrag V (2005). Burkitt lymphoma in adults: a prospective study of 72 patients treated with an adapted pediatric LMB protocol. Ann Oncol 16: 1928-1935.
591A. Divine M, Casassus P, Koscielny S, Bosq J, Moullet I, Lemaignan C, Stamberg J, Dupriez B, Najman A, Pico J (1999). Small noncleaved cell lymphoma. A prospective multicenter study of 51 adults treated with the LMB pediatric protocol. Blood 10: 523a.
592. Dixon N, Kishnani PS, Zimmerman S (2006). Clinical manifestations of hematologic and oncologic disorders in patients with Down syndrome. Am J Med Genet C Semin Med Genet 142: 149-157.
593. Djokic M, Le Beau MM, Swinnen LJ, Smith SM, Rubin CM, Anastasi J, Carlson KM (2006). Post-transplant lymphoproliferative disorder subtypes correlate with different recurring chromosomal abnormalities. Genes Chromosomes Cancer 45: 313-318.
594. Dobo I, Boiret N, Lippert E, Girodon F, Mossuz P, Donnard M, Campos L, Pineau D, Bascans E, Praloran V, Hermouet S (2004). A standardized endogenous megakaryocytic erythroid colony assay for the diagnosis of essential thrombocythemia. Haematologica 89: 1207-1212.
595. Dobo I, Donnard M, Girodon F, Mossuz P, Boiret N, Boukhari R, Allegraud A, Bascans E, Campos L, Pineau D, Turlure P, Praloran V, Hermouet S (2004). Standardization and comparison of endogenous erythroid colony assays performed with bone marrow or blood progenitors for the diagnosis of polycythemia vera. Hematol J 5: 161-167.
596. Doeden K, Molina-Kirsch H, Perez E, Warnke R, Sundram U (2007). Hydroa-like lymphoma with CD56 expression. J Cutan Pathol .:
597. Dogan A, Attygalle AD, Kyriakou C (2003). Angioimmunoblastic T-cell lymphoma. Br J Haematol 121: 681-691.
598. Dogan A, Burke JS, Goteri G, Stitson RN, Wotherspoon AC, Isaacson PG (2003). Micronodular T-cell/histiocyte-rich large B-cell lymphoma of the spleen: histology, immunophenotype, and differential diagnosis. Am J Surg Pathol 27: 903-911.
599. Dogan A, Du MQ, Aiello A, Diss TC, Ye HT, Pan LX, Isaacson PG (1998). Follicular lymphomas contain a clonally linked but phenotypically distinct neoplastic B-cell population in the interfollicular zone. Blood 91: 4708-4714.
600. Doglioni C, Wotherspoon AC, Moschini A, de Boni M, Isaacson PG (1992). High incidence of primary gastric lymphoma in northeastern Italy. Lancet 339: 834-835.
601. Dohner H, Stilgenbauer S, Benner A, Leupolt E, Krober A, Bullinger L, Dohner K, Bentz M, Lichter P (2000). Genomic aberrations and survival in chronic lymphocytic leukemia. N Engl J Med 343: 1910-1916.
602. Dohner K, Schlenk RF, Habdank M, Scholl C, Rucker FG, Corbacioglu A, Bullinger L, Frohling S, Dohner H (2005). Mutant nucleophosmin (NPM1) predicts favorable prognosis in younger adults with acute myeloid leukemia and normal cytogenetics: interaction with other gene mutations. Blood 106: 3740-3746.
603. Dohner K, Tobis K, Ulrich R, Frohling S, Benner A, Schlenk RF, Dohner H (2002). Prognostic significance of partial tandem duplications of the MLL gene in adult patients 16 to 60 years old with acute myeloid leukemia and normal cytogenetics: a study of the Acute Myeloid Leukemia Study Group Ulm. J Clin Oncol 20: 3254-3261.
604. Dong HY, Scadden DT, de Leval L, Tang Z, Isaacson PG, Harris NL (2005). Plasmablastic lymphoma in HIV-positive patients: an aggressive Epstein-Barr virus-associated extramedullary plasmacytic neoplasm. Am J Surg Pathol 29: 1633-1641.
605. Dorfman DM, Brown JA, Shahsafaei A, Freeman GJ (2006). Programmed death-1 (PD-1) is a marker of germinal center-associated T cells and angioimmunoblastic T-cell lymphoma. Am J Surg Pathol 30: 802-810.
606. Dotti G, Fiocchi R, Motta T, Facchinetti B, Chiodini B, Borleri GM, Gavazzeni G, Barbui T, Rambaldi A (1999). Primary effusion lymphoma after heart transplantation: a new entity associated with human herpesvirus-8. Leukemia 13: 664-670.
607. Douer D, Tallman MS (2005). Arsenic trioxide: new clinical experience with an old medication in hematologic malignancies. J Clin Oncol 23: 2396-2410.
608. Downing JR (1999). The AML1-ETO chimaeric transcription factor in acute myeloid leukaemia: biology and clinical significance. Br J Haematol 106: 296-308.
609. Doyle TJ, Venkatachalam KK, Maeda K, Saeed SM, Tilchen EJ (1983). Hodgkin's disease in renal transplant recipients. Cancer 51: 245-247.
610. Drayson M, Tang LX, Drew R, Mead GP, Carr-Smith H, Bradwell AR (2001). Serum free light-chain measurements for identifying and monitoring patients with nonsecretory multiple myeloma. Blood 97: 2900-2902.
611. Dreno B (2006). Standard and new treatments in cutaneous B-cell lymphomas. J Cutan Pathol 33 Suppl 1: 47-51.
612. Drenou B, Lamy T, Amiot L, Fardel O, Caulet-Maugendre S, Sasportes M, Diebold J, Le Prise PY, Fauchet R (1997). CD3- CD56+ non-Hodgkin's lymphomas with an aggressive behavior related to multidrug resistance. Blood 89: 2966-2974.
613. Drexler HG, Gignac SM, von Wasielewski R, Werner M, Dirks WG (2000). Pathobiology of NPM-ALK and variant fusion genes in anaplastic large cell lymphoma and other lymphomas. Leukemia 14: 1533-1559.
614. Droc C, Cualing HD, Kadin ME (2007). Need for an improved molecular/genetic classification for CD30+ lymphomas involving the skin. Cancer Control 14: 124-132.
615. Druker BJ, Guilhot F, O'Brien SG, Gathmann I, Kantarjian H, Gattermann N, Deininger MW, Silver RT, Goldman JM, Stone RM, Cervantes F, Hochhaus A, Powell BL, Gabrilove JL, Rousselot P, Reiffers J, Cornelissen JJ, Hughes T, Agis H, Fischer T, Verhoef G, Shepherd J, Saglio G, Gratwohl A, Nielsen JL, Radich JP, Simonsson B, Taylor K, Baccarani M, So C, Letvak L, Larson RA (2006). Five-year follow-up of patients receiving imatinib for chronic myeloid leukemia. N Engl J Med 355: 2408-2417.
616. Druker BJ, Talpaz M, Resta DJ, Peng B, Buchdunger E, Ford JM, Lydon NB, Kantarjian H, Capdeville R, Ohno-Jones S, Sawyers CL (2001). Efficacy and safety of a specific inhibitor of the BCR-ABL tyrosine kinase in chronic myeloid leukemia. N Engl J Med 344: 1031-1037.
617. Druker BJ, Tamura S, Buchdunger E, Ohno S, Segal GM, Fanning S, Zimmermann J, Lydon NB (1996). Effects of a selective inhibitor of the Abl tyrosine kinase on the growth of Bcr-Abl positive cells. Nat Med 2: 561-566.
617A. Du MQ, Bacon CM, Isaacson PG (2007). Kaposi sarcoma-associated herpesvirus/human herpesvirus 8 and lymphoproliferative disorders. J Clin Pathol 60: 1350-1357.
618. Du M, Diss TC, Xu C, Peng H, Isaacson PG, Pan L (1996). Ongoing mutation in MALT lymphoma immunoglobulin gene that antigen stimulation plays a role in the clonal expansion. Leukemia 10: 1190-1197.
618A. Du MQ, Diss TC, Liu H, Ye H, Hamoudi RA, Cabeçadas J, Dong HY, Harris NL, Chan JK, Rees JW, Dogan A, Isaacson PG (2002). KSHV- and EBV-associated germinotropic lymphoproliferative disorder. Blood 100:3415-3418.
618B. Du MQ, Diss TC, Xu CF, Wotherspoon AC, Isaacson PG, Pan LX (1997). Ongoing immunoglobulin gene mutations in mantle cell lymphomas. Br J Haematol. 96: 124-131.
619. Du MQ, Liu H, Diss TC, Ye H, Hamoudi RA, Dupin N, Meignin V, Oksenhendler E, Boshoff C, Isaacson PG (2001). Kaposi sarcoma-associated herpesvirus infects monotypic (IgM lambda) but polyclonal naive B cells in Castleman disease and associated lymphoproliferative disorders. Blood 97: 2130-2136.
620. Duchayne E, Fenneteau O, Pages MP, Sainty D, Arnoulet C, Dastugue N, Garand R, Flandrin G (2003). Acute megakaryoblastic leukaemia: a national clinical and biological study of 53 adult and childhood cases by the Groupe Francais d'Hematologie Cellulaire (GFHC). Leuk Lymphoma 44: 49-58.
621. Dufau JP, Le Tourneau A, Molina T, Le Houcq M, Claessens YE, Rio B, Delmer A, Diebold J (2000). Intravascular large B-cell lymphoma with bone marrow involvement at presentation and haemophagocytic syndrome: two

Western cases in favour of a specific variant. Histopathology 37: 509-512.
622. Dul JL, Argon Y (1990). A single amino acid substitution in the variable region of the light chain specifically blocks immunoglobulin secretion. Proc Natl Acad Sci U S A 87: 8135-8139.
623. Dunleavy K, Wilson WH, Jaffe ES (2007). Angioimmunoblastic T cell lymphoma: pathobiological insights and clinical implications. Curr Opin Hematol 14: 348-353.
624. Dunn-Walters DK, Boursier L, Spencer J, Isaacson PG (1998). Analysis of immunoglobulin genes in splenic marginal zone lymphoma suggests ongoing mutation. Hum Pathol 29: 585-593.
625. Dunphy CH, Gardner LJ, Grosso LE, Evans HL (2002). Flow cytometric immunophenotyping in posttransplant lymphoproliferative disorders. Am J Clin Pathol 117: 24-28.
626. Dunphy CH, Orton SO, Mantell J (2004). Relative contributions of enzyme cytochemistry and flow cytometric immunophenotyping to the evaluation of acute myeloid leukemias with a monocytic component and of flow cytometric immunophenotyping to the evaluation of absolute monocytoses. Am J Clin Pathol 122: 865-874.
627. Dupin N, Diss TL, Kellam P, Tulliez M, Du MQ, Sicard D, Weiss RA, Isaacson PG, Boshoff C (2000). HHV-8 is associated with a plasmablastic variant of Castleman disease that is linked to HHV-8-positive plasmablastic lymphoma. Blood 95: 1406-1412.
628. Dupin N, Fisher C, Kellam P, Ariad S, Tulliez M, Franck N, van Marck E, Salmon D, Gorin I, Escande JP, Weiss RA, Alitalo K, Boshoff C (1999). Distribution of human herpesvirus-8 latently infected cells in Kaposi's sarcoma, multicentric Castleman's disease, and primary effusion lymphoma. Proc Natl Acad Sci U S A 96: 4546-4551.
629. Duplantier JE, Seyama K, Day NK, Hitchcock R, Nelson RP, Ochs HD, Haraguchi S, Klemperer MR, Good RA (2001). Immunologic reconstitution following bone marrow transplantation for X-linked hyper IgM syndrome. Clin Immunol 98: 313-318.
630. Dupriez B, Morel P, Demory JL, Lai JL, Simon M, Plantier I, Bauters F (1996). Prognostic factors in agnogenic myeloid metaplasia: a report on 195 cases with a new scoring system. Blood 88: 1013-1018.
631. Dupuis J, Boye K, Martin N, Copie-Bergman C, Plonquet A, Fabiani B, Baglin AC, Haioun C, Delfau-Larue MH, Gaulard P (2006). Expression of CXCL13 by neoplastic cells in angioimmunoblastic T-cell lymphoma (AITL): a new diagnostic marker providing evidence that AITL derives from follicular helper T cells. Am J Surg Pathol 30: 490-494.
632. Dupuis J, Emile JF, Mounier N, Gisselbrecht C, Martin-Garcia N, Petrella T, Bouabdallah R, Berger F, Delmer A, Coiffier B, Reyes F, Gaulard P (2006). Prognostic significance of Epstein-Barr virus in nodal peripheral T-cell lymphoma, unspecified: A Groupe d'Etude des Lymphomes de l'Adulte (GELA) study. Blood 108: 4163-4169.
633. Durie BG, Salmon SE (1975). A clinical staging system for multiple myeloma. Correlation of measured myeloma cell mass with presenting clinical features, response to treatment, and survival. Cancer 36: 842-854.
634. Dyck PJ, Engelstad J, Dispenzieri A (2006). Vascular endothelial growth factor and POEMS. Neurology 66: 10-12.
635. Ebert BL, Pretz J, Bosco J, Chang CY, Tamayo P, Galili N, Raza A, Root DE, Attar E, Ellis SR, Golub TR (2008). Identification of RPS14 as a 5q- syndrome gene by RNA interference screen. Nature 451: 335-339.
636. Eck M, Schmausser B, Greiner A, Muller-Hermelink HK (2000). Helicobacter pylori in gastric mucosa-associated lymphoid tissue type lymphoma. Recent Results Cancer Res 156:9-18: 9-18.
636A. Ehlers A, Oker E, Bentink S, Lenze D, Stein H, Hummel M (2008). Histone acetylation and DNA demethylation of B cells result in a Hodgkin-like phenotype. Leukemia 22:835-841
637. Elenitoba-Johnson KS, Gascoyne RD, Lim MS, Chhanabai M, Jaffe ES, Raffeld M (1998). Homozygous deletions at chromosome 9p21 involving p16 and p15 are associated with histologic progression in follicle center lymphoma. Blood 91: 4677-4685.
638. Elenitoba-Johnson KS, Jaffe ES (1997). Lymphoproliferative disorders associated with congenital immunodeficiencies. Semin Diagn Pathol 14: 35-47.
639. Elenitoba-Johnson KS, Zarate-Osorno A, Meneses A, Krenacs L, Kingma DW, Raffeld M, Jaffe ES (1998). Cytotoxic granular protein expression, Epstein-Barr virus strain type, and latent membrane protein-1 oncogene deletions in nasal T-lymphocyte/natural killer cell lymphomas from Mexico. Mod Pathol 11: 754-761.
640. Elliott MA, Hanson CA, Dewald GW, Smoley SA, Lasho TL, Tefferi A (2005). WHO-defined chronic neutrophilic leukemia: a long-term analysis of 12 cases and a critical review of the literature. Leukemia 19: 313-317.
641. Ellis JT, Peterson P, Geller SA, Rappaport H (1986). Studies of the bone marrow in polycythemia vera and the evolution of myelofibrosis and second hematologic malignancies. Semin Hematol 23: 144-155.
642. Else M, Ruchlemer R, Osuji N, Del G, I, Matutes E, Woodman A, Wotherspoon A, Swansbury J, Dearden C, Catovsky D (2005). Long remissions in hairy cell leukemia with purine analogs: a report of 219 patients with a median follow-up of 12.5 years. Cancer 104: 2442-2448.
643. Elstrom RL, Andreadis C, Aqui NA, Ahya VN, Bloom RD, Brozena SC, Olthoff KM, Schuster SJ, Nasta SD, Stadtmauer EA, Tsai DE (2006). Treatment of PTLD with rituximab or chemotherapy. Am J Transplant 6: 569-576.
644. Emanuel PD, Bates LJ, Castleberry RP, Gualtieri RJ, Zuckerman KS (1991). Selective hypersensitivity to granulocyte-macrophage colony-stimulating factor by juvenile chronic myeloid leukemia hematopoietic progenitors. Blood 77: 925-929.
645. Engelhard M, Brittinger G, Huhn D, Gerhartz HH, Meusers P, Siegert W, Thiel E, Wilmanns W, Aydemir U, Bierwolf S, Griesser H, Tiemann M, Lennert K (1997). Subclassification of diffuse large B-cell lymphomas according to the Kiel classification: distinction of centroblastic and immunoblastic lymphomas is a significant prognostic risk factor. Blood 89: 2291-2297.
646. Engels EA, Pfeiffer RM, Goedert JJ, Virgo P, McNeel TS, Scoppa SM, Biggar RJ (2006). Trends in cancer risk among people with AIDS in the United States 1980-2002. AIDS 20: 1645-1654.
647. Engert A, Ballova V, Haverkamp H, Pfistner B, Josting A, Duhmke E, Muller-Hermelink K, Diehl V (2005). Hodgkin's lymphoma in elderly patients: a comprehensive retrospective analysis from the German Hodgkin's Study Group. J Clin Oncol 23: 5052-5060.
648. Epling-Burnette PK, Liu JH, Catlett-Falcone R, Turkson J, Oshiro M, Kothapalli R, Li Y, Wang JM, Yang-Yen HF, Karras J, Jove R, Loughran TP, Jr. (2001). Inhibition of STAT3 signaling leads to apoptosis of leukemic large granular lymphocytes and decreased Mcl-1 expression. J Clin Invest 107: 351-362.
649. Epling-Burnette PK, Painter JS, Chaurasia P, Bai F, Wei S, Djeu JY, Loughran TP, Jr. (2004). Dysregulated NK receptor expression in patients with lymphoproliferative disease of granular lymphocytes. Blood 103: 3431-3439.
650. Escribano L, Orfao A, Villarrubia J, Diaz-Agustin B, Cervero C, Rios A, Velasco JL, Ciudad J, Navarro JL, San Miguel JF (1998). Immunophenotypic characterization of human bone marrow mast cells. A flow cytometric study of normal and pathological bone marrow samples. Anal Cell Pathol 16: 151-159.
651. Estey E, Dohner H (2006). Acute myeloid leukaemia. Lancet 368: 1894-1907.
652. Evans PA, Pott C, Groenen PJ, Salles G, Davi F, Berger F, Garcia JF, Van Krieken JH, Pals S, Kluin P, Schuuring E, Spaargaren M, Boone E, Gonzalez D, Martinez B, Villuendas R, Gameiro P, Diss TC, Mills K, Morgan GJ, Carter GI, Milner BJ, Pearson D, Hummel M, Jung W, Ott M, Canioni D, Beldjord K, Bastard C, Delfau-Larue MH, van Dongen JJ, Molina TJ, Cabecadas J (2007). Significantly improved PCR-based clonality testing in B-cell malignancies by use of multiple immunoglobulin gene targets. Report of the BIOMED-2 Concerted Action BHM4-CT98-3936. Leukemia 21: 207-214.
653. Exner M, Thalhammer R, Kapiotis S, Mitterbauer G, Knobl P, Haas OA, Jager U, Schwarzinger I (2000). The "typical" immunophenotype of acute promyelocytic leukemia (APL-M3): does it prove true for the M3-variant? Cytometry 42: 106-109.
654. Facchetti F, Vermi W, Mason D, Colonna M (2003). The plasmacytoid monocyte/interferon producing cells. Virchows Arch 443: 703-717.
655. Facchetti F, Wolf-Peeters C, Kennes C, Rossi G, De Vos R, van den Oord JJ, Desmet VJ (1990). Leukemia-associated lymph node infiltrates of plasmacytoid monocytes (so-called plasmacytoid T-cells). Evidence for two distinct histological and immunophenotypical patterns. Am J Surg Pathol 14: 101-112.
656. Facer CA, Playfair JH (1989). Malaria, Epstein-Barr virus, and the genesis of lymphomas. Adv Cancer Res 53: 33-72.
657. Faderl S, Talpaz M, Estrov Z, Kantarjian HM (1999). Chronic myelogenous leukemia: biology and therapy. Ann Intern Med 131: 207-219.
658. Faguet GB, Barton BP, Smith LL, Garver FA (1977). Gamma heavy chain disease: clinical aspects and characterization of a deleted, noncovalently linked gamma1 heavy chain dimer (BAZ). Blood 49: 495-505.
659. Falini B (2001). Anaplastic large cell lymphoma: pathological, molecular and clinical features. Br J Haematol 114: 741-760.
660. Falini B, Bigerna B, Fizzotti M, Pulford K, Pileri SA, Delsol G, Carbone A, Paulli M, Magrini U, Menestrina F, Giardini R, Pilotti S, Mezzelani A, Ugolini B, Billi M, Pucciarini A, Pacini R, Pelicci PG, Flenghi L (1998). ALK expression defines a distinct group of T/null lymphomas ("ALK lymphomas") with a wide morphological spectrum. Am J Pathol 153: 875-886.
661. Falini B, Fizzotti M, Pucciarini A, Bigerna B, Marafioti T, Gambacorta M, Pacini R, Alunni C, Natali-Tanci L, Ugolini B, Sebastiani C, Cattoretti G, Pileri S, Dalla-Favera R, Stein H (2000). A monoclonal antibody (MUM1p) detects expression of the MUM1/IRF4 protein in a subset of germinal center B cells, plasma cells, and activated T cells. Blood 95: 2084-2092.
662. Falini B, Flenghi L, Fagioli M, Coco FL, Cordone I, Diverio D, Pasqualucci L, Biondi A, Riganelli D, Orleth A, Liso A, Martelli MF, Pelicci PG, Pileri S (1997). Immunocytochemical diagnosis of acute promyelocytic leukemia (M3) with the monoclonal antibody PG-M3 (anti-PML). Blood 90: 4046-4053.
662A. Falini B, Flenghi L, Pileri S, Gambacorta M, Bigerna B, Durkop H, Eitelbach F, Thiele J, Pacini R, Cavaliere A, et al (1993). PG-M1: a new monoclonal antibody directed against a fixative-resistant epitope on the macrophage-restricted form of the CD68 molecule. Am J Pathol 142: 1359-1372
663. Falini B, Lenze D, Hasserjian R, Coupland S, Jaehne D, Soupir C, Liso A, Martelli MP, Bolli N, Bacci F, Pettirossi V, Santucci A, Martelli MF, Pileri S, Stein H (2007). Cytoplasmic mutated nucleophosmin (NPM) defines the molecular status of a significant fraction of myeloid sarcomas. Leukemia 21: 1566-1570.
664. Falini B, Martelli MP, Bolli N, Bonasso R, Ghia E, Pallotta MT, Diverio D, Nicoletti I, Pacini R, Tabarrini A, Galletti BV, Mannucci R, Roti G, Rosati R, Specchia G, Liso A, Tiacci E, Alcalay M, Luzi L, Volorio S, Bernard L, Guarini A, Amadori S, Mandelli F, Pane F, Lo-Coco F, Saglio G, Pelicci PG, Martelli MF, Mecucci C (2006). Immunohistochemistry predicts nucleophosmin (NPM) mutations in acute myeloid leukemia. Blood 108: 1999-2005.
665. Falini B, Mecucci C, Saglio G, Lo-Coco F, Diverio D, Brown P, Pane F, Mancini M, Martelli MP, Pileri S, Haferlach T, Haferlach C, Schnittger S (2008). NPM1 mutations and cytoplasmic nucleophosmin are mutually exclusive of recurrent genetic abnormalities: a comparative analysis on 2562 patients with acute myeloid leukemia. Haematologica 93: 439-442.
666. Falini B, Mecucci C, Tiacci E, Alcalay M, Rosati R, Pasqualucci L, La Starza R, Diverio D, Colombo E, Santucci A, Bigerna B, Pacini R, Pucciarini A, Liso A, Vignetti M, Fazi P, Meani N, Pettirossi V, Saglio G, Mandelli F, Lo-Coco F, Pelicci PG, Martelli MF (2005). Cytoplasmic nucleophosmin in acute myelogenous leukemia with a normal karyotype. N Engl J Med 352: 254-266.
667. Falini B, Nicoletti I, Martelli MF, Mecucci C (2007). Acute myeloid leukemia carrying cytoplasmic/mutated nucleophosmin (NPMc+ AML): biologic and clinical features. Blood 109: 874-885.
668. Falini B, Pileri S, Zinzani PL, Carbone A, Zagonel V, Wolf-Peeters C, Verhoef G, Menestrina F, Todeschini G, Paulli M, Lazzarino M, Giardini R, Aiello A, Foss HD, Araujo I, Fizzotti M, Pelicci PG, Flenghi L, Martelli MF, Santucci A (1999). ALK+ lymphoma: clinico-pathological findings and outcome. Blood 93: 2697-2706.
669. Falini B, Pulford K, Pucciarini A, Carbone A, Wolf-Peeters C, Cordell J, Fizzotti M, Santucci A, Pelicci PG, Pileri S, Campo E, Ott G, Delsol G, Mason DY (1999). Lymphomas expressing ALK fusion protein(s) other than NPM-ALK. Blood 94: 3509-3515.
670. Falini B, Tiacci E, Liso A, Basso K, Sabattini E, Pacini R, Foa R, Pulsoni A, Dalla FR, Pileri S (2004). Simple diagnostic assay for hairy cell leukaemia by immunocytochemical detection of annexin A1 (ANXA1). Lancet 363: 1869-1870.
671. Fan Z, Natkunam Y, Bair E, Tibshirani R, Warnke RA (2003). Characterization of variant patterns of nodular lymphocyte predominant hodgkin lymphoma with immunohistologic and clinical correlation. Am J Surg Pathol 27: 1346-1356.
672. Farcet JP, Gaulard P, Marolleau JP, Le Couedic JP, Henni T, Gourdin MF, Divine M, Haioun C, Zafrani S, Goossens M (1990). Hepatosplenic T-cell lymphoma: sinusal/ sinusoidal localization of malignant cells expressing the T-cell receptor gamma delta. Blood 75: 2213-2219.

673. Favara BE, Feller AC, Pauli M, Jaffe ES, Weiss LM, Arico M, Bucsky P, Egeler RM, Elinder G, Gadner H, Gresik M, Henter JI, Imashuku S, Janka-Schaub G, Jaffe R, Ladisch S, Nezelof C, Pritchard J (1997). Contemporary classification of histiocytic disorders. The WHO Committee On Histiocytic/Reticulum Cell Proliferations. Reclassification Working Group of the Histiocyte Society. Med Pediatr Oncol 29: 157-166.

674. Favara BE, Jaffe R, Egeler RM (2002). Macrophage activation and hemophagocytic syndrome in langerhans cell histiocytosis: report of 30 cases. Pediatr Dev Pathol 5: 130-140.

675. Feiner HD (1988). Pathology of dysproteinemia: light chain amyloidosis, non-amyloid immunoglobulin deposition disease, cryoglobulinemia syndromes, and macroglobulinemia of Waldenstrom. Hum Pathol 19: 1255-1272.

675A. Feldman AL, Arber DA, Pittaluga S, Martinez A, Burke JS, Raffeld M, Camos M, Warnke R, Jaffe ES (2008). Clonally related follicular lymphomas and histiocytic/dendritic cell sarcomas: evidence for transdifferentiation of the follicular lymphoma clone. Blood 111: 5433-5439.

676. Feldman AL, Berthold F, Arceci RJ, Abramowsky C, Shehata BM, Mann KP, Lauer SJ, Pritchard J, Raffeld M, Jaffe ES (2005). Clonal relationship between precursor T-lymphoblastic leukaemia/lymphoma and Langerhans-cell histiocytosis. Lancet Oncol 6: 435-437.

677. Feldman AL, Minniti C, Santi M, Downing JR, Raffeld M, Jaffe ES (2004). Histiocytic sarcoma after acute lymphoblastic leukaemia: a common clonal origin. Lancet Oncol 5: 248-250.

678. Felgar RE, Macon WR, Kinney MC, Roberts S, Pasha T, Salhany KE (1997). TIA-1 expression in lymphoid neoplasms. Identification of subsets with cytotoxic T lymphocyte or natural killer cell differentiation. Am J Pathol 150: 1893-1900.

679. Felix CA (2000). Acute lymphoblastic leukemia in infants. In: Education Program Book. Education Program Book. American Society of Hematology: Washington, DC, pp. 294-302.

680. Felman P, Bryon PA, Gentilhomme O, Ffrench M, Charrin C, Espinouse D, Viala JJ (1988). The syndrome of abnormal chromatin clumping in leucocytes: a myelodysplastic disorder with proliferative features? Br J Haematol 70: 49-54.

681. Feltkamp CA, van Heerde P, Feltkamp-Vroom TM, Koudstaal J (1981). A malignant tumor arising from interdigitating cells; light microscopical, ultrastructural, immuno-and enzyme-histochemical characteristics. Virchows Arch [Pathol Anat] 393: 183-192.

682. Fenaux P, Beuscart R, Lai JL, Jouet JP, Bauters F (1988). Prognostic factors in adult chronic myelomonocytic leukemia: an analysis of 107 cases. J Clin Oncol 6: 1417-1424.

683. Fenaux P, Jouet JP, Zandecki M, Lai JL, Simon M, Pollet JP, Bauters F (1987). Chronic and subacute myelomonocytic leukaemia in the adult: a report of 60 cases with special reference to prognostic factors. Br J Haematol 65: 101-106.

684. Fenaux P, Morel P, Lai JL (1996). Cytogenetics of myelodysplastic syndromes. Semin Hematol 33: 127-138.

685. Fenaux P, Wang ZZ, Degos L (2007). Treatment of acute promyelocytic leukemia by retinoids. Curr Top Microbiol Immunol 313: 101-128.

686. Fermand JP, Brouet JC (1999). Heavy-chain diseases. Hematol Oncol Clin North Am 13: 1281-1294.

687. Fermand JP, Brouet JC, Danon F, Seligmann M (1989). Gamma heavy chain "disease": heterogeneity of the clinicopathologic features. Report of 16 cases and review of the literature. Medicine (Baltimore) 68: 321-335.

688. Fernandez V, Hartmann E, Ott G, Campo E, Rosenwald A (2005). Pathogenesis of mantle-cell lymphoma: all oncogenic roads lead to dysregulation of cell cycle and DNA damage response pathways. J Clin Oncol 23: 6364-6369.

689. Ferrando AA, Neuberg DS, Staunton J, Loh ML, Huard C, Raimondi SC, Behm FG, Pui CH, Downing JR, Gilliland DG, Lander ES, Golub TR, Look AT (2002). Gene expression signatures define novel oncogenic pathways in T cell acute lymphoblastic leukemia. Cancer Cell 1: 75-87.

690. Ferrara F, Morabito F, Martino B, Specchia G, Liso V, Nobile F, Boccuni P, Di Noto R, Pane F, Annunziata M, Schiavone EM, De Simone M, Guglielmi C, Del Vecchio L, Lo CF (2000). CD56 expression is an indicator of poor clinical outcome in patients with acute promyelocytic leukemia treated with simultaneous all-trans-retinoic acid and chemotherapy. J Clin Oncol 18: 1295-1300.

691. Ferrer A, Salaverria I, Bosch F, Villamor N, Rozman M, Bea S, Gine E, Lopez-Guillermo A, Campo E, Montserrat E (2007). Leukemic involvement is a common feature in mantle cell lymphoma. Cancer 109: 2473-2480.

692. Ferreri AJ, Campo E, Ambrosetti A, Ilariucci F, Seymour JF, Willemze R, Arrigoni G, Rossi G, Lopez-Guillermo A, Berti E, Eriksson M, Federico M, Cortelazzo S, Govi S, Frungillo N, Dell'Oro S, Lestani M, Asioli S, Pedrinis E, Ungari M, Motta T, Rossi R, Artusi T, Iuzzolino P, Zucca E, Cavalli F, Ponzoni M (2004). Anthracycline-based chemotherapy as primary treatment for intravascular lymphoma. Ann Oncol 15: 1215-1221.

693. Ferreri AJ, Campo E, Seymour JF, Willemze R, Ilariucci F, Ambrosetti A, Zucca E, Rossi G, Lopez-Guillermo A, Pavlovsky MA, Geerts ML, Candoni A, Lestani M, Asioli S, Milani M, Piris MA, Pileri S, Facchetti F, Cavalli F, Ponzoni M (2004). Intravascular lymphoma: clinical presentation, natural history, management and prognostic factors in a series of 38 cases, with special emphasis on the 'cutaneous variant'. Br J Haematol 127: 173-183.

694. Ferreri AJ, Dognini GP, Campo E, Willemze R, Seymour JF, Bairey O, Martelli M, De Renz AO, Doglioni C, Montalban C, Tedeschi A, Pavlovsky A, Morgan S, Uziel L, Ferracci M, Ascani S, Gianelli U, Patriarca C, Facchetti F, Dalla LA, Pertoldi B, Horvath B, Szomor A, Zucca E, Cavalli F, Ponzoni M (2007). Variations in clinical presentation, frequency of hemophagocytosis and clinical behavior of intravascular lymphoma diagnosed in different geographical regions. Haematologica 92: 486-492.

695. Ferreri AJ, Ponzoni M, Guidoboni M, Resti AG, Politi LS, Cortelazzo S, Demeter J, Zallio F, Palmas A, Muti G, Dognini GP, Pasini E, Lettini AA, Sacchetti F, De Conciliis C, Doglioni C, Dolcetti R (2006). Bacteria-eradicating therapy with doxycycline in ocular adnexal MALT lymphoma: a multicenter prospective trial. J Natl Cancer Inst 98: 1375-1382.

696. Ferringer T, Banks PM, Metcalf JS (2006). Langerhans cell sarcoma. Am J Dermatopathol 28: 36-39.

697. Ferry JA, Fung CY, Zukerberg L, Lucarelli MJ, Hasserjian RP, Preffer FI, Harris NL (2007). Lymphoma of the ocular adnexa: A study of 353 cases. Am J Surg Pathol 31: 170-184.

698. Ferry JA, Harris NL, Picker LJ, Weinberg DS, Rosales RK, Tapia J, Richardson EP, Jr. (1988). Intravascular lymphomatosis (malignant angioendotheliomatosis). A B-cell neoplasm expressing surface homing receptors. Mod Pathol 1: 444-452.

699. Ferry JA, Jacobson JO, Conti D, Delmonico F, Harris NL (1989). Lymphoproliferative disorders and hematologic malignancies following organ transplantation. Mod Pathol 2: 583-592.

700. Ferry JA, Zukerberg LR, Harris NL (1992). Florid progressive transformation of germinal centers. A syndrome affecting young men, without early progression to nodular lymphocyte predominance Hodgkin's disease. Am J Surg Pathol 16: 252-258.

700A. Feuerborn A, Möritz C, Von Bonin F, Dobbelstein M, Trümper L, Stürzenhofecker B, Kube D (2006). Dysfunctional p53 deletion mutants in cell lines derived from Hodgkin's lymphoma. Leuk Lymphoma 47:1932-1940.

701. Feuerhake F, Kutok JL, Monti S, Chen W, LaCasce AS, Cattoretti G, Kurtin P, Pinkus GS, de Leval L, Harris NL, Savage KJ, Neuberg D, Habermann TM, Dalla-Favera R, Golub TR, Aster JC, Shipp MA (2005). NFkappaB activity, function, and target-gene signatures in primary mediastinal large B-cell lymphoma and diffuse large B-cell lymphoma subtypes. Blood 106: 1392-1399.

702. Feuillard J, Jacob MC, Valensi F, Maynadie M, Gressin R, Chaperot L, Arnoulet C, Brignole-Baudouin F, Drenou B, Duchayne E, Falkenrodt A, Garand R, Homolle E, Husson B, Kuhlein E, Le Calvez G, Sainty D, Sotto MF, Trimoreau F, Bene MC (2002). Clinical and biologic features of CD4(+)CD56(+) malignancies. Blood 99: 1556-1563.

702A Fiedler W, Weh H, Zeller W. Translocation (14;18) and (8;22) in three patients with acute leukemia/lymphoma following centrocytic/centroblastic non-Hodgkin's lymphoma. Ann Hematol 1991; 63:282-287.

703. Fierro MT, Comessatti A, Quaglino P, Ortoncelli M, Osella AS, Ponti R, Novelli M, Bernengo MG (2006). Expression pattern of chemokine receptors and chemokine release in inflammatory erythroderma and Sezary syndrome. Dermatology 213: 284-292.

704. Finazzi G, Caruso V, Marchioli R, Capnist G, Chisesi T, Finelli C, Gugliotta L, Landolfi R, Kutti J, Gisslinger H, Marilus R, Patrono C, Pogliani EM, Randi ML, Villegas A, Tognoni G, Barbui T (2005). Acute leukemia in polycythemia vera: an analysis of 1638 patients enrolled in a prospective observational study. Blood 105: 2664-2670.

705. Finazzi G, Harrison C (2005). Essential thrombocythemia. Semin Hematol 42: 230-238.

706. Fink-Puches R, Zenahlik P, Back B, Smolle J, Kerl H, Cerroni L (2002). Primary cutaneous lymphomas: applicability of current classification schemes (European Organization for Research and Treatment of Cancer, World Health Organization) based on clinicopathologic features observed in a large group of patients. Blood 99: 800-805.

707. Finn LS, Viswanatha DS, Belasco JB, Snyder H, Huebner D, Sorbara L, Raffeld M, Jaffe ES, Salhany KE (1999). Primary follicular lymphoma of the testis in childhood. Cancer 85: 1626-1635.

708. Fioretos T, Strombeck B, Sandberg T, Johansson B, Billstrom R, Borg A, Nilsson PG, Van den BH, Hagemeijer A, Mitelman F, Hoglund M (1999). Isochromosome 17q in blast crisis of chronic myeloid leukemia and in other hematologic malignancies is the result of clustered breakpoints in 17p11 and is not associated with coding TP53 mutations. Blood 94: 225-232.

709. Flann S, Orchard GE, Wain EM, Russell-Jones R (2006). Three cases of lymphomatoid papulosis with a CD56+ immunophenotype. J Am Acad Dermatol 55: 903-906.

710. Flaum MA, Schooley RT, Fauci AS, Gralnick HR (1981). A clinicopathologic correlation of the idiopathic hypereosinophilic syndrome. I. Hematologic manifestations. Blood 58: 1012-1020.

711. Fletcher S, Abdalla S, Edwards M, Bain BJ (2007). Case 32. Eosinophilia: reactive or neoplastic? Leuk Lymphoma 48: 174-176.

712. Florena AM, Tripodo C, Iannitto E, Porcasi R, Ingrao S, Franco V (2004). Value of bone marrow biopsy in the diagnosis of essential thrombocythemia. Haematologica 89: 911-919.

713. Florian S, Esterbauer H, Binder T, Mullauer L, Haas OA, Sperr WR, Sillaber C, Valent P (2006). Systemic mastocytosis (SM) associated with chronic eosinophilic leukemia (SM-CEL): detection of FIP1L1/PDGFRalpha, classification by WHO criteria, and response to therapy with imatinib. Leuk Res 30: 1201-1205.

714. Flotho C, Steinemann D, Mullighan CG, Neale G, Mayer K, Kratz CP, Schlegelberger B, Downing JR, Niemeyer CM (2007). Genome-wide single-nucleotide polymorphism analysis in juvenile myelomonocytic leukemia identifies uniparental disomy surrounding the NF1 locus in cases associated with neurofibromatosis but not in cases with mutant RAS or PTPN11. Oncogene 26: 5816-5821.

715. Fonatsch C, Gudat H, Lengfelder E, Wandt H, Silling-Engelhardt G, Ludwig WD, Thiel E, Freund M, Bodenstein H, Schwieder G, *et al.* (1994). Correlation of cytogenetic findings with clinical features in 18 patients with inv(3)(q21q26) or t(3;3)(q21;q26). Leukemia 8: 1318-1326.

716. Fong CT, Brodeur GM (1987). Down's syndrome and leukemia: epidemiology, genetics, cytogenetics and mechanisms of leukemogenesis. Cancer Genet Cytogenet 28: 55-76.

717. Fonseca R, Bailey RJ, Ahmann GJ, Rajkumar SV, Hoyer JD, Lust JA, Kyle RA, Gertz MA, Greipp PR, Dewald GW (2002). Genomic abnormalities in monoclonal gammopathy of undetermined significance. Blood 100: 1417-1424.

718. Fonseca R, Barlogie B, Bataille R, Bastard C, Bergsagel PL, Chesi M, Davies FE, Drach J, Greipp PR, Kirsch IR, Kuehl WM, Hernandez JM, Minvielle S, Pilarski LM, Shaughnessy JD, Jr., Stewart AK, Avet-Loiseau H (2004). Genetics and cytogenetics of multiple myeloma: a workshop report. Cancer Res 64: 1546-1558.

719. Ford AM, Fasching K, Panzer-Grumayer ER, Koenig M, Haas OA, Greaves MF (2001). Origins of "late" relapse in childhood acute lymphoblastic leukemia with TEL-AML1 fusion genes. Blood 98: 558-564.

720. Ford AM, Pombo-de-Oliveira MS, McCarthy KP, MacLean JM, Carrico KC, Vincent RF, Greaves M (1997). Monoclonal origin of concordant T-cell malignancy in identical twins. Blood 89: 281-285.

721. Forestier E, Heim S, Blennow E, Borgstrom G, Holmgren G, Heinonen K, Johannsson J, Kerndrup G, Andersen MK, Lundin C, Nordgren A, Rosenquist R, Swolin B, Johansson B (2003). Cytogenetic abnormalities in childhood acute myeloid leukaemia: a Nordic series comprising all children enrolled in the NOPHO-93-AML trial between 1993 and 2001. Br J Haematol 121: 566-577.

722. Foss HD, Anagnostopoulos I, Araujo I, Assaf C, Demel G, Kummer JA, Hummel M, Stein H (1996). Anaplastic large-cell lymphomas of T-cell and null-cell phenotype express cytotoxic molecules. Blood 88: 4005-4011.

723. Foss HD, Reusch R, Demel G, Lenz G, Anagnostopoulos I, Hummel M, Stein H (1999). Frequent expression of the B-cell-specific acti-

vator protein in Reed-Sternberg cells of classical Hodgkin's disease provides further evidence for its B-cell origin. Blood 94: 3108-3113.
724. Fraga M, Brousset P, Schlaifer D, Payen C, Robert A, Rubie H, Huguet-Rigal F, Delsol G (1995). Bone marrow involvement in anaplastic large cell lymphoma. Immunohistochemical detection of minimal disease and its prognostic significance. Am J Clin Pathol 103: 82-89.
725. Fraga M, Sanchez-Verde L, Forteza J, Garcia-Rivero A, Piris MA (2002). T-cell/histiocyte-rich large B-cell lymphoma is a disseminated aggressive neoplasm: differential diagnosis from Hodgkin's lymphoma. Histopathology 41: 216-229.
726. Franchini G (1995). Molecular mechanisms of human T-cell leukemia/lymphotropic virus type I infection. Blood 86: 3619-3639.
727. Franco V, Florena AM, Campesi G (1996). Intrasinusoidal bone marrow infiltration: a possible hallmark of splenic lymphoma. Histopathology 29: 571-575.
728. Frangione B, Franklin EC (1973). Heavy chain diseases: clinical features and molecular significance of the disordered immunoglobulin structure. Semin Hematol 10: 53-64.
729. Frangione B, Franklin EC, Prelli F (1976). Mu heavy-chain disease—a defect in immunoglobulin assembly. Structural studies of the kappa chain. Scand J Immunol 5: 623-627.
730. Frank D, Cesarman E, Liu YF, Michler RE, Knowles DM (1995). Posttransplantation lymphoproliferative disorders frequently contain type A and not type B Epstein-Barr virus. Blood 85: 1396-1403.
731. Franke S, Wlodarska I, Maes B, Vandenberghe P, Achten R, Hagemeijer A, Wolf-Peeters C (2002). Comparative genomic hybridization pattern distinguishes T-cell/histiocyte-rich B-cell lymphoma from nodular lymphocyte predominance Hodgkin's lymphoma. Am J Pathol 161: 1861-1867.
732. Franklin EC, Kyle R, Seligmann M, Frangione B (1979). Correlation of protein structure and immunoglobulin gene organization in the light of two new deleted heavy chain disease proteins. Mol Immunol 16: 919-921.
732B. French DL, Laskov R, Scharff MD (1989). The role of somatic hypermutation in the generation of antibody diversity. Science 244: 1152-1157.
732A. French LE, Alcindor T, Shapiro M, McGinnis KS, Margolis DJ, Porter D, Leonard DG, Rook AH, Foss F (2002). Identification of amplified clonal T cell populations in the blood of patients with chronic graft-versus-host disease: positive correlation with response to photopheresis. Bone Marrow Transplant 30: 509-515.
733. Freud AG, Caligiuri MA (2006). Human natural killer cell development. Immunol Rev 214:56-72.
733A. Freyer DR, Kennedy R, Bostrom BC, Kohut G, Dehner LP (1996). Juvenile xanthogranuloma: forms of systemic disease and their clinical implications. J Pediatr 129: 227-237.
734. Friedmann D, Wechsler J, Delfau MH, Esteve E, Farcet JP, de Muret A, Parneix-Spake A, Vaillant L, Revuz J, Bagot M (1995). Primary cutaneous pleomorphic small T-cell lymphoma. A review of 11 cases. The French Study Group on Cutaneous Lymphomas. Arch Dermatol 131: 1009-1015.
735. Frizzera G, Hanto DW, Gajl-Peczalska KJ, Rosai J, McKenna RW, Sibley RK, Holahan KP, Lindquist LL (1981). Polymorphic diffuse B-cell hyperplasias and lymphomas in renal transplant recipients. Cancer Res 41: 4262-4279.
736. Froberg MK, Brunning RD, Dorion P, Litz CE, Torlakovic E (1998). Demonstration of clonality in neutrophils using FISH in a case of chronic neutrophilic leukemia. Leukemia 12: 623-626.
736A. Frohling S, Schlenk RF, Breitruck J, Benner A, Kreitmeier S, Tobis K, Dohner H, Dohner K (2002). Prognostic significance of activating FLT3 mutations in younger adults (16 to 60 years) with acute myeloid leukemia and normal cytogenetics: a study of the AML Study Group Ulm. Blood 100: 4372-4380.
737. Frohling S, Schlenk RF, Stolze I, Bihlmayr J, Benner A, Kreitmeier S, Tobis K, Dohner H, Dohner K (2004). CEBPA mutations in younger adults with acute myeloid leukemia and normal cytogenetics: prognostic relevance and analysis of cooperating mutations. J Clin Oncol 22: 624-633.
738. Fu K, Weisenburger DD, Greiner TC, Dave S, Wright G, Rosenwald A, Chiorazzi M, Iqbal J, Gesk S, Siebert R, De Jong D, Jaffe ES, Wilson WH, Delabie J, Ott G, Dave BJ, Sanger WG, Smith LM, Rimsza L, Braziel RM, Muller-Hermelink HK, Campo E, Gascoyne RD, Staudt LM, Chan WC (2005). Cyclin D1-negative mantle cell lymphoma: a clinicopathologic study based on gene expression profiling. Blood 106: 4315-4321.
739. Fukayama M, Ibuka T, Hayashi Y, Ooba T, Koike M, Mizutani S (1993). Epstein-Barr virus in pyothorax-associated pleural lymphoma. Am J Pathol 143: 1044-1049.
740. Gadner H, Grois N, Arico M, Broadbent V, Ceci A, Jakobson A, Komp D, Michaelis J, Nicholson S, Potschger U, Pritchard J, Ladisch S (2001). A randomized trial of treatment for multisystem Langerhans' cell histiocytosis. J Pediatr 138: 728-734.
741. Gaertner EM, Tsokos M, Derringer GA, Neuhauser TS, Arciero C, Andriko JA (2001). Interdigitating dendritic cell sarcoma. A report of four cases and review of the literature. Am J Clin Pathol 115: 589-597.
742. Gahn B, Haase D, Unterhalt M, Drescher M, Schoch C, Fonatsch C, Terstappen LW, Hiddemann W, Buchner T, Bennett JM, Wormann B (1996). De novo AML with dysplastic hematopoiesis: cytogenetic and prognostic significance. Leukemia 10: 946-951.
743. Gaidano G, Carbone A, Pastore C, Capello D, Migliazza A, Gloghini A, Roncella S, Ferrarini M, Saglio G, Dalla-Favera R (1997). Frequent mutation of the 5' noncoding region of the BCL-6 gene in acquired immunodeficiency syndrome-related non-Hodgkin's lymphomas. Blood 89: 3755-3762.
744. Gaidano G, Cerri M, Capello D, Berra E, Deambrogi C, Rossi D, Larocca LM, Campo E, Gloghini A, Tirelli U, Carbone A (2002). Molecular histogenesis of plasmablastic lymphoma of the oral cavity. Br J Haematol 119: 622-628.
745. Gale KB, Ford AM, Repp R, Borkhardt A, Keller C, Eden OB, Greaves MF (1997). Backtracking leukemia to birth: identification of clonotypic gene fusion sequences in neonatal blood spots. Proc Natl Acad Sci U S A 94: 13950-13954.
746. Gale RE, Green C, Allen C, Mead AJ, Burnett AK, Hills RK, Linch DC (2008). The impact of FLT3 internal tandem duplication mutant level, number, size and interaction with NPM1 mutations in a large cohort of young adult patients with acute myeloid leukemia. Blood 111: 2776-2784.
747. Gale RE, Hills R, Pizzey AR, Kottaridis PD, Swirsky D, Gilkes AF, Nugent E, Mills KI, Wheatley K, Solomon E, Burnett AK, Linch DC, Grimwade D (2005). Relationship between FLT3 mutation status, biologic characteristics, and response to targeted therapy in acute promyelocytic leukemia. Blood 106: 3768-3776.
748. Gallagher CJ, Gregory WM, Jones AE, Stansfeld AG, Richards MA, Dhaliwal HS, Malpas JS, Lister TA (1986). Follicular lymphoma: prognostic factors for response and survival. J Clin Oncol 4: 1470-1480.
748A Gallamini A, Hutchings M, Rigacci L, Specht L, Merli F, Hansen M, Patti C, Loft A, Di Raimondo F, D'Amore F, Biggi A, Vitolo U, Stelitano C, Sancetta R, Trentin L, Luminari S, Iannitto E, Viviani S, Pierri I, Levis A (2007). Early interim 2-[18F]fluoro-2-deoxy-D-glucose positron emission tomography is prognostically superior to international prognostic score in advanced-stage Hodgkin's lymphoma: a report from a joint Italian-Danish study. J Clin Oncol 25: 3746-3752.
749. Gallamini A, Stelitano C, Calvi R, Bellei M, Mattei D, Vitolo U, Morabito F, Martelli M, Brusamolino E, Iannitto E, Zaja F, Cortelazzo S, Rigacci L, Devizzi L, Todeschini G, Santini G, Brugiatelli M, Federico M (2004). Peripheral T-cell lymphoma unspecified (PTCL-U): a new prognostic model from a retrospective multicentric clinical study. Blood 103: 2474-2479.
750. Galton DA, Goldman JM, Wiltshaw E, Catovsky D, Henry K, Goldenberg GJ (1974). Prolymphocytic leukaemia. Br J Haematol 27: 7-23.
751. Gamis AS, Woods WG, Alonzo TA, Buxton A, Lange B, Barnard DR, Gold S, Smith FO (2003). Increased age at diagnosis has a significantly negative effect on outcome in children with Down syndrome and acute myeloid leukemia: a report from the Children's Cancer Group Study 2891. J Clin Oncol 21: 3415-3422.
752. Ganti AK, Weisenburger DD, Smith LM, Hans CP, Bociek RG, Bierman PJ, Vose JM, Armitage JO (2006). Patients with grade 3 follicular lymphoma have prolonged relapse-free survival following anthracycline-based chemotherapy: the Nebraska Lymphoma Study Group Experience. Ann Oncol 17: 920-927.
753. Garand R, Duchayne E, Blanchard D, Robillard N, Kuhlein E, Fenneteau O, Salomon-Nguyen F, Grange MJ, Rousselot P, Demur C (1995). Minimally differentiated erythroleukaemia (AML M6 'variant'): a rare subset of AML distinct from AML M6. Groupe Francais d'Hematologie Cellulaire. Br J Haematol 90: 868-875.
754. Garand R, Goasguen J, Brizard A, Buisine J, Charpentier A, Claisse JF, Duchayne E, Lagrange M, Segonds C, Troussard X, Flandrin G (1998). Indolent course as a relatively frequent presentation in T-prolymphocytic leukaemia. Groupe Francais d'Hematologie Cellulaire. Br J Haematol 103: 488-494.
754A. Garcia-Herrera A, Colomo L, Camos M, Carreras J, Balague O, Martinez A, Lopez-Guillermo A, Estrach T, Campo E (2008). Primary cutaneous small-medium CD4+ T-cell lymphomas. A heterogenous group of tumors with different clinicopathologic features and outcome. J Clin Oncol 26:3364-3371.
755. Garcia-Manero G, Faderl S, O'Brien S, Cortes J, Talpaz M, Kantarjian HM (2003). Chronic myelogenous leukemia: a review and update of therapeutic strategies. Cancer 98: 437-457.
756. Garcia-Montero AC, Jara-Acevedo M, Teodosio C, Sanchez ML, Nunez R, Prados A, Aldanondo I, Sanchez L, Dominguez M, Botana LM, Sanchez-Jimenez F, Sotlar K, Almeida J, Escribano L, Orfao A (2006). KIT mutation in mast cells and other bone marrow hematopoietic cell lineages in systemic mast cell disorders: a prospective study of the Spanish Network on Mastocytosis (REMA) in a series of 113 patients. Blood 108: 2366-2372.
757. Garcia-Sanz R, Orfao A, Gonzalez M, Tabernero MD, Blade J, Moro MJ, Fernandez-Calvo J, Sanz MA, Perez-Simon JA, Rasillo A, Miguel JF (1999). Primary plasma cell leukemia: clinical, immunophenotypic, DNA ploidy, and cytogenetic characteristics. Blood 93: 1032-1037.
758. Garcia JF, Mollejo M, Fraga M, Forteza J, Muniesa JA, Perez-Guillermo M, Perez-Seoane C, Rivera T, Ortega P, Piris MA (2005). Large B-cell lymphoma with Hodgkin's features. Histopathology 47: 101-110.
758A. Gardner RV, Velez MC, Ode DL, Lee JW, Correa H (2004). Gamma/delta T-cell lymphoma as a recurrent complication after transplantation. Leuk Lymphoma 45: 2355-2359.
759. Gascoyne RD, Adomat SA, Krajewski S, Krajewska M, Horsman DE, Tolcher AW, O'Reilly SE, Hoskins P, Coldman AJ, Reed JC, Connors JM (1997). Prognostic significance of Bcl-2 protein expression and Bcl-2 gene rearrangement in diffuse aggressive non-Hodgkin's lymphoma. Blood 90: 244-251.
760. Gascoyne RD, Aoun P, Wu D, Chhanabhai M, Skinnider BF, Greiner TC, Morris SW, Connors JM, Vose JM, Viswanatha DS, Coldman A, Weisenburger DD (1999). Prognostic significance of anaplastic lymphoma kinase (ALK) protein expression in adults with anaplastic large cell lymphoma. Blood 93: 3913-3921.
761. Gascoyne RD, Lamant L, Martin-Subero JI, Lestou VS, Harris NL, Muller-Hermelink HK, Seymour JF, Campbell LJ, Horsman DE, Auvigne I, Espinos E, Siebert R, Delsol G (2003). ALK-positive diffuse large B-cell lymphoma is associated with Clathrin-ALK rearrangements: report of 6 cases. Blood 102: 2568-2573.
762. Gattermann N, Billiet J, Kronenwett R, Zipperer E, Germing U, Nollet F, Criel A, Selleslag D (2007). High frequency of the JAK2 V617F mutation in patients with thrombocytosis (platelet count>600x109/L) and ringed sideroblasts more than 15% considered as MDS/MPD, unclassifiable. Blood 109: 1334-1335.
763. Gattermann N, Retzlaff S, Wang YL, Hofhaus G, Heinisch J, Aul C, Schneider W (1997). Heteroplasmic point mutations of mitochondrial DNA affecting subunit I of cytochrome c oxidase in two patients with acquired idiopathic sideroblastic anemia. Blood 90: 4961-4972.
764. Gaulard P, Belhadj K, Reyes F (2003). Gammadelta T-cell lymphomas. Semin Hematol 40: 233-243.
764A Gauwerky c, Hoxie J, Nowell P. Pre-B-cell leukemia with a t(8;14) and a t(14;18) translocation is preceded by follicular lymphoma. Oncogene 1988; 2:431-435.
765. Gavrilescu LC, Cross NCP, Van Etten RA (2006). Distinct leukemogenic activity and imatinib responsiveness of a BCR-PDGFRalpha fusion tyrosine kinase. Blood 108: Abstract 3634.
766. Gazzo S, Baseggio L, Coignet L, Poncet C, Morel D, Coiffier B, Felman P, Berger F, Salles G, Callet-Bauchu E (2003). Cytogenetic and molecular delineation of a region of chromosome 3q commonly gained in marginal zone B-cell lymphoma. Haematologica 88: 31-38.
767. Geary CG (2000). The story of chronic myeloid leukaemia. Br J Haematol 110: 2-11.
768. Geelen FA, Vermeer MH, Meijer CJ, Van der Putte SC, Kerkhof E, Kluin PM, Willemze R (1998). bcl-2 protein expression in primary cutaneous large B-cell lymphoma is site-related. J Clin Oncol 16: 2080-2085.
769. Geissinger E, Bonzheim I, Krenacs L, Roth S, Reimer P, Wilhelm M, Muller-Hermelink HK, Rudiger T (2006). Nodal peripheral T-cell lymphomas correspond to distinct mature T-cell populations. J Pathol 210: 172-180.
770. Geissinger E, Odenwald T, Lee SS, Bonzheim I, Roth S, Reimer P, Wilhelm M, Muller-Hermelink HK, Rudiger T (2004). Nodal peripheral T-cell lymphomas and, in particular,

their lymphoepithelioid (Lennert's) variant are often derived from CD8(+) cytotoxic T-cells. Virchows Arch 445: 334-343.
771. Geissmann F, Dieu-Nosjean MC, Dezutter C, Valladeau J, Kayal S, Leborgne M, Brousse N, Saeland S, Davoust J (2002). Accumulation of immature Langerhans cells in human lymph nodes draining chronically inflamed skin. J Exp Med 196: 417-430.
772. Geissmann F, Ruskone-Fourmestraux A, Hermine O, Bourquelot P, Belanger C, Audouin J, Delmer A, Macintyre EA, Varet B, Brousse N (1998). Homing receptor alpha4beta7 integrin expression predicts digestive tract involvement in mantle cell lymphoma. Am J Pathol 153: 1701-1705.
773. Gentile TC, Uner AH, Hutchison RE, Wright J, Ben Ezra J, Russell EC, Loughran TP, Jr. (1994). CD3+, CD56+ aggressive variant of large granular lymphocyte leukemia. Blood 84: 2315-2321.
774. George TI, Wrede JE, Bangs CD, Cherry AM, Warnke RA, Arber DA (2005). Low-grade B-Cell lymphomas with plasmacytic differentiation lack PAX5 gene rearrangements. J Mol Diagn 7: 346-351.
775. Georgii A, Buesche G, Kreft A (1998). The histopathology of chronic myeloproliferative diseases. Baillieres Clin Haematol 11: 721-749.
775B. Georgii A., Vykoupil KF, Buhr T, Choritz H, Dohler U, Kaloutsi V, Werner M (1990). Chronic myeloproliferative disorders in bone marrow biopsies. Pathol Res Pract 186: 3-27.
775D. Gerard-Marchant R, Hamlin I, Lennert K, Rilke F, Stansfeld AG, van Unnik JAM (1974). Classification of non-Hodgkin's Lymphomas. Lancet 2: 406-408.
775C. Gerdes J, Van Baarlen J, Pileri S, Schwarting R, Van Unnik JA, Stein H (1987). Tumor cell growth fraction in Hodgkin's disease. Am J Pathol 128: 390-393.
776. Germing U, Gattermann N, Aivado M, Hildebrandt B, Aul C (2000). Two types of acquired idiopathic sideroblastic anaemia (AISA): a time-tested distinction. Br J Haematol 108: 724-728.
777. Germing U, Gattermann N, Minning H, Heyll A, Aul C (1998). Problems in the classification of CMML—dysplastic versus proliferative type. Leuk Res 22: 871-878.
778. Germing U, Gattermann N, Strupp C, Aivado M, Aul C (2000). Validation of the WHO proposals for a new classification of primary myelodysplastic syndromes: a retrosepctive analysis of 1600 patients. Leuk Res 24: 983-992.
779. Germing U, Kundgen A, Gattermann N (2004). Risk assessment in chronic myelomonocytic leukemia (CMML). Leuk Lymphoma 45: 1311-1318.
780. Germing U, Strupp C, Knipp S, Kuendgen A, Giagounidis A, Hildebrandt B, Aul C, Haas R, Gattermann N, Bennett JM (2007). Chronic myelomonocytic leukemia in the light of the WHO proposals. Haematologica 92: 974-977.
781. Germing U, Strupp C, Kuendgen A, Aivado M, Giagounidis A, Hildebrandt B, Aul C, Haas R, Gattermann N (2006). Refractory anaemia with excess of blasts (RAEB): analysis of reclassification according to the WHO proposals. Br J Haematol 132: 162-167.
782. Germing U, Strupp C, Kuendgen A, Isa S, Knipp S, Hildebrandt B, Giagounidis A, Aul C, Gattermann N, Haas R (2006). Prospective validation of the WHO proposals for the classification of myelodysplastic syndromes. Haematologica 91: 1596-1604.
783. Germing U, Strupp C, Kundgen A, Bowen D, Aul C, Haas R, Gattermann N (2004). No increase in age-specific incidence of myelodysplastic syndromes. Haematologica 89: 905-910.
784. Gertz MA, Kyle RA (1990). Prognostic value of urinary protein in primary systemic amyloidosis (AL). Am J Clin Pathol 94: 313-317.
785. Gertz MA, Kyle RA (2003). Amyloidosis with IgM monoclonal gammopathies. Semin Oncol 30: 325-328.
786. Gertz MA, Kyle RA, Noel P (1993). Primary systemic amyloidosis: a rare complication of immunoglobulin M monoclonal gammopathies and Waldenstrom's macroglobulinemia. J Clin Oncol 11: 914-920.
787. Gertz MA, Lacy MQ, Dispenzieri A, Greipp PR, Litzow MR, Henderson KJ, Van Wier SA, Ahmann GJ, Fonseca R (2005). Clinical implications of t(11;14)(q13;q32), t(4;14)(p16.3;q32), and -17p13 in myeloma patients treated with high-dose therapy. Blood 106: 2837-2840.
788. Gesk S, Gascoyne RD, Schnitzer B, Bakshi N, Janssen D, Klapper W, Martin-Subero JI, Parwaresch R, Siebert R (2005). ALK-positive diffuse large B-cell lymphoma with ALK-Clathrin fusion belongs to the spectrum of pediatric lymphomas. Leukemia 19: 1839-1840.
789. Gesk S, Klapper W, Martin-Subero JI, Nagel I, Harder L, Fu K, Bernd HW, Weisenburger DD, Parwaresch R, Siebert R (2006). A chromosomal translocation in cyclin D1-negative/cyclin D2-positive mantle cell lymphoma fuses the CCND2 gene to the IGK locus. Blood 108: 1109-1110.
790. Ghia P, Guida G, Stella S, Gottardi D, Geuna M, Strola G, Scielzo C, Caligaris-Cappio F (2003). The pattern of CD38 expression defines a distinct subset of chronic lymphocytic leukemia (CLL) patients at risk of disease progression. Blood 101: 1262-1269.
791. Ghobrial IM, Habermann TM, Macon WR, Ristow KM, Larson TS, Walker RC, Ansell SM, Gores GJ, Stegall MD, McGregor CG (2005). Differences between early and late posttransplant lymphoproliferative disorders in solid organ transplant patients: are they two different diseases? Transplantation 79: 244-247.
792. Ghobrial IM, Habermann TM, Maurer MJ, Geyer SM, Ristow KM, Larson TS, Walker RC, Ansell SM, Macon WR, Gores GG, Stegall MD, McGregor CG (2005). Prognostic analysis for survival in adult solid organ transplant recipients with post-transplantation lymphoproliferative disorders. J Clin Oncol 23: 7574-7582.
793. Ghosh SK, Wood C, Boise LH, Mian AM, Deyev VV, Feuer G, Toomey NL, Shank NC, Cabral L, Barber GN, Harrington WJ, Jr. (2003). Potentiation of TRAIL-induced apoptosis in primary effusion lymphoma through azidothymidine-mediated inhibition of NF-kappa B. Blood 101: 2321-2327.
794. Giagounidis AA, Germing U, Haase S, Hildebrandt B, Schlegelberger B, Schoch C, Wilkens L, Heinsch M, Willems H, Aivado M, Aul C (2004). Clinical, morphological, cytogenetic, and prognostic features of patients with myelodysplastic syndromes and del(5q) including band q31. Leukemia 18: 113-119.
795. Giagounidis AA, Germing U, Strupp C, Hildebrandt B, Heinsch M, Aul C (2005). Prognosis of patients with del(5q) MDS and complex karyotype and the possible role of lenalidomide in this patient subgroup. Ann Hematol 84: 569-571.
796. Gianelli U, Vener C, Raviele PR, Moro A, Savi F, Annaloro C, Somalvico F, Radaelli F, Franco V, Deliliers GL (2006). Essential thrombocythemia or chronic idiopathic myelofibrosis? A single-center study based on hematopoietic bone marrow histology. Leuk Lymphoma 47: 1774-1781.
797. Gibson LE, Muller SA, Leiferman KM, Peters MS (1989). Follicular mucinosis: clinical and histopathologic study. J Am Acad Dermatol 20: 441-446.
798. Gidron A, Tallman MS (2006). Hairy cell leukemia: towards a curative strategy. Hematol Oncol Clin North Am 20: 1153-1162.
799. Gilmour KC, Cranston T, Jones A, Davies EG, Goldblatt D, Thrasher A, Kinnon C, Nichols KE, Gaspar HB (2000). Diagnosis of X-linked lymphoproliferative disease by analysis of SLAM-associated protein expression. Eur J Immunol 30: 1691-1697.
800. Gilmour KC, Gaspar HB (2003). Pathogenesis and diagnosis of X-linked lymphoproliferative disease. Expert Rev Mol Diagn 3: 549-561.
801. Girard T, Luquet-Besson I, Baran-Marszak F, Raphael M, Boue F (2005). HIV+ MALT lymphoma remission induced by highly active antiretroviral therapy alone. Eur J Haematol 74: 70-72.
802. Gisslinger H (2006). Update on diagnosis and management of essential thrombocythemia. Semin Thromb Hemost 32: 430-436.
803. Glas AM, Kersten MJ, Delahaye LJ, Witteveen AT, Kibbelaar RE, Velds A, Wessels LF, Joosten P, Kerkhoven RM, Bernards R, Van Krieken JH, Kluin PM, van't Veer LJ, De Jong D (2005). Gene expression profiling in follicular lymphoma to assess clinical aggressiveness and to guide the choice of treatment. Blood 105: 301-307.
804. Glas AM, Knoops L, Delahaye L, Kersten MJ, Kibbelaar RE, Wessels LA, van Laar R, Van Krieken JH, Baars JW, Raemaekers J, Kluin PM, van't Veer LJ, De Jong D (2007). Gene-expression and immunohistochemical study of specific T-cell subsets and accessory cell types in the transformation and prognosis of follicular lymphoma. J Clin Oncol 25: 390-398.
805. Glaser SL, Clarke CA, Gulley ML, Craig FE, DiGiuseppe JA, Dorfman RF, Mann RB, Ambinder RF (2003). Population-based patterns of human immunodeficiency virus-related Hodgkin lymphoma in the Greater San Francisco Bay Area, 1988-1998. Cancer 98: 300-309.
806. Glick JH, Barnes JM, Ezdinli EZ, Berard CW, Orlow EL, Bennett JM (1981). Nodular mixed lymphoma: results of a randomized trial failing to confirm prolonged disease-free survival with COPP chemotherapy. Blood 58: 920-925.
807. Glick JH, McFadden E, Costello W, Ezdinli E, Berard CW, Bennett JM (1982). Nodular histiocytic lymphoma: factors influencing prognosis and implications for aggressive chemotherapy. Cancer 49: 840-845.
808. Goemans BF, Zwaan CM, Miller M, Zimmermann M, Harlow A, Meshinchi S, Loonen AH, Hahlen K, Reinhardt D, Creutzig U, Kaspers GJ, Heinrich MC (2005). Mutations in KIT and RAS are frequent events in pediatric core-binding factor acute myeloid leukemia. Leukemia 19: 1536-1542.
809. Goldberg JM, Silverman LB, Levy DE, Dalton VK, Gelber RD, Lehmann L, Cohen HJ, Sallan SE, Asselin BL (2003). Childhood T-cell acute lymphoblastic leukemia: the Dana-Farber Cancer Institute acute lymphoblastic leukemia consortium experience. J Clin Oncol 21: 3616-3622.
810. Goldin LR, Pfeiffer RM, Li X, Hemminki K (2004). Familial risk of lymphoproliferative tumors in families of patients with chronic lymphocytic leukemia: results from the Swedish Family-Cancer Database. Blood 104: 1850-1854.
811. Golomb HM, Rowley JD, Vardiman JW, Testa JR, Butler A (1980). "Microgranular" acute promyelocytic leukemia: a distinct clinical, ultrastructural, and cytogenetic entity. Blood 55: 253-259.
812. Golub TR, Barker GF, Lovett M, Gilliland DG (1994). Fusion of PDGF receptor beta to a novel ets-like gene, tel, in chronic myelomonocytic leukemia with t(5;12) chromosomal translocation. Cell 77: 307-316.
813. Gono T, Yazaki M, Fushimi T, Suzuki T, Uehara T, Sano K, Kametani F, Ito N, Matsushita M, Nakamura S, Hoshii Y, Matsuda M, Ikeda S (2006). AH amyloidosis associated with lymphoplasmacytic lymphoma secreting a monoclonal gamma heavy chain carrying an unusual truncated D segment. Am J Kidney Dis 47: 908-914.
814. Gonzalez CL, Medeiros LJ, Braziel RM, Jaffe ES (1991). T-cell lymphoma involving subcutaneous tissue. A clinicopathologic entity commonly associated with hemophagocytic syndrome. Am J Surg Pathol 15: 17-27.
815. Gonzalez CL, Medeiros LJ, Jaffe ES (1991). Composite lymphoma. A clinicopathologic analysis of nine patients with Hodgkin's disease and B-cell non-Hodgkin's lymphoma. Am J Clin Pathol 96: 81-89.
816. Goodlad JR, Batstone PJ, Hamilton D, Hollowood K (2003). Follicular lymphoma with marginal zone differentiation: cytogenetic findings in support of a high-risk variant of follicular lymphoma. Histopathology 42: 292-298.
817. Goodlad JR, Hollowood K, Smith MA, Chan JK, Fletcher CD (1999). Primary juxtaarticular soft tissue lymphoma arising in the vicinity of inflamed joints in patients with rheumatoid arthritis. Histopathology 34: 199-204.
818. Goodlad JR, Krajewski AS, Batstone PJ, McKay P, White JM, Benton EC, Kavanagh GM, Lucraft HH (2002). Primary cutaneous follicular lymphoma: a clinicopathologic and molecular study of 16 cases in support of a distinct entity. Am J Surg Pathol 26: 733-741.
819. Goodlad JR, Krajewski AS, Batstone PJ, McKay P, White JM, Benton EC, Kavanagh GM, Lucraft HH (2003). Primary cutaneous diffuse large B-cell lymphoma: prognostic significance of clinicopathological subtypes. Am J Surg Pathol 27: 1538-1545.
820. Gopcsa L, Banyai A, Jakab K, Kormos L, Tamaska J, Matolcsy A, Gogolak P, Rajnavolgyi E, Paloczi K (2005). Extensive flow cytometric characterization of plasmacytoid dendritic cell leukemia cells. Eur J Haematol 75: 346-351.
821. Gordon MY, Goldman JM (1996). Cellular and molecular mechanisms in chronic myeloid leukaemia: biology and treatment. Br J Haematol 95: 10-20.
821A. Gordon S (2007). The macrophage: past, present and future. Eur J Immunol 37: S9-17.
821B. Gordon S, Taylor PR (2005). Monocyte and macrophage heterogeneity. Nat Rev Immunol 12: 953-964.
822. Gould VE, Warren WH, Faber LP, Kuhn C, Franke WW (1990). Malignant cells of epithelial phenotype limited to thoracic lymph nodes. Eur J Cancer 26: 1121-1126.
823. Goyal RK, McEvoy L, Wilson DB (1996). Hodgkin disease after renal transplantation in childhood. J Pediatr Hematol Oncol 18: 392-395.
824. Grange F, Bekkenk MW, Wechsler J, Meijer CJ, Cerroni L, Bernengo M, Bosq J, Hedelin G, Fink PR, van Vloten WA, Joly P, Bagot M, Willemze R (2001). Prognostic factors in primary cutaneous large B-cell lymphomas: a European multicenter study. J Clin Oncol 19: 3602-3610.
825. Grange F, Hedelin G, Joly P, Beylot-Barry M, D'Incan M, Delaunay M, Vaillant L, Avril MF, Bosq J, Wechsler J, Dalac S, Grosieux C, Franck N, Esteve E, Michel C, Bodemer C, Vergier B, Laroche L, Bagot M (1999). Prognostic factors in primary cutaneous lymphomas other than mycosis fungoides and the Sezary syndrome. The French Study Group on Cutaneous Lymphomas. Blood 93: 3637-3642.
826. Grange F, Petrella T, Beylot-Barry M,

Joly P, D'Incan M, Delaunay M, Machet L, Avril MF, Dalac S, Bernard P, Carlotti A, Esteve E, Vergier B, Dechelotte P, Cassagnau E, Courville P, Saiag P, Laroche L, Bagot M, Wechsler J (2004). Bcl-2 protein expression is the strongest independent prognostic factor of survival in primary cutaneous large B-cell lymphomas. Blood 103: 3662-3668.

827. Grasso JA, Myers TJ, Hines JD, Sullivan AL (1980). Energy-dispersive X-ray analysis of the mitochondria of sideroblastic anaemia. Br J Haematol 46: 57-72.

828. Gratwohl A, Brand R, Apperley J, Crawley C, Ruutu T, Corradini P, Carreras E, Devergie A, Guglielmi C, Kolb HJ, Niederwieser D (2006). Allogeneic hematopoietic stem cell transplantation for chronic myeloid leukemia in Europe 2006: transplant activity, long-term data and current results. An analysis by the Chronic Leukemia Working Party of the European Group for Blood and Marrow Transplantation (EBMT). Haematologica 91: 513-521.

829. Gratwohl A, Hermans J, Goldman JM, Arcese W, Carreras E, Devergie A, Frassoni F, Gahrton G, Kolb HJ, Niederwieser D, Ruutu T, Vernant JP, de Witte T, Apperley J (1998). Risk assessment for patients with chronic myeloid leukaemia before allogeneic blood or marrow transplantation. Chronic Leukemia Working Party of the European Group for Blood and Marrow Transplantation. Lancet 352: 1087-1092.

830. Graux C, Cools J, Michaux L, Vandenberghe P, Hagemeijer A (2006). Cytogenetics and molecular genetics of T-cell acute lymphoblastic leukemia: from thymocyte to lymphoblast. Leukemia 20: 1496-1510.

831. Gravel S, Delsol G, al Saati T (1998). Single-cell analysis of the t(14;18)(q32;q21) chromosomal translocation in Hodgkin's disease demonstrates the absence of this translocation in neoplastic Hodgkin and Reed-Sternberg cells. Blood 91: 2866-2874.

832. Greaves MF (2004). Biological models for leukaemia and lymphoma. IARC Sci Publ 157: 351-372.

833. Greenberg P, Cox C, LeBeau MM, Fenaux P, Morel P, Sanz G, Sanz M, Vallespi T, Hamblin T, Oscier D, Ohyashiki K, Toyama K, Aul C, Mufti G, Bennett J (1997). International scoring system for evaluating prognosis in myelodysplastic syndromes. Blood 89: 2079-2088.

833A. Greenberg P, Cox C, LeBeau MM, Fenaux P, Morel P, Sanz G, Sanz M, Vallespi T, Hamblin T, Oscier D, Ohyashiki K, Toyama K, Aul C, Mufti G, Bennett J (1998). Erratum. Blood 91:1100.

834. Greenberg PL, Young NS, Gattermann N (2002). Myelodysplastic syndromes. Hematology Am Soc Hematol Educ Program :136-61.: 136-161.

835. Greene ME, Mundschau G, Wechsler J, McDevitt M, Gamis A, Karp J, Gurbuxani S, Arceci R, Crispino JD (2003). Mutations in GATA1 in both transient myeloproliferative disorder and acute megakaryoblastic leukemia of Down syndrome. Blood Cells Mol Dis 31: 351-356.

836. Greer JP, Macon WR, Lamar RE, Wolff SN, Stein RS, Flexner JM, Collins RD, Cousar JB (1995). T-cell-rich B-cell lymphomas: diagnosis and response to therapy of 44 patients. J Clin Oncol 13: 1742-1750.

837. Gregg XT, Reddy V, Prchal JT (2002). Copper deficiency masquerading as myelodysplastic syndrome. Blood 100: 1493-1495.

837A. Greiner A, Tobollik S, Buettner M, Jungnickel B, Herrmann K, Kremmer E, Niedobitek G (2005). Differential expression of activation-induced cytidine deaminase (AID) in nodular lymphocyte-predominant and classical Hodgkin lymphoma. J Pathol 205: 541-547

838. Greiner TC, Gascoyne RD, Anderson ME, Kingma DW, Adomat SA, Said J, Jaffe ES (1996). Nodular lymphocyte-predominant Hodgkin's disease associated with large-cell lymphoma: analysis of Ig gene rearrangements by V-J polymerase chain reaction. Blood 88: 657-666.

839. Greiner TC, Moynihan MJ, Chan WC, Lytle DM, Pedersen A, Anderson JR, Weisenburger DD (1996). p53 mutations in mantle cell lymphoma are associated with variant cytology and predict a poor prognosis. Blood 87: 4302-4310.

840. Greipp PR, Leong T, Bennett JM, Gaillard JP, Klein B, Stewart JA, Oken MM, Kay NE, Van Ness B, Kyle RA (1998). Plasmablastic morphology—an independent prognostic factor with clinical and laboratory correlates: Eastern Cooperative Oncology Group (ECOG) myeloma trial E9486 report by the ECOG Myeloma Laboratory Group. Blood 91: 2501-2507.

841. Greipp PR, Lust JA, O'Fallon WM, Katzmann JA, Witzig TE, Kyle RA (1993). Plasma cell labeling index and beta 2-microglobulin predict survival independent of thymidine kinase and C-reactive protein in multiple myeloma. Blood 81: 3382-3387.

842. Greipp PR, San Miguel J, Durie BG, Crowley JJ, Barlogie B, Blade J, Boccadoro M, Child JA, Avet-Loiseau H, Kyle RA, Lahuerta JJ, Ludwig H, Morgan G, Powles R, Shimizu K, Shustik C, Sonneveld P, Tosi P, Turesson I, Westin J (2005). International staging system for multiple myeloma. J Clin Oncol 23: 3412-3420.

843. Griffin CA, Hawkins AL, Dvorak C, Henkle C, Ellingham T, Perlman EJ (1999). Recurrent involvement of 2p23 in inflammatory myofibroblastic tumors. Cancer Res 59: 2776-2780.

844. Griffin JH, Leung J, Bruner RJ, Caligiuri MA, Briesewitz R (2003). Discovery of a fusion kinase in EOL-1 cells and idiopathic hypereosinophilic syndrome. Proc Natl Acad Sci U S A 100: 7830-7835.

845. Grigg AP, Gascoyne RD, Phillips GL, Horsman DE (1993). Clinical, haematological and cytogenetic features in 24 patients with structural rearrangements of the Q arm of chromosome 3. Br J Haematol 83: 158-165.

846. Grimaldi JC, Meeker TC (1989). The t(5;14) chromosomal translocation in a case of acute lymphocytic leukemia joins the interleukin-3 gene to the immunoglobulin heavy chain gene. Blood 73: 2081-2085.

847. Grimwade D, Biondi A, Mozziconacci MJ, Hagemeijer A, Berger R, Neat M, Howe K, Dastugue N, Jansen J, Radford-Weiss I, Lo Coco F, Lessard M, Hernandez JM, Delabesse E, Head D, Liso V, Sainty D, Flandrin G, Solomon E, Birg F, Lafage-Pochitaloff M (2000). Characterization of acute promyelocytic leukemia cases lacking the classic t(15;17): results of the European Working Party. Groupe Francais de Cytogenetique Hematologique, Groupe de Francais d'Hematologie Cellulaire, UK Cancer Cytogenetics Group and BIOMED 1 European Community-Concerted Action "Molecular Cytogenetic Diagnosis in Haematological Malignancies". Blood 96: 1297-1308.

848. Grimwade D, Walker H, Oliver F, Wheatley K, Harrison C, Harrison G, Rees J, Hann I, Stevens R, Burnett A, Goldstone A (1998). The importance of diagnostic cytogenetics on outcome in AML: analysis of 1,612 patients entered into the MRC AML 10 trial. The Medical Research Council Adult and Children's Leukaemia Working Parties. Blood 92: 2322-2333.

849. Gritti C, Dastot H, Soulier J, Janin A, Daniel MT, Madani A, Grimber G, Briand P, Sigaux F, Stern MH (1998). Transgenic mice for MTCP1 develop T-cell prolymphocytic leukemia. Blood 92: 368-373.

850. Grogan TM, Durie BG, Spier CM, Richter L, Vela E (1989). Myelomonocytic antigen positive multiple myeloma. Blood 73: 763-769.

851. Grogg KL, Attygalle AD, Macon WR, Remstein ED, Kurtin PJ, Dogan A (2005). Angioimmunoblastic T-cell lymphoma: a neoplasm of germinal-center T-helper cells? Blood 106: 1501-1502.

852. Grogg KL, Attygalle AD, Macon WR, Remstein ED, Kurtin PJ, Dogan A (2006). Expression of CXCL13, a chemokine highly upregulated in germinal center T-helper cells, distinguishes angioimmunoblastic T-cell lymphoma from peripheral T-cell lymphoma, unspecified. Mod Pathol 19: 1101-1107.

853. Grogg KL, Lae ME, Kurtin PJ, Macon WR (2004). Clusterin expression distinguishes follicular dendritic cell tumors from other dendritic cell neoplasms: report of a novel follicular dendritic cell marker and clinicopathologic data on 12 additional follicular dendritic cell tumors and 6 additional interdigitating dendritic cell tumors. Am J Surg Pathol 28: 988-998.

854. Grogg KL, Macon WR, Kurtin PJ, Nascimento AG (2005). A survey of clusterin and fascin expression in sarcomas and spindle cell neoplasms: strong clusterin immunostaining is highly specific for follicular dendritic cell tumor. Mod Pathol 18: 260-266.

855. Gronbaek K, Straten PT, Ralfkiaer E, Ahrenkiel V, Andersen MK, Hansen NE, Zeuthen J, Hou-Jensen K, Guldberg P (1998). Somatic Fas mutations in non-Hodgkin's lymphoma: association with extranodal disease and autoimmunity. Blood 92: 3018-3024.

856. Gross TG, Bucuvalas JC, Park JR, Greiner TC, Hinrich SH, Kaufman SS, Langnas AN, McDonald RA, Ryckman FC, Shaw BW, Sudan DL, Lynch JC (2005). Low-dose chemotherapy for Epstein-Barr virus-positive post-transplantation lymphoproliferative disease in children after solid organ transplantation. J Clin Oncol 23: 6481-6488.

857. Grouard G, Rissoan MC, Filgueira L, Durand I, Banchereau J, Liu YJ (1997). The enigmatic plasmacytoid T cells develop into dendritic cells with interleukin (IL)-3 and CD40-ligand. J Exp Med 185: 1101-1111.

858. Gruszka-Westwood AM, Hamoudi RA, Matutes E, Tuset E, Catovsky D (2001). p53 abnormalities in splenic lymphoma with villous lymphocytes. Blood 97: 3552-3558.

859. Gruszka-Westwood AM, Matutes E, Coignet LJ, Wotherspoon A, Catovsky D (1999). The incidence of trisomy 3 in splenic lymphoma with villous lymphocytes: a study by FISH. Br J Haematol 104: 600-604.

860. Guikema JE, de Boer C, Haralambieva E, Smit LA, van Noesel CJ, Schuuring E, Kluin PM (2006). IGH switch breakpoints in Burkitt lymphoma: exclusive involvement of noncanonical class switch recombination. Genes Chromosomes Cancer 45: 808-819.

861. Guinee D, Jr., Jaffe E, Kingma D, Fishback N, Wallberg K, Krishnan J, Frizzera G, Travis W, Koss M (1994). Pulmonary lymphomatoid granulomatosis. Evidence for a proliferation of Epstein-Barr virus infected B-lymphocytes with a prominent T-cell component and vasculitis. Am J Surg Pathol 18: 753-764.

862. Guinee DG, Jr., Perkins SL, Travis WD, Holden JA, Tripp SR, Koss MN (1998). Proliferation and cellular phenotype in lymphomatoid granulomatosis: implications of a higher proliferation index in B cells. Am J Surg Pathol 22: 1093-1100.

863. Guitart J (2000). HIV-1 and an HTLV-II-associated cutaneous T-cell lymphoma. N Engl J Med 343: 303-304.

864. Guiter C, Dusanter-Fourt I, Copie-Bergman C, Boulland ML, Le Gouvello S, Gaulard P, Leroy K, Castellano F (2004). Constitutive STAT6 activation in primary mediastinal large B-cell lymphoma. Blood 104: 543-549.

865. Gupta R, Abdalla SH, Bain BJ (1999). Thrombocytosis with sideroblastic erythropoiesis: a mixed myeloproliferative myelodysplastic syndrome. Leuk Lymphoma 34: 615-619.

866. Gupta R, Soupir CP, Johari V, Hasserjian RP (2007). Myelodysplastic syndrome with isolated deletion of chromosome 20q: an indolent disease with minimal morphological dysplasia and frequent thrombocytopenic presentation. Br J Haematol 139: 265-268.

867. Haase D, Fonatsch C, Freund M, Wormann B, Bodenstein H, Bartels H, Stollmann-Gibbels B, Lengfelder E (1995). Cytogenetic findings in 179 patients with myelodysplastic syndromes. Ann Hematol 70: 171-187.

868. Hadzic N, Pagliuca A, Rela M, Portmann B, Jones A, Veys P, Heaton ND, Mufti GJ, Mieli-Vergani G (2000). Correction of the hyper-IgM syndrome after liver and bone marrow transplantation. N Engl J Med 342: 320-324.

869. Haferlach T, Schoch C, Loffler H, Gassmann W, Kern W, Schnittger S, Fonatsch C, Ludwig WD, Wuchter C, Schlegelberger B, Staib P, Reichle A, Kubica U, Eimermacher H, Balleisen L, Gruneisen A, Haase D, Aul C, Karow J, Lengfelder E, Wormann B, Heinecke A, Sauerland MC, Buchner T, Hiddemann W (2003). Morphologic dysplasia in de novo acute myeloid leukemia (AML) is related to unfavorable cytogenetics but has no independent prognostic relevance under the conditions of intensive induction therapy: results of a multiparameter analysis from the German AML Cooperative Group studies. J Clin Oncol 21: 256-265.

870. Haghighi B, Smoller BR, LeBoit PE, Warnke RA, Sander CA, Kohler S (2000). Pagetoid reticulosis (Woringer-Kolopp disease): an immunophenotypic, molecular, and clinicopathologic study. Mod Pathol 13: 502-510.

871. Hahtola S, Tuomela S, Elo L, Hakkinen T, Karenko L, Nedoszytko B, Heikkila H, Saarialho-Kere U, Roszkiewicz J, Aittokallio T, Lahesmaa R, Ranki A (2006). Th1 response and cytotoxicity genes are down-regulated in cutaneous T-cell lymphoma. Clin Cancer Res 12: 4812-4821.

872. Hallbook H, Gustafsson G, Smedmyr B, Soderhall S, Heyman M (2006). Treatment outcome in young adults and children >10 years of age with acute lymphoblastic leukemia in Sweden: a comparison between a pediatric protocol and an adult protocol. Cancer 107: 1551-1561.

873. Hallek M, Bergsagel PL, Anderson KC (1998). Multiple myeloma: increasing evidence for a multistep transformation process. Blood 91: 3-21.

873A. Hallek M, Cheson BD, Catovsky D, Caligaris-Cappio F, Dighiero G, Dohner H, Hillmen P, Keating MJ, Montserrat E, Rai KR, Kipps TJ (2008). Guidelines for the diagnosis and treatment of chronic lymphocytic leukemia: a report from the International Workshop on Chronic Lymphocytic Leukemia (IWCLL) updating the National Cancer Institute-Working Group (NCI-WG) 1996 guidelines. Blood 111: 5446-5456.

874. Hallermann C, Kaune KM, Gesk S, Martin-Subero JI, Gunawan B, Griesinger F, Vermeer MH, Santucci M, Pimpinelli N, Willemze R, Siebert R, Neumann C (2004). Molecular cytogenetic analysis of chromosomal breakpoints in the IGH, MYC, BCL6, and MALT1 gene loci in primary cutaneous B-cell lymphomas. J Invest Dermatol 123: 213-219.

875. Hallermann C, Kaune KM, Siebert R, Vermeer MH, Tensen CP, Willemze R, Gunawan B, Bertsch HP, Neumann C (2004). Chromosomal aberration patterns differ in subtypes of primary cutaneous B cell lymphomas. J Invest Dermatol 122: 1495-1502.

876. Hamblin TJ, Davis Z, Gardiner A, Oscier DG, Stevenson FK (1999). Unmutated Ig V(H) genes are associated with a more aggressive form of chronic lymphocytic leukemia. Blood 94: 1848-1854.

877. Hamilton-Dutoit SJ, Raphael M, Audouin J, Diebold J, Lisse I, Pedersen C, Oksenhendler E, Marelle L, Pallesen G (1993). In situ demonstration of Epstein-Barr virus small RNAs (EBER 1) in acquired immunodeficiency syndrome-related lymphomas: correlation with tumor morphology and primary site. Blood 82: 619-624.

878. Hammer RD, Glick AD, Greer JP, Collins RD, Cousar JB (1996). Splenic marginal zone lymphoma. A distinct B-cell neoplasm. Am J Surg Pathol 20: 613-626.

879. Han X, Bueso-Ramos CE (2007). Precursor T-cell acute lymphoblastic leukemia/lymphoblastic lymphoma and acute biphenotypic leukemias. Am J Clin Pathol 127: 528-544.

880. Hanamura I, Stewart JP, Huang Y, Zhan F, Santra M, Sawyer JR, Hollmig K, Zangarri M, Pineda-Roman M, van Rhee F, Cavallo F, Burington B, Crowley J, Tricot G, Barlogie B, Shaughnessy JD, Jr. (2006). Frequent gain of chromosome band 1q21 in plasma-cell dyscrasias detected by fluorescence in situ hybridization: incidence increases from MGUS to relapsed myeloma and is related to prognosis and disease progression following tandem stem-cell transplantation. Blood 108: 1724-1732.

880A. Hanna J, Markoulaki S, Schorderet P, Carey BW, Beard C, Wernig M, Creyghton MP, Steine EJ, Cassady JP, Foreman R, Lengner CJ, Dausman JA, Jaenisch R (2008). Direct reprogramming of terminally differentiated mature B lymphocytes to pluripotency. Cell 133: 250-264.

881. Hans CP, Weisenburger DD, Greiner TC, Chan WC, Aoun P, Cochran GT, Pan Z, Smith LM, Lynch JC, Bociek RG, Bierman PJ, Vose JM, Armitage JO (2005). Expression of PKC-beta or cyclin D2 predicts for inferior survival in diffuse large B-cell lymphoma. Mod Pathol 18: 1377-1384.

882. Hans CP, Weisenburger DD, Greiner TC, Gascoyne RD, Delabie J, Ott G, Muller-Hermelink HK, Campo E, Braziel RM, Jaffe ES, Pan Z, Farinha P, Smith LM, Falini B, Banham AH, Rosenwald A, Staudt LM, Connors JM, Armitage JO, Chan WC (2004). Confirmation of the molecular classification of diffuse large B-cell lymphoma by immunohistochemistry using a tissue microarray. Blood 103: 275-282.

883. Hans CP, Weisenburger DD, Vose JM, Hock LM, Lynch JC, Aoun P, Greiner TC, Chan WC, Bociek RG, Bierman PJ, Armitage JO (2003). A significant diffuse component predicts for inferior survival in grade 3 follicular lymphoma, but cytologic subtypes do not predict survival. Blood 101: 2363-2367.

884. Hansmann ML, Stein H, Fellbaum C, Hui PK, Parwaresch MR, Lennert K (1989). Nodular paragranuloma can transform into high-grade malignant lymphoma of B type. Hum Pathol 20: 1169-1175.

885. Hanson CA, Abaza M, Sheldon S, Ross CW, Schnitzer B, Stoolman LM (1993). Acute biphenotypic leukaemia: immunophenotypic and cytogenetic analysis. Br J Haematol 84: 49-60.

886. Hanson CA, Jaszcz W, Kersey JH, Astorga MG, Peterson BA, Gajl-Peczalska KJ, Frizzera G (1989). True histiocytic lymphoma: histopathologic, immunophenotypic and genotypic analysis. Br J Haematol 73: 187-198.

887. Hanto DW, Gajl-Peczalska KJ, Frizzera G, Arthur DC, Balfour HH, Jr., McClain K, Simmons RL, Najarian JS (1983). Epstein-Barr virus (EBV) induced polyclonal and monoclonal B-cell lymphoproliferative diseases occurring after renal transplantation. Clinical, pathologic, and virologic findings and implications for therapy. Ann Surg 198: 356-369.

888. Haque AK, Myers JL, Hudnall SD, Gelman BB, Lloyd RV, Payne D, Borucki M (1998). Pulmonary lymphomatoid granulomatosis in acquired immunodeficiency syndrome: lesions with Epstein-Barr virus infection. Mod Pathol 11: 347-356.

889. Haque T, Wilkie GM, Jones MM, Higgins CD, Urquhart G, Wingate P, Burns D, McAulay K, Turner M, Bellamy C, Amlot PL, Kelly D, MacGilchrist A, Gandhi MK, Swerdlow AJ, Crawford DH (2007). Allogeneic cytotoxic T-cell therapy for EBV-positive posttransplantation lymphoproliferative disease: results of a phase 2 multicenter clinical trial. Blood 110: 1123-1131.

890. Haralambieva E, Boerma EJ, van Imhoff GW, Rosati S, Schuuring E, Muller-Hermelink HK, Kluin PM, Ott G (2005). Clinical, immunophenotypic, and genetic analysis of adult lymphomas with morphologic features of Burkitt lymphoma. Am J Surg Pathol 29: 1086-1094.

891. Haralambieva E, Pulford KA, Lamant L, Pileri S, Roncador G, Gatter KC, Delsol G, Mason DY (2000). Anaplastic large-cell lymphomas of B-cell phenotype are anaplastic lymphoma kinase (ALK) negative and belong to the spectrum of diffuse large B-cell lymphomas. Br J Haematol 109: 584-591.

891A. Haralambieva E, Schuuring E, Rosati S, van Noesel C, Jansen P, Appel I, Guikema J, Wabinga H, Bleggi-Torres LF, Lam K., van den Berg BE, Mellink C, Zelderen-Bhola S, Kluin P (2004). Interphase fluorescence in situ hybridization for detection of 8q24/MYC breakpoints on routine histologic sections: validation in Burkitt lymphomas from three geographic regions. Genes Chromosomes Cancer 40:10-18

891B. Haralambieva E, Rosati S, van Noesel C, Boers E, van Marwijk Kooy M, Schuuring E, Kluin P (2004) Florid granulomatous reaction in Epstein-Barr virus-positive nonendemic Burkitt lymphomas: report of four cases. Am J Surg Pathol 28: 379-383.

892. Harif M, Barsaoui S, Benchekroun S, Boccon-Gibod L, Bouhas R, Doumbe P, El Haffaf Z, Khattab M, Ladjadj Y, Mallon B, Moreira C, Msefer-Alaoui F, Patte C, Rakotonirina G, Raphael M, Raquin MA, Tournade MF, Lemerle J (2005). [Treatment of childhood cancer in Africa. Preliminary results of the French-African paediatric oncology group]. Arch Pediatr 12: 851-853.

893. Harjunpaa A, Taskinen M, Nykter M, Karjalainen-Lindsberg ML, Nyman H, Monni O, Hemmer S, Yli-Harja O, Hautaniemi S, Meri S, Leppa S (2006). Differential gene expression in non-malignant tumour microenvironment is associated with outcome in follicular lymphoma patients treated with rituximab and CHOP. Br J Haematol 135: 33-42.

894. Harris MB, Shuster JJ, Carroll A, Look AT, Borowitz MJ, Crist WM, Nitschke R, Pullen J, Steuber CP, Land VJ (1992). Trisomy of leukemic cell chromosomes 4 and 10 identifies children with B-progenitor cell acute lymphoblastic leukemia with a very low risk of treatment failure: a Pediatric Oncology Group study. Blood 79: 3316-3324.

895. Harris NL, Demirjian Z (1991). Plasmacytoid T-zone cell proliferation in a patient with chronic myelomonocytic leukemia. Histologic and immunohistologic characterization. Am J Surg Pathol 15: 87-95.

896. Harris NL, Ferry JA, Swerdlow SH (1997). Posttransplant lymphoproliferative disorders: summary of Society for Hematopathology Workshop. Semin Diagn Pathol 14: 8-14.

896A. Harris NL, Horning SJ (2006). Burkitt's lymphoma--the message from microarrays. NEJM 354: 2495-2498.

897. Harris NL, Jaffe ES, Diebold J, Flandrin G, Muller-Hermelink HK, Vardiman J, Lister TA, Bloomfield CD (1999). World Health Organization classification of neoplastic diseases of the hematopoietic and lymphoid tissues: report of the Clinical Advisory Committee meeting-Airlie House, Virginia, November 1997. J Clin Oncol 17: 3835-3849.

898. Harris NL, Jaffe ES, Stein H, Banks PM, Chan JK, Cleary ML, Delsol G, Wolf-Peeters C, Falini B, Gatter KC (1994). A revised European-American classification of lymphoid neoplasms: a proposal from the International Lymphoma Study Group. Blood 84: 1361-1392.

899. Harris NL, Nadler LM, Bhan AK (1984). Immunohistologic characterization of two malignant lymphomas of germinal center type (centroblastic/centrocytic and centrocytic) with monoclonal antibodies. Follicular and diffuse lymphomas of small-cleaved-cell type are related but distinct entities. Am J Pathol 117: 262-272.

900. Harrison CJ, Moorman AV, Broadfield ZJ, Cheung KL, Harris RL, Reza JG, Robinson HM, Barber KE, Richards SM, Mitchell CD, Eden TO, Hann IM, Hill FG, Kinsey SE, Gibson BE, Lilleyman J, Vora A, Goldstone AH, Franklin IM, Durrant J, Martineau M (2004). Three distinct subgroups of hypodiploidy in acute lymphoblastic leukaemia. Br J Haematol 125: 552-559.

901. Harrison CN, Gale RE, Machin SJ, Linch DC (1999). A large proportion of patients with a diagnosis of essential thrombocythemia do not have a clonal disorder and may be at lower risk of thrombotic complications. Blood 93: 417-424.

902. Harrison CN, Green AR (2003). Essential thrombocythemia. Hematol Oncol Clin North Am 17: 1175-1190, vii.

903. Hart DN, Baker BW, Inglis MJ, Nimmo JC, Starling GC, Deacon E, Rowe M, Beard ME (1992). Epstein-Barr viral DNA in acute large granular lymphocyte (natural killer) leukemic cells. Blood 79: 2116-2123.

903A. Hartge P, Colt JS, Severson RK, Cerhan JR, Cozen W, Camann D, Zahm SH, Davis S (2005). Residential herbicide use and risk of non-Hodgkin lymphoma. Cancer Epidemiol Biomarkers Prev 14: 934-937.

904. Hasenclever D, Diehl V (1998). A prognostic score for advanced Hodgkin's disease. International Prognostic Factors Project on Advanced Hodgkin's Disease. N Engl J Med 339: 1506-1514.

905. Hasford J, Pfirrmann M, Hehlmann R, Allan NC, Baccarani M, Kluin-Nelemans JC, Alimena G, Steegmann JL, Ansari H (1998). A new prognostic score for survival of patients with chronic myeloid leukemia treated with interferon alfa. Writing Committee for the Collaborative CML Prognostic Factors Project Group. J Natl Cancer Inst 90: 850-858.

906. Hashimoto M, Yamashita Y, Mori N (2002). Immunohistochemical detection of CD79a expression in precursor T cell lymphoblastic lymphoma/leukaemias. J Pathol 197: 341-347.

907. Hasle H (1994). Myelodysplastic syndromes in childhood—classification, epidemiology, and treatment. Leuk Lymphoma 13: 11-26.

908. Hasle H, Niemeyer CM, Chessells JM, Baumann I, Bennett JM, Kerndrup G, Head DR (2003). A pediatric approach to the WHO classification of myelodysplastic and myeloproliferative diseases. Leukemia 17: 277-282.

909. Hasle H, Olesen G, Kerndrup G, Philip P, Jacobsen N (1996). Chronic neutrophil leukaemia in adolescence and young adulthood. Br J Haematol 94: 628-630.

910. Hasle H, Wadsworth LD, Massing BG, McBride M, Schultz KR (1999). A population-based study of childhood myelodysplastic syndrome in British Columbia, Canada. Br J Haematol 106: 1027-1032.

911. Hasserjian RP, Harris NL (2007). NK-cell lymphomas and leukemias: a spectrum of tumors with variable manifestations and immunophenotype. Am J Clin Pathol 127: 860-868.

912. Hayman SR, Bailey RJ, Jalal SM, Ahmann GJ, Dispenzieri A, Gertz MA, Greipp PR, Kyle RA, Lacy MQ, Rajkumar SV, Witzig TE, Lust JA, Fonseca R (2001). Translocations involving the immunoglobulin heavy-chain locus are possible early genetic events in patients with primary systemic amyloidosis. Blood 98: 2266-2268.

913. Head DR (1996). Revised classification of acute myeloid leukemia. Leukemia 10: 1826-1831.

914. Hebert J, Cayuela JM, Berkeley J, Sigaux F (1994). Candidate tumor-suppressor genes MTS1 (p16INK4A) and MTS2 (p15INK4B) display frequent homozygous deletions in primary cells from T- but not from B-cell lineage acute lymphoblastic leukemias. Blood 84: 4038-4044.

915. Heerema NA, Raimondi SC, Anderson JR, Biegel J, Camitta BM, Cooley LD, Gaynon PS, Hirsch B, Magenis RE, McGavran L, Patil S, Pettenati MJ, Pullen J, Rao K, Roulston D, Schneider NR, Shuster JJ, Sanger W, Sutcliffe MJ, van Tuinen P, Watson MS, Carroll AJ (2007). Specific extra chromosomes occur in a modal number dependent pattern in pediatric acute lymphoblastic leukemia. Genes Chromosomes Cancer 46: 684-693.

916. Hegewisch S, Mainzer K, Braumann D (1987). IgE myelomatosis. Presentation of a new case and summary of literature. Blut 55: 55-60.

916A. Heidemann BH, Clark VA (2001). Use of pre-emptive vasopressors for spinal anaesthesia-induced hypotension during Caesarean section. Br J Anaesth 87: 320-321.

917. Hemann MT, Bric A, Teruya-Feldstein J, Herbst A, Nilsson JA, Cordon-Cardo C, Cleveland JL, Tansey WP, Lowe SW (2005). Evasion of the p53 tumour surveillance network by tumour-derived MYC mutants. Nature 436: 807-811.

918. Henderson R, Spence L (2006). Down syndrome with myelodysplasia of megakaryoblastic lineage. Clin Lab Sci 19: 161-164.

918A. Herbst H, Dallenbach F, Hummel M, Niedobitek G, Pileri S, Müller-Lantzsch N, Stein H (1991). Epstein-Barr virus latent membrane protein expression in Hodgkin and Reed-Sternberg cells. Proc Natl Acad Sci U S A 88: 4766-4770.

919. Herbst H, Foss HD, Samol J, Araujo I, Klotzbach H, Krause H, Agathanggelou A, Niedobitek G, Stein H (1996). Frequent expression of interleukin-10 by Epstein-Barr virus-harboring tumor cells of Hodgkin's disease. Blood 87: 2918-2929.

919A. Herbst H, Niedobitek G, Kneba M, Hummel M, Finn T, Anagnostopoulos I, Bergholz M, Krieger G, Stein H (1990). High incidence of Epstein-Barr virus genomes in Hodgkin's disease. Am J Pathol 137: 13-18.

920. Herling M, Jones D (2007). CD4+/CD56+ hematodermic tumor: the fea-

tures of an evolving entity and its relationship to dendritic cells. Am J Clin Pathol 127: 687-700.

921. Herling M, Khoury JD, Washington LT, Duvic M, Keating MJ, Jones D (2004). A systematic approach to diagnosis of mature T-cell leukemias reveals heterogeneity among WHO categories. Blood 104: 328-335.

922. Herling M, Patel KA, Hsi ED, Chang KC, Rassidakis GZ, Ford R, Jones D (2007). TCL1 in B-cell tumors retains its normal b-cell pattern of regulation and is a marker of differentiation stage. Am J Surg Pathol 31: 1123-1129.

923. Herling M, Patel KA, Teitell MA, Konopleva M, Ravandi F, Kobayashi R, Jones D (2008). High TCL1 expression and intact T-cell receptor signaling define a hyperproliferative subset of T-cell prolymphocytic leukemia. Blood 111: 328-337.

924. Herling M, Teitell MA, Shen RR, Medeiros LJ, Jones D (2003). TCL1 expression in plasmacytoid dendritic cells (DC2s) and the related CD4+ CD56+ blastic tumors of skin. Blood 101: 5007-5009.

925. Hermine O, Haioun C, Lepage E, d'Agay MF, Briere J, Lavignac C, Fillet G, Salles G, Marolleau JP, Diebold J, Reyas F, Gaulard P (1996). Prognostic significance of bcl-2 protein expression in aggressive non-Hodgkin's lymphoma. Groupe d'Etude des Lymphomes de l'Adulte (GELA). Blood 87: 265-272.

926. Hermine O, Lefrere F, Bronowicki JP, Mariette X, Jondeau K, Eclache-Saudreau V, Delmas B, Valensi F, Cacoub P, Brechot C, Varet B, Troussard X (2002). Regression of splenic lymphoma with villous lymphocytes after treatment of hepatitis C virus infection. N Engl J Med 347: 89-94.

927. Hernandez Serrano RA, Arroyo I, Perez RJ, Quero J (1988). [Selection of infants at risk for sudden infant death syndrome]. An Esp Pediatr 29 Suppl 32:261-2.: 261-262.

928. Hernandez JM, del Canizo MC, Cuneo A, Garcia JL, Gutierrez NC, Gonzalez M, Castoldi G, San Miguel JF (2000). Clinical, hematological and cytogenetic characteristics of atypical chronic myeloid leukemia. Ann Oncol 11: 441-444.

929. Hernandez JM, Garcia JL, Gutierrez NC, Mollejo M, Martinez-Climent JA, Flores T, Gonzalez MB, Piris MA, San Miguel JF (2001). Novel genomic imbalances in B-cell splenic marginal zone lymphomas revealed by comparative genomic hybridization and cytogenetics. Am J Pathol 158: 1843-1850.

930. Hernandez L, Bea S, Pinyol M, Ott G, Katzenberger T, Rosenwald A, Bosch F, Lopez-Guillermo A, Delabie J, Colomer D, Montserrat E, Campo E (2005). CDK4 and MDM2 gene alterations mainly occur in highly proliferative and aggressive mantle cell lymphomas with wild-type INK4a/ARF locus. Cancer Res 65: 2199-2206.

931. Hernandez L, Pinyol M, Hernandez S, Bea S, Pulford K, Rosenwald A, Lamant L, Falini B, Ott G, Mason DY, Delsol G, Campo E (1999). TRK-fused gene (TFG) is a new partner of ALK in anaplastic large cell lymphoma producing two structurally different TFG-ALK translocations. Blood 94: 3265-3268.

932. Herndier BG, Sanchez HC, Chang KL, Chen YY, Weiss LM (1993). High prevalence of Epstein-Barr virus in the Reed-Sternberg cells of HIV-associated Hodgkin's disease. Am J Pathol 142: 1073-1079.

933. Hertel CB, Zhou XG, Hamilton-Dutoit SJ, Junker S (2002). Loss of B cell identity correlates with loss of B cell-specific transcription factors in Hodgkin/Reed-Sternberg cells of classical Hodgkin lymphoma. Oncogene 21: 4908-4920.

934. Herzenberg AM, Lien J, Magil AB

(1996). Monoclonal heavy chain (immunoglobulin G3) deposition disease: report of a case. Am J Kidney Dis 28: 128-131.

935. Heslop HE (2005). Biology and treatment of epstein-barr virus-associated non-hodgkin lymphomas. Hematology Am Soc Hematol Educ Program : 260-266.

936. Hess JL, Bodis S, Pinkus G, Silver B, Mauch P (1994). Histopathologic grading of nodular sclerosis Hodgkin's disease. Lack of prognostic significance in 254 surgically staged patients. Cancer 74: 708-714.

937. Hetet G, Dastot H, Baens M, Brizard A, Sigaux F, Grandchamp B, Stern MH (2000). Recurrent molecular deletion of the 12p13 region, centomeric to ETV6/TEL, in T-cell prolymphocytic leukemia. Hematol J 1: 42-47.

937A. Heuser M, Beutel G, Krauter J, Dohner K, von Neuhoff N, Schlegelberger B, Ganser A (2006). High meningioma 1 (MN1) expression as a predictor for poor outcome in acute myeloid leukemia with normal cytogenetics. Blood 108: 3898-3905.

938. Higgins JP, Warnke RA (1999). CD30 expression is common in mediastinal large B-cell lymphoma. Am J Clin Pathol 112: 241-247.

938A. Hinz M, Lemke P, Anagnostopoulos I, Hacker C, Krappmann D, Mathas S, Dörken B, Zenke M, Stein H, Scheidereit C (2002). Nuclear factor kappaB-dependent gene expression profiling of Hodgkin's disease tumor cells, pathogenetic significance, and link to constitutive signal transducer and activator of transcription 5a activity. J Exp Med 196: 605-617.

938B. Hinz M, Löser P, Mathas S, Krappmann D, Dörken B, Scheidereit C (2001). Constitutive NF-kappaB maintains high expression of a characteristic gene network, including CD40, CD86, and a set of antiapoptotic genes in Hodgkin/Reed-Sternberg cells. Blood 97: 2798-2807.

939. Hirose Y, Masaki Y, Sugai S (2002). Leukemic transformation with trisomy 8 in essential thrombocythemia: a report of four cases. Eur J Haematol 68: 112-116.

940. Hisada M, Chen BE, Jaffe ES, Travis LB (2007). Second cancer incidence and cause-specific mortality among 3104 patients with hairy cell leukemia: a population-based study. J Natl Cancer Inst 99: 215-222.

940A. Hisada M, Okayama A, Shioiri S, Spiegelman DL, Stuver SO, Mueller NE (1998). Risk factors for adult T-cell leukemia among carriers of human T-lymphotropic virus type I. Blood 92: 3557-61.

941. Hishima T, Oyaizu N, Fujii T, Tachikawa N, Ajisawa A, Negishi M, Nakamura T, Iwamoto A, Hayashi Y, Matsubara D, Sasao Y, Kimura S, Kikuchi Y, Teruya K, Yasuoka A, Oka S, Saito K, Mori S, Funata N, Sata T, Katano H (2006). Decrease in Epstein-Barr virus-positive AIDS-related lymphoma in the era of highly active antiretroviral therapy. Microbes Infect 8: 1301-1307.

942. Hitzler JK, Cheung J, Li Y, Scherer SW, Zipursky A (2003). GATA1 mutations in transient leukemia and acute megakaryoblastic leukemia of Down syndrome. Blood 101: 4301-4304.

943. Ho FC, Choy D, Loke SL, Kung IT, Fu KH, Liang R, Todd D, Khoo RK (1990). Polymorphic reticulosis and conventional lymphomas of the nose and upper aerodigestive tract: a clinicopathologic study of 70 cases, and immunophenotypic studies of 16 cases. Hum Pathol 21: 1041-1050.

944. Ho FC, Srivastava G, Loke SL, Fu KH, Leung BP, Liang R, Choy D (1990). Presence of Epstein-Barr virus DNA in nasal lymphomas of B and 'T' cell type. Hematol Oncol 8: 271-281.

944A. Hockenbery DM, Zutter M, Hickey W, Nahm M, Korsmeyer SJ (1991). BCL2 protein is

topographically restricted in tissues characterized by apoptotic cell death. Proc Natl Acad Sci U.S.A. 88: 6961-6965.

945. Hodges GF, Lenhardt TM, Cotelingam JD (1994). Bone marrow involvement in large-cell lymphoma. Prognostic implications of discordant disease. Am J Clin Pathol 101: 305-311.

946. Hodges KB, Collins RD, Greer JP, Kadin ME, Kinney MC (1999). Transformation of the small cell variant Ki-1+ lymphoma to anaplastic large cell lymphoma: pathologic and clinical features. Am J Surg Pathol 23: 49-58.

947. Hodgkin T (1832). On some morbid appearances of the absorbent glands and spleen. Med Chir Soc Tr 17: 68-

948. Hoefnagel JJ, Dijkman R, Basso K, Jansen PM, Hallermann C, Willemze R, Tensen CP, Vermeer MH (2005). Distinct types of primary cutaneous large B-cell lymphoma identified by gene expression profiling. Blood 105: 3671-3678.

949. Hoefnagel JJ, Vermeer MH, Jansen PM, Fleuren GJ, Meijer CJ, Willemze R (2003). Bcl-2, Bcl-6 and CD10 expression in cutaneous B-cell lymphoma: further support for a follicle centre cell origin and differential diagnostic significance. Br J Dermatol 149: 1183-1191.

950. Hoefnagel JJ, Vermeer MH, Jansen PM, Fleuren GJ, Meijer CJ, Willemze R (2003). Bcl-2, Bcl-6 and CD10 expression in cutaneous B-cell lymphoma: further support for a follicle centre cell origin and differential diagnostic significance. Br J Dermatol 149: 1183-1191.

951. Hoffman MA (2006). Clinical presentations and complications of hairy cell leukemia. Hematol Oncol Clin North Am 20: 1065-1073.

952. Hoffmann T, De Libero G, Colonna M, Wodnar-Filipowicz A, Passweg J, Favre G, Gratwohl A, Tichelli A (2000). Natural killer-type receptors for HLA class I antigens are clonally expressed in lymphoproliferative disorders of natural killer and T-cell type. Br J Haematol 110: 525-536.

953. Hofmann WJ, Momburg F, Moller P (1988). Thymic medullary cells expressing B lymphocyte antigens. Hum Pathol 19: 1280-1287.

954. Hoglund M, Sehn L, Connors JM, Gascoyne RD, Siebert R, Sall T, Mitelman F, Horsman DE (2004). Identification of cytogenetic subgroups and karyotypic pathways of clonal evolution in follicular lymphomas. Genes Chromosomes Cancer 39: 195-204.

955. Holland J, Trenkner DA, Wasserman TH, Fineberg B (1992). Plasmacytoma. Treatment results and conversion to myeloma. Cancer 69: 1513-1517.

956. Hollingsworth HC, Stetler-Stevenson M, Gagneten D, Kingma DW, Raffeld M, Jaffe ES (1994). Immunodeficiency-associated malignant lymphoma. Three cases showing genotypic evidence of both T- and B-cell lineages. Am J Surg Pathol 18: 1092-1101.

957. Hollowood K, Stamp G, Zouvani I, Fletcher CD (1995). Extranodal follicular dendritic cell sarcoma of the gastrointestinal tract. Morphologic, immunohistochemical and ultrastructural analysis of two cases. Am J Clin Pathol 103: 90-97.

958. Holm LE, Blomgren H, Lowhagen T (1985). Cancer risks in patients with chronic lymphocytic thyroiditis. N Engl J Med 312: 601-604.

959. Hongyo T, Hoshida Y, Nakatsuka S, Syaifudin M, Kojya S, Yang WI, Min YH, Chan H, Kim CH, Harabuchi Y, Himi T, Inuyama M, Aozasa K, Nomura T (2005). p53, K-ras, c-kit and beta-catenin gene mutations in sinonasal NK/T-cell lymphoma in Korea and Japan. Oncol Rep 13: 265-271.

960. Hongyo T, Kurooka M, Taniguchi E, Iuchi K, Nakajima Y, Aozasa K, Nomura T (1998). Frequent p53 mutations at dipyrimidine

sites in patients with pyothorax-associated lymphoma. Cancer Res 58: 1105-1107.

961. Honig GR, Suarez CR, Vida LN, Lu SJ, Liu ET (1998). Juvenile myelomonocytic leukemia (JMML) with the hematologic phenotype of severe beta thalassemia. Am J Hematol 58: 67-71.

962. Honorat JF, Ragab A, Lamant L, Delsol G, Ragab-Thomas J (2006). SHP1 tyrosine phosphatase negatively regulates NPM-ALK tyrosine kinase signaling. Blood 107: 4130-4138.

962A. Höpken UE, Foss HD, Meyer D, Hinz M, Leder K, Stein H, Lipp M (2002). Up-regulation of the chemokine receptor CCR7 in classical but not in lymphocyte-predominant Hodgkin disease correlates with distinct dissemination of neoplastic cells in lymphoid organs. Blood 99: 1109-1116

963. Horenstein MG, Nador RG, Chadburn A, Hyjek EM, Inghirami G, Knowles DM, Cesarman E (1997). Epstein-Barr virus latent gene expression in primary effusion lymphomas containing Kaposi's sarcoma-associated herpesvirus/human herpesvirus-8. Blood 90: 1186-1191.

964. Hornick JL, Jaffe ES, Fletcher CD (2004). Extranodal histiocytic sarcoma: clinicopathologic analysis of 14 cases of a rare epithelioid malignancy. Am J Surg Pathol 28: 1133-1144.

964A Horning SJ, Rosenberg SA (1984). The natural history of initially untreated low-grade non-Hodgkin's lymphomas. N Engl J Med 311: 1471-1475.

965. Horny HP, Kaiserling E (1988). Lymphoid cells and tissue mast cells of bone marrow lesions in systemic mastocytosis: a histological and immunohistological study. Br J Haematol 69: 449-455.

966. Horny HP, Kaiserling E, Campbell M, Parwaresch MR, Lennert K (1989). Liver findings in generalized mastocytosis. A clinicopathologic study. Cancer 63: 532-538.

967. Horny HP, Kaiserling E, Handgretinger R, Ruck P, Frank D, Weber R, Jaschonek KG, Waller HD (1995). Evidence for a lymphotropic nature of circulating plasmacytoid monocytes: findings from a case of CD56+ chronic myelomonocytic leukemia. Eur J Haematol 54: 209-216.

968. Horny HP, Kaiserling E, Parwaresch MR, Lennert K (1992). Lymph node findings in generalized mastocytosis. Histopathology 21: 439-446.

969. Horny HP, Lange K, Sotlar K, Valent P (2003). Increase of bone marrow lymphocytes in systemic mastocytosis: reactive lymphocytosis or malignant lymphoma? Immunohistochemical and molecular findings on routinely processed bone marrow biopsy specimens. J Clin Pathol 56: 575-578.

970. Horny HP, Parwaresch MR, Kaiserling E, Muller K, Olbermann M, Mainzer K, Lennert K (1986). Mast cell sarcoma of the larynx. J Clin Pathol 39: 596-602.

971. Horny HP, Parwaresch MR, Lennert K (1985). Bone marrow findings in systemic mastocytosis. Hum Pathol 16: 808-814.

972. Horny HP, Ruck M, Wehrmann M, Kaiserling E (1990). Blood findings in generalized mastocytosis: evidence of frequent simultaneous occurrence of myeloproliferative disorders. Br J Haematol 76: 186-193.

973. Horny HP, Ruck MT, Kaiserling E (1992). Spleen findings in generalized mastocytosis. A clinicopathologic study. Cancer 70: 459-468.

974. Horny HP, Sillaber C, Menke D, Kaiserling E, Wehrmann M, Stehberger B, Chott A, Lechner K, Lennert K, Valent P (1998). Diagnostic value of immunostaining for tryptase

in patients with mastocytosis. Am J Surg Pathol 22: 1132-1140.
975. Horny HP, Sotlar K, Sperr WR, Valent P (2004). Systemic mastocytosis with associated clonal haematological non-mast cell lineage diseases: a histopathological challenge. J Clin Pathol 57: 604-608.
976. Horny HP, Sotlar K, Stellmacher F, Krokowski M, Agis H, Schwartz LB, Valent P (2006). The tryptase positive compact round cell infiltrate of the bone marrow (TROCI-BM): a novel histopathological finding requiring the application of lineage specific markers. J Clin Pathol 59: 298-302.
977. Horny HP, Valent P (2001). Diagnosis of mastocytosis: general histopathological aspects, morphological criteria, and immunohistochemical findings. Leuk Res 25: 543-551.
978. Horny HP, Valent P (2002). Histopathological and immunohistochemical aspects of mastocytosis. Int Arch Allergy Immunol 127: 115-117.
979. Horsman DE, Gascoyne RD, Coupland RW, Coldman AJ, Adomat SA (1995). Comparison of cytogenetic analysis, southern analysis, and polymerase chain reaction for the detection of t(14; 18) in follicular lymphoma. Am J Clin Pathol 103: 472-478.
980. Hoshida Y, Hongyo T, Nakatsuka S, Nishiu M, Takakuwa T, Tomita Y, Nomura T, Aozasa K (2002). Gene mutations in lymphoproliferative disorders of T and NK/T cell phenotypes developing in renal transplant patients. Lab Invest 82: 257-264.
981. Hoshida Y, Li T, Dong Z, Tomita Y, Yamauchi A, Hanai J, Aozasa K (2001). Lymphoproliferative disorders in renal transplant patients in Japan. Int J Cancer 91: 869-875.
982. Hoshida Y, Xu JX, Fujita S, Nakamichi I, Ikeda J, Tomita Y, Nakatsuka S, Tamaru J, Iizuka A, Takeuchi T, Aozasa K (2007). Lymphoproliferative disorders in rheumatoid arthritis: clinicopathological analysis of 76 cases in relation to methotrexate medication. J Rheumatol 34: 322-331.
983. Howe RB, Porwit-MacDonald A, Wanat R, Tehranchi R, Hellstrom-Lindberg E (2004). The WHO classification of MDS does make a difference. Blood 103: 3265-3270.
984. Howell WM, Leung ST, Jones DB, Nakshabendi I, Hall MA, Lanchbury JS, Ciclitira PJ, Wright DH (1995). HLA-DRB, -DQA, and -DQB polymorphism in celiac disease and enteropathy-associated T-cell lymphoma. Common features and additional risk factors for malignancy. Hum Immunol 43: 29-37.
985. Hrusak O, Porwit-MacDonald A (2002). Antigen expression patterns reflecting genotype of acute leukemias. Leukemia 16: 1233-1258.
986. Hsi ED, Singleton TP, Swinnen L, Dunphy CH, Alkan S (2000). Mucosa-associated lymphoid tissue-type lymphomas occurring in post-transplantation patients. Am J Surg Pathol 24: 100-106.
987. Hsu SM, Jaffe ES (1984). Leu M1 and peanut agglutinin stain the neoplastic cells of Hodgkin's disease. Am J Clin Pathol 82: 29-32.
987A. Hu H (1987). Benzene-associated myelofibrosis. Ann Intern Med 106: 171-172.
988. Huang JZ, Sanger WG, Greiner TC, Staudt LM, Weisenburger DD, Pickering DL, Lynch JC, Armitage JO, Warnke RA, Alizadeh AA, Lossos IS, Levy R, Chan WC (2002). The t(14;18) defines a unique subset of diffuse large B-cell lymphoma with a germinal center B-cell gene expression profile. Blood 99: 2285-2290.
989. Huang KP, Weinstock MA, Clarke CA, McMillan A, Hoppe RT, Kim YH (2007). Second lymphomas and other malignant neoplasms in patients with mycosis fungoides and Sezary syndrome: evidence from population-based and clinical cohorts. Arch Dermatol 143: 45-50.
990. Huang Q, Chang KL, Gaal KK, Weiss LM (2005). An aggressive extranodal NK-cell lymphoma arising from indolent NK-cell lymphoproliferative disorder. Am J Surg Pathol 29: 1540-1543.
991. Huang WT, Chang KC, Huang GC, Hsiao JR, Chen HH, Chuang SS, Chen TY, Su WC, Tsao CJ (2005). Bone marrow that is positive for Epstein-Barr virus encoded RNA-1 by in situ hybridization is related with a poor prognosis in patients with extranodal natural killer/T-cell lymphoma, nasal type. Haematologica 90: 1063-1069.
992. Hudnall SD, Alperin JB, Petersen JR (2001). Composite nodular lymphocyte-predominance Hodgkin disease and gamma-heavy-chain disease: a case report and review of the literature. Arch Pathol Lab Med 125: 803-807.
992A Hummel M, Anagnostopoulos I, Dallenbach F, Korbjuhn P, Dimmler C, Stein H (1992). EBV infection patterns in Hodgkin's disease and normal lymphoid tissue: expression and cellular localization of EBV gene products. Br J Haematol 82: 689-694.
993. Hummel M, Anagnostopoulos I, Korbjuhn P, Stein H (1995). Epstein-Barr virus in B-cell non-Hodgkin's lymphomas: unexpected infection patterns and different infection incidence in low- and high-grade types. J Pathol 175: 263-271.
994. Hummel M, Bentink S, Berger H, Klapper W, Wessendorf S, Barth TF, Bernd HW, Cogliatti SB, Dierlamm J, Feller AC, Hansmann ML, Haralambieva E, Harder L, Hasenclever D, Kuhn M, Lenze D, Lichter P, Martin-Subero JI, Moller P, Muller-Hermelink HK, Ott G, Parwaresch RM, Pott C, Rosenwald A, Rosolowski M, Schwaenen C, Sturzenhofecker B, Szczepanowski M, Trautmann H, Wacker HH, Spang R, Loeffler M, Trumper L, Stein H, Siebert R (2006). A biologic definition of Burkitt's lymphoma from transcriptional and genomic profiling. N Engl J Med 354: 2419-2430.
994A. Hummel M, Tamaru J, Kalvelage B, Stein H (1994). Mantle cell (previously centrocytic) lymphomas express VH genes with no or very little somatic mutations like the physiologic cells of the follicle mantle. Blood 84: 403-407.
995. Hungness SI, Akin C (2007). Mastocytosis: advances in diagnosis and treatment. Curr Allergy Asthma Rep 7: 248-254.
996. Hurwitz CA, Raimondi SC, Head D, Krance R, Mirro J, Jr., Kalwinsky DK, Ayers GD, Behm FG (1992). Distinctive immunophenotypic features of t(8;21)(q22;q22) acute myeloblastic leukemia in children. Blood 80: 3182-3188.
997. Husby G, Blichfeldt P, Brinch L, Brandtzaeg P, Mellbye OJ, Sletten K, Stenstad T (1998). Chronic arthritis and gamma heavy chain disease: coincidence or pathogenic link? Scand J Rheumatol 27: 257-264.
998. Hussell T, Isaacson PG, Crabtree JE, Spencer J (1993). The response of cells from low-grade B-cell gastric lymphomas of mucosa-associated lymphoid tissue to Helicobacter pylori. Lancet 342: 571-574.
999. Hussong JW, Perkins SL, Schnitzer B, Hargreaves H, Frizzera G (1999). Extramedullary plasmacytoma. A form of marginal zone cell lymphoma? Am J Clin Pathol 111: 111-116.
1000. Ichikawa A, Kinoshita T, Watanabe T, Kato H, Nagai H, Tsushita K, Saito H, Hotta T (1997). Mutations of the p53 gene as a prognostic factor in aggressive B-cell lymphoma. N Engl J Med 337: 529-534.
1001. Ichinohasama R, Miura I, Kobayashi N, Saitoh Y, DeCoteau JF, Saiki Y, Mori S, Kadin ME, Ooya K (1998). Herpes virus type 8-negative primary effusion lymphoma associated with PAX-5 gene rearrangement and hepatitis C virus: a case report and review of the literature. Am J Surg Pathol 22: 1528-1537.
1002. Ikonomou IM, Tierens A, Troen G, Aamot HV, Heim S, Lauritzsen GF, Valerhaugen H, Delabie J (2006). Peripheral T-cell lymphoma with involvement of the expanded mantle zone. Virchows Arch 449: 78-87.
1003. Ilowite NT, Flignar CL, Ochs HD, Brichacek B, Harada S, Haas JE, Purtilo DT, Wedgwood RJ (1986). Pulmonary angiitis with atypical lymphoreticular infiltrates in Wiskott-Aldrich syndrome: possible relationship of lymphomatoid granulomatosis and EBV infection. Clin Immunol Immunopathol 41: 479-484.
1004. Imamura N, Kusunoki Y, Kawa-Ha K, Yumura K, Hara J, Oda K, Abe K, Dohy H, Inada T, Kajihara H (1990). Aggressive natural killer cell leukaemia/lymphoma: report of four cases and review of the literature. Possible existence of a new clinical entity originating from the third lineage of lymphoid cells. Br J Haematol 75: 49-59.
1004A. Inghirami G, Foitl DR, Sabichi A, Zhu BY, Knowles DM (1991). Autoantibody-associated cross-reactive idiotype-bearing human B lymphocytes: distribution and characterization, including Ig VH gene and CD5 antigen expression. Blood 78: 1503-1515.
1005. Ingram W, Lea NC, Cervera J, Germing U, Fenaux P, Cassinat B, Kiladjian JJ, Varkonyi J, Antunovic P, Westwood NB, Arno MJ, Mohamedali A, Gaken J, Kontou T, Czepulkowski BH, Twine NA, Tamaska J, Csomer J, Benedek S, Gattermann N, Zipperer E, Giagounidis A, Garcia-Casado Z, Sanz G, Mufti GJ (2006). The JAK2 V617F mutation identifies a subgroup of MDS patients with isolated deletion 5q and a proliferative bone marrow. Leukemia 20: 1319-1321.
1006. Inhorn RC, Aster JC, Roach SA, Slapak CA, Soiffer R, Tantravahi R, Stone RM (1995). A syndrome of lymphoblastic lymphoma, eosinophilia, and myeloid hyperplasia/malignancy associated with t(8;13)(p11;q11): description of a distinctive clinicopathologic entity. Blood 85: 1881-1887.
1007. Invernizzi R, Custodi P, de Fazio P, Bergamaschi G, Fenoglio C, Ricevuti G, Rosti V, Zambelli LM, Ascari E (1990). The syndrome of abnormal chromatin clumping in leucocytes: clinical and biological study of a case. Haematologica 75: 532-536.
1008. Inwald DP, Peters MJ, Walshe D, Jones A, Davies EG, Klein NJ (2000). Absence of platelet CD40L identifies patients with X-linked hyper IgM syndrome. Clin Exp Immunol 120: 499-502.
1009. Iqbal J, Neppalli VT, Wright G, Dave BJ, Horsman DE, Rosenwald A, Lynch J, Hans CP, Weisenburger DD, Greiner TC, Gascoyne RD, Campo E, Ott G, Muller-Hermelink HK, Delabie J, Jaffe ES, Grogan TM, Connors JM, Vose JM, Armitage JO, Staudt LM, Chan WC (2006). BCL2 expression is a prognostic marker for the activated B-cell-like type of diffuse large B-cell lymphoma. J Clin Oncol 24: 961-968.
1010. Irving JA, Mattman A, Lockitch G, Farrell K, Wadsworth LD (2003). Element of caution: a case of reversible cytopenias associated with excessive zinc supplementation. CMAJ 169: 129-131.
1011. Isaacson PG (1994). Gastrointestinal lymphoma. Hum Pathol 25: 1020-1029.
1011A. Isaacson PG (1996). Malignant lymphomas with a follicular growth pattern. Histopathology 28: 487-495.
1012. Isaacson PG, Dogan A, Price SK, Spencer J (1989). Immunoproliferative small-intestinal disease. An immunohistochemical study. Am J Surg Pathol 13: 1023-1033.
1013. Isaacson PG, Du MQ (2004). MALT lymphoma: from morphology to molecules. Nat Rev Cancer 4: 644-653.
1014. Isaacson PG, Matutes E, Burke M, Catovsky D (1994). The histopathology of splenic lymphoma with villous lymphocytes. Blood 84: 3828-3834.
1015. Isaacson PG, Norton AJ (eds.) (1994). Extranodal lymphomas. Churchill Livingstone: Edinburgh, London, Madrid, Melbourne, New York, Tokyo.
1016. Isaacson PG, Norton AJ, Addis BJ (1987). The human thymus contains a novel population of B lymphocytes. Lancet 2: 1488-1491.
1017. Isaacson PG, O'Connor NT, Spencer J, Bevan DH, Connolly CE, Kirkham N, Pollock DJ, Wainscoat JS, Stein H, Mason DY (1985). Malignant histiocytosis of the intestine: a T-cell lymphoma. Lancet 2: 688-691.
1018. Isaacson PG, Spencer J (1987). Malignant lymphoma of mucosa-associated lymphoid tissue. Histopathology 11: 445-462.
1019. Isaacson PG, Wotherspoon AC, Diss T, Pan LX (1991). Follicular colonization in B-cell lymphoma of mucosa-associated lymphoid tissue. Am J Surg Pathol 15: 819-828.
1020. Ishihara S, Ohshima K, Tokura Y, Yabuta R, Imaishi H, Wakiguchi H, Kurashige T, Kishimoto H, Katayama I, Okada S, Kawa-Ha K (1997). Hypersensitivity to mosquito bites conceals clonal lymphoproliferation of Epstein-Barr viral DNA-positive natural killer cells. Jpn J Cancer Res 88: 82-87.
1021. Ishihara S, Okada S, Wakiguchi H, Kurashige T, Hirai K, Kawa-Ha K (1997). Clonal lymphoproliferation following chronic active Epstein-Barr virus infection and hypersensitivity to mosquito bites. Am J Hematol 54: 276-281.
1022. Ishizawa S, Slovak ML, Popplewell L, Bedell V, Wrede JE, Carter NH, Snyder DS, Arber DA (2003). High frequency of pro-B acute lymphoblastic leukemia in adults with secondary leukemia with 11q23 abnormalities. Leukemia 17: 1091-1095.
1023. Isimbaldi G, Bandiera L, d'Amore ES, Conter V, Milani M, Mussolin L, Rosolen A (2006). ALK-positive plasmablastic B-cell lymphoma with the clathrin-ALK gene rearrangement. Pediatr Blood Cancer 46: 390-391.
1024. Iuchi K, Aozasa K, Yamamoto S, Mori T, Tajima K, Minato K, Mukai K, Komatsu H, Tagaki T, Kobashi Y. (1989). Non-Hodgkin's lymphoma of the pleural cavity developing from long-standing pyothorax. Summary of clinical and pathological findings in thirty-seven cases. Jpn J Clin Oncol 19: 249-257.
1025. Iuchi K, Sawamura K, Ichimiya A, Lee YE, Tada H, Mori T (1987). [A case of successfully resected giant hemangiomatous lesion in the thoracic cavity]. Nippon Kyobu Geka Gakkai Zasshi 35: 528-532.
1026. Ivanovski M, Silvestri F, Pozzato G, Anand S, Mazzaro C, Burrone OR, Efremov DG (1998). Somatic hypermutation, clonal diversity, and preferential expression of the VH 51p1/VL kv325 immunoglobulin gene combination in hepatitis C virus-associated immunocytomas. Blood 91: 2433-2442.
1027. Iwatsuki K, Xu Z, Ohtsuka M, Kaneko F (2000). Cutaneous lymphoproliferative disorders associated with Epstein-Barr virus infection: a clinical overview. J Dermatol Sci 22: 181-195.
1028. Izumi M, Mochizuki M, Kuroda M, Iwaya K, Mukai K (2002). Angiomyoid proliferative lesion: an unusual stroma-rich variant of Castleman's disease of hyaline-vascular type. Virchows Arch 441: 400-405.
1029. Jacknow G, Frizzera G, Gajl-Peczalska

K, Banks PM, Arthur DC, McGlave PB, Hurd DD (1985). Extramedullary presentation of the blast crisis of chronic myelogenous leukaemia. Br J Haematol 61: 225-236.

1030. Jackson A, Scarffe JH (1990). Prognostic significance of osteopenia and immunoparesis at presentation in patients with solitary myeloma of bone. Eur J Cancer 26: 363-371.

1030A. Jacob J, Kelsoe G, Rajewsky K, Weiss U (1991). Intraclonal generation of antibody mutants in germinal centres. Nature 354: 389-392.

1031. Jacob MC, Chaperot L, Mossuz P, Feuillard J, Valensi F, Leroux D, Bene MC, Bensa JC, Briere F, Plumas J (2003). CD4+ CD56+ lineage negative malignancies: a new entity developed from malignant early plasmacytoid dendritic cells. Haematologica 88: 941-955.

1032. Jaffe ES (1995). Nasal and nasal-type T/NK cell lymphoma: a unique form of lymphoma associated with the Epstein-Barr virus [comment]. Histopathology 27: 581-583.

1033. Jaffe ES (1995). Post-thymic T-cell lymphomas. In: Surgical Pathology of the Lymph Nodes and Related Organs (Major Problems in Pathology Series, Vol. 16) 2nd ed. W.B. Saunders Company: Philadelphia, pp. 360-364.

1034. Jaffe ES (2001). Anaplastic large cell lymphoma: the shifting sands of diagnostic hematopathology. Mod Pathol 14: 219-228.

1035. Jaffe ES (2006). Pathobiology of peripheral T-cell lymphomas. Hematology Am Soc Hematol Educ Program 126: 317-322.

1036. Jaffe ES, Blattner WA, Blayney DW, Bunn PA, Jr., Cossman J, Robert-Guroff M, Gallo RC (1984). The pathologic spectrum of adult T-cell leukemia/lymphoma in the United States. Human T-cell leukemia/lymphoma virus-associated lymphoid malignancies. Am J Surg Pathol 8: 263-275.

1037. Jaffe ES, Chan JK, Su IJ, Frizzera G, Mori S, Feller AC, Ho FC (1996). Report of the Workshop on Nasal and Related Extranodal Angiocentric T/Natural Killer Cell Lymphomas. Definitions, differential diagnosis, and epidemiology. Am J Surg Pathol 20: 103-111.

1038. Jaffe ES, Harris NL, Diebold J, Muller-Hermelink HK (1998). World Health Organization Classification of lymphomas: a work in progress. Ann Oncol 9 Suppl 5: S25-S30.

1039. Jaffe ES, Harris NL, Stein H, and Vardiman JW (eds.) (2001). Pathology and Genetics of Tumours of the Haematopoietic and Lymphoid Tissues. IARCPress: Lyon.

1040. Jaffe ES, Krenacs L, Raffeld M (2003). Classification of cytotoxic T-cell and natural killer cell lymphomas. Semin Hematol 40: 175-184.

1041. Jaffe ES, Puck JM, Jackson CE, Dale JK, Sneller MC, Fisher RE, Hsu AP, Lenardo MJ, Straus.S.E. (1999). Increased risk for diverse lymphomas in autoimmune lymphoproliferative syndrome (ALPS), an inherited disorder due to defective lymphocyte apoptosis. Blood 94: 597a.

1042. Jaffe ES, Wilson WH (1997). Lymphomatoid granulomatosis: pathogenesis, pathology and clinical implications. Cancer Surv 30:233-248..

1042B. Jaffe ES, Zarate-Osorno A, Kingma DW, Raffeld M, Medeiros LJ (1994). The interrelationship between Hodgkin's disease and non-Hodgkin's lymphomas. Ann Oncol 5: 7-11.

1042A. Jaffe R (2004). Liver involvement in the histiocytic disorders of childhood. Pediatr Dev Pathol 7: 214-225.

1043. Jahnke K, Thiel E, Martus P, Herrlinger U, Weller M, Fischer L, Korfel A (2006). Relapse of primary central nervous system lymphoma: clinical features, outcome and prognostic factors. J Neurooncol 80: 159-165.

1044. James C, Ugo V, Le Couedic JP, Staerk J, Delhommeau F, Lacout C, Garcon L, Raslova H, Berger R, Bennaceur-Griscelli A, Villeval JL, Constantinescu SN, Casadevall N, Vainchenker W (2005). A unique clonal JAK2 mutation leading to constitutive signalling causes polycythaemia vera. Nature 434: 1144-1148.

1045. Janka GE (2007). Hemophagocytic syndromes. Blood Rev 21: 245-253.

1045A. Janssen D, Fölster-Holst R, Harms D, Klapper W (2007). Clonality in juvenile xanthogranuloma Am J Surg Pathol 31:812-813.

1045B. Janssen D, Harms D (2005). Juvenile xanthogranuloma in childhood and adolescence: a clinicopathologic study of 129 patients from the Kiel pediatric tumor registry. Am J Surg Pathol 29:21-28.

1046. Janssen JW, Ludwig WD, Sterry W, Bartram CR (1993). SIL-TAL1 deletion in T-cell acute lymphoblastic leukemia. Leukemia 7: 1204-1210.

1047. Jantunen R, Juvonen E, Ikkala E, Oksanen K, Anttila P, Ruutu T (1999). Development of erythrocytosis in the course of essential thrombocythemia. Ann Hematol 78: 219-222.

1047A. Janz M, Hummel M, Truss M, Wollert-Wulf B, Mathas S, Jöhrens K, Hagemeier C, Bommert K, Stein H, Dörken B, Bargou RC (2006). Classical Hodgkin lymphoma is characterized by high constitutive expression of activating transcription factor 3 (ATF3), which promotes viability of Hodgkin/Reed-Sternberg cells. Blood 107: 2536-2539.

1048. Jares P, Campo E, Pinyol M, Bosch F, Miquel R, Fernandez PL, Sanchez-Beato M, Soler F, Perez-Losada A, Nayach I, Mallofre C, Piris MA, Montserrat E, Cardesa A (1996). Expression of retinoblastoma gene product (pRb) in mantle cell lymphomas. Correlation with cyclin D1 (PRAD1/CCND1) mRNA levels and proliferative activity. Am J Pathol 148: 1591-1600.

1048A. Jares P, Colomer D, Campo E (2007). Genetic and molecular pathogenesis of mantle cell lymphoma: perspectives for new targeted therapeutics. Nat Rev Cancer 7: 750-762.

1049. Jarviluoma A, Koopal S, Rasanen S, Makela TP, Ojala PM (2004). KSHV viral cyclin binds to p27KIP1 in primary effusion lymphomas. Blood 104: 3349-3354.

1050. Jasionowski TM, Hartung L, Greenwood JH, Perkins SL, Bahler DW (2003). Analysis of CD10+ hairy cell leukemia. Am J Clin Pathol 120: 228-235.

1051. Jaye DL, Geigerman CM, Herling M, Eastburn K, Waller EK, Jones D (2006). Expression of the plasmacytoid dendritic cell marker BDCA-2 supports a spectrum of maturation among CD4+ CD56+ hematodermic neoplasms. Mod Pathol 19: 1555-1562.

1052. Jemal A, Siegel R, Ward E, Murray T, Xu J, Thun MJ (2007). Cancer statistics, 2007. CA Cancer J Clin 57: 43-66.

1053. Jemal A, Tiwari RC, Murray T, Ghafoor A, Samuels A, Ward E, Feuer EJ, Thun MJ (2004). Cancer statistics, 2004. CA Cancer J Clin 54: 8-29.

1054. Jenkins RB, Tefferi A, Solberg LA, Jr., Dewald GW (1989). Acute leukemia with abnormal thrombopoiesis and inversions of chromosome 3. Cancer Genet Cytogenet 39: 167-179.

1055. Jensen MK, de Nully BP, Nielsen OJ, Hasselbalch HC (2000). Incidence, clinical features and outcome of essential thrombocythaemia in a well defined geographical area. Eur J Haematol 65: 132-139.

1056. Jerkeman M, Aman P, Cavallin-Stahl E, Torlakovic E, Akerman M, Mitelman F, Fioretos T (2002). Prognostic implications of BCL6 rearrangement in uniformly treated patients with diffuse large B-cell lymphoma—a Nordic Lymphoma Group study. Int J Oncol 20: 161-165.

1057. Jhala DN, Medeiros LJ, Lopez-Terrada D, Jhala NC, Krishnan B, Shahab I (2000). Neutrophil-rich anaplastic large cell lymphoma of T-cell lineage. A report of two cases arising in HIV-positive patients. Am J Clin Pathol 114: 478-482.

1058. Johan MF, Goodeve AC, Bowen DT, Frew ME, Reilly JT (2005). JAK2 V617F Mutation is uncommon in chronic myelomonocytic leukaemia. Br J Haematol 130: 968.

1059. Johansson P (2006). Epidemiology of the myeloproliferative disorders polycythemia vera and essential thrombocythemia. Semin Thromb Hemost 32: 171-173.

1060. Johansson P, Kutti J, Andreasson B, Safai-Kutti S, Vilen L, Wedel H, Ridell B (2004). Trends in the incidence of chronic Philadelphia chromosome negative (Ph-) myeloproliferative disorders in the city of Goteborg, Sweden, during 1983-99. J Intern Med 256: 161-165.

1061. Johnson LR, Nalesnik MA, Swerdlow SH (2006). Impact of Epstein-Barr virus in monomorphic B-cell posttransplant lymphoproliferative disorders: a histogenetic study. Am J Surg Pathol 30: 1604-1612.

1062. Johrens K, Stein H, Anagnostopoulos I (2007). T-bet transcription factor detection facilitates the diagnosis of minimal hairy cell leukemia infiltrates in bone marrow trephines. Am J Surg Pathol 31: 1181-1185.

1063. Jones AM, Gaspar HB (2000). Immunogenetics: changing the face of immunodeficiency. J Clin Pathol 53: 60-65.

1064. Jones AV, Kreil S, Zoi K, Waghorn K, Curtis C, Zhang L, Score J, Seear R, Chase AJ, Grand FH, White H, Zoi C, Loukopoulos D, Terpos E, Vervessou EC, Schultheis B, Emig M, Ernst T, Lengfelder E, Hehlmann R, Hochhaus A, Oscier D, Silver RT, Reiter A, Cross NC (2005). Widespread occurrence of the JAK2 V617F mutation in chronic myeloproliferative disorders. Blood 106: 2162-2168.

1065. Jones D, Amin M, Ordonez NG, Glassman AB, Hayes KJ, Medeiros LJ (2001). Reticulum cell sarcoma of lymph node with mixed dendritic and fibroblastic features. Mod Pathol 14: 1059-1067.

1066. Jones D, Ballestas ME, Kaye KM, Gulizia JM, Winters GL, Fletcher J, Scadden DT, Aster JC (1998). Primary-effusion lymphoma and Kaposi's sarcoma in a cardiac-transplant recipient. N Engl J Med 339: 444-449.

1067. Jones D, O'Hara C, Kraus MD, Perez-Atayde AR, Shahsafaei A, Wu L, Dorfman DM (2000). Expression pattern of T-cell-associated chemokine receptors and their chemokines correlates with specific subtypes of T-cell non-Hodgkin lymphoma. Blood 96: 685-690.

1068. Jones D, Vega F, Sarris AH, Medeiros LJ (2002). CD4-CD8-"Double-negative" cutaneous T-cell lymphomas share common histologic features and an aggressive clinical course. Am J Surg Pathol 26: 225-231.

1069. Jones JF, Shurin S, Abramowsky C, Tubbs RR, Sciotto CG, Wahl R, Sands J, Gottman D, Katz BZ, Sklar J (1988). T-cell lymphomas containing Epstein-Barr viral DNA in patients with chronic Epstein-Barr virus infections. N Engl J Med 318: 733-741.

1070. Jones SE, Fuks Z, Bull M, Kadin ME, Dorfman RF, Kaplan HS, Rosenberg SA, Kim H (1973). Non-Hodgkin's lymphomas. IV. Clinicopathologic correlation in 405 cases. Cancer 31: 806-823.

1070A. Joos S, Granzow M, Holtgreve-Grez H, Siebert R, Harder L, Martín-Subero JI, Wolf J, Adamowicz M, Barth TF, Lichter P, Jauch A (2003). Hodgkin's lymphoma cell lines are characterized by frequent aberrations on chromosomes 2p and 9p including REL and JAK2. Int J Cancer 103: 489-495.

1071. Joos S, Kupper M, Ohl S, von Bonin F, Mechtersheimer G, Bentz M, Marynen P, Moller P, Pfreundschuh M, Trumper L, Lichter P (2000). Genomic imbalances including amplification of the tyrosine kinase gene JAK2 in CD30+ Hodgkin cells. Cancer Res 60: 549-552.

1072. Joos S, Otano-Joos MI, Ziegler S, Bruderlein S, du MS, Bentz M, Moller P, Lichter P (1996). Primary mediastinal (thymic) B-cell lymphoma is characterized by gains of chromosomal material including 9p and amplification of the REL gene. Blood 87: 1571-1578.

1073. Jordan JH, Walchshofer S, Jurecka W, Mosberger I, Sperr WR, Wolff K, Chott A, Buhring HJ, Lechner K, Horny HP, Valent P (2001). Immunohistochemical properties of bone marrow mast cells in systemic mastocytosis: evidence for expression of CD2, CD117/Kit, and bcl-x(L). Hum Pathol 32: 545-552.

1073A. Jorgensen C, Legouffe MC, Perney P, Coste J, Tissot B, Segarra C, Bologna C, Bourrat L, Combe B, Blanc F, Sany J (1996). Sicca syndrome associated with hepatitis C virus infection. Arthritis Rheum 39: 1166-1171.

1074. Joseph G, Barker RL, Yuan B, Martin A, Medeiros J, Peiper SC (1994). Posttransplantation plasma cell dyscrasias. Cancer 74: 1959-1964.

1075. Joslin JM, Fernald AA, Tennant TR, Davis EM, Kogan SC, Anastasi J, Crispino JD, Le Beau MM (2007). Haploinsufficiency of EGR1, a candidate gene in the del(5q), leads to the development of myeloid disorders. Blood 110: 719-726.

1076. Josting A, Wolf J, Diehl V (2000). Hodgkin disease: prognostic factors and treatment strategies. Curr Opin Oncol 12: 403-411.

1077. Juneja SK, Imbert M, Jouault H, Scoazec JY, Sigaux F, Sultan C (1983). Haematological features of primary myelodysplastic syndromes (PMDS) at initial presentation: a study of 118 cases. J Clin Pathol 36: 1129-1135.

1078. Juneja SK, Imbert M, Sigaux F, Jouault H, Sultan C (1983). Prevalence and distribution of ringed sideroblasts in primary myelodysplastic syndromes. J Clin Pathol 36: 566-569.

1079. Kadin ME (2006). Pathobiology of CD30+ cutaneous T-cell lymphomas. J Cutan Pathol 33 Suppl 1: 10-17.

1080. Kadin ME, Agnarsson BA, Ellingsworth LR, Newcom SR (1990). Immunohistochemical evidence of a role for transforming growth factor beta in the pathogenesis of nodular sclerosing Hodgkin's disease. Am J Pathol 136: 1209-1214.

1080A. Kadin ME, Berard CW, Nanba K, Wakasa H (1983). Lymphoproliferative diseases in Japan and Western countries: Proceedings of the United States--Japan Seminar, September 6 and 7, 1982, in Seattle, Washington. Hum Pathol 14: 745-772

1081. Kadin ME, Liebowitz DN (1999). Cytokines and cytokine receptors in Hodgkin's disease. In: Hodgkin's Disease. Mauch P, Armitage JO, Diehl V, eds. Lippincott Williams & Wilkins: Philadelphia, pp. 139.

1082. Kagami Y, Suzuki R, Taji H, Yatabe Y, Takeuchi T, Maeda S, Kondo E, Kojima M, Motoori T, Mizoguchi Y, Okamoto M, Ohnishi K, Yamabe H, Seto M, Ogura M, Koshikawa T, Takahashi T, Kurita S, Morishima Y, Suchi T, Nakamura S (1999). Nodal cytotoxic lymphoma spectrum: a clinicopathologic study of 66 patients. Am J Surg Pathol 23: 1184-1200.

1083. Kako S, Kanda Y, Sato T, Goyama S, Noda N, Shoda E, Oshima K, Inoue M, Izutsu K, Watanabe T, Motokura T, Chiba S, Fukayama M, Kurokawa M (2007). Early relapse of JAK2 V617F-positive chronic neutrophilic leukemia with central nervous system

infiltration after unrelated bone marrow transplantation. Am J Hematol 82: 386-390.
1084. Kaleem Z, White G (2001). Diagnostic criteria for minimally differentiated acute myeloid leukemia (AML-M0). Evaluation and a proposal. Am J Clin Pathol 115: 876-884.
1085. Kambham N, Markowitz GS, Appel GB, Kleiner MJ, Aucouturier P, D'agati VD (1999). Heavy chain deposition disease: the disease spectrum. Am J Kidney Dis 33: 954-962.
1086. Kamel OW (2002). Iatrogenic lymphoproliferative disorders in non-transplantation settings. Recent Results Cancer Res 159: 19-26.
1087. Kamel OW, Gocke CD, Kell DL, Cleary ML, Warnke RA (1995). True histiocytic lymphoma: a study of 12 cases based on current definition. Leuk Lymphoma 18: 81-86.
1088. Kamel OW, van de Rijn M, LeBrun DP, Weiss LM, Warnke RA, Dorfman RF (1994). Lymphoid neoplasms in patients with rheumatoid arthritis and dermatomyositis: frequency of Epstein-Barr virus and other features associated with immunosuppression. Hum Pathol 25: 638-643.
1089. Kamel OW, van de RM, Weiss LM, Del Zoppo GJ, Hench PK, Robbins BA, Montgomery PG, Warnke RA, Dorfman RF (1993). Brief report: reversible lymphomas associated with Epstein-Barr virus occurring during methotrexate therapy for rheumatoid arthritis and dermatomyositis. N Engl J Med 328: 1317-1321.
1090. Kamel OW, Weiss LM, van de RM, Colby TV, Kingma DW, Jaffe ES (1996). Hodgkin's disease and lymphoproliferations resembling Hodgkin's disease in patients receiving long-term low-dose methotrexate therapy. Am J Surg Pathol 20: 1279-1287.
1091. Kanavaros P, de Bruin PC, Briere J, Meijer CJ, Gaulard P (1995). Epstein-Barr virus (EBV) in extranodal T-cell non-Hodgkin's lymphomas (T-NHL). Identification of nasal T-NHL as a distinct clinicopathological entity associated with EBV. Leuk Lymphoma 18: 27-34.
1092. Kanavaros P, Gaulard P, Charlotte F, Martin N, Ducos C, Lebezu M, Mason DY (1995). Discordant expression of immunoglobulin and its associated molecule mb-1/CD79a is frequently found in mediastinal large B cell lymphomas. Am J Pathol 146: 735-741.
1093. Kanavaros P, Lescs MC, Briere J, Divine M, Galateau F, Joab I, Bosq J, Farcet JP, Reyes F, Gaulard P (1993). Nasal T-cell lymphoma: a clinicopathologic entity associated with peculiar phenotype and with Epstein-Barr virus. Blood 81: 2688-2695.
1094. Kanegane H, Bhatia K, Gutierrez M, Kaneda H, Wada T, Yachie A, Seki H, Arai T, Kagimoto S, Okazaki M, Oh-ishi T, Moghaddam A, Wang F, Tosato G (1998). A syndrome of peripheral blood T-cell infection with Epstein-Barr virus (EBV) followed by EBV-positive T-cell lymphoma. Blood 91: 2085-2091.
1094A. Kanno H, Kojya S, Li T, Ohsawa M, Nakatsuka S, Miyaguchi M, Harabuchi Y, Aozasa K. (2000). Low frequency of HLA-A*0201 allele in patients with Epstein-Barr virus-positive nasal lymphomas with polymorphic reticulosis morphology. Int J Cancer 87: 195-199.
1095. Kanno H, Naka N, Yasunaga Y, Iuchi K, Yamauchi S, Hashimoto M, Aozasa K (1997). Production of the immunosuppressive cytokine interleukin-10 by Epstein-Barr-virus-expressing pyothorax-associated lymphoma: possible role in the development of overt lymphoma in immunocompetent hosts. Am J Pathol 150: 349-357.
1096. Kanno H, Nakatsuka S, Iuchi K, Aozasa K (2000). Sequences of cytotoxic T-lymphocyte epitopes in the Epstein-Barr virus (EBV) nuclear antigen-3B gene in a Japanese population with or without EBV-positive lymphoid malignancies. Int J Cancer 88: 626-632.
1097. Kanno H, Ohsawa M, Hashimoto M, Iuchi K, Nakajima Y, Aozasa K (1999). HLA-A alleles of patients with pyothorax-associated lymphoma: anti-Epstein-Barr virus (EBV) host immune responses during the development of EBV latent antigen-positive lymphomas. Int J Cancer 82: 630-634.
1098. Kanno H, Yasunaga Y, Iuchi K, Yamauchi S, Tatekawa T, Sugiyama H, Aozasa K (1996). Interleukin-6-mediated growth enhancement of cell lines derived from pyothorax-associated lymphoma. Lab Invest 75: 167-173.
1099. Kant JA, Hubbard SM, Longo DL, Simon RM, DeVita VT, Jaffe ES (1986). The pathologic and clinical heterogeneity of lymphocyte-depleted Hodgkin's disease. J Clin Oncol 4: 284-294.
1100. Kantarjian HM, Dixon D, Keating MJ, Talpaz M, Walters RS, McCredie KB, Freireich EJ (1988). Characteristics of accelerated disease in chronic myelogenous leukemia. Cancer 61: 1441-1446.
1101. Kantarjian HM, Keating MJ, Smith TL, Talpaz M, McCredie KB (1990). Proposal for a simple synthesis prognostic staging system in chronic myelogenous leukemia. Am J Med 88: 1-8.
1102. Kantarjian HM, McLaughlin P, Fuller LM, Dixon DO, Osborne BM, Cabanillas FF (1984). Follicular large cell lymphoma: analysis and prognostic factors in 62 patients. J Clin Oncol 2: 811-819.
1103. Kantarjian HM, Talpaz M, Giles F, O'Brien S, Cortes J (2006). New insights into the pathophysiology of chronic myeloid leukemia and imatinib resistance. Ann Intern 145: 913-923.
1104. Kanungo A, Medeiros LJ, Abruzzo LV, Lin P (2006). Lymphoid neoplasms associated with concurrent t(14;18) and 8q24/c-MYC translocation generally have a poor prognosis. Mod Pathol 19: 25-33.
1105. Kanzler H, Kuppers R, Hansmann ML, Rajewsky K (1996). Hodgkin and Reed-Sternberg cells in Hodgkin's disease represent the outgrowth of a dominant tumor clone derived from (crippled) germinal center B cells. J Exp Med 184: 1495-1505.
1106. Kapelushnik J, Ariad S, Benharroch D, Landau D, Moser A, Delsol G, Brousset P (2001). Post renal transplantation human herpesvirus 8-associated lymphoproliferative disorder and Kaposi's sarcoma. Br J Haematol 113: 425-428.
1107. Kaplan MA, Ferry JA, Harris NL, Jacobson JO (1994). Clonal analysis of posttransplant lymphoproliferative disorders, using both episomal Epstein-Barr virus and immunoglobulin genes as markers. Am J Clin Pathol 101: 590-596.
1108. Kapp U, Yeh WC, Patterson B, Elia AJ, Kagi D, Ho A, Hessel A, Tipsword M, Williams A, Mirtsos C, Itie A, Moyle M, Mak TW (1999). Interleukin 13 is secreted by and stimulates the growth of Hodgkin and Reed-Sternberg cells. J Exp Med 189: 1939-1946.
1109. Kardos G, Baumann I, Passmore SJ, Locatelli F, Hasle H, Schultz KR, Stary J, Schmitt-Graeff A, Fischer A, Harbott J, Chessells JM, Hann I, Fenu S, Rajnoldi AC, Kerndrup G, van Wering E, Rogge T, Nollke P, Niemeyer CM (2003). Refractory anemia in childhood: a retrospective analysis of 67 patients with particular reference to monosomy 7. Blood 102: 1997-2003.
1110. Kari L, Loboda A, Nebozhyn M, Rook AH, Vonderheid EC, Nichols C, Virok D, Chang C, Horng WH, Johnston J, Wysocka M, Showe MK, Showe LC (2003). Classification and prediction of survival in patients with the leukemic phase of cutaneous T cell lymphoma. J Exp Med 197: 1477-1488.
1111. Karube K, Guo Y, Suzumiya J, Sugita Y, Nomura Y, Yamamoto K, Shimizu K, Yoshida S, Komatani H, Takeshita M, Kikuchi M, Nakamura N, Takasu O, Arakawa F, Tagawa H, Seto M, Ohshima K (2007). CD10-MUM1+ follicular lymphoma lacks BCL2 gene translocation and shows characteristic biologic and clinical features. Blood 109: 3076-3079.
1112. Karube K, Ohshima K, Tsuchiya T, Yamaguchi T, Kawano R, Suzumiya J, Utsunomiya A, Harada M, Kikuchi M (2004). Expression of FoxP3, a key molecule in CD4CD25 regulatory T cells, in adult T-cell leukaemia/lymphoma cells. Br J Haematol 126: 81-84.
1113. Kasahara Y, Yachie A, Takei K, Kanegane C, Okada K, Ohta K, Seki H, Igarashi N, Maruhashi K, Katayama K, Katoh E, Terao G, Sakiyama Y, Koizumi S (2001). Differential cellular targets of Epstein-Barr virus (EBV) infection between acute EBV-associated hemophagocytic lymphohistiocytosis and chronic active EBV infection. Blood 98: 1882-1888.
1114. Kassan SS, Thomas TL, Moutsopoulos HM, Hoover R, Kimberly RP, Budman DR, Costa J, Decker JL, Chused TM (1978). Increased risk of lymphoma in sicca syndrome. Ann Intern Med 89: 888-892.
1115. Katakai T, Hara T, Lee JH, Gonda H, Sugai M, Shimizu A (2004). A novel reticular stromal structure in lymph node cortex: an immuno-platform for interactions among dendritic cells, T cells and B cells. Int Immunol 16: 1133-1142.
1116. Kato I, Tajima K, Suchi T, Aozasa K, Matsuzuka F, Kuma K, Tominaga S (1985). Chronic thyroiditis as a risk factor of B-cell lymphoma in the thyroid gland. Jpn J Cancer Res 76: 1085-1090.
1117. Kato K, Ohshima K, Ishihara S, Anzai K, Suzumiya J, Kikuchi M (1998). Elevated serum soluble Fas ligand in natural killer cell proliferative disorders. Br J Haematol 103: 1164-1166.
1118. Katzenberger T, Lohr A, Schwarz S, Dreyling M, Schoof J, Nickenig C, Stilgenbauer S, Kalla J, Ott MM, Muller-Hermelink HK, Ott G (2003). Genetic analysis of de novo CD5+ diffuse large B-cell lymphomas suggests an origin from a somatically mutated CD5+ progenitor B cell. Blood 101: 699-702.
1119. Katzenberger T, Ott G, Klein T, Kalla J, Muller-Hermelink HK, Ott MM (2004). Cytogenetic alterations affecting BCL6 are predominantly found in follicular lymphomas grade 3B with a diffuse large B-cell component. Am J Pathol 165: 481-490.
1120. Katzenberger T, Petzoldt C, Holler S, Mader U, Kalla J, Adam P, Ott MM, Muller-Hermelink HK, Rosenwald A, Ott G (2006). The Ki67 proliferation index is a quantitative indicator of clinical risk in mantle cell lymphoma. Blood 107: 3407.
1121. Katzenstein AL, Carrington CB, Liebow AA (1979). Lymphomatoid granulomatosis: a clinicopathologic study of 152 cases. Cancer 43: 360-373.
1122. Katzenstein AL, Peiper SC (1990). Detection of Epstein-Barr virus genomes in lymphomatoid granulomatosis: analysis of 29 cases by the polymerase chain reaction technique. Mod Pathol 3: 435-441.
1123. Katzmann JA, Abraham RS, Dispenzieri A, Lust JA, Kyle RA (2005). Diagnostic performance of quantitative kappa and lambda free light chain assays in clinical practice. Clin Chem 51: 878-881.
1124. Katzmann JA, Clark RJ, Rajkumar VS, Kyle RS (2003). Monoclonal free light chains in sera from healthy individuals: FLC MGUS. Clin Chem 49: pA24.
1125. Kaufmann H, Ackermann J, Baldia C, Nosslinger T, Wieser R, Seidl S, Sagaster V, Gisslinger H, Jager U, Pfeilstocker M, Zielinski C, Drach J (2004). Both IGH translocations and chromosome 13q deletions are early events in monoclonal gammopathy of undetermined significance and do not evolve during transition to multiple myeloma. Leukemia 18: 1879-1882.
1126. Kawa-Ha K, Ishihara S, Ninomiya T, Yumura-Yagi K, Hara J, Murayama F, Tawa A, Hirai K (1989). CD3-negative lymphoproliferative disease of granular lymphocytes containing Epstein-Barr viral DNA. J Clin Invest 84: 51-55.
1127. Kawamoto H (2006). A close developmental relationship between the lymphoid and myeloid lineages. Trends Immunol 27: 169-175.
1128. Kawano S, Tatsumi E, Yoneda N, Yamaguchi N, Goji J, Ito H, Nagai T, Nishikori M, Okamura A, Koiwai O (1995). Novel leukemic lymphoma with probable derivation from immature stage of natural killer (NK) lineage in an aged patient. Hematol Oncol 13: 1-11.
1129. Kay NE, O'Brien SM, Pettitt AR, Stilgenbauer S (2007). The role of prognostic factors in assessing 'high-risk' subgroups of patients with chronic lymphocytic leukemia. Leukemia 21: 1885-1891.
1130. Keating MJ, Cazin B, Coutre S, Birhiray R, Kovacsovics T, Langer W, Leber B, Maughan T, Rai K, Tjonnfjord G, Bekradda M, Itzhaki M, Herait P (2002). Campath-1H treatment of T-cell prolymphocytic leukemia in patients for whom at least one prior chemotherapy regimen has failed. J Clin Oncol 20: 205-213.
1131. Keats JJ, Fonseca R, Chesi M, Schop R, Baker A, Chng WJ, Van Wier S, Tiedemann R, Shi CX, Sebag M, Braggio E, Henry T, Zhu YX, Fogle H, Price-Troska T, Ahmann G, Mancini C, Brents LA, Kumar S, Greipp P, Dispenzieri A, Bryant B, Mulligan G, Bruhn L, Barrett M, Valdez R, Trent J, Stewart AK, Carpten J, Bergsagel PL (2007). Promiscuous mutations activate the noncanonical NF-kappaB pathway in multiple myeloma. Cancer Cell 12: 131-144.
1132. Keats JJ, Reiman T, Maxwell CA, Taylor BJ, Larratt LM, Mant MJ, Belch AR, Pilarski LM (2003). In multiple myeloma, t(4;14)(p16;q32) is an adverse prognostic factor irrespective of FGFR3 expression. Blood 101: 1520-1529.
1133. Keegan TH, Glaser SL, Clarke CA, Gulley ML, Craig FE, DiGiuseppe JA, Dorfman RF, Mann RB, Ambinder RF (2005). Epstein-Barr virus as a marker of survival after Hodgkin's lymphoma: a population-based study. J Clin Oncol 23: 7604-7613.
1134. Keene P, Mendelow B, Pinto MR, Bezwoda W, MacDougall L, Falkson G, Ruff P, Bernstein R (1987). Abnormalities of chromosome 12p13 and malignant proliferation of eosinophils: a nonrandom association. Br J Haematol 67: 25-31.
1135. Kelly A, Richards SJ, Sivakumaran M, Shiach C, Stewart AD, Roberts BE, Scott CS (1994). Clonality of CD3 negative large granular lymphocyte proliferations determined by PCR based X-inactivation studies. J Clin Pathol 47: 399-404.
1135A. Kelly LM, Gilliland DG (2002). Genetics of myeloid leukemias. Annu Rev Genomics Hum Genet 3: 179-198.
1136. Kennedy GA, Kay TD, Johnson DW, Hawley CM, Campbell SB, Isbel NM, Marlton P, Cobcroft R, Gill D, Cull G (2002). Neutrophil dysplasia characterised by a pseudo-Pelger-Huet anomaly occurring with the use of mycophenolate mofetil and ganciclovir following renal transplantation: a report of five cases.

Pathology 34: 263-266.
1137. Kern WF, Spier CM, Hanneman EH, Miller TP, Matzner M, Grogan TM (1992). Neural cell adhesion molecule-positive peripheral T-cell lymphoma: a rare variant with a propensity for unusual sites of involvement. Blood 79: 2432-2437.
1138. Khalidi HS, Brynes RK, Medeiros LJ, Chang KL, Slovak ML, Snyder DS, Arber DA (1998). The immunophenotype of blast transformation of chronic myelogenous leukemia: a high frequency of mixed lineage phenotype in "lymphoid" blasts and A comparison of morphologic, immunophenotypic, and molecular findings. Mod Pathol 11: 1211-1221.
1139. Khalidi HS, Chang KL, Medeiros LJ, Brynes RK, Slovak ML, Murata-Collins JL, Arber DA (1999). Acute lymphoblastic leukemia. Survey of immunophenotype, French-American-British classification, frequency of myeloid antigen expression, and karyotypic abnormalities in 210 pediatric and adult cases. Am J Clin Pathol 111: 467-476.
1140. Khoury H, Dalal BI, Nevill TJ, Horsman DE, Barnett MJ, Shepherd JD, Toze CL, Conneally EA, Sutherland HJ, Hogge DE, Nantel SH (2003). Acute myelogenous leukemia with t(8;21)—identification of a specific immunophenotype. Leuk Lymphoma 44: 1713-1718.
1141. Khoury JD, Jones D, Yared MA, Manning JT, Jr., Abruzzo LV, Hagemeister FB, Medeiros LJ (2004). Bone marrow involvement in patients with nodular lymphocyte predominant Hodgkin lymphoma. Am J Surg Pathol 28: 489-495.
1142. Khoury JD, Medeiros LJ, Manning JT, Sulak LE, Bueso-Ramos C, Jones D (2002). CD56(+) TdT(+) blastic natural killer cell tumor of the skin: a primitive systemic malignancy related to myelomonocytic leukemia. Cancer 94: 2401-2408.
1143. Kienle D, Krober A, Katzenberger T, Ott G, Leupolt E, Barth TF, Moller P, Benner A, Habermann A, Muller-Hermelink HK, Bentz M, Lichter P, Dohner H, Stilgenbauer S (2003). VH mutation status and VDJ rearrangement structure in mantle cell lymphoma: correlation with genomic aberrations, clinical characteristics, and outcome. Blood 102: 3003-3009.
1144. Kikuta H, Sakiyama Y, Matsumoto S, Oh-ishi T, Nakano T, Nagashima T, Oka T, Hironaka T, Hirai K (1993). Fatal Epstein-Barr virus-associated hemophagocytic syndrome. Blood 82: 3259-3264.
1145. Killick S, Matutes E, Powles RL, Hamblin M, Swansbury J, Treleaven JG, Zomas A, Atra A, Catovsky D (1999). Outcome of biphenotypic acute leukemia. Haematologica 84: 699-706.
1146. Kim BK, Surti U, Pandya A, Cohen J, Rabkin MS, Swerdlow SH (2005). Clinicopathologic, immunophenotypic, and molecular cytogenetic fluorescence in situ hybridization analysis of primary and secondary cutaneous follicular lymphomas. Am J Surg Pathol 29: 69-82.
1147. Kim Y, Weiss LM, Chen YY, Pullarkat V (2007). Distinct clonal origins of systemic mastocytosis and associated B-cell lymphoma. Leuk Res 31: 1749-1754.
1148. Kim YM, Ramirez JA, Mick JE, Giebler HA, Yan JP, Nyborg JK (2007). Molecular characterization of the Tax-containing HTLV-1 enhancer complex reveals a prominent role for CREB phosphorylation in Tax transactivation. J Biol Chem 282: 18750-18757.
1149. Kimura H, Hoshino Y, Kanegane H, Tsuge I, Okamura T, Kawa K, Morishima T (2001). Clinical and virologic characteristics of chronic active Epstein-Barr virus infection. Blood 98: 280-286.
1150. Kimura H, Morishima T, Kanegane H, Ohga S, Hoshino Y, Maeda A, Imai S, Okano M, Morio T, Yokota S, Tsuchiya S, Yachie A, Imashuku S, Kawa K, Wakiguchi H (2003). Prognostic factors for chronic active Epstein-Barr virus infection. J Infect Dis 187: 527-533.
1151. Kingma DW, Mueller BU, Frekko K, Sorbara LR, Wood LV, Katz D, Raffeld M, Jaffe ES (1999). Low-grade monoclonal Epstein-Barr virus-associated lymphoproliferative disorder of the brain presenting as human immunodeficiency virus-associated encephalopathy in a child with acquired immunodeficiency syndrome. Arch Pathol Lab Med 123: 83-87.
1152. Kinney MC, Collins RD, Greer JP, Whitlock JA, Sioutos N, Kadin ME (1993). A small-cell-predominant variant of primary Ki-1 (CD30)+ T-cell lymphoma. Am J Surg Pathol 17: 859-868.
1152A. Kipps TJ (1989). The CD5 B-cell. Adv Immunol 47: 117-185.
1153. Kipps TJ (2003). Immunobiology of chronic lymphocytic leukemia. Curr Opin Hematol 10: 312-318.
1154. Kiszewski AE, Alvarez-Mendoza A, Rios-Barrera VA, Hernandez-Pando R, Ruiz-Maldonado R (2007). Mastocytosis in children: clinicopathological study based on 35 cases. Histol Histopathol 22: 535-539.
1155. Kita K, Nakase K, Miwa H, Masuya M, Nishii K, Morita N, Takakura N, Otsuji A, Shirakawa S, Ueda T, *et al.* (1992). Phenotypical characteristics of acute myelocytic leukemia associated with the t(8;21)(q22;q22) chromosomal abnormality: frequent expression of immature B-cell antigen CD19 together with stem cell antigen CD34. Blood 80: 470-477.
1156. Kitano K, Ichikawa N, Mahbub B, Ueno M, Ito T, Shimodaira S, Kodaira H, Ishida F, Kobayashi H, Saito H, Okubo Y, Enokihara H, Kiyosawa K (1996). Eosinophilia associated with proliferation of CD(3+)4-(8-) alpha beta+ T cells with chromosome 16 anomalies. Br J Haematol 92: 315-317.
1157. Kjaeraas S, Husby G, Sletten K (2006). The amino acid sequence of an AL-protein, AL-KH, isolated from the heart of a patient with Waldenstroms macroglobulinemia and amyloidosis. Amyloid 13: 260-262.
1158. Klangby U, Okan I, Magnusson KP, Wendland M, Lind P, Wiman KG (1998). p16/INK4a and p15/INK4b gene methylation and absence of p16/INK4a mRNA and protein expression in Burkitt's lymphoma. Blood 91: 1680-1687.
1159. Klein U, Gloghini A, Gaidano G, Chadburn A, Cesarman E, Dalla-Favera R, Carbone A (2003). Gene expression profile analysis of AIDS-related primary effusion lymphoma (PEL) suggests a plasmablastic derivation and identifies PEL-specific transcripts. Blood 101: 4115-4121.
1160. Klein U, Tu Y, Stolovitzky GA, Mattioli M, Cattoretti G, Husson H, Freedman A, Inghirami G, Cro L, Baldini L, Neri A, Califano A, Dalla-Favera R (2001). Gene expression profiling of B cell chronic lymphocytic leukemia reveals a homogeneous phenotype related to memory B cells. J Exp Med 194: 1625-1638.
1161. Klemke CD, Mansmann U, Poenitz N, Dippel E, Goerdt S (2005). Prognostic factors and prediction of prognosis by the CTCL Severity Index in mycosis fungoides and Sezary syndrome. Br J Dermatol 153: 118-124.
1162. Klion AD, Noel P, Akin C, Law MA, Gilliland DG, Cools J, Metcalfe DD, Nutman TB (2003). Elevated serum tryptase levels identify a subset of patients with a myeloproliferative variant of idiopathic hypereosinophilic syndrome associated with tissue fibrosis, poor prognosis, and imatinib responsiveness. Blood 101: 4660-4666.
1163. Klion AD, Robyn J, Akin C, Noel P, Brown M, Law M, Metcalfe DD, Dunbar C, Nutman TB (2004). Molecular remission and reversal of myelofibrosis in response to imatinib mesylate treatment in patients with the myeloproliferative variant of hypereosinophilic syndrome. Blood 103: 473-478.
1164. Kluin-Nelemans HC, Buck G, le Cessie S, Richards S, Beverloo HB, Falkenburg JH, Littlewood T, Muus P, Bareford D, van der LH, Green AR, Roozendaal KJ, Milne AE, Chapman CS, Shepherd P (2004). Randomized comparison of low-dose versus high-dose interferon-alfa in chronic myeloid leukemia: prospective collaboration of 3 joint trials by the MRC and HOVON groups. Blood 103: 4408-4415.
1165. Knipp S, Strupp C, Gattermann N, Hildebrandt B, Schapira M, Giagounidis A, Aul C, Haas R, Germing U (2008). Presence of peripheral blasts in refractory anemia and refractory cytopenia with multilineage dysplasia predicts an unfavourable outcome. Leuk Res 32: 33-37.
1166. Knowles DM, Cesarman E, Chadburn A, Frizzera G, Chen J, Rose EA, Michler RE (1995). Correlative morphologic and molecular genetic analysis demonstrates three distinct categories of posttransplantation lymphoproliferative disorders. Blood 85: 552-565.
1167. Knowles DM, Inghirami G, Ubriaco A, Dalla-Favera R (1989). Molecular genetic analysis of three AIDS-associated neoplasms of uncertain lineage demonstrates their B-cell derivation and the possible pathogenetic role of the Epstein-Barr virus. Blood 73: 792-799.
1168. Knuutila S, Alitalo R, Ruutu T (1993). Power of the MAC (morphology-antibody-chromosomes) method in distinguishing reactive and clonal cells: report of a patient with acute lymphatic leukemia, eosinophilia, and t(5;14). Genes Chromosomes Cancer 8: 219-223.
1169. Ko YH, Ree HJ, Kim WS, Choi WH, Moon WS, Kim SW (2000). Clinicopathologic and genotypic study of extranodal nasal-type natural killer/T-cell lymphoma and natural killer precursor lymphoma among Koreans. Cancer 89: 2106-2116.
1170. Kodama K, Massone C, Chott A, Metze D, Kerl H, Cerroni L (2005). Primary cutaneous large B-cell lymphomas: clinicopathologic features, classification, and prognostic factors in a large series of patients. Blood 106: 2491-2497.
1171. Koduru PR, Raju K, Vadmal V, Menezes G, Shah S, Susin M, Kolitz J, Broome JD (1997). Correlation between mutation in P53, p53 expression, cytogenetics, histologic type, and survival in patients with B-cell non-Hodgkin's lymphoma. Blood 90: 4078-4091.
1172. Koeffler HP, Levine AM, Sparkes M, Sparkes RS (1980). Chronic myelocytic leukemia: eosinophils involved in the malignant clone. Blood 55: 1063-1065.
1173. Koeppen H, Newell K, Baunoch DA, Vardiman JW (1998). Morphologic bone marrow changes in patients with posttransplantation lymphoproliferative disorders. Am J Surg Pathol 22: 208-214.
1174. Koita H, Suzumiya J, Ohshima K, Takeshita M, Kimura N, Kikuchi M, Koono M (1997). Lymphoblastic lymphoma expressing natural killer cell phenotype with involvement of the mediastinum and nasal cavity. Am J Surg Pathol 21: 242-248.
1175. Koizumi K, Sawada K, Nishio M, Katagiri E, Fukae J, Fukada Y, Tarumi T, Notoya A, Shimizu T, Abe R, Kobayashi H, Koike T (1997). Effective high-dose chemotherapy followed by autologous peripheral blood stem cell transplantation in a patient with the aggressive form of cytophagic histiocytic panniculitis. Bone Marrow Transplant 20: 171-173.
1176. Kojima M, Nakamura S, Itoh H, Ohno Y, Masawa N, Joshita T, Suchi T (1999). Mast cell sarcoma with tissue eosinophilia arising in the ascending colon. Mod Pathol 12: 739-743.
1177. Kolde G, Brocker EB (1986). Multiple skin tumors of indeterminate cells in an adult. J Am Acad Dermatol 15: 591-597.
1178. Koldehoff M, Beelen DW, Trenschel R, Steckel NK, Peceny R, Ditschkowski M, Ottinger H, Elmaagacli AH (2004). Outcome of hematopoietic stem cell transplantation in patients with atypical chronic myeloid leukemia. Bone Marrow Transplant 34: 1047-1050.
1179. Komatsu H, Yoshida K, Seto M, Iida S, Aikawa T, Ueda R, Mikuni C (1993). Overexpression of PRAD1 in a mantle zone lymphoma patient with a t(11;22)(q13;q11) translocation. Br J Haematol 85: 427-429.
1179A. Kondo T, Kono H, Miyamoto N, Yoshida R, Toki H, Matsumoto I, Hara M, Inoue H, Inatsuki A, Funatsu T, et al (1989). Age- and sex-specific cumulative rate and risk of ATLL for HTLV-I carriers. Int J Cancer 43: 1061-1064.
1180. Konigsberg R, Ackermann J, Kaufmann H, Zojer N, Urbauer E, Kromer E, Jager U, Gisslinger H, Schreiber S, Heinz R, Ludwig H, Huber H, Drach J (2000). Deletions of chromosome 13q in monoclonal gammopathy of undetermined significance. Leukemia 14: 1975-1979.
1181. Konigsberg R, Zojer N, Ackermann J, Kromer E, Kittler H, Fritz E, Kaufmann H, Nosslinger T, Riedl L, Gisslinger H, Jager U, Simonitsch I, Heinz R, Ludwig H, Huber H, Drach J (2000). Predictive role of interphase cytogenetics for survival of patients with multiple myeloma. J Clin Oncol 18: 804-812.
1182. Koss MN, Hochholzer L, Langloss JM, Wehunt WD, Lazarus AA, Nichols PW (1986). Lymphomatoid granulomatosis: a clinicopathologic study of 42 patients. Pathology 18: 283-288.
1183. Koster A, Tromp HA, Raemaekers JM, Borm GF, Hebeda K, Mackenzie MA, Van Krieken JH (2007). The prognostic significance of the intra-follicular tumor cell proliferative rate in follicular lymphoma. Haematologica 92: 184-190.
1184. Kottaridis PD, Gale RE, Linch DC (2003). FLT3 mutations and leukaemia. Br J Haematol 122: 523-538.
1185. Kouides PA, Bennett JM (1996). Morphology and classification of the myelodysplastic syndromes and their pathologic variants. Semin Hematol 33: 95-110.
1186. Kralovics R, Passamonti F, Buser AS, Teo SS, Tiedt R, Passweg JR, Tichelli A, Cazzola M, Skoda RC (2005). A gain-of-function mutation of JAK2 in myeloproliferative disorders. N Engl J Med 352: 1779-1790.
1187. Kramer MH, Hermans J, Parker J, Krol AD, Kluin-Nelemans JC, Haak HL, van Groningen K, Van Krieken JH, De Jong D, Kluin PM (1996). Clinical significance of bcl2 and p53 protein expression in diffuse large B-cell lymphoma: a population-based study. J Clin Oncol 14: 2131-2138.
1188. Kramer MH, Hermans J, Wijburg E, Philippo K, Geelen E, Van Krieken JH, De Jong D, Maartense E, Schuuring E, Kluin PM (1998). Clinical relevance of BCL2, BCL6, and MYC rearrangements in diffuse large B-cell lymphoma. Blood 92: 3152-3162.
1188A. Kraus MD, Haley JC, Ruiz R, Essary L, Moran CA, Fletcher CD (2001). "Juvenile" xanthogranuloma: an immunophenotypic study with a reappraisal of histogenesis. Am J Dermatopathol 23: 104-111.
1189. Kreft A, Buche G, Ghalibafian M, Buhr T, Fischer T, Kirkpatrick CJ (2005). The incidence of myelofibrosis in essential thrombocythaemia, polycythaemia vera and chronic idiopathic myelofibrosis: a retrospective evaluation of sequential bone marrow biopsies. Acta

Haematol 113: 137-143.
1190. Kremer M, Spitzer M, Mandl-Weber S, Stecker K, Schmidt B, Hofler H, Quintanilla-Martinez L, Fend F (2003). Discordant bone marrow involvement in diffuse large B-cell lymphoma: comparative molecular analysis reveals a heterogeneous group of disorders. Lab Invest 83: 107-114.
1191. Krenacs L, Smyth MJ, Bagdi E, Krenacs T, Kopper L, Rudiger T, Zettl A, Muller-Hermelink HK, Jaffe ES, Raffeld M (2003). The serine protease granzyme M is preferentially expressed in NK-cell, gamma delta T-cell, and intestinal T-cell lymphomas: evidence of origin from lymphocytes involved in innate immunity. Blood 101: 3590-3593.
1191A. Krenacs L, Tiszalvicz L, Krenacs T, Boumsell L (1993). Immunohistochemical detection of CD1A antigen in formalin-fixed and paraffin embedded tissue sections with monoclonal antibody 010. J Pathol 171: 99-104.
1192. Krenacs L, Wellmann A, Sorbara L, Himmelmann AW, Bagdi E, Jaffe ES, Raffeld M (1997). Cytotoxic cell antigen expression in anaplastic large cell lymphomas of T- and null-cell type and Hodgkin's disease: evidence for distinct cellular origin. Blood 89: 980-989.
1193. Kriangkum J, Taylor BJ, Treon SP, Mant MJ, Belch AR, Pilarski LM (2004). Clonotypic IgM V/D/J sequence analysis in Waldenstrom macroglobulinemia suggests an unusual B-cell origin and an expansion of polyclonal B cells in peripheral blood. Blood 104: 2134-2142.
1194. Krishnan B, Matutes E, Dearden C (2006). Prolymphocytic leukemias. Semin Oncol 33: 257-263.
1195. Krishnan J, Wallberg K, Frizzera G (1994). T-cell-rich large B-cell lymphoma. A study of 30 cases, supporting its histologic heterogeneity and lack of clinical distinctiveness. Am J Surg Pathol 18: 455-465.
1196. Krober A, Bloehdorn J, Hafner S, Buhler A, Seiler T, Kienle D, Winkler D, Bangerter M, Schlenk RF, Benner A, Lichter P, Dohner H, Stilgenbauer S (2006). Additional genetic high-risk features such as 11q deletion, 17p deletion, and V3-21 usage characterize discordance of ZAP-70 and VH mutation status in chronic lymphocytic leukemia. J Clin Oncol 24: 969-975.
1197. Krober A, Seiler T, Benner A, Bullinger L, Bruckle E, Lichter P, Dohner H, Stilgenbauer S (2002). V(H) mutation status, CD38 expression level, genomic aberrations, and survival in chronic lymphocytic leukemia. Blood 100: 1410-1416.
1197A Kroft S, Domiati-Saad R, Finn W, et al. Precursor B-lymphblastic transformation of grade 1 follicle center lymphoma. Am J Clin Pathol 2000; 113:411-418.
1198. Krokowski M, Sotlar K, Krauth MT, Fodinger M, Valent P, Horny HP (2005). Delineation of patterns of bone marrow mast cell infiltration in systemic mastocytosis: value of CD25, correlation with subvariants of the disease, and separation from mast cell hyperplasia. Am J Clin Pathol 124: 560-568.
1199. Kuchenbauer F, Schoch C, Kern W, Hiddemann W, Haferlach T, Schnittger S (2005). Impact of FLT3 mutations and promyelocytic leukaemia-breakpoint on clinical characteristics and prognosis in acute promyelocytic leukaemia. Br J Haematol 130: 196-202.
1200. Kueck BD, Smith RE, Parkin J, Peterson LC, Hanson CA (1991). Eosinophilic leukemia: a myeloproliferative disorder distinct from the hypereosinophilic syndrome. Hematol Pathol 5: 195-205.
1201. Kuehl WM, Bergsagel PL (2002). Multiple myeloma: evolving genetic events and host interactions. Nat Rev Cancer 2: 175-187.
1202. Kumar S, Krenacs L, Medeiros J, Elenitoba-Johnson KS, Greiner TC, Sorbara L, Kingma DW, Raffeld M, Jaffe ES (1998). Subcutaneous panniculitic T-cell lymphoma is a tumor of cytotoxic T lymphocytes. Hum Pathol 29: 397-403.
1203. Kumar S, Krenacs L, Otsuki T, Kumar D, Harris CA, Wellmann A, Jaffe ES, Raffeld M (1996). bcl-1 rearrangement and cyclin D1 protein expression in multiple lymphomatous polyposis. Am J Clin Pathol 105: 737-743.
1204. Kummer JA, Vermeer MH, Dukers D, Meijer CJ, Willemze R (1997). Most primary cutaneous CD30-positive lymphoproliferative disorders have a CD4-positive cytotoxic T-cell phenotype. J Invest Dermatol 109: 636-640.
1205. Kuo TT, Shih LY, Tsang NM (2004). Nasal NK/T cell lymphoma in Taiwan: a clinicopathologic study of 22 cases, with analysis of histologic subtypes, Epstein-Barr virus LMP-1 gene association, and treatment modalities. Int J Surg Pathol 12: 375-387.
1205A. Küppers R, Klein U, Schwering I, Distler V, Bräuninger A, Cattoretti G, Tu Y, Stolovitzky GA, Califano A, Hansmann ML, Dalla-Favera R (2003). Identification of Hodgkin and Reed-Sternberg cell-specific genes by gene expression profiling. J Clin Invest 111: 529-537.
1206. Kurata M, Hasegawa M, Nakagawa Y, Abe S, Yamamoto K, Suzuki K, Kitagawa M (2006). Expression dynamics of drug resistance genes, multidrug resistance 1 (MDR1) and lung resistance protein (LRP) during the evolution of overt leukemia in myelodysplastic syndromes. Exp Mol Pathol 81: 249-254.
1207. Kurtin PJ, Dewald GW, Shields DJ, Hanson CA (1996). Hematologic disorders associated with deletions of chromosome 20q: a clinicopathologic study of 107 patients. Am J Clin Pathol 106: 680-688.
1208. Kurzrock R, Bueso-Ramos CE, Kantarjian H, Freireich E, Tucker SL, Siciliano M, Pilat S, Talpaz M (2001). BCR rearrangement-negative chronic myelogenous leukemia revisited. J Clin Oncol 19: 2915-2926.
1209. Kushner JP, Lee GR, Wintrobe MM, Cartwright GE (1971). Idiopathic refractory sideroblastic anemia: clinical and laboratory investigation of 17 patients and review of the literature. Medicine (Baltimore) 50: 139-159.
1210. Kussick SJ, Fromm JR, Rossini A, Li Y, Chang A, Norwood TH, Wood BL (2005). Four-color flow cytometry shows strong concordance with bone marrow morphology and cytogenetics in the evaluation for myelodysplasia. Am J Clin Pathol 124: 170-181.
1211. Kussick SJ, Kalnoski M, Braziel RM, Wood BL (2004). Prominent clonal B-cell populations identified by flow cytometry in histologically reactive lymphoid proliferations. Am J Clin Pathol 121: 464-472.
1212. Kussick SJ, Wood BL (2003). Four-color flow cytometry identifies virtually all cytogenetically abnormal bone marrow samples in the workup of non-CML myeloproliferative disorders. Am J Clin Pathol 120: 854-865.
1213. Kuze T, Nakamura N, Hashimoto Y, Sasaki Y, Abe M (2000). The characteristics of Epstein-Barr virus (EBV)-positive diffuse large B-cell lymphoma: comparison between EBV(+) and EBV(-) cases in Japanese population. Jpn J Cancer Res 91: 1233-1240.
1214. Kvasnicka HM, Thiele J (2004). Bone marrow angiogenesis: methods of quantification and changes evolving in chronic myeloproliferative disorders. Histol Histopathol 19: 1245-1260.
1215. Kvasnicka HM, Thiele J (2006). The impact of clinicopathological studies on staging and survival in essential thrombocythemia, chronic idiopathic myelofibrosis, and polycythemia rubra vera. Semin Thromb Hemost 32: 362-371.
1216. Kvasnicka HM, Thiele J (2007). Classification of ph-negative chronic myeloproliferative disorders - morphology as the yardstick of classification. Pathobiology 74: 63-71.
1217. Kvasnicka HM, Thiele J, Schmitt-Graeff A, Diehl V, Zankovich R, Niederle N, Leder LD, Schaefer HE (2001). Bone marrow features improve prognostic efficiency in multivariate risk classification of chronic-phase Ph(1+) chronic myelogenous leukemia: a multicenter trial. J Clin Oncol 19: 2994-3009.
1218. Kvasnicka HM, Thiele J, Schmitt-Graeff A, Diehl V, Zankovich R, Niederle N, Leder LD, Schaefer HE (2001). Prognostic impact of bone marrow erythropoietic precursor cells and myelofibrosis at diagnosis of Ph1+ chronic myelogenous leukaemia—a multicentre study on 495 patients. Br J Haematol 112: 727-739.
1219. Kvasnicka HM, Thiele J, Werden C, Zankovich R, Diehl V, Fischer R (1997). Prognostic factors in idiopathic (primary) osteomyelofibrosis. Cancer 80: 708-719.
1220. Kwong YL, Chan AC, Liang R, Chiang AK, Chim CS, Chan TK, Todd D, Ho FC (1997). CD56+ NK lymphomas: clinicopathological features and prognosis. Br J Haematol 97: 821-829.
1221. Kwong YL, Chan AC, Liang RH (1997). Natural killer cell lymphoma/leukemia: pathology and treatment. Hematol Oncol 15: 71-79.
1222. Kwong YL, Lam CC, Chan TM (2000). Post-transplantation lymphoproliferative disease of natural killer cell lineage: a clinicopathological and molecular analysis. Br J Haematol 110: 197-202.
1223. Kwong YL, Wong KF, Chan LC, Liang RH, Chan JK, Lin CK, Chan TK (1995). Large granular lymphocyte leukemia. A study of nine cases in a Chinese population. Am J Clin Pathol 103: 76-81.
1224. Kyle RA (1975). Multiple myeloma: review of 869 cases. Mayo Clin Proc 50: 29-40.
1225. Kyle RA, Gertz MA (1995). Primary systemic amyloidosis: clinical and laboratory features in 474 cases. Semin Hematol 32: 45-59.
1226. Kyle RA, Gertz MA, Witzig TE, Lust JA, Lacy MQ, Dispenzieri A, Fonseca R, Rajkumar SV, Offord JR, Larson DR, Plevak ME, Therneau TM, Greipp PR (2003). Review of 1027 patients with newly diagnosed multiple myeloma. Mayo Clin Proc 78: 21-33.
1227. Kyle RA, Greipp PR (1980). Smoldering multiple myeloma. N Engl J Med 302: 1347-1349.
1228. Kyle RA, Greipp PR, O'Fallon WM (1986). Primary systemic amyloidosis: multivariate analysis for prognostic factors in 168 cases. Blood 68: 220-224.
1229. Kyle RA, Rajkumar SV (2006). Monoclonal gammopathy of undetermined significance. Br J Haematol 134: 573-589.
1230. Kyle RA, Rajkumar SV, Therneau TM, Larson DR, Plevak MF, Melton LJ, III (2005). Prognostic factors and predictors of outcome of immunoglobulin M monoclonal gammopathy of undetermined significance. Clin Lymphoma 5: 257-260.
1231. Kyle RA, Remstein ED, Therneau TM, Dispenzieri A, Kurtin PJ, Hodnefield JM, Larson DR, Plevak MF, Jelinek DF, Fonseca R, Melton LJ, III, Rajkumar SV (2007). Clinical course and prognosis of smoldering (asymptomatic) multiple myeloma. N Engl J Med 356: 2582-2590.
1232. Kyle RA, Therneau TM, Rajkumar SV, Larson DR, Plevak MF, Offord JR, Dispenzieri A, Katzmann JA, Melton LJ, III (2006). Prevalence of monoclonal gammopathy of undetermined significance. N Engl J Med 354: 1362-1369.
1233. Kyle RA, Therneau TM, Rajkumar SV, Offord JR, Larson DR, Plevak MF, Melton LJ, III (2002). A long-term study of prognosis in monoclonal gammopathy of undetermined significance. N Engl J Med 346: 564-569.
1234. Kyle RA, Therneau TM, Rajkumar SV, Remstein ED, Offord JR, Larson DR, Plevak MF, Melton LJ, III (2003). Long-term follow-up of IgM monoclonal gammopathy of undetermined significance. Blood 102: 3759-3764.
1234A. Lachenal F, Berger F, Ghesquières H, Biron P, Hot A, Callet-Bauchu E, Chassagne C, Coiffier B, Durieu I, Rousset H, Salles G (2007). Angioimmunoblastic T-cell lymphoma: clinical and laboratory features at diagnosis in 77 patients. Medicine (Baltimore) 86: 282-292.
1235. Lae ME, Ahmed I, Macon WR (2002). Clusterin is widely expressed in systemic anaplastic large cell lymphoma but fails to differentiate primary from secondary cutaneous anaplastic large cell lymphoma. Am J Clin Pathol 118: 773-779.
1236. Lahortiga I, Vazquez I, Agirre X, Larrayoz MJ, Vizmanos JL, Gozzetti A, Calasanz MJ, Odero MD (2004). Molecular heterogeneity in AML/MDS patients with 3q21q26 rearrangements. Genes Chromosomes Cancer 40: 179-189.
1237. Lai JL, Preudhomme C, Zandecki M, Flactif M, Vanrumbeke M, Lepelley P, Wattel E, Fenaux P (1995). Myelodysplastic syndromes and acute myeloid leukemia with 17p deletion. An entity characterized by specific dysgranulopoiesis and a high incidence of P53 mutations. Leukemia 9: 370-381.
1238. Lai R, Arber DA, Chang KL, Wilson CS, Weiss LM (1998). Frequency of bcl-2 expression in non-Hodgkin's lymphoma: a study of 778 cases with comparison of marginal zone lymphoma and monocytoid B-cell hyperplasia. Mod Pathol 11: 864-869.
1239. Lai R, Weiss LM, Chang KL, Arber DA (1999). Frequency of CD43 expression in non-Hodgkin lymphoma. A survey of 742 cases and further characterization of rare CD43+ follicular lymphomas. Am J Clin Pathol 111: 488-494.
1240. Laiosa CV, Stadtfeld M, Graf T (2006). Determinants of lymphoid-myeloid lineage diversification. Annu Rev Immunol 24: 705-738.
1241. Lamant L, Dastugue N, Pulford K, Delsol G, Mariame B (1999). A new fusion gene TPM3-ALK in anaplastic large cell lymphoma created by a (1;2)(q25;p23) translocation. Blood 93: 3088-3095.
1242. Lamant L, de Reynies A, Duplantier MM, Rickman DS, Sabourdy F, Giuriato S, Brugieres L, Gaulard P, Espinos E, Delsol G (2007). Gene-expression profiling of systemic anaplastic large-cell lymphoma reveals differences based on ALK status and two distinct morphologic ALK+ subtypes. Blood 109: 2156-2164.
1243. Lamant L, Gascoyne RD, Duplantier MM, Armstrong F, Raghab A, Chhanabhai M, Rajcan-Separovic E, Raghab J, Delsol G, Espinos E (2003). Non-muscle myosin heavy chain (MYH9): a new partner fused to ALK in anaplastic large cell lymphoma. Genes Chromosomes Cancer 37: 427-432.
1244. Lamant L, Meggetto F, al Saati T, Brugieres L, de Paillerets BB, Dastugue N, Bernheim A, Rubie H, Terrier-Lacombe MJ, Robert A, Rigal F, Schlaifer D, Shiuta M, Mori S, Delsol G (1996). High incidence of the t(2;5)(p23;q35) translocation in anaplastic large cell lymphoma and its lack of detection in Hodgkin's disease. Comparison of cytogenetic analysis, reverse transcriptase-polymerase chain reaction, and P-80 immunostaining. Blood 87: 284-291.
1245. Lambertenghi-Deliliers G, Annaloro C, Oriani A, Soligo D (1992). Myelodysplastic syndrome associated with bone marrow fibrosis. Leuk Lymphoma 8: 51-55.
1246. Lambertenghi-Deliliers G, Orazi A,

Luksch R, Annaloro C, Soligo D (1991). Myelodysplastic syndrome with increased marrow fibrosis: a distinct clinico-pathological entity. Br J Haematol 78: 161-166.
1247. Lamy T, Loughran TP, Jr. (1999). Current concepts: large granular lymphocyte leukemia. Blood Rev 13: 230-240.
1248. Lamy T, Loughran TP, Jr. (2003). Clinical features of large granular lymphocyte leukemia. Semin Hematol 40: 185-195.
1248A. Lan Q, Zheng T, Chanock S, Zhang Y, Shen M, Wang SS, Berndt SI, Zahm SH, Holford TR, Leaderer B, Yeager M, Welch R, Hosgood D, Boyle P, Rothman N (2006). Genetic variants in caspase genes and susceptibility to non-Hodgkin lymphoma. Carcinogenesis 28: 823-827.
1249. Landgren O, Gridley G, Turesson I, Caporaso NE, Goldin LR, Baris D, Fears TR, Hoover RN, Linet MS (2006). Risk of monoclonal gammopathy of undetermined significance (MGUS) and subsequent multiple myeloma among African American and white veterans in the United States. Blood 107: 904-906.
1249A. Landis SH, Murray T, Bolden S, Wingo PA (1999). Cancer statistics, 1999. CA Cancer J Clin 49: 8-31.
1250. Lange BJ, Kobrinsky N, Barnard DR, Arthur DC, Buckley JD, Howells WB, Gold S, Sanders J, Neudorf S, Smith FO, Woods WG (1998). Distinctive demography, biology, and outcome of acute myeloid leukemia and myelodysplastic syndrome in children with Down syndrome: Children's Cancer Group Studies 2861 and 2891. Blood 91: 608-615.
1251. Langebrake C, Creutzig U, Reinhardt D (2005). Immunophenotype of Down syndrome acute myeloid leukemia and transient myeloproliferative disease differs significantly from other diseases with morphologically identical or similar blasts. Klin Padiatr 217: 126-134.
1252. Lanham S, Hamblin T, Oscier D, Ibbotson R, Stevenson F, Packham G (2003). Differential signaling via surface IgM is associated with VH gene mutational status and CD38 expression in chronic lymphocytic leukemia. Blood 101: 1087-1093.
1253. Lardelli P, Bookman MA, Sundeen J, Longo DL, Jaffe ES (1990). Lymphocytic lymphoma of intermediate differentiation. Morphologic and immunophenotypic spectrum and clinical correlations. Am J Surg Pathol 14: 752-763.
1254. Larson RA, Le Beau MM (2005). Therapy-related myeloid leukaemia: a model for leukemogenesis in humans. Chem Biol Interact 153-154:187-195.
1255. Larson RS, Scott MA, McCurley TL, Vnencak-Jones CL (1996). Microsatellite analysis of posttransplant lymphoproliferative disorders: determination of donor/recipient origin and identification of putative lymphomagenic mechanism. Cancer Res 56: 4378-4381.
1256. Laszewski MJ, Kemp JD, Goeken JA, Mitros FA, Platz CE, Dick FR (1990). Clonal immunoglobulin gene rearrangement in nodular lymphoid hyperplasia of the gastrointestinal tract associated with common variable immunodeficiency. Am J Clin Pathol 94: 338-343.
1257. Lazzarino M, Orlandi E, Paulli M, Strater J, Klersy C, Gianelli U, Gargantini L, Rousset MT, Gambacorta M, Marra E, Lavabre-Bertrand T, Magrini U, Manegold C, Bernasconi C, Moller P (1997). Treatment outcome and prognostic factors for primary mediastinal (thymic) B-cell lymphoma: a multicenter study of 106 patients. J Clin Oncol 15: 1646-1653.
1258. Le Beau MM (2001). Role of cytogenetics in the diagnosis and classification of hematopoietic neoplasms. In: Neoplastic Hematopathology. Knowles D, ed. Lippincott Williams and Wilkins: Philadelphia, pp. 319-418.
1259. Le Gouill S, Talmant P, Touzeau C, Moreau A, Garand R, Juge-Morineau N, Gaillard F, Gastinne T, Milpied N, Moreau P, Harousseau JL, Avet-Loiseau H (2007). The clinical presentation and prognosis of diffuse large B-cell lymphoma with t(14;18) and 8q24/c-MYC rearrangement. Haematologica 92: 1335-1342.
1260. Leblond V, Davi F, Charlotte F, Dorent R, Bitker MO, Sutton L, Gandjbakhch I, Binet JL, Raphael M (1998). Posttransplant lymphoproliferative disorders not associated with Epstein-Barr virus: a distinct entity? J Clin Oncol 16: 2052-2059.
1261. LeBoit PE (1994). Granulomatous slack skin. Dermatol Clin 12: 375-389.
1261A. LeBoit PE, Burg G, Weedon D, Sarasin A (2006). World Health Organization Classification of Tumours. Pathology and genetics of skin tumours. IARC, Lyon.
1262. LeBrun DP (2003). E2A basic helix-loop-helix transcription factors in human leukemia. Front Biosci 8: s206-222.
1263. Lechapt-Zalcman E, Challine D, Delfau-Larue MH, Haioun C, Desvaux D, Gaulard P (2001). Association of primary pleural effusion lymphoma of T-cell origin and human herpesvirus 8 in a human immunodeficiency virus-seronegative man. Arch Pathol Lab Med 125: 1246-1248.
1264. Lecuit M, Abachin E, Martin A, Poyart C, Pochart P, Suarez F, Bengoufa D, Feuillard J, Lavergne A, Gordon JI, Berche P, Guillevin L, Lortholary O (2004). Immunoproliferative small intestinal disease associated with Campylobacter jejuni. N Engl J Med 350: 239-248.
1265. Lee IJ, Kim SC, Kim HS, Bang D, Yang WI, Jung WH, Chi HS (1999). Paraneoplastic pemphigus associated with follicular dendritic cell sarcoma arising from Castleman's tumor. J Am Acad Dermatol 40: 294-297.
1266. Lee J, Suh C, Park YH, Ko YH, Bang SM, Lee JH, Lee DH, Huh J, Oh SY, Kwon HC, Kim HJ, Lee SI, Kim JH, Park J, Oh SJ, Kim K, Jung C, Park K, Kim WS (2006). Extranodal natural killer T-cell lymphoma, nasal-type: a prognostic model from a retrospective multicenter study. J Clin Oncol 24: 612-618.
1266A Lee JT, Innes DJ, Jr., Williams ME. Sequential bcl-2 and c-myc oncogene rearrangements associated with the clinical transformation of non-Hodgkin's lymphoma. J Clin Invest 1989; 84:1454-1459.
1267. Legrand O, Perrot JY, Simonin G, Baudard M, Cadiou M, Blanc C, Ramond S, Viguie F, Marie JP, Zittoun R (1998). Adult biphenotypic acute leukaemia: an entity with poor prognosis which is related to unfavourable cytogenetics and P-glycoprotein over-expression. Br J Haematol 100: 147-155.
1268. Leith CP, Kopecky KJ, Chen IM, Eijdems L, Slovak ML, McConnell TS, Head DR, Weick J, Grever MR, Appelbaum FR, Willman CL (1999). Frequency and clinical significance of the expression of the multidrug resistance proteins MDR1/P-glycoprotein, MRP1, and LRP in acute myeloid leukemia: a Southwest Oncology Group Study. Blood 94: 1086-1099.
1269. Leith CP, Kopecky KJ, Godwin J, McConnell T, Slovak ML, Chen IM, Head DR, Appelbaum FR, Willman CL (1997). Acute myeloid leukemia in the elderly: assessment of multidrug resistance (MDR1) and cytogenetics distinguishes biologic subgroups with remarkably distinct responses to standard chemotherapy. A Southwest Oncology Group study. Blood 89: 3323-3329.
1270. Leithauser F, Bauerle M, Huynh MQ, Moller P (2001). Isotype-switched immunoglobulin genes with a high load of somatic hypermutation and lack of ongoing mutational activity are prevalent in mediastinal B-cell lymphoma. Blood 98: 2762-2770.
1271. Leleu X, O'Connor K, Ho AW, Santos DD, Manning R, Xu L, Hatjiharissi E, Moreau AS, Branagan AR, Hunter ZR, Dimmock EA, Soumerai J, Patterson C, Ghobrial I, Treon SP (2007). Hepatitis C viral infection is not associated with Waldenstrom's macroglobulinemia. Am J Hematol 82: 83-84.
1272. Lengfelder E, Hochhaus A, Kronawitter U, Hoche D, Queisser W, Jahn-Eder M, Burkhardt R, Reiter A, Ansari H, Hehlmann R (1998). Should a platelet limit of 600 x 10(9)/l be used as a diagnostic criterion in essential thrombocythaemia? An analysis of the natural course including early stages. Br J Haematol 100: 15-23.
1273. Lennert K (eds.) (1978). Malignant Lymphomas other than Hodgkin's disease. Springer Verlag: New York.
1274. Lennert K, Feller AC (1992). Histopathology of non-Hodgkin's lymphomas. Springer Verlag: Berlin.
1275. Lennert K, Parwaresch MR (1979). Mast cells and mast cell neoplasia: a review. Histopathology 3: 349-365.
1276. Lennert K, Stein H, Kaiserling E (1975). Cytological and functional criteria for the classification of malignant lymphomata. Br J Cancer 31 SUPPL 2: 29-43.
1277. Lens D, De Schouwer PJ, Hamoudi RA, Abdul-Rauf M, Farahat N, Matutes E, Crook T, Dyer MJ, Catovsky D (1997). p53 abnormalities in B-cell prolymphocytic leukemia. Blood 89: 2015-2023.
1277A. Leoncini L, Spina D, Nyong'O A, Abinya O, Minacci C, Disanto A, De Luca F, de Vivo A, Sabattini E, Poggi S, Pileri S, Tosi P (1996).Neoplastic cells of Hodgkin's disease show differences in EBV expression between Kenya and Italy. Int J Cancer 65:781-784
1278. Leone G, Mele L, Pulsoni A, Equitani F, Pagano L (1999). The incidence of secondary leukemias. Haematologica 84: 937-945.
1279. Leroux D, Mugneret F, Callanan M, Radford-Weiss I, Dastugue N, Feuillard J, Le Mee F, Plessis G, Talmant P, Gachard N, Uettwiller F, Pages MP, Mozziconacci MJ, Eclache V, Sibille C, Avet-Loiseau H, Lafage-Pochitaloff M (2002). CD4(+), CD56(+) DC2 acute leukemia is characterized by recurrent clonal chromosomal changes affecting 6 major targets: a study of 21 cases by the Groupe Francais de Cytogenetique Hematologique. Blood 99: 4154-4159.
1280. Leroy H, Roumier C, Huyghe P, Biggio V, Fenaux P, Preudhomme C (2005). CEBPA point mutations in hematological malignancies. Leukemia 19: 329-334.
1281. Leroy K, Haioun C, Lepage E, Le Metayer N, Berger F, Labouyrie E, Meignin V, Petit B, Bastard C, Salles G, Gisselbrecht C, Reyes F, Gaulard P (2002). p53 gene mutations are associated with poor survival in low and low-intermediate risk diffuse large B-cell lymphomas. Ann Oncol 13: 1108-1115.
1282. Lessard M, Struski S, Leymarie V, Flandrin G, Lafage-Pochitaloff M, Mozziconacci MJ, Talmant P, Bastard C, Charrin C, Baranger L, Helias C, Cornillet-Lefebvre P, Mugneret F, Cabrol C, Pages MP, Fert-Ferret D, Nguyen-Khac F, Quilichini B, Barin C, Berger R (2005). Cytogenetic study of 75 erythroleukemias. Cancer Genet Cytogenet 163: 113-122.
1282A. Leulier F, Lemaitre B (2008). Toll-like receptors--taking an evolutionary approach. Nat Rev Genet 9:165-78.
1283. Levine AM (1993). AIDS-related malignancies: the emerging epidemic. J Natl Cancer Inst 85: 1382-1397.
1284. Levine EG, Arthur DC, Frizzera G, Peterson BA, Hurd DD, Bloomfield CD (1988). Cytogenetic abnormalities predict clinical outcome in non-Hodgkin lymphoma. Ann Intern Med 108: 14-20.
1285. Levine EG, Arthur DC, Machnicki J, Frizzera G, Hurd D, Peterson B, Gajl-Peczalska KJ, Bloomfield CD (1989). Four new recurring translocations in non-Hodgkin lymphoma. Blood 74: 1796-1800.
1285A. Levine PH, Blattner WA, Clark J, Tarone R, Maloney EM, Murphy EM, Gallo RC, Robert-Guroff M, Saxinger WC (1988). Geographic distribution of HTLV-I and identification of a new high-risk population. Int J Cancer 42: 7-12.
1286. Levine PH, Manns A, Jaffe ES, Colclough G, Cavallaro A, Reddy G, Blattner WA (1994). The effect of ethnic differences on the pattern of HTLV-I-associated T-cell leukemia/lymphoma (HATL) in the United States. Int J Cancer 56: 177-181.
1287. Levine RL, Loriaux M, Huntly BJ, Loh ML, Beran M, Stoffregen E, Berger R, Clark JJ, Willis SG, Nguyen KT, Flores NJ, Estey E, Gattermann N, Armstrong S, Look AT, Griffin JD, Bernard OA, Heinrich MC, Gilliland DG, Druker B, Deininger MW (2005). The JAK2V617F activating mutation occurs in chronic myelomonocytic leukemia and acute myeloid leukemia, but not in acute lymphoblastic leukemia or chronic lymphocytic leukemia. Blood 106: 3377-3379.
1287A. Levine RL, Pardanani A, Tefferi A, Gilliland DG (2007). Role of JAK2 in the pathogenesis and therapy of myeloproliferative disorders. Nat Rev Cancer 7: 673-683.
1288. Levine RL, Wadleigh M, Cools J, Ebert BL, Wernig G, Huntly BJ, Boggon TJ, Wlodarska I, Clark JJ, Moore S, Adelsperger J, Koo S, Lee JC, Gabriel S, Mercher T, D'Andrea A, Frohling S, Dohner K, Marynen P, Vandenberghe P, Mesa RA, Tefferi A, Griffin JD, Eck MJ, Sellers WR, Meyerson M, Golub TR, Lee SJ, Gilliland DG (2005). Activating mutation in the tyrosine kinase JAK2 in polycythemia vera, essential thrombocythemia, and myeloid metaplasia with myelofibrosis. Cancer Cell 7: 387-397.
1289. Lewis EB (1963). Leukemia, multiple myeloma and anaplastic anemia in American Radiologists. Science 142: 1492-1494.
1290. Li C, Inagaki H, Kuo TT, Hu S, Okabe M, Eimoto T (2003). Primary cutaneous marginal zone B-cell lymphoma: a molecular and clinicopathologic study of 24 asian cases. Am J Surg Pathol 27: 1061-1069.
1291. Li JY, Gaillard F, Moreau A, Harousseau JL, Laboisse C, Milpied N, Bataille R, Avet-Loiseau H (1999). Detection of translocation t(11;14)(q13;q32) in mantle cell lymphoma by fluorescence in situ hybridization. Am J Pathol 154: 1449-1452.
1292. Li WV, Kapadia SB, Sonmez-Alpan E, Swerdlow SH (1996). Immunohistochemical characterization of mast cell disease in paraffin sections using tryptase, CD68, myeloperoxidase, lysozyme, and CD20 antibodies. Mod Pathol 9: 982-988.
1293. Liang R, Todd D, Chan TK, Chiu E, Lie A, Kwong YL, Choy D, Ho FC (1995). Treatment outcome and prognostic factors for primary nasal lymphoma. J Clin Oncol 13: 666-670.
1294. Licht JD (2001). AML1 and the AML1-ETO fusion protein in the pathogenesis of t(8;21) AML. Oncogene 20: 5660-5679.
1295. Lichtman MA, Segel GB (2005). Uncommon phenotypes of acute myelogenous leukemia: basophilic, mast cell, eosinophilic, and myeloid dendritic cell subtypes: a review. Blood Cells Mol Dis 35: 370-383.
1296. Liebross RH, Ha CS, Cox JD, Weber D, Delasalle K, Alexanian R (1998). Solitary bone

plasmacytoma: outcome and prognostic factors following radiotherapy. Int J Radiat Oncol Biol Phys 41: 1063-1067.
1297. Lierman E, Folens C, Stover EH, Mentens N, Van Miegroet H, Scheers W, Boogaerts M, Vandenberghe P, Marynen P, Cools J (2006). Sorafenib is a potent inhibitor of FIP1L1-PDGFRalpha and the imatinib-resistant FIP1L1-PDGFRalpha T674I mutant. Blood 108: 1374-1376.
1298. Lightfoot J, Hitzler JK, Zipursky A, Albert M, Macgregor PF (2004). Distinct gene signatures of transient and acute megakaryoblastic leukemia in Down syndrome. Leukemia 18: 1617-1623.
1299. Lim MS, Beaty M, Sorbara L, Cheng RZ, Pittaluga S, Raffeld M, Jaffe ES (2002). T-cell/histiocyte-rich large B-cell lymphoma: a heterogeneous entity with derivation from germinal center B cells. Am J Surg Pathol 26: 1458-1466.
1300. Lim MS, Straus SE, Dale JK, Fleisher TA, Stetler-Stevenson M, Strober W, Sneller MC, Puck JM, Lenardo MJ, Elenitoba-Johnson KS, Lin AY, Raffeld M, Jaffe ES (1998). Pathological findings in human autoimmune lymphoproliferative syndrome. Am J Pathol 153: 1541-1550.
1301. Lim ST, Karim R, Tulpule A, Nathwani BN, Levine AM (2005). Prognostic factors in HIV-related diffuse large-cell lymphoma: before versus after highly active antiretroviral therapy. J Clin Oncol 23: 8477-8482.
1302. Lim ZY, Killick S, Germing U, Cavenagh J, Culligan D, Bacigalupo A, Marsh J, Mufti GJ (2007). Low IPSS score and bone marrow hypocellularity in MDS patients predict hematological responses to antithymocyte globulin. Leukemia 21: 1436-1441.
1303. Lima M, Almeida J, Dos Anjos TM, Alguero Md MC, Santos AH, Balanzategui A, Queiros ML, Barcena P, Izarra A, Fonseca S, Bueno C, Justica B, Gonzalez M, San Miguel JF, Orfao A (2003). TCRalphabeta+/CD4+ large granular lymphocytosis: a new clonal T-cell lymphoproliferative disorder. Am J Pathol 163: 763-771.
1304. Lima M, Almeida J, Montero AG, Teixeira MA, Queiros ML, Santos AH, Balanzategui A, Estevinho A, Alguero MC, Barcena P, Fonseca S, Amorim ML, Cabeda JM, Pinho L, Gonzalez M, San Miguel J, Justica B, Orfao A (2004). Clinicobiological, immunophenotypic, and molecular characteristics of monoclonal CD56-/+dim chronic natural killer cell large granular lymphocytosis. Am J Pathol 165: 1117-1127.
1305. Lin CH, Kuo KT, Chuang SS, Kuo SH, Chang JH, Chang KC, Hsu HC, Tien HF, Cheng AL (2006). Comparison of the expression and prognostic significance of differentiation markers between diffuse large B-cell lymphoma of central nervous system origin and peripheral nodal origin. Clin Cancer Res 12: 1152-1156.
1306. Lin CW, Liu TY, Chen SU, Wang KT, Medeiros LJ, Hsu SM (2005). CD94 1A transcripts characterize lymphoblastic lymphoma/leukemia of immature natural killer cell origin with distinct clinical features. Blood 106: 3567-3574.
1307. Lin CW, O'Brien S, Faber J, Manshouri T, Romaguera J, Huh YO, Kantarjian H, Keating M, Albitar M (1999). De novo CD5+ Burkitt lymphoma/leukemia. Am J Clin Pathol 112: 828-835.
1308. Lin LI, Chen CY, Lin DT, Tsay W, Tang JL, Yeh YC, Shen HL, Su FH, Yao M, Huang SY, Tien HF (2005). Characterization of CEBPA mutations in acute myeloid leukemia: most patients with CEBPA mutations have biallelic mutations and show a distinct immunophenotype of the leukemic cells. Clin Cancer Res 11: 1372-1379.
1309. Lin O, Frizzera G (1997). Angiomyoid and follicular dendritic cell proliferative lesions in Castleman's disease of hyaline-vascular type: a study of 10 cases. Am J Surg Pathol 21: 1295-1306.
1310. Lin P, Jones D, Dorfman DM, Medeiros LJ (2000). Precursor B-cell lymphoblastic lymphoma: a predominantly extranodal tumor with low propensity for leukemic involvement. Am J Surg Pathol 24: 1480-1490.
1311. Lin P, Mansoor A, Bueso-Ramos C, Hao S, Lai R, Medeiros LJ (2003). Diffuse large B-cell lymphoma occurring in patients with lymphoplasmacytic lymphoma/Waldenstrom macroglobulinemia. Clinicopathologic features of 12 cases. Am J Clin Pathol 120: 246-253.
1312. Lin P, Owens R, Tricot G, Wilson CS (2004). Flow cytometric immunophenotypic analysis of 306 cases of multiple myeloma. Am J Clin Pathol 121: 482-488.
1313. Lindfors KK, Meyer JE, Dedrick CG, Hassell LA, Harris NL (1985). Thymic cysts in mediastinal Hodgkin disease. Radiology 156: 37-41.
1314. Lindstrom MS, Wiman KG (2002). Role of genetic and epigenetic changes in Burkitt lymphoma. Semin Cancer Biol 12: 381-387.
1315. Linet MS, Harlow SD, McLaughlin JK (1987). A case-control study of multiple myeloma in whites: chronic antigenic stimulation, occupation, and drug use. Cancer Res 47: 2978-2981.
1316. Lipford E, Wright JJ, Urba W, Whang-Peng J, Kirsch IR, Raffeld M, Cossman J, Longo DL, Bakhshi A, Korsmeyer SJ (1987). Refinement of lymphoma cytogenetics by the chromosome 18q21 major breakpoint region. Blood 70: 1816-1823.
1317. Lipford EH, Jr., Margolick JB, Longo DL, Fauci AS, Jaffe ES (1988). Angiocentric immunoproliferative lesions: a clinicopathologic spectrum of post-thymic T-cell proliferations. Blood 72: 1674-1681.
1318. Liso A, Capello D, Marafioti T, Tiacci E, Cerri M, Distler V, Paulli M, Carbone A, Delsol G, Campo E, Pileri S, Pasqualucci L, Gaidano G, Falini B (2006). Aberrant somatic hypermutation in tumor cells of nodular-lymphocyte-predominant and classic Hodgkin lymphoma. Blood 108: 1013-1020.
1319. Liso A, Tiacci E, Binazzi R, Pulford K, Benedetti R, Carotti A, Aversa F, Falini B (2004). Haploidentical peripheral-blood stem-cell transplantation for ALK-positive anaplastic large-cell lymphoma. Lancet Oncol 5: 127-128.
1320. List A, Dewald G, Bennett J, Giagounidis A, Raza A, Feldman E, Powell B, Greenberg P, Thomas D, Stone R, Reeder C, Wride K, Patin J, Schmidt M, Zeldis J, Knight R (2006). Lenalidomide in the myelodysplastic syndrome with chromosome 5q deletion. N Engl J Med 355: 1456-1465.
1320A. Liu D, Shimonov J, Primanneni S, Lai Y, Ahmed T, Seiter K (2007). t(8;14;18): a 3-way chromosome translocation in two patients with Burkitt's lymphoma/leukemia. Mol Cancer : 6: 35.
1320B. Lister TA, Crowther D, SutcliffeSB, Glatstein E, Canellos GP, Young RC, Rosenberg SA, Coltman CA, Tubiana M (1989). Report of a committee convened to discuss the evaluation and staging of patients with Hodgkin's disease: Cotswolds meeting. J Clin Oncol 7: 1630-1636.
1321. Liu H, Ruskon-Fourmestraux A, Lavergne-Slove A, Ye H, Molina T, Bouhnik Y, Hamoudi RA, Diss TC, Dogan A, Megraud F, Rambaud JC, Du MQ, Isaacson PG (2001). Resistance of t(11;18) positive gastric mucosa-associated lymphoid tissue lymphoma to Helicobacter pylori eradication therapy. Lancet 357: 39-40.
1322. Liu HL, Hoppe RT, Kohler S, Harvell JD, Reddy S, Kim YH (2003). CD30+ cutaneous lymphoproliferative disorders: the Stanford experience in lymphomatoid papulosis and primary cutaneous anaplastic large cell lymphoma. J Am Acad Dermatol 49: 1049-1058.
1323. Liu JH, Wei S, Lamy T, Epling-Burnette PK, Starkebaum G, Djeu JY, Loughran TP (2000). Chronic neutropenia mediated by fas ligand. Blood 95: 3219-3222.
1324. Liu TX, Becker MW, Jelinek J, Wu WS, Deng M, Mikhalkevich N, Hsu K, Bloomfield CD, Stone RM, DeAngelo DJ, Galinsky IA, Issa JP, Clarke MF, Look AT (2007). Chromosome 5q deletion and epigenetic suppression of the gene encoding alpha-catenin (CTNNA1) in myeloid cell transformation. Nat Med 13: 78-83.
1325. Liu YJ (2005). IPC: professional type 1 interferon-producing cells and plasmacytoid dendritic cell precursors. Annu Rev Immunol 23: 275-306.
1325A. Liu YJ, Zhang J, Lane PJ, Chan EY, MacLennan IC (1991). Sites of specific B cell activation in primary and secondary responses to T cell-dependent and T cell-independent antigens. Eur J Immunol 21: 2951-2962.
1326. Locatelli F, Nollke P, Zecca M, Korthof E, Lanino E, Peters C, Pession A, Kabisch H, Uderzo C, Bonfim CS, Bader P, Dilloo D, Stary J, Fischer A, Revesz T, Fuhrer M, Hasle H, Trebo M, van den Heuvel-Eibrink MM, Fenu S, Strahm B, Giorgiani G, Bonora MR, Duffner U, Niemeyer CM (2005). Hematopoietic stem cell transplantation (HSCT) in children with juvenile myelomonocytic leukemia (JMML): results of the EWOG-MDS/EBMT trial. Blood 105: 410-419.
1327. Locker J, Nalesnik M (1989). Molecular genetic analysis of lymphoid tumors arising after organ transplantation. Am J Pathol 135: 977-987.
1328. Loddenkemper C, Anagnostopoulos I, Hummel M, Johrens-Leder K, Foss HD, Jundt F, Wirth T, Dorken B, Stein H (2004). Differential Emu enhancer activity and expression of BOB.1/OBF.1, Oct2, PU.1, and immunoglobulin in reactive B-cell populations, B-cell non-Hodgkin lymphomas, and Hodgkin lymphomas. J Pathol 202: 60-69.
1329. Loh ML, Vattikuti S, Schubbert S, Reynolds MG, Carlson E, Lieuw KH, Cheng JW, Lee CM, Stokoe D, Bonifas JM, Curtiss NP, Gotlib J, Meshinchi S, Le Beau MM, Emanuel PD, Shannon KM (2004). Mutations in PTPN11 implicate the SHP-2 phosphatase in leukemogenesis. Blood 103: 2325-2331.
1329A. Lones MA, Cairo MS, Perkins SL (2000). T-cell-rich large B-cell lymphoma in children and adolescents: a clinicopathologic report of six cases from the Children's Cancer Group Study CCG-5961. Cancer 88: 2378-2386.
1330. Lones MA, Mishalani S, Shintaku IP, Weiss LM, Nichols WS, Said JW (1995). Changes in tonsils and adenoids in children with posttransplant lymphoproliferative disorder: report of three cases with early involvement of Waldeyer's ring. Hum Pathol 26: 525-530.
1331. Longley BJ, Tyrrell L, Lu SZ, Ma YS, Langley K, Ding TG, Duffy T, Jacobs P, Tang LH, Modlin I (1996). Somatic c-KIT activating mutation in urticaria pigmentosa and aggressive mastocytosis: establishment of clonality in a human mast cell neoplasm. Nat Genet 12: 312-314.
1332. Longley BJ, Jr., Metcalfe DD, Tharp M, Wang X, Tyrrell L, Lu SZ, Heitjan D, Ma Y (1999). Activating and dominant inactivating c-KIT catalytic domain mutations in distinct clinical forms of human mastocytosis. Proc Natl Acad Sci U S A 96: 1609-1614.
1333. Longley BJ, Jr., Morganroth GS, Tyrrell L, Ding TG, Anderson DM, Williams DE, Halaban R (1993). Altered metabolism of mast-cell growth factor (c-kit ligand) in cutaneous mastocytosis. N Engl J Med 328: 1302-1307.
1334. Longley J, Duffy TP, Kohn S (1995). The mast cell and mast cell disease. J Am Acad Dermatol 32: 545-561.
1335. Longo DL, Young RC, Hubbard SM, Wesley M, Fisher RI, Jaffe E, Berard C, DeVita VT, Jr. (1984). Prolonged initial remission in patients with nodular mixed lymphoma. Ann Intern Med 100: 651-656.
1336. Lopez-Guillermo A, Cid J, Salar A, Lopez A, Montalban C, Castrillo JM, Gonzalez M, Ribera JM, Brunet S, Garcia-Conde J, Fernandez dS, Bosch F, Montserrat E (1998). Peripheral T-cell lymphomas: initial features, natural history, and prognostic factors in a series of 174 patients diagnosed according to the R.E.A.L. Classification. Ann Oncol 9: 849-855.
1337. Lorsbach RB, Shay-Seymore D, Moore J, Banks PM, Hasserjian RP, Sandlund JT, Behm FG (2002). Clinicopathologic analysis of follicular lymphoma occurring in children. Blood 99: 1959-1964.
1338. Lossos IS, Alizadeh AA, Diehn M, Warnke R, Thorstenson Y, Oefner PJ, Brown PO, Botstein D, Levy R (2002). Transformation of follicular lymphoma to diffuse large-cell lymphoma: alternative patterns with increased or decreased expression of c-myc and its regulated genes. Proc Natl Acad Sci U S A 99: 8886-8891.
1339. Lossos IS, Morgensztern D (2006). Prognostic biomarkers in diffuse large B-cell lymphoma. J Clin Oncol 24: 995-1007.
1340. Loughran TP, Jr., Zambello R, Ashley R, Guderian J, Pellenz M, Semenzato G, Starkebaum G (1993). Failure to detect Epstein-Barr virus DNA in peripheral blood mononuclear cells of most patients with large granular lymphocyte leukemia. Blood 81: 2723-2727.
1341. Louie DC, Offit K, Jaslow R, Parsa NZ, Murty VV, Schluger A, Chaganti RS (1995). p53 overexpression as a marker of poor prognosis in mantle cell lymphomas with t(11;14)(q13;q32). Blood 86: 2892-2899.
1342. Lucio P, Gaipa G, van Lochem EG, van Wering ER, Porwit-MacDonald A, Faria T, Bjorklund E, Biondi A, van den Beemd MW, Baars E, Vidriales B, Parreira A, van Dongen JJ, San Miguel JF, Orfao A (2001). BIOMED-I concerted action report: flow cytometric immunophenotyping of precursor B-ALL with standardized triple-stainings. BIOMED-1 Concerted Action Investigation of Minimal Residual Disease in Acute Leukemia: International Standardization and Clinical Evaluation. Leukemia 15: 1185-1192.
1343. Luk IS, Shek TW, Tang VW, Ng WF (1999). Interdigitating dendritic cell tumor of the testis: a novel testicular spindle cell neoplasm. Am J Surg Pathol 23: 1141-1148.
1344. Lukes R, Butler J, Hicks E (1966). Natural history of Hodgkin's disease as related to its patholgical picture. Cancer 19: 317-344.
1344A. Lukes RJ, Collins RD (1974). Immunologic characterization of human malignant lymphomas. Cancer 34: 1488-1503.
1344B. Lukes RJ, Collins RD (1992). Tumors of the Haematopoietic system. Washington: AFIP.
1345. Lukes RJ, Craver L, Hall T, Rappaport H, Ruben P (1966). Report of the nomenclature committee. Cancer Res 26: 1311.
1346. Luna-Fineman S, Shannon KM, Atwater SK, Davis J, Masterson M, Ortega J, Sanders J, Steinherz P, Weinberg V, Lange BJ (1999). Myelodysplastic and myeloproliferative disorders of childhood: a study of 167 patients. Blood 93: 459-466.
1347. Lundberg LG, Lerner R, Sundelin P, Rogers R, Folkman J, Palmblad J (2000). Bone marrow in polycythemia vera, chronic myelocyt-

ic leukemia, and myelofibrosis has an increased vascularity. Am J Pathol 157: 15-19.

1348. Lundell R, Hartung L, Hill S, Perkins SL, Bahler DW (2005). T-cell large granular lymphocyte leukemias have multiple phenotypic abnormalities involving pan-T-cell antigens and receptors for MHC molecules. Am J Clin Pathol 124: 937-946.

1349. Luppi M, Barozzi P, Santagostino G, Trovato R, Schulz TF, Marasca R, Bottalico D, Bignardi L, Torelli G (2000). Molecular evidence of organ-related transmission of Kaposi sarcoma-associated herpesvirus or human herpesvirus-8 in transplant patients. Blood 96: 3279-3281.

1350. Luppi M, Marasca R, Morselli M, Barozzi P, Torelli G (1994). Clonal nature of hypereosinophilic syndrome. Blood 84: 349-350.

1351. Ma X, Does M, Raza A, Mayne ST (2007). Myelodysplastic syndromes: incidence and survival in the United States. Cancer 109: 1536-1542.

1352. Ma Z, Morris SW, Valentine V, Li M, Herbrick JA, Cui X, Bouman D, Li Y, Mehta PK, Nizetic D, Kaneko Y, Chan GC, Chan LC, Squire J, Scherer SW, Hitzler JK (2001). Fusion of two novel genes, RBM15 and MKL1, in the t(1;22)(p13;q13) of acute megakaryoblastic leukemia. Nat Genet 28: 220-221.

1353. Maartense E, Kramer MH, le Cessie S, Kluin-Nelemans JC, Kluin PM, Snijder S, Noordijk EM (2004). Lack of prognostic significance of BCL2 and p53 protein overexpression in elderly patients with diffuse large B-cell non-Hodgkin's lymphoma: results from a population-based non-Hodgkin's lymphoma registry. Leuk Lymphoma 45: 101-107.

1354. Macdonald D, Reiter A, Cross NC (2002). The 8p11 myeloproliferative syndrome: a distinct clinical entity caused by constitutive activation of FGFR1. Acta Haematol 107: 101-107.

1355. Mackey AC, Green L, Liang LC, Dinndorf P, Avigan M (2007). Hepatosplenic T cell lymphoma associated with infliximab use in young patients treated for inflammatory bowel disease. J Pediatr Gastroenterol Nutr 44: 265-267.

1355A. MacLennan IC (1994). Germinal centers. Annu Rev Immunol 12: 117-139.

1356. Maclennan KA, Bennett MH, Vaughan HB, Vaughan HG (1992). Diagnosis and grading of nodular sclerosing Hodgkin's disease: a study of 2190 patients. Int Rev Exp Pathol 33: 27-51.

1356A. MacLennan IC, Liu YJ, Oldfield S, Zhang J, Lane PJ (1990). The evolution of B-cell clones. Curr Top Microbiol Immunol 159: 37-63.

1357. Macon WR, Levy NB, Kurtin PJ, Salhany KE, Elkhalifa MY, Casey TT, Craig FE, Vnencak-Jones CL, Gulley ML, Park JP, Cousar JB (2001). Hepatosplenic alphabeta T-cell lymphomas: a report of 14 cases and comparison with hepatosplenic gammadelta T-cell lymphomas. Am J Surg Pathol 25: 285-296.

1358. Macon WR, Williams ME, Greer JP, Cousar JB (1995). Paracortical nodular T-cell lymphoma. Identification of an unusual variant of peripheral T-cell lymphoma. Am J Surg Pathol 19: 297-303.

1359. Macpherson N, Lesack D, Klasa R, Horsman D, Connors JM, Barnett M, Gascoyne RD (1999). Small noncleaved, non-Burkitt's (Burkit-Like) lymphoma: cytogenetics predict outcome and reflect clinical presentation. J Clin Oncol 17: 1558-1567.

1360. Maeda K, Matsuda M, Suzuki H, Saitoh HA (2002). Immunohistochemical recognition of human follicular dendritic cells (FDCs) in routinely processed paraffin sections. J Histochem Cytochem 50: 1475-1486.

1361. Maeda T, Murata K, Fukushima T, Sugahara K, Tsuruda K, Anami M, Onimaru Y,

Tsukasaki K, Tomonaga M, Moriuchi R, Hasegawa H, Yamada Y, Kamihira S (2005). A novel plasmacytoid dendritic cell line, CAL-1, established from a patient with blastic natural killer cell lymphoma. Int J Hematol 81: 148-154.

1361A. Maes B, Anastasopoulou A, Kluin-Nelemans JC, Teodorovic I, Achten R, Carbone A, De Wolf-Peeters C (2007). Among diffuse large B-cell lymphomas, T-cell-rich/histiocyte-rich BCL and CD30+ anaplastic B-cell subtypes exhibit distinct clinical features. Ann Oncol 12: 853-858.

1362. Magalhaes IQ, Splendore A, Emerenciano M, Figueiredo A, Ferrari I, Pombo-de-Oliveira MS (2006). GATA1 mutations in acute leukemia in children with Down syndrome. Cancer Genet Cytogenet 166: 112-116.

1363. Magrath IT, Janus C, Edwards BK, Spiegel R, Jaffe ES, Berard CW, Miliauskas J, Morris K, Barnwell R (1984). An effective therapy for both undifferentiated (including Burkitt's) lymphomas and lymphoblastic lymphomas in children and young adults. Blood 63: 1102-1111.

1364. Magrath IT, Sariban E (1985). Clinical features of Burkitt's lymphoma in the USA. IARC Sci Publ 60: 119-127.

1365. Magro CM, Crowson AN, Kovatich AJ, Burns F (2001). Lupus profundus, indeterminate lymphocytic lobular panniculitis and subcutaneous T-cell lymphoma: a spectrum of subcuticular T-cell lymphoid dyscrasia. J Cutan Pathol 28: 235-247.

1366. Magro CM, Crowson AN, Morrison C, Merati K, Porcu P, Wright ED (2006). CD8+ lymphomatoid papulosis and its differential diagnosis. Am J Clin Pathol 125: 490-501.

1367. Maitra A, McKenna RW, Weinberg AG, Schneider NR, Kroft SH (2001). Precursor B-cell lymphoblastic lymphoma. A study of nine cases lacking blood and bone marrow involvement and review of the literature. Am J Clin Pathol 115: 868-875.

1368. Majlis A, Pugh WC, Rodriguez MA, Benedict WF, Cabanillas F (1997). Mantle cell lymphoma: correlation of clinical outcome and biologic features with three histologic variants. J Clin Oncol 15: 1664-1671.

1369. Makishima H, Ito T, Momose K, Nakazawa H, Shimodaira S, Kamijo Y, Nakazawa Y, Ichikawa N, Ueno M, Kobayashi H, Kitano K, Saito H, Kiyosawa K, Ishida F (2007). Chemokine system and tissue infiltration in aggressive NK-cell leukemia. Leuk Res 31: 1237-1245.

1370. Malcovati L, Germing U, Kuendgen A, Della Porta MG, Pascutto C, Invernizzi R, Giagounidis A, Hildebrandt B, Bernasconi P, Knipp S, Strupp C, Lazzarino M, Aul C, Cazzola M (2007). Time-dependent prognostic scoring system for predicting survival and leukemic evolution in myelodysplastic syndromes. J Clin Oncol 25: 3503-3510.

1371. Malcovati L, Porta MG, Pascutto C, Invernizzi R, Boni M, Travaglino E, Passamonti F, Arcaini L, Maffioli M, Bernasconi P, Lazzarino M, Cazzola M (2005). Prognostic factors and life expectancy in myelodysplastic syndromes classified according to WHO criteria: a basis for clinical decision making. J Clin Oncol 23: 7594-7603.

1372. Maljaei SH, Brito-Babapulle V, Hiorns LR, Catovsky D (1998). Abnormalities of chromosomes 8, 11, 14, and X in T-prolymphocytic leukemia studied by fluorescence in situ hybridization. Cancer Genet Cytogenet 103: 110-116.

1373. Mallett RB, Matutes E, Catovsky D, MacLennan K, Mortimer PS, Holden CA (1995). Cutaneous infiltration in T-cell prolymphocytic leukaemia. Br J Dermatol 132: 263-266.

1374. Malpas J, Bergsagel D, Kyle R,

Anderson K (eds.) (2004). Myeloma: Biology and Management. 3rd edition. Saunders: Philadelphia.

1375. Malyukova A, Dohda T, von der Lehr N, Akhondi S, Corcoran M, Heyman M, Spruck C, Grander D, Lendahl U, Sangfelt O (2007). The tumor suppressor gene hCDC4 is frequently mutated in human T-cell acute lymphoblastic leukemia with functional consequences for Notch signaling. Cancer Res 67: 5611-5616.

1376. Manabe A, Yoshimasu T, Ebihara Y, Yagasaki H, Wada M, Ishikawa K, Hara J, Koike K, Moritake H, Park YD, Tsuji K, Nakahata T (2004). Viral infections in juvenile myelomonocytic leukemia: prevalence and clinical implications. J Pediatr Hematol Oncol 26: 636-641.

1377. Manaloor EJ, Neiman RS, Heilman DK, Albitar M, Casey T, Vattuone T, Kotylo P, Orazi A (2000). Immunohistochemistry can be used to subtype acute myeloid leukemia in routinely processed bone marrow biopsy specimens. Comparison with flow cytometry. Am J Clin Pathol 113: 814-822.

1378. Mann RB, Berard CW (1983). Criteria for the cytologic subclassification of follicular lymphomas: a proposed alternative method. Hematol Oncol 1: 187-192.

1379. Mansoor A, Medeiros LJ, Weber DM, Alexanian R, Hayes K, Jones D, Lai R, Glassman A, Bueso-Ramos CE (2001). Cytogenetic findings in lymphoplasmacytic lymphoma/Waldenstrom macroglobulinemia. Chromosomal abnormalities are associated with the polymorphous subtype and an aggressive clinical course. Am J Clin Pathol 116: 543-549.

1380. Mantadakis E, Shannon KM, Singer DA, Finklestein J, Chan KW, Hilden JM, Sandler ES (1999). Transient monosomy 7: a case series in children and review of the literature. Cancer 85: 2655-2661.

1381. Mao X, Lillington D, Scarisbrick JJ, Mitchell T, Czepulkowski B, Russell-Jones R, Young B, Whittaker SJ (2002). Molecular cytogenetic analysis of cutaneous T-cell lymphomas: identification of common genetic alterations in Sezary syndrome and mycosis fungoides. Br J Dermatol 147: 464-475.

1382. Mao X, Lillington DM, Czepulkowski B, Russell-Jones R, Young BD, Whittaker S (2003). Molecular cytogenetic characterization of Sezary syndrome. Genes Chromosomes Cancer 36: 250-260.

1383. Mao X, Orchard G, Lillington DM, Russell-Jones R, Young BD, Whittaker S (2003). Genetic alterations in primary cutaneous CD30+ anaplastic large cell lymphoma. Genes Chromosomes Cancer 37: 176-185.

1384. Mao X, Orchard G, Lillington DM, Russell-Jones R, Young BD, Whittaker SJ (2003). Amplification and overexpression of JUNB is associated with primary cutaneous T-cell lymphomas. Blood 101: 1513-1519.

1385. Mao Z, Quintanilla-Martinez L, Raffeld M, Richter M, Krugmann J, Burek C, Hartmann E, Rudiger TH, Jaffe ES, Muller-Hermelink HK, Ott G, Fend F, Rosenwald A (2007). IgVH mutational status and clonality analysis of Richter's transformation. Am J Surg Pathol. 32:1605-1614.

1386. Marafioti T, Paterson JC, Ballabio E, Reichard KK, Tedoldi S, Hollowood K, Dictor M, Hansmann ML, Pileri SA, Dyer MJ, Sozzani S, Dikic I, Shaw SA, Petrella T, Stein H, Isaacson PG, Facchetti F, Mason DY (2008). Novel markers of normal and neoplastic human plasmacytoid dendritic cells. Blood 111: 3778-3792.

1387. Marafioti T, Hummel M, Anagnostopoulos I, Foss HD, Falini B, Delsol G, Isaacson PG, Pileri S, Stein H (1997). Origin of nodular lymphocyte-predominant Hodgkin's disease from a clonal expansion of highly

mutated germinal-center B cells. N Engl J Med 337: 453-458.

1387A. Marafioti T, Hummel M, Anagnostopoulos I, Foss HD, Huhn D, Stein H (1999). Classical Hodgkin's disease and follicular lymphoma originating from the same germinal center B cell. J Clin Oncol 17: 3804-3809.

1388. Marafioti T, Hummel M, Foss HD, Laumen H, Korbjuhn P, Anagnostopoulos I, Lammert H, Demel G, Theil J, Wirth T, Stein H (2000). Hodgkin and reed-sternberg cells represent an expansion of a single clone originating from a germinal center B-cell with functional immunoglobulin gene rearrangements but defective immunoglobulin transcription. Blood 95: 1443-1450.

1388A. Marafioti T, Pozzobon M, Hansmann ML, Delsol G, Pileri SA, Mason DY (2003). Expression of intracellular signaling molecules in classical and lymphocyte predominance Hodgkin disease. Blood 103: 188-193.

1389. Marchioli R, Finazzi G, Landolfi R, Kutti J, Gisslinger H, Patrono C, Marilus R, Villegas A, Tognoni G, Barbui T (2005). Vascular and neoplastic risk in a large cohort of patients with polycythemia vera. J Clin Oncol 23: 2224-2232.

1390. Marcucci G, Mrózek K, Ruppert AS, Maharry K, Kolitz JE, Moore JO, Mayer RJ, Pettenati MJ, Powell BL, Edwards CG, Sterling LJ, Vardiman JW, Schiffer CA, Carroll AJ, Larson RA, Bloomfield CD (2005). Prognostic factors and outcome of core binding factor acute myeloid leukemia patients with t(8;21) differ from those of patients with inv(16): a Cancer and Leukemia Group B study. J Clin Oncol 23: 5705-5717.

1390A. Marcucci G, Baldus CD, Ruppert AS, Radmacher MD, Mrózek K, Whitman SP, Kolitz JE, Edwards CG, Vardiman JW, Powell BL, Baer MR, Moore JO, Perrotti D, Caligiuri MA, Carroll AJ, Larson RA, de la Chapelle CA, Bloomfield CD (2005). Overexpression of the ETS-related gene, ERG, predicts a worse outcome in acute myeloid leukemia with normal karyotype: a Cancer and Leukemia Group B study. J Clin Oncol 23: 9234-9242.

1390B. Marcucci G, Maharry K, Whitman SP, Vukosavljevic T, Paschka P, Langer C, Mrózek K, Baldus CD, Carroll AJ, Powell BL, Kolitz JE, Larson RA, Bloomfield CD (2007). High expression levels of the ETS-related gene, ERG, predict adverse outcome and improve molecular risk-based classification of cytogenetically normal acute myeloid leukemia: a Cancer and Leukemia Group B Study. J Clin Oncol 25: 3337-3343.

1391. Maric I, Robyn J, Metcalfe DD, Fay MP, Carter M, Wilson T, Fu W, Stoddard J, Scott L, Hartsell M, Kirshenbaum A, Akin C, Nutman TB, Noel P, Klion AD (2007). KIT D816V-associated systemic mastocytosis with eosinophilia and FIP1L1/PDGFRA-associated chronic eosinophilic leukemia are distinct entities. J Allergy Clin Immunol 120: 680-687.

1392. Mariette X, Cazals-Hatem D, Warszawki J, Liote F, Balandraud N, Sibilia J (2002). Lymphomas in rheumatoid arthritis patients treated with methotrexate: a 3-year prospective study in France. Blood 99: 3909-3915.

1393. Marlton P, Keating M, Kantarjian H, Pierce S, O'Brien S, Freireich EJ, Estey E (1995). Cytogenetic and clinical correlates in AML patients with abnormalities of chromosome 16. Leukemia 9: 965-971.

1394. Martelli MP, Manes N, Pettirossi V, Liso A, Pacini R, Mannucci R, Zei T, Bolli N, di Raimondo F, Specchia G, Nicoletti I, Martelli MF, Falini B (2008). Absence of nucleophosmin leukaemic mutants in B and T cells from AML with NPM1 mutations: implications for the cell of origin of NPMc+ AML. Leukemia 22: 195-198.

1395. Marti GE, Rawstron AC, Ghia P, Hillmen P, Houlston RS, Kay N, Schleinitz TA, Caporaso N (2005). Diagnostic criteria for monoclonal B-cell lymphocytosis. Br J Haematol 130: 325-332.
1396. Martiat P, Michaux JL, Rodhain J (1991). Philadelphia-negative (Ph-) chronic myeloid leukemia (CML): comparison with Ph+ CML and chronic myelomonocytic leukemia. The Groupe Francais de Cytogenetique Hematologique. Blood 78: 205-211.
1397. Martin A, Baran-Marzak F, El Mansouri S, Legendre C, Leblond V, Charlotte F, Davi F, Canioni D, Raphael M (2000). Expression of p16/INK4a in posttransplantation lymphoproliferative disorders. Am J Pathol 156: 1573-1579.
1398. Martin A, Capron F, Liguory-Brunaud MD, De Frejacques C, Pluot M, Diebold J (1994). Epstein-Barr virus-associated primary malignant lymphomas of the pleural cavity occurring in longstanding pleural chronic inflammation. Hum Pathol 25: 1314-1318.
1399. Martin A, Flaman JM, Frebourg T, Davi F, El Mansouri S, Amouroux J, Raphael M (1998). Functional analysis of the p53 protein in AIDS-related non-Hodgkin's lymphomas and polymorphic lymphoproliferations. Br J Haematol 101: 311-317.
1400. Martin AR, Weisenburger DD, Chan WC, Ruby EI, Anderson JR, Vose JM, Bierman PJ, Bast MA, Daley DT, Armitage JO (1995). Prognostic value of cellular proliferation and histologic grade in follicular lymphoma. Blood 85: 3671-3678.
1401. Martin PL, Look AT, Schnell S, Harris MB, Pullen J, Shuster JJ, Carroll AJ, Pettenati MJ, Rao PN (1996). Comparison of fluorescence in situ hybridization, cytogenetic analysis, and DNA index analysis to detect chromosomes 4 and 10 aneuploidy in pediatric acute lymphoblastic leukemia: a Pediatric Oncology Group study. J Pediatr Hematol Oncol 18: 113-121.
1401A. Martín-Subero JI, Klapper W, Sotnikova A, Callet-Bauchu E, Harder L, Bastard C, Schmitz R, Grohmann S, Höppner J, Riemke J, Barth TF, Berger F, Bernd HW, Claviez A, Gesk S, Frank GA, Kaplanskaya IB, Möller P, Parwaresch RM, Rüdiger T, Stein H, Küppers R, Hansmann ML, Siebert R; Deutsche Krebshilfe Network Project Molecular Mechanisms in Malignant Lymphomas (2006). Chromosomal breakpoints affecting immunoglobulin loci are recurrent in Hodgkin and Reed-Sternberg cells of classical Hodgkin lymphoma. Cancer Res 66: 10332-10338.
1402. Martinez-Climent JA, Vizcarra E, Benet I, Marugan I, Terol MJ, Solano C, Arbona C, Tormo M, Comes AM, Garcia-Conde J (1998). Cytogenetic response induced by interferon alpha in the myeloproliferative disorder with eosinophilia, T cell lymphoma and the chromosomal translocation t(8;13)(p11;q12). Leukemia 12: 999-1000.
1403. Martinez A, Pittaluga S, Villamor N, Colomer D, Rozman M, Raffeld M, Montserrat E, Campo E, Jaffe ES (2004). Clonal T-cell populations and increased risk for cytotoxic T-cell lymphomas in B-CLL patients: clinicopathologic observations and molecular analysis. Am J Surg Pathol 28: 849-858.
1404. Marzano AV, Ghislanzoni M, Gianelli U, Caputo R, Alessi E, Berti E (2005). Fatal CD8+ epidermotropic cytotoxic primary cutaneous T-cell lymphoma with multiorgan involvement. Dermatology 211: 281-285.
1405. Marzano AV, Vezzoli P, Mariotti F, Boneschi V, Caputo R, Berti E (2005). Paraneoplastic pemphigus associated with follicular dendritic cell sarcoma and Castleman disease. Br J Dermatol 153: 214-215.
1406. Maschek H, Georgii A, Kaloutsi V, Werner M, Bandecar K, Kressel MG, Choritz H, Freund M, Hufnagl D (1992). Myelofibrosis in primary myelodysplastic syndromes: a retrospective study of 352 patients. Eur J Haematol 48: 208-214.
1406A. Mason DY, Banks PM, Chan J, Cleary ML, Delsol G, de Wolf Peeters C, Falini B, Gatter K, Grogan TM, Harris NL, et al. (1994) Nodular lymphocyte predominance Hodgkin's disease. A distinct clinicopathological entity. Am J Surg Pathol 18: 526-530.
1407. Mason DY, Bastard C, Rimokh R, Dastugue N, Huret JL, Kristoffersson U, Magaud JP, Nezelof C, Tilly H, Vannier JP (1990). CD30-positive large cell lymphomas ('Ki-1 lymphoma') are associated with a chromosomal translocation involving 5q35. Br J Haematol 74: 161-168.
1408. Mason DY, Pulford KA, Bischof D, Kuefer MU, Butler LH, Lamant L, Delsol G, Morris SW (1998). Nucleolar localization of the nucleophosmin-anaplastic lymphoma kinase is not required for malignant transformation. Cancer Res 58: 1057-1062.
1409. Massey GV, Zipursky A, Chang MN, Doyle JJ, Nasim S, Taub JW, Ravindranath Y, Dahl G, Weinstein HJ (2006). A prospective study of the natural history of transient leukemia (TL) in neonates with Down syndrome (DS): Children's Oncology Group (COG) study POG-9481. Blood 107: 4606-4613.
1410. Massone C, Chott A, Metze D, Kerl K, Citarella L, Vale E, Kerl H, Cerroni L (2004). Subcutaneous, blastic natural killer (NK), NK/T-cell, and other cytotoxic lymphomas of the skin: a morphologic, immunophenotypic, and molecular study of 50 patients. Am J Surg Pathol 28: 719-735.
1411. Massone C, Kodama K, Kerl H, Cerroni L (2005). Histopathologic features of early (patch) lesions of mycosis fungoides: a morphologic study on 745 biopsy specimens from 427 patients. Am J Surg Pathol 29: 550-560.
1412. Massone C, Kodama K, Salmhofer W, Abe R, Shimizu H, Parodi A, Kerl H, Cerroni L (2005). Lupus erythematosus panniculitis (lupus profundus): clinical, histopathological, and molecular analysis of nine cases. J Cutan Pathol 32: 396-404.
1413. Massone C, Lozzi GP, Egberts F, Fink-Puches R, Cota C, Kerl H, Cerroni L (2006). The protean spectrum of non-Hodgkin lymphomas with prominent involvement of subcutaneous fat. J Cutan Pathol 33: 418-425.
1414. Mastovich S, Ratech H, Ware RE, Moore JO, Borowitz MJ (1994). Hepatosplenic T-cell lymphoma: an unusual case of a gamma delta T-cell lymphoma with a blast-like terminal transformation. Hum Pathol 25: 102-108.
1414A. Masuko K, Kato S, Hagihara M, Tsuchida F, Takemoto Y, Izawa K, Kato T, Yamamori S, Mizushima Y, Nishioka K, Tsuji K, Yamamoto K. (1996). Stable clonal expansion of T cells induced by bone marrow transplantation. Blood 87: 789-799.
1415. Matano S, Nakamura S, Kobayashi K, Yoshida T, Matsuda T, Sugimoto T (1997). Deletion of the long arm of chromosome 20 in a patient with chronic neutrophilic leukemia: cytogenetic findings in chronic neutrophilic leukemia. Am J Hematol 54: 72-75.
1416. Mateo M, Mollejo M, Villuendas R, Algara P, Sanchez-Beato M, Martinez P, Piris MA (1999). 7q31-32 allelic loss is a frequent finding in splenic marginal zone lymphoma. Am J Pathol 154: 1583-1589.
1416A. Mathas S, Janz M, Hummel F, Hummel M, Wollert-Wulf B, Lusatis S, Anagnostopoulos I, Lietz A, Sigvardsson M, Jundt F, Jöhrens K, Bommert K, Stein H, Dörken B (2006). Intrinsic inhibition of transcription factor E2A by HLH proteins ABF-1 and Id2 mediates reprogramming of neoplastic B cells in Hodgkin lymphoma. Nat Immunol 7: 207-215
1416B. Mathas S, Hinz M, Anagnostopoulos I, Krappmann D, Lietz A, Jundt F, Bommert K, Mechta-Grigoriou F, Stein H, Dörken B, Scheidereit C (2002). Aberrantly expressed c-Jun and JunB are a hallmark of Hodgkin lymphoma cells, stimulate proliferation and synergize with NF-kappa B. Embo J 21: 4104-4113.
1417. Mathew P, Tefferi A, Dewald GW, Goldberg SL, Su J, Hoagland HC, Noel P (1993). The 5q- syndrome: a single-institution study of 43 consecutive patients. Blood 81: 1040-1045.
1418. Matolcsy A, Chadburn A, Knowles DM (1995). De novo CD5-positive and Richter's syndrome-associated diffuse large B cell lymphomas are genotypically distinct. Am J Pathol 147: 207-216.
1419. Matolcsy A, Nador RG, Cesarman E, Knowles DM (1998). Immunoglobulin VH gene mutational analysis suggests that primary effusion lymphomas derive from different stages of B cell maturation. Am J Pathol 153: 1609-1614.
1420. Matsuda A, Germing U, Jinnai I, Iwanaga M, Misumi M, Kuendgen A, Strupp C, Miyazaki Y, Tsushima H, Sakai M, Bessho M, Gattermann N, Aul C, Tomonaga M (2007). Improvement of criteria for refractory cytopenia with multilineage dysplasia according to the WHO classification based on prognostic significance of morphological features in patients with refractory anemia according to the FAB classification. Leukemia 21: 678-686.
1421. Matsushima AY, Strauchen JA, Lee G, Scigliano E, Hale EE, Weisse MT, Burstein D, Kamel O, Moore PS, Chang Y (1999). Posttransplantation plasmacytic proliferations related to Kaposi's sarcoma-associated herpesvirus. Am J Surg Pathol 23: 1393-1400.
1422. Matthes T, Rustin P, Trachsel H, Darbellay R, Costaridou S, Xaidara A, Rideau A, Beris P (2006). Different pathophysiological mechanisms of intramitochondrial iron accumulation in acquired and congenital sideroblastic anemia caused by mitochondrial DNA deletion. Eur J Haematol 77: 169-174.
1423. Matutes E (2006). Immunophenotyping and differential diagnosis of hairy cell leukemia. Hematol Oncol Clin North Am 20: 1051-1063.
1424. Matutes E, Brito-Babapulle V, Swansbury J, Ellis J, Morilla R, Dearden C, Sempere A, Catovsky D (1991). Clinical and laboratory features of 78 cases of T-prolymphocytic leukemia. Blood 78: 3269-3274.
1425. Matutes E, Crockard AD, O'Brien M, Catovsky D (1983). Ultrastructural cytochemistry of chronic T-cell leukaemias. A study with four acid hydrolases. Histochem J 15: 895-909.
1426. Matutes E, Garcia TJ, O'Brien M, Catovsky D (1986). The morphological spectrum of T-prolymphocytic leukaemia. Br J Haematol 64: 111-124.
1427. Matutes E, Morilla R, Farahat N, Carbonell F, Swansbury J, Dyer M, Catovsky D (1997). Definition of acute biphenotypic leukemia. Haematologica 82: 64-66.
1428. Matutes E, Morilla R, Owusu-Ankomah K, Houlihan A, Catovsky D (1994). The immunophenotype of splenic lymphoma with villous lymphocytes and its relevance to the differential diagnosis with other B-cell disorders. Blood 83: 1558-1562.
1429. Matutes E, Oscier D, Garcia-Marco J, Ellis J, Copplestone A, Gillingham R, Hamblin T, Lens D, Swansbury GJ, Catovsky D (1996). Trisomy 12 defines a group of CLL with atypical morphology: correlation between cytogenetic, clinical and laboratory features in 544 patients. Br J Haematol 92: 382-388.
1429A. Matutes E, Oscier D, Montalban C, Berger F, Callet-Bauchu E, Dogan A, Felman P, Franco V, Iannitto E, Mollejo M, Papadaki T, Remstein ED, Salar A, Solé F, Stamatopoulos K, Thieblemont C, Traverse-Glehen A, Wotherspoon A, Coiffier B, Piris MA (2008). Splenic marginal zone lymphoma proposals for a revision of diagnostic, staging and therapeutic criteria. Leukemia 22: 487-495.
1430. Matutes E, Owusu-Ankomah K, Morilla R, Garcia MJ, Houlihan A, Que TH, Catovsky D (1994). The immunological profile of B-cell disorders and proposal of a scoring system for the diagnosis of CLL. Leukemia 8: 1640-1645.
1431. Matutes E, Wotherspoon A, Catovsky D (2003). The variant form of hairy-cell leukaemia. Best Pract Res Clin Haematol 16: 41-56.
1432. Mauch P, Armitage JO, Diehl V (eds.) (1999). Hodgkin's Disease. Lippincott Williams & Wilkins: Philadelphia.
1433. Mauritzson N, Albin M, Rylander L, Billstrom R, Ahlgren T, Mikoczy Z, Bjork J, Stromberg U, Nilsson PG, Mitelman F, Hagmar L, Johansson B (2002). Pooled analysis of clinical and cytogenetic features in treatment-related and de novo adult acute myeloid leukemia and myelodysplastic syndromes based on a consecutive series of 761 patients analyzed 1976-1993 and on 5098 unselected cases reported in the literature 1974-2001. Leukemia 16: 2366-2378.
1434. Mazzaro C, Franzin F, Tulissi P, Pussini E, Crovatto M, Carniello GS, Efremov DG, Burrone O, Santini G, Pozzato G (1996). Regression of monoclonal B-cell expansion in patients affected by mixed cryoglobulinemia responsive to alpha-interferon therapy. Cancer 77: 2604-2613.
1435. Mc Lornan DP, Percy MJ, Jones AV, Cross NC, Mc Mullin MF (2005). Chronic neutrophilic leukemia with an associated V617F JAK2 tyrosine kinase mutation. Haematologica 90: 1696-1697.
1436. McClain KL, Leach CT, Jenson HB, Joshi VV, Pollock BH, Hutchison RE, Murphy SB (2000). Molecular and virologic characteristics of lymphoid malignancies in children with AIDS. J Acquir Immune Defic Syndr 23: 152-159.
1437. McClure RF, Dewald GW, Hoyer JD, Hanson CA (1999). Isolated isochromosome 17q: a distinct type of mixed myeloproliferative disorder/myelodysplastic syndrome with an aggressive clinical course. Br J Haematol 106: 445-454.
1438. McClure RF, Remstein ED, Macon WR, Dewald GW, Habermann TM, Hoering A, Kurtin PJ (2005). Adult B-cell lymphomas with burkitt-like morphology are phenotypically and genotypically heterogeneous with aggressive clinical behavior. Am J Surg Pathol 29: 1652-1660.
1438A. McDonnell TJ, Deane N, Platt FM, Nunez G, Jaeger U, McKearn JP, Korsmeyer SJ (1989). bcl-2-immunoglobulin transgenic mice demonstrate extended B cell survival and follicular lymphoproliferation. Cell 57: 79-88.
1439. McElwaine S, Mulligan C, Groet J, Spinelli M, Rinaldi A, Denyer G, Mensah A, Cavani S, Baldo C, Dagna-Bricarelli F, Hann I, Basso G, Cotter FE, Nizetic D (2004). Microarray transcript profiling distinguishes the transient from the acute type of megakaryoblastic leukaemia (M7) in Down's syndrome, revealing PRAME as a specific discriminating marker. Br J Haematol 125: 729-742.
1440. McGregor JM, Crook T, Fraser-Andrews EA, Rozycka M, Crossland S, Brooks L, Whittaker SJ (1999). Spectrum of p53 gene mutations suggests a possible role for ultraviolet radiation in the pathogenesis of advanced cutaneous lymphomas. J Invest Dermatol 112: 317-321.
1441. McKenna RW, Parkin J, Kersey JH, Gajl-Peczalska KJ, Peterson L, Brunning RD (1977). Chronic lymphoproliferative disorder

with unusual clinical, morphologic, ultrastructural and membrane surface marker characteristics. Am J Med 62: 588-596.
1442. McKenna RW, Washington LT, Aquino DB, Picker LJ, Kroft SH (2001). Immunophenotypic analysis of hematogones (B-lymphocyte precursors) in 662 consecutive bone marrow specimens by 4-color flow cytometry. Blood 98: 2498-2507.
1443. McLaughlin P, Fuller LM, Velasquez WS, Butler JJ, Hagemeister FB, Sullivan-Halley JA, Dixon DO (1987). Stage III follicular lymphoma: durable remissions with a combined chemotherapy-radiotherapy regimen. J Clin Oncol 5: 867-874.
1444. McManus DT, Catherwood MA, Carey PD, Cuthbert RJ, Alexander HD (2004). ALK-positive diffuse large B-cell lymphoma of the stomach associated with a clathrin-ALK rearrangement. Hum Pathol 35: 1285-1288.
1445. McMullin MF, Bareford D, Campbell P, Green AR, Harrison C, Hunt B, Oscier D, Polkey MI, Reilly JT, Rosenthal E, Ryan K, Pearson TC, Wilkins B (2005). Guidelines for the diagnosis, investigation and management of polycythaemia/erythrocytosis. Br J Haematol 130: 174-195.
1446. McNiff JM, Cooper D, Howe G, Crotty PL, Tallini G, Crouch J, Eisen RN (1996). Lymphomatoid granulomatosis of the skin and lung. An angiocentric T-cell-rich B-cell lymphoproliferative disorder. Arch Dermatol 132: 1464-1470.
1447. Mead AJ, Linch DC, Hills RK, Wheatley K, Burnett AK, Gale RE (2007). FLT3 tyrosine kinase domain mutations are biologically distinct from and have a significantly more favorable prognosis than FLT3 internal tandem duplications in patients with acute myeloid leukemia. Blood 110: 1262-1270.
1448. Medeiros LJ, Peiper SC, Elwood L, Yano T, Raffeld M, Jaffe ES (1991). Angiocentric immunoproliferative lesions: a molecular analysis of eight cases. Hum Pathol 22: 1150-1157.
1449. Meech SJ, McGavran L, Odom LF, Liang X, Meltesen L, Gump J, Wei Q, Carlsen S, Hunger SP (2001). Unusual childhood extramedullary hematologic malignancy with natural killer cell properties that contains tropomyosin 4—anaplastic lymphoma kinase gene fusion. Blood 98: 1209-1216.
1450. Meeker TC, Hardy D, Willman C, Hogan T, Abrams J (1990). Activation of the interleukin-3 gene by chromosome translocation in acute lymphocytic leukemia with eosinophilia. Blood 76: 285-289.
1450A. Mele A, Pulsoni A, Bianco E, Musto P, Szklo A, Sanpaolo MG, Iannitto E, De Renzo A, Martino B, Liso V, Andrizzi C, Pusterla S, Dore F, Maresca M, Rapicetta M, Marcucci F, Mandelli F, Franceschi S (2003). Hepatitis C virus and B-cell non-Hodgkin lymphomas: an Italian multicenter case-control study. Blood 102: 996-999.
1451. Melendez B, Diaz-Uriarte R, Cuadros M, Martinez-Ramirez A, Fernandez-Piqueras J, Dopazo A, Cigudosa JC, Rivas C, Dopazo J, Martinez-Delgado B, Benitez J (2004). Gene expression analysis of chromosomal regions with gain or loss of genetic material detected by comparative genomic hybridization. Genes Chromosomes Cancer 41: 353-365.
1452. Melnick A, Licht JD (1999). Deconstructing a disease: RARalpha, its fusion partners, and their roles in the pathogenesis of acute promyelocytic leukemia. Blood 93: 3167-3215.
1453. Melnyk A, Rodriguez A, Pugh WC, Cabanillas F (1997). Evaluation of the Revised European-American Lymphoma classification confirms the clinical relevance of immunophenotype in 560 cases of aggressive non-Hodgkin's lymphoma. Blood 89: 4514-4520.
1454. Melo JV (1996). The diversity of BCR-ABL fusion proteins and their relationship to leukemia phenotype. Blood 88: 2375-2384.
1455. Melo JV, Barnes DJ (2007). Chronic myeloid leukaemia as a model of disease evolution in human cancer. Nat Rev Cancer 7: 441-453.
1456. Melo JV, Catovsky D, Galton DA (1986). The relationship between chronic lymphocytic leukaemia and prolymphocytic leukaemia. I. Clinical and laboratory features of 300 patients and characterization of an intermediate group. Br J Haematol 63: 377-387.
1457. Melo JV, Hegde U, Parreira A, Thompson I, Lampert IA, Catovsky D (1987). Splenic B cell lymphoma with circulating villous lymphocytes: differential diagnosis of B cell leukaemias with large spleens. J Clin Pathol 40: 642-651.
1458. Melo JV, Myint H, Galton DA, Goldman JM (1994). P190BCR-ABL chronic myeloid leukaemia: the missing link with chronic myelomonocytic leukaemia? Leukemia 8: 208-211.
1459. Melzner I, Bucur AJ, Bruderlein S, Dorsch K, Hasel C, Barth TF, Leithauser F, Moller P (2005). Biallelic mutation of SOCS-1 impairs JAK2 degradation and sustains phospho-JAK2 action in the MedB-1 mediastinal lymphoma line. Blood 105: 2535-2542.
1459A. Melzner I, Weniger MA, Menz CK, Möller P (2006). Absence of the JAK2 V617F activating mutation in classical Hodgkin lymphoma and primary mediastinal B-cell lymphoma. Leukaemia 20: 157-158.
1460. Menke DM, Horny HP, Griesser H, Tiemann M, Katzmann JA, Kaiserling E, Parwaresch R, Kyle RA (2001). Primary lymph node plasmacytomas (plasmacytic lymphomas). Am J Clin Pathol 115: 119-126.
1461. Mercher T, Coniat MB, Monni R, Mauchauffe M, Nguyen KF, Gressin L, Mugneret F, Leblanc T, Dastugue N, Berger R, Bernard OA (2001). Involvement of a human gene related to the Drosophila spen gene in the recurrent t(1;22) translocation of acute megakaryocytic leukemia. Proc Natl Acad Sci U S A 98: 5776-5779.
1462. Merlini G, Stone MJ (2006). Dangerous small B-cell clones. Blood 108: 2520-2530.
1463. Mesa RA, Hanson CA, Rajkumar SV, Schroeder G, Tefferi A (2000). Evaluation and clinical correlations of bone marrow angiogenesis in myelofibrosis with myeloid metaplasia. Blood 96: 3374-3380.
1464. Mesa RA, Verstovsek S, Cervantes F, Barosi G, Reilly JT, Dupriez B, Levine R, Bousse-Kerdiles MC, Wadleigh M, Campbell PJ, Silver RT, Vannucchi AM, Deeg HJ, Gisslinger H, Thomas D, Odenike O, Solberg LA, Gotlib J, Hexner E, Nimer SD, Kantarjian H, Orazi A, Vardiman JW, Thiele J, Tefferi A (2007). Primary myelofibrosis (PMF), post polycythemia vera myelofibrosis (post-PV MF), post essential thrombocythemia myelofibrosis (post-ET MF), blast phase PMF (PMF-BP): Consensus on terminology by the international working group for myelofibrosis research and treatment (IWG-MRT). Leuk Res 31: 737-740.
1465. Metcalfe DD (1991). Classification and diagnosis of mastocytosis: current status. J Invest Dermatol 96: 2S-4S.
1466. Metcalfe DD (1991). The liver, spleen, and lymph nodes in mastocytosis. J Invest Dermatol 96: 45S-46S.
1467. Metchnikoff E (eds.) (1968). Lectures on the comparative pathology of inflammation. Reprint of the 1893 English translation. New York.
1467A. Metchnikoff E (1883). Untersuchungen uber die intracellulare Verdauung bei wirbellosen Thieren. Arb Zoologischen Inst Univ Wien 5: 141.
1468. Metter GE, Nathwani BN, Burke JS, Winberg CD, Mann RB, Barcos M, Kjeldsberg CR, Whitcomb CC, Dixon DO, Miller TP (1985). Morphological subclassification of follicular lymphoma: variability of diagnoses among hematopathologists, a collaborative study between the Repository Center and Pathology Panel for Lymphoma Clinical Studies. J Clin Oncol 3: 25-38.
1469. Metzgeroth G, Walz C, Score J, Siebert R, Schnittger S, Haferlach C, Popp H, Haferlach T, Erben P, Mix J, Muller MC, Beneke H, Muller L, Del Valle F, Aulitzky WE, Wittkowsky G, Schmitz N, Schulte C, Muller-Hermelink K, Hodges E, Whittaker SJ, Diecker F, Dohner H, Schuld P, Hehlmann R, Hochhaus A, Cross NC, Reiter A (2007). Recurrent finding of the FIP1L1-PDGFRA fusion gene in eosinophilia-associated acute myeloid leukemia and lymphoblastic T-cell lymphoma. Leukemia 21: 1183-1188.
1470. Meyer C, Schneider B, Jakob S, Strehl S, Attarbaschi A, Schnittger S, Schoch C, Jansen MW, van Dongen JJ, Den Boer ML, Pieters R, Ennas MG, Angelucci E, Koehl U, Greil J, Griesinger F, Zur Stadt U, Eckert C, Szczepanski T, Niggli FK, Schafer BW, Kempski H, Brady HJ, Zuna J, Trka J, Nigro LL, Biondi A, Delabesse E, Macintyre E, Stanulla M, Schrappe M, Haas OA, Burmeister T, Dingermann T, Klingebiel T, Marschalek R (2006). The MLL recombinome of acute leukemias. Leukemia 20: 777-784.
1471. Michaux JL, Martiat P (1993). Chronic myelomonocytic leukaemia (CMML)—a myelodysplastic or myeloproliferative syndrome? Leuk Lymphoma 9: 35-41.
1472. Michels SD, McKenna RW, Arthur DC, Brunning RD (1985). Therapy-related acute myeloid leukemia and myelodysplastic syndrome: a clinical and morphologic study of 65 cases. Blood 65: 1364-1372.
1473. Michiels JJ, van Genderen PJ, Lindemans J, van Vliet HH (1996). Erythromelalgic, thrombotic and hemorrhagic manifestations in 50 cases of thrombocythemia. Leuk Lymphoma 22 Suppl 1: 47-56.
1474. Michor F (2007). Chronic myeloid leukemia blast crisis arises from progenitors. Stem Cells 25: 1114-1118.
1475. Miettinen M, Fletcher CD, Lasota J (1993). True histiocytic lymphoma of small intestine. Analysis of two S-100 protein-positive cases with features of interdigitating reticulum cell sarcoma. Am J Clin Pathol 100: 285-292.
1476. Miettinen M, Franssila KO, Saxen E (1983). Hodgkin's disease, lymphocytic predominance nodular. Increased risk for subsequent non-Hodgkin's lymphomas. Cancer 51: 2293-2300.
1477. Miles DK, Freedman MH, Stephens K, Pallavicini M, Sievers EL, Weaver M, Grunberger T, Thompson P, Shannon KM (1996). Patterns of hematopoietic lineage involvement in children with neurofibromatosis type 1 and malignant myeloid disorders. Blood 88: 4314-4320.
1478. Miller TP, Grogan TM, Dahlberg S, Spier CM, Braziel RM, Banks PM, Foucar K, Kjeldsberg CR, Levy N, Nathwani BN (1994). Prognostic significance of the Ki-67-associated proliferative antigen in aggressive non-Hodgkin's lymphomas: a prospective Southwest Oncology Group trial. Blood 83: 1460-1466.
1479. Miller TP, Lippman SM, Spier CM, Slymen DJ, Grogan TM (1988). HLA-DR (Ia) immune phenotype predicts outcome for patients with diffuse large cell lymphoma. J Clin Invest 82: 370-372.
1479A. Mills J, et al (2008). A 44-year-old man with fatigue and lesions in the pituitary and cerebellum. N Engl J Med (in press)
1480. Minkov M, Grois N, Heitger A, Potschger U, Westermeier T, Gadner H (2002). Response to initial treatment of multisystem Langerhans cell histiocytosis: an important prognostic indicator. Med Pediatr Oncol 39: 581-585.
1481. Minkov M, Potschger U, Grois N, Gadner H, Dworzak MN (2007). Bone marrow assessment in Langerhans cell histiocytosis. Pediatr Blood Cancer 49: 694-698.
1482. Minkov M, Prosch H, Steiner M, Grois N, Potschger U, Kaatsch P, Janka-Schaub G, Gadner H (2005). Langerhans cell histiocytosis in neonates. Pediatr Blood Cancer 45: 802-807.
1483. Miralles GD, O'Fallon JR, Talley NJ (1992). Plasma-cell dyscrasia with polyneuropathy. The spectrum of POEMS syndrome. N Engl J Med 327: 1919-1923.
1484. Miranda RN, Esparza AR, Sambandam S, Medeiros LJ (1994). Systemic mast cell disease presenting with peripheral blood eosinophilia. Hum Pathol 25: 727-730.
1485. Mirza I, Macpherson N, Paproski S, Gascoyne RD, Yang B, Finn WG, Hsi ED (2002). Primary cutaneous follicular lymphoma: an assessment of clinical, histopathologic, immunophenotypic, and molecular features. J Clin Oncol 20: 647-655.
1486. Misdraji J, Fernandez dC, Ferry JA (1997). Follicle center lymphoma of the ampulla of Vater presenting with jaundice: report of a case. Am J Surg Pathol 21: 484-488.
1487. Mitelman F (1993). The cytogenetic scenario of chronic myeloid leukemia. Leuk Lymphoma 11 Suppl 1: 11-15.
1488. Mitelman F, Levan G, Nilsson PG, Brandt L (1976). Non-random karyotypic evolution in chronic myeloid leukemia. Int J Cancer 18: 24-30.
1489. Mitsiades CS, McMillin DW, Klippel S, Hideshima T, Chauhan D, Richardson PG, Munshi NC, Anderson KC (2007). The role of the bone marrow microenvironment in the pathophysiology of myeloma and its significance in the development of more effective therapies. Hematol Oncol Clin North Am 21: 1007-1034 vii-viii.
1490. Mittal K, Neri A, Feiner H, Schinella R, Alfonso F (1990). Lymphomatoid granulomatosis in the acquired immunodeficiency syndrome. Evidence of Epstein-Barr virus infection and B-cell clonal selection without myc rearrangement. Cancer 65: 1345-1349.
1491. Mitus AJ, Stein R, Rappeport JM, Antin JH, Weinstein HJ, Alper CA, Smith BR (1989). Monoclonal and oligoclonal gammopathy after bone marrow transplantation. Blood 74: 2764-2768.
1492. Miwa H, Takakuwa T, Nakatsuka S, Tomita Y, Iuchi K, Aozasa K (2002). DNA sequences of the immunoglobulin heavy chain variable region gene in pyothorax-associated lymphoma. Oncology 62: 241-250.
1493. Miyazaki Y, Kuriyama K, Miyawaki S, Ohtake S, Sakamaki H, Matsuo T, Emi N, Kobayashi T, Matsushima T, Shinagawa K, Ohno R, Tomonaga M (2003). Cytogenetic heterogeneity of acute myeloid leukaemia (AML) with trilineage dysplasia: Japan Adult Leukaemia Study Group-AML 92 study. Br J Haematol 120: 56-62.
1494. Moldenhauer G, Popov SW, Wotschke B, Bruderlein S, Riedl P, Fissolo N, Schirmbeck R, Ritz O, Moller P, Leithauser F (2006). AID expression identifies interfollicular large B cells as putative precursors of mature B-cell malignancies. Blood 107: 2470-2473.
1495. Molina A, Lombard C, Donlon T, Bangs

CD, Dorfman RF (1990). Immunohistochemical and cytogenetic studies indicate that malignant angioendotheliomatosis is a primary intravascular (angiotropic) lymphoma. Cancer 66: 474-479.
1495A. Mollejo M, Algara P, Mateo MS, Menárguez J, Pascual E, Fresno MF, Camacho FI, Piris MA (2003). Large B-cell lymphoma presenting in the spleen: identification of different clinicopathologic conditions. Am J Surg Pathol 27: 895-902.
1496. Mollejo M, Algara P, Mateo MS, Sanchez-Beato M, Lloret E, Medina MT, Piris MA (2002). Splenic small B-cell lymphoma with predominant red pulp involvement: a diffuse variant of splenic marginal zone lymphoma? Histopathology 40: 22-30.
1497. Mollejo M, Menarguez J, Lloret E, Sanchez A, Campo E, Algara P, Cristobal E, Sanchez E, Piris MA (1995). Splenic marginal zone lymphoma: a distinctive type of low-grade B-cell lymphoma. A clinicopathological study of 13 cases. Am J Surg Pathol 19: 1146-1157.
1498. Moller P, Herrmann B, Moldenhauer G, Momburg F (1987). Defective expression of MHC class I antigens is frequent in B-cell lymphomas of high-grade malignancy. Int J Cancer 40: 32-39.
1499. Moller P, Lammler B, Eberlein-Gonska M, Feichter GE, Hofmann WJ, Schmitteckert H, Otto HF (1986). Primary mediastinal clear cell lymphoma of B-cell type. Virchows Arch A Pathol Anat Histopathol 409: 79-92.
1500. Moller P, Moldenhauer G, Momburg F, Lammler B, Eberlein-Gonska M, Kiesel S, Dorken B (1987). Mediastinal lymphoma of clear cell type is a tumor corresponding to terminal steps of B cell differentiation. Blood 69: 1087-1095.
1501. Monda L, Warnke R, Rosai J (1986). A primary lymph node malignancy with features suggestive of dendritic reticulum cell differentiation. A report of 4 cases. Am J Pathol 122: 562-572.
1502. Montalban C, Santon A, Boixeda D, Redondo C, Alvarez I, Calleja JL, de Argila CM, Bellas C (2001). Treatment of low grade gastric mucosa-associated lymphoid tissue lymphoma in stage I with Helicobacter pylori eradication. Long-term results after sequential histologic and molecular follow-up. Haematologica 86: 609-617.
1503. Montesinos-Rongen M, Kuppers R, Schluter D, Spieker T, Van Roost D, Schaller C, Reifenberger G, Wiestler OD, Deckert-Schluter M (1999). Primary central nervous system lymphomas are derived from germinal-center B cells and show a preferential usage of the V4-34 gene segment. Am J Pathol 155: 2077-2086.
1504. Montesinos-Rongen M, Roers A, Kuppers R, Rajewsky K, Hansmann ML (1999). Mutation of the p53 gene is not a typical feature of Hodgkin and Reed-Sternberg cells in Hodgkin's disease. Blood 94: 1755-1760.
1505. Montesinos-Rongen M, Van Roost D, Schaller C, Wiestler OD, Deckert M (2004). Primary diffuse large B-cell lymphomas of the central nervous system are targeted by aberrant somatic hypermutation. Blood 103: 1869-1875.
1506. Monteverde A, Sabattini E, Poggi S, Ballare M, Bertoncelli MC, de Vivo A, Briskomatis A, Roncador G, Falini B, Pileri SA (1995). Bone marrow findings further support the hypothesis that essential mixed cryoglobulinemia type II is characterized by a monoclonal B-cell proliferation. Leuk Lymphoma 20: 119-124.
1507. Monti S, Savage KJ, Kutok JL, Feuerhake F, Kurtin P, Mihm M, Wu B, Pasqualucci L, Neuberg D, Aguiar RC, Dal Cin P, Ladd C, Pinkus GS, Salles G, Harris NL, Dalla-Favera R, Habermann TM, Aster JC, Golub TR, Shipp MA (2005). Molecular profiling of diffuse large B-cell lymphoma identifies robust subtypes including one characterized by host inflammatory response. Blood 105: 1851-1861.
1508. Montoto S, Lopez-Guillermo A, Colomer D, Esteve J, Bosch F, Ferrer A, Villamor N, Moreno C, Campo E, Montserrat E (2003). Incidence and clinical significance of bcl-2/IgH rearrangements in follicular lymphoma. Leuk Lymphoma 44: 71-76.
1509. Montserrat E, Villamor N, Reverter JC, Brugues RM, Tassies D, Bosch F, Aguilar JL, Vives-Corrons JL, Rozman M, Rozma C (1996). Bone marrow assessment in B-cell chronic lymphocytic leukaemia: aspirate or biopsy? A comparative study in 258 patients. Br J Haematol 93: 111-116.
1510. Moorman AV, Richards SM, Robinson HM, Strefford JC, Gibson BE, Kinsey SE, Eden TO, Vora AJ, Mitchell CD, Harrison CJ (2007). Prognosis of children with acute lymphoblastic leukemia (ALL) and intrachromosomal amplification of chromosome 21 (iAMP21). Blood 109: 2327-2330.
1511. Moreau EJ, Matutes E, A'Hern RP, Morilla AM, Morilla RM, Owusu-Ankomah KA, Seon BK, Catovsky D (1997). Improvement of the chronic lymphocytic leukemia scoring system with the monoclonal antibody SN8 (CD79b). Am J Clin Pathol 108: 378-382.
1512. Morel P, Lepage E, Brice P, Dupriez B, d'Agay MF, Fenaux P, Gosselin B, Bauters F, Gisselbrecht C (1992). Prognosis and treatment of lymphoblastic lymphoma in adults: a report on 80 patients. J Clin Oncol 10: 1078-1085.
1513. Morerio C, Acquila M, Rosanda C, Rapella A, Dufour C, Locatelli F, Maserati E, Pasquali F, Panarello C (2004). HCMOGT-1 is a novel fusion partner to PDGFRB in juvenile myelomonocytic leukemia with t(5;17)(q33;p11.2). Cancer Res 64: 2649-2651.
1514. Mori H, Colman SM, Xiao Z, Ford AM, Healy LE, Donaldson C, Hows JM, Navarrete C, Greaves M (2002). Chromosome translocations and covert leukemic clones are generated during normal fetal development. Proc Natl Acad Sci U S A 99: 8242-8247.
1515. Mori N, Yamashita Y, Tsuzuki T, Nakayama A, Nakazawa M, Hasegawa Y, Kojima H, Nagasawa T (2000). Lymphomatous features of aggressive NK cell leukaemia/lymphoma with massive necrosis, haemophagocytosis and EB virus infection. Histopathology 37: 363-371.
1516. Mori N, Yatabe Y, Narita M, Kobayashi T, Asai J (1996). Pyothorax-associated lymphoma. An unusual case with biphenotypic character of T and B cells. Am J Surg Pathol 20: 760-766.
1517. Morice WG (2007). The immunophenotypic attributes of NK cells and NK-cell lineage lymphoproliferative disorders. Am J Clin Pathol 127: 881-886.
1518. Morice WG, Hodnefield JM, Kurtin PJ, Hanson CA (2004). An unusual case of leukemic mantle cell lymphoma with a blastoid component showing loss of CD5 and aberrant expression of CD10. Am J Clin Pathol 122: 122-127.
1519. Morice WG, Jevremovic D, Hanson CA (2007). The expression of the novel cytotoxic protein granzyme M by large granular lymphocytic leukaemias of both T-cell and NK-cell lineage: an unexpected finding with implications regarding the pathobiology of these disorders. Br J Haematol 137: 237-239.
1520. Morice WG, Kurtin PJ, Leibson PJ, Tefferi A, Hanson CA (2003). Demonstration of aberrant T-cell and natural killer-cell antigen expression in all cases of granular lymphocytic leukaemia. Br J Haematol 120: 1026-1036.
1521. Morice WG, Kurtin PJ, Tefferi A, Hanson CA (2002). Distinct bone marrow findings in T-cell granular lymphocytic leukemia revealed by paraffin section immunoperoxidase stains for CD8, TIA-1, and granzyme B. Blood 99: 268-274.
1522. Morice WG, Macon WR, Dogan A, Hanson CA, Kurtin PJ (2006). NK-cell-associated receptor expression in hepatosplenic T-cell lymphoma, insights into pathogenesis. Leukemia 20: 883-886.
1523. Morice WG, Rodriguez FJ, Hoyer JD, Kurtin PJ (2005). Diffuse large B-cell lymphoma with distinctive patterns of splenic and bone marrow involvement: clinicopathologic features of two cases. Mod Pathol 18: 495-502.
1524. Morra E, Cesana C, Klersy C, Varettoni M, Cavanna L, Canesi B, Tresoldi E, Barbarano L, Lazzarino M (2003). Predictive variables for malignant transformation in 452 patients with asymptomatic IgM monoclonal gammopathy. Semin Oncol 30: 172-177.
1525. Morris SW, Kirstein MN, Valentine MB, Dittmer KG, Shapiro DN, Saltman DL, Look AT (1994). Fusion of a kinase gene, ALK, to a nucleolar protein gene, NPM, in non-Hodgkin's lymphoma. Science 263: 1281-1284.
1525A. Morton LM, Wang SS, Devesa SS, Hartge P, Weisenburger DD, Linet MS (2006). Lymphoma incidence patterns by WHO subtype in the United States, 1992-2001. Blood 107: 265-276.
1526. Moskowitz CH, Zelenetz AD, Kewalramani T, Hamlin P, Lessac-Chenen S, Houldsworth J, Olshen A, Chaganti R, Nimer S, Teruya-Feldstein J (2005). Cell of origin, germinal center versus nongerminal center, determined by immunohistochemistry on tissue microarray, does not correlate with outcome in patients with relapsed and refractory DLBCL. Blood 106: 3383-3385.
1527. Mossuz P, Girodon F, Donnard M, Latger-Cannard V, Dobo I, Boiret N, Lecron JC, Binquet C, Barro C, Hermouet S, Praloran V (2004). Diagnostic value of serum erythropoietin level in patients with absolute erythrocytosis. Haematologica 89: 1194-1198.
1528. Mounier N, Briere J, Gisselbrecht C, Emile JF, Lederlin P, Sebban C, Berger F, Bosly A, Morel P, Tilly H, Bouabdallah R, Reyes F, Gaulard P, Coiffier B (2003). Rituximab plus CHOP (R-CHOP) overcomes bcl-2—associated resistance to chemotherapy in elderly patients with diffuse large B-cell lymphoma (DLBCL). Blood 101: 4279-4284.
1529. Mounier N, Briere J, Gisselbrecht C, Reyes F, Gaulard P, Coiffier B (2006). Estimating the impact of rituximab on bcl-2-associated resistance to CHOP in elderly patients with diffuse large B-cell lymphoma. Haematologica 91: 715-716.
1529A. Mourad N, Mounier N, Briere J, Raffoux E, Delmer A, Feller A, Meijer CJ, Emile JF, Bouabdallah R, Bosly A, Diebold J, Haioun C, Coiffier B, Gisselbrecht C, Gaulard P (2008). Clinical, biological and pathological features in 157 patients with angioimmunoblastic T-cell lymphoma treated within the Groupe d'Etude des Lymphomes de l'Adulte (GELA) trials. Blood 111: 4463-4470..
1530. Mrózek K, Heinonen K, de la Chapelle A, Bloomfield CD (1997). Clinical significance of cytogenetics in acute myeloid leukemia. Semin Oncol 24: 17-31.
1531. Mrózek K, Heinonen K, Lawrence D, Carroll AJ, Koduru PR, Rao KW, Strout MP, Hutchison RE, Moore JO, Mayer RJ, Schiffer CA, Bloomfield CD (1997). Adult patients with de novo acute myeloid leukemia and t(9; 11)(p22; q23) have a superior outcome to patients with other translocations involving band 11q23: a cancer and leukemia group B study. Blood 90: 4532-4538.
1531A. Mrózek K, Bloomfield CD (2006). Chromosome aberrations, gene mutations and expression changes, and prognosis in adult acute myeloid leukemia. Hematology Am Soc Hematol Educ Program: 169-77
1532. Mrózek K, Marcucci G, Paschka P, Whitman SP, Bloomfield CD (2007). Clinical relevance of mutations and gene-expression changes in adult acute myeloid leukemia with normal cytogenetics: are we ready for a prognostically prioritized molecular classification? Blood 109: 431-448.
1533. Mrózek K, Prior TW, Edwards C, Marcucci G, Carroll AJ, Snyder PJ, Koduru PR, Theil KS, Pettenati MJ, Archer KJ, Caligiuri MA, Vardiman JW, Kolitz JE, Larson RA, Bloomfield CD (2001). Comparison of cytogenetic and molecular genetic detection of t(8;21) and inv(16) in a prospective series of adults with de novo acute myeloid leukemia: a Cancer and Leukemia Group B Study. J Clin Oncol 19: 2482-2492.
1534. Muehleck SD, McKenna RW, Arthur DC, Parkin JL, Brunning RD (1984). Transformation of chronic myelogenous leukemia: clinical, morphologic, and cytogenetic features. Am J Clin Pathol 82: 1-14.
1535. Mueller NC, Grufferman (1999). The epidemiology of Hodgkin's disease. In: Hodgkin's Disease. Mauch P, Armitage JO, Diehl V, eds. Lippincott Williams & Wilkins: Philadelphia, pp. 61.
1536. Mufti GJ (2004). Pathobiology, classification, and diagnosis of myelodysplastic syndrome. Best Pract Res Clin Haematol 17: 543-557.
1537. Mullaney BP, Ng VL, Herndier BG, McGrath MS, Pallavicini MG (2000). Comparative genomic analyses of primary effusion lymphoma. Arch Pathol Lab Med 124: 824-826.
1538. Mulligan SP, Matutes E, Dearden C, Catovsky D (1991). Splenic lymphoma with villous lymphocytes: natural history and response to therapy in 50 cases. Br J Haematol 78: 206-209.
1539. Mullighan CG, Kennedy A, Zhou X, Radtke I, Phillips LA, Shurtleff SA, Downing JR (2007). Pediatric acute myeloid leukemia with NPM1 mutations is characterized by a gene expression profile with dysregulated HOX gene expression distinct from MLL-rearranged leukemias. Leukemia 21: 2000-2009.
1540. Munn SE, McGregor JM, Jones A, Amlot P, Rustin MH, Russell JR, Whittaker S (1996). Clinical and pathological heterogeneity in cutaneous gamma-delta T-cell lymphoma: a report of three cases and a review of the literature. Br J Dermatol 135: 976-981.
1540A. Munshi NC, Digumarthy S, Rahermtullah A (2008). Case 13-2008 - A 46-year old man with rheumatoid arthritis and lymphadenopathy. N Engl J Med 358: 1838-1848.
1541. Munoz L, Nomdedeu JF, Villamor N, Guardia R, Colomer D, Ribera JM, Torres JP, Berlanga JJ, Fernandez C, Llorente A, Queipo de Llano MP, Sanchez JM, Brunet S, Sierra J (2003). Acute myeloid leukemia with MLL rearrangements: clinicobiological features, prognostic impact and value of flow cytometry in the detection of residual leukemic cells. Leukemia 17: 76-82.
1542. Murakami I, Gogusev J, Fournet JC, Glorion C, Jaubert F (2002). Detection of molecular cytogenetic aberrations in langerhans cell histiocytosis of bone. Hum Pathol 33: 555-560.
1543. Muramatsu M, Akasaka T, Kadowaki N, Ohno H, Fukuhara S, Okuma M (1997). Rearrangement of the BCL6 gene in B-cell lymphoid neoplasms. Leukemia 11 Suppl 3: 318-320.
1544. Murase T, Nakamura S, Kawauchi K,

Matsuzaki H, Sakai C, Inaba T, Nasu K, Tashiro K, Suchi T, Saito H (2000). An Asian variant of intravascular large B-cell lymphoma: clinical, pathological and cytogenetic approaches to diffuse large B-cell lymphoma associated with haemophagocytic syndrome. Br J Haematol 111: 826-834.

1545. Murase T, Yamaguchi M, Suzuki R, Okamoto M, Sato Y, Tamaru J, Kojima M, Miura I, Mori N, Yoshino T, Nakamura S (2007). Intravascular large B-cell lymphoma (IVLBCL): a clinicopathologic study of 96 cases with special reference to the immunophenotypic heterogeneity of CD5. Blood 109: 478-485.

1546. Muris JJ, Cillessen SA, Vos W, van Houdt IS, Kummer JA, Van Krieken JH, Jiwa NM, Jansen PM, Kluin-Nelemans HC, Ossenkoppele GJ, Gundy C, Meijer CJ, Oudejans JJ (2005). Immunohistochemical profiling of caspase signaling pathways predicts clinical response to chemotherapy in primary nodal diffuse large B-cell lymphomas. Blood 105: 2916-2923.

1547. Muris JJ, Meijer CJ, Vos W, Van Krieken JH, Jiwa NM, Ossenkoppele GJ, Oudejans JJ (2006). Immunohistochemical profiling based on Bcl-2, CD10 and MUM1 expression improves risk stratification in patients with primary nodal diffuse large B cell lymphoma. J Pathol 208: 714-723.

1548. Murphy S (1999). Diagnostic criteria and prognosis in polycythemia vera and essential thrombocythemia. Semin Hematol 36: 9-13.

1549. Murphy S, Peterson P, Iland H, Laszlo J (1997). Experience of the Polycythemia Vera Study Group with essential thrombocythemia: a final report on diagnostic criteria, survival, and leukemic transition by treatment. Semin Hematol 34: 29-39.

1550. Murphy SB (1978). Childhood non-Hodgkin's lymphoma. N Engl J Med 299: 1446-1448.

1551. Murphy SB, Hustu HO (1980). A randomized trial of combined modality therapy of childhood non-Hodgkin's lymphoma. Cancer 45: 630-637.

1552. Murray A, Cuevas EC, Jones DB, Wright DH (1995). Study of the immunohistochemistry and T cell clonality of enteropathy-associated T cell lymphoma. Am J Pathol 146: 509-519.

1553. Muschen M, Rajewsky K, Brauninger A, Baur AS, Oudejans JJ, Roers A, Hansmann ML, Kuppers R (2000). Rare occurrence of classical Hodgkin's disease as a T cell lymphoma. J Exp Med 191: 387-394.

1554. Nachman JB, Heerema NA, Sather H, Camitta B, Forestier E, Harrison CJ, Dastugue N, Schrappe M, Pui CH, Basso G, Silverman LB, Janka-Schaub GE (2007). Outcome of treatment in children with hypodiploid acute lymphoblastic leukemia. Blood 110: 1112-1115.

1555. Nador RG, Cesarman E, Chadburn A, Dawson DB, Ansari MQ, Sald J, Knowles DM (1996). Primary effusion lymphoma: a distinct clinicopathologic entity associated with the Kaposi's sarcoma-associated herpes virus. Blood 88: 645-656.

1556. Nador RG, Chadburn A, Gundappa G, Cesarman E, Said JW, Knowles DM (2003). Human immunodeficiency virus (HIV)-associated polymorphic lymphoproliferative disorders. Am J Surg Pathol 27: 293-302.

1557. Nagata H, Worobec AS, Oh CK, Chowdhury BA, Tannenbaum S, Suzuki Y, Metcalfe DD (1995). Identification of a point mutation in the catalytic domain of the protooncogene c-kit in peripheral blood mononuclear cells of patients who have mastocytosis with an associated hematologic disorder. Proc Natl Acad Sci U S A 92: 10560-10564.

1558. Nair C, Chopra H, Shinde S, Barbhaya S, Kumar A, Dhond S, Yejamanam B, Sapre R, Chougule A, Advani S (1995). Immunophenotype and ultrastructural studies in blast crisis of chronic myeloid leukemia. Leuk Lymphoma 19: 309-313.

1559. Najean Y, Triebel F, Dresch C (1981). Pure erythrocytosis: reappraisal of a study of 51 cases. Am J Hematol 10: 129-136.

1560. Nakajima Y, Waku M, Kojima A, Sato Y, Miyanaga S (1996). [Prognosis of the surgical treatment for non-Hodgkin lymphoma originating from chronic tuberculous empyema—analysis of 11 cases with pleuropneumonectomy]. Nippon Kyobu Geka Gakkai Zasshi 44: 484-492.

1561. Nakamura F, Tatsumi E, Tani K, Kumagai S, Kosaka Y, Sano K, Nakamura H, Nesumi N, Abe T, Koiwai O (1996). Coexpression of cell-surface immunoglobulin (sIg), terminal deoxynucleotidyl transferase (TdT) and recombination activating gene 1 (RAG-1): two cases and derived cell lines. Leukemia 10: 1159-1163.

1561A. Nakamura N, Ohshima K, Abe M, Osamura Y (2007). Demonstration of chimeric DNA of bcl-2 and immunoglobulin heavy chain in follicular lymphoma and subsequent Hodgkin lymphoma from the same patient. J Clin Exp Hematop 47: 9-13.

1562. Nakamura S, Aoyagi K, Furuse M, Suekane H, Matsumoto T, Yao T, Sakai Y, Fuchigami T, Yamamoto I, Tsuneyoshi M, Fujishima M (1998). B-cell monoclonality precedes the development of gastric MALT lymphoma in Helicobacter pylori-associated chronic gastritis. Am J Pathol 152: 1271-1279.

1563. Nakamura S, Hara K, Suchi T, Ito M, Ikeda H, Nagahama M, Nakayama A, Nakagawa A, Kaneshima H, Asai J (1988). Interdigitating cell sarcoma. A morphologic, immunohistologic, and enzyme-histochemical study. Cancer 61: 562-568.

1564. Nakamura S, Koshikawa T, Kitoh K, Nakayama A, Yamakawa M, Imai Y, Ishii K, Fujita M, Suchi T (1994). Interdigitating cell sarcoma: a morphologic and immunologic study of lymph node lesions in four cases. Pathol Int 44: 374-386.

1565. Nakamura S, Shiota M, Nakagawa A, Yatabe Y, Kojima M, Motoori T, Suzuki R, Kagami Y, Ogura M, Morishima Y, Mizoguchi Y, Okamoto M, Seto M, Koshikawa T, Mori S, Suchi T (1997). Anaplastic large cell lymphoma: a distinct molecular pathologic entity: a reappraisal with special reference to p80(NPM/ALK) expression. Am J Surg Pathol 21: 1420-1432.

1566. Nakamura S, Yao T, Aoyagi K, Iida M, Fujishima M, Tsuneyoshi M (1997). Helicobacter pylori and primary gastric lymphoma. A histopathologic and immunohistochemical analysis of 237 patients. Cancer 79: 3-11.

1567. Nakashima Y, Tagawa H, Suzuki R, Karnan S, Karube K, Ohshima K, Muta K, Nawata H, Morishima Y, Nakamura S, Seto M (2005). Genome-wide array-based comparative genomic hybridization of natural killer cell lymphoma/leukemia: different genomic alteration patterns of aggressive NK-cell leukemia and extranodal Nk/T-cell lymphoma, nasal type. Genes Chromosomes Cancer 44: 247-255.

1568. Nakatsuka S, Yao M, Hoshida Y, Yamamoto S, Iuchi K, Aozasa K (2002). Pyothorax-associated lymphoma: a review of 106 cases. J Clin Oncol 20: 4255-4260.

1569. Nalesnik MA, Jaffe R, Starzl TE, Demetris AJ, Porter K, Burnham JA, Makowka L, Ho M, Locker J (1988). The pathology of posttransplant lymphoproliferative disorders occurring in the setting of cyclosporine A-prednisone immunosuppression. Am J Pathol 133: 173-192.

1570. Nalesnik MA, Randhawa P, Demetris AJ, Casavilla A, Fung JJ, Locker J (1993). Lymphoma resembling Hodgkin disease after posttransplant lymphoproliferative disorder in a liver transplant recipient. Cancer 72: 2568-2573.

1571. Narducci MG, Scala E, Bresin A, Caprini E, Picchio MC, Remotti D, Ragone G, Nasorri F, Frontani M, Arcelli D, Volinia S, Lombardo GA, Baliva G, Napolitano M, Russo G (2006). Skin homing of Sezary cells involves SDF-1-CXCR4 signaling and down-regulation of CD26/dipeptidylpeptidase IV. Blood 107: 1108-1115.

1572. Narimatsu H, Ota Y, Kami M, Takeuchi K, Suzuki R, Matsuo K, Matsumura T, Yuji K, Kishi Y, Hamaki T, Sawada U, Miyata S, Sasaki T, Tobinai K, Kawabata M, Atsuta Y, Tanaka Y, Ueda R, Nakamura S (2007). Clinicopathological features of pyothorax-associated lymphoma; a retrospective survey involving 98 patients. Ann Oncol 18: 122-128.

1573. Narumi H, Kojima K, Matsuo Y, Shikata H, Sekiya K, Niiya T, Bando S, Niiya H, Azuma T, Yakushijin Y, Sakai I, Yasukawa M, Fujita S (2004). T-cell large granular lymphocytic leukemia occurring after autologous peripheral blood stem cell transplantation. Bone Marrow Transplant 33: 99-101.

1574. Nascimento AF, Pinkus JL, Pinkus GS (2004). Clusterin, a marker for anaplastic large cell lymphoma immunohistochemical profile in hematopoietic and nonhematopoietic malignant neoplasms. Am J Clin Pathol 121: 709-717.

1575. Nash R, McSweeney P, Zambello R, Semenzato G, Loughran TP, Jr. (1993). Clonal studies of CD3- lymphoproliferative disease of granular lymphocytes. Blood 81: 2363-2368.

1576. Nash RA, Dansey R, Storek J, Georges GE, Bowen JD, Holmberg LA, Kraft GH, Mayes MD, McDonagh KT, Chen CS, Dipersio J, Lemaistre CF, Pavletic S, Sullivan KM, Sunderhaus J, Furst DE, McSweeney PA (2003). Epstein-Barr virus-associated post-transplantation lymphoproliferative disorder after high-dose immunosuppressive therapy and autologous CD34-selected hematopoietic stem cell transplantation for severe autoimmune diseases. Biol Blood Marrow Transplant 9: 583-591.

1577. Nathwani BN, Anderson JR, Armitage JO, Cavalli F, Diebold J, Drachenberg MR, Harris NL, MacLennan KA, Muller-Hermelink HK, Ullrich FA, Weisenburger DD (1999). Clinical significance of follicular lymphoma with monocytoid B cells. Non-Hodgkin's Lymphoma Classification Project. Hum Pathol 30: 263-268.

1578. Nathwani BN, Anderson JR, Armitage JO, Cavalli F, Diebold J, Drachenberg MR, Harris NL, MacLennan KA, Muller-Hermelink HK, Ullrich FA, Weisenburger DD (1999). Marginal zone B-cell lymphoma: A clinical comparison of nodal and mucosa-associated lymphoid tissue types. Non-Hodgkin's Lymphoma Classification Project. J Clin Oncol 17: 2486-2492.

1579. Nathwani BN, Metter GE, Miller TP, Burke JS, Mann RB, Barcos M, Kjeldsberg CR, Dixon DO, Winberg CD, Whitcomb CC (1986). What should be the morphologic criteria for the subdivision of follicular lymphomas? Blood 68: 837-845.

1580. Natkunam Y, Farinha P, Hsi ED, Hans CP, Tibshirani R, Sehn LH, Connors JM, Gratzinger D, Rosado M, Zhao S, Pohlman B, Wongchaowart N, Bast M, Avigdor A, Schiby G, Nagler A, Byrne GE, Levy R, Gascoyne RD, Lossos IS (2008). LMO2 protein expression predicts survival in patients with diffuse large B-cell lymphoma treated with anthracycline-based chemotherapy with and without rituximab. J Clin Oncol 26: 447-454.

1581. Natkunam Y, Warnke RA, Haghighi B, Su LD, Le Boit PE, Kim YH, Kohler S (2000). Co-expression of CD56 and CD30 in lymphomas with primary presentation in the skin: clinicopathologic, immunohistochemical and molecular analyses of seven cases. J Cutan Pathol 27: 392-399.

1582. Nava VE, Jaffe ES (2005). The pathology of NK-cell lymphomas and leukemias. Adv Anat Pathol 12: 27-34.

1582A. Navarro JT, Ribera JM, Mate JL, Granada I, Juncà J, Batlle M, Millá F, Feliu E (2003). Hepatosplenic T-gammadelta lymphoma in a patient with Crohn's disease treated with azathioprine. Leuk Lymphoma 44: 531-533.

1583. Navas IC, Ortiz-Romero PL, Villuendas R, Martinez P, Garcia C, Gomez E, Rodriguez JL, Garcia D, Vanaclocha F, Iglesias L, Piris MA, Algara P (2000). p16(INK4a) gene alterations are frequent in lesions of mycosis fungoides. Am J Pathol 156: 1565-1572.

1584. Navid F, Mosijczuk AD, Head DR, Borowitz MJ, Carroll AJ, Brandt JM, Link MP, Rozans MK, Thomas GA, Schwenn MR, Shields DJ, Vietti TJ, Pullen DJ (1999). Acute lymphoblastic leukemia with the (8;14)(q24;q32) translocation and FAB L3 morphology associated with a B-precursor immunophenotype: the Pediatric Oncology Group experience. Leukemia 13: 135-141.

1585. Neiman RS, Rosen PJ, Lukes RJ (1973). Lymphocyte-depletion Hodgkin's disease. A clinicopathological entity. N Engl J Med 288: 751-755.

1586. Nelson BP, Nalesnik MA, Bahler DW, Locker J, Fung JJ, Swerdlow SH (2000). Epstein-Barr virus-negative post-transplant lymphoproliferative disorders: a distinct entity? Am J Surg Pathol 24: 375-385.

1587. Neubauer A, Thiede C, Morgner A, Alpen B, Ritter M, Neubauer B, Wundisch T, Ehninger G, Stolte M, Bayerdorffer E (1997). Cure of Helicobacter pylori infection and duration of remission of low-grade gastric mucosa-associated lymphoid tissue lymphoma. J Natl Cancer Inst 89: 1350-1355.

1588. Neuwirtova R, Mocikova K, Musilova J, Jelinek J, Havlicek F, Michalova K, Adamkov M (1996). Mixed myelodysplastic and myeloproliferative syndromes. Leuk Res 20: 717-726.

1589. Ng CS, Lo ST, Chan JK, Chan WC (1997). CD56+ putative natural killer cell lymphomas: production of cytolytic effectors and related proteins mediating tumor cell apoptosis? Hum Pathol 28: 1276-1282.

1590. Ng SB, Lai KW, Murugaya S, Lee KM, Loong SL, Fook-Chong S, Tao M, Sng I (2004). Nasal-type extranodal natural killer/T-cell lymphomas: a clinicopathologic and genotypic study of 42 cases in Singapore. Mod Pathol 17: 1097-1107.

1591. Nguyen DT, Diamond LW, Hansmann ML, Hell K, Fischer R (1994). Follicular dendritic cell sarcoma. Identification by monoclonal antibodies in paraffin sections. Appl Immunohistochem 2: 60-64.

1592. Ni H, Barosi G, Rondelli D, Hoffman R (2005). Studies of the site and distribution of CD34+ cells in idiopathic myelofibrosis. Am J Clin Pathol 123: 833-839.

1593. Nicholls PK, Stanley MA (2000). The immunology of animal papillomaviruses. Vet Immunol Immunopathol 73: 101-127.

1594. Nichols CR, Roth BJ, Heerema N, Griep J, Tricot G (1990). Hematologic neoplasia associated with primary mediastinal germ-cell tumors. N Engl J Med 322: 1425-1429.

1595. Niemeyer CM, Arico M, Basso G, Biondi A, Cantu RA, Creutzig U, Haas O, Harbott J, Hasle H, Kerndrup G, Locatelli F, Mann G, Stollmann-Gibbels B, Veer-Korthof ET, van Wering E, Zimmermann M (1997).

Chronic myelomonocytic leukemia in childhood: a retrospective analysis of 110 cases. European Working Group on Myelodysplastic Syndromes in Childhood (EWOG-MDS). Blood 89: 3534-3543.
1595A. Niemeyer CM, Baumann I (2008). Myelodysplastic syndrome in children and adolescents. Semin Hematol 45: 60-70.
1596. Niemeyer CM, Fenu S, Hasle H, Mann G, Stary J, van Wering E (1998). Responce: Differentiating juvenile myelomonocytic leukemia from infectious disease. Blood 91: 365-366.
1597. Nieters A, Kallinowski B, Brennan P, Ott M, Maynadie M, Benavente Y, Foretova L, Cocco PL, Staines A, Vornanen M, Whitby D, Boffetta P, Becker N, De Sanjose S (2006). Hepatitis C and risk of lymphoma: results of the European multicenter case-control study EPI-LYMPH. Gastroenterology 131: 1879-1886.
1598. Niitsu N, Okamoto M, Nakamura N, Nakamine H, Aoki S, Hirano M, Miura I (2007). Prognostic impact of chromosomal alteration of 3q27 on nodal B-cell lymphoma: correlation with histology, immunophenotype, karyotype, and clinical outcome in 329 consecutive patients. Leuk Res 31: 1191-1197.
1599. Nishiu M, Tomita Y, Nakatsuka S, Takakuwa T, Iizuka N, Hoshida Y, Ikeda J, Iuchi K, Yanagawa R, Nakamura Y, Aozasa K (2004). Distinct pattern of gene expression in pyothorax-associated lymphoma (PAL), a lymphoma developing in long-standing inflammation. Cancer Sci 95: 828-834.
1600. Nitta Y, Iwatsuki K, Kimura H, Kojima S, Morishima T, Tsuji K, Oono T (2005). Fatal natural killer cell lymphoma arising in a patient with a crop of Epstein-Barr virus-associated disorders. Eur J Dermatol 15: 503-506.
1601. Nizze H, Cogliatti SB, von Schilling C, Feller AC, Lennert K (1991). Monocytoid B-cell lymphoma: morphological variants and relationship to low-grade B-cell lymphoma of the mucosa-associated lymphoid tissue. Histopathology 18: 403-414.
1602. Nodit L, Bahler DW, Jacobs SA, Locker J, Swerdlow SH (2003). Indolent mantle cell lymphoma with nodal involvement and mutated immunoglobulin heavy chain genes. Hum Pathol 34: 1030-1034.
1603. Nogova L, Reineke T, Brillant C, Sieniawski M, Rudiger T, Josting A, Bredenfeld H, Skripnitchenko R, Muller RP, Muller-Hermelink HK, Diehl V, Engert A (2008). Lymphocyte-predominant and classical Hodgkin's lymphoma: a comprehensive analysis from the German Hodgkin Study Group. J Clin Oncol 26: 434-439.
1604. Nonami A, Yokoyama T, Takeshita M, Ohshima K, Kubota A, Okamura S (2004). Human herpes virus 8-negative primary effusion lymphoma (PEL) in a patient after repeated chylous ascites and chylothorax. Intern Med 43: 236-242.
1605. Norton AJ, Matthews J, Pappa V, Shamash J, Love S, Rohatiner AZ, Lister TA (1995). Mantle cell lymphoma: natural history defined in a serially biopsied population over a 20-year period. Ann Oncol 6: 249-256.
1606. Notarangelo L, Casanova JL, Conley ME, Chapel H, Fischer A, Puck J, Roifman C, Seger R, Geha RS (2006). Primary immunodeficiency diseases: an update from the International Union of Immunological Societies Primary Immunodeficiency Diseases Classification Committee Meeting in Budapest, 2005. J Allergy Clin Immunol 117: 883-896.
1607. Nowell PC, Hungerford DA (1960). A minutre chromosome in human chronic granulocytic leukemia. Science 132: 1497-1500.
1608. Nowicki MO, Pawlowski P, Fischer T, Hess G, Pawlowski T, Skorski T (2003). Chronic myelogenous leukemia molecular signature. Oncogene 22: 3952-3963.
1609. Nucifora G, Laricchia-Robbio L, Senyuk V (2006). EVI1 and hematopoietic disorders: history and perspectives. Gene 368: 1-11.
1609A. Nunez G, London L, Hockenbery D, Alexander M, McKearn JP, Korsmeyer SJ (1990). Deregulated Bcl-2 gene expression selectively prolongs survival of growth factor-deprived hemopoietic cell lines. J Immunol 144: 3602-3610.
1610. Nyman H, Adde M, Karjalainen-Lindsberg ML, Taskinen M, Berglund M, Amini RM, Blomqvist C, Enblad G, Leppa S (2007). Prognostic impact of immunohistochemically defined germinal center phenotype in diffuse large B-cell lymphoma patients treated with immunochemotherapy. Blood 109: 4930-4935.
1611. O'Briain DS, Kennedy MJ, Daly PA, O'Brien AA, Tanner WA, Rogers P, Lawlor E (1989). Multiple lymphomatous polyposis of the gastrointestinal tract. A clinicopathologically distinctive form of non-Hodgkin's lymphoma of B-cell centrocytic type. Am J Surg Pathol 13: 691-699.
1612. O'Conor GT (1963). Significant aspects of childhood lymphoma in Africa. Cancer Res 23: 1514-1518.
1613. O'Malley DP, Kim YS, Perkins SL, Baldridge L, Juliar BE, Orazi A (2005). Morphologic and immunohistochemical evaluation of splenic hematopoietic proliferations in neoplastic and benign disorders. Mod Pathol 18: 1550-1561.
1614. O'Malley DP, Vance GH, Orazi A (2005). Chronic lymphocytic leukemia/small lymphocytic lymphoma with trisomy 12 and focal cyclin d1 expression: a potential diagnostic pitfall. Arch Pathol Lab Med 129: 92-95.
1615. O'Neil J, Shank J, Cusson N, Murre C, Kelliher M (2004). TAL1/SCL induces leukemia by inhibiting the transcriptional activity of E47/HEB. Cancer Cell 5: 587-596.
1616. O'Shea JJ, Jaffe ES, Lane HC, MacDermott RP, Fauci AS (1987). Peripheral T cell lymphoma presenting as hypereosinophilia with vasculitis. Clinical, pathologic, and immunologic features. Am J Med 82: 539-545.
1617. Ocio EM, Schop RF, Gonzalez B, Van Wier SA, Hernandez-Rivas JM, Gutierrez NC, Garcia-Sanz R, Moro MJ, Aguilera C, Hernandez J, Xu R, Greipp PR, Dispenzieri A, Jalal SM, Lacy MQ, Gonzalez-Paz N, Gertz MA, San Miguel JF, Fonseca R (2007). 6q deletion in Waldenstrom macroglobulinemia is associated with features of adverse prognosis. Br J Haematol 136: 80-86.
1618. Ocqueteau M, Orfao A, Almeida J, Blade J, Gonzalez M, Garcia-Sanz R, Lopez-Berges C, Moro MJ, Hernandez J, Escribano L, Caballero D, Rozman M, San Miguel JF (1998). Immunophenotypic characterization of plasma cells from monoclonal gammopathy of undetermined significance patients. Implications for the differential diagnosis between MGUS and multiple myeloma. Am J Pathol 152: 1655-1665.
1619. Odame I, Li P, Lau L, Doda W, Noseworthy M, Babyn P, Weitzman S (2006). Pulmonary Langerhans cell histiocytosis: a variable disease in childhood. Pediatr Blood Cancer 47: 889-893.
1620. Offit K, Lo CF, Louie DC, Parsa NZ, Leung D, Portlock C, Ye BH, Lista F, Filippa DA, Rosenbaum A (1994). Rearrangement of the bcl-6 gene as a prognostic marker in diffuse large-cell lymphoma. N Engl J Med 331: 74-80.
1621. Offit K, Parsa NZ, Gaidano G, Filippa DA, Louie D, Pan D, Jhanwar SC, Dalla-Favera R, Chaganti RS (1993). 6q deletions define distinct clinico-pathologic subsets of non-Hodgkin's lymphoma. Blood 82: 2157-2162.
1622. Ogata K, Kishikawa Y, Satoh C, Tamura H, Dan K, Hayashi A (2006). Diagnostic application of flow cytometric characteristics of CD34+ cells in low-grade myelodysplastic syndromes. Blood 108: 1037-1044.
1623. Ogata K, Nakamura K, Yokose N, Tamura H, Tachibana M, Taniguchi O, Iwakiri R, Hayashi T, Sakamaki H, Murai Y, Tohyama K, Tomoyasu S, Nonaka Y, Mori M, Dan K, Yoshida Y (2002). Clinical significance of phenotypic features of blasts in patients with myelodysplastic syndrome. Blood 100: 3887-3896.
1624. Ohmine K, Ota J, Ueda M, Ueno S, Yoshida K, Yamashita Y, Kirito K, Imagawa S, Nakamura Y, Saito K, Akutsu M, Mitani K, Kano Y, Komatsu N, Ozawa K, Mano H (2001). Characterization of stage progression in chronic myeloid leukemia by DNA microarray with purified hematopoietic stem cells. Oncogene 20: 8249-8257.
1625. Ohnishi H, Kandabashi K, Maeda Y, Kawamura M, Watanabe T (2006). Chronic eosinophilic leukaemia with FIP1L1-PDGFRA fusion and T6741 mutation that evolved from Langerhans cell histiocytosis with eosinophilia after chemotherapy. Br J Haematol 134: 547-549.
1626. Ohno H, Fukuhara S (1997). Significance of rearrangement of the BCL6 gene in B-cell lymphoid neoplasms. Leuk Lymphoma 27: 53-63.
1627. Ohno T, Stribley JA, Wu G, Hinrichs SH, Weisenburger DD, Chan WC (1997). Clonality in nodular lymphocyte-predominant Hodgkin's disease. N Engl J Med 337: 459-465.
1628. Ohno Y, Amakawa R, Fukuhara S, Huang CR, Kamesaki H, Amano H, Imanaka T, Takahashi Y, Arita Y, Uchiyama T (1989). Acute transformation of chronic large granular lymphocyte leukemia associated with additional chromosome abnormality. Cancer 64: 63-67.
1629. Ohsawa M, Tomita Y, Kanno H, Iuchi K, Kawabata Y, Nakajima Y, Komatsu H, Mukai K, Shimoyama M, Aozasa K (1995). Role of Epstein-Barr virus in pleural lymphomagenesis. Mod Pathol 8: 848-853.
1630. Ohshima K (2007). Pathological features of diseases associated with human T-cell leukemia virus type I. Cancer Sci 98: 772-778.
1631. Ohshima K, Mukai Y, Shiraki H, Suzumiya J, Tashiro K, Kikuchi M (1997). Clonal integration and expression of human T-cell lymphotropic virus type I in carriers detected by polymerase chain reaction and inverse PCR. Am J Hematol 54: 306-312.
1632. Ohshima K, Suzumiya J, Kato A, Tashiro K, Kikuchi M (1997). Clonal HTLV-I-infected CD4+ T-lymphocytes and non-clonal non-HTLV-I-infected giant cells in incipient ATLL with Hodgkin-like histologic features. Int J Cancer 72: 592-598.
1633. Ohshima K, Suzumiya J, Sato K, Kanda M, Simazaki T, Kawasaki C, Haraoka S, Kikuchi M (1999). Survival of patients with HTLV-I-associated lymph node lesions. J Pathol 189: 539-545.
1634. Ohshima K, Suzumiya J, Shimazaki K, Kato A, Tanaka T, Kanda M, Kikuchi M (1997). Nasal T/NK cell lymphomas commonly express perforin and Fas ligand: important mediators of tissue damage. Histopathology 31: 444-450.
1635. Okamura T, Kinukawa N, Niho Y, Mizoguchi H (2001). Primary chronic myelofibrosis: clinical and prognostic evaluation in 336 Japanese patients. Int J Hematol 73: 194-198.
1636. Okano M, Matsumoto S, Osato T, Sakiyama Y, Thiele GM, Purtilo DT (1991). Severe chronic active Epstein-Barr virus infection syndrome. Clin Microbiol Rev 4: 129-135.
1637. Oki Y, Kantarjian HM, Zhou X, Cortes J, Faderl S, Verstovsek S, O'Brien S, Koller C, Beran M, Bekele BN, Pierce S, Thomas D, Ravandi F, Wierda WG, Giles F, Ferrajoli A, Jabbour E, Keating MJ, Bueso-Ramos CE, Estey E, Garcia-Manero G (2006). Adult acute megakaryocytic leukemia: an analysis of 37 patients treated at M.D. Anderson Cancer Center. Blood 107: 880-884.
1638. Oksenhendler E, Boulanger E, Galicier L, Du MQ, Dupin N, Diss TC, Hamoudi R, Daniel MT, Agbalika F, Boshoff C, Clauvel JP, Isaacson PG, Meignin V (2002). High incidence of Kaposi sarcoma-associated herpesvirus-related non-Hodgkin lymphoma in patients with HIV infection and multicentric Castleman disease. Blood 99: 2331-2336.
1639. Okuda T, Sakamoto S, Deguchi T, Misawa S, Kashima K, Yoshihara T, Ikushima S, Hibi S, Imashuku S (1991). Hemophagocytic syndrome associated with aggressive natural killer cell leukemia. Am J Hematol 38: 321-323.
1640. Okun DB, Tanaka KR (1978). Leukocyte alkaline phosphatase. Am J Hematol 4: 293-299.
1641. Olney HJ, Le Beau MM (2007). Evaluation of recurring cytogenetic abnormalities in the treatment of myelodysplastic syndromes. Leuk Res 31: 427-434.
1642. Olsen E, Vonderheid E, Pimpinelli N, Willemze R, Kim Y, Knobler R, Zackheim H, Duvic M, Estrach T, Lamberg S, Wood G, Dummer R, Ranki A, Burg G, Heald P, Pittelkow M, Bernengo MG, Sterry W, Laroche L, Trautinger F, Whittaker S (2007). Revisions to the staging and classification of mycosis fungoides and Sezary syndrome: a proposal of the International Society for Cutaneous Lymphomas (ISCL) and the cutaneous lymphoma task force of the European Organization of Research and Treatment of Cancer (EORTC). Blood 110: 1713-1722.
1643. Olteanu H, Wang HY, Chen W, McKenna RW, Karandikar NJ (2007). Immunophenotypic identification of high-risk monoclonal gammopathy of undetermined significance. Mod Pathol 20: 255A.
1644. Onciu M, Behm FG, Downing JR, Shurtleff SA, Raimondi SC, Ma Z, Morris SW, Kennedy W, Jones SC, Sandlund JT (2003). ALK-positive plasmablastic B-cell lymphoma with expression of the NPM-ALK fusion transcript: report of 2 cases. Blood 102: 2642-2644.
1645. Onida F, Kantarjian HM, Smith TL, Ball G, Keating MJ, Estey EH, Glassman AB, Albitar M, Kwari MI, Beran M (2002). Prognostic factors and scoring systems in chronic myelomonocytic leukemia: a retrospective analysis of 213 patients. Blood 99: 840-849.
1646. Opelz G, Dohler B (2004). Lymphomas after solid organ transplantation: a collaborative transplant study report. Am J Transplant 4: 222-230.
1647. Orazi A (2007). Histopathology in the diagnosis and classification of acute myeloid leukemia, myelodysplastic syndromes, and myelodysplastic/myeloproliferative diseases. Pathobiology 74: 97-114.
1648. Orazi A, Albitar M, Heerema NA, Haskins S, Neiman RS (1997). Hypoplastic myelodysplastic syndromes can be distinguished from acquired aplastic anemia by CD34 and PCNA immunostaining of bone marrow biopsy specimens. Am J Clin Pathol 107: 268-274.
1649. Orazi A, Chiu R, O'Malley DP, Czader M, Allen SL, An C, Vance GH (2006). Chronic myelomonocytic leukemia: The role of bone marrow biopsy immunohistology. Mod Pathol 19: 1536-1545.
1650. Orazi A, Neiman RS, Cualing H, Heerema NA, John K (1994). CD34 immunostaining of bone marrow biopsy specimens is a reliable way to classify the phases of chronic myeloid leukemia. Am J Clin Pathol 101: 426-428.
1651. Orazi A, O'Malley DP, Jiang J, Vance

GH, Thomas J, Czader M, Fang W, An C, Banks PM (2005). Acute panmyelosis with myelofibrosis: an entity distinct from acute megakaryoblastic leukemia. Mod Pathol 18: 603-614.

1652. Orchard J, Garand R, Davis Z, Babbage G, Sahota S, Matutes E, Catovsky D, Thomas PW, Avet-Loiseau H, Oscier D (2003). A subset of t(11;14) lymphoma with mantle cell features displays mutated IgVH genes and includes patients with good prognosis, nonnodal disease. Blood 101: 4975-4981.

1653. Orchard JA, Ibbotson RE, Davis Z, Wiestner A, Rosenwald A, Thomas PW, Hamblin TJ, Staudt LM, Oscier DG (2004). ZAP-70 expression and prognosis in chronic lymphocytic leukaemia. Lancet 363: 105-111.

1654. Orfao A, Chillon MC, Bortoluci AM, Lopez-Berges MC, Garcia-Sanz R, Gonzalez M, Tabernero MD, Garcia-Marcos MA, Rasillo AI, Hernandez-Rivas J, San Miguel JF (1999). The flow cytometric pattern of CD34, CD15 and CD13 expression in acute myeloblastic leukemia is highly characteristic of the presence of PML-RARalpha gene rearrangements. Haematologica 84: 405-412.

1655. Orfao A, Escribano L, Villarrubia J, Velasco JL, Cervero C, Ciudad J, Navarro JL, San Miguel JF (1996). Flow cytometric analysis of mast cells from normal and pathological human bone marrow samples: identification and enumeration. Am J Pathol 149: 1493-1499.

1656. Orfao A, Garcia-Montero AC, Sanchez L, Escribano L (2007). Recent advances in the understanding of mastocytosis: the role of KIT mutations. Br J Haematol 138: 12-30.

1656A. Ortonne N, Dupuis J, Plonquet A, Martin N, Copie-Bergman C, Bagot M, Delfau-Larue MH, Gaulier A, Haioun C, Wechsler J, Gaulard P (2007). Characterization of CXCL13+ neoplastic t cells in cutaneous lesions of angioimmunoblastic T-cell lymphoma (AITL). Am J Surg Pathol 31: 1068-1076.

1657. Osborne BM, Butler JJ, Gresik MV (1992). Progressive transformation of germinal centers: comparison of 23 pediatric patients to the adult population. Mod Pathol 5: 135-140.

1658. Oscier DG, Thompsett A, Zhu D, Stevenson FK (1997). Differential rates of somatic hypermutation in V(H) genes among subsets of chronic lymphocytic leukemia defined by chromosomal abnormalities. Blood 89: 4153-4160.

1659. Oshimi K (1996). Lymphoproliferative disorders of natural killer cells. Int J Hematol 63: 279-290.

1660. Oshimi K (2007). Progress in understanding and managing natural killer-cell malignancies. Br J Haematol 139: 532-544.

1661. Oshimi K, Yamada O, Kaneko T, Nishinarita S, Iizuka Y, Urabe A, Inamori T, Asano S, Takahashi S, Hattori M (1993). Laboratory findings and clinical courses of 33 patients with granular lymphocyte-proliferative disorders. Leukemia 7: 782-788.

1662. Osuji N, Beiske K, Randen U, Matutes E, Tjonnfjord G, Catovsky D, Wotherspoon A (2007). Characteristic appearances of the bone marrow in T-cell large granular lymphocyte leukaemia. Histopathology 50: 547-554.

1663. Osuji N, Matutes E, Catovsky D, Lampert I, Wotherspoon A (2005). Histopathology of the spleen in T-cell large granular lymphocyte leukemia and T-cell prolymphocytic leukemia: a comparative review. Am J Surg Pathol 29: 935-941.

1664. Osuji N, Matutes E, Tjonnfjord G, Grech H, Del G, I, Wotherspoon A, Swansbury JG, Catovsky D (2006). T-cell large granular lymphocyte leukemia: A report on the treatment of 29 patients and a review of the literature. Cancer 107: 570-578.

1665. Otsuki T, Kumar S, Ensoli B, Kingma DW, Yano T, Stetler-Stevenson M, Jaffe ES, Raffeld M (1996). Detection of HHV-8/KSHV DNA sequences in AIDS-associated extranodal lymphoid malignancies. Leukemia 10: 1358-1362.

1666. Ott G, Kalla J, Ott MM, Schryen B, Katzenberger T, Muller JG, Muller-Hermelink HK (1997). Blastoid variants of mantle cell lymphoma: frequent bcl-1 rearrangements at the major translocation cluster region and tetraploid chromosome clones. Blood 89: 1421-1429.

1667. Ott G, Katzenberger T, Greiner A, Kalla J, Rosenwald A, Heinrich U, Ott MM, Muller-Hermelink HK (1997). The t(11;18)(q21;q21) chromosome translocation is a frequent and specific aberration in low-grade but not high-grade malignant non-Hodgkin's lymphomas of the mucosa-associated lymphoid tissue (MALT-) type. Cancer Res 57: 3944-3948.

1668. Ott G, Katzenberger T, Lohr A, Kindelberger S, Rudiger T, Wilhelm M, Kalla J, Rosenwald A, Muller JG, Ott MM, Muller-Hermelink HK (2002). Cytomorphologic, immunohistochemical, and cytogenetic profiles of follicular lymphoma: 2 types of follicular lymphoma grade 3. Blood 99: 3806-3812.

1669. Ott MM, Rosenwald A, Katzenberger T, Dreyling M, Krumdiek AK, Kalla J, Greiner A, Ott G, Muller-Hermelink HK (2000). Marginal zone B-cell lymphomas (MZBL) arising at different sites represent different biological entities. Genes Chromosomes Cancer 28: 380-386.

1670. Ottensmeier CH, Thompsett AR, Zhu D, Wilkins BS, Sweetenham JW, Stevenson FK (1998). Analysis of VH genes in follicular and diffuse lymphoma shows ongoing somatic mutation and multiple isotype transcripts in early disease with changes during disease progression. Blood 91: 4292-4299.

1671. Owaidah TM, Al Beihany A, Iqbal MA, Elkum N, Roberts GT (2006). Cytogenetics, molecular and ultrastructural characteristics of biphenotypic acute leukemia identified by the EGIL scoring system. Leukemia 20: 620-626.

1672. Owen RG, Barrans SL, Richards SJ, O'Connor SJ, Child JA, Parapia LA, Morgan GJ, Jack AS (2001). Waldenstrom macroglobulinemia. Development of diagnostic criteria and identification of prognostic factors. Am J Clin Pathol 116: 420-428.

1673. Owen RG, Treon SP, Al Katib A, Fonseca R, Greipp PR, McMaster ML, Morra E, Pangalis GA, San Miguel JF, Branagan AR, Dimopoulos MA (2003). Clinicopathological definition of Waldenstrom's macroglobulinemia: consensus panel recommendations from the Second International Workshop on Waldenstrom's Macroglobulinemia. Semin Oncol 30: 110-115.

1674. Oyama T, Ichimura K, Suzuki R, Suzumiya J, Ohshima K, Yatabe Y, Yokoi T, Kojima M, Kamiya Y, Taji H, Kagami Y, Ogura M, Saito H, Morishima Y, Nakamura S (2003). Senile EBV+ B-cell lymphoproliferative disorders: a clinicopathologic study of 22 patients. Am J Surg Pathol 27: 16-26.

1675. Oyama T, Yamamoto K, Asano N, Oshiro A, Suzuki R, Kagami Y, Morishima Y, Takeuchi K, Izumo T, Mori S, Ohshima K, Suzumiya J, Nakamura N, Abe M, Ichimura K, Sato Y, Yoshino T, Naoe T, Shimoyama Y, Kamiya K, Kinoshita T, Nakamura S (2007). Age-related EBV-associated B-cell lymphoproliferative disorders constitute a distinct clinicopathologic group: a study of 96 patients. Clin Cancer Res 13: 5124-5132.

1676. Oyarzo MP, Lin P, Glassman A, Bueso-Ramos CE, Luthra R, Medeiros LJ (2004). Acute myeloid leukemia with t(6;9)(p23;q34) is associated with dysplasia and a high frequency of flt3 gene mutations. Am J Clin Pathol 122:

348-358.

1677. Paietta E, Ferrando AA, Neuberg D, Bennett JM, Racevskis J, Lazarus H, Dewald G, Rowe JM, Wiernik PH, Tallman MS, Look AT (2004). Activating FLT3 mutations in CD117/KIT(+) T-cell acute lymphoblastic leukemias. Blood 104: 558-560.

1678. Paietta E, Goloubeva O, Neuberg D, Bennett JM, Gallagher R, Racevskis J, Dewald G, Wiernik PH, Tallman MS (2004). A surrogate marker profile for PML/RAR alpha expressing acute promyelocytic leukemia and the association of immunophenotypic markers with morphologic and molecular subtypes. Cytometry B Clin Cytom 59: 1-9.

1679. Paietta E, Racevskis J, Neuberg D, Rowe JM, Goldstone AH, Wiernik PH (1997). Expression of CD25 (interleukin-2 receptor alpha chain) in adult acute lymphoblastic leukemia predicts for the presence of BCR/ABL fusion transcripts: results of a preliminary laboratory analysis of ECOG/MRC Intergroup Study E2993. Eastern Cooperative Oncology Group/Medical Research Council. Leukemia 11: 1887-1890.

1680. Pal S, Sullivan DG, Kim S, Lai KK, Kae J, Cotler SJ, Carithers RL, Jr., Wood BL, Perkins JD, Gretch DR (2006). Productive replication of hepatitis C virus in perihepatic lymph nodes in vivo: implications of HCV lymphotropism. Gastroenterology 130: 1107-1116.

1681. Palutke M, Tabaczka P, Mirchandani I, Goldfarb S (1981). Lymphocytic lymphoma simulating hairy cell leukemia: a consideration of reliable and unreliable diagnostic features. Cancer 48: 2047-2055.

1682. Panani AD (2006). Cytogenetic findings in untreated patients with essential thrombocythemia. In Vivo 20: 381-384.

1683. Pandolfi F, Loughran TP, Jr., Starkebaum G, Chisesi T, Barbui T, Chan WC, Brouet JC, De Rossi G, McKenna RW, Salsano F (1990). Clinical course and prognosis of the lymphoproliferative disease of granular lymphocytes. A multicenter study. Cancer 65: 341-348.

1684. Pane F, Frigeri F, Camera A, Sindona M, Brighel F, Martinelli V, Luciano L, Selleri C, Del Vecchio L, Rotoli B, Salvatore F (1996). Complete phenotypic and genotypic lineage switch in a Philadelphia chromosome-positive acute lymphoblastic leukemia. Leukemia 10: 741-745.

1685. Pane F, Frigeri F, Sindona M, Luciano L, Ferrara F, Cimino R, Meloni G, Saglio G, Salvatore F, Rotoli B (1996). Neutrophilic-chronic myeloid leukemia: a distinct disease with a specific molecular marker (BCR/ABL with C3/A2 junction). Blood 88: 2410-2414.

1686. Paquette RL, Landaw EM, Pierre RV, Kahan J, Lubbert M, Lazcano O, Isaac G, McCormick F, Koeffler HP (1993). N-ras mutations are associated with poor prognosis and increased risk of leukemia in myelodysplastic syndrome. Blood 82: 590-599.

1687. Pardanani A, Akin C, Valent P (2006). Pathogenesis, clinical features, and treatment advances in mastocytosis. Best Pract Res Clin Haematol 19: 595-615.

1688. Pardanani A, Brockman SR, Paternoster SF, Flynn HC, Ketterling RP, Lasho TL, Ho CL, Li CY, Dewald GW, Tefferi A (2004). FIP1L1-PDGFRA fusion: prevalence and clinicopathologic correlates in 89 consecutive patients with moderate to severe eosinophilia. Blood 104: 3038-3045.

1689. Pardanani AD, Levine RL, Lasho T, Pikman Y, Mesa RA, Wadleigh M, Steensma DP, Elliott MA, Wolanskyj AP, Hogan WJ, McClure RF, Litzow MR, Gilliland DG, Tefferi A (2006). MPL515 mutations in myeloproliferative and other myeloid disorders: a study of 1182 patients. Blood 108: 3472-3476.

1690. Park S, Lee J, Ko YH, Han A, Jun HJ, Lee SC, Hwang IG, Park YH, Ahn JS, Jung CW, Kim K, Ahn YC, Kang WK, Park K, Kim WS (2007). The impact of Epstein-Barr virus status on clinical outcome in diffuse large B-cell lymphoma. Blood 110: 972-978.

1690A. Parkin DM, Pisani P, Ferlay J (1999). Global cancer statistics. CA Cancer J Clin 49: 33-64.

1691. Parkin JL, Arthur DC, Abramson CS, McKenna RW, Kersey JH, Heideman RL, Brunning RD (1982). Acute leukemia associated with the t(4;11) chromosome rearrangement: ultrastructural and immunologic characteristics. Blood 60: 1321-1331.

1692. Parreira L, Tavares dC, Hibbin JA, Marsh JC, Marcus RE, Babapulle VB, Spry CJ, Goldman JM, Catovsky D (1986). Chromosome and cell culture studies in eosinophilic leukaemia. Br J Haematol 62: 659-669.

1693. Parry-Jones N, Matutes E, Morilla R, Brito-Babapulle V, Wotherspoon A, Swansbury GJ, Catovsky D (2007). Cytogenetic abnormalities additional to t(11;14) correlate with clinical features in leukaemic presentation of mantle cell lymphoma, and may influence prognosis: a study of 60 cases by FISH. Br J Haematol 137: 117-124.

1694. Parwaresch MR, Horny HP, Lennert K (1985). Tissue mast cells in health and disease. Pathol Res Pract 179: 439-461.

1695. Pascal V, Schleinitz N, Brunet C, Ravet S, Bonnet E, Lafarge X, Touinssi M, Reviron D, Viallard JF, Moreau JF, Dechanet-Merville J, Blanco P, Harle JR, Sampol J, Vivier E, Dignat-George F, Paul P (2004). Comparative analysis of NK cell subset distribution in normal and lymphoproliferative disease of granular lymphocyte conditions. Eur J Immunol 34: 2930-2940.

1696. Paschka P, Marcucci G, Ruppert AS, Mrózek K, Chen H, Kittles RA, Vukosavljevic T, Perrotti D, Vardiman JW, Carroll AJ, Kolitz JE, Larson RA, Bloomfield CD (2006). Adverse prognostic significance of KIT mutations in adult acute myeloid leukemia with inv(16) and t(8;21): a Cancer and Leukemia Group B Study. J Clin Oncol 24: 3904-3911.

1696A. Paschka P, Marcucci G, Ruppert AS, Whitman SP, Mrózek K, Maharry K, Langer C, Baldus CD, Zhao W, Powell BL, Baer MR, Carroll AJ, Caligiuri MA, Kolitz JE, Larson RA, Bloomfield CD (2008). Wilms tumor 1 gene mutations independently predict poor outcome in adults with cytogenetically normal acute leukemia: A Cancer and Leukemia Group B study. J Clin Oncol, in press.

1697. Pasqualetti P, Festuccia V, Collacciani A, Casale R (1997). The natural history of monoclonal gammopathy of undetermined significance. A 5- to 20-year follow-up of 263 cases. Acta Haematol 97: 174-179.

1698. Pasqualucci L, Liso A, Martelli MP, Bolli N, Pacini R, Tabarrini A, Carini M, Bigerna B, Pucciarini A, Mannucci R, Nicoletti I, Tiacci E, Meloni G, Specchia G, Cantore N, Di Raimondo F, Pileri S, Mecucci C, Mandelli F, Martelli MF, Falini B (2006). Mutated nucleophosmin detects clonal multilineage involvement in acute myeloid leukemia: Impact on WHO classification. Blood 108: 4146-4155.

1698A. Pasqualucci L, Migliazza A, Fracchiolla N, William C, Neri A, Baldini L, Chaganti RS, Klein U, Kuppers R, Rajewsky K, Dalla-Favera R (1998). BCL-6 mutations in normal germinal center B cells: evidence of somatic hypermutation acting outside Ig loci. Proc Natl Acad Sci USA 95: 11816-11821.

1699. Pasqualucci L, Neumeister P, Goossens T, Nanjangud G, Chaganti RS, Kuppers R, Dalla-Favera R (2001). Hypermutation of multiple proto-oncogenes in B-cell diffuse large-cell lymphomas. Nature

412: 341-346.
1700. Passamonti F, Malabarba L, Orlandi E, Barate C, Canevari A, Brusamolino E, Bonfichi M, Arcaini L, Caberlon S, Pascutto C, Lazzarino M (2003). Polycythemia vera in young patients: a study on the long-term risk of thrombosis, myelofibrosis and leukemia. Haematologica 88: 13-18.
1701. Passamonti F, Rumi E, Arcaini L, Castagnola C, Lunghi M, Bernasconi P, Giovanni Della PM, Columbo N, Pascutto C, Cazzola M, Lazzarino M (2005). Leukemic transformation of polycythemia vera: a single center study of 23 patients. Cancer 104: 1032-1036.
1702. Passamonti F, Rumi E, Pungolino E, Malabarba L, Bertazzoni P, Valentini M, Orlandi E, Arcaini L, Brusamolino E, Pascutto C, Cazzola M, Morra E, Lazzarino M (2004). Life expectancy and prognostic factors for survival in patients with polycythemia vera and essential thrombocythemia. Am J Med 117: 755-761.
1703. Passamonti F, Vanelli L, Malabarba L, Rumi E, Pungolino E, Malcovati L, Pascutto C, Morra E, Lazzarino M, Cazzola M (2003). Clinical utility of the absolute number of circulating CD34-positive cells in patients with chronic myeloproliferative disorders. Haematologica 88: 1123-1129.
1704. Passmore SJ, Chessells JM, Kempski H, Hann IM, Brownbill PA, Stiller CA (2003). Paediatric myelodysplastic syndromes and juvenile myelomonocytic leukaemia in the UK: a population-based study of incidence and survival. Br J Haematol 121: 758-767.
1705. Passmore SJ, Hann IM, Stiller CA, Ramani P, Swansbury GJ, Gibbons B, Reeves BR, Chessells JM (1995). Pediatric myelodysplasia: a study of 68 children and a new prognostic scoring system. Blood 85: 1742-1750.
1706. Patel BB, Mohamed AN, Schiffer CA (2006). "Acute myelogenous leukemia like" translocations in CML blast crisis: two new cases of inv(16)/t(16;16) and a review of the literature. Leuk Res 30: 225-232.
1707. Patsalides AD, Atac G, Hedge U, Janik J, Grant N, Jaffe ES, Dwyer A, Patronas NJ, Wilson WH (2005). Lymphomatoid granulomatosis: abnormalities of the brain at MR imaging. Radiology 237: 265-273.
1708. Patte C, Auperin A, Gerrard M, Michon J, Pinkerton R, Sposto R, Weston C, Raphael M, Perkins SL, McCarthy K, Cairo MS (2007). Results of the randomized international FAB/LMB96 trial for intermediate risk B-cell non-Hodgkin lymphoma in children and adolescents: it is possible to reduce treatment for the early responding patients. Blood 109: 2773-2780.
1709. Paul C, Le Tourneau A, Cayuela JM, Devidas A, Robert C, Molinie V, Dubertret L (1997). Epstein-Barr virus-associated lymphoproliferative disease during methotrexate therapy for psoriasis. Arch Dermatol 133: 867-871.
1710. Paulli M, Berti E (2004). Cutaneous T-cell lymphomas (including rare subtypes). Current concepts. II. Haematologica 89: 1372-1388.
1711. Paulli M, Berti E, Rosso R, Boveri E, Kindl S, Klersy C, Lazzarino M, Borroni G, Menestrina F, Santucci M (1995). CD30/Ki-1-positive lymphoproliferative disorders of the skin—clinicopathologic correlation and statistical analysis of 86 cases: a multicentric study from the European Organization for Research and Treatment of Cancer Cutaneous Lymphoma Project Group. J Clin Oncol 13: 1343-1354.
1712. Paulli M, Strater J, Gianelli U, Rousset MT, Gambacorta M, Orlandi E, Klersy C, Lavabre-Bertrand T, Morra E, Manegold C, Lazzarino M, Magrini U, Moller P (1999). Mediastinal B-cell lymphoma: a study of its histomorphologic spectrum based on 109 cases. Hum Pathol 30: 178-187.
1713. Pawson R, Matutes E, Brito-Babapulle V, Maljaie H, Hedges M, Mercieca J, Dyer M, Catovsky D (1997). Sezary cell leukaemia: a distinct T cell disorder or a variant form of T prolymphocytic leukaemia? Leukemia 11: 1009-1013.
1714. Pearson MG, Vardiman JW, Le Beau MM, Rowley JD, Schwartz S, Kerman SL, Cohen MM, Fleischman EW, Prigogina EL (1985). Increased numbers of marrow basophils may be associated with a t(6;9) in ANLL. Am J Hematol 18: 393-403.
1715. Pearson TC, Wetherley-Mein G (1979). The course and complications of idiopathic erythrocytosis. Clin Lab Haematol 1: 189-196.
1716. Pedersen-Bjergaard J, Christiansen DH, Desta F, Andersen MK (2006). Alternative genetic pathways and cooperating genetic abnormalities in the pathogenesis of therapy-related myelodysplasia and acute myeloid leukemia. Leukemia 20: 1943-1949.
1717. Peh SC, Kim LH, Poppema S (2002). Frequent presence of subtype A virus in Epstein-Barr virus-associated malignancies. Pathology 34: 446-450.
1718. Pekarsky Y, Hallas C, Isobe M, Russo G, Croce CM (1999). Abnormalities at 14q32.1 in T cell malignancies involve two oncogenes. Proc Natl Acad Sci U S A 96: 2949-2951.
1719. Pellat-Deceunynck C, Barille S, Jego G, Puthier D, Robillard N, Pineau D, Rapp MJ, Harousseau JL, Amiot M, Bataille R (1998). The absence of CD56 (NCAM) on malignant plasma cells is a hallmark of plasma cell leukemia and of a special subset of multiple myeloma. Leukemia 12: 1977-1982.
1720. Pellegrino B, Terrier-Lacombe MJ, Oberlin O, Leblanc T, Perel Y, Bertrand Y, Beard C, Edan C, Schmitt C, Plantaz D, Pacquement H, Vannier JP, Lambilliote C, Couillault G, Babin-Boilletot A, Thuret I, Demeocq F, Leverger G, Delsol G, Landman-Parker J (2003). Lymphocyte-predominant Hodgkin's lymphoma in children: therapeutic abstention after initial lymph node resection—a Study of the French Society of Pediatric Oncology. J Clin Oncol 21: 2948-2952.
1721. Pellet P, Berger R, Bernheim A, Brouet JC, Tsapis A (1989). Molecular analysis of a t(9;14)(p11;q32) translocation occurring in a case of human alpha heavy chain disease. Oncogene 4: 653-657.
1722. Peloponese JM, Jr., Kinjo T, Jeang KT (2007). Human T-cell leukemia virus type 1 Tax and cellular transformation. Int J Hematol 86: 101-106.
1723. Penn I (1991). The changing pattern of posttransplant malignancies. Transplant Proc 23: 1101-1103.
1724. Perez-Ordonez B, Erlandson RA, Rosai J (1996). Follicular dendritic cell tumor: report of 13 additional cases of a distinctive entity. Am J Surg Pathol 20: 944-955.
1725. Perez-Ordonez B, Rosai J (1998). Follicular dendritic cell tumor: review of the entity. Semin Diagn Pathol 15: 144-154.
1726. Perez-Persona E, Vidriales MB, Mateo G, Garcia-Sanz R, Mateos MV, de Coca AG, Galende J, Martin-Nunez G, Alonso JM, de Las HN, Hernandez JM, Martin A, Lopez-Berges C, Orfao A, San Miguel JF (2007). New criteria to identify risk of progression in monoclonal gammopathy of uncertain significance and smoldering multiple myeloma based on multiparameter flow cytometry analysis of bone marrow plasma cells. Blood 110: 2586-2592.
1727. Perrone T, Frizzera G, Rosai J (1986). Mediastinal diffuse large-cell lymphoma with sclerosis. A clinicopathologic study of 60 cases. Am J Surg Pathol 10: 176-191.
1728. Pescarmona E, De S, V, Pistilli A, Pacchiarotti A, Martelli M, Guglielmi C, Mandelli F, Baroni CD, Le Coco F (1997). Pathogenetic and clinical implications of Bcl-6 and Bcl-2 gene configuration in nodal diffuse large B-cell lymphomas. J Pathol 183: 281-286.
1729. Peters AM, Kohfink B, Martin H, Griesinger F, Wormann B, Gahr M, Roesler J (1999). Defective apoptosis due to a point mutation in the death domain of CD95 associated with autoimmune lymphoproliferative syndrome, T-cell lymphoma, and Hodgkin's disease. Exp Hematol 27: 868-874.
1730. Peterson LC, Bloomfield CD, Brunning RD (1976). Blast crisis as an initial or terminal manifestation of chronic myeloid leukemia. A study of 28 patients. Am J Med 60: 209-220.
1731. Peterson LC, Brown BA, Crosson JT, Mladenovic J (1986). Application of the immunoperoxidase technic to bone marrow trephine biopsies in the classification of patients with monoclonal gammopathies. Am J Clin Pathol 85: 688-693.
1732. Peterson LC, Parkin JL, Arthur DC, Brunning RD (1991). Acute basophilic leukemia. A clinical, morphologic, and cytogenetic study of eight cases. Am J Clin Pathol 96: 160-170.
1733. Peterson LF, Zhang DE (2004). The 8;21 translocation in leukemogenesis. Oncogene 23: 4255-4262.
1734. Petitjean B, Jardin F, Joly B, Martin-Garcia N, Tilly H, Picquenot JM, Briere J, Danel C, Mehaut S, Abd-Al-Samad I, Copie-Bergman C, Delfau-Larue MH, Gaulard P (2002). Pyothorax-associated lymphoma: a peculiar clinicopathologic entity derived from B cells at late stage of differentiation and with occasional aberrant dual B- and T-cell phenotype. Am J Surg Pathol 26: 724-732.
1735. Petrella T, Bagot M, Willemze R, Beylot-Barry M, Vergier B, Delaunay M, Meijer CJ, Courville P, Joly P, Grange F, de Muret A, Machet L, Dompmartin A, Bosq J, Durlach A, Bernard P, Dalac S, Dechelotte P, D'Incan M, Wechsler J, Teitell MA (2005). Blastic NK-cell lymphomas (agranular CD4+CD56+ hematodermic neoplasms): a review. Am J Clin Pathol 123: 662-675.
1736. Petrella T, Comeau MR, Maynadie M, Couillault G, de Muret A, Maliszewski CR, Dalac S, Durlach A, Galibert L (2002). 'Agranular CD4+ CD56+ hematodermic neoplasm' (blastic NK-cell lymphoma) originates from a population of CD56+ precursor cells related to plasmacytoid monocytes. Am J Surg Pathol 26: 852-862.
1737. Petrella T, Dalac S, Maynadie M, Mugneret F, Thomine E, Courville P, Joly P, Lenormand B, Arnould L, Wechsler J, Bagot M, Rieux C, Bosq J, Avril MF, Bernheim A, Molina T, Devidas A, Delfau-Larue MH, Gaulard P, Lambert D (1999). CD4+ CD56+ cutaneous neoplasms: a distinct hematological entity? Groupe Francais d'Etude des Lymphomes Cutanes (GFELC). Am J Surg Pathol 23: 137-146.
1738. Petrella T, Delfau-Larue MH, Caillot D, Morcillo JL, Casasnovas O, Portier H, Gaulard P, Farcet JP, Arnould L (1996). Nasopharyngeal lymphomas: further evidence for a natural killer cell origin. Hum Pathol 27: 827-833.
1739. Petrella T, Meijer CJ, Dalac S, Willemze R, Maynadie M, Machet L, Casasnovas O, Vergier B, Teitell MA (2004). TCL1 and CLA expression in agranular CD4/CD56 hematodermic neoplasms (blastic NK-cell lymphomas) and leukemia cutis. Am J Clin Pathol 122: 307-313.
1739A. Piccaluga PP, Agostinelli C, Califano A, Rossi M, Basso K, Zupo S, Went P, Klein U, Zinzani PL, Baccarani M, Dalla Favera R, Pileri SA (2007). Gene expression analysis of peripheral T cell lymphoma, unspecified, reveals distinct profiles and new potential therapeutic targets. J Clin Invest 117: 823-834.
1740. Piccaluga PP, Agostinelli C, Righi S, Zinzani PL, Pileri SA (2007). Expression of CD52 in peripheral T-cell lymphoma. Haematologica 92: 566-567.
1741. Piccaluga PP, Ascani S, Agostinelli C, Paolini S, Laterza C, Papayannidis C, Martinelli G, Visani G, Baccarani M, Pileri SA (2007). Myeloid sarcoma of liver: an unusual cause of jaundice. Report of three cases and review of literature. Histopathology 50: 802-805.
1742. Pileri SA, Ascani S, Cox MC, Campidelli C, Bacci F, Piccioli M, Piccaluga PP, Agostinelli C, Asioli S, Novero D, Bisceglia M, Ponzoni M, Gentile A, Rinaldi P, Franco V, Vincelli D, Pileri A, Jr., Gasbarra R, Falini B, Zinzani PL, Baccarani M (2007). Myeloid sarcoma: clinico-pathologic, phenotypic and cytogenetic analysis of 92 adult patients. Leukemia 21: 340-350.
1743. Pileri SA, Ascani S, Leoncini L, Sabattini E, Zinzani PL, Piccaluga PP, Pileri A, Jr., Giunti M, Falini B, Bolis GB, Stein H (2002). Hodgkin's lymphoma: the pathologist's viewpoint. J Clin Pathol 55: 162-176.
1744. Pileri SA, Gaidano G, Zinzani PL, Falini B, Gaulard P, Zucca E, Pieri F, Berra E, Sabattini E, Ascani S, Piccioli M, Johnson PW, Giardini R, Pescarmona E, Novero D, Piccaluga PP, Marafioti T, Alonso MA, Cavalli F (2003). Primary mediastinal B-cell lymphoma: high frequency of BCL-6 mutations and consistent expression of the transcription factors OCT-2, BOB.1, and PU.1 in the absence of immunoglobulins. Am J Pathol 162: 243-253.
1745. Pileri SA, Grogan TM, Harris NL, Banks P, Campo E, Chan JK, Favera R, Delsol G, De Wolf PC, Falini B, Gascoyne RD, Gaulard P, Gatter KC, Isaacson PG, Jaffe ES, Kluin P, Knowles DM, Mason DY, Mori S, Muller-Hermelink HK, Piris MA, Ralfkiaer E, Stein H, Su IJ, Warnke RA, Weiss LM (2002). Tumors of histiocytes and accessory dendritic cells. An immunohistochemical approach to classification from the International Lymphoma Study Group based on 61 cases. Histopathology 41: 1-29.
1746. Pileri SA, Pulford K, Mori S, Mason DY, Sabattini E, Roncador G, Piccioli M, Ceccarelli C, Piccaluga PP, Santini D, Leone O, Stein H, Falini B (1997). Frequent expression of the NPM-ALK chimeric fusion protein in anaplastic large-cell lymphoma, lympho-histiocytic type. Am J Pathol 150: 1207-1211.
1747. Pilichowska ME, Fleming MD, Pinkus JL, Pinkus GS (2007). CD4+/CD56+ hematodermic neoplasm ("blastic natural killer cell lymphoma"): neoplastic cells express the immature dendritic cell marker BDCA-2 and produce interferon. Am J Clin Pathol 128: 445-453.
1748. Pillay K, Solomon R, Daubenton JD, Sinclair-Smith CC (2004). Interdigitating dendritic cell sarcoma: a report of four paediatric cases and review of the literature. Histopathology 44: 283-291.
1749. Pilozzi E, Muller-Hermelink HK, Falini B, Wolf-Peeters C, Fidler C, Gatter K, Wainscoat J (1999). Gene rearrangements in T-cell lymphoblastic lymphoma. J Pathol 188: 267-270.
1750. Pilozzi E, Pulford K, Jones M, Muller-Hermelink HK, Falini B, Ralfkiaer E, Pileri S, Pezzella F, Wolf-Peeters C, Arber D, Stein H, Mason D, Gatter K (1998). Co-expression of CD79a (JCB117) and CD3 by lymphoblastic lymphoma. J Pathol 186: 140-143.
1751. Pinkel D (1998). Differentiating juvenile

myelomonocytic leukemia from infectious disease. Blood 91: 365-367.
1752. Pinkus GS, Said JW (1985). Hodgkin's disease, lymphocyte predominance type, nodular—a distinct entity? Unique staining profile for L&H variants of Reed-Sternberg cells defined by monoclonal antibodies to leukocyte common antigen, granulocyte-specific antigen, and B-cell-specific antigen. Am J Pathol 118: 1-6.
1753. Pinkus GS, Said JW (1988). Hodgkin's disease, lymphocyte predominance type, nodular—further evidence for a B cell derivation. L & H variants of Reed-Sternberg cells express L26, a pan B cell marker. Am J Pathol 133: 211-217.
1754. Pinto A, Hutchison RE, Grant LH, Trevenen CL, Berard CW (1990). Follicular lymphomas in pediatric patients. Mod Pathol 3: 308-313.
1755. Pinyol M, Bea S, Pla L, Ribrag V, Bosq J, Rosenwald A, Campo E, Jares P (2007). Inactivation of RB1 in mantle-cell lymphoma detected by nonsense-mediated mRNA decay pathway inhibition and microarray analysis. Blood 109: 5422-5429.
1756. Pinyol M, Cobo F, Bea S, Jares P, Nayach I, Fernandez PL, Montserrat E, Cardesa A, Campo E (1998). p16(INK4a) gene inactivation by deletions, mutations, and hypermethylation is associated with transformed and aggressive variants of non-Hodgkin's lymphomas. Blood 91: 2977-2984.
1757. Pinyol M, Hernandez L, Cazorla M, Balbin M, Jares P, Fernandez PL, Montserrat E, Cardesa A, Lopez-Otin C, Campo E (1997). Deletions and loss of expression of p16INK4a and p21Waf1 genes are associated with aggressive variants of mantle cell lymphomas. Blood 89: 272-280.
1758. Piris M, Brown DC, Gatter KC, Mason DY (1990). CD30 expression in non-Hodgkin's lymphoma. Histopathology 17: 211-218.
1759. Pitman SD, Huang Q, Zuppan CW, Rowsell EH, Cao JD, Berdeja JG, Weiss LM, Wang J (2006). Hodgkin lymphoma-like posttransplant lymphoproliferative disorder (HL-like PTLD) simulates monomorphic B-cell PTLD both clinically and pathologically. Am J Surg Pathol 30: 470-476.
1760. Pittaluga S, Ayoubi TA, Wlodarska I, Stul M, Cassiman JJ, Mecucci C, Van den BH, Van De Ven WJ, Wolf-Peeters C (1996). BCL-6 expression in reactive lymphoid tissue and in B-cell non-Hodgkin's lymphomas. J Pathol 179: 145-150.
1761. Pittaluga S, Verhoef G, Criel A, Maes A, Nuyts J, Boogaerts M, De Wolf PC (1996). Prognostic significance of bone marrow trephine and peripheral blood smears in 55 patients with mantle cell lymphoma. Leuk Lymphoma 21: 115-125.
1762. Pittaluga S, Wiodarska I, Pulford K, Campo E, Morris SW, Van den BH, Wolf-Peeters C (1997). The monoclonal antibody ALK1 identifies a distinct morphological subtype of anaplastic large cell lymphoma associated with 2p23/ALK rearrangements. Am J Pathol 151: 343-351.
1763. Piva R, Pellegrino E, Mattioli M, Agnelli L, Lombardi L, Boccalatte F, Costa G, Ruggeri BA, Cheng M, Chiarle R, Palestro G, Neri A, Inghirami G (2006). Functional validation of the anaplastic lymphoma kinase signature identifies CEBPB and BCL2A1 as critical target genes. J Clin Invest 116: 3171-3182.
1764. Poirel HA, Bernheim A, Schneider A, Meddeb M, Choquet S, Leblond V, Charlotte F, Davi F, Canioni D, Macintyre E, Mamzer-Bruneel MF, Hirsch I, Hermine O, Martin A, Cornillet-Lefebvre P, Patey M, Toupance O, Kemeny JL, Deteix P, Raphael M (2005). Characteristic pattern of chromosomal imbalances in posttransplantation lymphoproliferative disorders: correlation with histopathological subcategories and EBV status. Transplantation 80: 176-184.
1765. Ponti R, Quaglino P, Novelli M, Fierro MT, Comessatti A, Peroni A, Bonello L, Bernengo MG (2005). T-cell receptor gamma gene rearrangement by multiplex polymerase chain reaction/heteroduplex analysis in patients with cutaneous T-cell lymphoma (mycosis fungoides/Sezary syndrome) and benign inflammatory disease: correlation with clinical, histological and immunophenotypical findings. Br J Dermatol 153: 565-573.
1766. Ponzoni M, Arrigoni G, Gould VE, Del Curto B, Maggioni M, Scapinello A, Paolino S, Cassisa A, Patriarca C (2000). Lack of CD 29 (beta1 integrin) and CD 54 (ICAM-1) adhesion molecules in intravascular lymphomatosis. Hum Pathol 31: 220-226.
1767. Ponzoni M, Berger F, Chassagne-Clement C, Tinguely M, Jouvet A, Ferreri AJ, Dell'Oro S, Terreni MR, Doglioni C, Weis J, Cerati M, Milani M, Iuzzolino P, Motta T, Carbone A, Pedrinis E, Sanchez J, Blay JY, Reni M, Conconi A, Bertoni F, Zucca E, Cavalli F, Borisch B (2007). Reactive perivascular T-cell infiltrate predicts survival in primary central nervous system B-cell lymphomas. Br J Haematol 138: 316-323.
1768. Ponzoni M, Ferreri AJ (2006). Intravascular lymphoma: a neoplasm of 'homeless' lymphocytes? Hematol Oncol 24: 105-112.
1769. Ponzoni M, Ferreri AJ, Campo E, Facchetti F, Mazzucchelli L, Yoshino T, Murase T, Pileri SA, Doglioni C, Zucca E, Cavalli F, Nakamura S (2007). Definition, diagnosis, and management of intravascular large B-cell lymphoma: proposals and perspectives from an international consensus meeting. J Clin Oncol 25: 3168-3173.
1770. Popovici C, Zhang B, Gregoire MJ, Jonveaux P, Lafage-Pochitaloff M, Birnbaum D, Pebusque MJ (1999). The t(6;8)(q27;p11) translocation in a stem cell myeloproliferative disorder fuses a novel gene, FOP, to fibroblast growth factor receptor 1. Blood 93: 1381-1389.
1771. Poppema S (1980). The diversity of the immunohistological staining pattern of Sternberg-Reed cells. J Histochem Cytochem 28: 788-791.
1772. Poppema S (1989). The nature of the lymphocytes surrounding Reed-Sternberg cells in nodular lymphocyte predominance and in other types of Hodgkin's disease. Am J Pathol 135: 351-357.
1773. Porcu P, Neiman RS, Orazi A (1999). Splenectomy in agnogenic myeloid metaplasia. Blood 93: 2132-2134.
1774. Portlock CS, Donnelly GB, Qin J, Straus D, Yahalom J, Zelenetz A, Noy A, O'Connor O, Horwitz S, Moskowitz C, Filippa DA (2004). Adverse prognostic significance of CD20 positive Reed-Sternberg cells in classical Hodgkin's disease. Br J Haematol 125: 701-708.
1775. Porwit-MacDonald A, Janossy G, Ivory K, Swirsky D, Peters R, Wheatley K, Walker H, Turker A, Goldstone AH, Burnett A (1996). Leukemia-associated changes identified by quantitative flow cytometry. IV. CD34 overexpression in acute myelogenous leukemia M2 with t(8;21). Blood 87: 1162-1169.
1775A. Pozzato G, Mazzaro C, Crovatto M, Modolo ML, Ceselli S, Mazzi G, Sulfaro S, Franzin F, Tulissi P, Moretti M (1994). Low-grade malignant lymphoma, hepatitis C virus infection, and mixed cryoglobulinemia. Blood 84: 3047-3053.
1776. Pozzi C, D'Amico M, Fogazzi GB, Curioni S, Ferrario F, Pasquali S, Quattrocchio G, Rollino C, Segagni S, Locatelli F (2003). Light chain deposition disease with renal involvement: clinical characteristics and prognostic factors. Am J Kidney Dis 42: 1154-1163.
1777. Prakash S, Fountaine T, Raffeld M, Jaffe ES, Pittaluga S (2006). IgD positive L&H cells identify a unique subset of nodular lymphocyte predominant Hodgkin lymphoma. Am J Surg Pathol 30: 585-592.
1778. Prchal JT (2001). Pathogenetic mechanisms of polycythemia vera and congenital polycythemic disorders. Semin Hematol 38: 10-20.
1779. Preud'Homme JL, Aucouturier P, Touchard G, Striker L, Khamlichi AA, Rocca A, Denoroy L, Cogne M (1994). Monoclonal immunoglobulin deposition disease (Randall type). Relationship with structural abnormalities of immunoglobulin chains. Kidney Int 46: 965-972.
1780. Preudhomme C, Sagot C, Boissel N, Cayuela JM, Tigaud I, de Botton S, Thomas X, Raffoux E, Lamandin C, Castaigne S, Fenaux P, Dombret H (2002). Favorable prognostic significance of CEBPA mutations in patients with de novo acute myeloid leukemia: a study from the Acute Leukemia French Association (ALFA). Blood 100: 2717-2723.
1780A. Prevot S, Hamilton-Dutoit S, Audouin J, Walter P, Pallesen G, Diebold J (1992). Analysis of African Burkitt's and high-grade B cell non-Burkitt's lymphoma for Epstein-Barr virus genomes using in situ hybridization. Br J Haematol 80: 27-32.
1781. Price SK (1990). Immunoproliferative small intestinal disease: a study of 13 cases with alpha heavy-chain disease. Histopathology 17: 7-17.
1782. Provencio M, Espana P, Millan I, Yebra M, Sanchez AC, de la TA, Bonilla F, Regueiro CA, de Letona JM (2004). Prognostic factors in Hodgkin's disease. Leuk Lymphoma 45: 1133-1139.
1783. Przybylski GK, Wu H, Macon WR, Finan J, Leonard DG, Felgar RE, DiGiuseppe JA, Nowell PC, Swerdlow SH, Kadin ME, Wasik MA, Salhany KE (2000). Hepatosplenic and subcutaneous panniculitis-like gamma/delta T cell lymphomas are derived from different Vdelta subsets of gamma/delta T lymphocytes. J Mol Diagn 2: 11-19.
1784. Pui CH, Schrappe M, Ribeiro RC, Niemeyer CM (2004). Childhood and adolescent lymphoid and myeloid leukemia. Hematology Am Soc Hematol Educ Program :118-45.: 118-145.
1785. Pulford K, Lamant L, Espinos E, Jiang Q, Xue L, Turturro F, Delsol G, Morris SW (2004). The emerging normal and disease-related roles of anaplastic lymphoma kinase. Cell Mol Life Sci 61: 2939-2953.
1786. Pulford K, Lamant L, Morris SW, Butler LH, Wood KM, Stroud D, Delsol G, Mason DY (1997). Detection of anaplastic lymphoma kinase (ALK) and nucleolar protein nucleophosmin (NPM)-ALK proteins in normal and neoplastic cells with the monoclonal antibody ALK1. Blood 89: 1394-1404.
1787. Pulsipher MA, Adams RH, Asch J, Petersen FB (2004). Successful treatment of JMML relapsed after unrelated allogeneic transplant with cytoreduction followed by DLI and interferon-alpha: evidence for a graft-versus-leukemia effect in non-monosomy-7 JMML. Bone Marrow Transplant 33: 113-115.
1788. Purtilo DT, Strobach RS, Okano M, Davis JR (1992). Epstein-Barr virus-associated lymphoproliferative disorders. Lab Invest 67: 5-23.
1789. Qin Y, Greiner A, Trunk MJ, Schmausser B, Ott MM, Muller-Hermelink HK (1995). Somatic hypermutation in low-grade mucosa-associated lymphoid tissue-type B-cell lymphoma. Blood 86: 3528-3534.
1790. Quarterman MJ, Lesher JL, Jr., Davis LS, Pantazis CG, Mullins S (1995). Rapidly progressive CD8-positive cutaneous T-cell lymphoma with tongue involvement. Am J Dermatopathol 17: 287-291.
1791. Quinn ER, Chan CH, Hadlock KG, Foung SK, Flint M, Levy S (2001). The B-cell receptor of a hepatitis C virus (HCV)-associated non-Hodgkin lymphoma binds the viral E2 envelope protein, implicating HCV in lymphomagenesis. Blood 98: 3745-3749.
1792. Quintana PG, Kapadia SB, Bahler DW, Johnson JT, Swerdlow SH (1997). Salivary gland lymphoid infiltrates associated with lymphoepithelial lesions: a clinicopathologic, immunophenotypic, and genotypic study. Hum Pathol 28: 850-861.
1793. Quintanilla-Martinez L, Davies-Hill T, Fend F, Calzada-Wack J, Sorbara L, Campo E, Jaffe ES, Raffeld M (2003). Sequestration of p27Kip1 protein by cyclin D1 in typical and blastic variants of mantle cell lymphoma (MCL): implications for pathogenesis. Blood 101: 3181-3187.
1794. Quintanilla-Martinez L, Fend F, Moguel LR, Spilove L, Beaty MW, Kingma DW, Raffeld M, Jaffe ES (1999). Peripheral T-cell lymphoma with Reed-Sternberg-like cells of B-cell phenotype and genotype associated with Epstein-Barr virus infection. Am J Surg Pathol 23: 1233-1240.
1795. Quintanilla-Martinez L, Franklin JL, Guerrero I, Krenacs L, Naresh KN, Rama-Rao C, Bhatia K, Raffeld M, Magrath IT (1999). Histological and immunophenotypic profile of nasal NK/T cell lymphomas from Peru: high prevalence of p53 overexpression. Hum Pathol 30: 849-855.
1796. Quintanilla-Martinez L, Kremer M, Keller G, Nathrath M, Gamboa-Dominguez A, Meneses A, Luna-Contreras L, Cabras A, Hoefler H, Mohar A, Fend F (2001). p53 Mutations in nasal natural killer/T-cell lymphoma from Mexico: association with large cell morphology and advanced disease. Am J Pathol 159: 2095-2105.
1797. Quintanilla-Martinez L, Kumar S, Fend F, Reyes E, Teruya-Feldstein J, Kingma DW, Sorbara L, Raffeld M, Straus SE, Jaffe ES (2000). Fulminant EBV(+) T-cell lymphoproliferative disorder following acute/chronic EBV infection: a distinct clinicopathologic syndrome. Blood 96: 443-451.
1798. Quintanilla-Martinez L, Pittaluga S, Miething C, Klier M, Rudelius M, Davies-Hill T, Anastasov N, Martinez A, Vivero A, Duyster J, Jaffe ES, Fend F, Raffeld M (2006). NPM-ALK-dependent expression of the transcription factor CCAAT/enhancer binding protein beta in ALK-positive anaplastic large cell lymphoma. Blood 108: 2029-2036.
1799. Rabbani GR, Phyliky RL, Tefferi A (1999). A long-term study of patients with chronic natural killer cell lymphocytosis. Br J Haematol 106: 960-966.
1800. Radaelli F, Mazza R, Curioni E, Ciani A, Pomati M, Maiolo AT (2002). Acute megakaryocytic leukemia in essential thrombocythemia: an unusual evolution? Eur J Haematol 69: 108-111.
1801. Radaszkiewicz T, Dragosics B, Bauer P (1992). Gastrointestinal malignant lymphomas of the mucosa-associated lymphoid tissue: factors relevant to prognosis. Gastroenterology 102: 1628-1638.
1802. Raderer M, Streubel B, Woehrer S, Puespoek A, Jaeger U, Formanek M, Chott A (2005). High relapse rate in patients with MALT lymphoma warrants lifelong follow-up. Clin Cancer Res 11: 3349-3352.
1803. Radich JP, Dai H, Mao M, Oehler V, Schelter J, Druker B, Sawyers C, Shah N, Stock W, Willman CL, Friend S, Linsley PS

(2006). Gene expression changes associated with progression and response in chronic myeloid leukemia. Proc Natl Acad Sci U S A 103: 2794-2799.
1803A Raffeld M, Wright JJ, Lipford E, et al. Clonal evolution of t(14;18) follicular lymphomas demonstrated by immunoglobulin genes and the 18q21 major breakpoint region. Cancer Res 1987; 47:2537-2542.
1804. Rahemtullah A, Reichard KK, Preffer FI, Harris NL, Hasserjian RP (2006). A double-positive CD4+CD8+ T-cell population is commonly found in nodular lymphocyte predominant Hodgkin lymphoma. Am J Clin Pathol 126: 805-814.
1805. Rai KR, Sawitsky A, Cronkite EP, Chanana AD, Levy RN, Pasternack BS (1975). Clinical staging of chronic lymphocytic leukemia. Blood 46: 219-234.
1806. Raimondi SC, Pui CH, Hancock ML, Behm FG, Filatov L, Rivera GK (1996). Heterogeneity of hyperdiploid (51-67) childhood acute lymphoblastic leukemia. Leukemia 10: 213-224.
1807. Rainey JJ, Omenah D, Sumba PO, Moormann AM, Rochford R, Wilson ML (2007). Spatial clustering of endemic Burkitt's lymphoma in high-risk regions of Kenya. Int J Cancer 120: 121-127.
1808. Rajkumar SV, Greipp PR (1999). Prognostic factors in multiple myeloma. Hematol Oncol Clin North Am 13: 1295-314, xi.
1809. Ralfkiaer E (1991). Immunohistological markers for the diagnosis of cutaneous lymphomas. Semin Diagn Pathol 8: 62-72.
1810. Ralfkiaer E, Delsol G, O'Connor NT, Brandtzaeg P, Brousset P, Vejlsgaard GL, Mason DY (1990). Malignant lymphomas of true histiocytic origin. A clinical, histological, immunophenotypic and genotypic study. J Pathol 160: 9-17.
1811. Ralfkiaer E, Wolff-Sneedorff A, Thomsen K, Geisler C, Vejlsgaard GL (1992). T-cell receptor gamma delta-positive peripheral T-cell lymphomas presenting in the skin: a clinical, histological and immunophenotypic study. Exp Dermatol 1: 31-36.
1812. Ramot B, Shahin N, Bubis JJ (1965). Malabsorption syndrome in lymphoma of small intestine. A study of 13 cases. Isr Med J 47: 221-226.
1813. Ramsay AD, Smith WJ, Isaacson PG (1988). T-cell-rich B-cell lymphoma. Am J Surg Pathol 12: 433-443.
1814. Randall RE, Williamson WC, Mullinax F, Tung MY, Still WJ (1976). Manifestations of systemic light chain deposition. Am J Med 60: 293-299.
1815. Randi ML, Putti MC, Fabris F, Sainati L, Zanesco L, Girolami A (2000). Features of essential thrombocythaemia in childhood: a study of five children. Br J Haematol 108: 86-89.
1816. Randolph GJ, Angeli V, Swartz MA (2005). Dendritic-cell trafficking to lymph nodes through lymphatic vessels. Nat Rev Immunol 5: 617-628.
1817. Ranganathan S, Webber S, Ahuja S, Jaffe R (2004). Hodgkin-like posttransplant lymphoproliferative disorder in children: does it differ from posttransplant Hodgkin lymphoma? Pediatr Dev Pathol 7: 348-360.
1818. Raphael M, Gentilhomme O, Tulliez M, Byron PA, Diebold J (1991). Histopathologic features of high-grade non-Hodgkin's lymphomas in acquired immunodeficiency syndrome. The French Study Group of Pathology for Human Immunodeficiency Virus-Associated Tumors. Arch Pathol Lab Med 115: 15-20.
1819. Raphael MM, Audouin J, Lamine M, Delecluse HJ, Vuillaume M, Lenoir GM, Gisselbrecht C, Lennert K, Diebold J (1994). Immunophenotypic and genotypic analysis of acquired immunodeficiency syndrome-related non-Hodgkin's lymphomas. Correlation with histologic features in 36 cases. French Study Group of Pathology for HIV-Associated Tumors. Am J Clin Pathol 101: 773-782.
1819A Rappaport H, Berard CW, Butler JJ, Dorfman RF, Lukes RJ, Thomas LB (1971) Report of the Committee on Histopathological Criteria Contributing to Staging of Hodgkin's Disease. Cancer Res 31: 1864-1865.
1819B. Rappaport H (1966). Tumors of the Haematopoietic system. Washington DC: AFIP.
1820. Rappaport H, Winter W, Hicks E (1956). Follicular lymphoma. A re-evaluation of its position in the scheme of malignant lymphoma, based on a survey of 253 cases. Cancer 9: 792-821.
1821. Rasmussen T, Kuehl M, Lodahl M, Johnsen HE, Dahl IM (2005). Possible roles for activating RAS mutations in the MGUS to MM transition and in the intramedullary to extramedullary transition in some plasma cell tumors. Blood 105: 317-323.
1822. Rassenti LZ, Huynh L, Toy TL, Chen L, Keating MJ, Gribben JG, Neuberg DS, Flinn IW, Rai KR, Byrd JC, Kay NE, Greaves A, Weiss A, Kipps TJ (2004). ZAP-70 compared with immunoglobulin heavy-chain gene mutation status as a predictor of disease progression in chronic lymphocytic leukemia. N Engl J Med 351: 893-901.
1823. Rawstron AC, Green MJ, Kuzmicki A, Kennedy B, Fenton JA, Evans PA, O'Connor SJ, Richards SJ, Morgan GJ, Jack AS, Hillmen P (2002). Monoclonal B lymphocytes with the characteristics of "indolent" chronic lymphocytic leukemia are present in 3.5% of adults with normal blood counts. Blood 100: 635-639.
1824. Raza A, Buonamici S, Lisak L, Tahir S, Li D, Imran M, Chaudary NI, Pervaiz H, Gallegos JA, Alvi MI, Mumtaz M, Gezer S, Venugopal P, Reddy P, Galili N, Candoni A, Singer J, Nucifora G (2004). Arsenic trioxide and thalidomide combination produces multi-lineage hematological responses in myelodysplastic syndromes patients, particularly in those with high pre-therapy EVI1 expression. Leuk Res 28: 791-803.
1825. Reardon DA, Hanson CA, Roth MS, Castle VP (1994). Lineage switch in Philadelphia chromosome-positive acute lymphoblastic leukemia. Cancer 73: 1526-1532.
1826. Redaelli A, Bell C, Casagrande J, Stephens J, Botteman M, Laskin B, Pashos C (2004). Clinical and epidemiologic burden of chronic myelogenous leukemia. Expert Rev Anticancer Ther 4: 85-96.
1827. Redaelli A, Laskin BL, Stephens JM, Botteman MF, Pashos CL (2005). A systematic literature review of the clinical and epidemiological burden of acute lymphoblastic leukaemia (ALL). Eur J Cancer Care (Engl) 14: 53-62.
1828. Ree HJ, Kadin ME, Kikuchi M, Ko YH, Go JH, Suzumiya J, Kim DS (1998). Angioimmunoblastic lymphoma (AILD-type T-cell lymphoma) with hyperplastic germinal centers. Am J Surg Pathol 22: 643-655.
1828A. Reed JC (2008). Bcl-2-family proteins and hematologic malignancies: history and future prospects. Blood 111: 3322-30.
1829. Regev A, Stark P, Blickstein D, Lahav M (1997). Thrombotic complications in essential thrombocythemia with relatively low platelet counts. Am J Hematol 56: 168-172.
1830. Reichard KK, Burks EJ, Foucar MK, Wilson CS, Viswanatha DS, Hozier JC, Larson RS (2005). CD4(+) CD56(+) lineage-negative malignancies are rare tumors of plasmacytoid dendritic cells. Am J Surg Pathol 29: 1274-1283.
1831. Reichard KK, McKenna RW, Kroft SH (2007). ALK-positive diffuse large B-cell lymphoma: report of four cases and review of the literature. Mod Pathol 20: 310-319.
1832. Reilly JT (2002). Cytogenetic and molecular genetic aspects of idiopathic myelofibrosis. Acta Haematol 108: 113-119.
1832A. Reilly JT (2005). Cytogenetic and molecular genetic abnormalities in agnogenic myeloid metaplasia. Semin Oncol 32:359-364.
1833. Reiter A, Walz C, Watmore A, Schoch C, Blau I, Schlegelberger B, Berger U, Telford N, Aruliah S, Yin JA, Vanstraelen D, Barker HF, Taylor PC, O'Driscoll A, Benedetti F, Rudolph C, Kolb HJ, Hochhaus A, Hehlmann R, Chase A, Cross NC (2005). The t(8;9)(p22;p24) is a recurrent abnormality in chronic and acute leukemia that fuses PCM1 to JAK2. Cancer Res 65: 2662-2667.
1834. Reiter E, Greinix H, Rabitsch W, Keil F, Schwarzinger I, Jaeger U, Lechner K, Worel N, Streubel B, Fonatsch C, Mitterbauer G, Kalhs P (2000). Low curative potential of bone marrow transplantation for highly aggressive acute myelogenous leukemia with inversioin inv (3)(q21q26) or homologous translocation t(3;3) (q21;q26). Ann Hematol 79: 374-377.
1835. Remacha AF, Nomdedeu JF, Puget G, Estivill C, Sarda MP, Canals C, Aventin A (2006). Occurrence of the JAK2 V617F mutation in the WHO provisional entity: myelodysplastic/myeloproliferative disease, unclassifiable-refractory anemia with ringed sideroblasts associated with marked thrombocytosis. Haematologica 91: 719-720.
1836. Remstein ED, Dogan A, Einerson RR, Paternoster SF, Fink SR, Law M, Dewald GW, Kurtin PJ (2006). The incidence and anatomic site specificity of chromosomal translocations in primary extranodal marginal zone B-cell lymphoma of mucosa-associated lymphoid tissue (MALT lymphoma) in North America. Am J Surg Pathol 30: 1546-1553.
1837. Remstein ED, James CD, Kurtin PJ (2000). Incidence and subtype specificity of API2-MALT1 fusion translocations in extranodal, nodal, and splenic marginal zone lymphomas. Am J Pathol 156: 1183-1188.
1838. Renne C, Martin-Subero JI, Hansmann ML, Siebert R (2005). Molecular cytogenetic analyses of immunoglobulin loci in nodular lymphocyte predominant Hodgkin's lymphoma reveal a recurrent IGH-BCL6 juxtaposition. J Mol Diagn 7: 352-356.
1839. Renneville A, Quesnel B, Charpentier A, Terriou L, Crinquette A, Lai JL, Cossement C, Lionne-Huyghe P, Rose C, Bauters F, Preudhomme C (2006). High occurrence of JAK2 V617 mutation in refractory anemia with ringed sideroblasts associated with marked thrombocytosis. Leukemia 20: 2067-2070.
1840. Riccardi A, Gobbi PG, Ucci G, Bertoloni D, Luoni R, Rutigliano L, Ascari E (1991). Changing clinical presentation of multiple myeloma. Eur J Cancer 27: 1401-1405.
1841. Rice L, Popat U (2005). Every case of essential thrombocythemia should be tested for the Philadelphia chromosome. Am J Hematol 78: 71-73.
1842. Richard P, Vassallo J, Valmary S, Missoury R, Delsol G, Brousset P (2006). "In situ-like" mantle cell lymphoma: a report of two cases. J Clin Pathol 59: 995-996.
1843. Riemersma SA, Jordanova ES, Schop RF, Philippo K, Looijenga LH, Schuuring E, Kluin PM (2000). Extensive genetic alterations of the HLA region, including homozygous deletions of HLA class II genes in B-cell lymphomas arising in immune-privileged sites. Blood 96: 3569-3577.
1844. Ries LA, *et al.* (eds.) (2004). SEER Cancer Statistics Review, 1975-2001. National Cancer Institute: Bethesda, MD.
1845. Ries LA, Kosary CL, Hankey BF et al.(eds.) (1999). SEER Cancer Statistics Review, 1973-1996. National Cancer Institute: Bethesda, MD.
1846. Rimsza LM, Roberts RA, Miller TP, Unger JM, LeBlanc M, Braziel RM, Weisenberger DD, Chan WC, Muller-Hermelink HK, Jaffe ES, Gascoyne RD, Campo E, Fuchs DA, Spier CM, Fisher RI, Delabie J, Rosenwald A, Staudt LM, Grogan TM (2004). Loss of MHC class II gene and protein expression in diffuse large B-cell lymphoma is related to decreased tumor immunosurveillance and poor patient survival regardless of other prognostic factors: a follow-up study from the Leukemia and Lymphoma Molecular Profiling Project. Blood 103: 4251-4258.
1847. Rinaldi A, Kwee I, Poretti G, Mensah A, Pruneri G, Capello D, Rossi D, Zucca E, Ponzoni M, Catapano C, Tibiletti MG, Paulli M, Gaidano G, Bertoni F (2006). Comparative genome-wide profiling of post-transplant lymphoproliferative disorders and diffuse large B-cell lymphomas. Br J Haematol 134: 27-36.
1847A. Ripp JA, Loiue DC, Chan W, Nawaz H, Portlock CS (2002). T-cell rich B-cell lymphoma: clinical distinctiveness and response to treatment in 45 patients. Leuk Lymphoma 43: 1573-1580.
1848. Ritz O, Leithauser F, Hasel C, Bruderlein S, Ushmorov A, Moller P, Wirth T (2005). Downregulation of internal enhancer activity contributes to abnormally low immunoglobulin expression in the MedB-1 mediastinal B-cell lymphoma cell line. J Pathol 205: 336-348.
1849. Rizvi MA, Evens AM, Tallman MS, Nelson BP, Rosen ST (2006). T-cell non-Hodgkin lymphoma. Blood 107: 1255-1264.
1850. Robak T (2006). Current treatment options in hairy cell leukemia and hairy cell leukemia variant. Cancer Treat Rev 32: 365-376.
1851. Robertson LE, Redman JR, Butler JJ, Osborne BM, Velasquez WS, McLaughlin P, Swan F, Rodriguez MA, Hagemeister FB, Fuller LM, . (1991). Discordant bone marrow involvement in diffuse large-cell lymphoma: a distinct clinical-pathologic entity associated with a continuous risk of relapse. J Clin Oncol 9: 236-242.
1852. Robertson PB, Neiman RS, Worapongpaiboon S, John K, Orazi A (1997). 013 (CD99) positivity in hematologic proliferations correlates with TdT positivity. Mod Pathol 10: 277-282.
1853. Robetorye RS, Bohling SD, Medeiros LJ, Elenitoba-Johnson KS (2000). Follicular lymphoma with monocytoid B-cell proliferation: molecular assessment of the clonal relationship between the follicular and monocytoid B-cell components. Lab Invest 80: 1593-1599.
1854. Robyn J, Lemery S, McCoy JP, Kubofcik J, Kim YJ, Pack S, Nutman TB, Dunbar C, Klion AD (2006). Multilineage involvement of the fusion gene in patients with FIP1L1/PDGFRA-positive hypereosinophilic syndrome. Br J Haematol 132: 286-292.
1855. Rochford R, Cannon MJ, Moormann AM (2005). Endemic Burkitt's lymphoma: a polymicrobial disease? Nat Rev Microbiol 3: 182-187.
1856. Rodig SJ, Abramson JS, Pinkus GS, Treon SP, Dorfman DM, Dong HY, Shipp MA, Kutok JL (2006). Heterogeneous CD52 expression among hematologic neoplasms: implications for the use of alemtuzumab (CAMPATH-1H). Clin Cancer Res 12: 7174-7179.
1857. Rodig SJ, Savage KJ, LaCasce AS, Weng AP, Harris NL, Shipp MA, Hsi ED, Gascoyne RD, Kutok JL (2007). Expression of TRAF1 and nuclear c-Rel distinguishes primary mediastinal large cell lymphoma from other

types of diffuse large B-cell lymphoma. Am J Surg Pathol 31: 106-112.

1858. Rodig SJ, Vergilio JA, Shahsafaei A, Dorfman DM (2008). Characteristic Expression Patterns of TCL1, CD38, and CD44 Identify Aggressive Lymphomas Harboring a MYC Translocation. Am J Surg Pathol 32: 113-122.

1859. Rodriguez-Jurado R, Vidaurri-de la Cruz H, Duran-Mckinster C, Ruiz-Maldonado R (2003). Indeterminate cell histiocytosis. Clinical and pathologic study in a pediatric patient. Arch Pathol Lab Med 127: 748-751.

1860. Rodriguez J, McLaughlin P, Hagemeister FB, Fayad L, Rodriguez MA, Santiago M, Hess M, Romaguera J, Cabanillas F (1999). Follicular large cell lymphoma: an aggressive lymphoma that often presents with favorable prognostic features. Blood 93: 2202-2207.

1861. Rodriguez J, Pugh WC, Cabanillas F (1993). T-cell-rich B-cell lymphoma. Blood 82: 1586-1589.

1862. Rodriguez J, Romaguera JE, Katz RL, Said J, Cabanillas F (2001). Primary effusion lymphoma in an HIV-negative patient with no serologic evidence of Kaposi's sarcoma virus. Leuk Lymphoma 41: 185-189.

1862A. Roncador G, Garcia JF, Garcia JF, Maestre L, Lucas E, Menarguez J, Ohshima K, Nakamura S, Banham AH, Piris MA (2005). FOXP3, a selective marker for a subset of adult T-cell leukaemia/lymphoma. Leukemia 19: 2247-2253.

1863. Rosales CM, Lin P, Mansoor A, Bueso-Ramos C, Medeiros LJ (2001). Lympho-plasmacytic lymphoma/Waldenstrom macro-globulinemia associated with Hodgkin disease. A report of two cases. Am J Clin Pathol 116: 34-40.

1864. Rosati S, Mick R, Xu F, Stonys E, Le Beau MM, Larson R, Vardiman JW (1996). Refractory cytopenia with multilineage dysplasia: further characterization of an 'unclassifiable' myelodysplastic syndrome. Leukemia 10: 20-26.

1865. Rosenberg AS, Morgan MB (2001). Cutaneous indeterminate cell histiocytosis: a new spindle cell variant resembling dendritic cell sarcoma. J Cutan Pathol 28: 531-537.

1866. Rosenberg CL, Wong E, Petty EM, Bale AE, Tsujimoto Y, Harris NL, Arnold A (1991). PRAD1, a candidate BCL1 oncogene: mapping and expression in centrocytic lymphoma. Proc Natl Acad Sci U S A 88: 9638-9642.

1867. Rosenwald A, Alizadeh AA, Widhopf G, Simon R, Davis RE, Yu X, Yang L, Pickeral OK, Rassenti LZ, Powell J, Botstein D, Byrd JC, Grever MR, Cheson BD, Chiorazzi N, Wilson WH, Kipps TJ, Brown PO, Staudt LM (2001). Relation of gene expression phenotype to immunoglobulin mutation genotype in B cell chronic lymphocytic leukemia. J Exp Med 194: 1639-1647.

1868. Rosenwald A, Ott G, Pulford K, Katzenberger T, Kuhl J, Kalla J, Ott MM, Mason DY, Muller-Hermelink HK (1999). t(1;2)(q21;p23) and t(2;3)(p23;q21): two novel variant transloca-tions of the t(2;5)(p23;q35) in anaplastic large cell lymphoma. Blood 94: 362-364.

1869. Rosenwald A, Wright G, Chan WC, Connors JM, Campo E, Fisher RI, Gascoyne RD, Muller-Hermelink HK, Smeland EB, Giltnane JM, Hurt EM, Zhao H, Averett L, Yang L, Wilson WH, Jaffe ES, Simon R, Klausner RD, Powell J, Duffey PL, Longo DL, Greiner TC, Weisenburger DD, Sanger WG, Dave BJ, Lynch JC, Vose J, Armitage JO, Montserrat E, Lopez-Guillermo A, Grogan TM, Miller TP, LeBlanc M, Ott G, Kvaloy S, Delabie J, Holte H, Krajci P, Stokke T, Staudt LM (2002). The use of molecular profiling to predict survival after chemotherapy for diffuse large-B-cell lym-phoma. N Engl J Med 346: 1937-1947.

1870. Rosenwald A, Wright G, Leroy K, Yu X, Gaulard P, Gascoyne RD, Chan WC, Zhao T, Haioun C, Greiner TC, Weisenburger DD, Lynch JC, Vose J, Armitage JO, Smeland EB, Kvaloy S, Holte H, Delabie J, Campo E, Montserrat E, Lopez-Guillermo A, Ott G, Muller-Hermelink HK, Connors JM, Braziel R, Grogan TM, Fisher RI, Miller TP, LeBlanc M, Chiorazzi M, Zhao H, Yang L, Powell J, Wilson WH, Jaffe ES, Simon R, Klausner RD, Staudt LM (2003). Molecular diagnosis of primary mediastinal B cell lymphoma identifies a clinically favorable subgroup of diffuse large B cell lymphoma relat-ed to Hodgkin lymphoma. J Exp Med 198: 851-862.

1871. Rosenwald A, Wright G, Wiestner A, Chan WC, Connors JM, Campo E, Gascoyne RD, Grogan TM, Muller-Hermelink HK, Smeland EB, Chiorazzi M, Giltnane JM, Hurt EM, Zhao H, Averett L, Henrickson S, Yang L, Powell J, Wilson WH, Jaffe ES, Simon R, Klausner RD, Montserrat E, Bosch F, Greiner TC, Weisenburger DD, Sanger WG, Dave BJ, Lynch JC, Vose J, Armitage JO, Fisher RI, Miller TP, LeBlanc M, Ott G, Kvaloy S, Holte H, Delabie J, Staudt LM (2003). The proliferation gene expression signature is a quantitative integrator of oncogenic events that predicts sur-vival in mantle cell lymphoma. Cancer Cell 3: 185-197.

1872. Rosh JR, Gross T, Mamula P, Griffiths A, Hyams J (2007). Hepatosplenic T-cell lym-phoma in adolescents and young adults with Crohn's disease: a cautionary tale? Inflamm Bowel Dis 13: 1024-1030.

1872A. Rosier RN, Kattapuram S, Rosenberg AE (2000). Case 9-2000- A 41-Year-Old Man with Multiple Bony Lesions and Adjacent Soft-Tissue Masses. N Engl J Med 342: 875-83

1873. Rossbach HC (2006). Familial infantile myelofibrosis as an autosomal recessive disor-der: preponderance among children from Saudi Arabia. Pediatr Hematol Oncol 23: 453-454.

1874. Rossi G, Donisi A, Casari S, Re A, Cadeo G, Carosi G (1999). The International Prognostic Index can be used as a guide to treatment decisions regarding patients with human immunodeficiency virus-related sys-temic non-Hodgkin lymphoma. Cancer 86: 2391-2397.

1875. Rostagno A, Frizzera G, Ylagan L, Kumar A, Ghiso J, Gallo G (2002). Tumoral non-amyloidotic monoclonal immunoglobulin light chain deposits ('aggregoma'): presenting feature of B-cell dyscrasia in three cases with immunohistochemical and biochemical analy-ses. Br J Haematol 119: 62-69.

1876. Roulland S, Lebailly P, Roussel G, Briand M, Cappellen D, Pottier D, Hardouin A, Troussard X, Bastard C, Henry-Amar M, Gauduchon P (2003). BCL-2/JH translocation in peripheral blood lymphocytes of unexposed individuals: lack of seasonal variations in fre-quency and molecular features. Int J Cancer 104: 695-698.

1877. Roulland S, Navarro JM, Grenot P, Milili M, Agopian J, Montpellier B, Gauduchon P, Lebailly P, Schiff C, Nadel B (2006). Follicular lymphoma-like B cells in healthy individuals: a novel intermediate step in early lymphomagen-esis. J Exp Med 203: 2425-2431.

1878. Roullet MR, Cornfield DB (2006). Large natural killer cell lymphoma arising from an indolent natural killer cell large granular lym-phocyte proliferation. Arch Pathol Lab Med 130: 1712-1714.

1879. Roumiantsev S, Krause DS, Neumann CA, Dimitri CA, Asiedu F, Cross NC, Van Etten RA (2004). Distinct stem cell myeloprolifera-tive/T lymphoma syndromes induced by ZNF198-FGFR1 and BCR-FGFR1 fusion genes from 8p11 translocations. Cancer Cell 5: 287-298.

1880. Roumier C, Eclache V, Imbert M, Davi F, Macintyre E, Garand R, Talmant P, Lepelley P, Lai JL, Casasnovas O, Maynadie M, Mugneret F, Bilhou-Naberra C, Valensi F, Radford I, Mozziconacci MJ, Arnoulet C, Duchayne E, Dastugue N, Cornillet P, Daliphard S, Garnache F, Boudjerra N, Jouault H, Fenneteau O, Pedron B, Berger R, Flandrin G, Fenaux P, Preudhomme C (2003). M0 AML, clinical and biologic features of the disease, including AML1 gene mutations: a report of 59 cases by the Groupe Francais d'Hematologie Cellulaire (GFHC) and the Groupe Francais de Cytogenetique Hematologique (GFCH). Blood 101: 1277-1283.

1881. Rousselet MC, Francois S, Croue A, Maigre M, Saint-Andre JP, Ifrah N (1994). A lymph node interdigitating reticulum cell sarco-ma. Arch Pathol Lab Med 118: 183-188.

1882. Rowe D, Cotterill SJ, Ross FM, Bunyan DJ, Vickers SJ, Bryon J, McMullan DJ, Griffiths MJ, Reilly JT, Vandenberghe EA, Wilson G, Watmore AE, Bown NP (2000). Cytogenetically cryptic AML1-ETO and CBF beta-MYH11 gene rearrangements: incidence in 412 cases of acute myeloid leukaemia. Br J Haematol 111: 1051-1056.

1883. Rowe M, Rowe DT, Gregory CD, Young LS, Farrell PJ, Rupani H, Rickinson AB (1987). Differences in B cell growth phenotype reflect novel patterns of Epstein-Barr virus latent gene expression in Burkitt's lymphoma cells. EMBO J 6: 2743-2751.

1884. Rowley JD (1973). Letter: A new con-sistent chromosomal abnormality in chronic myelogenous leukaemia identified by quinacrine fluorescence and Giemsa staining. Nature 243: 290-293.

1885. Rowley JD (1988). Chromosome stud-ies in the non-Hodgkin's lymphomas: the role of the 14;18 translocation. J Clin Oncol 6: 919-925.

1886. Rowley JD, Olney HJ (2002). International workshop on the relationship of prior therapy to balanced chromosome aberra-tions in therapy-related myelodysplastic syn-dromes and acute leukemia: overview report. Genes Chromosomes Cancer 33: 331-345.

1887. Rowlings PA, Curtis RE, Passweg JR, Deeg HJ, Socie G, Travis LB, Kingma DW, Jaffe ES, Sobocinski KA, Horowitz MM (1999). Increased incidence of Hodgkin's disease after allogeneic bone marrow transplantation. J Clin Oncol 17: 3122-3127.

1888. Rozman C, Montserrat E (1995). Chronic lymphocytic leukemia. N Engl J Med 333: 1052-1057.

1889. Rubenstein JL, Fridlyand J, Shen A, Aldape K, Ginzinger D, Batchelor T, Treseler P, Berger M, McDermott M, Prados M, Karch J, Okada C, Hyun W, Parikh S, Haqq C, Shuman M (2006). Gene expression and angiotropism in primary CNS lymphoma. Blood 107: 3716-3723.

1890. Rubio-Moscardo F, Climent J, Siebert R, Piris MA, Martin-Subero JI, Nielander I, Garcia-Conde J, Dyer MJ, Terol MJ, Pinkel D, Martinez-Climent JA (2005). Mantle-cell lym-phoma genotypes identified with CGH to BAC microarrays define a leukemic subgroup of dis-ease and predict patient outcome. Blood 105: 4445-4454.

1891. Rubnitz JE, Raimondi SC, Tong X, Srivastava DK, Razzouk BI, Shurtleff SA, Downing JR, Pui CH, Ribeiro RC, Behm FG (2002). Favorable impact of the t(9;11) in child-hood acute myeloid leukemia. J Clin Oncol 20: 2302-2309.

1892. Ruchlemer R, Parry-Jones N, Brito-Babapulle V, Attolico I, Wotherspoon AC, Matutes E, Catovsky D (2004). B-prolympho-cytic leukaemia with t(11;14) revisited: a splenomegalic form of mantle cell lymphoma evolving with leukaemia. Br J Haematol 125: 330-336.

1893. Ruco LP, Gearing AJ, Pigott R, Pomponi D, Burgio VL, Cafolla A, Baiocchini A, Baroni CD (1991). Expression of ICAM-1, VCAM-1 and ELAM-1 in angiofollicular lymph node hyperplasia (Castleman's disease): evi-dence for dysplasia of follicular dendritic reticu-lum cells. Histopathology 19: 523-528.

1894. Rudiger T, Ichinohasama R, Ott MM, Muller-Deubert S, Miura I, Ott G, Muller-Hermelink HK (2000). Peripheral T-cell lym-phoma with distinct perifollicular growth pattern: a distinct subtype of T-cell lymphoma? Am J Surg Pathol 24: 117-122.

1895. Rudiger T, Jaffe ES, Delsol G, Dewolf-Peeters C, Gascoyne RD, Georgii A, Harris NL, Kadin ME, MacLennan KA, Poppema S, Stein H, Weiss LE, Muller-Hermelink HK (1998). Workshop report on Hodgkin's disease and related diseases ('grey zone' lymphoma). Ann Oncol 9 Suppl 5: S31-S38.

1896. Rudiger T, Weisenburger DD, Anderson JR, Armitage JO, Diebold J, MacLennan KA, Nathwani BN, Ullrich F, Muller-Hermelink HK (2002). Peripheral T-cell lym-phoma (excluding anaplastic large-cell lym-phoma): results from the Non-Hodgkin's Lymphoma Classification Project. Ann Oncol 13: 140-149.

1897. Ruggeri M, Tosetto A, Frezzato M, Rodeghiero F (2003). The rate of progression to polycythemia vera or essential thrombo-cythemia in patients with erythrocytosis or thrombocytosis. Ann Intern Med 139: 470-475.

1898. Ruiz A, Reischl U, Swerdlow SH, Hartke M, Streubel B, Procop G, Tubbs RR, Cook JR (2007). Extranodal marginal zone B-cell lymphomas of the ocular adnexa: multipa-rameter analysis of 34 cases including inter-phase molecular cytogenetics and PCR for Chlamydia psittaci. Am J Surg Pathol 31: 792-802.

1899. Rund D, Krichevsky S, Bar-Cohen S, Goldschmidt N, Kedmi M, Malik E, Gural A, Shafran-Tikva S, Ben Neriah S, Ben Yehuda D (2005). Therapy-related leukemia: clinical char-acteristics and analysis of new molecular risk factors in 96 adult patients. Leukemia 19: 1919-1928.

1900. Ruskone-Fourmestraux A, Delmer A, Lavergne A, Molina T, Brousse N, Audouin J, Rambaud JC (1997). Multiple lymphomatous polyposis of the gastrointestinal tract: prospec-tive clinicopathologic study of 31 cases. Groupe D'etude des Lymphomes Digestifs. Gastroenterology 112: 7-16.

1901. Ruskova A, Thula R, Chan G (2004). Aggressive Natural Killer-Cell Leukemia: report of five cases and review of the literature. Leuk Lymphoma 45: 2427-2438.

1902. Ryder J, Wang X, Bao L, Gross SA, Hua F, Irons RD (2007). Aggressive natural killer cell leukemia: report of a Chinese series and review of the literature. Int J Hematol 85: 18-25.

1903. Sacchi S, Vinci G, Gugliotta L, Rupoli S, Gargantini L, Martinelli V, Baravelli S, Lazzarino M, Finazzi G (2000). Diagnosis of essential thrombocythemia at platelet counts between 400 and 600x10(9)/L. Gruppo Italiano Malattie Mieloproliferative Croniche(GIMMC). Haematologica 85: 492-495.

1904. Saez AI, Saez AJ, Artiga MJ, Perez-Rosado A, Camacho FI, Diez A, Garcia JF, Fraga M, Bosch R, Rodriguez-Pinilla SM, Mollejo M, Romero C, Sanchez-Verde L, Pollan M, Piris MA (2004). Building an outcome pre-dictor model for diffuse large B-cell lymphoma.

Am J Pathol 164: 613-622.

1905. Saffer H, Wahed A, Rassidakis GZ, Medeiros LJ (2002). Clusterin expression in malignant lymphomas: a survey of 266 cases. Mod Pathol 15: 1221-1226.

1906. Safley AM, Sebastian S, Collins TS, Tirado CA, Stenzel TT, Gong JZ, Goodman BK (2004). Molecular and cytogenetic characterization of a novel translocation t(4;22) involving the breakpoint cluster region and platelet-derived growth factor receptor-alpha genes in a patient with atypical chronic myeloid leukemia. Genes Chromosomes Cancer 40: 44-50.

1907. Saglio G, Pane F, Gottardi E, Frigeri F, Buonaiuto MR, Guerrasio A, de Micheli D, Parziale A, Fornaci MN, Martinelli G, Salvatore F (1996). Consistent amounts of acute leukemia-associated P190BCR/ABL transcripts are expressed by chronic myelogenous leukemia patients at diagnosis. Blood 87: 1075-1080.

1908. Sahara N, Takeshita A, Shigeno K, Fujisawa S, Takeshita K, Naito K, Ihara M, Ono T, Tamashima S, Nara K, Ohnishi K, Ohno R (2002). Clinicopathological and prognostic characteristics of CD56-negative multiple myeloma. Br J Haematol 117: 882-885.

1909. Said JW (2007). Immunodeficiency-related Hodgkin lymphoma and its mimics. Adv Anat Pathol 14: 189-194.

1910. Said JW, Shintaku IP, Asou H, deVos S, Baker J, Hanson G, Cesarman E, Nador R, Koeffler HP (1999). Herpesvirus 8 inclusions in primary effusion lymphoma: report of a unique case with T-cell phenotype. Arch Pathol Lab Med 123: 257-260.

1911. Said JW, Tasaka T, Takeuchi S, Asou H, de Vos S, Cesarman E, Knowles DM, Koeffler HP (1996). Primary effusion lymphoma in women: report of two cases of Kaposi's sarcoma herpes virus-associated effusion-based lymphoma in human immunodeficiency virus-negative women. Blood 88: 3124-3128.

1912. Said W, Chien K, Takeuchi S, Tasaka T, Asou H, Cho SK, de Vos S, Cesarman E, Knowles DM, Koeffler HP (1996). Kaposi's sarcoma-associated herpesvirus (KSHV or HHV8) in primary effusion lymphoma: ultrastructural demonstration of herpesvirus in lymphoma cells. Blood 87: 4937-4943.

1913. Saikia T, Advani S, Dasgupta A, Ramakrishnan G, Nair C, Gladstone B, Kumar MS, Badrinath Y, Dhond S (1988). Characterisation of blast cells during blastic phase of chronic myeloid leukaemia by immunophenotyping—experience in 60 patients. Leuk Res 12: 499-506.

1913A. Sainati L, Matutes E, Mulligan S, de Olivera MP, Rani S, Lampert IA, Catovsky D (1990). A variant form of hairy cell leukemia resistant to alpha-interferon: clinical and phenotypic characteristics of 17 patients. Blood 76: 157-162.

1914. Sainty D, Liso V, Cantu-Rajnoldi A, Head D, Mozziconacci MJ, Arnoulet C, Benattar L, Fenu S, Mancini M, Duchayne E, Mahon FX, Gutierrez N, Birg F, Biondi A, Grimwade D, Lafage-Pochitaloff M, Hagemeijer A, Flandrin G (2000). A new morphologic classification system for acute promyelocytic leukemia distinguishes cases with underlying PLZF/RARA gene rearrangements. Groupe Francais de Cytogenetique Hematologique, UK Cancer Cytogenetics Group and BIOMED 1 European Community-Concerted Action Molecular Cytogenetic Diagnosis in Haematological Malignancies. Blood 96: 1287-1296.

1914A. Saito M, Gao J, Basso K, Kitagawa Y, Smith PM, Bhagat G, Pernis A, Pasqualucci L, Dalla-Favera R (2007). A signaling pathway mediating downregulation of BCL6 in germinal center B cells is blocked by BCL6 gene alter-

ations in B cell lymphoma. Cancel Cell 12: 280-292.

1915. Salar A, Fernandez dS, Romagosa V, Domingo-Claros A, Gonzalez-Barca E, Pera J, Climent J, Granena A (1998). Diffuse large B-cell lymphoma: is morphologic subdivision useful in clinical management? Eur J Haematol 60: 202-208.

1916. Salar A, Juanpere N, Bellosillo B, Domingo-Domenech E, Espinet B, Seoane A, Romagosa V, Gonzalez-Barca E, Panades A, Pedro C, Nieto M, Abella E, Sole F, Ariza A, Fernandez-Sevilla A, Besses C, Serrano S (2006). Gastrointestinal involvement in mantle cell lymphoma: a prospective clinic, endoscopic, and pathologic study. Am J Surg Pathol 30: 1274-1280.

1917. Salaverria I, Perez-Galan P, Colomer D, Campo E (2006). Mantle cell lymphoma: from pathology and molecular pathogenesis to new therapeutic perspectives. Haematologica 91: 11-16.

1918. Salaverria I, Zettl A, Bea S, Moreno V, Valls J, Hartmann E, Ott G, Wright G, Lopez-Guillermo A, Chan WC, Weisenburger DD, Gascoyne RD, Grogan TM, Delabie J, Jaffe ES, Montserrat E, Muller-Hermelink HK, Staudt LM, Rosenwald A, Campo E (2007). Specific secondary genetic alterations in mantle cell lymphoma provide prognostic information independent of the gene expression-based proliferation signature. J Clin Oncol 25: 1216-1222.

1919. Salhany KE, Macon WR, Choi JK, Elenitsas R, Lessin SR, Felgar RE, Wilson DM, Przybylski GK, Lister J, Wasik MA, Swerdlow SH (1998). Subcutaneous panniculitis-like T-cell lymphoma: clinicopathologic, immunophenotypic, and genotypic analysis of alpha/beta and gamma/delta subtypes. Am J Surg Pathol 22: 881-893.

1920. Salloum E, Cooper DL, Howe G, Lacy J, Tallini G, Crouch J, Schultz M, Murren J (1996). Spontaneous regression of lymphoproliferative disorders in patients treated with methotrexate for rheumatoid arthritis and other rheumatic diseases. J Clin Oncol 14: 1943-1949.

1921. Salmi TT, Collin P, Korponay-Szabo IR, Laurila K, Partanen J, Huhtala H, Kiraly R, Lorand L, Reunala T, Maki M, Kaukinen K (2006). Endomysial antibody-negative coeliac disease: clinical characteristics and intestinal autoantibody deposits. Gut 55: 1746-1753.

1922. Salomon-Nguyen F, Valensi F, Troussard X, Flandrin G (1996). The value of the monoclonal antibody, DBA44, in the diagnosis of B-lymphoid disorders. Leuk Res 20: 909-913.

1923. Salaverria I, Bea S, Lopez-Guillermo A, Lespinet V, Pinyol M, Burkhardt B, Lamant L, Zettl A, Horsman D, Gascoyne R, Ott G, Siebert R, Delsol G, Campo E (2008). Genomic profiling reveals different genetic aberrations in systemic ALK-positive and ALK-negative anaplastic large cell lymphomas. Br J Haematol. 140: 516-526.

1924. Samoszuk M, Nansen L (1990). Detection of interleukin-5 messenger RNA in Reed-Sternberg cells of Hodgkin's disease with eosinophilia. Blood 75: 13-16.

1925. Sanchez-Beato M, Saez AI, Navas IC, Algara P, Sol MM, Villuendas R, Camacho F, Sanchez-Aguilera A, Sanchez E, Piris MA (2001). Overall survival in aggressive B-cell lymphomas is dependent on the accumulation of alterations in p53, p16, and p27. Am J Pathol 159: 205-213.

1926. Sandberg Y, Almeida J, Gonzalez M, Lima M, Barcena P, Szczepanski T, Gastel-Mol EJ, Wind H, Balanzategui A, van Dongen JJ, Miguel JF, Orfao A, Langerak AW (2006). TCRgammadelta+ large granular lymphocyte

leukemias reflect the spectrum of normal antigen-selected TCRgammadelta+ T-cells. Leukemia 20: 505-513.

1927. Sander B, Middel P, Gunawan B, Schulten HJ, Baum F, Golas MM, Schulze F, Grabbe E, Parwaresch R, Fuzesi L (2007). Follicular dendritic cell sarcoma of the spleen. Hum Pathol 38: 668-672.

1928. Sander CA, Jaffe ES, Gebhardt FC, Yano T, Medeiros LJ (1992). Mediastinal lymphoblastic lymphoma with an immature B-cell immunophenotype. Am J Surg Pathol 16: 300-305.

1929. Sander CA, Medeiros LJ, Weiss LM, Yano T, Sneller MC, Jaffe ES (1992). Lymphoproliferative lesions in patients with common variable immunodeficiency syndrome. Am J Surg Pathol 16: 1170-1182.

1930. Sander CA, Yano T, Clark HM, Harris C, Longo DL, Jaffe ES, Raffeld M (1993). p53 mutation is associated with progression in follicular lymphomas. Blood 82: 1994-2004.

1931. Sanderson CJ (1992). Interleukin-5, eosinophils, and disease. Blood 79: 3101-3109.

1931A. Sangüeza OP, Salmon JK, White CR Jr, Beckstead JH (1995). Juvenile xanthogranuloma: a clinical, histopathologic and immunohistochemical study. J Cutan Pathol 22: 327-335.

1932. Sansonno D, De Vita S, Cornacchiulo V, Carbone A, Boiocchi M, Dammacco F (1996). Detection and distribution of hepatitis C virus-related proteins in lymph nodes of patients with type II mixed cryoglobulinemia and neoplastic or non-neoplastic lymphoproliferation. Blood 88: 4638-4645.

1933. Santucci M, Pimpinelli N, Arganini L (1991). Primary cutaneous B-cell lymphoma: a unique type of low-grade lymphoma. Clinicopathologic and immunologic study of 83 cases. Cancer 67: 2311-2326.

1934. Santucci M, Pimpinelli N, Massi D, Kadin ME, Meijer CJ, Muller-Hermelink HK, Paulli M, Wechsler J, Willemze R, Audring H, Bernengo MG, Cerroni L, Chimenti S, Chott A, Diaz-Perez JL, Dippel E, Duncan LM, Feller AC, Geerts ML, Hallermann C, Kempf W, Russell-Jones R, Sander C, Berti E (2003). Cytotoxic/natural killer cell cutaneous lymphomas. Report of EORTC Cutaneous Lymphoma Task Force Workshop. Cancer 97: 610-627.

1934A. Sargent RL, Cook JR, Aguilera NI, Surti U, Abbondanzo SL, Gollin SM, Swerdlow SH (2008). Fluorescence immunophenotypic and interphase cytogenetic characterization of nodal lymphoplasmacytic lymphoma. Am J Surg Pathol. In press.

1935. Sarris A, Jhanwar S, Cabanillas F (1999). Cytogenetics of Hodgkin's disease. In: Hodgkin's Disease. Mauch P, Armitage JO, Diehl V, eds. Lippincott Williams & Wilkins: Philadelphia, pp. 195.

1936. Sasajima Y, Yamabe H, Kobashi Y, Hirai K, Mori S (1993). High expression of the Epstein-Barr virus latent protein EB nuclear antigen-2 on pyothorax-associated lymphomas. Am J Pathol 143: 1280-1285.

1937. Sasaki H, Manabe A, Kojima S, Tsuchida M, Hayashi Y, Ikuta K, Okamura I, Koike K, Ohara A, Ishii E, Komada Y, Hibi S, Nakahata T (2001). Myelodysplastic syndrome in childhood: a retrospective study of 189 patients in Japan. Leukemia 15: 1713-1720.

1938. Sashida G, Takaku TI, Shoji N, Nishimaki J, Ito Y, Miyazawa K, Kimura Y, Ohyashiki JH, Ohyashiki K (2003). Clinico-hematologic features of myelodysplastic syndrome presenting as isolated thrombocytopenia: an entity with a relatively favorable prognosis. Leuk Lymphoma 44: 653-658.

1939. Sato Y, Ichimura K, Tanaka T, Takata K, Morito T, Sato H, Kondo E, Yanai H, Ohara

N, Oka T, Yoshino T (2008). Duodenal follicular lymphomas share common characteristics with mucosa-associated lymphoid tissue lymphomas. J Clin Pathol 61: 377-381.

1940. Satou Y, Yasunaga J, Yoshida M, Matsuoka M (2006). HTLV-I basic leucine zipper factor gene mRNA supports proliferation of adult T cell leukemia cells. Proc Natl Acad Sci U S A 103: 720-725.

1940A. Sausville EA, Worsham GF, Matthews MJ, Makuch RW, Fischmann AB, Schechter GP, Gazdar AF, Bunn PA (1985). Histologic assessment of lymph nodes in mycosis fungoides/Sezary syndrome (cutaneous T-cell lymphoma): clinical correlations and prognostic import of a new classification system. Hum Pathol 16: 1098-1109.

1941. Savage DG, Szydlo RM, Chase A, Apperley JF, Goldman JM (1997). Bone marrow transplantation for chronic myeloid leukaemia: the effects of differing criteria for defining chronic phase on probabilities of survival and relapse. Br J Haematol 99: 30-35.

1942. Savage DG, Szydlo RM, Goldman JM (1997). Clinical features at diagnosis in 430 patients with chronic myeloid leukaemia seen at a referral centre over a 16-year period. Br J Haematol 96: 111-116.

1943. Savage KJ, Al Rajhi N, Voss N, Paltiel C, Klasa R, Gascoyne RD, Connors JM (2006). Favorable outcome of primary mediastinal large B-cell lymphoma in a single institution: the British Columbia experience. Ann Oncol 17: 123-130.

1943A. Savage KJ, Harris NL, Vose JM, Ullrich F, Jaffe ES, Connors JM, Rimsza L, Pileri SA, Chhanabhai M, Gascoyne RD, Armitage JO, Weisenburger DD (2008). ALK-negative anaplastic large cell lymphoma (ALCL) is clinically and immunophenotypically different from both ALK-positive ALCL and peripheral T-cell lymphoma, not otherwise specified: report from the International Peripheral T-cell Lymphoma Project. Blood 111: 5496-5504..

1944. Savage KJ, Monti S, Kutok JL, Cattoretti G, Neuberg D, de Leval L, Kurtin P, Dal Cin P, Ladd C, Feuerhake F, Aguiar RC, Li S, Salles G, Berger F, Jing W, Pinkus GS, Habermann T, Dalla-Favera R, Harris NL, Aster JC, Golub TR, Shipp MA (2003). The molecular signature of mediastinal large B-cell lymphoma differs from that of other diffuse large B-cell lymphomas and shares features with classical Hodgkin lymphoma. Blood 102: 3871-3879.

1945. Savilo E, Campo E, Mollejo M, Pinyol M, Piris MA, Zukerberg LR, Yang WI, Koelliker DD, Nguyen PL, Harris NL (1998). Absence of cyclin D1 protein expression in splenic marginal zone lymphoma. Mod Pathol 11: 601-606.

1946. Savoldo B, Goss JA, Hammer MM, Zhang L, Lopez T, Gee AP, Lin YF, Quiros-Tejeira RE, Reinke P, Schubert S, Gottschalk S, Finegold MJ, Brenner MK, Rooney CM, Heslop HE (2006). Treatment of solid organ transplant recipients with autologous Epstein Barr virus-specific cytotoxic T lymphocytes (CTLs). Blood 108: 2942-2949.

1947. Sawyer JR, Waldron JA, Jagannath S, Barlogie B (1995). Cytogenetic findings in 200 patients with multiple myeloma. Cancer Genet Cytogenet 82: 41-49.

1948. Sawyers CL (1999). Chronic myeloid leukemia. N Engl J Med 340: 1330-1340.

1949. Scandura JM, Boccuni P, Cammenga J, Nimer SD (2002). Transcription factor fusions in acute leukemia: variations on a theme. Oncogene 21: 3422-3444.

1950. Scarabello A, Leinweber B, Ardigo M, Rutten A, Feller AC, Kerl H, Cerroni L (2002). Cutaneous lymphomas with prominent granulomatous reaction: a potential pitfall in the histopathologic diagnosis of cutaneous T- and

B-cell lymphomas. Am J Surg Pathol 26: 1259-1268.

1951. Scarisbrick JJ, Woolford AJ, Calonje E, Photiou A, Ferreira S, Orchard G, Russell-Jones R, Whittaker SJ (2002). Frequent abnormalities of the p15 and p16 genes in mycosis fungoides and sezary syndrome. J Invest Dermatol 118: 493-499.

1952. Scarisbrick JJ, Woolford AJ, Russell-Jones R, Whittaker SJ (2000). Loss of heterozygosity on 10q and microsatellite instability in advanced stages of primary cutaneous T-cell lymphoma and possible association with homozygous deletion of PTEN. Blood 95: 2937-2942.

1953. Scarpa A, Moore PS, Rigaud G, Inghirami G, Montresor M, Menegazzi M, Todeschini G, Menestrina F (1999). Molecular features of primary mediastinal B-cell lymphoma: involvement of p16INK4A, p53 and c-myc. Br J Haematol 107: 106-113.

1954. Schade AE, Wlodarski MW, Maciejewski JP (2006). Pathophysiology defined by altered signal transduction pathways: the role of JAK-STAT and PI3K signaling in leukemic large granular lymphocytes. Cell Cycle 5: 2571-2574.

1955. Schafer AI (2004). Thrombocytosis. N Engl J Med 350: 1211-1219.

1956. Schaffner C, Idler I, Stilgenbauer S, Dohner H, Lichter P (2000). Mantle cell lymphoma is characterized by inactivation of the ATM gene. Proc Natl Acad Sci U S A 97: 2773-2778.

1957. Schaffner C, Stilgenbauer S, Rappold GA, Dohner H, Lichter P (1999). Somatic ATM mutations indicate a pathogenic role of ATM in B-cell chronic lymphocytic leukemia. Blood 94: 748-753.

1958. Scheck O, Horny HP, Ruck P, Schmelzle R, Kaiserling E (1987). Solitary mastocytoma of the eyelid. A case report with special reference to the immunocytology of human tissue mast cells, and a review of the literature. Virchows Arch A Pathol Anat Histopathol 412: 31-36.

1958A. Scheffer E, Meijer CJ, van Vloten WA (1980). Dermatopathic lymphadenopathy and lymph node involvement in mycosis fungoides. Cancer 45: 137-148

1959. Scheffer E, Meijer CJ, van Vloten WA, Willemze R (1986). A histologic study of lymph nodes from patients with the Sezary syndrome. Cancer 57: 2375-2380.

1960. Schlegelberger B, Weber-Matthiesen K, Himmler A, Bartels H, Sonnen R, Kuse R, Feller AC, Grote W (1994). Cytogenetic findings and results of combined immunophenotyping and karyotyping in Hodgkin's disease. Leukemia 8: 72-80.

1961. Schlegelberger B, Zhang Y, Weber-Matthiesen K, Grote W (1994). Detection of aberrant clones in nearly all cases of angioimmunoblastic lymphadenopathy with dysproteinemia-type T-cell lymphoma by combined interphase and metaphase cytogenetics. Blood 84: 2640-2648.

1962. Schlenk RF, Benner A, Krauter J, Buchner T, Sauerland C, Ehninger G, Schaich M, Mohr B, Niederwieser D, Krahl R, Pasold R, Dohner K, Ganser A, Dohner H, Heil G (2004). Individual patient data-based meta-analysis of patients aged 16 to 60 years with core binding factor acute myeloid leukemia: a survey of the German Acute Myeloid Leukemia Intergroup. J Clin Oncol 22: 3741-3750.

1962A. Schlenk RF, Döhner K, Krauter J, Fröhling S, Corbacioglu A, Bullinger L, Habdank M, Späth D, Morgan M, Benner A, Schlegelberger B, Heil G, Ganser A, Döhner H; German-Austrian Acute Myeloid Leukemia Study Group (2008). Mutations and treatment

outcome in cytogenetically normal acute myeloid leukemia. NEJM 358:1909-1918.

1963. Schlette E, Bueso-Ramos C, Giles F, Glassman A, Hayes K, Medeiros LJ (2001). Mature B-cell leukemias with more than 55% prolymphocytes. A heterogeneous group that includes an unusual variant of mantle cell lymphoma. Am J Clin Pathol 115: 571-581.

1964. Schmid C, Pan L, Diss T, Isaacson PG (1991). Expression of B-cell antigens by Hodgkin's and Reed-Sternberg cells. Am J Pathol 139: 701-707.

1965. Schmid C, Sargent C, Isaacson PG (1991). L and H cells of nodular lymphocyte predominant Hodgkin's disease show immunoglobulin light-chain restriction. Am J Pathol 139: 1281-1289.

1966. Schmitt-Graeff A, Thiele J, Zuk I, Kvasnicka HM (2002). Essential thrombocythemia with ringed sideroblasts: a heterogeneous spectrum of diseases, but not a distinct entity. Haematologica 87: 392-399.

1967. Schmitt C, Balogh B, Grundt A, Buchholtz C, Leo A, Benner A, Hensel M, Ho AD, Leo E (2006). The bcl-2/IgH rearrangement in a population of 204 healthy individuals: occurrence, age and gender distribution, breakpoints, and detection method validity. Leuk Res 30: 745-750.

1968. Schmitz LL, McClure JS, Litz CE, Dayton V, Weisdorf DJ, Parkin JL, Brunning RD (1994). Morphologic and quantitative changes in blood and marrow cells following growth factor therapy. Am J Clin Pathol 101: 67-75.

1969. Schnittger S, Bacher U, Haferlach C, Dengler R, Krober A, Kern W, Haferlach T (2008). Detection of an MPLW515 mutation in a case with features of both essential thrombocythemia and refractory anemia with ringed sideroblasts and thrombocytosis. Leukemia 22: 453-455.

1969A. Schnittger S, Kohl TM, Haferlach T, Kern W, Hiddemann W, Spiekermann K, Schoch C (2006). KIT-D816 mutations in AML1-ETO-positive AML are associated with impaired event-free and overall survival. Blood 107: 1791-1799.

1970. Schnittger S, Schoch C, Kern W, Mecucci C, Tschulik C, Martelli MF, Haferlach T, Hiddemann W, Falini B (2005). Nucleophosmin gene mutations are predictors of favorable prognosis in acute myelogenous leukemia with a normal karyotype. Blood 106: 3733-3739.

1971. Schooley RT, Flaum MA, Gralnick HR, Fauci AS (1981). A clinicopathologic correlation of the idiopathic hypereosinophilic syndrome. II. Clinical manifestations. Blood 58: 1021-1026.

1972. Schop RF, Van Wier SA, Xu R, Ghobrial I, Ahmann GJ, Greipp PR, Kyle RA, Dispenzieri A, Lacy MQ, Rajkumar SV, Gertz MA, Fonseca R (2006). 6q deletion discriminates Waldenstrom macroglobulinemia from IgM monoclonal gammopathy of undetermined significance. Cancer Genet Cytogenet 169: 150-153.

1973. Schraders M, De Jong D, Kluin P, Groenen P, van Krieken H (2005). Lack of Bcl-2 expression in follicular lymphoma may be caused by mutations in the BCL2 gene or by absence of the t(14;18) translocation. J Pathol 205: 329-335.

1973A. Schrager JA, Pittaluga S, Raffeld M, Jaffe ES (2005) Granulomatous reaction in Burkitt lymphoma: correlation with EBV positivity and clinical outcome..Am J Surg Pathol 29:1115-1116.

1974. Schubbert S, Zenker M, Rowe SL, Boll S, Klein C, Bollag G, van dB, I, Musante L, Kalscheuer V, Wehner LE, Nguyen H, West B, Zhang KY, Sistermans E, Rauch A, Niemeyer CM, Shannon K, Kratz CP (2006). Germline

KRAS mutations cause Noonan syndrome. Nat Genet 38: 331-336.

1975. Schultz KR, Bowman P, Slayton WB, Aledo A, Devidas M, Sather H, Borowitz MJ, Davies S, Trigg M, Pasut B, Jorstad D, Elsinger T, Burden L, Wang C, Rutledge R, Gaynon P, Carroll A, Heerema N, Winick N, Hunger S, Carroll WL, Camitta B (2007). Improved Early Event Free Survival (EFS) in Children with Philadelphia Chromosome-Positive (Ph+) Acute Lymphoblastic Leukemia (ALL) with Intensive Imatinib In Combination With High Dose Chemotherapy: Children's Oncology Group (COG) Study AALL0031. Blood 110: 776.

1976. Schultz KR, Pullen DJ, Sather HN, Shuster JJ, Devidas M, Borowitz MJ, Carroll AJ, Heerema NA, Rubnitz JE, Loh ML, Raetz EA, Winick NJ, Hunger SP, Carroll WL, Gaynon PS, Camitta BM (2007). Risk- and response-based classification of childhood B-precursor acute lymphoblastic leukemia: a combined analysis of prognostic markers from the Pediatric Oncology Group (POG) and Children's Cancer Group (CCG). Blood 109: 926-935.

1976A. Schwarting R, Gerdes J, Dürkop H, Falini B, Pileri S, Stein H (1989). BER-H2: a new anti-Ki-1 (CD30) monoclonal antibody directed at a formol-resistant epitope. Blood 74: 1678-1689

1977. Schwartz LB, Sakai K, Bradford TR, Ren S, Zweiman B, Worobec AS, Metcalfe DD (1995). The alpha form of human tryptase is the predominant type present in blood at baseline in normal subjects and is elevated in those with systemic mastocytosis. J Clin Invest 96: 2702-2710.

1977A. Schwering I, Bräuninger A, Klein U, Jungnickel B, Tinguely M, Diehl V, Hansmann ML, Dalla-Favera R, Rajewsky K, Küppers R (2003). Loss of the B-lineage-specific gene expression program in Hodgkin and Reed-Sternberg cells of Hodgkin lymphoma. Blood 101:1505-1512.

1978. Schwyzer R, Sherman GG, Cohn RJ, Poole JE, Willem P (1998). Granulocytic sarcoma in children with acute myeloblastic leukemia and t(8;21). Med Pediatr Oncol 31: 144-149.

1979. Score J, Curtis C, Waghorn K, Stalder M, Jotterand M, Grand FH, Cross NC (2006). Identification of a novel imatinib responsive KIF5B-PDGFRA fusion gene following screening for PDGFRA overexpression in patients with hypereosinophilia. Leukemia 20: 827-832.

1980. Scott AA, Head DR, Kopecky KJ, Appelbaum FR, Theil KS, Grever MR, Chen IM, Whittaker MH, Griffith BB, Licht JD (1994). HLA-DR-, CD33+, CD56+, CD16- myeloid/natural killer cell acute leukemia: a previously unrecognized form of acute leukemia potentially misdiagnosed as French-American-British acute myeloid leukemia-M3. Blood 84: 244-255.

1981. Scott LM, Tong W, Levine RL, Scott MA, Beer PA, Stratton MR, Futreal PA, Erber WN, McMullin MF, Harrison CN, Warren AJ, Gilliland DG, Lodish HF, Green AR (2007). JAK2 exon 12 mutations in polycythemia vera and idiopathic erythrocytosis. N Engl J Med 356: 459-468.

1982. Scquizzato E, Teramo A, Miorin M, Facco M, Piazza F, Noventa F, Trentin L, Agostini C, Zambello R, Semenzato G (2007). Genotypic evaluation of killer immunoglobulin-like receptors in NK-type lymphoproliferative disease of granular lymphocytes. Leukemia 21: 1060-1069.

1983. Secker-Walker LM, Mehta A, Bain B (1995). Abnormalities of 3q21 and 3q26 in myeloid malignancy: a United Kingdom Cancer Cytogenetic Group study. Br J Haematol 91:

490-501.

1984. Secker-Walker LM, Moorman AV, Bain BJ, Mehta AB (1998). Secondary acute leukemia and myelodysplastic syndrome with 11q23 abnormalities. EU Concerted Action 11q23 Workshop. Leukemia 12: 840-844.

1984A. Sedelies KA, Sayers TJ, Edwards KM, Chen W, Pellicci DG, Godfrey DI, Trapani JA (2004). Discordant regulation of granzyme H and granzyme B expression in human lymphocytes. J Biol Chem 279: 26581-26587.

1985. Sehn LH, Berry B, Chhanabhai M, Fitzgerald C, Gill K, Hoskins P, Klasa R, Savage KJ, Shenkier T, Sutherland J, Gascoyne RD, Connors JM (2007). The revised International Prognostic Index (R-IPI) is a better predictor of outcome than the standard IPI for patients with diffuse large B-cell lymphoma treated with R-CHOP. Blood 109: 1857-1861.

1986. Seiler T, Dohner H, Stilgenbauer S (2006). Risk stratification in chronic lymphocytic leukemia. Semin Oncol 33: 186-194.

1987. Seitz V, Hummel M, Marafioti T, Anagnostopoulos I, Assaf C, Stein H (2000). Detection of clonal T-cell receptor gamma-chain gene rearrangements in Reed-Sternberg cells of classic Hodgkin disease. Blood 95: 3020-3024.

1988. Seligmann M (1975). Immuno-histochemical, clinical and pathological features of alpha-heavy chain disease. Arch Intern Med 135: 78-82.

1989. Seligmann M, Mihaesco E, Preud'Homme JL, Danon F, Brouet JC (1979). Heavy chain diseases: current findings and concepts. Immunol Rev 48: 145-167.

1990. Sellick GS, Lubbe SJ, Matutes E, Catovsky D, Houlston RS (2007). Microsatellite instability indicative of defects in the major mismatch repair genes is rare in patients with B-cell chronic lymphocytic leukemia: Evaluation with disease stage and family history. Leuk Lymphoma 48: 1320-1322.

1991. Selves J, Meggetto F, Brousset P, Voigt JJ, Pradere B, Grasset D, Icart J, Mariame B, Knecht H, Delsol G (1996). Inflammatory pseudotumor of the liver. Evidence for follicular dendritic reticulum cell proliferation associated with clonal Epstein-Barr virus. Am J Surg Pathol 20: 747-753.

1992. Semenzato G, Zambello R, Starkebaum G, Oshimi K, Loughran TP, Jr. (1997). The lymphoproliferative disease of granular lymphocytes: updated criteria for diagnosis. Blood 89: 256-260.

1993. Senff NJ, Hoefnagel JJ, Jansen PM, Vermeer MH, van Baarlen J, Blokx WA, Canninga-van Dijk MR, Geerts ML, Hebeda KM, Kluin PM, Lam KH, Meijer CJ, Willemze R (2007). Reclassification of 300 primary cutaneous B-Cell lymphomas according to the new WHO-EORTC classification for cutaneous lymphomas: comparison with previous classifications and identification of prognostic markers. J Clin Oncol 25: 1581-1587.

1994. Serpell LC, Sunde M, Blake CC (1997). The molecular basis of amyloidosis. Cell Mol Life Sci 53: 871-887.

1995. Seto M, Yamamoto K, Iida S, Akao Y, Utsumi KR, Kubonishi I, Miyoshi I, Ohtsuki T, Yawata Y, Namba M, . (1992). Gene rearrangement and overexpression of PRAD1 in lymphoid malignancy with t(11;14)(q13;q32) translocation. Oncogene 7: 1401-1406.

1996. Shabrawi-Caelen L, Kerl H, Cerroni L (2004). Lymphomatoid papulosis: reappraisal of clinicopathologic presentation and classification into subtypes A, B, and C. Arch Dermatol 140: 441-447.

1997. Shannon KM, O'Connell P, Martin GA, Paderanga D, Olson K, Dinndorf P, McCormick F (1994). Loss of the normal NF1 allele from the

bone marrow of children with type 1 neurofibromatosis and malignant myeloid disorders. N Engl J Med 330: 597-601.
1998. Shapiro RS, McClain K, Frizzera G, Gajl-Peczalska KJ, Kersey JH, Blazar BR, Arthur DC, Patton DF, Greenberg JS, Burke B (1988). Epstein-Barr virus associated B cell lymphoproliferative disorders following bone marrow transplantation. Blood 71: 1234-1243.
1999. Sharpe RW, Bethel KJ (2006). Hairy cell leukemia: diagnostic pathology. Hematol Oncol Clin North Am 20: 1023-1049.
2000. Shaughnessy J, Jacobson J, Sawyer J, McCoy J, Fassas A, Zhan F, Bumm K, Epstein J, Anaissie E, Jagannath S, Vesole D, Siegel D, Desikan R, Munshi N, Badros A, Tian E, Zangari M, Tricot G, Crowley J, Barlogie B (2003). Continuous absence of metaphase-defined cytogenetic abnormalities, especially of chromosome 13 and hypodiploidy, ensures long-term survival in multiple myeloma treated with Total Therapy I: interpretation in the context of global gene expression. Blood 101: 3849-3856.
2001. Shaughnessy JD, Jr., Zhan F, Burington BE, Huang Y, Colla S, Hanamura I, Stewart JP, Kordsmeier B, Randolph C, Williams DR, Xiao Y, Xu H, Epstein J, Anaissie E, Krishna SG, Cottler-Fox M, Hollmig K, Mohiuddin A, Pineda-Roman M, Tricot G, van Rhee F, Sawyer J, Alsayed Y, Walker R, Zangari M, Crowley J, Barlogie B (2007). A validated gene expression model of high-risk multiple myeloma is defined by deregulated expression of genes mapping to chromosome 1. Blood 109: 2276-2284.
2002. Shen L, Liang AC, Lu L, Au WY, Kwong YL, Liang RH, Srivastava G (2002). Frequent deletion of Fas gene sequences encoding death and transmembrane domains in nasal natural killer/T-cell lymphoma. Am J Pathol 161: 2123-2131.
2003. Shepherd PC, Ganesan TS, Galton DA (1987). Haematological classification of the chronic myeloid leukaemias. Baillieres Clin Haematol 1: 887-906.
2004. Shi G, Weh HJ, Duhrsen U, Zeller W, Hossfeld DK (1997). Chromosomal abnormality inv(3)(q21q26) associated with multilineage hematopoietic progenitor cells in hematopoietic malignancies. Cancer Genet Cytogenet 96: 58-63.
2005. Shia J, Teruya-Feldstein J, Pan D, Hegde A, Klimstra DS, Chaganti RS, Qin J, Portlock CS, Filippa DA (2002). Primary follicular lymphoma of the gastrointestinal tract: a clinical and pathologic study of 26 cases. Am J Surg Pathol 26: 216-224.
2006. Shigesada K, van de Sluis B, Liu PP (2004). Mechanism of leukemogenesis by the inv(16) chimeric gene CBFB/PEBP2B-MHY11. Oncogene 23: 4297-4307.
2007. Shih LY, Lee CT (1994). Identification of masked polycythemia vera from patients with idiopathic marked thrombocytosis by endogenous erythroid colony assay. Blood 83: 744-748.
2008. Shih LY, Liang DC, Fu JF, Wu JH, Wang PN, Lin TL, Dunn P, Kuo MC, Tang TC, Lin TH, Lai CL (2006). Characterization of fusion partner genes in 114 patients with de novo acute myeloid leukemia and MLL rearrangement. Leukemia 20: 218-223.
2009. Shimabukuro-Vornhagen A, Haverkamp H, Engert A, Balleisen L, Majunke P, Heil G, Eich HT, Stein H, Diehl V, Josting A (2005). Lymphocyte-rich classical Hodgkin's lymphoma: clinical presentation and treatment outcome in 100 patients treated within German Hodgkin's Study Group trials. J Clin Oncol 23: 5739-5745.
2009A. Shimada A, Taki T, Tabuchi K, Tawa A, Horibe K, Tsuchida M, Hanada R, Tsukimoto I, Hayashi Y (2006). KIT mutations, and not FLT3 internal tandem duplication, are strongly associated with a poor prognosis in pediatric acute myeloid leukemia with t(8;21): a study of the Japanese Childhood AML Cooperative Study Group. Blood 107: 1806-1809.
2010. Shimoyama M (1991). Diagnostic criteria and classification of clinical subtypes of adult T-cell leukaemia-lymphoma. A report from the Lymphoma Study Group (1984-87). Br J Haematol 79: 428-437.
2011. Shimoyama Y, Oyama T, Asano N, Oshiro A, Suzuki R, Kagami Y, Morishima Y, Nakamura S (2006). Senile Epstein-Barr virus-associated B-cell lymphoproliferative disorders: a mini review. J Clin Exp Hematop 46: 1-4.
2012. Shiong YS, Lian JD, Lin CY, Shu KH, Lu YS, Chou G (1992). Epstein-Barr virus-associated T-cell lymphoma of the maxillary sinus in a renal transplant recipient. Transplant Proc 24: 1929-1931.
2013. Shiota M, Nakamura S, Ichinohasama R, Abe M, Akagi T, Takeshita M, Mori N, Fujimoto J, Miyauchi J, Mikata A (1995). Anaplastic large cell lymphomas expressing the novel chimeric protein p80NPM/ALK: a distinct clinicopathologic entity. Blood 86: 1954-1960.
2014. Shiramizu B, Barriga F, Neequaye J, Jafri A, Dalla-Favera R, Neri A, Guttierez M, Levine P, Magrath I (1991). Patterns of chromosomal breakpoint locations in Burkitt's lymphoma: relevance to geography and Epstein-Barr virus association. Blood 77: 1516-1526.
2015. Shiseki M, Kitagawa Y, Wang YH, Yoshinaga K, Kondo T, Kuroiwa H (2007). Lack of nucleophosmin mutation in patients with myelodysplastic syndrome and acute myeloid leukemia with chromosome 5 abnormalities. Leukaemia and Lymphoma 48: 2141-2144.
2016. Shivakumar L, Armitage JO (2006). Bcl-2 gene expression as a predictor of outcome in diffuse large B-cell lymphoma. Clin Lymphoma Myeloma 6: 455-457.
2017. Shou Y, Martelli ML, Gabrea A, Qi Y, Brents LA, Roschke A, Dewald G, Kirsch IR, Bergsagel PL, Kuehl WM (2000). Diverse karyotypic abnormalities of the c-myc locus associated with c-myc dysregulation and tumor progression in multiple myeloma. Proc Natl Acad Sci U S A 97: 228-233.
2018. Sibaud V, Beylot-Barry M, Thiebaut R, Parrens M, Vergier B, Delaunay M, Beylot C, Chene G, Ferrer J, de Mascarel A, Dubus P, Merlio JP (2003). Bone marrow histopathologic and molecular staging in epidermotropic T-cell lymphomas. Am J Clin Pathol 119: 414-423.
2019. Sidoroff A, Zelger B, Steiner H, Smith N (1996). Indeterminate cell histiocytosis—a clinicopathological entity with features of both X- and non-X histiocytosis. Br J Dermatol 134: 525-532.
2020. Siebert JD, Ambinder RF, Napoli VM, Quintanilla-Martinez L, Banks PM, Gulley ML (1995). Human immunodeficiency virus-associated Hodgkin's disease contains latent, not replicative, Epstein-Barr virus. Hum Pathol 26: 1191-1195.
2021. Siegert W, Nerl C, Agthe A, Engelhard M, Brittinger G, Tiemann M, Lennert K, Huhn D (1995). Angioimmunoblastic lymphadenopathy (AILD)-type T-cell lymphoma: prognostic impact of clinical observations and laboratory findings at presentation. The Kiel Lymphoma Study Group. Ann Oncol 6: 659-664.
2022. Silver RT, Woolf SH, Hehlmann R, Appelbaum FR, Anderson J, Bennett C, Goldman JM, Guilhot F, Kantarjian HM, Lichtin AE, Talpaz M, Tura S (1999). An evidence-based analysis of the effect of busulfan, hydroxyurea, interferon, and allogeneic bone marrow transplantation in treating the chronic phase of chronic myeloid leukemia: developed for the American Society of Hematology. Blood 94: 1517-1536.
2023. Silverman LB, Sallan SE (2003). Newly diagnosed childhood acute lymphoblastic leukemia: update on prognostic factors and treatment. Curr Opin Hematol 10: 290-296.
2024. Simon HU, Plotz SG, Dummer R, Blaser K (1999). Abnormal clones of T cells producing interleukin-5 in idiopathic eosinophilia. N Engl J Med 341: 1112-1120.
2025. Simonelli C, Spina M, Cinelli R, Talamini R, Tedeschi R, Gloghini A, Vaccher E, Carbone A, Tirelli U (2003). Clinical features and outcome of primary effusion lymphoma in HIV-infected patients: a single-institution study. J Clin Oncol 21: 3948-3954.
2026. Singh ZN, Huo D, Anastasi J, Smith SM, Karrison T, Le Beau MM, Larson RA, Vardiman JW (2007). Therapy-related myelodysplastic syndrome: morphologic subclassification may not be clinically relevant. Am J Clin Pathol 127: 197-205.
2027. Siu LL, Chan JK, Wong KF, Kwong YL (2002). Specific patterns of gene methylation in natural killer cell lymphomas : p73 is consistently involved. Am J Pathol 160: 59-66.
2028. Siu LL, Chan V, Chan JK, Wong KF, Liang R, Kwong YL (2000). Consistent patterns of allelic loss in natural killer cell lymphoma. Am J Pathol 157: 1803-1809.
2029. Siu LL, Wong KF, Chan JK, Kwong YL (1999). Comparative genomic hybridization analysis of natural killer cell lymphoma/leukemia. Recognition of consistent patterns of genetic alterations. Am J Pathol 155: 1419-1425.
2030. Skinnider BF, Connors JM, Sutcliffe SB, Gascoyne RD (1999). Anaplastic large cell lymphoma: a clinicopathologic analysis. Hematol Oncol 17: 137-148.
2030A. Skinnider BF, Elia AJ, Gascoyne RD, Patterson B, Trumper L, Kapp U, Mak TW (2002). Signal transducer and activator of transcription 6 is frequently activated in Hodgkin and Reed-Sternberg cells of Hodgkin lymphoma. Blood 99: 618-26.
2031. Skinnider BF, Elia AJ, Gascoyne RD, Trumper LH, von Bonin F, Kapp U, Patterson B, Snow BE, Mak TW (2001). Interleukin 13 and interleukin 13 receptor are frequently expressed by hodgkin and reed-sternberg cells of hodgkin lymphoma. Blood 97: 250-255.
2032. Skoda R, Prchal JT (2005). Lessons from familial myeloproliferative disorders. Semin Hematol 42: 266-273.
2033. Sloand EM, Mainwaring L, Fuhrer M, Ramkissoon S, Risitano AM, Keyvanafar K, Lu J, Basu A, Barrett AJ, Young NS (2005). Preferential suppression of trisomy 8 compared with normal hematopoietic cell growth by autologous lymphocytes in patients with trisomy 8 myelodysplastic syndrome. Blood 106: 841-851.
2034. Slovak ML, Bedell V, Popplewell L, Arber DA, Schoch C, Slater R (2002). 21q22 balanced chromosome aberrations in therapy-related hematopoietic disorders: report from an international workshop. Genes Chromosomes Cancer 33: 379-394.
2035. Slovak ML, Gundacker H, Bloomfield CD, Dewald G, Appelbaum FR, Larson RA, Tallman MS, Bennett JM, Stirewalt DL, Meshinchi S, Willman CL, Ravindranath Y, Alonzo TA, Carroll AJ, Raimondi SC, Heerema NA (2006). A retrospective study of 69 patients with t(6;9)(p23;q34) AML emphasizes the need for a prospective, multicenter initiative for rare 'poor prognosis' myeloid malignancies. Leukemia 20: 1295-1297.
2036. Slovak ML, Kopecky KJ, Cassileth PA, Harrington DH, Theil KS, Mohamed A, Paietta E, Willman CL, Head DR, Rowe JM, Forman SJ, Appelbaum FR (2000). Karyotypic analysis predicts outcome of preremission and postremission therapy in adult acute myeloid leukemia: a southwest oncology Group/Eastern cooperative oncology group study. Blood 96: 4075-4083.
2037. Smith DB, Harris M, Gowland E, Chang J, Scarffe JH (1986). Non-secretory multiple myeloma: a report of 13 cases with a review of the literature. Hematol Oncol 4: 307-313.
2038. Smith JR, Braziel RM, Paoletti S, Lipp M, Uguccioni M, Rosenbaum JT (2003). Expression of B-cell-attracting chemokine 1 (CXCL13) by malignant lymphocytes and vascular endothelium in primary central nervous system lymphoma. Blood 101: 815-821.
2039. Smith MA, Reis LA, Gurnew JG *et al.* (eds.) (1995). Cancer incidence and survival among children and adolescents: United States SEER program 1975-1995. National Cancer Institute, SEER Program: Bethesda, MD.
2040. Smith ML, Cavenagh JD, Lister TA, Fitzgibbon J (2004). Mutation of CEBPA in familial acute myeloid leukemia. N Engl J Med 351: 2403-2407.
2041. Smith SM, Le Beau MM, Huo D, Karrison T, Sobecks RM, Anastasi J, Vardiman JW, Rowley JD, Larson RA (2003). Clinical-cytogenetic associations in 306 patients with therapy-related myelodysplasia and myeloid leukemia: the University of Chicago series. Blood 102: 43-52.
2042. Sneller MC, Wang J, Dale JK, Strober W, Middelton LA, Choi Y, Fleisher TA, Lim MS, Jaffe ES, Puck JM, Lenardo MJ, Straus SE (1997). Clincial, immunologic, and genetic features of an autoimmune lymphoproliferative syndrome associated with abnormal lymphocyte apoptosis. Blood 89: 1341-1348.
2043. Sohn SK, Jung JT, Kim DH, Kim JG, Kwak EK, Park T, Shin DG, Sohn KR, Lee KB (2003). Prognostic significance of bcl-2, bax, and p53 expression in diffuse large B-cell lymphoma. Am J Hematol 73: 101-107.
2043A. Sojka DK, Huang YH, Fowell DJ (2008). Mechanisms of regulatory T-cell suppression - a diverse arsenal for a moving target. Immunology 124: 13-22.
2044. Sokal JE, Cox EB, Baccarani M, Tura S, Gomez GA, Robertson JE, Tso CY, Braun TJ, Clarkson BD, Cervantes F, *et al.* (1984). Prognostic discrimination in "good-risk" chronic granulocytic leukemia. Blood 63: 789-799.
2045. Sokal JE, Sheerin KA (1986). Decreased stainable marrow iron in chronic granulocytic leukemia. Am J Med 81: 395-399.
2046. Sokolowska-Wojdylo M, Wenzel J, Gaffal E, Steitz J, Roszkiewicz J, Bieber T, Tuting T (2005). Absence of CD26 expression on skin-homing CLA+ CD4+ T lymphocytes in peripheral blood is a highly sensitive marker for early diagnosis and therapeutic monitoring of patients with Sezary syndrome. Clin Exp Dermatol 30: 702-706.
2047. Solal-Celigny P, Desaint B, Herrera A, Chastang C, Amar M, Vroclans M, Brousse N, Mancilla F, Renoux M, Bernard JF (1984). Chronic myelomonocytic leukemia according to FAB classification: analysis of 35 cases. Blood 63: 634-638.
2048. Solal-Celigny P, Roy P, Colombat P, White J, Armitage JO, Arranz-Saez R, Au WY, Bellei M, Brice P, Caballero D, Coiffier B, Conde-Garcia E, Doyen C, Federico M, Fisher RI, Garcia-Conde JF, Guglielmi C, Hagenbeek A, Haioun C, LeBlanc M, Lister AT, Lopez-Guillermo A, McLaughlin P, Milpied N, Morel P, Mounier N, Proctor SJ, Rohatiner A, Smith P, Soubeyran P, Tilly H, Vitolo U, Zinzani PL, Zucca E, Montserrat E (2004). Follicular lymphoma international prognostic index. Blood 104: 1258-1265.

2049. Soler J, Bordes R, Ortuno F, Montagud M, Martorell J, Pons C, Nomdedeu J, Lopez-Lopez JJ, Prat J, Rutllant M (1994). Aggressive natural killer cell leukaemia/lymphoma in two patients with lethal midline granuloma. Br J Haematol 86: 659-662.
2050. Soligo D, Delia D, Oriani A, Cattoretti G, Orazi A, Bertolli V, Quirici N, Deliliers GL (1991). Identification of CD34+ cells in normal and pathological bone marrow biopsies by QBEND10 monoclonal antibody. Leukemia 5: 1026-1030.
2051. Sommer VH, Clemmensen OJ, Nielsen O, Wasik M, Lovato P, Brender C, Eriksen KW, Woetmann A, Kaestel CG, Nissen MH, Ropke C, Skov S, Odum N (2004). In vivo activation of STAT3 in cutaneous T-cell lymphoma. Evidence for an antiapoptotic function of STAT3. Leukemia 18: 1288-1295.
2052. Song SY, Kim WS, Ko YH, Kim K, Lee MH, Park K (2002). Aggressive natural killer cell leukemia: clinical features and treatment outcome. Haematologica 87: 1343-1345.
2053. Sordillo PP, Epremian B, Koziner B, Lacher M, Lieberman P (1982). Lymphomatoid granulomatosis: an analysis of clinical and immunologic characteristics. Cancer 49: 2070-2076.
2054. Soriano AO, Thompson MA, Admirand JH, Fayad LE, Rodriguez AM, Romaguera JE, Hagemeister FB, Pro B (2007). Follicular dendritic cell sarcoma: A report of 14 cases and a review of the literature. Am J Hematol 82: 725-728.
2055. Soter NA (2000). Mastocytosis and the skin. Hematol Oncol Clin North Am 14: 537-555.
2056. Sotlar K, Fridrich C, Mall A, Jaussi R, Bultmann B, Valent P, Horny HP (2002). Detection of c-kit point mutation Asp-816 —> Val in microdissected pooled single mast cells and leukemic cells in a patient with systemic mastocytosis and concomitant chronic myelomonocytic leukemia. Leuk Res 26: 979-984.
2057. Sotlar K, Horny HP, Simonitsch I, Krokowski M, Aichberger KJ, Mayerhofer M, Printz D, Fritsch G, Valent P (2004). CD25 indicates the neoplastic phenotype of mast cells: a novel immunohistochemical marker for the diagnosis of systemic mastocytosis (SM) in routinely processed bone marrow biopsy specimens. Am J Surg Pathol 28: 1319-1325.
2058. Soubrier MJ, Dubost JJ, Sauvezie BJ (1994). POEMS syndrome: a study of 25 cases and a review of the literature. French Study Group on POEMS Syndrome. Am J Med 97: 543-553.
2059. Soumelis V, Liu YJ (2006). From plasmacytoid to dendritic cell: morphological and functional switches during plasmacytoid predendritic cell differentiation. Eur J Immunol 36: 2286-2292.
2060. Soussain C, Patte C, Ostronoff M, Delmer A, Rigal-Huguet F, Cambier N, Leprise PY, Francois S, Cony-Makhoul P, Harousseau JL (1995). Small noncleaved cell lymphoma and leukemia in adults. A retrospective study of 65 adults treated with the LMB pediatric protocols. Blood 85: 664-674.
2061. Soutar R, Lucraft H, Jackson G, Reece A, Bird J, Low E, Samson D (2004). Guidelines on the diagnosis and management of solitary plasmacytoma of bone and solitary extramedullary plasmacytoma. Br J Haematol 124: 717-726.
2062. Specht L, Hasenclever D (1999). Prognostic factors of Hodgkin's disease. In: Hodgkin's Disease. Mauch P, Armitage JO, Diehl V, eds. Lippincott Williams & Wilkins: Philadelphia, pp. 295.
2063. Speck NA, Gilliland DG (2002). Core-binding factors in haematopoiesis and leukaemia. Nat Rev Cancer 2: 502-513.
2064. Spencer J, Cerf-Bensussan N, Jarry A, Brousse N, Guy-Grand D, Krajewski AS, Isaacson PG (1988). Enteropathy-associated T cell lymphoma (malignant histiocytosis of the intestine) is recognized by a monoclonal antibody (HML-1) that defines a membrane molecule on human mucosal lymphocytes. Am J Pathol 132: 1-5.
2064A. Spencer J, Finn T, Pulford KA, Mason DY, Isaacson PG (1985). The human gut contains a novel population of B lymphocytes which resemble marginal zone cells. Clin Exp Immunol 62: 607-612.
2065. Sperr WR, Drach J, Hauswirth AW, Ackermann J, Mitterbauer M, Mitterbauer G, Foedinger M, Fonatsch C, Simonitsch-Klupp I, Kalhs P, Valent P (2005). Myelomastocytic leukemia: evidence for the origin of mast cells from the leukemic clone and eradication by allogeneic stem cell transplantation. Clin Cancer Res 11: 6787-6792.
2066. Sperr WR, Walchshofer S, Horny HP, Fodinger M, Simonitsch I, Fritsche-Polanz R, Schwarzinger I, Tschachler E, Sillaber C, Hagen W, Geissler K, Chott A, Lechner K, Valent P (1998). Systemic mastocytosis associated with acute myeloid leukaemia: report of two cases and detection of the c-kit mutation Asp-816 to Val. Br J Haematol 103: 740-749.
2067. Spiers AS, Bain BJ, Turner JE (1977). The peripheral blood in chronic granulocytic leukaemia. Study of 50 untreated Philadelphia-positive cases. Scand J Haematol 18: 25-38.
2068. Spina M, Vaccher E, Nasti G, Tirelli U (2000). Human immunodeficiency virus-associated Hodgkin's disease. Semin Oncol 27: 480-488.
2069. Spiro IJ, Yandell DW, Li C, Saini S, Ferry J, Powelson J, Katkov WN, Cosimi AB (1993). Brief report: lymphoma of donor origin occurring in the porta hepatis of a transplanted liver. N Engl J Med 329: 27-29.
2070. Spits H, Lanier LL, Phillips JH (1995). Development of human T and natural killer cells. Blood 85: 2654-2670.
2070A. Spits H, Blom B, Jaleco AC, Weijer K, Verschuren MC, van Dongen JJ, Heemskerk MH, Res PC (1998). Early stages in the development of human T, natural killer and thymic dendritic cells. Immunol Rev 165: 75-86.
2071. Spivak JL (2002). Polycythemia vera: myths, mechanisms, and management. Blood 100: 4272-4290.
2072. Spry CJ, Davies J, Tai PC, Olsen EG, Oakley CM, Goodwin JF (1983). Clinical features of fifteen patients with the hypereosinophilic syndrome. Q J Med 52: 1-22.
2073. Srinivas SK, Sample JT, Sixbey JW (1998). Spontaneous loss of viral episomes accompanying Epstein-Barr virus reactivation in a Burkitt's lymphoma cell line. J Infect Dis 177: 1705-1709.
2074. Staal-Viliare A, Latger-Cannard V, Rault JP, Didion J, Gregoire MJ, Bologna S, Witz B, Jonveaux P, Lecompte T, Rio Y (2006). [A case of de novo acute basophilic leukaemia: diagnostic criteria and review of the literature]. Ann Biol Clin (Paris) 64: 361-365.
2075. Stachurski D, Miron PM, Al Homsi S, Hutchinson L, Lee HN, Woda B, Wang SA (2007). Anaplastic lymphoma kinase-positive diffuse large B-cell lymphoma with a complex karyotype and cryptic 3' ALK gene insertion to chromosome 4 q22-24. Hum Pathol 38: 940-945.
2076. Standen GR, Jasani B, Wagstaff M, Wardrop CA (1990). Chronic neutrophilic leukemia and multiple myeloma. An association with lambda light chain expression. Cancer 66: 162-166.
2077. Standen GR, Steers FJ, Jones L (1993). Clonality of chronic neutrophilic leukaemia associated with myeloma: analysis using the X-linked probe M27 beta. J Clin Pathol 46: 297-298.
2078. Stanley M, McKenna RW, Ellinger G, Brunning RD (1985). Classification of 358 cases of Acute Myeloid Leukemia by FAB criteria: analysis of clinical and morphologic features. In: Chronic and acute leukemias in adults, Bloomfield CD (ed.) Martinus Nijhoff Publishers: Boston, pp 147-174.
2078A. Stansfeld AG, Diebold J, Noel H et al. Updated Kiel classification for lymphomas. Lancet 1: 292-293
2079. Stark B, Resnitzky P, Jeison M, Luria D, Blau O, Avigad S, Shaft D, Kodman Y, Gobuzov R, Ash S (1995). A distinct subtype of M4/M5 acute myeloblastic leukemia (AML) associated with t(8:16)(p11:p13), in a patient with the variant t(8:19)(p11:q13)—case report and review of the literature. Leuk Res 19: 367-379.
2079A. Starý J, Baumann I, Creutzig U, Harbott J, Michalova K, Niemeyer C (2008). Getting the numbers straight in pediatric MDS: distribution of subtypes after exclusion of down syndrome. Pediatr Blood Cancer 50: 435-436.
2080. Starzl TE, Nalesnik MA, Porter KA, Ho M, Iwatsuki S, Griffith BP, Rosenthal JT, Hakala TR, Shaw BW, Jr., Hardesty RL (1984). Reversibility of lymphomas and lymphoproliferative lesions developing under cyclosporin-steroid therapy. Lancet 1: 583-587.
2081. Steensma DP, Caudill JS, Pardanani A, McClure RF, Lasho TL, Tefferi A (2006). MPL W515 and JAK2 V617 mutation analysis in patients with refractory anemia with ringed sideroblasts and an elevated platelet count. Haematologica 91: ECR57.
2082. Steensma DP, Dewald GW, Lasho TL, Powell HL, McClure RF, Levine RL, Gilliland DG, Tefferi A (2005). The JAK2 V617F activating tyrosine kinase mutation is an infrequent event in both "atypical" myeloproliferative disorders and myelodysplastic syndromes. Blood 106: 1207-1209.
2083. Steensma DP, Hanson CA, Letendre L, Tefferi A (2001). Myelodysplasia with fibrosis: a distinct entity? Leuk Res 25: 829-838.
2084. Steensma DP, Hecksel KA, Porcher JC, Lasho TL (2007). Candidate gene mutation analysis in idiopathic acquired sideroblastic anemia (refractory anemia with ringed sideroblasts). Leuk Res 31: 623-628.
2085. Steer EJ, Cross NC (2002). Myeloproliferative disorders with translocations of chromosome 5q31-35: role of the platelet-derived growth factor receptor Beta. Acta Haematol 107: 113-122.
2086. Stein H, Diehl V, Marafioti T, Jox A, Wolf J, Hummel M (1999). The nature of Reed-Sternberg cells, Lymphocytic and Histiocytic cells and their molecular biology in Hodgkin's disease. In: Hodgkin's Disease. Mauch P, Armitage JO, Diehl V, eds. Lippincott Williams & Wilkins: Philadelphia, pp. 121.
2087. Stein H, Foss HD, Durkop H, Marafioti T, Delsol G, Pulford K, Pileri S, Falini B (2000). CD30(+) anaplastic large cell lymphoma: a review of its histopathologic, genetic, and clinical features. Blood 96: 3681-3695.
2088. Stein H, Gerdes J, Kirchner H, Schaadt M, Diehl V (1981). Hodgkin and Sternberg-Reed cell antigen(s) detected by an antiserum to a cell line (L428) derived from Hodgkin's disease. Int J Cancer 28: 425-429.
2089. Stein H, Hansmann ML, Lennert K, Brandtzaeg P, Gatter KC, Mason DY (1986). Reed-Sternberg and Hodgkin cells in lymphocyte-predominant Hodgkin's disease of nodular subtype contain J chain. Am J Clin Pathol 86: 292-297.
2090. Stein H, Marafioti T, Foss HD, Laumen H, Hummel M, Anagnostopoulos I, Wirth T, Demel G, Falini B (2001). Down-regulation of BOB.1/OBF.1 and Oct2 in classical Hodgkin disease but not in lymphocyte predominant Hodgkin disease correlates with immunoglobulin transcription. Blood 97: 496-501.
2091. Stein H, Mason DY, Gerdes J, O'Connor N, Wainscoat J, Pallesen G, Gatter K, Falini B, Delsol G, Lemke H (1985). The expression of the Hodgkin's disease associated antigen Ki-1 in reactive and neoplastic lymphoid tissue: evidence that Reed-Sternberg cells and histiocytic malignancies are derived from activated lymphoid cells. Blood 66: 848-858.
2092. Stein H, Uchanska-Ziegler B, Gerdes J, Ziegler A, Wernet P (1982). Hodgkin and Sternberg-Reed cells contain antigens specific to late cells of granulopoiesis. Int J Cancer 29: 283-290.
2093. Steinherz PG, Gaynon PS, Breneman JC, Cherlow JM, Grossman NJ, Kersey JH, Johnstone HS, Sather HN, Trigg ME, Chappell R, Hammond D, Bleyer WA (1996). Cytoreduction and prognosis in acute lymphoblastic leukemia—the importance of early marrow response: report from the Childrens Cancer Group. J Clin Oncol 14: 389-398.
2094. Steinman RM, Hemmi H (2006). Dendritic cells: translating innate to adaptive immunity. Curr Top Microbiol Immunol 311: 17-58.
2095. Stellmacher F, Sotlar K, Balleisen L, Valent P, Horny HP (2004). Bone marrow mastocytosis associated with IgM kappa plasma cell myeloma. Leuk Lymphoma 45: 801-805.
2096. Stephens K, Weaver M, Leppig KA, Maruyama K, Emanuel PD, Le Beau MM, Shannon KM (2006). Interstitial uniparental isodisomy at clustered breakpoint intervals is a frequent mechanism of NF1 inactivation in myeloid malignancies. Blood 108: 1684-1689.
2097. Stern MH, Soulier J, Rosenzwajg M, Nakahara K, Canki-Klain N, Aurias A, Sigaux F, Kirsch IR (1993). MTCP-1: a novel gene on the human chromosome Xq28 translocated to the T cell receptor alpha/delta locus in mature T cell proliferations. Oncogene 8: 2475-2483.
2098. Sterry W, Siebel A, Mielke V (1992). HTLV-1-negative pleomorphic T-cell lymphoma of the skin: the clinicopathological correlations and natural history of 15 patients. Br J Dermatol 126: 456-462.
2099. Stewart AK, Bergsagel PL, Greipp PR, Dispenzieri A, Gertz MA, Hayman SR, Kumar S, Lacy MQ, Lust JA, Russell SJ, Witzig TE, Zeldenrust SR, Dingli D, Reeder CB, Roy V, Kyle RA, Rajkumar SV, Fonseca R (2007). A practical guide to defining high-risk myeloma for clinical trials, patient counseling and choice of therapy. Leukemia 21: 529-534.
2099A. Stewart BW, Kleihues P (2003). World Cancer Report. IARC Press.
2100. Stilgenbauer S, Schaffner C, Litterst A, Liebisch P, Gilad S, Bar-Shira A, James MR, Lichter P, Dohner H (1997). Biallelic mutations in the ATM gene in T-prolymphocytic leukemia. Nat Med 3: 1155-1159.
2101. Stiller CA, Chessells JM, Fitchett M (1994). Neurofibromatosis and childhood leukaemia/lymphoma: a population-based UKCCSG study. Br J Cancer 70: 969-972.
2102. Storniolo AM, Moloney WC, Rosenthal DS, Cox C, Bennett JM (1990). Chronic myelomonocytic leukemia. Leukemia 4: 766-770.
2103. Stover EH, Chen J, Lee BH, Cools J, McDowell E, Adelsperger J, Cullen D, Coburn A, Moore SA, Okabe R, Fabbro D, Manley PW, Griffin JD, Gilliland DG (2005). The small molecule tyrosine kinase inhibitor AMN107 inhibits TEL-PDGFRbeta and FIP1L1-PDGFRalpha in

vitro and in vivo. Blood 106: 3206-3213.
2104. Strahm B, Locatelli F, Bader P, Ehlert K, Kremens B, Zintl F, Fuhrer M, Stachel D, Sykora KW, Sedlacek P, Baumann I, Niemeyer CM (2007). Reduced intensity conditioning in unrelated donor transplantation for refractory cytopenia in childhood. Bone Marrow Transplant 40: 329-333.
2105. Strasser-Weippl K, Steurer M, Kees M, Augustin F, Tzankov A, Dirnhofer S, Fiegl M, Simonitsch-Klupp I, Zojer N, Gisslinger H, Ludwig H (2006). Age and hemoglobin level emerge as most important clinical prognostic parameters in patients with osteomyelofibrosis: introduction of a simplified prognostic score. Leuk Lymphoma 47: 441-450.
2106. Strauchen JA (2001). Indolent T-lymphoblastic proliferation: report of a case with an 11-year history and association with myasthenia gravis. Am J Surg Pathol 25: 411-415.
2107. Straus SE (1988). The chronic mononucleosis syndrome. J Infect Dis 157: 405-412.
2108. Straus SE, Jaffe ES, Puck JM, Dale JK, Elkon KB, Rosen-Wolff A, Peters AM, Sneller MC, Hallahan CW, Wang J, Fischer RE, Jackson CM, Lin AY, Baumler C, Siegert E, Marx A, Vaishnaw AK, Grodzicky T, Fleisher TA, Lenardo MJ (2001). The development of lymphomas in families with autoimmune lymphoproliferative syndrome with germline Fas mutations and defective lymphocyte apoptosis. Blood 98: 194-200.
2109. Streeter RR, Presant CA, Reinhard E (1977). Prognostic significance of thrombocytosis in idiopathic sideroblastic anemia. Blood 50: 427-432.
2109A. Streubel B, Huber D, Wohrer S, Chott A, Raderer M (2004). Frequency of chromosomal aberrations involving MALT1 in mucosa-associated lymphoid tissue lymphoma in patients with Sjogren's syndrome. Clin Cancer Res 10: 476-480.
2110. Streubel B, Simonitsch-Klupp I, Mullauer L, Lamprecht A, Huber D, Siebert R, Stolte M, Trautinger F, Lukas J, Puspok A, Formanek M, Assanasen T, Muller-Hermelink HK, Cerroni L, Raderer M, Chott A (2004). Variable frequencies of MALT lymphoma-associated genetic aberrations in MALT lymphomas of different sites. Leukemia 18: 1722-1726.
2111. Streubel B, Vinatzer U, Lamprecht A, Raderer M, Chott A (2005). T(3;14)(p14.1;q32) involving IGH and FOXP1 is a novel recurrent chromosomal aberration in MALT lymphoma. Leukemia 19: 652-658.
2112. Streubel B, Vinatzer U, Willheim M, Raderer M, Chott A (2006). Novel t(5;9)(q33;q22) fuses ITK to SYK in unspecified peripheral T-cell lymphoma. Leukemia 20: 313-318.
2112A. Stewart BW, Kleihues P (2003). World Cancer Report. IARC Press.
2113. Strom SS, Gu Y, Gruschkus SK, Pierce SA, Estey EH (2005). Risk factors of myelodysplastic syndromes: a case-control study. Leukemia 19: 1912-1918.
2113A. Strom SS, Velez-Bravo V, Estey EH (2008). Epidemiology of myelodysplastic syndromes. Semin Hematol 45: 8-13.
2114. Strupp C, Gattermann N, Giagounidis A, Aul C, Hildebrandt B, Haas R, Germing U (2003). Refractory anemia with excess of blasts in transformation: analysis of reclassification according to the WHO proposals. Leuk Res 27: 397-404.
2115. Su IJ, Chen RL, Lin DT, Lin KS, Chen CC (1994). Epstein-Barr virus (EBV) infects T lymphocytes in childhood EBV-associated hemophagocytic syndrome in Taiwan. Am J Pathol 144: 1219-1225.
2116. Su MW, Dorocicz I, Dragowska WH, Ho V, Li G, Voss N, Gascoyne R, Zhou Y (2003). Aberrant expression of T-plastin in Sezary cells. Cancer Res 63: 7122-7127.
2117. Suarez F, Wlodarska I, Rigal-Huguet F, Mempel M, Martin-Garcia N, Farcet JP, Delsol G, Gaulard P (2000). Hepatosplenic alphabeta T-cell lymphoma: an unusual case with clinical, histologic, and cytogenetic features of gammadelta hepatosplenic T-cell lymphoma. Am J Surg Pathol 24: 1027-1032.
2118. Sugimoto K, Hirano N, Toyoshima H, Chiba S, Mano H, Takaku F, Yazaki Y, Hirai H (1993). Mutations of the p53 gene in myelodysplastic syndrome (MDS) and MDS-derived leukemia. Blood 81: 3022-3026.
2119. Sulak LE, Clare CN, Morale BA, Hansen KL, Montiel MM (1990). Biphenotypic acute leukemia in adults. Am J Clin Pathol 94: 54-58.
2120. Sultan C, Sigaux F, Imbert M, Reyes F (1981). Acute myelodysplasia with myelofibrosis: a report of eight cases. Br J Haematol 49: 11-16.
2120A. Summers K, Stevens J, Kakkas I, Smith M, Smith LL, Macdougall F, Cavenagh J, Bonnet D, Young BD, Lister TA, Fitzgibbon J (2007). Wilms' tumour 1 mutations are associated with FLT3-ITD and failure of standard induction chemotherapy in patients with normal karyotype AML. Leukemia 21: 550-551.
2121. Summers KE, Goff LK, Wilson AG, Gupta RK, Lister TA, Fitzgibbon J (2001). Frequency of the Bcl-2/IgH rearrangement in normal individuals: implications for the monitoring of disease in patients with follicular lymphoma. J Clin Oncol 19: 420-424.
2122. Sun X, Chang KC, Abruzzo LV, Lai R, Younes A, Jones D (2003). Epidermal growth factor receptor expression in follicular dendritic cells: a shared feature of follicular dendritic cell sarcoma and Castleman's disease. Hum Pathol 34: 835-840.
2123. Sutcliffe MJ, Shuster JJ, Sather HN, Camitta BM, Pullen J, Schultz KR, Borowitz MJ, Gaynon PS, Carroll AJ, Heerema NA (2005). High concordance from independent studies by the Children's Cancer Group (CCG) and Pediatric Oncology Group (POG) associating favorable prognosis with combined trisomies 4, 10, and 17 in children with NCI Standard-Risk B-precursor Acute Lymphoblastic Leukemia: a Children's Oncology Group (COG) initiative. Leukemia 19: 734-740.
2124. Suvajdzic N, Marisavljevic D, Kraguljac N, Pantic M, Djordjevic V, Jankovic G, Cemerikic-Martinovic V, Colovic M (2004). Acute panmyelosis with myelofibrosis: clinical, immunophenotypic and cytogenetic study of twelve cases. Leuk Lymphoma 45: 1873-1879.
2125. Suzukawa K, Parganas E, Gajjar A, Abe T, Takahashi S, Tani K, Asano S, Asou H, Kamada N, Yokota J, *et al.* (1994). Identification of a breakpoint cluster region 3' of the ribophorin I gene at 3q21 associated with the transcriptional activation of the EVI1 gene in acute myelogenous leukemias with inv(3)(q21q26). Blood 84: 2681-2688.
2126. Suzuki H, Asano H, Ohashi H, Kinoshita T, Murate T, Saito H, Hotta T (1999). Clonality analysis of refractory anemia with ring sideroblasts: simultaneous study of clonality and cytochemistry of bone marrow progenitors. Leukemia 13: 130-134.
2127. Suzuki K, Ohshima K, Karube K, Suzumiya J, Ohga S, Ishihara S, Tamura K, Kikuchi M (2004). Clinicopathological states of Epstein-Barr virus-associated T/NK-cell lymphoproliferative disorders (severe chronic active EBV infection) of children and young adults. Int J Oncol 24: 1165-1174.
2128. Suzuki R, Suzumiya J, Nakamura S, Aoki S, Notoya A, Ozaki S, Gondo H, Hino N, Mori H, Sugimori H, Kawa K, Oshimi K (2004). Aggressive natural killer-cell leukemia revisited: large granular lymphocyte leukemia of cytotoxic NK cells. Leukemia 18: 763-770.
2129. Suzuki R, Yamamoto K, Seto M, Kagami Y, Ogura M, Yatabe Y, Suchi T, Kodera Y, Morishima Y, Takahashi T, Saito H, Ueda R, Nakamura S (1997). CD7+ and CD56+ myeloid/natural killer cell precursor acute leukemia: a distinct hematolymphoid disease entity. Blood 90: 2417-2428.
2130. Suzumiya J, Ohshima K, Takeshita M, Kanda M, Kawasaki C, Kimura N, Tamura K, Kikuchi M (1999). Nasal lymphomas in Japan: a high prevalence of Epstein-Barr virus type A and deletion within the latent membrane protein gene. Leuk Lymphoma 35: 567-578.
2131. Sweet DL, Golomb HM, Rowley JD, Vardiman JM (1979). Acute myelogenous leukemia and thrombocythemia associated with an abnormality of chromosome no. 3. Cancer Genet Cytogenet 1: 33-37.
2132. Swerdlow SH (2004). Pediatric follicular lymphomas, marginal zone lymphomas, and marginal zone hyperplasia. Am J Clin Pathol 122 Suppl: S98-109.
2133. Swerdlow SH (2007). T-cell and NK-cell posttransplantation lymphoproliferative disorders. Am J Clin Pathol 127: 887-895.
2134. Swerdlow SH, Habeshaw JA, Murray LJ, Dhaliwal HS, Lister TA, Stansfeld AG (1983). Centrocytic lymphoma: a distinct clinicopathologic and immunologic entity. A multiparameter study of 18 cases at diagnosis and relapse. Am J Pathol 113: 181-197.
2135. Swerdlow SH, Utz GL, Williams ME (1993). Bcl-2 protein in centrocytic lymphoma; a paraffin section study. Leukemia 7: 1456-1458.
2136. Swerdlow SH, Williams ME (2002). From centrocytic to mantle cell lymphoma: a clinicopathologic and molecular review of 3 decades. Hum Pathol 33: 7-20.
2137. Swerdlow SH, Yang WI, Zukerberg LR, Harris NL, Arnold A, Williams ME (1995). Expression of cyclin D1 protein in centrocytic/mantle cell lymphomas with and without rearrangement of the BCL1/cyclin D1 gene. Hum Pathol 26: 999-1004.
2138. Szczepanski T, Pongers-Willemse MJ, Langerak AW, Harts WA, Wijkhuijs AJ, van Wering ER, van Dongen JJ (1999). Ig heavy chain gene rearrangements in T-cell acute lymphoblastic leukemia exhibit predominant DH6-19 and DH7-27 gene usage, can result in complete V-D-J rearrangements, and are rare in T-cell receptor alpha beta lineage. Blood 93: 4079-4085.
2139. Szpurka H, Tiu R, Murugesan G, Aboudola S, Hsi ED, Theil KS, Sekeres MA, Maciejewski JP (2006). Refractory anemia with ringed sideroblasts associated with marked thrombocytosis (RARS-T), another myeloproliferative condition characterized by JAK2 V617F mutation. Blood 108: 2173-2181.
2140. Taddesse-Heath L, Pittaluga S, Sorbara L, Bussey M, Raffeld M, Jaffe ES (2003). Marginal zone B-cell lymphoma in children and young adults. Am J Surg Pathol 27: 522-531.
2141. Taegtmeyer AB, Halil O, Bell AD, Carby M, Cummins D, Banner NR (2005). Neutrophil dysplasia (acquired pseudo-pelger anomaly) caused by ganciclovir. Transplantation 80: 127-130.
2142. Tagawa H, Suguro M, Tsuzuki S, Matsuo K, Karnan S, Ohshima K, Okamoto M, Morishima Y, Nakamura S, Seto M (2005). Comparison of genome profiles for identification of distinct subgroups of diffuse large B-cell lymphoma. Blood 106: 1770-1777.
2143. Tai YC, Kim LH, Peh SC (2004). High frequency of EBV association and 30-bp deletion in the LMP-1 gene in CD56 lymphomas of the upper aerodigestive tract. Pathol Int 54: 158-166.
2144. Tajima K, Hinuma Y (1992). Epidemiology of HTLV-I/II in Japan and the world. In: Advances in Adult T-Cell Leukemia and HTLV-I Research (Gann Monograph on Cancer Research). Takatsuki K, Hinuma Y, Yoshida M, eds. Japan Scientific Societies Press: Tokyo, pp. 129-149.
2145. Takahashi E, Kajimoto K, Fukatsu T, Yoshida M, Eimoto T, Nakamura S (2005). Intravascular large T-cell lymphoma: a case report of CD30-positive and ALK-negative anaplastic type with cytotoxic molecule expression. Virchows Arch 447: 1000-1006.
2146. Takakuwa T, Ham MF, Luo WJ, Nakatsuka S, Daibata M, Aozasa K (2006). Loss of expression of Epstein-Barr virus nuclear antigen-2 correlates with a poor prognosis in cases of pyothorax-associated lymphoma. Int J Cancer 118: 2782-2789.
2147. Takakuwa T, Luo WJ, Ham MF, Mizuki M, Iuchi K, Aozasa K (2003). Establishment and characterization of unique cell lines derived from pyothorax-associated lymphoma which develops in long-standing pyothorax and is strongly associated with Epstein-Barr virus infection. Cancer Sci 94: 858-863.
2148. Takatsuki K, Yamaguchi K, Watanabe T, Mochizuki M (1992). Adult T-cell leukemia and HTLV-1 related disease. Gann mono Can Res 32: 1-15.
2149. Takeshita M, Akamatsu M, Ohshima K, Kobari S, Kikuchi M, Suzumiya J, Uike N, Okamura T (1995). CD30 (Ki-1) expression in adult T-cell leukaemia/lymphoma is associated with distinctive immunohistological and clinical characteristics. Histopathology 26: 539-546.
2150. Talal N, Sokoloff L, Barth WF (1967). Extrasalivary lymphoid abnormalities in Sjogren's syndrome (reticulum cell sarcoma, "pseudolymphoma," macroglobulinemia). Am J Med 43: 50-65.
2151. Talaulikar D, Dahlstrom JE, Shadbolt B, McNiven M, Broomfield A, Pidcock M (2007). Occult bone marrow involvement in patients with diffuse large B-cell lymphoma: results of a pilot study. Pathology 39: 580-585.
2152. Tallman MS, Andersen JW, Schiffer CA, Appelbaum FR, Feusner JH, Ogden A, Shepherd L, Willman C, Bloomfield CD, Rowe JM, Wiernik PH (1997). All-trans-retinoic acid in acute promyelocytic leukemia. N Engl J Med 337: 1021-1028.
2153. Tallman MS, Kim HT, Paietta E, Bennett JM, Dewald G, Cassileth PA, Wiernik PH, Rowe JM (2004). Acute monocytic leukemia (French-American-British classification M5) does not have a worse prognosis than other subtypes of acute myeloid leukemia: a report from the Eastern Cooperative Oncology Group. J Clin Oncol 22: 1276-1286.
2154. Tamaska J, Adam E, Kozma A, Gopcsa L, Andrikovics H, Tordai A, Halm G, Bereczki L, Bagdi E, Krenacs L (2006). Hepatosplenic gammadelta T-cell lymphoma with ring chromosome 7, an isochromosome 7q equivalent clonal chromosomal aberration. Virchows Arch 449: 479-483.
2155. Tan BT, Warnke RA, Arber DA (2006). The frequency of B- and T-cell gene rearrangements and epstein-barr virus in T-cell lymphomas: a comparison between angioimmunoblastic T-cell lymphoma and peripheral T-cell lymphoma, unspecified with and without associated B-cell proliferations. J Mol Diagn 8: 466-475.
2156. Tanaka M, Suda T, Haze K, Nakamura N, Sato K, Kimura F, Motoyoshi K, Mizuki M, Tagawa S, Ohga S, Hatake K, Drummond AH,

Nagata S (1996). Fas ligand in human serum. Nat Med 2: 317-322.
2157. Tanaka Y, Kurata M, Togami K, Fujita H, Watanabe N, Matsushita A, Maeda A, Nagai K, Sada A, Matsui T, Takahashi T (2006). Chronic eosinophilic leukemia with the FIP1L1-PDGFRalpha fusion gene in a patient with a history of combination chemotherapy. Int J Hematol 83: 152-155.
2158. Tangye SG, Phillips JH, Lanier LL, Nichols KE (2000). Functional requirement for SAP in 2B4-mediated activation of human natural killer cells as revealed by the X-linked lymphoproliferative syndrome. J Immunol 165: 2932-2936.
2159. Taniere P, Thivolet-Bejui F, Vitrey D, Isaac S, Loire R, Cordier JF, Berger F (1998). Lymphomatoid granulomatosis—a report on four cases: evidence for B phenotype of the tumoral cells. Eur Respir J 12: 102-106.
2160. Tao J, Valderrama E (1999). Epstein-Barr virus-associated polymorphic B-cell lymphoproliferative disorders in the lungs of children with AIDS: a report of two cases. Am J Surg Pathol 23: 560-566.
2161. Tao Q, Robertson KD, Manns A, Hildesheim A, Ambinder RF (1998). Epstein-Barr virus (EBV) in endemic Burkitt's lymphoma: molecular analysis of primary tumor tissue. Blood 91: 1373-1381.
2162. Tartaglia M, Niemeyer CM, Fragale A, Song X, Buechner J, Jung A, Hahlen K, Hasle H, Licht JD, Gelb BD (2003). Somatic mutations in PTPN11 in juvenile myelomonocytic leukemia, myelodysplastic syndromes and acute myeloid leukemia. Nat Genet 34: 148-150.
2163. Tashiro H, Shirasaki R, Noguchi M, Gotoh M, Kawasugi K, Shirafuji N (2006). Molecular analysis of chronic eosinophilic leukemia with t(4;10) showing good response to imatinib mesylate. Int J Hematol 83: 433-438.
2164. Taylor AM, Metcalfe JA, Thick J, Mak YF (1996). Leukemia and lymphoma in ataxia telangiectasia. Blood 87: 423-438.
2165. Tcheng WY, Said J, Hall T, Al Akash S, Malogolowkin M, Feig SA (2006). Post-transplant multiple myeloma in a pediatric renal transplant patient. Pediatr Blood Cancer 47: 218-223.
2166. Tedeschi A, Barate C, Minola E, Morra E (2007). Cryoglobulinemia. Blood Rev 21: 183-200.
2167. Tefferi A (2000). Myelofibrosis with myeloid metaplasia. N Engl J Med 342: 1255-1265.
2168. Tefferi A (2006). The diagnosis of polycythemia vera: new tests and old dictums. Best Pract Res Clin Haematol 19: 455-469.
2169. Tefferi A, Elliott MA, Pardanani A (2006). Atypical myeloproliferative disorders: diagnosis and management. Mayo Clin Proc 81: 553-563.
2170. Tefferi A, Hoagland HC, Therneau TM, Pierre RV (1989). Chronic myelomonocytic leukemia: natural history and prognostic determinants. Mayo Clin Proc 64: 1246-1254.
2171. Tefferi A, Lasho TL, Gilliland G (2005). JAK2 mutations in myeloproliferative disorders. N Engl J Med 353: 1416-1417.
2172. Tefferi A, Lasho TL, Schwager SM, Steensma DP, Mesa RA, Li CY, Wadleigh M, Gary GD (2005). The JAK2(V617F) tyrosine kinase mutation in myelofibrosis with myeloid metaplasia: lineage specificity and clinical correlates. Br J Haematol 131: 320-328.
2173. Tefferi A, Li CY, Witzig TE, Dhodapkar MV, Okuno SH, Phyliky RL (1994). Chronic natural killer cell lymphocytosis: a descriptive clinical study. Blood 84: 2721-2725.
2174. Tefferi A, Mesa RA, Schroeder G, Hanson CA, Li CY, Dewald GW (2001). Cytogenetic findings and their clinical relevance in myelofibrosis with myeloid metaplasia. Br J Haematol 113: 763-771.
2175. Tefferi A, Murphy S (2001). Current opinion in essential thrombocythemia: pathogenesis, diagnosis, and management. Blood Rev 15: 121-131.
2176. Tefferi A, Pardanani A (2004). Clinical, genetic, and therapeutic insights into systemic mast cell disease. Curr Opin Hematol 11: 58-64.
2177. Tefferi A, Thiele J, Orazi A, Kvasnicka HM, Barbui T, Hanson CA, Barosi G, Verstovsek S, Birgegard G, Mesa R, Reilly JT, Gisslinger H, Vannucchi AM, Cervantes F, Finazzi G, Hoffman R, Gilliland DG, Bloomfield CD, Vardiman JW (2007). Proposals and rationale for revision of the World Health Organization diagnostic criteria for polycythemia vera, essential thrombocythemia, and primary myelofibrosis: recommendations from an ad hoc international expert panel. Blood 110: 1092-1097.
2178. Tehranchi R, Invernizzi R, Grandien A, Zhivotovsky B, Fadeel B, Forsblom AM, Travaglino E, Samuelsson J, Hast R, Nilsson L, Cazzola M, Wibom R, Hellstrom-Lindberg E (2005). Aberrant mitochondrial iron distribution and maturation arrest characterize early erythroid precursors in low-risk myelodysplastic syndromes. Blood 106: 247-253.
2179. Teitell MA, Lones MA, Perkins SL, Sanger WG, Cairo MS, Said JW (2005). TCL1 expression and Epstein-Barr virus status in pediatric Burkitt lymphoma. Am J Clin Pathol 124: 569-575.
2180. ten Berge RL, de Bruin PC, Oudejans JJ, Ossenkoppele GJ, van d, V, Meijer CJ (2003). ALK-negative anaplastic large-cell lymphoma demonstrates similar poor prognosis to peripheral T-cell lymphoma, unspecified. Histopathology 43: 462-469.
2181. ten Berge RL, Oudejans JJ, Ossenkoppele GJ, Meijer CJ (2003). ALK-negative systemic anaplastic large cell lymphoma: differential diagnostic and prognostic aspects—a review. J Pathol 200: 4-15.
2182. ten Berge RL, Oudejans JJ, Ossenkoppele GJ, Pulford K, Willemze R, Falini B, Chott A, Meijer CJ (2000). ALK expression in extranodal anaplastic large cell lymphoma favours systemic disease with (primary) nodal involvement and a good prognosis and occurs before dissemination. J Clin Pathol 53: 445-450.
2183. Terre C, Nguyen-Khac F, Barin C, Mozziconacci MJ, Eclache V, Leonard C, Chapiro E, Farhat H, Bouyon A, Rousselot P, Choquet S, Spentchian M, Dubreuil P, Leblond V, Castaigne S (2006). Trisomy 4, a new chromosomal abnormality in Waldenstrom's macroglobulinemia: a study of 39 cases. Leukemia 20: 1634-1636.
2184. Teruya-Feldstein J, Chiao E, Filippa DA, Lin O, Comenzo R, Coleman M, Portlock C, Noy A (2004). CD20-negative large-cell lymphoma with plasmablastic features: a clinically heterogenous spectrum in both HIV-positive and -negative patients. Ann Oncol 15: 1673-1679.
2185. Teruya-Feldstein J, Jaffe ES, Burd PR, Kanegane H, Kingma DW, Wilson WH, Longo DL, Tosato G (1997). The role of Mig, the monokine induced by interferon-gamma, and IP-10, the interferon-gamma-inducible protein-10, in tissue necrosis and vascular damage associated with Epstein-Barr virus-positive lymphoproliferative disease. Blood 90: 4099-4105.
2186. Teruya-Feldstein J, Jaffe ES, Burd PR, Kingma DW, Setsuda JE, Tosato G (1999). Differential chemokine expression in tissues involved by Hodgkin's disease: direct correlation of eotaxin expression and tissue eosinophilia. Blood 93: 2463-2470.
2187. Teruya-Feldstein J, Temeck BK, Sloas MM, Kingma DW, Raffeld M, Pass HI, Mueller B, Jaffe ES (1995). Pulmonary malignant lymphoma of mucosa-associated lymphoid tissue (MALT) arising in a pediatric HIV-positive patient. Am J Surg Pathol 19: 357-363.
2188. Teruya-Feldstein J, Zauber P, Setsuda JE, Berman EL, Sorbara L, Raffeld M, Tosato G, Jaffe ES (1998). Expression of human herpesvirus-8 oncogene and cytokine homologues in an HIV-seronegative patient with multicentric Castleman's disease and primary effusion lymphoma. Lab Invest 78: 1637-1642.
2189. Testoni N, Borsaru G, Martinelli G, Carboni C, Ruggeri D, Ottaviani E, Pelliconi S, Ricci P, Pastano R, Visani G, Zaccaria A, Tura S (1999). 3q21 and 3q26 cytogenetic abnormalities in acute myeloblastic leukemia: biological and clinical features. Haematologica 84: 690-694.
2190. Thangavelu M, Finn WG, Yelavarthi KK, Roenigk HH, Jr., Samuelson E, Peterson L, Kuzel TM, Rosen ST (1997). Recurring structural chromosome abnormalities in peripheral blood lymphocytes of patients with mycosis fungoides/Sezary syndrome. Blood 89: 3371-3377.
2191. Thangavelu M, Olopade O, Beckman E, Vardiman JW, Larson RA, McKeithan TW, Le Beau MM, Rowley JD (1990). Clinical, morphologic, and cytogenetic characteristics of patients with lymphoid malignancies characterized by both t(14;18)(q32;q21) and t(8;14)(q24;q32) or t(8;22)(q24;q11). Genes Chromosomes Cancer 2: 147-158.
2192. Thelander EF, Walsh SH, Thorselius M, Laurell A, Landgren O, Larsson C, Rosenquist R, Lagercrantz S (2005). Mantle cell lymphomas with clonal immunoglobulin V(H)3-21 gene rearrangements exhibit fewer genomic imbalances than mantle cell lymphomas utilizing other immunoglobulin V(H) genes. Mod Pathol 18: 331-339.
2193. Thieblemont C, Bastion Y, Berger F, Rieux C, Salles G, Dumontet C, Felman P, Coiffier B (1997). Mucosa-associated lymphoid tissue gastrointestinal and nongastrointestinal lymphoma behavior: analysis of 108 patients. J Clin Oncol 15: 1624-1630.
2194. Thieblemont C, Berger F, Dumontet C, Moullet I, Bouafia F, Felman P, Salles G, Coiffier B (2000). Mucosa-associated lymphoid tissue lymphoma is a disseminated disease in one third of 158 patients analyzed. Blood 95: 802-806.
2195. Thieblemont C, Felman P, Berger F, Dumontet C, Arnaud P, Hequet O, Arcache J, Callet-Bauchu E, Salles G, Coiffier B (2002). Treatment of splenic marginal zone B-cell lymphoma: an analysis of 81 patients. Clin Lymphoma 3: 41-47.
2196. Thieblemont C, Felman P, Callet-Bauchu E, Traverse-Glehen A, Salles G, Berger F, Coiffier B (2003). Splenic marginal-zone lymphoma: a distinct clinical and pathological entity. Lancet Oncol 4: 95-103.
2197. Thieblemont C, Nasser V, Felman P, Leroy K, Gazzo S, Callet-Bauchu E, Loriod B, Granjeaud S, Gaulard P, Haioun C, Traverse-Glehen A, Baseggio L, Bertucci F, Birnbaum D, Magrangeas F, Minvielle S, Avet-Loiseau H, Salles G, Coiffier B, Berger F, Houlgatte R (2004). Small lymphocytic lymphoma, marginal zone B-cell lymphoma, and mantle cell lymphoma exhibit distinct gene-expression profiles allowing molecular diagnosis. Blood 103: 2727-2737.
2198. Thiede C, Koch S, Creutzig E, Steudel C, Illmer T, Schaich M, Ehninger G (2006). Prevalence and prognostic impact of NPM1 mutations in 1485 adult patients with acute myeloid leukemia (AML). Blood 107: 4011-4020.
2199. Thiele J, Bennewitz FG, Bertsch HP, Falk S, Fischer R, Stutte HJ (1993). Splenic haematopoiesis in primary (idiopathic) osteomyelofibrosis: immunohistochemical and morphometric evaluation of proliferative activity of erytro- and endoreduplicative capacity of megakaryopoiesis (PCNA- and Ki-67 staining). Virchows Arch B Cell Pathol Incl Mol Pathol 64: 281-286.
2200. Thiele J, Kvasnicka HM (2003). Chronic myeloproliferative disorders with thrombocythemia: a comparative study of two classification systems (PVSG, WHO) on 839 patients. Ann Hematol 82: 148-152.
2201. Thiele J, Kvasnicka HM (2003). Diagnostic differentiation of essential thrombocythaemia from thrombocythaemias associated with chronic idiopathic myelofibrosis by discriminate analysis of bone marrow features—a clinicopathological study on 272 patients. Histol Histopathol 18: 93-102.
2202. Thiele J, Kvasnicka HM (2004). Prefibrotic chronic idiopathic myelofibrosis—a diagnostic enigma? Acta Haematol 111: 155-159.
2203. Thiele J, Kvasnicka HM (2005). Diagnostic impact of bone marrow histopathology in polycythemia vera (PV). Histol Histopathol 20: 317-328.
2204. Thiele J, Kvasnicka HM (2005). Hematopathologic findings in chronic idiopathic myelofibrosis. Semin Oncol 32: 380-394.
2205. Thiele J, Kvasnicka HM (2006). Clinicopathological criteria for differential diagnosis of thrombocythemias in various myeloproliferative disorders. Semin Thromb Hemost 32: 219-230.
2206. Thiele J, Kvasnicka HM (2007). Myelofibrosis - What's in a Name?. Consensus on Definition and EUMNET Grading. Pathobiology 74: 89-96.
2207. Thiele J, Kvasnicka HM, Beelen DW, Zirbes TK, Jung F, Reske D, Leder LD, Schaefer UW (2000). Relevance and dynamics of myelofibrosis regarding hematopoietic reconstitution after allogeneic bone marrow transplantation in chronic myelogenous leukemia—a single center experience on 160 patients. Bone Marrow Transplant 26: 275-281.
2208. Thiele J, Kvasnicka HM, Czieslick C (2002). CD34+ progenitor cells in idiopathic (primary) myelofibrosis: a comparative quantification between spleen and bone marrow tissue. Ann Hematol 81: 86-89.
2209. Thiele J, Kvasnicka HM, Diehl V (2005). Bone marrow CD34+ progenitor cells in Philadelphia chromosome-negative chronic myeloproliferative disorders—a clinicopathological study on 575 patients. Leuk Lymphoma 46: 709-715.
2210. Thiele J, Kvasnicka HM, Diehl V (2005). Initial (latent) polycythemia vera with thrombocytosis mimicking essential thrombocythemia. Acta Haematol 113: 213-219.
2211. Thiele J, Kvasnicka HM, Diehl V (2005). Standardization of bone marrow features—does it work in hematopathology for histological discrimination of different disease patterns? Histol Histopathol 20: 633-644.
2212. Thiele J, Kvasnicka HM, Diehl V, Fischer R, Michiels J (1999). Clinicopathological diagnosis and differential criteria of thrombocythemias in various myeloproliferative disorders by histopathology, histochemistry and immunostaining from bone marrow biopsies. Leuk Lymphoma 33: 207-218.
2213. Thiele J, Kvasnicka HM, Dietrich H, Stein G, Hann M, Kaminski A, Rathjen N, Metz KA, Beelen DW, Ditschkowski M, Zander A, Kroeger N (2005). Dynamics of bone marrow changes in patients with chronic idiopathic

myelofibrosis following allogeneic stem cell transplantation. Histol Histopathol 20: 879-889.
2214. Thiele J, Kvasnicka HM, Facchetti F, Franco V, van der WJ, Orazi A (2005). European consensus on grading bone marrow fibrosis and assessment of cellularity. Haematologica 90: 1128-1132.
2215. Thiele J, Kvasnicka HM, Fischer R (1999). Bone marrow histopathology in chronic myelogenous leukemia (CML)—evaluation of distinctive features with clinical impact. Histol Histopathol 14: 1241-1256.
2216. Thiele J, Kvasnicka HM, Orazi A (2005). Bone marrow histopathology in myeloproliferative disorders—current diagnostic approach. Semin Hematol 42: 184-195.
2217. Thiele J, Kvasnicka HM, Schmitt-Graeff A, Diehl V (2003). Bone marrow histopathology following cytoreductive therapy in chronic idiopathic myelofibrosis. Histopathology 43: 470-479.
2218. Thiele J, Kvasnicka HM, Schmitt-Graeff A, Diehl V (2003). Dynamics of fibrosis in chronic idiopathic (primary) myelofibrosis during therapy: a follow-up study on 309 patients. Leuk Lymphoma 44: 949-953.
2219. Thiele J, Kvasnicka HM, Schmitt-Graeff A, Kriener S, Engels K, Staib P, Griesshammer M, Waller CF, Ottmann OG, Hansmann ML (2004). Effects of the tyrosine kinase inhibitor imatinib mesylate (STI571) on bone marrow features in patients with chronic myelogenous leukemia. Histol Histopathol 19: 1277-1288.
2220. Thiele J, Kvasnicka HM, Schmitt-Graeff A, Zankovich R, Diehl V (2002). Follow-up examinations including sequential bone marrow biopsies in essential thrombocythemia (ET): a retrospective clinicopathological study of 120 patients. Am J Hematol 70: 283-291.
2221. Thiele J, Kvasnicka HM, Schmitt-Graeff A, Zirbes TK, Birnbaum F, Kressmann C, Melguizo-Grahmann M, Frackenpohl H, Sprungmann C, Leder LD, Diehl V, Zankovich R, Schaefer HE, Niederle N, Fischer R (2000). Bone marrow features and clinical findings in chronic myeloid leukemia—a comparative, multicenter, immunohistological and morphometric study on 614 patients. Leuk Lymphoma 36: 295-308.
2222. Thiele J, Kvasnicka HM, Vardiman J (2006). Bone marrow histopathology in the diagnosis of chronic myeloproliferative disorders: a forgotten pearl. Best Pract Res Clin Haematol 19: 413-437.
2223. Thiele J, Kvasnicka HM, Zankovich R, Diehl V (2000). Relevance of bone marrow features in the differential diagnosis between essential thrombocythemia and early stage idiopathic myelofibrosis. Haematologica 85: 1126-1134.
2224. Thiele J, Kvasnicka HM, Zankovich R, Diehl V (2001). The value of bone marrow histology in differentiating between early stage Polycythemia vera and secondary (reactive) Polycythemias. Haematologica 86: 368-374.
2225. Thiele J, Kvasnicka HM, Zerhusen G, Vardiman J, Diehl V, Luebbert M, Schmitt-Graeff A (2004). Acute panmyelosis with myelofibrosis: a clinicopathological study on 46 patients including histochemistry of bone marrow biopsies and follow-up. Ann Hematol 83: 513-521.
2226. Thiele J, Quitmann H, Wagner S, Fischer R (1991). Dysmegakaryopoiesis in myelodysplastic syndromes (MDS): an immunomorphometric study of bone marrow trephine biopsy specimens. J Clin Pathol 44: 300-305.
2227. Thiele J, Schmitz B, Fuchs R, Kvasnicka HM, Lorenzen J, Fischer R (1998). Detection of the bcr/abl gene in bone marrow macrophages in CML and alterations during interferon therapy—a fluorescence in situ hybridization study on trephine biopsies. J Pathol 186: 331-335.
2228. Thiele J, Windecker R, Kvasnicka HM, Titius BR, Zankovich R, Fischer R (1994). Erythropoiesis in primary (idiopathic) osteomyelofibrosis: quantification, PCNA-reactivity, and prognostic impact. Am J Hematol 46: 36-42.
2229. Thomas DA, Faderl S, O'Brien S, Bueso-Ramos C, Cortes J, Garcia-Manero G, Giles FJ, Verstovsek S, Wierda WG, Pierce SA, Shan J, Brandt M, Hagemeister FB, Keating MJ, Cabanillas F, Kantarjian H (2006). Chemoimmunotherapy with hyper-CVAD plus rituximab for the treatment of adult Burkitt and Burkitt-type lymphoma or acute lymphoblastic leukemia. Cancer 106: 1569-1580.
2230. Thomas E, Brewster DH, Black RJ, Macfarlane GJ (2000). Risk of malignancy among patients with rheumatic conditions. Int J Cancer 88: 497-502.
2231. Thompson MA, Stumph J, Henrickson SE, Rosenwald A, Wang Q, Olson S, Brandt SJ, Roberts J, Zhang X, Shyr Y, Kinney MC (2005). Differential gene expression in anaplastic lymphoma kinase-positive and anaplastic lymphoma kinase-negative anaplastic large cell lymphomas. Hum Pathol 36: 494-504.
2232. Thorley-Lawson DA, Gross A (2004). Persistence of the Epstein-Barr virus and the origins of associated lymphomas. N Engl J Med 350: 1328-1337.
2233. Thorns C, Bastian B, Pinkel D, Roydasgupta R, Fridlyand J, Merz H, Krokowski M, Bernd HW, Feller AC (2007). Chromosomal aberrations in angioimmunoblastic T-cell lymphoma and peripheral T-cell lymphoma unspecified: A matrix-based CGH approach. Genes Chromosomes Cancer 46: 37-44.
2234. Thornton PD, Bellas C, Santon A, Shah G, Pocock C, Wotherspoon AC, Matutes E, Catovsky D (2005). Richter's transformation of chronic lymphocytic leukemia. The possible role of fludarabine and the Epstein-Barr virus in its pathogenesis. Leuk Res 29: 389-395.
2235. Tiacci E, Liso A, Piris M, Falini B (2006). Evolving concepts in the pathogenesis of hairy-cell leukaemia. Nat Rev Cancer 6: 437-448.
2236. Tiacci E, Pileri S, Orleth A, Pacini R, Tabarrini A, Frenguelli F, Liso A, Diverio D, Lo-Coco F, Falini B (2004). PAX5 expression in acute leukemias: higher B-lineage specificity than CD79a and selective association with t(8;21)-acute myelogenous leukemia. Cancer Res 64: 7399-7404.
2236A. Tiemann M, Riener MO, Claviez A, Meyer U, Dorffel W, Reiter A, Parwaresch R (2005). Proliferation rate and outcome in children with T-cell rich B-cell lymphoma: a clinicopathologic study from the NHL-BFM-study group. Leuk Lymphoma 46: 1295-1300.
2237. Tiemann M, Schrader C, Klapper W, Dreyling MH, Campo E, Norton A, Berger F, Kluin P, Ott G, Pileri S, Pedrinis E, Feller AC, Merz H, Janssen D, Hansmann ML, Krieken H, Moller P, Stein H, Unterhalt M, Hiddemann W, Parwaresch R (2005). Histopathology, cell proliferation indices and clinical outcome in 304 patients with mantle cell lymphoma (MCL): a clinicopathological study from the European MCL Network. Br J Haematol 131: 29-38.
2238. Tien HF, Su IJ, Tang JL, Liu MC, Lee FY, Chen YC, Chuang SM (1997). Clonal chromosomal abnormalities as direct evidence for clonality in nasal T/natural killer cell lymphomas. Br J Haematol 97: 621-625.
2239. Tilly H, Rossi A, Stamatoullas A, Lenormand B, Bigorgne C, Kunlin A, Monconduit M, Bastard C (1994). Prognostic value of chromosomal abnormalities in follicular lymphoma. Blood 84: 1043-1049.
2240. Timar B, Fulop Z, Csernus B, Angster C, Bognar A, Szepesi A, Kopper L, Matolcsy A (2004). Relationship between the mutational status of VH genes and pathogenesis of diffuse large B-cell lymphoma in Richter's syndrome. Leukemia 18: 326-330.
2241. Tinguely M, Vonlanthen R, Muller E, Dommann-Scherrer CC, Schneider J, Laissue JA, Borisch B (1998). Hodgkin's disease-like lymphoproliferative disorders in patients with different underlying immunodeficiency states. Mod Pathol 11: 307-312.
2242. Titgemeyer C, Grois N, Minkov M, Flucher-Wolfram B, Gatterer-Menz I, Gadner H (2001). Pattern and course of single-system disease in Langerhans cell histiocytosis data from the DAL-HX 83- and 90-study. Med Pediatr Oncol 37: 108-114.
2243. Tobin G (2007). The immunoglobulin genes: structure and specificity in chronic lymphocytic leukemia. Leuk Lymphoma 48: 1081-1086.
2244. Tobin G, Thunberg U, Johnson A, Thorn I, Soderberg O, Hultdin M, Botling J, Enblad G, Sallstrom J, Sundstrom C, Roos G, Rosenquist R (2002). Somatically mutated Ig V(H)3-21 genes characterize a new subset of chronic lymphocytic leukemia. Blood 99: 2262-2264.
2245. Tokita K, Maki K, Tadokoro J, Nakamura Y, Arai Y, Sasaki K, Eguchi-Ishimae M, Eguchi M, Mitani K (2007). Chronic idiopathic myelofibrosis expressing a novel type of TEL-PDGFRB chimaera responded to imatinib mesylate therapy. Leukemia 21: 190-192.
2246. Tolksdorf G, Stein H, Lennert K (1980). Morphological and immunological definition of a malignant lymphoma derived from germinal-centre cells with cleaved nuclei (centrocytes). Br J Cancer 41: 168-182.
2247. Tomita S, Mori KL, Sakajiri S, Oshimi K (2003). B-cell marker negative (CD7+, CD19-) Epstein-Barr virus-related pyothorax-associated lymphoma with rearrangement in the JH gene. Leuk Lymphoma 44: 727-730.
2248. Tomita Y, Ohsawa M, Qiu K, Hashimoto M, Yang WI, Kim GE, Aozasa K (1997). Epstein-Barr virus in lymphoproliferative diseases in the sino-nasal region: close association with CD56+ immunophenotype and polymorphic-reticulosis morphology. Int J Cancer 70: 9-13.
2249. Tordjman R, Macintyre E, Emile JF, Valensi F, Ribrag V, Burtin ML, Varet B, Brousse N, Hermine O (1996). Aggressive acute CD3+. Leukemia 10: 1514-1519.
2250. Torlakovic E, Nielsen S, Vyberg M (2005). Antibody selection in immunohistochemical detection of cyclin D1 in mantle cell lymphoma. Am J Clin Pathol 124: 782-789.
2250A. Torlakovic E, Tierens A, Dang HD, Delabie J (2001). The transcription factor PU.1, necessary for B-cell development is expressed in lymphocyte predominance, but not classical Hodgkin's disease. Am J Pathol 159: 1807-1814.
2251. Torlakovic E, Torlakovic G, Nguyen PL, Brunning RD, Delabie J (2002). The value of anti-pax-5 immunostaining in routinely fixed and paraffin-embedded sections: a novel pan pre-B and B-cell marker. Am J Surg Pathol 26: 1343-1350.
2252. Torlakovic EE, Aamot HV, Heim S (2006). A marginal zone phenotype in follicular lymphoma with t(14;18) is associated with secondary cytogenetic aberrations typical of marginal zone lymphoma. J Pathol 209: 258-264.
2253. Toro JR, Beaty M, Sorbara L, Turner ML, White J, Kingma DW, Raffeld M, Jaffe ES (2000). gamma delta T-cell lymphoma of the skin: a clinical, microscopic, and molecular study. Arch Dermatol 136: 1024-1032.
2254. Toro JR, Liewehr DJ, Pabby N, Sorbara L, Raffeld M, Steinberg SM, Jaffe ES (2003). Gamma-delta T-cell phenotype is associated with significantly decreased survival in cutaneous T-cell lymphoma. Blood 101: 3407-3412.
2255. Tort F, Camacho E, Bosch F, Harris NL, Montserrat E, Campo E (2004). Familial lymphoid neoplasms in patients with mantle cell lymphoma. Haematologica 89: 314-319.
2256. Tort F, Pinyol M, Pulford K, Roncador G, Hernandez L, Nayach I, Kluin-Nelemans HC, Kluin P, Touriol C, Delsol G, Mason D, Campo E (2001). Molecular characterization of a new ALK translocation involving moesin (MSN-ALK) in anaplastic large cell lymphoma. Lab Invest 81: 419-426.
2257. Touhy EA (1920). A case of splenomegaly with polymorphonuclear neutrophil hyperleukocytosis. Am J Med Sci 160: 18-25.
2258. Touriol C, Greenland C, Lamant L, Pulford K, Bernard F, Rousset T, Mason DY, Delsol G (2000). Further demonstration of the diversity of chromosomal changes involving 2p23 in ALK-positive lymphoma: 2 cases expressing ALK kinase fused to CLTCL (clathrin chain polypeptide-like). Blood 95: 3204-3207.
2259. Tournilhac O, Santos DD, Xu L, Kutok J, Tai YT, Le Gouill S, Catley L, Hunter Z, Branagan AR, Boyce JA, Munshi N, Anderson KC, Treon SP (2006). Mast cells in Waldenstrom's macroglobulinemia support lymphoplasmacytic cell growth through CD154/CD40 signaling. Ann Oncol 17: 1275-1282.
2260. Toyama K, Ohyashiki K, Yoshida Y, Abe T, Asano S, Hirai H, Hirashima K, Hotta T, Kuramoto A, Kuriya S (1993). Clinical implications of chromosomal abnormalities in 401 patients with myelodysplastic syndromes: a multicentric study in Japan. Leukemia 7: 499-508.
2261. Tracey L, Villuendas R, Dotor AM, Spiteri I, Ortiz P, Garcia JF, Peralto JL, Lawler M, Piris MA (2003). Mycosis fungoides shows concurrent deregulation of multiple genes involved in the TNF signaling pathway: an expression profile study. Blood 102: 1042-1050.
2262. Traverse-Glehen A, Baseggio L, Callet-Bauchu E, Morel D, Gazzo S, Ffrench M, Verney A, Rolland D, Thieblemont C, Magaud JP, Salles G, Coiffier B, Berger F, Felman P (2008). Splenic red pulp lymphoma with numerous basophilic villous lymphocytes: a distinct clinico-pathological and molecular entity? Blood 111: 2253-2260.
2263. Traverse-Glehen A, Davi F, Ben Simon E, Callet-Bauchu E, Felman P, Baseggio L, Gazzo S, Thieblemont C, Charlot C, Coiffier B, Berger F, Salles G (2005). Analysis of VH genes in marginal zone lymphoma reveals marked heterogeneity between splenic and nodal tumors and suggests the existence of clonal selection. Haematologica 90: 470-478.
2264. Traverse-Glehen A, Felman P, Callet-Bauchu E, Gazzo S, Baseggio L, Bryon PA, Thieblemont C, Coiffier B, Salles G, Berger F (2006). A clinicopathological study of nodal marginal zone B-cell lymphoma. A report on 21 cases. Histopathology 48: 162-173.
2265. Traverse-Glehen A, Pittaluga S, Gaulard P, Sorbara L, Alonso MA, Raffeld M, Jaffe ES (2005). Mediastinal gray zone lymphoma: the missing link between classic Hodgkin's lymphoma and mediastinal large B-cell lymphoma. Am J Surg Pathol 29: 1411-1421.
2266. Trempat P, Villalva C, Laurent G, Armstrong F, Delsol G, Dastugue N, Brousset P

(2003). Chronic myeloproliferative disorders with rearrangement of the platelet-derived growth factor alpha receptor: a new clinical target for STI571/Glivec. Oncogene 22: 5702-5706.

2267. Treon SP, Hunter ZR, Aggarwal A, Ewen EP, Masota S, Lee C, Santos DD, Hatjiharissi E, Xu L, Leleu X, Tournilhac O, Patterson CJ, Manning R, Branagan AR, Morton CC (2006). Characterization of familial Waldenstrom's macroglobulinemia. Ann Oncol 17: 488-494.

2268. Trinei M, Lanfrancone L, Campo E, Pulford K, Mason DY, Pelicci PG, Falini B (2000). A new variant anaplastic lymphoma kinase (ALK)-fusion protein (ATIC-ALK) in a case of ALK-positive anaplastic large cell lymphoma. Cancer Res 60: 793-798.

2269. Trofe J, Buell JF, Beebe TM, Hanaway MJ, First MR, Alloway RR, Gross TG, Succop P, Woodle ES (2005). Analysis of factors that influence survival with post-transplant lymphoproliferative disorder in renal transplant recipients: the Israel Penn International Transplant Tumor Registry experience. Am J Transplant 5: 775-780.

2270. Trotter MJ, Whittaker SJ, Orchard GE, Smith NP (1997). Cutaneous histopathology of Sezary syndrome: a study of 41 cases with a proven circulating T-cell clone. J Cutan Pathol 24: 286-291.

2271. Tsang P, Cesarman E, Chadburn A, Liu YF, Knowles DM (1996). Molecular characterization of primary mediastinal B cell lymphoma. Am J Pathol 148: 2017-2025.

2272. Tsang RW, Gospodarowicz MK, Pintilie M, Bezjak A, Wells W, Hodgson DC, Stewart AK (2001). Solitary plasmacytoma treated with radiotherapy: impact of tumor size on outcome. Int J Radiat Oncol Biol Phys 50: 113-120.

2273. Tsang WY, Chan JK, Ng CS, Pau MY (1996). Utility of a paraffin section-reactive CD56 antibody (123C3) for characterization and diagnosis of lymphomas. Am J Surg Pathol 20: 202-210.

2273A. Tsirigotis P, Economopoulos T, Rontogianni D, Dervenoulas J, Papageorgiou E, Bollas G, Mantzios G, Kalantzis D, Koumarianou A, Raptis S (2001). T-cell-rich B-cell lymphoma. Analysis of clinical features, response to treatment, survival and comparison with diffuse large B-cell lymphoma. Oncology. 61: 257-264.

2273B. Tsukamoto Y, Katsunobu Y, Omura Y, Maeda I, Hirai M, Teshima H, Konishi Y (2006). Subcutaneous panniculitis-like T-cell lymphoma: succesful initial treatment with prednisolone and cyclosporin A. Intern Med 45: 21-24.

2274. Tsukasaki K, Tsushima H, Yamamura M, Hata T, Murata K, Maeda T, Atogami S, Sohda H, Momita S, Ideda S, Katamine S, Yamada Y, Kamihira S, Tomonaga M (1997). Integration patterns of HTLV-I provirus in relation to the clinical course of ATL: frequent clonal change at crisis from indolent disease. Blood 89: 948-956.

2275. Tzankov A, Krugmann J, Fend F, Fischhofer M, Greil R, Dirnhofer S (2003). Prognostic significance of CD20 expression in classical Hodgkin lymphoma: a clinicopathological study of 119 cases. Clin Cancer Res 9: 1381-1386.

2276. Uccini S, Monardo F, Stoppacciaro A, Gradilone A, Agliano AM, Faggioni A, Manzari V, Vago L, Costanzi G, Ruco LP, . (1990). High frequency of Epstein-Barr virus genome detection in Hodgkin's disease of HIV-positive patients. Int J Cancer 46: 581-585.

2277. Uckun FM, Sather HN, Gaynon PS, Arthur DC, Trigg ME, Tubergen DG, Nachman J, Steinherz PG, Sensel MG, Reaman GH (1997). Clinical features and treatment outcome of children with myeloid antigen positive acute lymphoblastic leukemia: a report from the Children's Cancer Group. Blood 90: 28-35.

2278. Ueda C, Nishikori M, Kitawaki T, Uchiyama T, Ohno H (2004). Coexistent rearrangements of c-MYC, BCL2, and BCL6 genes in a diffuse large B-cell lymphoma. Int J Hematol 79: 52-54.

2279. Urosevic M, Conrad C, Kamarashev J, Asagoe K, Cozzio A, Burg G, Dummer R (2005). CD4+CD56+ hematodermic neoplasms bear a plasmacytoid dendritic cell phenotype. Hum Pathol 36: 1020-1024.

2280. Vaandrager JW, Schuuring E, Raap T, Philippo K, Kleiverda K, Kluin P (2000). Interphase FISH detection of BCL2 rearrangement in follicular lymphoma using breakpoint-flanking probes. Genes Chromosomes Cancer 27: 85-94.

2281. Vaandrager JW, Schuuring E, Zwikstra E, De Boer CJ, Kleiverda KK, Van Krieken JH, Kluin-Nelemans HC, van Ommen GJ, Raap AK, Kluin PM (1996). Direct visualization of dispersed 11q13 chromosomal translocations in mantle cell lymphoma by multicolor DNA fiber fluorescence in situ hybridization. Blood 88: 1177-1182.

2282. Vaghefi P, Martin A, Prevot S, Charlotte F, Camilleri-Broet S, Barli E, Davi F, Gabarre J, Raphael M, Poirel HA (2006). Genomic imbalances in AIDS-related lymphomas: relation with tumoral Epstein-Barr virus status. AIDS 20: 2285-2291.

2283. Vaishampayan UN, Mohamed AN, Dugan MC, Bloom RE, Palutke M (2001). Blastic mantle cell lymphoma associated with Burkitt-type translocation and hypodiploidy. Br J Haematol 115: 66-68.

2284. Vakiani E, Nandula SV, Subramaniyam S, Keller CE, Alobeid B, Murty VV, Bhagat G (2007). Cytogenetic analysis of B-cell post-transplant lymphoproliferations validates the World Health Organization classification and suggests inclusion of florid follicular hyperplasia as a precursor lesion. Hum Pathol 38: 315-325.

2285. Valbuena JR, Medeiros LJ, Rassidakis GZ, Hao S, Wu CD, Chen L, Lin P (2006). Expression of B cell-specific activator protein/PAX5 in acute myeloid leukemia with t(8;21)(q22;q22). Am J Clin Pathol 126: 235-240.

2286. Valent P, Akin C, Escribano L, Fodinger M, Hartmann K, Brockow K, Castells M, Sperr WR, Kluin-Nelemans HC, Hamdy NA, Lortholary O, Robyn J, van Doormaal J, Sotlar K, Hauswirth AW, Arock M, Hermine O, Hellmann A, Triggiani M, Niedoszytko M, Schwartz LB, Orfao A, Horny HP, Metcalfe DD (2007). Standards and standardization in mastocytosis: consensus statements on diagnostics, treatment recommendations and response criteria. Eur J Clin Invest 37: 435-453.

2287. Valent P, Akin C, Metcalfe DD (2007). FIP1L1/PDGFRA is a molecular marker of chronic eosinophilic leukaemia but not for systemic mastocytosis. Eur J Clin Invest 37: 153-154.

2288. Valent P, Akin C, Sperr WR, Horny HP, Arock M, Lechner K, Bennett JM, Metcalfe DD (2003). Diagnosis and treatment of systemic mastocytosis: state of the art. Br J Haematol 122: 695-717.

2289. Valent P, Akin C, Sperr WR, Horny HP, Metcalfe DD (2002). Smouldering mastocytosis: a novel subtype of systemic mastocytosis with slow progression. Int Arch Allergy Immunol 127: 137-139.

2290. Valent P, Horny HP, Escribano L, Longley BJ, Li CY, Schwartz LB, Marone G, Nunez R, Akin C, Sotlar K, Sperr WR, Wolff K, Brunning RD, Parwaresch MR, Austen KF, Lennert K, Metcalfe DD, Vardiman JW, Bennett JM (2001). Diagnostic criteria and classification of mastocytosis: a consensus proposal. Leuk Res 25: 603-625.

2291. van den Bosch CA (2004). Is endemic Burkitt's lymphoma an alliance between three infections and a tumour promoter? Lancet Oncol 5: 738-746.

2292. van den Heuvel-Eibrink MM (2007). Paroxysmal nocturnal hemoglobinuria in children. Paediatr Drugs 9: 11-16.

2293. van den Berg A, Visser L, Poppema S (1999). High expression of the CC chemokine TARC in Reed-Sternberg cells. A possible explanation for the characteristic T-cell infiltratein Hodgkin's lymphoma. Am J Pathol 154: 1685-1691.

2293A. van den Oord JJ, Wolf-Peeters C, Desmet VJ (1986). The marginal zone in the human reactive lymph node. Am J Clin Pathol 86: 475-479.

2293B. van den Oord JJ, Wolf-Peeters C, Desmet VJ (1989). Marginal zone lymphocytes in the lymph node. Hum Pathol 20: 1225-1227.

2294. van der Velden VH, Bruggemann M, Hoogeveen PG, de Bie M, Hart PG, Raff T, Pfeifer H, Luschen S, Szczepanski T, van Wering ER, Kneba M, van Dongen JJ (2004). TCRB gene rearrangements in childhood and adult precursor-B-ALL: frequency, applicability as MRD-PCR target, and stability between diagnosis and relapse. Leukemia 18: 1971-1980.

2295. van Dongen JJ, Seriu T, Panzer-Grumayer ER, Biondi A, Pongers-Willemse MJ, Corral L, Stolz F, Schrappe M, Masera G, Kamps WA, Gadner H, van Wering ER, Ludwig WD, Basso G, de Bruijn MA, Cazzaniga G, Hettinger K, van der Does-van den Berg, Hop WC, Riehm H, Bartram CR (1998). Prognostic value of minimal residual disease in acute lymphoblastic leukaemia in childhood. Lancet 352: 1731-1738.

2296. van Doorn R, Dijkman R, Vermeer MH, Out-Luiting JJ, van der Raaij-Helmer EM, Willemze R, Tensen CP (2004). Aberrant expression of the tyrosine kinase receptor EphA4 and the transcription factor twist in Sezary syndrome identified by gene expression analysis. Cancer Res 64: 5578-5586.

2297. van Doorn R, Scheffer E, Willemze R (2002). Follicular mycosis fungoides, a distinct disease entity with or without associated follicular mucinosis: a clinicopathologic and follow-up study of 51 patients. Arch Dermatol 138: 191-198.

2298. van Doorn R, Van Haselen CW, Voorst Vader PC, Geerts ML, Heule F, de Rie M, Steijlen PM, Dekker SK, van Vloten WA, Willemze R (2000). Mycosis fungoides: disease evolution and prognosis of 309 Dutch patients. Arch Dermatol 136: 504-510.

2298A. Van Gool SW, Delabie J, Vandenberghe P, Coorevits L, De Wolf-Peeters C, Ceuppens JL (1997). Expression of B7-2 (CD86) molecules by Reed-Sternberg cells of Hodgkin's disease. Leukaemia 11: 846-851.

2299. van Gorp J, Weiping L, Jacobse K, Liu YH, Li FY, De Weger RA, Li G (1994). Epstein-Barr virus in nasal T-cell lymphomas (polymorphic reticulosis/midline malignant reticulosis) in western China. J Pathol 173: 81-87.

2300. Van Haselen CW, Toonstra J, van der Putte SJ, van Dongen JJ, van Hees CL, van Vloten WA (1998). Granulomatous slack skin. Report of three patients with an updated review of the literature. Dermatology 196: 382-391.

2301. van Imhoff GW, Boerma EJ, van der HB, Schuuring E, Verdonck LF, Kluin-Nelemans HC, Kluin PM (2006). Prognostic impact of germinal center-associated proteins and chromosomal breakpoints in poor-risk diffuse large B-cell lymphoma. J Clin Oncol 24: 4135-4142.

2302. Van Krieken JH (2004). Lymphoproliferative disease associated with immune deficiency in children. Am J Clin Pathol 122 Suppl: S122-S127.

2302A. Van Krieken JH, von Schilling C, Kluin PM, Lennert K (1989). Splenic marginal zone lymphocytes and related cells in the lymph node: a morphologic and immunohistochemical study. Hum Pathol 20: 320-325.

2303. Van Neer FJ, Toonstra J, Voorst Vader PC, Willemze R, van Vloten WA (2001). Lymphomatoid papulosis in children: a study of 10 children registered by the Dutch Cutaneous Lymphoma Working Group. Br J Dermatol 144: 351-354.

2304. van Nierop K, de Groot C (2002). Human follicular dendritic cells: function, origin and development. Semin Immunol 14: 251-257.

2305. Van Overbeke L, Ectors N, Tack J (2005). What is the role of celiac disease in enteropathy-type intestinal lymphoma? A retrospective study of nine cases. Acta Gastroenterol Belg 68: 419-423.

2306. van Rhee F, Hochhaus A, Lin F, Melo JV, Goldman JM, Cross NC (1996). p190 BCR-ABL mRNA is expressed at low levels in p210-positive chronic myeloid and acute lymphoblastic leukemias. Blood 87: 5213-5217.

2307. van Spronsen DJ, Vrints LW, Hofstra G, Crommelin MA, Coebergh JW, Breed WP (1997). Disappearance of prognostic significance of histopathological grading of nodular sclerosing Hodgkin's disease for unselected patients, 1972-92. Br J Haematol 96: 322-327.

2308. Vandenberghe E, Wolf-Peeters C, van den Oord J, Wlodarska I, Delabie J, Stul M, Thomas J, Michaux JL, Mecucci C, Cassiman JJ, . (1991). Translocation (11;14): a cytogenetic anomaly associated with B-cell lymphomas of non-follicle centre cell lineage. J Pathol 163: 13-18.

2309. Vandenberghe P, Wlodarska I, Michaux L, Zachee P, Boogaerts M, Vanstraelen D, Herregods MC, Van Hoof A, Selleslag D, Roufosse F, Maerevoet M, Verhoef G, Cools J, Gilliland DG, Hagemeijer A, Marynen P (2004). Clinical and molecular features of FIP1L1-PDF-GRA (+) chronic eosinophilic leukemias. Leukemia 18: 734-742.

2310. Vardiman JW (2003). The new World Health Organization classification of myeloid neoplasms: Q&A with James W. Vardiman, MD. Clin Adv Hematol Oncol 1: 18, 21-

2311. Vardiman JW (2004). Myelodysplastic/myeloproliferative diseases. Cancer Treat Res 121: 13-43.

2312. Vardiman JW (2006). Hematopathological concepts and controversies in the diagnosis and classification of myelodysplastic syndromes. Hematology Am Soc Hematol Educ Program 199-204.

2313. Vargas H, Mouzakes J, Purdy SS, Cohn AS, Parnes SM (2002). Follicular dendritic cell tumor: an aggressive head and neck tumor. Am J Otolaryngol 23: 93-98.

2314. Varon R, Vissinga C, Platzer M, Cerosaletti KM, Chrzanowska KH, Saar K, Beckmann G, Seemanova E, Cooper PR, Nowak NJ, Stumm M, Weemaes CM, Gatti RA, Wilson RK, Digweed M, Rosenthal A, Sperling K, Concannon P, Reis A (1998). Nibrin, a novel DNA double-strand break repair protein, is mutated in Nijmegen breakage syndrome. Cell 93: 467-476.

2315. Vasef MA, Zaatari GS, Chan WC, Sun NC, Weiss LM, Brynes RK (1995). Dendritic cell tumors associated with low-grade B-cell malignancies. Report of three cases. Am J Clin Pathol 104: 696-701.

2316. Vassallo J, Lamant L, Brugieres L, Gaillard F, Campo E, Brousset P, Delsol G

(2006). ALK-positive anaplastic large cell lymphoma mimicking nodular sclerosis Hodgkin's lymphoma: report of 10 cases. Am J Surg Pathol 30: 223-229.
2317. Vassallo J, Paes RP, Soares FA, Menezes Y, Aldred V, Ribeiro KC, Alves AC (2005). Histological classification of 1,025 cases of Hodgkin's lymphoma from the State of Sao Paulo, Brazil. Sao Paulo Med J 123: 134-136.
2318. Veelken H, Vik DS, Schulte MJ, Martens UM, Finke J, Schmitt-Graeff A (2007). Immunophenotype as prognostic factor for diffuse large B-cell lymphoma in patients undergoing clinical risk-adapted therapy. Ann Oncol 18: 931-939.
2319. Vega F, Chang CC, Medeiros LJ, Udden MM, Cho-Vega JH, Lau CC, Finch CJ, Vilchez RA, McGregor D, Jorgensen JL (2005). Plasmablastic lymphomas and plasmablastic plasma cell myelomas have nearly identical immunophenotypic profiles. Mod Pathol 18: 806-815.
2320. Vega F, Coombes KR, Thomazy VA, Patel K, Lang W, Jones D (2006). Tissue-specific function of lymph node fibroblastic reticulum cells. Pathobiology 73: 71-81.
2321. Vega F, Medeiros LJ, Bueso-Ramos C, Jones D, Lai R, Luthra R, Abruzzo LV (2001). Hepatosplenic gamma/delta T-cell lymphoma in bone marrow. A sinusoidal neoplasm with blastic cytologic features. Am J Clin Pathol 116: 410-419.
2322. Vega F, Medeiros LJ, Gaulard P (2007). Hepatosplenic and other gammadelta T-cell lymphomas. Am J Clin Pathol 127: 869-880.
2323. Velankar MM, Nathwani BN, Schlutz MJ, Bain LA, Arber DA, Slovak ML, Weiss LM (1999). Indolent T-lymphoblastic proliferation: report of a case with a 16-year course without cytotoxic therapy. Am J Surg Pathol 23: 977-981.
2324. Venditti A, Del Poeta G, Buccisano F, Tamburini A, Cox-Froncillo MC, Aronica G, Bruno A, Del Moro B, Epiceno AM, Battaglia A, Forte L, Postorino M, Cordero V, Santinelli S, Amadori S (1998). Prognostic relevance of the expression of Tdt and CD7 in 335 cases of acute myeloid leukemia. Leukemia 12: 1056-1063.
2325. Vener C, Soligo D, Berti E, Gianelli U, Servida F, Ceretti E, Caputo R, Passoni E, Lambertenghi DG (2007). Indeterminate cell histiocytosis in association with later occurrence of acute myeloblastic leukaemia. Br J Dermatol 156: 1357-1361.
2326. Veneri D, Aqel H, Franchini M, Meneghini V, Krampera M (2004). Prevalence of hepatitis C virus infection in IgM-type monoclonal gammopathy of uncertain significance and Waldenstrom macroglobulinemia. Am J Hematol 77: 421.
2327. Verburgh E, Achten R, Louw VJ, Brusselmans C, Delforge M, Boogaerts M, Hagemeijer A, Vandenberghe P, Verhoef G (2007). A new disease categorization of low-grade myelodysplastic syndromes based on the expression of cytopenia and dysplasia in one versus more than one lineage improves on the WHO classification. Leukemia 21: 668-677.
2328. Verburgh E, Achten R, Maes B, Hagemeijer A, Boogaerts M, Wolf-Peeters C, Verhoef G (2003). Additional prognostic value of bone marrow histology in patients subclassified according to the International Prognostic Scoring System for myelodysplastic syndromes. J Clin Oncol 21: 273-282.
2329. Vergier B, Belaud-Rotureau MA, Benassy MN, Beylot-Barry M, Dubus P, Delaunay M, Garroste JC, Taine L, Merlio JP (2004). Neoplastic cells do not carry bcl2-JH rearrangements detected in a subset of primary cutaneous follicle center B-cell lymphomas. Am J Surg Pathol 28: 748-755.
2330. Vergier B, de Muret A, Beylot-Barry M, Vaillant L, Ekouevi D, Chene G, Carlotti A, Franck N, Dechelotte P, Souteyrand P, Courville P, Joly P, Delaunay M, Bagot M, Grange F, Fraitag S, Bosq J, Petrella T, Durlach A, de Mascarel A, Merlio JP, Wechsler J (2000). Transformation of mycosis fungoides: clinicopathological and prognostic features of 45 cases. French Study Group of Cutaneious Lymphomas. Blood 95: 2212-2218.
2331. Verhaak RG, Goudswaard CS, van Putten W, Bijl MA, Sanders MA, Hugens W, Uitterlinden AG, Erpelinck CA, Delwel R, Lowenberg B, Valk PJ (2005). Mutations in nucleophosmin (NPM1) in acute myeloid leukemia (AML): association with other gene abnormalities and previously established gene expression signatures and their favorable prognostic significance. Blood 106: 3747-3754.
2332. Verkarre V, Romana SP, Cellier C, Asnafi V, Mention JJ, Barbe U, Nusbaum S, Hermine O, Macintyre E, Brousse N, Cerf-Bensussan N, Radford-Weiss I (2003). Recurrent partial trisomy 1q22-q44 in clonal intraepithelial lymphocytes in refractory celiac sprue. Gastroenterology 125: 40-46.
2333. Vermeer MH, Geelen FA, Kummer JA, Meijer CJ, Willemze R (1999). Expression of cytotoxic proteins by neoplastic T cells in mycosis fungoides increases with progression from plaque stage to tumor stage disease. Am J Pathol 154: 1203-1210.
2334. Vermeer MH, Geelen FA, Van Haselen CW, Voorst Vader PC, Geerts ML, van Vloten WA, Willemze R (1996). Primary cutaneous large B-cell lymphomas of the legs. A distinct type of cutaneous B-cell lymphoma with an intermediate prognosis. Dutch Cutaneous Lymphoma Working Group. Arch Dermatol 132: 1304-1308.
2335. Vermi W, Facchetti F, Rosati S, Vergoni F, Rossi E, Festa S, Remotti D, Grigolato P, Massarelli G, Frizzera G (2004). Nodal and extranodal tumor-forming accumulation of plasmacytoid monocytes/interferon-producing cells associated with myeloid disorders. Am J Surg Pathol 28: 585-595.
2335A. Vidal AU, Gessain A, Yoshida M, Mahieux R, Nishioka K, Tekaia F, Rosen L, De Thé G (1994). Molecular epidemiology of HTLV type I in Japan: evidence for two distinct ancestral lineages with a particular geographical distribution. AIDS Res Hum Retroviruses 10: 1557-1566.
2336. Vie H, Chevalier S, Garand R, Moisan JP, Praloran V, Devilder MC, Moreau JF, Soulillou JP (1989). Clonal expansion of lymphocytes bearing the gamma delta T-cell receptor in a patient with large granular lymphocyte disorder. Blood 74: 285-290.
2337. Vijay A, Gertz MA (2007). Waldenstrom macroglobulinemia. Blood 109: 5096-5103.
2338. Virgilio L, Lazzeri C, Bichi R, Nibu K, Narducci MG, Russo G, Rothstein JL, Croce CM (1998). Deregulated expression of TCL1 causes T cell leukemia in mice. Proc Natl Acad Sci U S A 95: 3885-3889.
2339. Vitolo U, Gaidano G, Botto B, Volpe G, Audisio E, Bertini M, Calvi R, Freilone R, Novero D, Orsucci L, Pastore C, Capello D, Parvis G, Sacco C, Zagonel V, Carbone A, Mazza U, Palestro G, Saglio G, Resegotti L (1998). Rearrangements of bcl-6, bcl-2, c-myc and 6q deletion in B-diffuse large-cell lymphoma: clinical relevance in 71 patients. Ann Oncol 9: 55-61.
2340. Vizmanos JL, Hernandez R, Vidal MJ, Larrayoz MJ, Odero MD, Marin J, Ardanaz MT, Calasanz MJ, Cross NC (2004). Clinical variability of patients with the t(6;8)(q27;p12) and FGFR1OP-FGFR1 fusion: two further cases. Hematol J 5: 534-537.
2341. von den Driesch P, Coors EA (2002). Localized cutaneous small to medium-sized pleomorphic T-cell lymphoma: a report of 3 cases stable for years. J Am Acad Dermatol 46: 531-535.
2341A. von Wasielewski S, Franklin J, Fischer R, Hübner K, Hansmann ML, Diehl V, Georgii A, von Wasielewski R (2003). Nodular sclerosing Hodgkin disease: new grading predicts prognosis in intermediate and advanced stages. Blood 101:4063-4069.
2342. Vonderheid EC, Pena J, Nowell P (2006). Sezary cell counts in erythrodermic cutaneous T-cell lymphoma: implications for prognosis and staging. Leuk Lymphoma 47: 1841-1856.
2343. Voorhees PM, Carder KA, Smith SV, Ayscue LH, Rao KW, Dunphy CH (2004). Follicular lymphoma with a burkitt translocation—predictor of an aggressive clinical course: a case report and review of the literature. Arch Pathol Lab Med 128: 210-213.
2344. Vorechovsky I, Luo L, Dyer MJ, Catovsky D, Amlot PL, Yaxley JC, Foroni L, Hammarstrom L, Webster AD, Yuille MA (1997). Clustering of missense mutations in the ataxia-telangiectasia gene in a sporadic T-cell leukaemia. Nat Genet 17: 96-99.
2345. Vos JA, Abbondanzo SL, Barekman CL, Andriko JW, Miettinen M, Aguilera NS (2005). Histiocytic sarcoma: a study of five cases including the histiocyte marker CD163. Mod Pathol 18: 693-704.
2346. Vose JM, Bierman PJ, Lynch JC, Weisenburger DD, Kessinger A, Chan WC, Greiner TC, Armitage JO (1998). Effect of follicularity on autologous transplantation for large-cell non-Hodgkin's lymphoma. J Clin Oncol 16: 844-849.
2347. Vyas P, Crispino JD (2007). Molecular insights into Down syndrome-associated leukemia. Curr Opin Pediatr 19: 9-14.
2348. Waggott W, Delsol G, Jarret RF, Mason DY, Gatter KC, Boultwood J, Wainscoat JS (1997). NPM-ALK gene fusion and Hodgkin's disease. Blood 90: 1712-1713.
2349. Wagner SD, Martinelli V, Luzzatto L (1994). Similar patterns of V kappa gene usage but different degrees of somatic mutation in hairy cell leukemia, prolymphocytic leukemia, Waldenstrom's macroglobulinemia, and myeloma. Blood 83: 3647-3653.
2350. Wahner-Roedler DL, Kyle RA (1992). Mu-heavy chain disease: presentation as a benign monoclonal gammopathy. Am J Hematol 40: 56-60.
2351. Wahner-Roedler DL, Kyle RA (1998). Heavy chain disease. In: Myeloma, Biology and Management. Malpas JA, Bergsagel DE, Kyle RA, Anderson KC, eds. Oxford University Press: New York, pp. 604-638.
2352. Wahner-Roedler DL, Witzig TE, Loehrer LL, Kyle RA (2003). Gamma-heavy chain disease: review of 23 cases. Medicine (Baltimore) 82: 236-250.
2353. Walts AE, Shintaku IP, Said JW (1990). Diagnosis of malignant lymphoma in effusions from patients with AIDS by gene rearrangement. Am J Clin Pathol 94: 170-175.
2354. Walz C, Curtis C, Schnittger S, Schultheis B, Metzgeroth G, Schoch C, Lengfelder E, Erben P, Muller MC, Haferlach T, Hochhaus A, Hehlmann R, Cross NC, Reiter A (2006). Transient response to imatinib in a chronic eosinophilic leukemia associated with ins(9;4)(q33;q12q25) and a CDK5RAP2-PDGFRA fusion gene. Genes Chromosomes Cancer 45: 950-956.
2355. Walz C, Metzgeroth G, Haferlach C, Schmitt-Graeff A, Fabarius A, Hagen V, Prummer O, Rauh S, Hehlmann R, Hochhaus A, Cross NC, Reiter A (2007). Characterization of three new imatinib-responsive fusion genes in chronic myeloproliferative disorders generated by disruption of the platelet-derived growth factor receptor beta gene. Haematologica 92: 163-169.
2356. Wandt H, Schakel U, Kroschinsky F, Prange-Krex G, Mohr B, Thiede C, Pascheberg U, Soucek S, Schaich M, Ehninger G (2008). Multilineage dysplasia according to the World Health Organisation (WHO) classification in acute myeloid leukemia (AML) has no correlation with age and no independent prognostic relevance as analysed in 1766 patients. Blood 111: 1855-1861.
2357. Wang J, Bu DF, Li T, Zheng R, Zhang BX, Chen XX, Zhu XJ (2005). Autoantibody production from a thymoma and a follicular dendritic cell sarcoma associated with paraneoplastic pemphigus. Br J Dermatol 153: 558-564.
2358. Wang SA, Hasserjian RP, Loew JM, Sechman EV, Jones D, Hao S, Liu Q, Zhao W, Mehdi M, Galili N, Woda B, Raza A (2006). Refractory anemia with ringed sideroblasts associated with marked thrombocytosis harbors JAK2 mutation and shows overlapping myeloproliferative and myelodysplastic features. Leukemia 20: 1641-1644.
2358A. Wang SA, Olson N, Zukerberg L, Harris NL (2006). Splenic marginal zone lymphoma with micronodular T-cell rich B-cell lymphoma. Am J Surg Pathol 30: 128-132.
2358B. Wang SA, Wang L, Hochberg EP, Muzikansky A, Harris NL, Hasserjian RP (2005). Low histologic grade follicular lymphoma with high proliferation index: morphologic and clinical features. Am J Surg Pathol 29: 1490-1496.
2358C. Wang SS, Cozen W, Cerhan JR, Colt JS, Morton LM, Engels EA, Davis S, Severson RK, Rothman N, Chanock SJ, Hartge P (2007). Immune mechanisms in non-Hodgkin lymphoma: joint effects of the TNF G308A and IL10 T3575A polymorphisms with non-Hodgkin lymphoma risk factors. Cancer Res 67: 5042-5054.
2359. Warnke RA, Jones D, Hsi ED (2007). Morphologic and immunophenotypic variants of nodal T-cell lymphomas and T-cell lymphoma mimics. Am J Clin Pathol 127: 511-527.
2360. Warnke RA, Kim H, Fuks Z, Dorfman RF (1977). The coexistence of nodular and diffuse patterns in nodular non-Hodgkin's lymphomas: significance and clinicopathologic correlation. Cancer 40: 1229-1233.
2361. Warren HS, Christiansen FT, Witt CS (2003). Functional inhibitory human leucocyte antigen class I receptors on natural killer (NK) cells in patients with chronic NK lymphocytosis. Br J Haematol 121: 793-804.
2362. Washington LT, Doherty D, Glassman A, Martins J, Ibrahim S, Lai R (2002). Myeloid disorders with deletion of 5q as the sole karyotypic abnormality: the clinical and pathologic spectrum. Leuk Lymphoma 43: 761-765.
2363. Watanabe O, Maruyama I, Arimura K, Kitajima I, Arimura H, Hanatani M, Matsuo K, Arisato T, Osame M (1998). Overproduction of vascular endothelial growth factor/vascular permeability factor is causative in Crow-Fukase (POEMS) syndrome. Muscle Nerve 21: 1390-1397.
2364. Watanuki-Miyauchi R, Kojima Y, Tsurumi H, Hara T, Goto N, Kasahara S, Saio M, Moriwaki H, Takami T (2005). Expression of survivin and of antigen detected by a novel monoclonal antibody, T332, is associated with outcome of diffuse large B-cell lymphoma and its subtypes. Pathol Int 55: 324-330.
2365. Webb D, Roberts I, Vyas P (2007). Haematology of Down syndrome. Arch Dis

Child Fetal Neonatal Ed 92: F503-F507.
2366. Webber SA (1999). Post-transplant lymphoproliferative disorders: a preventable complication of solid organ transplantation? Pediatr Transplant 3: 95-99.
2367. Webber SA, Naftel DC, Fricker FJ, Olesnevich P, Blume ED, Addonizio L, Kirklin JK, Canter CE (2006). Lymphoproliferative disorders after paediatric heart transplantation: a multi-institutional study. Lancet 367: 233-239.
2368. Weber T, Weber RG, Kaulich K, Actor B, Meyer-Puttlitz B, Lampel S, Buschges R, Weigel R, Deckert-Schluter M, Schmiedek P, Reifenberger G, Lichter P (2000). Characteristic chromosomal imbalances in primary central nervous system lymphomas of the diffuse large B-cell type. Brain Pathol 10: 73-84.
2369. Weinreb M, Day PJ, Niggli F, Green EK, Nyong'o AO, Othieno-Abinya NA, Riyat MS, Raafat F, Mann JR (1996). The consistent association between Epstein-Barr virus and Hodgkin's disease in children in Kenya. Blood 87: 3828-3836.
2370. Weinreb M, Day PJ, Niggli F, Powell JE, Raafat F, Hesseling PB, Schneider JW, Hartley PS, Tzortzatou-Stathopoulou F, Khalek ER, Mangoud A, El Safy UR, Madanat F, Al Sheyyab M, Mpofu C, Revesz T, Rafii R, Tiedemann K, Waters KD, Barrantes JC, Nyongo A, Riyat MS, Mann JR (1996). The role of Epstein-Barr virus in Hodgkin's disease from different geographical areas. Arch Dis Child 74: 27-31.
2371. Weir EG, Ali Ansari-Lari M, Batista DA, Griffin CA, Fuller S, Smith BD, Borowitz MJ (2007). Acute bilineal leukemia: a rare disease with poor outcome. Leukemia 21: 2264-2270.
2372. Weir EG, Cowan K, LeBeau P, Borowitz MJ (1999). A limited antibody panel can distinguish B-precursor acute lymphoblastic leukemia from normal B precursors with four color flow cytometry: implications for residual disease detection. Leukemia 13: 558-567.
2373. Weisberg E, Manley PW, Cowan-Jacob SW, Hochhaus A, Griffin JD (2007). Second generation inhibitors of BCR-ABL for the treatment of imatinib-resistant chronic myeloid leukaemia. Nat Rev Cancer 7: 345-356.
2374. Weisenburger DD, Anderson J, Armitage J, et al (1998). Grading of follicular lymphoma: diagnostic accuracy, reproducibility, and clinical relevance. Mod Pathol 11: 142a-
2374A. Weiss LM (2000). Epstein-Barr virus and Hodgkin's disease. Curr Oncol Rep 2: 199-204.
2375. Weiss LM, Berry GJ, Dorfman RF, Banks P, Kaiserling E, Curtis J, Rosai J, Warnke RA (1990). Spindle cell neoplasms of lymph nodes of probable reticulum cell lineage. True reticulum cell sarcoma? Am J Surg Pathol 14: 405-414.
2376. Weiss LM, Bindl JM, Picozzi VJ, Link MP, Warnke RA (1986). Lymphoblastic lymphoma: an immunophenotype study of 26 cases with comparison to T cell acute lymphoblastic leukemia. Blood 67: 474-478.
2377. Weiss LM, Jaffe ES, Liu XF, Chen YY, Shibata D, Medeiros LJ (1992). Detection and localization of Epstein-Barr viral genomes in angioimmunoblastic lymphadenopathy and angioimmunoblastic lymphadenopathy-like lymphoma. Blood 79: 1789-1795.
2377A. Weiss LM, Movahed LA, Warnke RA, Sklar J (1989). Detection of Epstein-Barr viral genomes in Reed-Sternberg cells of Hodgkin's disease. N EJM 320: 502-506.
2378. Weiss LM, Strickler JG, Dorfman RF, Horning SJ, Warnke RA, Sklar J (1986). Clonal T-cell populations in angioimmunoblastic lymphadenopathy and angioimmunoblastic lymphadenopathy-like lymphoma. Am J Pathol 122: 392-397.
2379. Weiss LM, Warnke RA, Sklar J, Cleary ML (1987). Molecular analysis of the t(14;18) chromosomal translocation in malignant lymphomas. N Engl J Med 317: 1185-1189.
2380. Weissmann DJ, Ferry JA, Harris NL, Louis DN, Delmonico F, Spiro I (1995). Posttransplantation lymphoproliferative disorders in solid organ recipients are predominantly aggressive tumors of host origin. Am J Clin Pathol 103: 748-755.
2381. Weitzman S, Greenberg ML, Thorner P (1991). Treatment of non-Hodgkin's lymphoma in childhood. by PH Wiernik, GP Canellos, RA Kyle, Schiffer CA. 1 vol. 2nd ed. . New York 1991. In: Neoplastic diseases of blood. Neoplastic diseases of blood. Churchill Livingstone: New York, pp. 753-768.
2381A. Weitzman S, Jaffe R (2005). Uncommon histiocytic disorders: the non-Langerhans cell histiocytoses. Pediatr Blood Cancer 45: 256-264.
2382. Weller PF, Bubley GJ (1994). The idiopathic hypereosinophilic syndrome. Blood 83: 2759-2779.
2383. Wellmann A, Thieblemont C, Pittaluga S, Sakai A, Jaffe ES, Siebert P, Raffeld M (2000). Detection of differentially expressed genes in lymphomas using cDNA arrays: identification of clusterin as a new diagnostic marker for anaplastic large-cell lymphomas. Blood 96: 398-404.
2384. Wendum D, Sebban C, Gaulard P, Coiffier B, Tilly H, Cazals D, Boehn A, Casasnovas RO, Bouabdallah R, Jaubert J, Ferrant A, Diebold J, de Mascarel A, Gisselbrecht C (1997). Follicular large-cell lymphoma treated with intensive chemotherapy: an analysis of 89 cases included in the LNH87 trial and comparison with the outcome of diffuse large B-cell lymphoma. Groupe d'Etude des Lymphomes de l'Adulte. J Clin Oncol 15: 1654-1663.
2385. Weng AP, Ferrando AA, Lee W, Morris JP, Silverman LB, Sanchez-Irizarry C, Blacklow SC, Look AT, Aster JC (2004). Activating mutations of NOTCH1 in human T cell acute lymphoblastic leukemia. Science 306: 269-271.
2386. Weng AP, Millholland JM, Yashiro-Ohtani Y, Arcangeli ML, Lau A, Wai C, Del Bianco C, Rodriguez CG, Sai H, Tobias J, Li Y, Wolfe MS, Shachaf C, Felsher D, Blacklow SC, Pear WS, Aster JC (2006). c-Myc is an important direct target of Notch1 in T-cell acute lymphoblastic leukemia/lymphoma. Genes Dev 20: 2096-2109.
2387. Weniger MA, Gesk S, Ehrlich S, Martin-Subero JI, Dyer MJ, Siebert R, Moller P, Barth TF (2007). Gains of REL in primary mediastinal B-cell lymphoma coincide with nuclear accumulation of REL protein. Genes Chromosomes Cancer 46: 406-415.
2388. Weniger MA, Melzner I, Menz CK, Wegener S, Bucur AJ, Dorsch K, Mattfeldt T, Barth TF, Moller P (2006). Mutations of the tumor suppressor gene SOCS-1 in classical Hodgkin lymphoma are frequent and associated with nuclear phospho-STAT5 accumulation. Oncogene 25: 2679-2684.
2389. Weniger MA, Pulford K, Gesk S, Ehrlich S, Banham AH, Lyne L, Martin-Subero JI, Siebert R, Dyer MJ, Moller P, Barth TF (2006). Gains of the proto-oncogene BCL11A and nuclear accumulation of BCL11A(XL) protein are frequent in primary mediastinal B-cell lymphoma. Leukemia 20: 1880-1882.
2390. Went P, Agostinelli C, Gallamini A, Piccaluga PP, Ascani S, Sabattini E, Bacci F, Falini B, Motta T, Paulli M, Artusi T, Piccioli M, Zinzani PL, Pileri SA (2006). Marker expression in peripheral T-cell lymphoma: a proposed clinical-pathologic prognostic score. J Clin Oncol 24: 2472-2479.
2391. Went P, Ascani S, Strom E, Brorson SH, Musso M, Zinzani PL, Falini B, Dirnhofer S, Pileri S (2004). Nodal marginal-zone lymphoma associated with monoclonal light-chain and heavy-chain deposition disease. Lancet Oncol 5: 381-383.
2392. Went PT, Zimpfer A, Pehrs AC, Sabattini E, Pileri SA, Maurer R, Terracciano L, Tzankov A, Sauter G, Dirnhofer S (2005). High specificity of combined TRAP and DBA.44 expression for hairy cell leukemia. Am J Surg Pathol 29: 474-478.
2393. Wessendorf S, Barth TF, Viardot A, Mueller A, Kestler HA, Kohlhammer H, Lichter P, Bentz M, Dohner H, Moller P, Schwaenen C (2007). Further delineation of chromosomal consensus regions in primary mediastinal B-cell lymphomas: an analysis of 37 tumor samples using high-resolution genomic profiling (array-CGH). Leukemia 21: 2463-2469.
2394. Westwood NB, Gruszka-Westwood AM, Pearson CE, Delord CF, Green AR, Huntly BJ, Lakhani A, McMullin MF, Pearson TC (2000). The incidences of trisomy 8, trisomy 9 and D20S108 deletion in polycythaemia vera: an analysis of blood granulocytes using interphase fluorescence in situ hybridization. Br J Haematol 110: 839-846.
2394A. Whitman SP, Archer KJ, Feng L, Baldus C, Becknell B, Carlson BD, Carroll AJ, Mrózek K, Vardiman JW, George SL, Kolitz JE, Larson RA, Bloomfield CD, Caligiuri MA (2001). Absence of the wild-type allele predicts poor prognosis in adult de novo acute myeloid leukemia with normal cytogenetics and the internal tandem duplication of FLT3: a cancer and leukemia group B study. Cancer Res 61: 7233-7239
2395. Whitman SP, Ruppert AS, Marcucci G, Mrózek K, Paschka P, Langer C, Baldus CD, Wen J, Vukosavljevic T, Powell BL, Carroll AJ, Kolitz JE, Larson RA, Caligiuri MA, Bloomfield CD (2007). Long-term disease-free survivors with cytogenetically normal acute myeloid leukemia and MLL partial tandem duplication: a Cancer and Leukemia Group B study. Blood 109: 5164-5167.
2396. Whitman SP, Ruppert AS, Radmacher MD, Mrózek K, Paschka P, Langer C, Baldus CD, Wen J, Racke F, Powell BL, Kolitz JE, Larson RA, Caligiuri MA, Marcucci G, Bloomfield CD (2008). FLT3 D835/I836 mutations are associated with poor disease-free survival and a distinct gene-expression signature among younger adults with de novo cytogenetically normal acute myeloid leukemia lacking FLT3 Internal tandem duplications. Blood 111: 1552-1559.
2397. Whittaker SJ, Smith NP (1992). Diagnostic value of T-cell receptor beta gene rearrangement analysis on peripheral blood lymphocytes of patients with erythroderma. J Invest Dermatol 99: 361-362.
2398. Whittaker SJ, Smith NP, Jones RR, Luzzatto L (1991). Analysis of beta, gamma, and delta T-cell receptor genes in mycosis fungoides and Sezary syndrome. Cancer 68: 1572-1582.
2399. Wickert RS, Weisenburger DD, Tierens A, Greiner TC, Chan WC (1995). Clonal relationship between lymphocytic predominance Hodgkin's disease and concurrent or subsequent large-cell lymphoma of B lineage. Blood 86: 2312-2320.
2400. Wiemels JL, Cazzaniga G, Daniotti M, Eden OB, Addison GM, Masera G, Saha V, Biondi A, Greaves MF (1999). Prenatal origin of acute lymphoblastic leukaemia in children. Lancet 354: 1499-1503.
2401. Wiestner A, Padosch SA, Ghilardi N, Cesar JM, Odriozola J, Shapiro A, Skoda RC (2000). Hereditary thrombocythaemia is a genetically heterogeneous disorder: exclusion of TPO and MPL in two families with hereditary thrombocythaemia. Br J Haematol 110: 104-109.
2402. Wiestner A, Rosenwald A, Barry TS, Wright G, Davis RE, Henrickson SE, Zhao H, Ibbotson RE, Orchard JA, Davis Z, Stetler-Stevenson M, Raffeld M, Arthur DC, Marti GE, Wilson WH, Hamblin TJ, Oscier DG, Staudt LM (2003). ZAP-70 expression identifies a chronic lymphocytic leukemia subtype with unmutated immunoglobulin genes, inferior clinical outcome, and distinct gene expression profile. Blood 101: 4944-4951.
2403. Wilder RB, Ha CS, Cox JD, Weber D, Delasalle K, Alexanian R (2002). Persistence of myeloma protein for more than one year after radiotherapy is an adverse prognostic factor in solitary plasmacytoma of bone. Cancer 94: 1532-1537.
2404. Wilks S (1856). Cases of lardaceous disease and some allied affections, with remarks. Guy's Hosp Rep 17: 103.
2405. Wilks S (1856). Enlargement of the lymphatic glands and spleen (or, Hodgkin's disease) with remarks. Guy's Hosp Rep 11: 56.
2406. Willemse MJ, Seriu T, Hettinger K, d'Aniello E, Hop WC, Panzer-Grumayer ER, Biondi A, Schrappe M, Kamps WA, Masera G, Gadner H, Riehm H, Bartram CR, van Dongen JJ (2002). Detection of minimal residual disease identifies differences in treatment response between T-ALL and precursor B-ALL. Blood 99: 4386-4393.
2407. Willemze R, Jaffe ES, Burg G, Cerroni L, Berti E, Swerdlow SH, Ralfkiaer E, Chimenti S, Diaz-Perez JL, Duncan LM, Grange F, Harris NL, Kempf W, Kerl H, Kurrer M, Knobler R, Pimpinelli N, Sander C, Santucci M, Sterry W, Vermeer MH, Wechsler J, Whittaker S, Meijer CJ (2005). WHO-EORTC classification for cutaneous lymphomas. Blood 105: 3768-3785.
2408. Willemze R, Jansen PM, Cerroni L, Berti E, Santucci M, Assaf C, Canninga-van Dijk MR, Carlotti A, Geerts ML, Hahtola S, Hummel M, Jeskanen L, Kempf W, Massone C, Ortiz-Romero PL, Paulli M, Petrella T, Ranki A, Rodriguez Peralto JL, Robson A, Senff NJ, Vermeer MH, Wechsler J, Whittaker S, Meijer CJ (2007). Subcutaneous panniculitis-like T-cell lymphoma: definition, classification and prognostic factors. An EORTC Cutaneous Lymphoma Group study of 83 cases. Blood 111: 838-845.
2409. Willemze R, Kerl H, Sterry W, Berti E, Cerroni L, Chimenti S, Diaz-Perez JL, Geerts ML, Goos M, Knobler R, Ralfkiaer E, Santucci M, Smith N, Wechsler J, van Vloten WA, Meijer CJ (1997). EORTC classification for primary cutaneous lymphomas: a proposal from the Cutaneous Lymphoma Study Group of the European Organization for Research and Treatment of Cancer. Blood 90: 354-371.
2410. Williams ME, Swerdlow SH, Rosenberg CL, Arnold A (1993). Chromosome 11 translocation breakpoints at the PRAD1/cyclin D1 gene locus in centrocytic lymphoma. Leukemia 7: 241-245.
2411. Williams ME, Westermann CD, Swerdlow SH (1990). Genotypic characterization of centrocytic lymphoma: frequent rearrangement of the chromosome 11 bcl-1 locus. Blood 76: 1387-1391.
2412. Williams ME, Whitefield M, Swerdlow SH (1997). Analysis of the cyclin-dependent kinase inhibitors p18 and p19 in mantle-cell lymphoma and chronic lymphocytic leukemia. Ann Oncol 8 Suppl 2: 71-73.
2413. Williams ME, Woytowitz D, Finkelstein SD, Swerdlow SH (1995). MTS1/MTS2 (p15/p16) deletions and p53 mutations in mantle cell (centrocytic) lymphoma. Blood 86: 747a-

2414. Williamson PJ, Kruger AR, Reynolds PJ, Hamblin TJ, Oscier DG (1994). Establishing the incidence of myelodysplastic syndrome. Br J Haematol 87: 743-745.
2415. Willis MS, McKenna RW, Peterson LC, Coad JE, Kroft SH (2005). Low blast count myeloid disorders with Auer rods: a clinicopathologic analysis of 9 cases. Am J Clin Pathol 124: 191-198.
2416. Willis TG, Jadayel DM, Du MQ, Peng H, Perry AR, Abdul-Rauf M, Price H, Karran L, Majekodunmi O, Wlodarska I, Pan L, Crook T, Hamoudi R, Isaacson PG, Dyer MJ (1999). Bcl10 is involved in t(1;14)(p22;q32) of MALT B cell lymphoma and mutated in multiple tumor types. Cell 96: 35-45.
2417. Willman CL (1998). Molecular genetic features of myelodysplastic syndromes (MDS). Leukemia 12 Suppl 1: S2-S6.
2418. Willman CL, Busque L, Griffith BB, Favara BE, McClain KL, Duncan MH, Gilliland DG (1994). Langerhans'-cell histiocytosis (histiocytosis X)—a clonal proliferative disease. N Engl J Med 331: 154-160.
2419. Wilson MS, Weiss LM, Gatter KC, Mason DY, Dorfman RF, Warnke RA (1990). Malignant histiocytosis. A reassessment of cases previously reported in 1975 based on paraffin section immunophenotyping studies. Cancer 66: 530-536.
2420. Wilson WH, Kingma DW, Raffeld M, Wittes RE, Jaffe ES (1996). Association of lymphomatoid granulomatosis with Epstein-Barr viral infection of B lymphocytes and response to interferon-alpha 2b. Blood 87: 4531-4537.
2421. Wilson WH, Teruya-Feldstein J, Fest T, Harris C, Steinberg SM, Jaffe ES, Raffeld M (1997). Relationship of p53, bcl-2, and tumor proliferation to clinical drug resistance in non-Hodgkin's lymphomas. Blood 89: 601-609.
2422. Wimazal F, Fonatsch C, Thalhammer R, Schwarzinger I, Mullauer L, Sperr WR, Bennett JM, Valent P (2007). Idiopathic cytopenia of undetermined significance (ICUS) versus low risk MDS: The diagnostic interface. Leuk Res 31: 1461-1468.
2423. Winter JN, Weller EA, Horning SJ, Krajewska M, Variakojis D, Habermann TM, Fisher RI, Kurtin PJ, Macon WR, Chhanabhai M, Felgar RE, Hsi ED, Medeiros LJ, Weick JK, Reed JC, Gascoyne RD (2006). Prognostic significance of Bcl-6 protein expression in DLBCL treated with CHOP or R-CHOP: a prospective correlative study. Blood 107: 4207-4213.
2424. Witkiewicz A, Raghunath P, Wasik A, Junkins-Hopkins JM, Jones D, Zhang Q, Odum N, Wasik MA (2007). Loss of SHP-1 tyrosine phosphatase expression correlates with the advanced stages of cutaneous T-cell lymphoma. Hum Pathol 38: 462-467.
2425. Wlodarska I, Martin-Garcia N, Achten R, Wolf-Peeters C, Pauwels P, Tulliez M, de Mascarel A, Briere J, Patey M, Hagemeijer A, Gaulard P (2002). Fluorescence in situ hybridization study of chromosome 7 aberrations in hepatosplenic T-cell lymphoma: isochromosome 7q as a common abnormality accumulating in forms with features of cytologic progression. Genes Chromosomes Cancer 33: 243-251.
2426. Wlodarska I, Stul M, Wolf-Peeters C, Hagemeijer A (2004). Heterogeneity of BCL6 rearrangements in nodular lymphocyte predominant Hodgkin's lymphoma. Haematologica 89: 965-972.
2427. Wlodarska I, Wolf-Peeters C, Falini B, Verhoef G, Morris SW, Hagemeijer A, Van den BH (1998). The cryptic inv(2)(p23q35) defines a new molecular genetic subtype of ALK-positive anaplastic large-cell lymphoma. Blood 92: 2688-2695.
2428. Wlodarski MW, O'Keefe C, Howe EC, Risitano AM, Rodriguez A, Warshawsky I, Loughran TP, Jr., Maciejewski JP (2005). Pathologic clonal cytotoxic T-cell responses: nonrandom nature of the T-cell-receptor restriction in large granular lymphocyte leukemia. Blood 106: 2769-2780.
2429. Wohrer S, Streubel B, Bartsch R, Chott A, Raderer M (2004). Monoclonal immunoglobulin production is a frequent event in patients with mucosa-associated lymphoid tissue lymphoma. Clin Cancer Res 10: 7179-7181.
2430. Wolanskyj AP, Schwager SM, McClure RF, Larson DR, Tefferi A (2006). Essential thrombocythemia beyond the first decade: life expectancy, long-term complication rates, and prognostic factors. Mayo Clin Proc 81: 159-166.
2431. Wolf-Peeters C, Achten R (2000). Anaplastic large cell lymphoma: what's in a name? J Clin Pathol 53: 407-408.
2432. Wolf-Peeters C, Achten R (2000). gammadelta T-cell lymphomas: a homogeneous entity? Histopathology 36: 294-305.
2433. Wolf BC, Kumar A, Vera JC, Neiman RS (1986). Bone marrow morphology and immunology in systemic amyloidosis. Am J Clin Pathol 86: 84-88.
2434. Wolf T, Brodt HR, Fichtlscherer S, Mantzsch K, Hoelzer D, Helm EB, Mitrou PS, Chow KU (2005). Changing incidence and prognostic factors of survival in AIDS-related non-Hodgkin's lymphoma in the era of highly active antiretroviral therapy (HAART). Leuk Lymphoma 46: 207-215.
2435. Wolfe F, Michaud K (2007). The effect of methotrexate and anti-tumor necrosis factor therapy on the risk of lymphoma in rheumatoid arthritis in 19,562 patients during 89,710 person-years of observation. Arthritis Rheum 56: 1433-1439.
2436. Wolff K, Komar M, Petzelbauer P (2001). Clinical and histopathological aspects of cutaneous mastocytosis. Leuk Res 25: 519-528.
2437. Wong KF, Chan JK, Cheung MM, So JC (2001). Bone marrow involvement by nasal NK cell lymphoma at diagnosis is uncommon. Am J Clin Pathol 115: 266-270.
2438. Wong KF, Chan JK, Ng CS, Lee KC, Tsang WY, Cheung MM (1992). CD56 (NKH1)-positive hematolymphoid malignancies: an aggressive neoplasm featuring frequent cutaneous/mucosal involvement, cytoplasmic azurophilic granules, and angiocentricity. Hum Pathol 23: 798-804.
2439. Wong KF, So CC, Chan JK (2002). Nucleolated variant of mantle cell lymphoma with leukemic manifestations mimicking prolymphocytic leukemia. Am J Clin Pathol 117: 246-251.
2440. Wong KF, Zhang YM, Chan JK (1999). Cytogenetic abnormalities in natural killer cell lymphoma/leukaemia—is there a consistent pattern? Leuk Lymphoma 34: 241-250.
2441. Wood GS, Hu CH, Beckstead JH, Turner RR, Winkelmann RK (1985). The indeterminate cell proliferative disorder: report of a case manifesting as an unusual cutaneous histiocytosis. J Dermatol Surg Oncol 11: 1111-1119.
2442. Woodlock TJ, Seshi B, Sham RL, Cyran EM, Bennett JM (1994). Use of cell surface antigen phenotype in guiding therapeutic decisions in chronic myelomonocytic leukemia. Leuk Res 18: 173-181.
2443. Worsley A, Oscier DG, Stevens J, Darlow S, Figes A, Mufti GJ, Hamblin TJ (1988). Prognostic features of chronic myelomonocytic leukaemia: a modified Bournemouth score gives the best prediction of survival. Br J Haematol 68: 17-21.
2444. Wotherspoon AC, Doglioni C, Diss TC, Pan L, Moschini A, de Boni M, Isaacson PG (1993). Regression of primary low-grade B-cell gastric lymphoma of mucosa-associated lymphoid tissue type after eradication of Helicobacter pylori. Lancet 342: 575-577.
2445. Wotherspoon AC, Ortiz-Hidalgo C, Falzon MR, Isaacson PG (1991). Helicobacter pylori-associated gastritis and primary B-cell gastric lymphoma. Lancet 338: 1175-1176.
2446. Wotherspoon AC, Soosay GN, Diss TC, Isaacson PG (1990). Low-grade primary B-cell lymphoma of the lung. An immunohistochemical, molecular, and cytogenetic study of a single case. Am J Clin Pathol 94: 655-660.
2447. Wright DH (1971). Burkitt's lymphoma: a review of the pathology, immunology and possible aetiological factors. Pathology annual. In: SC Sommers. Pathology annual., ed. Appleton-Century-Crofts: New York, pp. 337-363.
2448. Wright DH (1997). Enteropathy associated T cell lymphoma. Cancer Surv 30: 249-261.
2449. Wright G, Tan B, Rosenwald A, Hurt EH, Wiestner A, Staudt LM (2003). A gene expression-based method to diagnose clinically distinct subgroups of diffuse large B cell lymphoma. Proc Natl Acad Sci U S A 100: 9991-9996.
2450. Wu CD, Wickert RS, Williamson JE, Sun NC, Brynes RK, Chan WC (1999). Using fluorescence-based human androgen receptor gene assay to analyze the clonality of microdissected dendritic cell tumors. Am J Clin Pathol 111: 105-110.
2451. Wu H, Wasik MA, Przybylski G, Finan J, Haynes B, Moore H, Leonard DG, Montone KT, Naji A, Nowell PC, Kamoun M, Tomaszewski JE, Salhany KE (2000). Hepatosplenic gamma-delta T-cell lymphoma as a late-onset posttransplant lymphoproliferative disorder in renal transplant recipients. Am J Clin Pathol 113: 487-496.
2452. Wu SS, Brady K, Anderson JJ, Vezina R, Skinner M, Neiman RS, Wolf BC (1991). The predictive value of bone marrow morphologic characteristics and immunostaining in primary (AL) amyloidosis. Am J Clin Pathol 96: 95-99.
2453. Wu TT, Swerdlow SH, Locker J, Bahler D, Randhawa P, Yunis EJ, Dickman PS, Nalesnik MA (1996). Recurrent Epstein-Barr virus-associated lesions in organ transplant recipients. Hum Pathol 27: 157-164.
2454. Wu Y, Slovak ML, Snyder DS, Arber DA (2006). Coexistence of inversion 16 and the Philadelphia chromosome in acute and chronic myeloid leukemias : report of six cases and review of literature. Am J Clin Pathol 125: 260-266.
2455. Wu YH, Chen HC, Hsiao PF, Tu MI, Lin YC, Wang TY (2007). Hydroa vacciniforme-like Epstein-Barr virus-associated monoclonal T-lymphoproliferative disorder in a child. Int J Dermatol 46: 1081-1086.
2456. Wuchter C, Harbott J, Schoch C, Schnittger S, Borkhardt A, Karawajew L, Ratei R, Ruppert V, Haferlach T, Creutzig U, Dorken B, Ludwig WD (2000). Detection of acute leukemia cells with mixed lineage leukemia (MLL) gene rearrangements by flow cytometry using monoclonal antibody 7.1. Leukemia 14: 1232-1238.
2457. Wundisch T, Neubauer A, Stolte M, Ritter M, Thiede C (2003). B-cell monoclonality is associated with lymphoid follicles in gastritis. Am J Surg Pathol 27: 882-887.
2458. Xu Y, Dolan MM, Nguyen PL (2003). Diagnostic significance of detecting dysgranulopoiesis in chronic myeloid leukemia. Am J Clin Pathol 120: 778-784.
2459. Xu Y, McKenna RW, Karandikar NJ, Pildain AJ, Kroft SH (2005). Flow cytometric analysis of monocytes as a tool for distinguishing chronic myelomonocytic leukemia from reactive monocytosis. Am J Clin Pathol 124: 799-806.
2460. Ya-In C, Brandwein J, Pantalony D, Chang H (2005). Hairy cell leukemia variant with features of intrasinusoidal bone marrow involvement. Arch Pathol Lab Med 129: 395-398.
2461. Yam LT, Yam CF, Li CY (1980). Eosinophilia in systemic mastocytosis. Am J Clin Pathol 73: 48-54.
2462. Yamaguchi K (1994). Human T-lymphotropic virus type I in Japan. Lancet 343: 213-216.
2463. Yamaguchi M, Seto M, Okamoto M, Ichinohasama R, Nakamura N, Yoshino T, Suzumiya J, Murase T, Miura I, Akasaka T, Tamaru J, Suzuki R, Kagami Y, Hirano M, Morishima Y, Ueda R, Shiku H, Nakamura S (2002). De novo CD5+ diffuse large B-cell lymphoma: a clinicopathologic study of 109 patients. Blood 99: 815-821.
2463A. Yamamoto JF, Goodman MT (2008). Patterns of leukemia incidence in the United States by subtype and demographic characteristics, 1997-2002. Cancer Causes Control 19: 379-390.
2464. Yamamura M, Yamada Y, Momita S, Kamihira S, Tomonaga M (1998). Circulating interleukin-6 levels are elevated in adult T-cell leukaemia/lymphoma patients and correlate with adverse clinical features and survival. Br J Haematol 100: 129-134.
2465. Yanada M, Suzuki M, Kawashima K, Kiyoi H, Kinoshita T, Emi N, Saito H, Naoe T (2005). Long-term outcomes for unselected patients with acute myeloid leukemia categorized according to the World Health Organization classification: a single-center experience. Eur J Haematol 74: 418-423.
2466. Yanagisawa K, Ohminami H, Sato M, Takada K, Hasegawa H, Yasukawa M, Fujita S (1998). Neoplastic involvement of granulocytic lineage, not granulocytic-monocytic, monocytic, or erythrocytic lineage, in a patient with chronic neutrophilic leukemia. Am J Hematol 57: 221-224.
2467. Yang WI, Zukerberg LR, Motokura T, Arnold A, Harris NL (1994). Cyclin D1 (Bcl-1, PRAD1) protein expression in low-grade B-cell lymphomas and reactive hyperplasia. Am J Pathol 145: 86-96.
2468. Yano T, Sander CA, Clark HM, Dolezal MV, Jaffe ES, Raffeld M (1993). Clustered mutations in the second exon of the MYC gene in sporadic Burkitt's lymphoma. Oncogene 8: 2741-2748.
2468A Yano T, Jaffe ES, Longo DL, Raffeld M. MYC rearrangements in histologically progressed follicular lymphomas. Blood 1992; 80:758-767.
2469. Yeoh EJ, Ross ME, Shurtleff SA, Williams WK, Patel D, Mahfouz R, Behm FG, Raimondi SC, Relling MV, Patel A, Cheng C, Campana D, Wilkins D, Zhou X, Li J, Liu H, Pui CH, Evans WE, Naeve C, Wong L, Downing JR (2002). Classification, subtype discovery, and prediction of outcome in pediatric acute lymphoblastic leukemia by gene expression profiling. Cancer Cell 1: 133-143.
2470. Yin CC, Medeiros LJ, Cromwell CC, Mehta AP, Lin P, Luthra R, Abruzzo LV (2007). Sequence analysis proves clonal identity in five patients with typical and blastoid mantle cell lymphoma. Mod Pathol 20: 1-7.
2471. Yoshimi A, Baumann I, Fuhrer M, Bergstrasser E, Gobel U, Sykora KW, Klingebiel T, Gross-Wieltsch U, van den Heuvel-Eibrink MM, Fischer A, Nollke P, Niemeyer C (2007). Immunosuppressive therapy with anti-thymocyte globulin and cyclosporine A in selected children with hypoplastic refractory cytopenia. Haematologica 92: 397-400.
2472. Yoshino T, Miyake K, Ichimura K,

2472. Mannami T, Ohara N, Hamazaki S, Akagi T (2000). Increased incidence of follicular lymphoma in the duodenum. Am J Surg Pathol 24: 688-693.

2473. Yoshino T, Nakamura S, Matsuno Y, Ochiai A, Yokoi T, Kitadai Y, Suzumiya J, Tobinai K, Kobayashi Y, Oda I, Mera K, Ohtsu A, Ishikura S (2006). Epstein-Barr virus involvement is a predictive factor for the resistance to chemoradiotherapy of gastric diffuse large B-cell lymphoma. Cancer Sci 97: 163-166.

2474. You W, Weisbrot IM (1979). Chronic neutrophilic leukemia. Report of two cases and review of the literature. Am J Clin Pathol 72: 233-242.

2475. Young KH, Chan WC, Fu K, Iqbal J, Sanger WG, Ratashak A, Greiner TC, Weisenburger DD (2006). Mantle cell lymphoma with plasma cell differentiation. Am J Surg Pathol 30: 954-961.

2476. Young KH, Weisenburger DD, Dave BJ, Smith L, Sanger W, Iqbal J, Campo E, Delabie J, Gascoyne RD, Ott G, Rimsza L, Muller-Hermelink HK, Jaffe ES, Rosenwald A, Staudt LM, Chan WC, Greiner TC (2007). Mutations in the DNA-binding codons of TP53, which are associated with decreased expression of TRAILreceptor-2, predict for poor survival in diffuse large B-cell lymphoma. Blood 110: 4396-4405.

2477. Young NS (2006). Pathophysiologic mechanisms in acquired aplastic anemia. Hematology Am Soc Hematol Educ Program: 72-77.

2478. Young NS, Calado RT, Scheinberg P (2006). Current concepts in the pathophysiology and treatment of aplastic anemia. Blood 108: 2509-2519.

2479. Yousem SA, Colby TV, Chen YY, Chen WG, Weiss LM (2001). Pulmonary Langerhans' cell histiocytosis: molecular analysis of clonality. Am J Surg Pathol 25: 630-636.

2480. Yu RC, Chu C, Buluwela L, Chu AC (1994). Clonal proliferation of Langerhans cells in Langerhans cell histiocytosis. Lancet 343: 767-768.

2481. Yunis JJ, Mayer MG, Arnesen MA, Aeppli DP, Oken MM, Frizzera G (1989). bcl-2 and other genomic alterations in the prognosis of large-cell lymphoma. N Engl J Med 320: 1047-1054.

2482. Zambello R, Falco M, Della CM, Trentin L, Carollo D, Castriconi R, Cannas G, Carlomagno S, Cabrelle A, Lamy T, Agostini C, Moretta A, Semenzato G, Vitale M (2003). Expression and function of KIR and natural cytotoxicity receptors in NK-type lymphoproliferative diseases of granular lymphocytes. Blood 102: 1797-1805.

2483. Zambello R, Loughran TP, Jr., Trentin L, Pontisso P, Battistella L, Raimondi R, Facco M, Sancetta R, Agostini C, Pizzolo G (1995). Serologic and molecular evidence for a possible pathogenetic role of viral infection in CD3-negative natural killer-type lymphoproliferative disease of granular lymphocytes. Leukemia 9: 1207-1211.

2484. Zambello R, Loughran TP, Jr., Trentin L, Rassu M, Facco M, Bortolin M, Nash R, Agostini C, Semenzato G (1997). Spontaneous resolution of p58/EB6 antigen restricted NK-type lymphoproliferative disease of granular lymphocytes: role of Epstein Barr virus infection. Br J Haematol 99: 215-221.

2485. Zambello R, Trentin L, Ciccone E, Bulian P, Agostini C, Moretta A, Moretta L, Semenzato G (1993). Phenotypic diversity of natural killer (NK) populations in patients with NK-type lymphoproliferative disease of granular lymphocytes. Blood 81: 2381-2385.

2486. Zangwill SD, Hsu DT, Kichuk MR, Garvin JH, Stolar CJ, Haddad J, Jr., Stylianos S, Michler RE, Chadburn A, Knowles DM, Addonizio LJ (1998). Incidence and outcome of primary Epstein-Barr virus infection and lymphoproliferative disease in pediatric heart transplant recipients. J Heart Lung Transplant 17: 1161-1166.

2487. Zarate-Osorno A, Medeiros LJ, Longo DL, Jaffe ES (1992). Non-Hodgkin's lymphomas arising in patients successfully treated for Hodgkin's disease. A clinical, histologic, and immunophenotypic study of 14 cases. Am J Surg Pathol 16: 885-895.

2487A. Zelenetz AD (2206) Mantle cell lymphoma: an update on management. Ann Oncol 17: iv12-14.

2488. Zelent A, Guidez F, Melnick A, Waxman S, Licht JD (2001). Translocations of the RARalpha gene in acute promyelocytic leukemia. Oncogene 20: 7186-7203.

2488A. Zelger B, Cerio R, Orchard G, Wilson-Jones E (1994). Juvenile and adult xanthogranuloma. A histological and immunohistochemical comparison. Am J Surg Pathol 18:126-135.

2489. Zeller B, Gustafsson G, Forestier E, Abrahamsson J, Clausen N, Heldrup J, Hovi L, Jonmundsson G, Lie SO, Glomstein A, Hasle H (2005). Acute leukaemia in children with Down syndrome: a population-based Nordic study. Br J Haematol 128: 797-804.

2490. Zettl A, Lee SS, Rudiger T, Starostik P, Marino M, Kirchner T, Ott M, Muller-Hermelink HK, Ott G (2002). Epstein-Barr virus-associated B-cell lymphoproliferative disorders in angioimmunoblastic T-cell lymphoma and peripheral T-cell lymphoma, unspecified. Am J Clin Pathol 117: 368-379.

2491. Zettl A, Ott G, Makulik A, Katzenberger T, Starostik P, Eichler T, Puppe B, Bentz M, Muller-Hermelink HK, Chott A (2002). Chromosomal gains at 9q characterize enteropathy-type T-cell lymphoma. Am J Pathol 161: 1635-1645.

2492. Zettl A, Rudiger T, Konrad MA, Chott A, Simonitsch-Klupp I, Sonnen R, Muller-Hermelink HK, Ott G (2004). Genomic profiling of peripheral T-cell lymphoma, unspecified, and anaplastic large T-cell lymphoma delineates novel recurrent chromosomal alterations. Am J Pathol 164: 1837-1848.

2493. Zettl A, Rudiger T, Marx A, Muller-Hermelink HK, Ott G (2005). Composite marginal zone B-cell lymphoma and classical Hodgkin's lymphoma: a clinicopathological study of 12 cases. Histopathology 46: 217-228.

2494. Zettl A, Rudiger T, Muller-Hermelink HK (2007). [Enteropathy type T-cell lymphomas: pathology and pathogenesis.]. Pathologe 28: 59-64.

2495. Zhan F, Huang Y, Colla S, Stewart JP, Hanamura I, Gupta S, Epstein J, Yaccoby S, Sawyer J, Burington B, Anaissie E, Hollmig K, Pineda-Roman M, Tricot G, van Rhee F, Walker R, Zangari M, Crowley J, Barlogie B, Shaughnessy JD, Jr. (2006). The molecular classification of multiple myeloma. Blood 108: 2020-2028.

2496. Zhang A, Ohshima K, Sato K, Kanda M, Suzumiya J, Shimazaki K, Kawasaki C, Kikuchi M (1999). Prognostic clinicopathologic factors, including immunologic expression in diffuse large B-cell lymphomas. Pathol Int 49: 1043-1052.

2496A. Zhang Y, Sanjose SD, Bracci PM, Morton LM, Wang R, Brennan P, Hartge P, Boffetta P, Becker N, Maynadie M, Foretova L, Cocco P, Staines A, Holford T, Holly EA, Nieters A, Benavente Y, Bernstein L, Zahm SH, Zheng T (2008). Personal use of hair dye and the risk of certain subtypes of non-Hodgkin lymphoma. Am J Epidemiol 167: 1321-1331.

2497. Zhu D, Oscier DG, Stevenson FK (1995). Splenic lymphoma with villous lymphocytes involves B cells with extensively mutated Ig heavy chain variable region genes. Blood 85: 1603-1607.

2498. Zhu YM, Zhao WL, Fu JF, Shi JY, Pan Q, Hu J, Gao XD, Chen B, Li JM, Xiong SM, Gu LJ, Tang JY, Liang H, Jiang H, Xue YQ, Shen ZX, Chen Z, Chen SJ (2006). NOTCH1 mutations in T-cell acute lymphoblastic leukemia: prognostic significance and implication in multifactorial leukemogenesis. Clin Cancer Res 12: 3043-3049.

2499. Zinzani PL, Bendandi M, Martelli M, Falini B, Sabattini E, Amadori S, Gherlinzoni F, Martelli MF, Mandelli F, Tura S, Pileri SA (1996). Anaplastic large-cell lymphoma: clinical and prognostic evaluation of 90 adult patients. J Clin Oncol 14: 955-962.

2500. Zinzani PL, Martelli M, Bertini M, Gianni AM, Devizzi L, Federico M, Pangalis G, Michels J, Zucca E, Cantonetti M, Cortelazzo S, Wotherspoon A, Ferreri AJ, Zaja F, Lauria F, De Renzo A, Liberati MA, Falini B, Balzarotti M, Calderoni A, Zaccaria A, Gentilini P, Fattori PP, Pavone E, Angelopoulou MK, Alinari L, Brugiatelli M, Di Renzo N, Bonifazi F, Pileri SA, Cavalli F (2002). Induction chemotherapy strategies for primary mediastinal large B-cell lymphoma with sclerosis: a retrospective multinational study on 426 previously untreated patients. Haematologica 87: 1258-1264.

2501. Zinzani PL, Martelli M, Magagnoli M, Zaccaria A, Ronconi F, Cantonetti M, Bocchia M, Marra R, Gobbi M, Falini B, Gherlinzoni F, Moretti L, De Renzo A, Mazza P, Pavone E, Sabattini E, Amendola A, Bendandi M, Pileri SA, Mandelli F, Tura S (1998). Anaplastic large cell lymphoma Hodgkin's-like: a randomized trial of ABVD versus MACOP-B with and without radiation therapy. Blood 92: 790-794.

2502. Zinzani PL, Quaglino P, Pimpinelli N, Berti E, Baliva G, Rupoli S, Martelli M, Alaibac M, Borroni G, Chimenti S, Alterini R, Alinari L, Fierro MT, Cappello N, Pileri A, Soligo D, Paulli M, Pileri S, Santucci M, Bernengo MG (2006). Prognostic factors in primary cutaneous B-cell lymphoma: the Italian Study Group for Cutaneous Lymphomas. J Clin Oncol 24: 1376-1382.

2503. Zipursky A, Brown EJ, Christensen H, Doyle J (1999). Transient myeloproliferative disorder (transient leukemia) and hematologic manifestations of Down syndrome. Clin Lab Med 19: 157-67, vii.

2504. Zittoun R, Rea D, Ngoc LH, Ramond S (1994). Chronic neutrophilic leukemia. A study of four cases. Ann Hematol 68: 55-60.

2505. Zu Y, Steinberg SM, Campo E, Hans CP, Weisenburger DD, Braziel RM, Delabie J, Gascoyne RD, Muller-Hermelink HK, Pittaluga S, Raffeld M, Chan WC, Jaffe ES (2005). Validation of tissue microarray immunohistochemistry staining and interpretation in diffuse large B-cell lymphoma. Leuk Lymphoma 46: 693-701.

2506. Zuckerman E, Zuckerman T, Levine AM, Douer D, Gutekunst K, Mizokami M, Qian DG, Velankar M, Nathwani BN, Fong TL (1997). Hepatitis C virus infection in patients with B-cell non-Hodgkin lymphoma. Ann Intern Med 127: 423-428.

2507. Zukerberg LR, Collins AB, Ferry JA, Harris NL (1991). Coexpression of CD15 and CD20 by Reed-Sternberg cells in Hodgkin's disease. Am J Pathol 139: 475-483.

2508. Zukerberg LR, Medeiros LJ, Ferry JA, Harris NL (1993). Diffuse low-grade B-cell lymphomas. Four clinically distinct subtypes defined by a combination of morphologic and immunophenotypic features. Am J Clin Pathol 100: 373-385.

2509. Zukerberg LR, Yang WI, Arnold A, Harris NL (1995). Cyclin D1 expression in non-Hodgkin's lymphomas. Detection by immunohistochemistry. Am J Clin Pathol 103: 756-760.

2510. Zutter MM, Martin PJ, Sale GE, Shulman HM, Fisher L, Thomas ED, Durnam DM (1988). Epstein-Barr virus lymphoproliferation after bone marrow transplantation. Blood 72: 520-529.

2510A. Zvulunov A, Barak Y, Metzker A (1995). Juvenile xanthogranuloma, neurofibromatosis, and juvenile chronic myelogenous leukemia. World statistical analysis. Arch Dermatol 131: 904-908.

Subject Index

α naphthyl acetate esterase, 21, 78, 83

α naphthyl butyrate esterase, 21, 78

Amegakaryocytic thrombocytopenia, 106, 107

AML, *see* Acute myeloid leukaemia

AML (megakaryoblastic) with t(1;22)(p13;q13), 29, 30

AML with balanced translocations/ inversions, 110

AML with cytoplasmic nucleophosmin, 120

AML with inv(3)(q21q26.2), 29, 30, *116-117*, 125

AML with t(15;17)(q22;q12), 112

AML1, 36, 104, 111, 131, 170, 172

AMM, 44

Amyloidoma, 210

Amyloidosis, primary, 200, *209-211*

Anaplastic large cell lymphoma, 162, 163, 234, 255, 289, 290, 294, 301, 306, *312-319*, 328, 349, 355

Anaplastic large cell lymphoma, ALK-negative, *317-319*

Anaplastic large cell lymphoma, ALK-positive, *312-316*

Anaplastic large cell lymphoma, "common pattern", 312, 313

Anaplastic large cell lymphoma, "composite pattern", 313

Anaplastic large cell lymphoma, "Hodgkin-like pattern", 313

Anaplastic large cell lymphoma, hypo-cellular, 313, 315

Anaplastic large cell lymphoma, "lymphohistiocytic pattern", 313

Anaplastic large cell lymphoma, "small cell pattern", 313

Anaplastic large cell lymphoma, primary cutaneous, *300-301*

Anaplastic lymphoma kinase, *see* ALK

Annexin A1, 192, 193

Angiocentric immunoproliferative lesion, 285

Angiocentric T-cell lymphoma, 285

Angioimmunoblastic T-cell lymphoma, 162, 163, 166, 177, 196, 283, 307, 308, *309-311*, 351

Angiolymphoid hyperplasia, 52

Angiotropic large cell lymphoma, 252

Anisopoikilocytosis, 45, 100, 105, 138, 143

Ann Arbor staging system, 322

Ann Arbor staging system, Cotswald revision, 322

Annexin A1 (ANXA1), 160, 186, 189, 190

API2/MALT1, 163

Aplastic anaemia in childhood, 106

Arsenic trioxide, 114, 117

Artemis, 339

Asymptomatic (smoldering) plasma cell myeloma, 202

Ataxia-telangiectasia, 271, 336, 339

ATM (ataxia telangiectasia mutated), 182, 231, 271, 336, 338, 339

ATRA, 30, 113, 114

Atypical chronic myeloid leukaemia, 26, 38, 52, 71, 85

Atypical chronic myeloid leukaemia, BCR-ABL1 negative, *80-81*

Auer rods, 78, 83, 89, 91, 92, 97, 100, 101, 110, 112-115, 130-133, 135

Autoimmune lymphoproliferative syndrome, 165, 336, 339

B

B acute lymphoblastic leukaemia, 150, *168-170*

B lymphoblastic leukaemia, 26, 165, 168

B lymphoblastic leukaemia/lymphoblastic lymphoma, not otherwise specified, *168-170*

B Lymphoblastic leukaemia/lymphoma with hyperdiploidy, *173-174*

B Lymphoblastic leukaemia/lymphoma with hypodiploidy, *174*

B Lymphoblastic leukaemia/lymphoma with recurrent genetic abnormalities, *171-175*

B Lymphoblastic leukaemia/ lymphoma with t(1;19) (q23;p13.3); E2A-PBX1 (TCF3-PBX1), *175*

B Lymphoblastic leukaemia/lymphoma with t(5;14)(q31;q32); IL3-IGH, *174-175*

B Lymphoblastic leukaemia/lymphoma with t(9;22)(q34;q11.2); BCR-ABL1, *171*

B Lymphoblastic leukaemia/lymphoma with t(12;21) (p13;q22); TEL-AML1 (ETV6-RUNX1), *172-173*

B Lymphoblastic leukaemia/lymphoma with t(v;11q23); MLL rearranged, *171-172*

Basic leucine zipper factor, 281

B-cell lymphoma, unclassifiable, with features intermediate between DLBCL and Burkitt lymphoma, 234, *265-266*

B-cell lymphoma, unclassifiable, with features intermediate between DLBCL and classical Hodgkin lymphoma, 234, *267-268*

B-cell prolymphocytic leukaemia, 181, *183-184*

Basket cells, 181

BCL2, 14, 15, 159, 160, 163, 186, 195, 219, 223-227, 231, 235, 236, 238, 241, 242, 250, 251, 264-266, 315

BCL6, 159, 160, 162, 163, 186, 219, 223, 224, 227, 231, 235-237, 241, 242, 244, 250, 251, 261, 264-266, 307, 315, 316, 324, 325, 340, 347, 348

BCL10, 195, 217

BCR, 15, 23-27, 32, 35, 36, 38, 39, 43, 44, 47, 48, 50-53, 64, 65, 69-71, 73, 76, 79-82, 84-86, 138, 151, 152, 171, 180, 182, 237, 251

BCR-ABL1, 15, 24-27, 32, 35, 36, 38, 39, 43, 44, 47, 48, 50-53, 64, 65, 69-71, 76, 79-86, 138, 151, 152, 171

BDCA-2/CD303, 146

Bence Jones protein, 197, 205

Benign cephalic histiocytosis, 366

Benign monoclonal gammopathy, 200

ßF1, 287, 304

Bilineal leukaemia, 150

Biphenotypic leukaemia, 150, 151, 154

Birbeck granule, 357, 358, 360, 362, 364, 365

Blast phase, 23, 24, 30, 32, 65, 112, 117, 138, 151, 152

Blastic natural killer leukaemia/lymphoma, 145

Blastic NK-cell lymphoma, 145

Blastic plasmacytoid dendritic cell neoplasm, 29, 15, 141, *145-147*

Blastoid mantle cell lymphoma, 229, 233

BMI1, 231

BOB.1, 251, 267, 324, 326, 328

Body cavity based lymphoma, 260

Borrelia burgdorferi, 166, 214

Budd-Chiari syndrome, 41, 48

Bullous mastocytosis, 55

Burkitt leukaemia variant, 263

Burkitt leukaemia/lymphoma, 168

Burkitt lymphoma, 141, 160, 163, 165, 166, 176, 233, 235, *262-264*, 266, 337-340, 343, 348, 351

Burkitt-like lymphoma, 265, 266

C

C/EBPβ, 315, 316

CAE, 21, 57, 79, 130, 132, 134-136, 138, 140

CALM-AF10, 178

Campylobacter jejuni, 166, 198, 214

Canale-Smith syndrome, 339

Carcinoma showing thymus-like element (CASTLE), 364

Castleman disease, 213, 258, 309, 355, 363

CBFA, 111, 112

CBFB, 28, 29, 111, 112

CBFB-MYH11, 29, 111, 112

CCAAT/enhancer binding protein, 118

cCD22, 131, 151

cCD79a, 131, 151

CCND1, 14, 186, 195, 206, 229, 231

CCND3, 206

CD1a, 161, 177, 270, 355, 357, 358, 362, 364-366

CD2, 56, 57, 62, 70, 72, 79, 112, 113, 131, 132, 146, 154, 161, 163, 177, 246, 270, 274, 277, 279, 283, 287, 297, 299, 300, 303, 304, 310, 315, 318, 326

CD3, 23, 146, 150, 154, 158, 161-163, 177, 224, 238, 246, 248, 254, 267, 270, 271, 273, 274, 277, 279, 283, 287, 290, 293, 294, 297, 299-301, 303, 304, 306, 308, 310, 314, 318, 324, 326, 338, 343, 364

CD4, 79, 112, 114, 131-134, 140, 142, 144, 146, 161-163, 177, 224, 246, 248, 255, 262, 267, 270-273, 279, 280, 283, 287, 290, 293, 294, 297, 298, 300, 301, 303-308, 310, 311, 315, 318, 324, 325, 336-338, 340, 349, 355, 357, 360, 365

CD4 positive, primary cutaneous small/ medium T-cell lymphoma, *304-305*

CD5, 79, 146, 154, 158, 160-163, 177, 180, 181, 183, 186, 189, 192, 195, 197, 216, 217, 219, 223, 227, 231, 234-236, 238, 253, 273, 274, 283, 287, 290, 293, 297, 299, 300, 303, 304, 306-308, 310, 315, 318, 338

CD7, 23, 101, 116, 122, 125, 128, 131-134, 137, 142, 144, 146, 154, 161, 163, 177, 246, 270, 271, 273, 274, 283, 287, 290, 297, 299, 303, 304, 306-308

CD8, 161-163, 177, 237, 248, 270, 271, 273, 274, 278, 280, 283, 287, 289-291, 293-295, 297, 298, 300, 301, 303, 304, 306-308, 310, 315, 318, 324, 325, 336-338, 349

CD8 positive cytotoxic T-cell lymphoma, rimary cutaneous aggressive epidermotropic, *303-304*

CD9, 23, 61, 138, 173, 175

CD10, 150-152, 159, 160, 162-164, 169, 171, 174, 181, 186, 189, 192, 195, 197, 205, 216, 217, 219, 223, 225, 227, 231, 235, 236, 241, 242, 244, 250, 253, 264, 266, 267, 306, 307, 311, 348

CD11b, 23, 101, 112-114, 121, 122, 131-134, 138, 277

CD14, 23, 61, 79, 81, 112, 114, 121, 122, 131-134, 141, 142, 144, 150, 366

CD15, 61, 79, 101, 110, 112, 113, 116, 122, 131-134, 142, 144, 152, 172, 238, 244, 248, 250, 267, 300, 306, 307, 315, 319, 324, 326, 327, 333, 347, 349, 351, 357

CD16, 61, 146, 155, 161, 163, 273, 274, 276, 277, 287, 355

CD19, 110, 131, 132, 146, 150-152, 169, 171, 174, 181, 183, 195, 201, 205, 223, 235, 250, 261, 264, 266, 338, 348

CD20, 15, 146, 153, 160, 169, 173, 181, 183, 186, 189, 190, 192, 195, 199, 205, 208, 216, 223, 227, 235-237, 241, 242, 244, 246, 248, 250, 254, 255, 259, 264, 266-268, 306, 307, 324, 326, 328, 333, 338, 344, 347-349, 351, 364

CD21, 162, 216, 220, 221, 224, 227, 311, 324, 333, 355, 357, 362, 364, 365

CD22, 138, 150, 152, 169, 181, 183, 189, 190, 193, 195, 223, 235, 241, 250, 264, 266

CD23, 70, 160, 180-182, 186, 192, 195, 216, 219, 221, 224, 231, 250, 311, 362, 364, 365

CD25, 56, 57, 60-62, 70, 72, 138, 163, 171, 189, 190, 192, 195, 283, 287, 306, 315, 338

CD26, 299

CD27, 259

CD30, 140, 163, 164, 235, 238, 244, 246, 248, 250, 254, 255, 257, 261, 267, 283, 287, 290, 297, 298, 300, 301, 304, 306, 307, 312-315, 317-319, 324, 326-328, 333, 334, 338, 342, 347-349, 351, 355, 360, 362, 364, 365

CD30-positive lymphoproliferative disorders, primary cutaneous, *300-301*

CD33, 23, 61, 79, 101, 110, 112-114, 116, 117, 121, 122, 125, 128, 131-134, 137, 138, 141,142, 144, 146, 150, 153, 169, 171, 177, 357

CD34, 20, 23, 34, 44, 45, 47, 65, 79, 92, 96, 100, 101, 105-107, 110, 112-114, 116, 117, 121, 122, 125, 128, 130-135, 137, 138, 140, 142, 144, 146, 151, 169, 173, 175, 362, 364

CD35, 216, 227, 311, 355, 357, 362, 364, 365

CD38, 101, 116, 125, 131, 146, 151, 160, 169, 182, 192, 195, 201, 205, 235, 256, 259, 264

CD40, 160, 336, 339

CD40L, 324, 339

CD41, 105, 106, 116, 117, 136, 139, 142, 144

CD43, 79, 146, 160, 181, 186, 216, 219, 223, 224, 227, 231, 255, 264, 287, 306, 315, 318, 326

CD45, 61, 117, 137, 169, 173, 254, 255, 261, 267, 315, 324, 326, 327, 339, 349, 357, 359, 362, 364, 365

CD52, 205, 270, 271, 306, 307

CD54, 250, 253

CD56, 23, 79, 101, 111, 113, 114, 122, 125, 128, 131, 132, 134, 140, 142, 144-146, 155, 158, 161-164, 177, 201, 203, 205, 257, 274, 277, 279, 280, 287, 289-291, 293-295, 300, 303, 306, 307

CD57, 161-163, 224, 255, 273, 274, 277, 287, 324, 325, 338

CD61, 23, 101, 105, 106, 116, 117, 136, 139, 140, 142, 144

CD64, 79, 112-114, 116, 122, 131-134, 150, 355

CD68, 61, 79, 121, 133, 134, 140, 146, 238, 315, 327, 355, 357, 359, 362, 364-366

CD71, 92, 135, 142, 144

CD77, 264

CD79a, 110, 146, 150-152, 160, 169, 177, 181, 183, 186, 195, 205, 216, 223, 227, 235, 241, 242, 244, 246, 250, 251, 254, 256, 259, 266, 267, 307, 324, 326, 328, 338, 348, 364

CD94/NKG2, 273, 275

CD99, 140, 177

CD103, 160, 186, 189, 192, 195, 290

CD105, 92

CD117, 57, 59, 61, 62, 92, 101, 107, 112-114, 116, 131-135, 138, 140-142, 144, 146, 150, 153, 171, 177, 205

CD123, 79, 138, 140, 146, 189, 192, 355

CD134, 324

CD138, 160, 195, 197, 201, 204, 205, 235, 238, 246, 254, 256, 259, 328, 348

CD161, 155, 275

CD163, 79, 133, 134, 141, 355, 357, 365, 366

CDK4, 178, 231

CDK6, 186

CDKN2A, 178, 228, 241, 242, 298, 349

CDKN2B, 228, 242

CEBPA, 23, 28-30, 118-120, 122, 123, 125, 126

CEL, *see* Chronic eosinophilic leukaemia

Cell types,

- doughnut, 312

- clear, 306

- flame, 205

- Gaucher-like, 205

- hallmark, 312, 313, 317

- hand-mirror, 169

- Hodgkin, 238, 247, 326, 327, 329

- L&H, 323

Monomorphic T/NK-cell PTLD, 349

Morula cells, 205

Mott cells, 205

MPL, 23, 25, 44, 47, 50, 64, 86

MPN, *see* Myeloproliferative neoplasms

MPO, *see* Myeloperoxidase

M-protein, 200-203, 205, 207-213

MSN, 315

Mu heavy chain disease, *197-198*

Multicentric Castleman disease, 166, 234, 260

Multicentric Castleman disease, large B-cell lymphoma arising in HHV8-associated, 234, *258*

Multiple lymphomatous polyposis, 229

Multiple myeloma, 38, 202

Myasthenia gravis, 196

MYC, 14, 36, 177, 178, 206, 224, 225, 231, 235, 237, 241, 242, 251, 262-266, 289, 290, 325, 340, 348

Mycosis fungoides, 294, *296-298*

Mycosis fungoides, folliculotropic variant, 298

Mycosis fungoides, ISCL-EORTC staging system, 296

Myelodysplasia, 24, 28-30, 34, 43, 49, 65, 76, 81, 91, 101, 104, 106, 115, 124, 125, 128, 130, 131, 136, 138, 145, 356

Myelodysplastic syndrome (MDS), 15, 18, 19, 22, 23, 25-30, 39, 43, 44, 48-50, 53, 57, 59, 71, 76, 77, 79, 85, 86, *87-108*, 110, 116, 118, 124, 125, 127-129, 135, 136, 139-141, 143, 144, 150

Myelodysplastic syndrome with 5q deletion, 102

Myelodysplastic syndrome with isolated del(5q), 27, *102*

Myelodysplastic syndrome, NOS, 103

Myelodysplastic syndrome, therapy-related, 127

Myelodysplastic syndrome, unclassifiable, 27, *103*

Myelodysplastic/myeloproliferative neoplasms (MDS/MPN), 18, 19, 22, 23, 25-30, *75-86*, 79, 85, 86, 91, 102, 124, 127-129, 140

Myelodysplastic/myeloproliferative neoplasm, unclassifiable, *85-86*

Myelodysplastic/myeloproliferative neoplasms, therapy-related, 127

Myelofibrosis, 19, 24, 37, 42, 44, 46, 48, 64, 65, 71, 86, 92, 101, 137, 138

Myelofibrosis, primary, *44-47*

Myelofibrosis/sclerosis with myeloid metaplasia, 44

Myeloid and lymphoid neoplasms with FGFR1 abnormalities, 26, *72-73*

Myeloid and lymphoid neoplasms with PDGFRA rearrangement, 26, *68-71*

Myeloid and lymphoid neoplasms with PDGFRB rearrangement, 26, *71-72*

Myeloid leukaemia associated with Down syndrome, 29, *143-144*

Myeloid proliferations related to Down syndrome, 29, 30, *142-144*

Myeloid sarcoma, 28-30, 47, 73, 110, 111, 118, 122, *140-141*

Myelomastocytic leukaemia, 56

Myelomatosis, 202

Myeloperoxidase (MPO), 20, 21, 23, 35, 57, 83, 107, 110, 112-114, 116, 117, 121, 122, 130-132, 134-136, 138, 140, 141, 144, 146, 150, 151, 155, 169, 357, 362, 364

Myeloproliferative disease, 23, 25, 38, 82

Myeloproliferative neoplasm, unclassifiable, *64-65*, 85

Myeloproliferative neoplasms (MPN), 23, *31-66*

Myeloproliferative variant of the hypereosinophilic syndrome, 69

Myofibroblasts, 355, 365

N

Naphthol-ASD-chloroacetate esterase, 21, 33, 34, 41, 45, 49, 57, 76, 78, 83, 105, 112, 130, 140

Naphthol-butyrate esterase, 145

Nasal type T-cell lymphomas, 146

Natural killer cell lymphoblastic leukaemia/lymphoma, *155*

NBS1, 339

Neurofibromin, 84

Neutrophil alkaline phosphatase, 35, 39

NF1, 23, 26, 82, 84, 366

NFκB, 162, 163, 206, 329

NG2, 114, 172

Nibrin, 339

Nijmegen breakage syndrome, 336, 339

NK-cell leukaemia, aggressive, *276-277*

NK-cell LGL lymphocytosis, 274

NK-cell lineage granular lymphocyte proliferative disorder, 274

Nodal marginal zone B-cell lymphoma, 218

Nodal marginal zone lymphoma, 166, *218-219*, 308

Nodal marginal zone lymphoma, paediatric, *219*

Nodular lymphocyte predominant Hodgkin lymphoma, 322, *323-325*

Nodular sclerosis classical Hodgkin lymphoma, 165, 267, 313, 322, 326, 327, *330*, 331, 334, 341

Non-myelomatous gammopathy, 200

Non-secretory myeloma, 200, 203

Non-specific esterase, 20, 21, 112-114, 122, 132-134, 136, 138, 140, 169, 354

Noonan syndrome, 82

NOTCH1, 178

NPM1, 23, 28-30, 114, 118-122, 125, 126, 141

NPM-ALK, 254, 314-316

NPMc+ AML, 120

NRAS, 23, 26, 28, 81, 84, 111, 118, 201, 206

Nuclear matrix associated gene, 114

Nucleophosmin, 114, 118, 120, 314, 315

NUMA1, 114

NUP214, 115, 116

O

OCT-2, 251, 267

Onychodystrophy, 299

Osseous plasmacytoma, 208

Osteosclerosis, 42

Osteosclerotic myeloma, 200, *212-213*

OTT, 117

P

p16^{INK4a}, 36, 224, 241, 251, 264, 298, 299, 349

p18^{INK4c}, 206, 231

p190, 32, 35, 79, 171

p210, 35, 79, 171

p230, 35, 39

Paediatric follicular lymphoma, 225

Paediatric nodal marginal zone lymphoma, *219*

Pagetoid reticulosis, 298

Pancytopenia, 89, 94, 103, 106, 115, 124, 138, 188, 252, 279, 339, 356, 360

Panmyelosis, 42

Pappenheimer body, 98

Parafollicular B-cell lymphoma, 218

Paraneoplastic pemphigus, 363

Paroxysmal nocturnal haemoglobinuria, 91, 106, 107

Randall disease, 211

RARA, 28, 30, 113, 114

RARS, *see* Refractory anaemia with ring sideroblasts

RARS-T, *see* Refractory anaemia with ring sideroblasts and thrombocytosis

RB1, 36, 147, 206, 231

RBM15-MKL1, 30, 117

RBTN1, 177

RBTN2, 177

RCC, *see* Refractory cytopenia of childhood

Reed-Sternberg cells, 182, 234, 238, 243, 244, 247, 250, 261, 300, 301, 306, 308, 310, 313, 322, 326, 327, 330, 331, 337, 347-349, 364

Refractory anaemia, 27, 49, 65, 85, 88-91, 94-97, 99, 103, 104, 124, 125, 132

Refractory anaemia of childhood, 104

Refractory anaemia with excess blasts (RAEB), 23, 27, 89-94, 96, 98-99, *100-101*, 104,136, 139

Refractory anaemia with ring sideroblasts (RARS), 27, 49, 65, 85, 86, 88, 89, 94, *96-97*, 104

Refractory anaemia with ring sideroblasts and thrombocytosis (RARS-T), 26, 27, 49, 65, *85-86*

Refractory anaemia with unilineage dysplasia, 88

Refractory cytopenia of childhood (RCC), 27, *104-107*, 143

Refractory cytopenia with multilineage dysplasia, 89, 90, 97, *98-99*, 100, 103, 106

Refractory cytopenia with unilineage dysplasia, 89-90, *94-95*, 100, 103

Refractory neutropenia, 89, 90, 94, 95

Refractory thrombocytopenia, 27, 89-91, 94, 95

Regressing atypical histiocytosis, 355

Restrictive cardiomegaly, 51

Restrictive cardiomyopathy, 69

Reticulin fibrosis, 33, 44, 48, 49, 59, 60, 100, 101,189, 193, 273

Reticulin/collagen fibrosis, 60

Reticulohistiocytoma of the dorsum, 227

Reticulohistiocytosis, 354

Retinoic acid receptor α, 113

Rhabdomyosarcoma, 137, 315

Rheumatoid arthritis, 196, 245, 350

Rituximab, 190, 193, 236, 255

Rosai-Dorfman disease, 354

RPN1-EVI1, 30, 116

RUNX1, 23, 28, 29, 62, 110, 111, 112, 128, 131, 172

RUNX1-RUNX1T1, 29, 110, 111

RUNX1T1 (ETO), 111

RUNX2, 147

Russell body, 205, 210

S

S100, 355, 358, 362, 364-366

sCD23, 182

Sclerosing cholangitis, 359, 366

Sea-blue histiocytes, 33

Seckel syndrome, 107

Senile EBV-associated B-cell lymphoproliferative disorder, 243

SerpinA1, 315, 316

Severe combined immunodeficiency, 336

Sézary cells, 299

Sézary syndrome, 296, 297, *299*, 349

Sezary syndrome, ISCL-EORTC staging system, 296

SHP1, 315

SHP2, 82

Shwachmann-Diamond syndrome, 88, 107

Signal transducer and activator of transcription, 24

Sjögren syndrome, 196, 215, 219

SLE, 196, 294

SLVL, 185, 186

Small lymphocytic lymphoma, *180-182* 216, 217, 229, 233, 339, 351

Small round cell tumours, 141

Smudge cells, 181

SOC-1, 329

SOCS1, 236, 251

Solitary mastocytoma of skin, 54, 57

Solitary plasmacytoma of bone, 200, *208*

Somatic hypermutation, 158, 159, 182, 186, 190, 192, 195, 197, 201, 205, 207, 217, 228, 231, 235, 241, 250, 258, 264, 325, 329, 347, 348, 349

Sorafenib, 70

Splenic B-cell lymphoma with villous lymphocytes, 191

Splenic diffuse red pulp small B-cell lymphoma, *191-192*

Splenic lymphoma with circulating villous lymphocytes, 185

Splenic lymphoma/leukaemia, unclassifiable, *191-193*

Splenic marginal zone lymphoma, 160, 164, 166, 183, *185-187*, 189-191

Splenic marginal zone lymphoma, diffuse variant, 191

Splenic red pulp lymphoma with numerous basophilic villous lymphocytes, 191

Spoke wheel, chromatin pattern, 205

Sporadic fatal infectious mononucleosis, 278

Stabilin-1, 366

Starry sky pattern, 78, 169, 176, 214, 229, 264-266

STAT, 24, 251, 329

Stem cell acute leukaemia, 151

Strongyloidiasis, 282

Subcutaneous panniculitis-like T-cell lymphoma, 163, *294-295*, 302, 355

Syncytial variant, nodular sclerosis classical Hodgkin lymphoma, 330

Syndrome of abnormal chromatin clumping, 81

Systemic EBV+ T-cell lymphoproliferative disease of childhood, *278-280*

Systemic lupus erythematosus, 196, 294

Systemic mastocytosis, 25, 52-55, 57, *58-61*, 70

Systemic mastocytosis with associated haematological clonal non-mast cell disorder, 54

T

T lymphoblastic leukaemia/lymphoma, 161, 165, *176-178*

T-bet, 189, 190

T-cell chronic lymphocytic leukemia, 270

T-cell large granular lymphocytic leukaemia, 163, *272-273*

T-cell prolymphocytic leukaemia, 163, *270-271*, 337

T-cell rich large B-cell lymphoma, 238, 323, 326

T-cell/histiocyte-rich large B-cell lymphoma, 234, *238-239*, 325

T-cell receptor (TCR), 112, 131, 146, 151, 158, 161-164, 169, 176-178, 249. 261, 270, 273, 275, 277, 279, 280, 283, 287, 290, 293-295, 297, 299-301, 303, 304, 307, 311, 315, 318, 319, 328, 329, 336, 338, 339, 348, 349, 357, 358, 362, 364, 366

T-cell-rich B-cell lymphoma, 238